VOLUME FIVE

CAMPBELL'S
OPERATIVE ORTHOPAEDICS

VOLUME FIVE

Eighth Edition

CAMPBELL'S OPERATIVE ORTHOPAEDICS

Edited by

A.H. CRENSHAW, M.D.

Editorial assistance by

KAY DAUGHERTY

Art coordination by

CHARLES CURRO

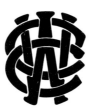

with over 7900 illustrations

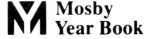

St. Louis   Baltimore   Boston   Chicago   London   Philadelphia   Sydney   Toronto

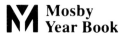

Mosby
Year Book
Dedicated to Publishing Excellence

Editor: Eugenia A. Klein
Managing Editor: Kathryn H. Falk
Editorial assistance by: Robin Sutter and Diane Schindler
Project Manager: Gayle May Morris
Production Editors: Deborah Vogel, Sheila Walker,
  Donna L. Walls, Mary Cusick Drone, and Judith Bange
Book and Cover Design: Gail Morey Hudson

EIGHTH EDITION

Previous editions copyrighted 1939, 1949, 1956, 1963, 1971, 1980, 1987

Printed in the United States of America

Mosby–Year Book, Inc.
11830 Westline Industrial Drive, St. Louis, Missouri 63146

Library of Congress Cataloging in Publication Data

Campbell's operative orthopaedics / edited by A.H. Crenshaw;
  editorial assistance by Kay Daugherty; art coordination by Charles
  Curro.— 8th ed.
      p.   cm.
    Includes bibliographical references and indexes.
    ISBN 0-8016-1096-6
    1. Orthopedic surgery.   I. Crenshaw, A.H. (Andrew Hoyt), 1920-
.   II. Daugherty, Kay.   III. Campbell, Willis C. (Willis Cohoon),
1880-1941.   IV. Title: Operative orthopaedics.
    [DNLM: 1. Orthopedics.   WE 168 C1921]
RD731.C32   1991
617.3 — dc20
DNLM/DLC
for Library of Congress   91-29931
                                                        CIP

92 93 94 95 96 CL/UN/MV 9 8 7 6 5 4 3 2 1

Contributors

JAMES H. BEATY, M.D.

Chapters 42, 43, 44, and 47

Associate Professor, University of Tennessee–Campbell Clinic Department of Orthopaedic Surgery, University of Tennessee, Memphis; Chief, Tennessee Crippled Children's Service; Associate Chief of Pediatric Orthopaedics, LeBonheur Children's Medical Center; Active Staff, Campbell Clinic, Inc., Baptist Memorial Hospitals, Regional Medical Center at Memphis, Veterans' Administration Medical Center

JAMES H. CALANDRUCCIO, M.D.

Chapter 70

Instructor, University of Tennessee–Campbell Clinic Department of Orthopaedic Surgery, University of Tennessee, Memphis; Active Staff, Campbell Clinics, Inc., Baptist Memorial Hospitals, University of Tennessee–William F. Bowld Hospital, Veterans' Administration Hospital, LeBonnheur Children's Medical Center

S. TERRY CANALE, M.D.

Chapters 26, 32, and 40

Professor, University of Tennessee–Campbell Clinic Department of Orthopaedic Surgery, University of Tennessee, Memphis; Chief of Pediatric Orthopaedics, LeBonnheur Children's Medical Center; Active Staff, Campbell Clinic, Inc., Baptist Memorial Hospital; Consultant Staff, Regional Medical Center at Memphis, Veterans' Administration Medical Center

PETER G. CARNESALE, M.D.

Chapters 7 through 12

Clinical Associate Professor, University of Tennessee–Campbell Clinic Department of Orthopaedic Surgery, University of Tennessee, Memphis; Chief of Orthopaedics, Veterans' Administration Medical Center; Active Staff, Campbell Clinic, Inc., Baptist Memorial Hospital, Regional Medical Center at Memphis; Consultant Staff, LeBonheur Children's Medical Center, St. Joseph Hospital, St. Jude Children's Research Hospital, Methodist Hospitals

A.H. CRENSHAW, M.D.

Chapter 1

Clinical Professor, University of Tennessee–Campbell Clinic Department of Orthopaedic Surgery, University of Tennessee, Memphis; Emeritus Staff, Campbell Clinic, Inc.

ANDREW H. CRENSHAW, JR., M.D.

Chapters 2, 25, and 34

Assistant Professor, University of Tennessee–Campbell Clinic Department of Orthopaedic Surgery, University of Tennessee, Memphis; Active Staff, Campbell Clinic, Inc., Baptist Memorial Hospitals, Regional Medical Center at Memphis, Veterans' Administration Medical Center; Associate Staff, LeBonnheur Children's Medical Center; Consultant Staff, University of Tennessee–William F. Bowld Hospital; Courtesy Staff, Baptist Memorial Hospital–Germantown

JOSEPH P. DUTKOWSKY, M.D.

Chapter 41

Assistant Professor and Director of Laboratory Research, University of Tennessee–Campbell Clinic Department of Orthopaedic Surgery, University of Tennessee, Memphis; Active Staff, Campbell Clinic, University of Tennessee–William F. Bowld Hospital, LeBonheur Children's Medical Center, Regional Medical Center at Memphis, Veterans' Administration Hospital, Baptist Memorial Hospitals; Consultant Staff, St. Jude Children's Research Hospital, St. Joseph Hospital

ALLEN S. EDMONSON, M.D.

Chapters 81 and 82

Clinical Professor, University of Tennessee–Campbell Clinic Department of Orthopaedic Surgery; Assistant Dean, University of Tennessee, Memphis; Director of Graduate Medical Education, Baptist Memorial Hospital; Active Staff, Campbell Clinic, Inc., Regional Medical Center at Memphis; Consultant Staff, Methodist Hospital, St. Francis Hospital, St. Joseph Hospital, Veterans' Administration Medical Center; LeBonheur Children's Medical Center

BARNEY L. FREEMAN III, M.D.

Chapters 30, 31, and 83

Clinical Associate Professor, University of Tennessee–Campbell Clinic Department of Orthopaedic Surgery, University of Tennessee, Memphis; Active Staff, Campbell Clinic, Inc., Baptist Memorial Hospitals, Regional Medical Center at Memphis; Consultant Staff, LeBonheur Children's Medical Center, Methodist Hospital, Germantown Community Hospital–Methodist Hospital East, St. Francis Hospital, Veterans' Administration Medical Center

STANLEY C. GRAVES, M.D.

Chapter 58

Instructor, University of Tennessee–Campbell Clinic Department of Orthopaedic Surgery, University of Tennessee, Memphis; Active Staff, Campbell Clinic, Inc., Baptist Memorial Hospitals, University of Tennessee–William F. Bowld Hospital, Regional Medical Center at Memphis

JAMES W. HARKESS, M.D.

Chapters 14 and 16

Assistant Professor, University of Tennessee–Campbell Clinic Department of Orthopaedic Surgery, University of Tennessee, Memphis; Active Staff, Campbell Clinic, Inc., Regional Medical Center at Memphis, University of Tennessee–William F. Bowld Hospital, LeBonheur Children's Medical Center, Veterans' Administration Medical Center, Baptist Memorial Hospitals

MARK T. JOBE, M.D.

Chapters 45, 49, 69, 70, 71, 73, 74, 75, and 77

Instructor, University of Tennessee–Campbell Clinic Department of Orthopaedic Surgery, University of Tennessee, Memphis; Active Staff, Campbell Clinic, Inc., Baptist Memorial Hospitals, University of Tennessee–William F. Bowld Hospital, Regional Medical Center at Memphis, LeBonheur Children's Medical Center, Veterans' Administration Medical Center

E. JEFF JUSTIS, JR., M.D.

Chapters 13 and 64

Clinical Associate Professor, University of Tennessee–Campbell Clinic Department of Orthopaedic Surgery, University of Tennessee, Memphis; Active Staff, Campbell Clinic, Inc., Baptist Memorial Hospital, Regional Medical Center at Memphis; Consultant Staff, Arlington Developmental Center, LeBonheur Children's Medical Center, Veterans' Administration Medical Center; Courtesy Staff, Methodist Hospital; Consultant to the Surgeon General, United States Air Force; Consultant Staff in Hand Surgery, Mississippi and Tennessee Crippled Children's Services

DAVID G. LAVELLE, M.D.

Chapter 29

Assistant Professor, University of Tennessee–Campbell Clinic Department of Orthopaedic Surgery, University of Tennessee, Memphis; Active Staff, Campbell Clinic, Inc., Baptist Memorial Hospials, Regional Medical Center at Memphis, University of Tennessee–William F. Bowld Hospital; Consultant Staff, LeBonheur Children's Medical Center, Veterans' Administration Medical Center

MARVIN R. LEVENTHAL, M.D.

Chapters 79 and 80

Assistant Professor, University of Tennessee–Campbell Clinic Department of Orthopaedic Surgery, University of Tennessee, Memphis; Active Staff, Campbell Clinic, Inc., Baptist Memorial Hospitals, Regional Medical Center at Memphis, LeBonheur Children's Medical Center, University of Tennessee–William F. Bowld Hospital; Consultant Staff, Veterans' Administration Medical Center

LEE W. MILFORD, M.D.

Chapter 69

Clinical Professor, University of Tennessee–Campbell Clinic Department of Orthopaedic Surgery, University of Tennessee, Memphis; Emeritus Staff, Campbell Clinic, Inc.

ROBERT H. MILLER III, M.D.

Chapters 35, 36, and 37

Assistant Professor, University of Tennessee–Campbell Clinic Department of Orthopaedic Surgery, University of Tennessee, Memphis; Active Staff, Campbell Clinic, Inc., Baptist Memorial Hospitals, Regional Medical Center at Memphis, University of Tennessee–William F. Bowld Hospital, Veterans' Administration Medical Center

BARRY B. PHILLIPS, M.D.

Chapters 38 and 39

Instructor, University of Tennessee–Campbell Clinic Department of Orthopaedic Surgery, University of Tennessee, Memphis; Active Staff, Campbell Clinic, Inc., Baptist Memorial Hospitals, Regional Medical Center at Memphis; Courtesy Staff, LeBonheur Children's Medical Center

E. GREER RICHARDSON, M.D.

Chapters 50 through 60

Associate Professor, University of Tennessee–Campbell Clinic Department of Orthopaedic Surgery, University of Tennessee, Memphis; Active Staff, Campbell Clinic, Inc., Baptist Memorial Hospitals, Regional Medical Center at Memphis; Consultant Staff, University of Tennessee–William F. Bowld Hospital, Veterans' Administration Medical Center; Courtesy Staff, LeBonheur Children's Medical Center

THOMAS A. RUSSELL, M.D.

Chapters 22, 24, and 27

Associate Professor, University of Tennessee–Campbell Clinic Department of Orthopaedic Surgery, University of Tennessee,

Memphis; Active Staff, Campbell Clinic, Inc., Baptist Memorial Hospitals, Regional Medical Center at Memphis, University of Tennessee–William F. Bowld Hospital; Consultant Staff, Veterans' Administration Medical Center, LeBonheur Children's Medical Center

FRED P. SAGE, M.D.

Chapters 46 and 48

Clinical Professor, University of Tennessee–Campbell Clinic Department of Orthopaedic Surgery, University of Tennessee, Memphis; Active Staff, Campbell Clinic, Inc., Baptist Memorial Hospitals, Regional Medical Center at Memphis, LeBonheur Children's Medical Center, Methodist Hospitals

T. DAVID SISK, M.D.

Chapters 17 and 33

Professor and Acting Chairman, University of Tennessee–Campbell Clinic Department of Orthopaedic Surgery, University of Tennessee, Memphis; Active Staff, Campbell Clinic, Inc., Baptist Memorial Hospitals, LeBonheur Children's Medical Center, Methodist Hospitals, Regional Medical Center at Memphis, University of Tennessee–William F. Bowld Hospital

J. CHARLES TAYLOR, M.D.

Chapters 23 and 28

Assistant Professor, University of Tennessee–Campbell Clinic Department of Orthopaedic Surgery, University of Tennessee, Memphis; Active Staff, Campbell Clinic, Inc., Baptist Memorial Hospitals, Regional Medical Center at Memphis, University of Tennessee–William F. Bowld Hospital, LeBonheur Children's Medical Center, Veterans' Administration Medical Center

ROBERT E. TOOMS, M.D.

Chapters 14, 15, 18, 19, 20, and 21

Professor, University of Tennessee–Campbell Clinic Department of Orthopaedic Surgery, University of Tennessee, Memphis; Chief of Staff, Campbell Clinic, Inc.; Active Staff, Baptist Memorial Hospitals, LeBonheur Children's Medical Center, Regional Medical Center at Memphis; Medical Director, University of Tennessee Rehabilitation Engineering Center; Medical Director, Regional Spinal Cord Center; Chief, Memphis Child Amputee Clinic and St. Jude Children's Research Hospital Amputee Clinic

WILLIAM C. WARNER, JR., M.D.

Chapters 3 through 6

Instructor, University of Tennessee–Campbell Clinic Department of Orthopaedic Surgery, University of Tennessee, Memphis; Chief, Mississippi Crippled Children's Service; Active Staff, Campbell Clinic, Inc., Baptist Memorial Hospitals, LeBonheur Children's Medical Center, Veterans' Administration Medical Center, University of Tennessee–William F. Bowld Hospital

GEORGE W. WOOD II, M.D.

Chapters 84, 85, and 86

Clinical Associate Professor, University of Tennessee–Campbell Clinic Department of Orthopaedic Surgery, University of Tennessee, Memphis; Active Staff, Campbell Clinic, Inc., Baptist Memorial Hospitals, Regional Medical Center at Memphis; Consultant Staff, LeBonheur Children's Medical Center, Veteran's Administration Medical Center, University of Tennessee–William F. Bowld Hospital

PHILLIP E. WRIGHT II, M.D.

Chapters 17, 45, 49, 61, 62, 63, 65, 66, 67, 68, 72, 74, 76, and 78

Associate Professor, Director of Hand Fellowship, and Director of Orthopaedic Microsurgery, University of Tennessee–Campbell Clinic Department of Orthopaedic Surgery, University of Tennessee, Memphis; Chief of Hand Surgery Service, Regional Medical Center at Memphis; Active Staff, Campbell Clinic, Inc., Baptist Memorial Hospitals, University of Tennessee–William F. Bowld Hospital, Veterans' Administration Medical Center

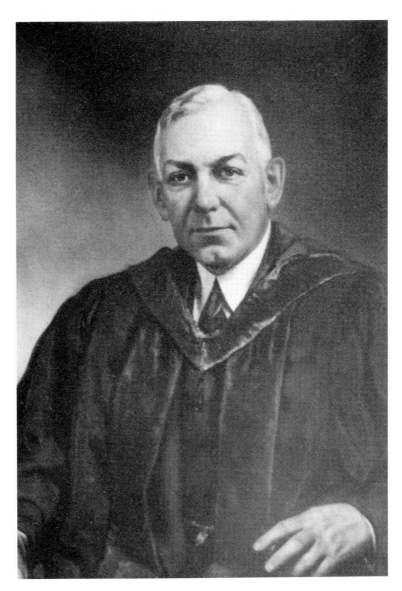

WILLIS C. CAMPBELL, M.D.

1880-1941

Preface to Eighth Edition

Many new methods and techniques in orthopaedic surgery have been developed or refined during the last 5 to 6 years; those of importance to practicing orthopaedic surgeons are included in this eighth edition.

All chapters have been revised and brought up-to-date. All are written by members of the staff of the Campbell Clinic. Several authors, some new to this edition, have had much experience in a busy, Level 1 trauma center, and this experience is reflected in the discussions on fresh fractures, delayed unions, nonunions, microsurgery, and other subjects.

The format of this edition is essentially the same as for the last edition. The discussions on the foot have been expanded into 11 chapters and on the hand into 18. A total of 86 chapters have been grouped into 18 parts for better presentation. Over 2300 illustrations are new or totally redrawn.

We have continued to use almost entirely the method

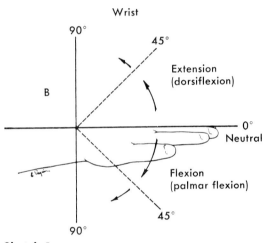

Sketch 1

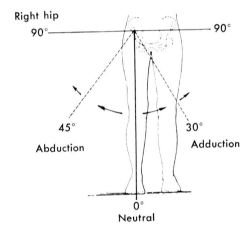

Sketch 2

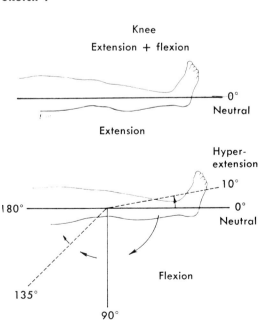

Sketch 3

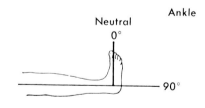

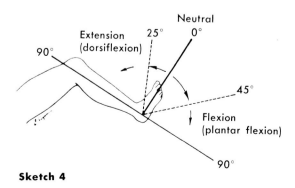

Sketch 4

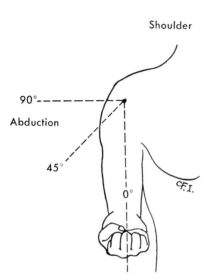

Sketch 5

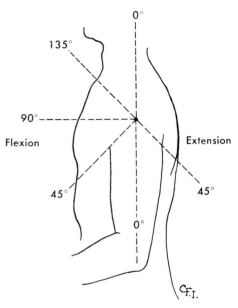

Sketch 6

of measuring joint motion advocated by the American Academy of Orthopaedic Surgeons. The neutral position is 0 degrees instead of 180 degrees as in the first three editions (see sketches 1 through 4*). For the shoulder, however, the method of the Academy seems too complicated for adoption here. Although the neutral position is 0 degrees as for other joints, the direction of movement in adduction, abduction, flexion, and extension is the same as that used in previous editions (see sketches 5 and 6).

Reproduced by courtesy of the American Academy of Orthopaedic Surgeons.

The editor and members of the staff wish to thank Charlie Curro, Art Director, and artists, Richard Fritzler, Sarah C. McQueen, and Rick Mendius, for their artwork for this edition. Marlene DenHouter, John Klausmeyer, and Mary Stewart also contributed illustrations, and Dan Ralph provided photographic services.

I wish to especially thank Kay Daugherty, our medical editor, for her skillful help with the manuscript; without her help this revision would not have been possible. I wish also to thank Joan Crowson, medical librarian, for her help with references, and Eugenia Klein, Kathy Falk, Robin Sutter, and Deborah Vogel at Mosby–Year Book, Inc. for their encouragement and expert assistance.

A.H. Crenshaw, M.D.

Preface to First Edition

The title of this book, *Operative Orthopedics,* is not intended to convey the impression that the chief or most important method of treatment of orthopaedic affections is open surgery. Although many orthopaedic affections are best treated by operative measures alone, the majority are successfully treated by more conservative means. Further, such measures are often essential adjuncts either before or after operation.

This volume has been written to meet the current need for a comprehensive work on operative orthopedics, not only for the specialist, but also for many industrial and general surgeons who are doing excellent work in some branches of orthopedic surgery, and are making valuable contributions to this field.

The evolution of orthopedic surgery has been exceedingly slow as compared to that of surgery in general. Not until aseptic technic had been materially refined was surgery of the bones and joints feasible. The statement is often made that the World War afforded the experience which made possible the rapid development or orthopedic surgery during the past two decades. The surgery of the war, however, was chiefly the surgery of sepsis; there was little of the refined asepsis which is required in reconstruction surgery. Undoubtedly, the demonstration during the war of the necessity and importance of this field led many able men to specialize in orthopedics, and to them considerable credit is due for its subsequent progress.

No classification of orthopedic affections is entirely satisfactory; consequently, any arrangement of operative procedures is subject to similar criticism. With the exception of the chapters on Arthroplasty and Arthrodesis, operations described in this text are grouped together according to their applicability to a given affection. This involves less repetition as to generalities of etiology, pathology, and treatment than would be necessary in a classification according to anatomic location. Operative procedures appropriate to two or more affections are described in the discussion of the one wherein they are most commonly employed.

To overcome the too widespread conception of orthopedic surgery as a purely mechanical equation, an effort is made in the first chapter of this book to correlate the mechanical, surgical, and physiologic principles of orthopedic practice, and throughout the book to emphasize the practical application of these physiologic principles. A special chapter has been written on surgical technic,

for the purpose of stressing certain details in preparation and aftertreatment which vary to some extent from those described in works on general surgery. A thorough knowledge of these phases of treatment is a requisite to success. To avoid constant repetition, chapters have been included on apparatus and on surgical approaches; repeated reference is made to these chapters. The after treatment is given in detail for practically all operative technics. This is a most essential, yet too often neglected, factor in the success of any surgical treatment.

In giving the position or range of motion of a joint, only one system has been followed: with the exception of the ankle and wrist, the joint is in neutral position when parallel with the long axis of the body in the anteroposterior and lateral planes. As the joint proceeds from the neutral position in any direction, the number of degrees in which such movement is recorded decreases progressively from 180 to 170, 160, and so on, to the anatomic limit of motion in that particular direction. To illustrate, complete extension of the knee is 180 degrees; when the joint is flexed 30 degrees, the position is recorded as the angle formed between the component parts of the joint, i.e., the leg and thigh, or 150 degrees. Flexion to a right angle is 90 degrees, and full flexion 30 degrees. In the wrist, the joint is at 180 degrees, or in the neutral position, when midway between supination and pronation, and flexion and extension. In the ankle joint, motion is recorded as follows: the extreme of dorsiflexion, 75 degrees; right angle, 90 degrees; and the extreme of plantar flexion, 140 degrees.

In some instances, the exact end results have been given, to the best of our knowledge. So many factors are involved in any one condition, that a survey of end results can be of only questionable value unless the minute details of each case are considered. Following arthroplasty of the knee, for example, one must consider the etiology, pathology, position of the ankylosed joint, the structure of the bones comprising the joint, the distribution of the ankylosis, and the age of the patient, in estimating the end result in each case. Further, a true survey should include the results of *all* patients treated over a period of *many* years, and should be made by the surgeon himself, rather than by a group of assistants, or by correspondence.

In our private clinic and the hospitals with which we are associated, a sufficient amount of material on every phase of orthopedic surgery has been accumulated during the past twenty years or more to justify an evaluation of the various procedures. From this personal experience, we also feel that definite conclusions may be drawn in regard to the indications, contraindications, complications, and other considerations entering into orthopedic treatment. In all surgical cases, mature judgment is required for the selection of the most appropriate procedure. With this in mind, the technics which have proved most efficient in the author's experience have been given preference in the text. In addition, after a comprehensive search of the literature, operative measures have been selected which in the judgment of the author are most practicable.

Although no attempt has been made to produce an atlas of orthopedic surgery, an effort has been made to describe those procedures which conform to mechanical and physiologic principles and will meet all individual requirements. In any work of this nature, there are sins of omission; also, many surgeons in the same field may arrive independently at the same conclusions and devise identical procedures. We have endeavored, however, to give credit where credit was due. If there are errors, correction will gladly be made. In some of the chapters we have drawn heavily from authoritative articles on special subjects; the author gratefully acknowledges his indebtedness for this material. He also wishes to thank those authors who have so graciously granted permission for the reproduction of original drawings.

In conclusion, I cannot too deeply express my sincere appreciation and gratitude to my associate, Dr. Hugh Smith, who has untiringly and most efficiently devoted practically all of his time during the past two years to collaboration with me in the compilation and preparation of material, which alone has made this work possible. I also desire to express appreciation to Dr. J.S. Speed for his collaboration on the sections on Spastic Cerebral Paralysis and Peripheral Nerve Injuries to Dr. Harold Boyd for anatomic dissections verifying all surgical approaches described, and for his assistance in preparing the chapter on this subject; to Dr. Don Slocum for his aid in the preparation of the chapter on Physiology and Pathology; to Mrs. Allene Jefferson for her efficient editorial services, and to Mr. Ivan Summers and Mr. Charles Ingram for their excellent illustrations.

Willis C. Campbell
1939

Contents

Color Plates

PART XVII

THE HAND

CHAPTER 61

Basic Surgical Technique and Aftercare

PHILLIP E. WRIGHT II*

PREOPERATIVE PLANNING

Before arranging for any operation it is important for the patient and the surgeon to have realistic expectations about its outcome. The patient should understand the options; the alternatives to surgery; the expected outcome with and without surgical treatment; the potential risks, hazards, and benefits of the surgery; the nature of the incisions; the potential need for incisions to be made on other parts of the body for the harvesting of grafts; and the possible use of internal fixation, drains, and other types of implants such as those used in silicone arthroplasty. The nature of immobilization after surgery, including the use of splints and casts, also should be understood by the patient, and he should understand that recovery and rehabilitation might be prolonged, especially after major reconstructive procedures on the hand.

As part of the preoperative preparation the patient is instructed to keep his hands clean for several days before surgery and to avoid skin injury to minimize the potential for infection. If he develops cuts or skin infections, the operation should be delayed. Although the skin of the hand and upper extremity will be thoroughly prepared in the operating room, the limb should be scrubbed with an antiseptic soap (iodophors and chlorhexidine derivatives are effective). If the fingernails are long or dirty, they should be cleaned and trimmed to remove potential sources of bacterial contamination.

ARRANGEMENT AND ROUTINE IN OPERATING ROOM

Because surgical results depend considerably on the skill, judgment, and precise work of the surgeon, it is im-

portant to keep intraoperative distractions to a minimum. Disorganization, fatigue, and uncertainty decrease efficiency of the operating team. It is important for the surgeon to establish a standard routine that is followed regularly (Fig. 61-1). Each assistant can then depend on this routine. The activities of the assistants in following this routine should not be disrupted by the surgeon with irregular, unexpected, or inconsistent demands. A standard routine makes it possible for assistants to know what is expected of them at each step in the operation and allows them to perform without hesitation, delay, or wasted motion.

The operating room should always be quiet and pleasant. When a local anesthetic is being used and the patient is awake, loud or inappropriate noises or bursts of conversation may alarm the patient and should be avoided.

The stool on which the surgeon sits should be firm and comfortable and absolutely stable. It should allow the surgeon to sit with the knees almost level with the hips, the feet resting flat on the floor without strain. The working surface of the operating hand table should be at elbow height to provide a comfortable support for the forearms. If the light is directed from above the surgeon's left shoulder (for a right-handed surgeon), it will shine directly on the operative field and shadows are avoided.

Seated opposite the surgeon, the assistant should view the operative field from 8 to 10 cm higher than the surgeon to allow him to see clearly without bending forward and obstructing the surgeon's view. Although mechanical hand holders are available, none are as good as a motivated and well-trained assistant. It is especially helpful for the assistant to be familiar with each procedure. Usually the primary duty of the assistant is to hold the patient's hand stable, secure, and motionless, retract-

*Revision of chapter by Lee W. Milford, M.D.

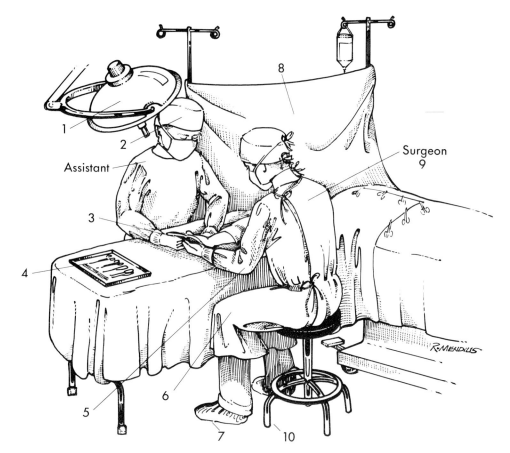

Fig. 61-1 Standard routine is used in operating room, regardless of procedure being performed. Light *(1)* passes over surgeon's left shoulder. Assistant's head *(2)* is 7.5 to 10 cm higher than surgeon's. Assistant holds patient's hand *(3)* firm and motionless. Basic instruments *(4)* are always arranged in same order. Surgeon's elbows *(5)* rest on study table; knees *(6)* are almost level with hips; and feet *(7)* rest flat on floor. Vertical draping *(8)* prevents contamination of operative field by patient's face or by anesthesiologist. Surgeon holds back *(9)* comfortably erect and sits on a stool *(10)* that is firm and absolutely stable. See Fig. 62-1 for a description of hand table.

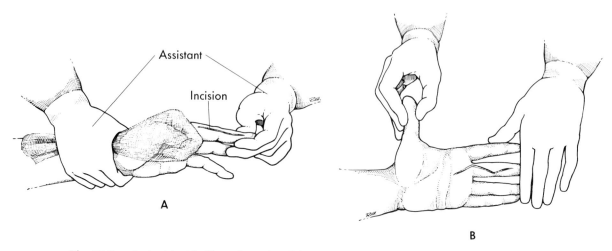

Fig. 61-2 **A,** Assistant holds patient's hand firm and motionless and exposes operative field for a midlateral digital incision. **B,** Ideal position for assistant to stabilize patient's hand as surgeon makes zigzag incision.

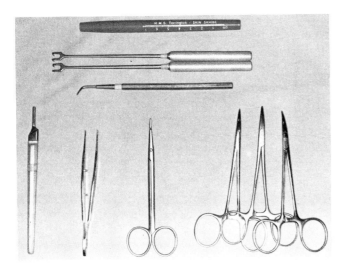

Fig. 61-3 Basic instruments for any surgical procedure on hand. Octagonal-shaped knife handle is preferable to flat handle because knife is more commonly held by precision pinch in hand surgery. Instruments are knife handle, small rat-tooth forceps, dissecting scissors, small hemostats, ruler-marking pencil, double-hook Lovejoy retractors, and probe.

ing the fingers to present to the surgeon the best access to the operative field (Fig. 61-2).

The hand operating table should be stable and immobile. Room should be sufficient for the patient's hand and for resting the elbows and forearms of the surgeon and assistant, thus minimizing muscle fatigue. For most procedures, the surgeon should sit on the axillary side of the involved extremity, allowing the anatomy of either hand to be seen in the same relative position. Some procedures on the dorsum of the hand and wrist may be performed more easily from the cephalic side. If the surgeon changes sides, it is important to keep in mind the change in routine to avoid anatomic disorientation.

The tray holding the basic instruments should be placed on a shelf extending from the operating table, level with the working surface. The instruments should always be arranged in the same order (Fig. 61-3). This arrangement allows the surgeon to save time by routinely reaching for instruments from the basic tray. With practice this can be done without the surgeon looking at the instruments.

Using the so-called "drop" technique, the surgeon discards an instrument after using it, and the nurse returns it to its place on the tray. The discarded knife, tissue forceps, and dissecting scissors that are used constantly are not retrieved by the nurse unless requested be the surgeon. Special instruments should be readily available on another large table so that they can be quickly handed to the surgeon on request. Additional knife blades and special sutures and needles also should be immediately available.

Choice of Anesthetic

Drugs used for local and regional anesthesia should become effective within a few minutes after injection, should cause no local irritation, and should have low systemic toxicity. Lidocaine seems to fulfill these requirements. For regional blocks, a total of up to 50 ml of 1% solution is the recommended safe dosage in a 70 kg adult. Mepivacaine (Carbocaine) acts longer but may be slower in onset and has been found to have about the same toxicity. The recommended dosage is up to 40 ml of 1% solution in a 70 kg adult. Bupivacaine (Marcaine) is preferred by many in replantation surgery, because it is effective for 8 hours or more. It can be used for axillary brachial block to avoid the use of a general anesthesic.

Unsatisfactory anesthesia for operations on the hand and upper extremity will prevent the surgeon from accomplishing his goals and will likely compromise the result of surgery. For accurate and precise work the part must be motionless, the procedure should be completely painless, and the patient should be comfortable. All anesthetic techniques carry some risks, and the selection of the technique depends on the needs of the patient and the preferences of the surgeon and anesthesiologist. The selection should be part of the preoperative planning.

At times general anesthesia is preferred. Factors that favor the use of this type of anesthesia include extensive and prolonged hand and upper extremity operations, performance of procedures on other parts of the body (chest, abdomen, or harvesting of various tissue grafts), extensive operations in young children, the presence of infection in a region that would preclude injecting a local anesthetic agent, and the preference of a particularly uneasy or anxious patient.

Regional anesthesia has many advantages in hand and upper extremity surgery. Satisfactory regional anesthesia can be achieved for emergency procedures performed on patients with a full stomach; in these situations and in elective operations, a regional anesthetic will block vasoconstrictive afferent impulses from the surgical wound and also avoid some of the unpleasant postoperative complications of general anesthesia. Outpatient surgery can be safely performed under regional anesthetic blocks, and the need for postoperative nursing care is decreased. A regional anesthesia may permit operations to be done on the hand and upper extremity in patients with unstable cardiac or severe pulmonary or renal problems that would create an increased risk under general anesthesia.

Regional anesthesia is less satisfactory in children or extremely nervous, anxious, or uncooperative adults. It probably should be avoided in patients with documented allergies to local anesthetic agents and in those taking anticoagulants. A regional anesthetic agent may be difficult to administer in patients with contractures or involvement of joints that limit positioning of the limb for satisfactory blocks and in those whose veins or blood pressure evaluation does not allow the use of the intrave- nous technique. Care should be taken when administer- ing regional anesthetic agents to avoid complications such as overdosage, intravascular injection (when doing nerve blocks), pneumothorax (when doing supraclavicu- lar brachial plexus blocks), and the dissemination of in- fection.

For operations on the hand and upper extremity four methods of regional anesthesia are in widespread use. They are (1) brachial plexus blocks using the inter- scalene, axillary, or supraclavicular approach; (2) intra- venous regional blocks; (3) peripheral nerve blocks dis- tal to the axilla, including blocks of the median, radial, ulnar, and digital nerves; and (4) local infiltration of an- esthetic agents. It is helpful to have the patient satisfacto- rily sedated before surgery. The use of regional anesthe- sia requires that sufficient time be allowed in the imme- diate period before surgery for preparation of the patient, for the administration of the regional anesthetic agents, and for the anesthetic to become effective before making the skin incision. In many situations, especially in elec- tive operations, simple nerve blocks at the wrist or fin- gers require little premedication.

BRACHIAL PLEXUS BLOCKS. The traditional ap- proaches for administering anesthesia to the major com- ponents of the brachial plexus include the axillary, inter- scalene, and supraclavicular routes. The axillary and in- terscalene approaches are probably the most commonly used and are probably somewhat safer than the supra- clavicular route, which carries the risk of a low incidence (1% to 5%) of pneumothorax. Dysesthesias and "brachi- algia" may persist after brachial plexus blocks and the patient should understand this before the block. It also might create difficulty in patients who require fine ma- nipulation of the hands in their occupation (surgeons, technicians, artists, musicians). The axillary brachial plexus block will provide satisfactory anesthesia for most procedures distal to the elbow. Local infiltration in a ring around the proximal arm within the subcutaneous tis- sues will prevent pain from tourniquet pressure caused by blocking of the intercostobrachial nerve. The use of the interscalene brachial plexus block allows operations to be done more proximally in the extremity; satisfactory anesthesia for shoulder operations has been described using this route. The axillary and interscalene ap- proaches are generally preferred over the supraclavicular

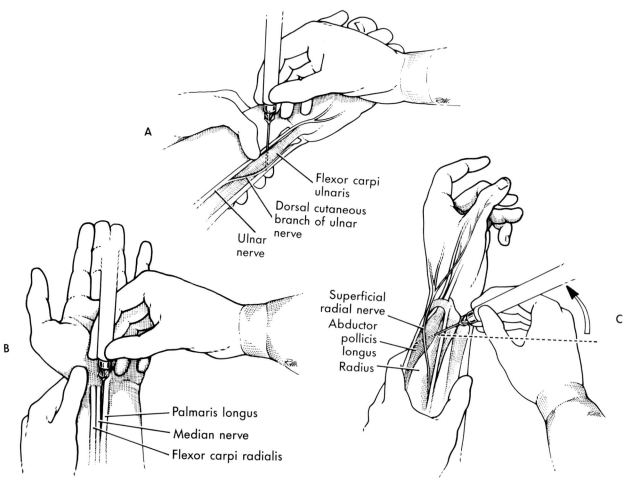

Fig. 61-4 Technique of peripheral nerve blocks. **A,** Ulnar nerve, superficial branch. **B,** Me- dian nerve. **C,** Superficial radial nerve. (From Abadir AR. In Omer GE Jr and Spinner M: Man- agement of peripheral nerve problems, Philadelphia, 1980, WB Saunders Co.)

approach because of their relative ease of administration and the minimal risk of significant complications.

Contraindications to axillary brachial plexus block include infection in the axilla, axillary lymphadenopathy, and malignancy.

INTRAVENOUS REGIONAL ANESTHETIC. The intravenous regional anesthesia technique using a double (Bier's) tourniquet is useful, especially for procedures of relatively short duration (60 to 90 minutes). A specially designed double tourniquet is used. The patient should be satisfactorily premedicated and intravenous infusion should be in place in the contralateral arm. The usual anesthetic agent is lidocaine. In most situations, approximately 30 to 60 ml of 0.5% lidocaine will provide sufficient and safe anesthesia. Satisfactory anesthesia can be obtained in a short period of time. As the more proximal tourniquet becomes uncomfortable, the distal tourniquet is inflated and *then* the proximal tourniquet is deflated. The tourniquet is left inflated for a minimum of 30 minutes after injection of the anesthetic agent into the extremity. In the usual situation, the limb is exsanguinated, the proximal tourniquet is inflated to a safe level (usually 250 to 300 mm Hg), and using sterile technique the anesthesiologist intravenously introduces the previously determined volume of anesthetic agent. The limb is then prepared and the drapes are applied. Haas and Landeen found that wrapping of the limb following exsanguination and intravenous infiltration of the local anesthetic agent helped in dispersal of the agent. They found no premedication to be necessary and that a Penrose drain applied about the wrist provided a dry operative field. Reported reactions during intravenous regional anesthesia include cardiac arrhythmias (bradycardia and cardiac arrest), unconsciousness, vertigo, and nystagmus.

PERIPHERAL NERVE BLOCKS. The median, radial, and ulnar nerves may be blocked at the elbow and wrist, and these blocks are extremely helpful for brief procedures (Fig. 61-4). A tourniquet may not be required or may be used for a short period of time, usually 30 minutes or less. It is essential to know the location of the respective nerves before attempting regional blocks. Blocks at the wrist may be especially useful for procedures such as tenolyses and capsulotomies because motion of the fingers may be observed during surgery. Although a tourniquet may be used briefly, the patient can be kept comfortable; a tourniquet may be used longer than 30 minutes if the patient is adequately sedated.

DIGITAL NERVE BLOCKS. Digital nerve blocks provide excellent anesthesia for procedures on the fingers (Fig. 61-5). Rarely is a tourniquet required. If hemostasis is required, traditionally a Penrose drain or a French rubber catheter applied about the finger has provided satisfactory and safe ischemia. At times, especially in the elderly

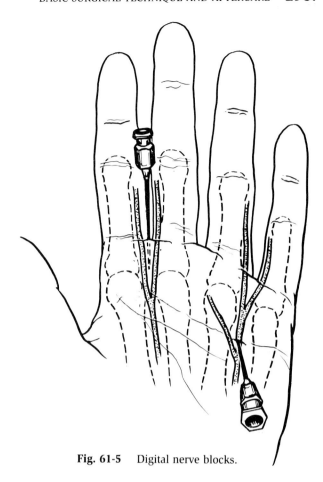

Fig. 61-5 Digital nerve blocks.

and those with vascular disorders in the fingers (Raynaud's disease, atherosclerosis, diabetes) vascular insufficiency may develop in the digit and care should be taken when using digital tourniquets in these patients. Usually perineural injection around the digital nerves proximal to the finger web spaces is a safer technique than injection of the nerves at the base of the fingers. Because ischemia may develop after injection of an anesthetic agent in a circle around the base of the finger, this technique should be avoided. The use of epinephrine in the local anesthetic agent also should be avoided.

LOCAL INFILTRATION. Local infiltration of an anesthetic agent is used for conditions that do not require deep, extensive dissection. This method is satisfactory for trigger digit release, small scar revision, and excision of benign masses from the skin and subcutaneous tissues of the foream, hand, and fingers.

Preparation and Draping for Elective Surgery

Regardless of the operation to be done, the method of preparing and draping the upper extremity and hand should be the same. This helps to standardize the routine and allows movement about the operative field while minimizing the risk of bacterial contamination. The preparation of other areas for graft donor sites varies

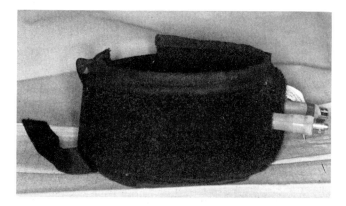

Fig. 61-6 Tourniquet of appropriate size with a Velcro fastener that eliminates buckle seems to be safer and more efficient.

depending on the requirements of the procedure. If skin, tendon, bone, nerve, or other grafts are required, the patient should be positioned to allow easy access to those specific areas. Care should be taken to pad and protect neurovascular structures. The electrocautery grounding pads should be attached in a safe and secure manner. Usually the hand and forearm are scrubbed before the time of the surgery. After the patient arrives in the operating room, the hair is removed from the areas where skin incisions will be made on the hand, forearm, and elsewhere as needed. The tourniquet (Fig. 61-6) is applied to the forearm; however, it is not inflated until all preparations have been completed. After the patient has been satisfactorily anesthetized, the hand and forearm are scrubbed by an assistant while the surgeon scrubs his own hands. The surgeon then puts on gloves and prepares the skin with an antiseptic solution of choice. Iodophor soaps and skin preparation solutions and combinations of chlorhexidine and alcohol have been found to be effective. Wetting the padding beneath the tourniquet with these solution should be avoided to minimize skin reactions. Then a waterproof sheet is placed on the well-padded hand surgery table, followed by a sterile drape-sheet. Combinations of sterile towels and sheets are then applied, leaving exposed the upper extremity and hand and other areas that may require access during the operation. The gloves used in preparation of the surgical field are removed and the surgeon puts on a gown and gloves and seats himself, usually on the axillary side of the forearm as previously noted. The operating lights are adjusted, and the skin incisions are outlined with a skin marking pencil or with methylene blue and applicator sticks. Only after the preparation and draping have been completed is the extremity exsanguinated with an elastic bandage.

Tourniquet

A bloodless field is essential for accurate dissection to avoid damaging small vital structures. The inherent dangers of tourniquet use are ischemia and its complications, including muscle contracture and nerve paralysis. Because the pressure may be more reliably monitored and controlled with a pneumatic tourniquet, complications are believed to be less likely with this type than with an elastic or rubber bandage tourniquet. Regardless of the tourniquet used, disproportionate or prolonged edema, stiffness, diminished sensibility, and weakness or paralysis, temporary or permanent, may result.

When operations are performed with the patient under local anesthesia and last less than 30 minutes, an elastic (Martin) bandage will provide sufficient hemostasis and may be used safely. Wrapping of the bandage is begun at the fingertips and proceeds proximally on the forearm. It is applied in layers overlapping less than 5 to 6 mm. When the midforearm is reached, four or five layers of the elastic are overlapped. Wrinkles are avoided. The pressure is increased with each layer so that only moderate stretching is needed. The bandage is then unwrapped beginning distally from the hand up to the midforearm. The overlapped layers in the midforearm are left in place until the operation is finished. For some procedures done with local infiltration or wrist block anesthesia, a pneumatic tourniquet may be used rather than an elastic wrap tourniquet. The tourniquet may be applied above or just below the elbow and left inflated up to 30 minutes without extreme discomfort.

Improvements in pressure control and calibration design have resulted in the development of "automatic" pneumatic tourniquets that allow the setting of pressures within a safe range and for specific periods of time. Alarms notify the surgeon and anesthesiologist when the preset time has passed. Pneumatic tourniquets are available in several widths with Velcro strap fasteners. There is no absolute rule as to how long a tourniquet may safely remain inflated on the arm. The reports of most authors, especially Wilgis, suggest that the "recovery time" or revascularization time between periods of tourniquet inflation is related to the length of time the tourniquet has been inflated (Table 61-1). In practice, the usual limit is considered to be 1 to 1½ hours. If this limit is exceeded, the risk of paralysis may be increased. Usually, if the operation lasts more than 1½ hours, the tourniquet is released for at least 15 minutes and the limb is elevated with minimal compression applied to the incisions with sterile dressings. The limb is again exsanguinated with an elastic wrap, and the tourniquet is reinflated.

The usual procedure for tourniquet application involves first the application of several layers of cotton sheet wadding wrapped smoothly about the middle of the upper arm near the axilla. The tourniquet is smoothly applied by the surgeon or an experienced assistant. Wrinkles are avoided because their presence may cause blisters and pinching of the skin with necrosis. The limb is exsanguinated either by elevation for 2 to 5 minutes or by wrapping with a Martin elastic bandage

Table 61-1   Tourniquet time and revascularization

Tourniquet time	No.	pH range	Mean	Po$_2$ range (mm Hg)	Mean (mm Hg)	Pco$_2$ range (mm Hg)	Mean (mm Hg)
Preinflation		7.38-7.42	7.40	40-50	45	35-40	38
½ hr	50	7.29-7.35	7.31	22-27	24	45-53	50
1 hr	40	7.15-7.22	7.19	19-22	20	60-66	62
1½ hr	26	7.02-7.10	7.04	6-16	10	80-88	85
2 hr	12	6.88-6.96	6.90	0-6	4	92-110	104

From Wilgis EFS: J Bone Joint Surg 53-A:1343, 1971.

about 10 cm wide beginning at the fingertips and proceeding to just distal to the tourniquet. With automatic tourniquets, inflation is usually rapid enough to avoid trapping excessive blood in the arm during inflation. Wrapping of the limb should be avoided in patients with infections in the limb or in whom malignant tumors are suspected. The tourniquet inflation pressure generally should not exceed 300 mm Hg for adults and 250 mm Hg or lower for children. The wider cuffs minimize focal compression of nerves beneath the cuff; however, smaller cuffs are required for children. Neimkin and Smith found that a double tourniquet on the upper arm with alternating sites of pressure at hourly intervals permitted safe use of the tourniquet for periods of up to 3½ hours in some patients.

Once the tourniquet is released, both it and the underlying cotton wrapping (sheet wadding) should be immediately removed to avoid venous congestion.

Flatt has emphasized the need to check the calibration of the pressure indicator gauge of older design tourniquets with a mercury manometer. He also reports that extreme pressures caused by a faulty gauge even over a short period of time may produce nerve damage that requires weeks for recovery.

Instruments

For the accurate work required in hand surgery, instruments with small points are necessary; the handles, however, should be large enough to allow a firm, secure grip.

The four basic instruments are the knife, the small forceps, the dissecting scissors, and the mosquito hemostat (see Fig. 61-3). The knife blade, which should be firmly attached to the handle, is changed often. The knife should be used for most dissection, to avoid tearing through the tissues with a blunt instrument. The forceps should be carefully checked before surgery for cleanliness and precision of closure, since this instrument will touch the tissues most often. The scissors should have sharp double points, preferably curved, to dissect neurovascular bundles. Instruments used for fine surgery on soft tissues are shown in Figs. 61-7 to 61-10.

A mosquito hemostat or small forceps is preferred for

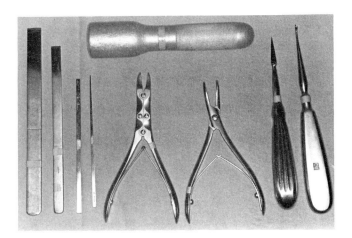

Fig. 61-7   Instruments for small bone surgery include osteotomes, bone cutter, rongeur, awl, small curet, and small hammer.

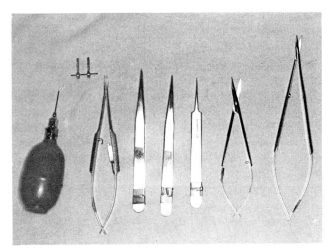

Fig. 61-8   Instruments useful in microvascular and digital nerve surgery include small irrigation bulb, microvascular clamp, microneedle holder, pickups, and scissors of assorted lengths.

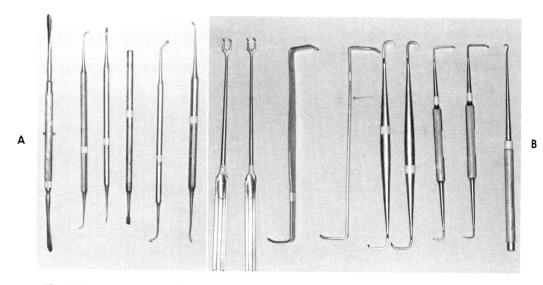

Fig. 61-9 **A,** Certain dental instruments are often useful for dissection of ligaments and bone. **B,** Retractors of numerous designs have been used in hand surgery, but modified tonsil prong *(left)* has proved to be the most useful.

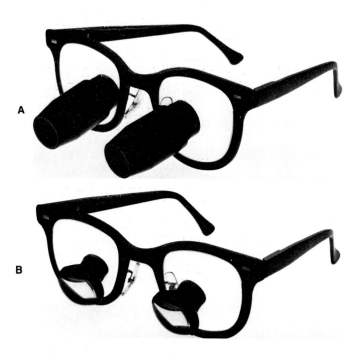

Fig. 61-10 Magnifying glasses for fine surgery on soft tissues. **A,** It is possible to achieve magnification up to 6× with magnification lens on glasses frame. However, magnification lens becomes too heavy for mounting if more than 6× magnification is needed. **B,** Magnification lens set within corrective lens is easy to use with magnification and pupillary distance set for individual surgeon.

clamping vessels because they cause minimal tissue damage. Vessels should be clamped as seen, even when a tourniquet is used. An electric cautery, especially of the bipolar type, is helpful. Retractors should be of the small single- or double-hook type and should have handles long enough to keep the assistant's hands out of the surgeon's working area. Small self-retaining retractors also are useful in certain situations.

For drilling holes in bone, small steel twist drill points provided in most surgical drill sets are satisfactory. Drill points with a 2 mm diameter or small sharp-pointed Kirschner wires may be required. Air- or battery-powered drills allow precise placement of drill holes and wires. Needle holders with narrow noses and smooth jaws are used for tying the finest suture material. Sufficient varieties of wire and synthetic sutures are available to meet the needs in managing tissues of all types. Most sutures are available with swaged, straight, or curved needles.

BASIC SKIN TECHNIQUES
Incisions

As long as certain principles are observed, skin incisions can be made anywhere on the hand and not only in or near major skin creases (Figs. 61-11 and 61-12). In fact, incisions within deep creases should be avoided. Here subcutaneous fat is thin, and moisture tends to accumulate, macerating the skin edges. An incision should be long enough to expose the deep structures without excessive stretching of the skin edges; greater exposure is possible if the skin and subcutaneous fat are dissected

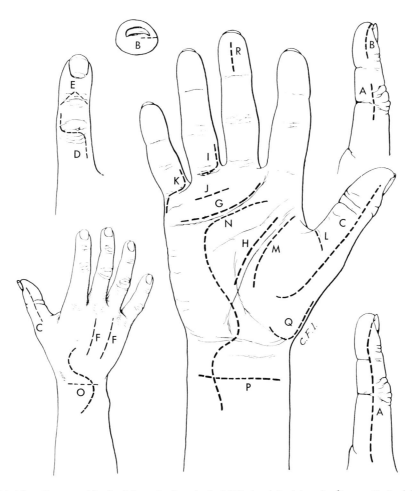

Fig. 61-11   Correct skin incisions in hand. *A,* Midlateral incision in finger. *B,* Incision for draining felon. *C,* Midlateral incision in thumb. *D,* Incision to expose central slip of extensor tendon. *E,* Inverted V incision for arthrodesis of distal interphalangeal joint. *F,* Incision to expose metacarpal shaft. *G,* Incision to expose palmar fascia distally. *H,* Incision to expose structures in middle of palm. *I,* L incision of base of finger. *J,* Short transverse incision to expose flexor tendon sheath. *K,* S incision in base of finger. *L,* Incision to expose proximal end of flexor tendon sheath of thumb. *M,* Incision to expose structures in thenar eminence. *N,* Extensive palmar and wrist incision. *O,* Incisions in dorsum of wrist. *P,* Transverse incision in volar surface of wrist. *Q,* Incision in base of thumb. *R,* Alternate incision to drain a felon. (Modified from Bunnell S: J Bone Joint Surg 14:27, 1932; and Bruner JM: Br J Plast Surg 4:48, 1951.)

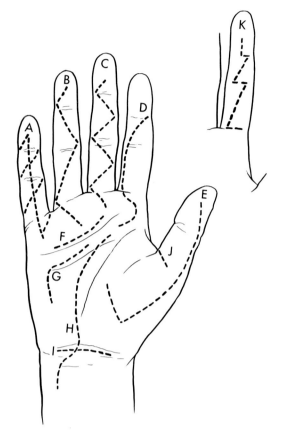

Fig. 61-12 Additional correct skin incisions in hand. *A,* Z-plasty incision often used in Dupuytren's contracture (McGregor). *B* and *C,* Zigzag incisions for Dupuytren's contracture or exposure of flexor tendon sheath. *D,* Volar flap incision. *E,* Incision to expose structures in volar side of the thumb and thenar area. *F,* Incision in distal palm for trigger finger or other affections of proximal tendon sheath. *G,* Incision to form flap over hypothenar area. *H,* Incision to expose structures in middle of palm; it may be extended proximally into wrist. *I,* Short transverse incision in volar surface of wrist. *J,* Short transverse incision to release trigger thumb.

from the underlying fascia. The tissue beneath the skin incision is usually converted into a mobile oval or elliptic opening. The placement of an incision applies only to the skin; entries into deeper structures are made according to their anatomy and may be opposite in direction to those made in the skin. For example, while the skin incision over the radial surface of the wrist in de Quervain's disease may be transverse, the underlying incision in the stenosed sheath is longitudinal.

Generally, shorter incisions may suffice on the dorsum of the hand because here the skin is more mobile. For example, through a 7.5 cm lazy-S longitudinal incision on the middorsum of the wrist, structures can be exposed from the extreme radial side of the wrist to the extreme ulnar side or from the tendon of the extensor pollicis brevis to that of the extensor carpi ulnaris.

Rarely should an incision be made in a straight line. If gently curved, the scar is less noticeable and usually

conforms better to natural lines. A curved incision can also later be extended with freer choice of direction. Exposure is usually better on the concave side of a semicircular incision; an S-shaped incision provides even more exposure.

Parallel or nearly parallel incisions that are too close together or too long should be avoided, because healing may be slow or skin necrosis may even develop because of impairment of the blood supply. Scars that adhere to the underlying structures, especially bone, should be avoided if possible. The offset incision is helpful: the first incision is carried through the skin and subcutaneous fat, and after a flap is undermined on one side, the deep approach is made through the fascia and muscle parallel with but offset from the skin incision.

The plane of motion of a part is approximately perpendicular to the long axis of skin creases. Therefore an incision should not cross a crease at or near a right angle, since the resulting scar, being in the line of tension created by motion, will hypertrophy; indeed, it may limit motion, since a mature scar will not stretch like skin. Although true elsewhere in the body, this principle is more important when dealing with the hand, especially the fingers because the development of contractures creates such significant impairment to function.

At times incisions may be outlined on the skin with a sterile skin pencil, especially if multiple incisions are needed. They may then be made without hesitation, thus saving time after the tourniquet is inflated.

FINGER INCISIONS. A basic and versatile finger incision, the midlateral, has sometimes been misunderstood because of poor drawings and illustrations. With this incision the neurovascular bundle may be carried volarward with the volar flap of the incision, or it may be left in place by carrying the dissection superficial to it.

To carry the neurovascular bundle volarward, begin the incision on the midlateral aspect of the finger at the level of the proximal finger crease and carry it distally to the proximal interphalangeal joint just dorsal to the flexor skin crease; continue it distally along the middle phalanx, again dorsal to the distal flexor skin crease, and proceed toward the lateral edge of the fingernail (Fig. 61-13). Since flexor skin creases extend slightly over halfway around the finger, the incision is in fact slightly posterolateral. Develop the dorsal flap a little to aid in closure of the incision. On the radial sides of the index and middle fingers and the ulnar side of the little finger is a dorsal branch of the digital nerve that should be preserved when possible (Fig. 61-14). Develop the volar flap by continuing into the subcutaneous fat over the proximal and middle phalanges, but since fat is scanty over the proximal interphalangeal joint, be careful not to enter it by mistake. Immediately after incising the fat, carry the dissection volarward deep to the neurovascular bundle and expose the tendon sheath. The sheath can then be incised, or the neurovascular bundle can be exposed

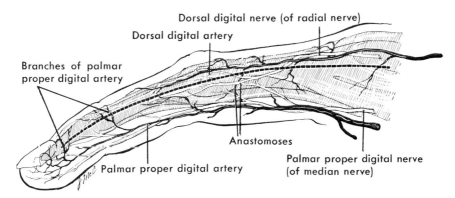

Fig. 61-13   Midlateral skin incision in finger extending from metacarpophalangeal joint to lateral edge of nail. To avoid flexor skin creases, it is placed slightly posterolateral. (Modified from Anson JB and Maddock WG: Callander's surgical anatomy, ed 3, Philadelphia, 1952, WB Saunders Co.)

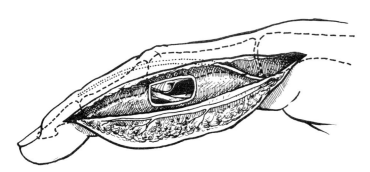

Fig. 61-14   Midlateral approach especially to expose flexor tendon sheath. On radial sides of index and middle fingers and on ulnar side of little finger is dorsal branch of digital nerve that should be preserved if possible. Volar flap containing neurovascular bundle has been developed and reflected. Window has been cut in sheath to show relations of flexor tendons.

by further dissection (Fig. 61-15). The opposite neurovascular bundle can also be exposed because of its anterolateral position.

For the second basic midlateral incision, the skin flap is developed superficial to the neurovascular bundle. Make the same midlateral skin incision, but just distal to the distal flexor skin crease carry the incision obliquely into the pulp of the finger. As the volar skin flap is developed through the subcutaneous fat, carefully isolate the neurovascular bundle; it can best be found at the middle of the middle phalanx. Then expose the bundle by dissecting the fat from its volar surface and expose the flexor tendon sheath by carrying the dissection toward the bone. If necessary, the skin flap can be developed further by dissecting into the depths of the pulp distally, being careful not to disturb the nerves and arteries, and by extending the incision into the palm proximally.

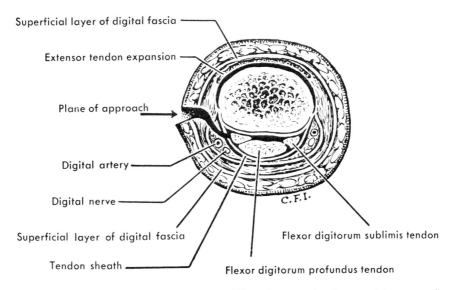

Fig. 61-15   Cross section of finger to show midlateral approach when used to expose flexor tendons.

Using the principles just outlined and illustrated, many less extensive exposures of the finger are possible.

Surprisingly, new incisions and approaches are still being described that allow more direct access to deep structures. The popular volar zigzag finger incision (see Fig. 61-12, *B* and *C*) does not require mobilizing either neurovascular bundle and directly exposes the volar surface of the flexor tendon sheath. However, when used on a contracted skin surface it tends to straighten out and result in a more linear scar than is desirable; here multiple Z-plasty incisions are more satisfactory. In either type of incision, care must be taken to protect the neurovascular bundles.

The volar midline oblique incision (see Fig. 61-12) is useful for a variety of procedures and often can be used instead of a volar zigzag incision. It generally is safe and easily closed. The incision crosses the flexion creases in the volar pulp transversely and slightly obliquely, allowing approach to the flexor sheath in the midline of the finger between the neurovascular bundles.

THUMB INCISIONS. Midlateral incisions described for the fingers are also suitable for the thumb; the radial side is more accessible, and an incision here can be extended by curving its proximal end at the midmetacarpal area and creating a flap on the palmar surface of the thumb (see Fig. 61-11, *C*). Care should be taken to avoid the dorsal branch of the superficial radial nerve to the radial side of the thumb. This incision may be used for tendon grafts without an additional palmar incision, since the flap can be developed sufficiently to expose most of the flexor surface of the thumb. Fat is scanty on the lateral aspects of the distal joint of the thumb, and the volar plate of the capsule may be opened by mistake when seeking the flexor tendon sheath.

When a transverse incision for trigger thumb is made at the level of the metacarpophalangeal joint, the two digital nerves of the thumb, located to either side of the flexor tendon as in the fingers, must be carefully avoided (see Fig. 61-11, *L*).

PALMAR INCISIONS. As a rule, distal palmar incisions are transverse; in the proximal palm they tend to be more longitudinal, with the distal end curving radially and paralleling the closest major skin crease, but at any desired distance from it. An incision of any desired length may be made across the palm, provided that the underlying digital nerves and other vital structures are protected. After the skin and underlying fat are incised, the latter is dissected from the palmar fascia and is carried with the skin flaps. It may be desirable, although tedious, to preserve small vessels perforating the palmar fascia if wide undermining of the skin flaps is necessary; otherwise most of the vital structures are deep to the palmar fascia. In the distal palm, structures lying between the metacarpal heads are not protected by the palmar fascia. After the skin flaps are retracted, the fascia can be

incised in any direction necessary for ample exposure; excision of the fascia may be desirable. The tendons and, parallel to them, the neurovascular bundles are then seen. The superficial volar arch can be ligated and cut at one end if deeper exposure is required. Incisions in the more proximal palm should parallel the thenar crease; however, when extended proximal to the wrist, they should not cross the flexor wrist creases at a right angle. The most important structure in the thenar area is the recurrent branch (motor) of the median nerve, which should be exposed and protected if its exact location is in doubt. In addition, care should be taken to avoid injury to the palmar cutaneous branch of the median nerve, lying near the base of the thumb to the radial side of the flexor carpi radialis.

Basic Skin Closure Techniques*

Early closure but not necessarily immediate closure of all hand wounds lessens the chances of infection and excessive scarring, which may destroy the gliding mechanism essential to hand movements. Immediate coverage is imperative when bone, cartilage, and tendon are laid bare, for without it these structures will not survive. Whenever possible, direct suture of the skin without tension is the best method of closure. On the dorsum of the hand or wrist this is sometimes possible even after considerable loss of the mobile skin by extending the wrist to relieve tension; care should be taken, though, not to hyperextend the metacarpophalangeal joints (Fig. 61-16). When a large defect here is closed in this man-

---

*Also see discussion of considerations for skin closure, p. 2988.

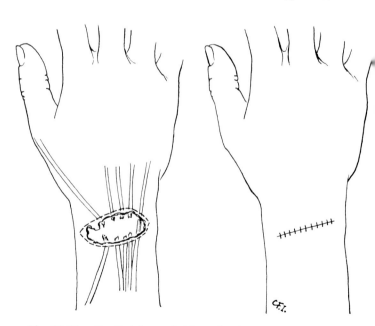

Fig. 61-16 Small defects of skin and subcutaneous tissue on dorsum of hand or wrist can be closed after wrist has been extended to relieve tension. This closure may require a graft later to permit wrist flexion while making a fist.

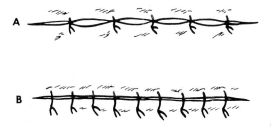

Fig. 61-17 **A,** Skin has been closed by an insufficient number of sutures placed too superficially and too close to skin edges. **B,** Skin has been closed by sufficient number of sutures placed more deeply and well away from skin edges.

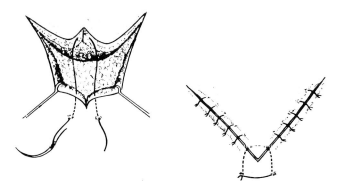

Fig. 61-18 Apical stitch is useful for suturing sharp angle in laceration or in elective flap.

ner, flexion of the wrist and fingers will be limited, and replacement of skin by grafting may be necessary later. The advantages of primary closure by direct suture are jeopardized unless each suture is accurately and patiently placed, for not just the epidermis, but each plane of tissue should meet its corresponding plane. Placing sutures too few in number and too close to the skin edges in attempting a "plastic closure" jeopardizes satisfactory wound closure: the underlying tissues heal poorly, the skin edges tend to separate between the sutures, and necrosis occurs around the sutures (Fig. 61-17). The apical stitch is extremely useful for suturing a sharp angle in a laceration or in an elective flap, since it holds effectively without embarrassing the circulation at the apex (Fig. 61-18). At times a dog-ear of redundant tissue is left after closure of a wound with uneven edges. This dog-ear may be excised one side at a time after splitting it down the middle to create two triangles; each triangle is then excised at its base. The line of excision of

one side is used to mark the line of excision of the other. Another method of excising a dog-ear is shown in Fig. 61-19.

When closure without excessive tension by direct suture is impossible, some type of skin graft must be chosen without prolonged delay, usually within about 5 days. The types of skin grafts most frequently used are described in Chapter 62.

Z-PLASTY. The Z-plasty is an application of the transposition type of local flap; suitably constructed skin flaps are brought from adjacent areas to release a contracture. Typically, a Z-plasty produces a gain in length along the central limb and the central limb undergoes a change in orientation. Its primary use is in the release of a long, narrow contracture surrounded by tissue mobile enough to allow some shifting and manipulation without the

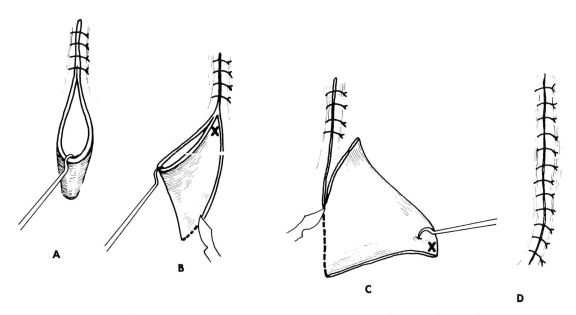

Fig. 61-19 Method of excising dog-ear. **A,** Fold of skin has been caught at its apex by a hook. **B,** Fold has been retracted to one side and skin is being incised along base of fold on opposite side; point X will form apex of flap. **C,** Skin has been unfolded and resulting flap is being excised. **D,** Skin closure has been completed.

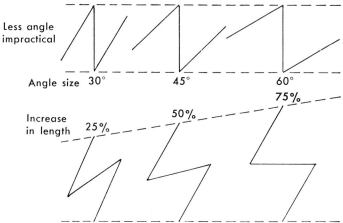

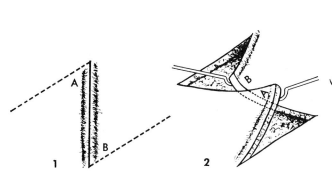

Fig. 61-20   Angles permissible in performing Z-plasties. Angle that central limb of Z makes with each of other two limbs should be between 45 and 60 degrees. When angle is less than 45 degrees, blood supply to flap is impaired; when more than 60 degrees, flaps cannot be transposed without severe tension.

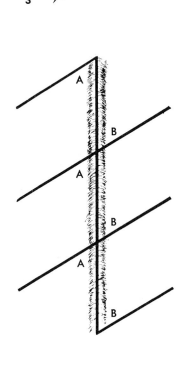

Fig. 61-21   Simple Z-plasty to release a long narrow contracture. *1,* Central limb of Z *(solid line)* is to be made among line of contracture, and other two limbs *(broken lines)* are to be made where shown. *2,* Incisions have been made and flaps are being shifted. *3,* Flaps have been sutured in their new positions. Note apical stitches at *A* and *B*.

danger of necrosis from impaired blood supply. The Z-plasty should not be used in attempting to close a wide fusiform defect. Nor should the Z-plasty be used in the primary closure of a wound unless the wound consists only of a laceration similar to a surgical incision.

■ *TECHNIQUE (Fig. 61-20).* **Make the central limb of the Z along the line of the contracture to be released (Fig. 61-21). Now make the other two limbs of the Z equal in length to that of the central limb; the angle between each limb and the central limb must be equal to each other and is usually about 60 degrees. An increase in this angle will not allow transposition of the flap without severe tension; a decrease makes the Z less effective in releasing tension and impairs the blood supply to each flap. Handle the points of the flaps with care, since they are most likely to undergo necrosis; suture each point with an apical stitch. Multiple Z-plasties (Figs. 61-22 and 61-23) may be used when a scar is too long to allow correction with one Z-plasty and when the scars re-**

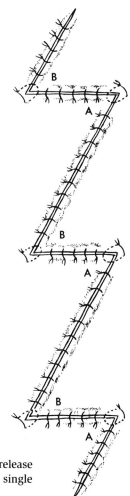

Fig. 61-22   Multiple Z-plasties to release scar too long to be released by single Z-plasty.

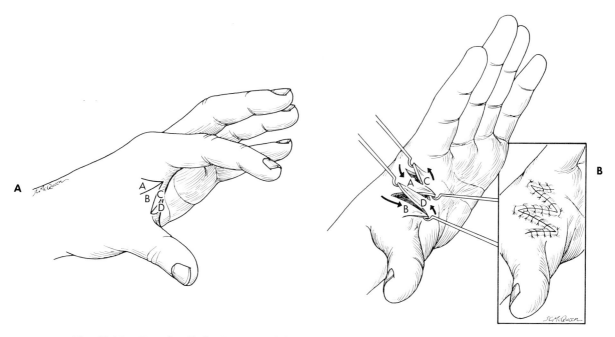

Fig. 61-23 Four-flap Z-plasties are useful in reducing first web contractures secondary to narrow linear scar and with normal elastic surrounding tissue. **A,** Outline of flaps. **B,** Flaps are rotated. *Inset,* Flaps are sutured in place.

sulting from the rotation of the flaps will be in a more desirable position.

• • •

McGregor has modified the standard multiple Z-plasty for use in the fixed palmar skin of the hand and fingers (see Fig. 61-12, *A*). The length of its limbs may be varied, making adjoining flaps larger or smaller as desired; however, the length of the limbs of each individual Z must be equal. The oblique limbs are curved to broaden the tips of the flaps, thus increasing their blood supply. On the finger the oblique limbs end in the flexor skin creases; then when the flaps are shifted, the oblique limbs become transverse and fall within the creases (Fig. 61-24).

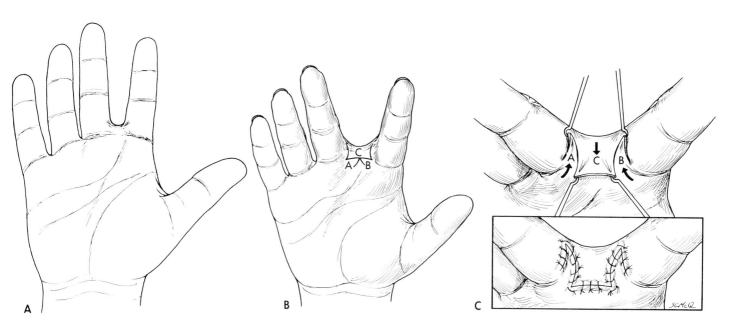

Fig. 61-24 To correct linear contracture of second, third, or fourth web caused by only a narrow scar, a dorsal flap may be fashioned using technique shown. **A,** Web contracture. **B,** Flaps are outlined. **C,** Flaps are rotated in place. *Inset,* Flaps are sutured.

CARE AFTER SURGERY

Care after surgery must be managed intelligently so that tissues are allowed to heal and functions of the affected part are restored as rapidly as possible. That care begins with the application of the dressing. The routine dressing is applied as follows. A closely woven patch of gauze impregnated with Xeroform or Adaptic is placed over each incision. Granulation tissue cannot grow through this material and cause it to adhere; the gauze also prevents the wound from becoming macerated. Then after the hand has been positioned properly, cotton sponges or synthetic (Acrilan) sponges that have been moistened in saline or glycerin solution are carefully placed around it. Moist sponges conform to the contours of the hand more accurately and distribute pressure more evenly than do dry ones. They also promote absorption of blood because they prevent blood from collecting and drying at the wound. Next a roll of cotton or synthetic sheet wadding is wrapped around the hand and forearm. Finally an appropriate splint, usually plaster, is applied and is held in position with a roll of 2-inch (5 cm) or 3-inch (7.5 cm) gauze bandage. Splints and bandages on children tend to slip distally but can be controlled effectively by applying a long arm splint or cast

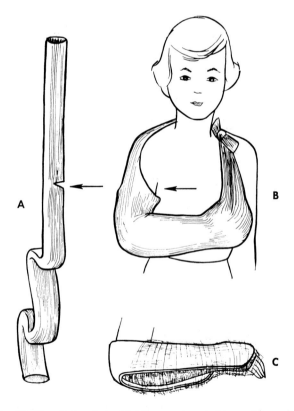

Fig. 61-25   Tube of stockinette may be used to enclose entire extremity of child after surgery. It prevents contamination of dressing and wound. **A** and **B,** Tube is opened *(arrows),* is slipped on extremity, and is tied around neck. **C,** Plaster splint to immobilize forearm and wrist is prevented from slipping distally by including elbow.

and a tube of stockinette that encloses the entire extremity (Fig. 61-25). Immediately before the tourniquet is removed, the hand is kept constantly elevated to prevent edema and hemorrhage after surgery. Elevation should be maintained for at least 48 hours; this can be done by positioning the hand on a pillow resting on the chest, by light overhead suspension that elevates the hand and forearm while the elbow rests on the bed (Fig. 61-26, *A*), or by using a preformed rubber sponge block (Fig. 61-26, *B*).

Bed rest for 3 days or more is strongly recommended after major surgery on the hand. Body activity increases edema of the hand, and merely supporting it in a sling while the patient is ambulatory is not effective. Fingers not splinted should be exercised. The shoulder is likely to become stiff, especially in older patients, and should be abducted and elevated toward the head several times daily; this is easily remembered if done at each mealtime.

Sutures of nylon or steel may not require removal until the splint is discarded, usually at 3 or 4 weeks; therefore complete redressing may be unnecessary unless hematoma or infection is suspected, and in these instances the dressing should be opened as needed, and the splint should be reapplied. Even when no complications are suspected, it is safe to inspect the wound at about 7 days. This avoids unpleasant surprises and allows timely management of unexpected infection or skin necrosis.

When extensor tendons have been sutured, immobilization is necessary for 4 weeks, and then gentle active exercises are begun, but the hand is supported between exercise periods until the fifth or sixth week. After flexor tendon repairs, early protected motion may be started. Usually splint immobilization is necessary for 3 weeks, and then splint-protected active exercises are begun; exercises against moderate resistance are begun during the fifth to sixth week. When tendons have been transferred, immobilization is necessary for 3 to 4 weeks; active motion is then begun, but some type of wrist support is continued until the fifth or sixth week.

Active use of the hand is the most effective way to reestablish motion after surgery. The use of splints, hand blocks, and putty is valuable. Physical therapy and occupational therapy are helpful because they result in purposeful movement and a sense of accomplishment and prevent the boredom that is frequent when a patient is requested to repeat a single motion dozens of times. Often the best therapy is the patient's usual work, and if possible he should be offered the opportunity to return to it as part of the treatment, even if on a limited basis. The return to the activities of daily living and work seems also to have a beneficial psychologic effect.

Applying excessive heat to the hand while it is held dependent or passive manipulation of joints by the patient, therapist, or surgeon is always contraindicated. Two points are especially important in the care after surgery. First, the patient should never be sent to a physical

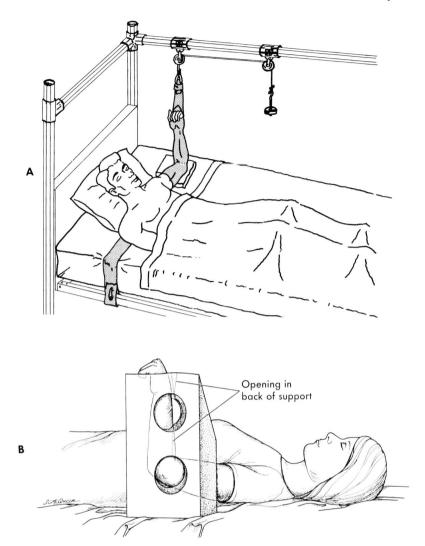

Fig. 61-26   **A,** Tube of stockinette and traction may be used to elevate hand and forearm after surgery. Tube is opened, is slipped on extremity, and is carried across bed beneath shoulders. At level of palm it is opened again to allow motion of digits. One end of stockinette is attached to mattress frame and the other to traction apparatus. **B,** Preformed rubber sponge block is also useful for elevating hand postoperatively while in bed. It was originally designed for postoperative foot protection. Although hand, forearm, and elbow are contained within block, they are not constricted. It is a mobile elevator so patient may take it home for nighttime use.

therapist without specific written orders describing the exact treatment requested; the therapist cannot be expected to prescribe treatment, and when orders are not specific, the hand may be treated in a hot whirlpool bath in the dependent position. This feels good at the time, but edema and stiffness usually develop later. Second, the patient should not be required to carry out movements of the hand that are markedly painful. The cause of pain should be sought, and if necessary the part should be splinted.

These general principles of care after surgery are as important as the surgery itself; neglect of them will disrupt the results of the finest surgical skill.

SPLINTING

Splinting may have one of three purposes: (1) to immobilize all or part of the hand in a position that will promote healing and prevent deformity, (2) to correct an existing deformity and promote function in that part, and (3) to supply power to compensate for weakness, especially in muscles affected by peripheral nerve palsy. Splints may function to prevent motion (static splints) or to assist motion (dynamic splints).

Immobilizing splints are most frequently used after an operation for a limited time only or intermittently to ensure correct position of joints and to relax muscles; they are also used to prevent further deformity, as in the arthritic hand. The splint should permit unaffected parts to function as normally as possible. They should be comfortable and light. A splint maker should be available for making technical adjustments requiring special skills, but the patient should be able to apply the splint, remove it, and make minor adjustments. The patient should thoroughly understand the reason for wearing it and should be convinced of its value. As treatment progresses, faithful use of the splint can be determined by observing the patient's skill in applying and removing it.

Some of the more useful splints are illustrated in Figs. 61-27 to 61-35.

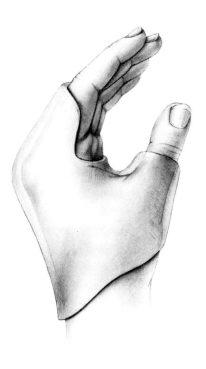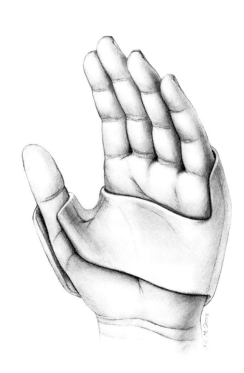

Fig. 61-27 Splint is comfortable and has very low profile, which encourages wearing while recovery is progressing in median-ulnar nerve palsies. It permits pinch and some grasping while maintaining metacarpophalangeal joints in slight flexion. It blocks metacarpophalangeal joint extension and thus prevents clawing.

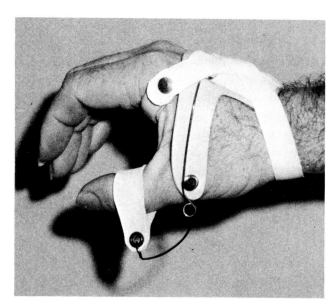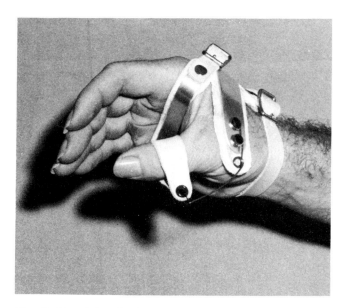

Fig. 61-28 Splint for low median nerve palsy dynamically holds thumb in abduction, extension, and opposition, thus preventing an adduction contracture of thumb. It is light and compact. (Courtesy Dr. George E Omer, Jr.)

Fig. 61-29 Splint for low median nerve palsy functions like splint shown in Fig. 61-28. However, it is made of metal instead of plastic. (Courtesy Dr. George E Omer, Jr.)

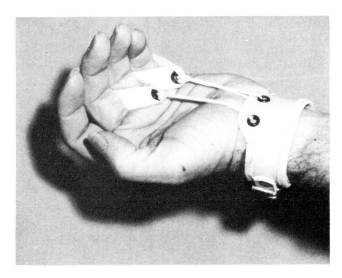

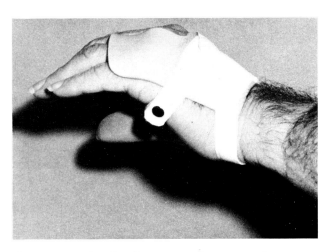

Fig. 61-30 Splint for ulnar nerve palsy dynamically forces metacarpophalangeal joints of ring and little fingers into flexion. Part of palm is covered by rubber bands, which is a disadvantage. (Courtesy Dr. George E Omer, Jr.)

Fig. 61-31 Splint for ulnar nerve palsy prevents hyperextension deformity of metacarpophalangeal joints of ring and little fingers. Further, it conforms to shape of transverse metacarpal arch and has no attachments that hinder function of hand. (Courtesy Dr. George E Omer, Jr.)

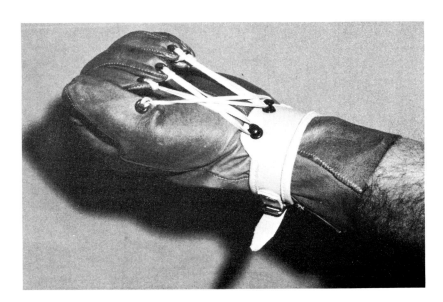

Fig. 61-32 Flexor glove dynamically forces fingers into flexion, exerting continuous force on proximal interphalangeal and metacarpophalangeal joints. Sometimes it also flexes wrist when proximal eyelets are too far proximal, and when desirable, it may be applied over volar wrist splint. (Courtesy Dr. George E Omer, Jr.)

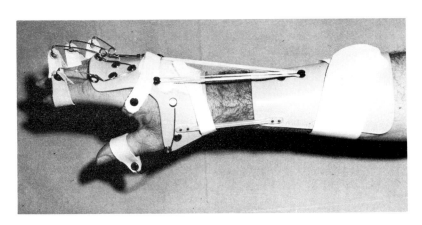

Fig. 61-33 Splint for high radial nerve palsy dynamically splints wrist and digits in extension. Further, it is light and pliable and has none of large outriggers usually employed to extend digits. (Courtesy Dr. George E Omer, Jr.)

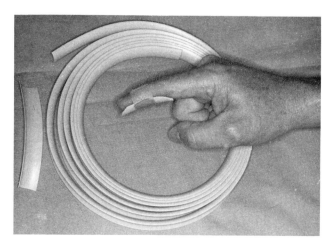

Fig. 61-34 Preformed plastic gutter splints for digits are easily adjustable in length and support soft tissue or fracture healing.

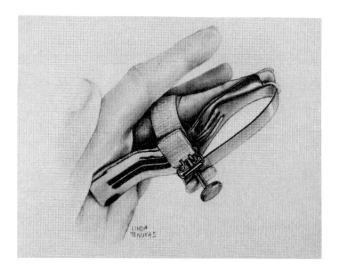

Fig. 61-35 Joint-Jack finger splint. (Courtesy Joint-Jack Co, Glastonbury, Connecticut.)

The Joint-Jack, a splint that gradually extends the contracted proximal interphalangeal joint, has been designed by Kirk Watson (Fig. 61-35). The tension is gradually increased by a screw in conjunction with a strap. It is used only intermittently. The patient should be cautioned about possible skin pressure problems that may occur over the proximal interphalangeal joint.

REFERENCES
General
Boyes JH: Operative technique in surgery of the hand, AAOS Instr Course Lect 9:181, 1952.

Chase RA: Surgery of the hand. I. N Engl J Med 287:1174, 1972.

Chase RA: Surgery of the hand. II. N Engl J Med 287:1227, 1972.

Gordon L and Buncke HJ: Universal microsurgical operating table, J Hand Surg 3:101, 1978.

Howard LD Jr, Pratt DR, and Bunnell S: The use of compound F (Hydrocortone) in operative and non-operative conditions of the hand, J Bone Joint Surg 35 A:994, 1953.

Jones KG, Marmor L, and Lankford LL: An overview on new procedures in surgery of the hand, Clin Orthop 99:154, 1974.

Kelikian H: The crippled hand, AAOS Instr Course Lect 14:163, 1957.

Ketchum LD et al: A clinical study of forces generated by the intrinsic muscles of the index finger and the extrinsic flexor and extensor muscles of the hand, J Hand Surg 3:571, 1978.

Kilgore ES and Newmeyer WL: In favor of standing to do hand surgery, J Hand Surg 2:326, 1977.

Lunseth PA, Burton RI, and Braun RM: Continuous suction drainage in hand surgery, J Hand Surg 4:193, 1979.

McGregor IA: Fundamental techniques of plastic surgery and their surgical applications, Edinburgh, 1960, E & S Livingstone, Ltd.

Peters CR and Kleinert HE: Office and emergency room care of the injured hand, South Med J 69:53, 1976.

Rank BK and Wakefield AR: Surgery of repair as applied to hand injuries, Baltimore, 1960, Williams & Wilkins.

Rob C and Smith R, editors: Operative surgery: orthopaedics and plastic surgery, vol 1, part X Hand, Philadelphia, 1959, FA Davis Co.

Tanzer RC: Prevention of postoperative hematoma in surgery of the hand: the use of the "compression suture," J Bone Joint Surg 34-A:797, 1952.

Verdan C: Basic principles in surgery of the hand, Surg Clin North Am 47:355, 1967.

Walker PS, Davidson W, and Erkman MJ: An apparatus to assess function of the hand, J Hand Surg 3:189, 1978.

Anesthesia
Abadir A: Anesthesia for hand surgery, Orthop Clin North Am 2:205, 1970.

Adams JP, Dealy EJ, and Kenmore PI: Intravenous regional anesthesia in hand surgery, J Bone Joint Surg 46-A:811, 1964.

Burnham PJ: Regional block at the wrist of the great nerves of the hand, JAMA 167:847, 1958.

Haas LM and Landeen FH: Improved intravenous regional anesthesia for surgery of the hand, wrist, and forearm: the second trap technique, J Hand Surg 3:194, 1978.

Hunter JM, Schneider LH, Dumont J, and Erickson JC III: A dynamic approach to problems of hand function using local anesthesia supplemented by intravenous fentanyl-droperidol, Clin Orthop 104:112, 1974.

Kasdan ML et al: Axillary block anesthesia for surgery of the hand, Plast Reconstr Surg 46:256, 1970.

Vatashsky E et al: Anesthesia in a hand surgery unit, J Hand Surg 5:495, 1980.

Instruments
Barron JN: Instruments for hand surgery, Hand 6:211, 1974.

Tegtmeier RE: Self-retaining retractors for hand surgery, Plast Reconstr Surg 53:495, 1974.

Incisions
Burnham PJ: A new incision for amputation of the index finger and its metacarpal, Am J Surg 97:331, 1959.

Skin closure
McGregor IA: The Z-plasty in hand surgery, J Bone Joint Surg 49-B:448, 1967.

Postoperative management
Bruner JM: Problems of postoperative position and motion in surgery of the hand, J Bone Joint Surg 35-A:355, 1953.

Tourniquet
Bolton CF and McFarlane RM: Human pneumatic tourniquet paralysis, Neurology 28:787, 1978.

Bruner JM: Safety factors in the use of the pneumatic tourniquet for hemostasis in surgery of the hand, J Bone Joint Surg 33-A:221, 1951.

Denny-Brown D and Brenner C: Paralysis of nerve induced by direct pressure and by tourniquet, Arch Neurol Psychiatr 51:1, 1944.

Dery R, Pelletier J, and Jacques A: Metabolic changes induced in the limb during tourniquet ischemia, Can Anaesth Soc J 12:367, 1965.

Eckhoff NL: Tourniquet paralysis: a plea for the extended use of the pneumatic tourniquet, Lancet 2:343, 1931.

Flatt AE: Tourniquet time in hand surgery, Arch Surg 104:190, 1972.

Klenerman L: The tourniquet in surgery, J Bone Joint Surg 44-B:937, 1962.

Klenerman L, Biswas M, and Hulands GH: Systemic and local effects of the application of a tourniquet, J Bone Joint Surg 62-B:385, 1980.

Middleton RWD and Varian JP: Tourniquet paralysis, Aust NZ J Surg 44:124, 1974.

Miller SH et al: The acute effects of tourniquet ischemia on tissue and blood gas tensions in the primate limb, J Hand Surg 3:11, 1978.

Miller SH et al: Effects of tourniquet ischemia and postischemic edema on muscle metabolism, J Hand Surg 4:547, 1979.

Neimkin RJ and Smith RJ: Double tourniquet with linked mercury manometers for hand surgery, J Hand Surg 8:938, 1983.

Ochoa J, Fowler TJ, and Gilliatt RW: Anatomical changes in peripheral nerves compressed by a pneumatic tourniquet, J Anat 113:433, 1972.

Paletta FX, Willman V, and Ship AG: Prolonged tourniquet ischemia of extremities, J Bone Joint Surg 42-A:945, 1960.

Patterson S and Klenerman L: The effect of pneumatic tourniquets on the ultra structure of skeletal muscle, J Bone Joint Surg 61-B:178, 1979.

Price AJ, Jones NAG, and Webb PJ: Do tourniquets prevent deep vein thrombosis? J Bone Joint Surg 62-B:529, 1980.

Rorabeck CH: Tourniquet induced nerve ischemia: an experimental investigation, J Trauma 20:280, 1980.

Rudge P: Tourniquet paralysis with prolonged conduction block, J Bone Joint Surg 56-B:716, 1974.

Solonen KA, Tarkkanen L, and Narvanen S: Metabolic changes in the upper limb during tourniquet ischemia, Acta Orthop Scand 39:20, 1968.

Thomassen EH: An improved method for application of the pneumatic tourniquet on extremities, Clin Orthop 103:99, 1974.

Tountas CP and Bergman RA: Tourniquet ischemia: ultrastructural and histochemical observations of ischemic human muscle and of monkey muscle and nerve, J Hand Surg 2:31, 1977.

Wilgis EFS: Observations on the effects of tourniquet ischemia, J Bone Joint Surg 53-A:1343, 1971.

Splinting

Bunnell S: Spring splint to supinate or pronate the hand, J Bone Joint Surg 31-A:664, 1949.

Bunnell S and Howard LD Jr: Additional elastic hand splints, J Bone Joint Surg 32-A:226, 1950.

Fess RE and Philips C: Hand splinting: principles and methods, ed 2, St Louis, 1986, Mosby–Year Book, Inc.

Kent H: Functional brace for the paralyzed hand: a preliminary report, J Bone Joint Surg 36-A:1082, 1954.

Ketchum LD, Hibbard A, and Hassanein KM: Follow-up report on the electrically driven hand splint, J Hand Surg 4:474, 1979.

Littler JW and Tobin WJ: Thumb abduction splint, J Bone Joint Surg 30-A:240, 1948.

Nickel V, Perry J, and Garrett AL: Development of useful function in the severely paralyzed hand, J Bone Joint Surg 45-A:933, 1963.

Peacock EE Jr: Dynamic splinting for the prevention and correction of hand deformities: a simple and inexpensive method, J Bone Joint Surg 34-A:789, 1952.

Schottstaedt ER and Robinson GB: Functional bracing of the arm. II. J Bone Joint Surg 38-A:841, 1956.

Stewart JE: A plastic opponens splint for the thumb, J Bone Joint Surg 30-A:783, 1948.

Strong ML: A new method of extension-block splinting for the proximal interphalangeal joint: preliminary report, J Hand Surg 5:606, 1980.

Thomas FB: An improved splint for radial (musculospiral) nerve paralysis, J Bone Joint Surg 33-B:272, 1951.

Weber ER and Davis J: Rehabilitation following hand surgery, Orthop Clin North Am 9:529, 1978.

Zide BM, Bevin AG, and Hollis LI: Examples of simply fabricated custom-made splints for the hand, J Hand Surg 6:35, 1981.

Anatomy

Albright JA and Linburg RM: Common variations of the radial wrist extensors, J Hand Surg 3:134, 1978.

Anson JB and Maddock WG: Callander's surgical anatomy, ed 3, Philadelphia, 1952, WB Saunders Co.

Ashby BS: Hypertrophy of the palmaris longus muscle: report of a case, J Bone Joint Surg 46-B:230, 1964.

Bowers WH et al: The proximal interphalangeal joint volar plate. I. An anatomical and biomechanical study, J Hand Surg 5:79, 1980.

Bunnell S: Surgery of the hand, eds 2 and 3, Philadelphia, 1948, 1956, JB Lippincott Co.

Chase RA: Surgical anatomy of the hand, Surg Clin North Am 44:1349, 1964.

Conway H, and Stark RB: Arterial vascularization of the soft tissues of the hand, J Bone Joint Surg 36-A:1238, 1954.

Culver JE Jr: Extensor pollicis and indicis communis tendon: a rare anatomic variation revisited, J Hand Surg 5:548, 1980.

Durksen F: Anomalous lumbrical muscles in the hand: a case report, J Hand Surg 3:550, 1978.

Engber WD and Gmeiner JG: Palmar cutaneous branch of the ulnar nerve, J Hand Surg 5:26, 1980.

Eyler DL and Markee JE: The anatomy and function of the intrinsic musculature of the fingers, J Bone Joint Surg 36-A:1, 1954.

Flatt AF: Kinesiology of the hand, AAOS Instr Course Lect 18:266, 1961.

Furnas DW: Muscle-tendon variations in the flexor compartment of the wrist, Plast Reconstr Surg 36:320, 1965.

Kaplan EB: Embryological development of the tendinous apparatus of the fingers: relation to function, J Bone Joint Surg 32-A:820, 1950.

Kaplan EB: Functional and surgical anatomy of the hand, Philadelphia, 1953, JB Lippincott Co.

Kisner WH: Double sublimis tendon to fifth finger with absence of profundus, Plast Reconstr Surg 65:229, 1980.

Landsmeer JMF: The coordination of finger-joint motions, J Bone Joint Surg 45-A:1654, 1963.

Lassa R and Shrewsbury MM: A variation in the path of the deep motor branch of the ulnar nerve at the wrist, J Bone Joint Surg 57-A:990, 1975.

Linburg RM and Comstock BE: Anomalous tendon slips from the flexor pollicis longus to the flexor digitorum profundus, J Hand Surg 4:79, 1979.

Littler JW: The physiology and dynamic function of the hand, Surg Clin North Am 40:259, 1960.

Littler JW: The finger extensor mechanism, Surg Clin North Am 47:415, 1967.

McFarlane RM: Observations on the functional anatomy of the intrinsic muscles of the thumb, J Bone Joint Surg 44-A:1073, 1962.

Micks JE, Reswick JB, and Hager DL: The mechanism of the intrinsic minus finger: a biomechanical study, J Hand Surg 3:333, 1978.

Moes RJ: Andreas Vasalius and the anatomy of the upper extremity, J Hand Surg 1:23, 1976.

Ochiai N, et al: Vascular anatomy of flexor tendons. I. Vincular system and blood supply of the profundus tendon in the digital sheath, J Hand Surg 4:321, 1979.

Parks BJ and Horner RL: Medical and surgical importance of the arterial blood supply of the thumb, J Hand Surg 3:383, 1978.

Resnick D: Roentgenographic anatomy of the tendon sheaths of the hand and wrist: tenography, Am J Roentgenol Radium Ther Nucl Med 124:44, 1975.

Schenck RR: Variations of the extensor tendons of the fingers: surgical significance, J Bone Joint Surg 46-A:103, 1964.

Shrewsbury MM and Johnson RK: A systemic study of the oblique retinacular ligament of the human finger: its structure and function, J Hand Surg 2:194, 1977.

Shrewsbury MM and Johnson RK: Ligaments of the distal interphalangeal joint and the mallet position, J Hand Surg 5:214, 1980.

Tubiana R and Valentin P: The physiology of the extension of the fingers, Surg Clin North Am 44:897, 1964.

Vichare NA: Anomalous muscle belly of the flexor digitorum superficialis: report of a case, J Bone Joint Surg 52-B:757, 1970.

Wallace WA and Coupland RE: Variations in the nerves of the thumb and index finger, J Bone Joint Surg 57-B:491, 1975.

Winkleman NZ: Aberrant sensory branch of the median nerve to the third web space: a case report, J Hand Surg 5:566, 1980.

Acute Injuries

PHILLIP E. WRIGHT II*

For the acutely injured hand, the purpose of treatment is to restore its function. It is necessary to prevent infection, salvage injured parts, and promote primary healing. Nerves and tendons may be repaired in the primary phase of care, but this is secondary in importance to thorough cleansing and debridement, correct stabilization of fractures and dislocations, and wound closure or coverage with skin grafts or skin flaps. Through patient history and examination the surgeon must personally appraise the injury to decide what primary procedures can be done safely and what later secondary procedures may be necessary.

HISTORY

The history should provide accurately and concisely the following information: (1) the exact time of injury (to determine the interval before treatment); (2) the first aid measures given and by whom and where; (3) the nature, amount, and time of receiving any medication; (4) the exact mechanism of injury (to determine the amount of crushing, contamination, and blood loss); (5) the nature, time, and amount of food and liquid taken by the patient (information necessary for selection of the anesthetic); and (6) the patient's age, occupation, place of employment, handedness, and general health status. General, vague, nonspecific statements are best avoided.

FIRST AID

The patient's initial evaluation includes an assessment of other potentially serious or life-threatening injuries. Open hand wounds should be covered immediately with a sterile dressing to prevent further contamination. When the wound is severe and bleeding, the hand should be elevated with the patient lying supine; if bleeding is not controlled by elevation alone, manual or digital pressure must be applied to the wound through the dressing. Bleeding may be quickly controlled by removing an improperly applied tourniquet; rarely is a tourniquet necessary. At times, it may be helpful to elevate the arm and control bleeding with a pneumatic tourniquet or blood pressure cuff inflated to 100 to 150 mm Hg greater than the systolic pressure. The tourniquet should be deflated as soon as bleeding is controlled.

Do not use hemostats and ligatures to control bleeding in the emergency department because this may damage the vessels and nerves, thereby interfering with later repair.

FIRST EXAMINATION

With the patient supine and as comfortable as possible, the wound is examined in two stages. The first examination is made before surgery, but under sterile conditions; masks should cover the faces of the examiner and, when possible, the patient. Sterile instruments and gloves are used. The purpose of this examination is to estimate the size of the wound and determine the extent of

*Revision of chapter by Lee W. Milford, M.D.

skin loss and injury to the deep structures. Probing the depth of the wound rarely is helpful. The viability of the skin and any gross positional deformity are noted. The wound is then covered, and examination is attempted to help determine what deep structures are functioning; *each one of these structures must be considered damaged until proved otherwise.* To lessen the chance of error, the assessment of each tissue should be orderly; attention is first directed to the circulation and skin and then to bones, tendons, and nerves.

The condition of the skin is assessed constantly so that a timely choice can be made between primary closure by direct skin suture or by appropriate skin grafts or flaps.

Roentgenograms of an injured hand are made routinely to reveal fractures, dislocations, or foreign bodies.

Careful assessments for severed tendons and nerves are done next. The techniques for these evaluations are found in detail in Chapters 63 and 65, respectively.

From this first examination the surgeon should obtain some idea about the extent of injury and what procedures will be necessary. A final decision is withheld until the second examination is done during surgery. The patient's general medical condition is evaluated. Antibiotics, sedation, blood transfusions, tetanus prophylaxis, and other measures are provided as indicated. Before sedatives or narcotics are given, the patient should be advised as to the extent of his injuries, the general plan of treatment, and the prognosis, especially with regard to any possible amputation. He should also be forewarned when skin grafts, or distant skin flaps are anticipated.

Anesthesia

A regional block or general anesthetic may be selected, depending on the patient's age and general condition, the severity of the injury, the interval since the last ingestion of food or drink, and whether a distant flap will be necessary (see Chapter 61 for more details).

Tourniquet

A tourniquet is necessary while the wound is being cleansed and inspected and while the deep structures are being repaired. When the viability of an area of skin is questionable because of a crushing or avulsing injury, a tourniquet should be used as briefly as possible. When there is a large wound with fractures, elevation of the hand for 2 minutes is better than wrapping it with a Martin bandage before inflation of the tourniquet. This prevents further crushing and displacement of fracture fragments (for more information on the tourniquet, see Chapter 61).

Cleansing and Draping of Hand

After the patient or the part is anesthetized and the tourniquet is applied, the first aid dressing is removed and a sterile pad is placed over the major wound. The uninvolved skin surrounding the wound is shaved. The hand is held over a drain basin and scrubbed with antiseptic soap and water to above the elbow. The nails and nail beds are cleansed, and the nails are trimmed. Next, the wound is exposed and irrigated with normal saline solution (Fig. 62-1). Usually antiseptics are not used in the wound because of the potential tissue toxicity. The wound is irrigated with normal saline, either poured or through a pulsating lavage apparatus to provide a stream with enough force to loosen small foreign particles and to remove large hematomas. A gloved finger may be placed in the wound to loosen hematomas or to palpate the bones, but the depths of the wound should not be rubbed with a sponge or brush. Small bleeding vessels, which are sometimes more easily seen under water, are clamped with mosquito hemostats and cauterized. Small flaps and tags of devitalized fat and fascia seen floating in the solution may be removed at their bases. Nerve ends are not debrided. Ragged skin edges may be trimmed, but complete excision of the edges of the wound usually is not necessary in the hand.

As the deeper parts of the wound are cleaned, they are carefully searched for foreign materials, especially if there is suspicion that they contain broken glass, wood, or pieces of glove, or when the wound has been caused by a gunshot. Cleaning should not be hurried and often may take up half of the total operating time; it must be thorough to help prevent infection. Primary healing without infection is necessary to limit the scar and to allow additional early reconstruction, if needed. When the cleaning is complete, all instruments, gloves, and drapes used during this process are discarded, and the hand is redraped (see Chapter 61 for the details of draping and of the routine in the operating room).

SECOND EXAMINATION

After a diligent effort has been made to convert the contaminated wound into a clean one in the operating room, the wound is examined again. The tissues in the depths of the wound, including exposed bones, tendons, and nerves, are assessed in an orderly anatomic manner to avoid error; the skin is also carefully examined. Only after an accurate assessment of the damage can correct decisions be made as to which structures may be repaired primarily. Bones and joints are inspected to assess bone loss, the extent of periosteal stripping, and fracture stability. This evaluation allows estimation of potential bone healing and the advisability of early joint motion after internal fixation of fractures. Suspected damage to tendons and nerves must now be confirmed by direct vision since the conclusions drawn from the first examination may be wrong; usually the damage has been underestimated. Passive finger motion often delivers severed tendons into the wound. Small hematomas seen within synovial sheaths may be indications of further tendon injury. Evaluating the skin damage is most important because primary closure may depend on this evaluation. Frequently some skin appears to be lost when actually it

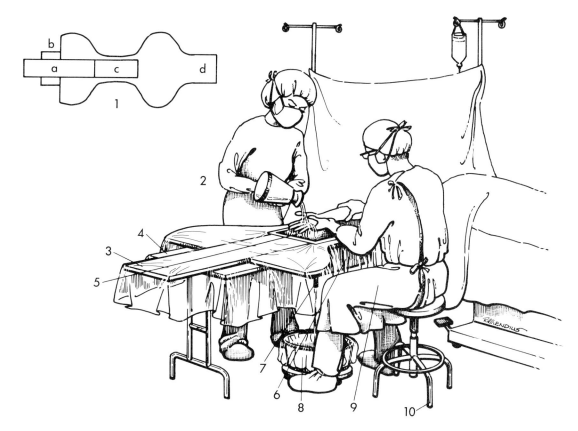

Fig. 62-1 Hand table and routine of cleansing hand. *1,* View of table from above. Movable panel, *a,* has been pushed to left so that pan may be inserted at *c.* When panel, *a,* has been pushed to right and table has been draped, basic instruments are placed on shelf, *b.* End of table, *d,* is placed beneath patient. *2,* Assistant irrigates open wound with normal saline solution. *3,* Movable panel has been pushed to left. *4,* Shelf on which basic instruments will be placed. *5,* Plastic sheet in which hole has been made to receive pan has been spread over table. *6,* Pan has been inserted to receive irrigating solution. *7,* Drainpipe in bottom of pan. *8,* Bucket into which irrigation solution flows from pan. *9,* Surgeon is seated comfortably on stool, *10,* which is firm and stable.

has only retracted; this is especially true of L-shaped wounds on the dorsum of the hand. When skin is crushed or flaps of skin are avulsed, the possibility of necrosis must be seriously considered. Releasing the tourniquet may be necessary for accurate evaluation. A valuable sign that skin is viable is a pink blush immediately after release of the tourniquet. The extent of bleeding from the skin edges, the color of the skin immediately after compression, and the amount of undermining of the skin edges must all be observed. Necrosis, infection, and scarring may all occur when flaps of doubtful viability are retained. The extent of skin loss from the injury itself and after surgical excision of nonviable flaps must be evaluated, and plans must be made for complete coverage.

CONSIDERATIONS FOR AMPUTATION

Considerations for amputation are discussed in Chapter 69.

ORDER OF TISSUE REPAIR

To set priorities for repair of each tissue is important. After the wound is cleaned, the bony architecture must be reestablished immediately if possible (see Chapter 64) or within a few days after the wound becomes clean; otherwise, the soft tissues will contract, making their repair difficult or impossible without grafting. Even though definitive closure may not be possible, the bony architecture should be reestablished. It is preferable to close the wound within the first 5 days. If the injury and wound conditions permit, tendons and nerves should be repaired at the time of primary or secondary skin closure. It is easier to suture the tendons and then repair the nerves than to attempt to suture the nerves first and maintain their continuity while manipulating the hand to suture the tendons. While awaiting repair, nerves will contract, especially in the fingers and palm. Therefore consideration should be given to tagging the nerve ends with a small suture, not necessarily together, but to the soft tissues of the palm. If repairs of nerve and tendons are delayed, repair or reconstructions may be carried out later. See Chapters 63 and 65 for additional discussions of nerve and tendon repair and reconstruction.

ARTERIAL INJURIES

When either the radial or ulnar artery alone is lacerated at the wrist level or more distally, the circulation in the hand usually remains sufficient. Even when both arteries are lacerated, the prognosis for survival of the hand is excellent in young people, good in those in early middle age, and fair in those who are older; in these circumstances circulation through collateral vessels or an uninjured patent median artery or both may be adequate. Even in older patients, repairing the radial or ulnar artery at the wrist is optional. It may be argued that circulation obtained by repair of the artery, even though temporary, may be sufficient to sustain the hand while the collateral circulation is developing. Repair of arteries and veins distal to the wrist usually results in survival of severely impaired or amputated digits. This requires knowledge and skill in microsurgical technique (Chapter 49). Also see the discussion on ulnar tunnel syndrome in Chapter 76.

CONSIDERATIONS FOR SKIN CLOSURE

Primary skin closure is desirable and usually can be done in all sharply incised, "tidy" wounds. The purpose of primary skin closure is to obtain early healing and to avoid infection, granulation tissue, edema, and excessive scar production. Misjudgment may lead to delayed healing as a result of hematoma, swelling, and infection, any of which may require reopening the wound for drainage or additional debridement. Certain wounds should never be closed primarily; these include the severely contaminated or crush wounds caused by farm machinery, human bites, tornado missiles, and augers. High-velocity missile wounds, other war wounds, and wounds contaminated with animal or human feces or fertilizer also should not be closed primarily.

When in doubt, the wound should be left open after careful debridement using an anesthetic. Within about 24 to 48 hours the wound should be reinspected, and if it is sufficiently clean, it can be closed by direct suture or by skin graft. If possible, a wound should be closed within about 5 days of injury. Generally, a wound should not be left open to granulate and heal by secondary intention unless it cannot be made sufficiently clean to allow skin grafting or closure.

METHODS AND INDICATIONS FOR SKIN CLOSURE
Direct Suture

Unless severely contaminated or crushed, every wound of the hand (except those mentioned previously) should be closed primarily, because healing by primary intention is the desired result. As stated previously, most *incised* wounds can be closed by simple direct suture of the skin. Usually, the subcutaneous tissue is not sutured separately, but care should be taken to avoid inversion of the skin edges. Careful hemostasis is necessary. Closure is easier when all viable skin edges have been preserved during the initial cleansing.

Skin Grafts

Wounds with distally attached flaps may have enough skin for primary closure but not enough venous drainage for the skin to survive. This deficient drainage causes engorgement and venous distention and finally thrombosis and necrosis; the color of the flap changes from a deep blue to purple and then to black. The retrograde flap is often the result of a crushing or tearing injury, and the very nature of this injury even further jeopardizes the survival of the flap. Such a flap on the dorsal surface of the hand or forearm is less likely to survive than one on the palm (Fig. 62-2). When there is doubt, the skin should be excised and replaced with a split graft (p. 2990).

When skin is lost without exposing deep structures, such as nerves, tendons, joints, or cortical bone, it should be replaced immediately with either a split-thickness graft or occasionally with a full-thickness one. A skin defect on the dorsal surface of the hand may be converted to a transverse elliptical one and closed in a trans-

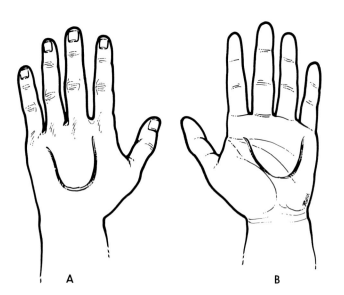

Fig. 62-2 Flap attached distally on dorsum of hand, **A,** is less likely to survive than is similar one on palm, **B.**

verse line. Because of the mobility of the dorsal hand skin, this type of closure is possible here and is made easier when the wrist is dorsiflexed.

Skin Flaps

When a skin defect exposes deep structures, a split-thickness or full-thickness skin graft is insufficient coverage for nerves, tendons, and cortical bone. These structures will not readily support a skin graft and require good nutrition to survive. A skin flap graft is necessary to provide subcutaneous tissue for coverage and for sufficient nutrition. This flap may be a local one, but usually it is obtained from a distance, either as a pedicle flap or a free tissue transfer.

Coverage of Specific Areas with Flaps

A large skin defect on the dorsum of a finger that exposes tendons not covered with paratenon should be covered with a flap. Frequently a double local flap can be constructed by rotating a proximally based local flap on one side and a distally based local flap on the other side of the defect to cover the exposed tendon. The donor defects are covered with split grafts. When multiple fingers are involved or when there is a need for larger area coverage, a subpectoral flap may be in order. Thick subcutaneous fat, as is found on the lower abdomen, is not preferred on a flap, especially on the finger.

Skin defects on the volar surface of a finger that expose tendons may be covered with a cross finger flap. The flap is raised from the dorsal surface of an adjacent finger and extends from the midline of one of its lateral surfaces to that of the other; the flap is a little wider than the defect it is to cover. Although such a flap from the dorsal surface of one finger may be used to cover a defect on the volar surface of another, the reverse is never indicated. The use of flaps for amputations of the fingertip and thumb are discussed in Chapter 69.

Skin defects on the palm or dorsum of the hand that expose vital structures may be covered with a local rotation flap, a flap from an adjacent unsalvageable finger, a flap from the opposite forearm or upper arm, or a flap from the abdomen, depending on the size of the defect and the presence and location of any associated injuries. Although cross-arm and cross-forearm flaps provide good skin, immobilizing both upper extremities is a disadvantage. An abdominal flap from the same side allows the most comfortable position of the arm. To ensure survival of the random pattern flap (since it must be applied immediately), its base should be as wide as its length. The length-to-width ratio may exceed 3:1 with axial pattern flaps such as the groin pedicle flap. The donor area and the raw part of the flap that will not make contact with the defect should be covered with split-thickness skin grafts. A local rotation flap is unlikely to survive, however, if undermining of the skin is extensive, espe-

cially if the skin is already crushed or contused from the injury. A filleted finger makes an excellent pedicle graft when this technique is applicable (Fig. 62-3). In some situations, free tissue transfer by microvascular technique will provide the best coverage (Chapter 49).

Management of the Donor Area

There are several acceptable methods for treating the donor area. In one, the donor area is dressed with one layer of finely woven nylon or silk gauze. When the dressing prevents drying, the donor area tends to become macerated and secondary infection and necrosis may occur, and this area may itself require skin grafting later. Otherwise the part is left uncovered, and drying of the area is encouraged. In another technique, a synthetic adhesive film is placed over the donor site. Serum and blood accumulate daily for 1 to 2 days and the film is changed. After about 7 to 10 days this can be removed and the area is left open, usually with satisfactory heal-

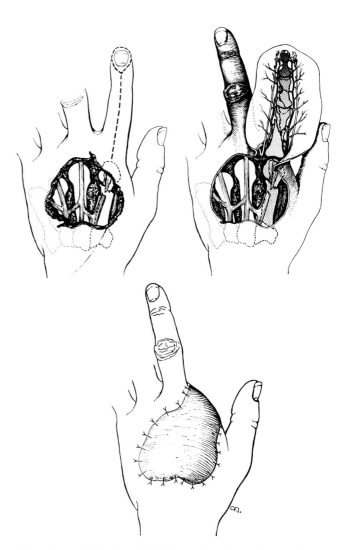

Fig. 62-3 Filleted graft fashioned from finger (see text).

ing. Bed sheets should be kept off the donor site with a bed cradle support.

GRAFTS AND FLAPS
Free Grafts

When free skin grafts are to be obtained, it is well to remember that "the thinner the graft the better the take" and yet when the graft is expected to be permanent, "the thicker the graft the better the function." A thick graft is better able to withstand friction and constant use than a thin one and will contract only about 10%; a thin graft may contract 50% to 75%. For the graft to survive, it must reestablish its nutrition before death of its entire thickness occurs; great care is therefore needed, both in operative technique and in aftercare, to ensure that it remains undisturbed and in direct contact with the recipient area during healing. This takes careful planning, especially in children. The graft will not survive if a hematoma separates it from the underlying vascular bed; rarely will it survive a gross infection. For primary coverage of acute wounds, free skin grafts are usually of thin or medium thickness. They will not easily survive on bare cortical bone, bare tendon, or bare cartilage. Full-thickness free skin grafts are not often used on the hand; but such a graft or a thick split graft may be useful for the palmar surface because it contains elastic tissue and in growing children will contract less and will tend to accommodate with growth. Since the survival of a full-thickness graft is so uncertain, it is best used only in elective surgery for skin coverage in the palm; it should rarely be used in acute injuries, with the possible exception of the fingertips. The so-called "pinch grafts" are no longer used.

Split-thickness Skin Grafts

Frequently only a small or postage stamp graft is needed, and it may be obtained within the same operative field from the forearm; however, taking a graft from this area is undesirable in children and women because it will leave a slight scar. More suitable donor areas for these and larger grafts are the anterior and lateral aspects of the thigh and the medial aspect of the arm just inferior to the axilla. In some older women skin is available inferior to a pendulous breast without leaving a readily visible scar.

OBTAINING GRAFTS WITH RAZOR BLADE

■ *TECHNIQUE.* A small skin graft easily may be cut with an ordinary new razor blade held in a hemostat. Lubricate the surface of the skin with a drop of mineral oil and keep it taut with a tongue blade. Hold the side of the razor blade almost parallel to the skin with the edge of the blade in contact with it. Cut the split graft with to-and-fro motions of the

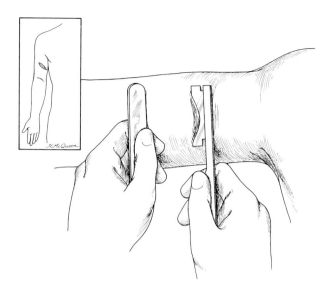

Fig. 62-4   Technique of removing split-thickness skin graft from flexor surface above elbow with Weck knife. This permits hiding scar at donor site much more effectively than if extensor surfaces distal to elbow were used.

blade; take care not to consciously force the blade forward, since it will automatically advance with the to-and-fro motions. A Weck knife (Fig. 62-4) is an instrument that refines this technique.

OBTAINING SKIN GRAFTS WITH DERMATOME

■ *TECHNIQUE.* Two types of mechanical dermatomes are in widespread use for split-thickness grafts: the powered (electrical or pneumatic) and the manual (drum) dermatomes. The electrically powered dermatomes, such as the Stryker, Brown, or Padgett, are not hard to assemble and use; an inexperienced operator can cut consistently good grafts up to 7.5 cm wide. Skin glue is not required, but light lubrication of the skin with mineral oil or petroleum jelly is helpful. Bony prominences are not satisfactory donor sites with these dermatomes. The Reese drum dermatome does require skin glue and must be operated with precision, but it is excellent for cutting grafts more than 7.5 cm wide. Usually it more accurately controls the thickness of the grafts. Three suggestions are offered in the use of this dermatome: (1) stretch the rubber tape tightly on the drum, (2) wait at least 3 minutes for the glue to dry before applying the dermatome to the skin, and (3) rotate the drum slowly and lift up gently while cutting the graft.

When using either type of dermatome, cut the graft somewhat larger than the recipient area.

APPLYING SPLIT-THICKNESS GRAFTS

■ *TECHNIQUE.* The recipient area must have a vascular bed and be free of active bleeding and gross infection. If the recipient area is not suitable, prepara-

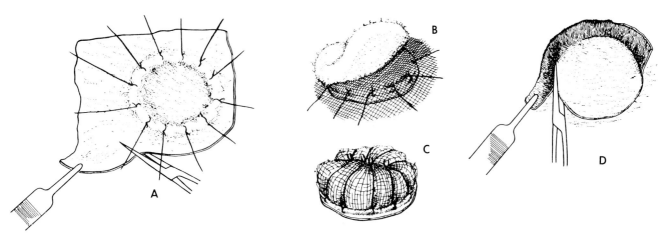

Fig. 62-5 Technique of applying split-thickness graft. **A,** Graft has been sutured over defect and redundant edges of graft are being trimmed. **B,** Sheet of finely meshed gauze and pack of moist cotton or gauze have been placed over graft. **C,** Sutures have been tied over pack. **D,** Necrotic edges of graft are being trimmed away after graft has healed.

tion may require several days of enzymatic debridement, multiple dressing changes, and surgical debridement to remove dead and infected material. Meshing of the graft is helpful if a large area is to be covered. Meshing also allows the free drainage of serum and blood from beneath the graft (Fig. 62-5, *B*). Place the graft on the recipient area without trimming or excessive handling. The graft border may be attached with sutures or skin staples to secure it in its new position. Then trim the redundant edge (Fig. 62-5, *A*). When suturing the graft in place, it is much easier to insert a small curved needle first through the graft and then through the skin around the recipient area than to do the reverse.

A stent dressing may be applied, or finely meshed nonadherent gauze (Xeroform or Adaptic) may be placed over the graft and held in place with a bulky dressing secured by circumferential conforming gauze and when necessary may be covered by a thin layer of plaster for splinting. The dressing is usually changed after about a week; any necrotic graft is then removed and a fresh dressing is applied. When an area of necrosis is large, regrafting may be necessary. When a slough is anticipated or when another procedure is planned in which a split-thickness graft will be used, a graft larger than needed initially may be cut and refrigerated at between 0° and 5° C in a Ringer's solution or in a saline solution to which penicillin has been added; it can then be used at any later time up to 21 days.

Free Full-thickness Grafts

When a full-thickness graft is used, the recipient area must be free of infection and hemostasis must be complete. Preferred donor areas include the groin or the medial aspect of the arm where the skin is thin and where

the defect created by removing the graft may be closed by undermining and suturing the skin edges (Fig. 62-6).

Sometimes an associated injury makes a detached piece of skin and underlying fat available; in this instance the skin may be stabilized on a dermatome drum and a full-thickness graft excised from the fat.

■ *TECHNIQUE.* Make a pattern on sterile tape or gauze of the area to be covered. Using this pattern, outline the anticipated graft on the donor area with methylene blue or a skin marker. It should be slightly larger than the pattern to allow for the necessary margin in suturing and for shrinkage. Remove the

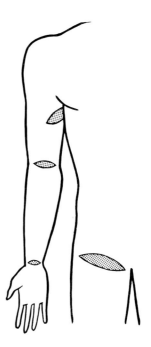

Fig. 62-6 Sites from which to obtain full-thickness skin grafts. Groin or medial apsect of arm is preferable (see text).

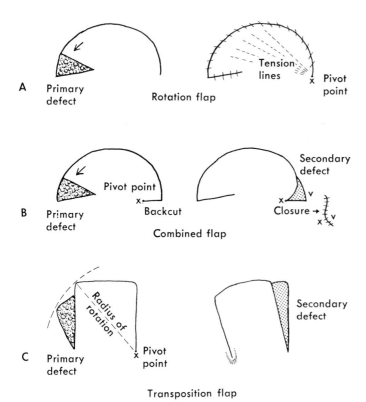

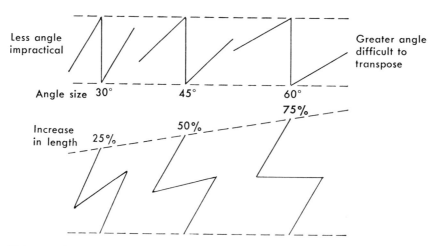

Fig. 62-7 Principles of three types of local flaps. In each type, defect to be covered is converted into triangular one. Flap may be rotated, **A,** transposed, **C,** or both, **B. B,** Backcut in combined flap decreases tension on flap but also decreases blood supply to flap; defect created by this backcut is closed as shown. **C,** Defect created by transposing flap must be covered with split-thickness graft. (Redrawn from Rank BK and Wakefiled AR: Surgery of repair as applied to hand injuries, Baltimore, 1960, Williams & Wilkins, and from McGregor IA: Fundamental techniques of plastic surgery and their surgical applications, Edinburgh, 1960, E & S Livingstone, Ltd.)

graft with a sharp knife by dissection between the fat and the skin; do not take any fat with the graft. Suture it in place and excise the redundant edges. Apply a stent dressing and support the hand with a plaster splint for at least 7 to 10 days before redressing. At that time dark blisters of the superficial layer of the graft may be seen, but this usually does not indicate deep necrosis.

Flap Grafts

A flap graft may be used in the primary closure of a hand wound or in a secondary procedure to replace scars, skin of poor quality, or necrotic skin. It may be obtained locally or from a distant part. When the area to be covered is small, a local flap may be indicated, like one of those shown in Fig. 62-7, or a Z-plasty, as shown in Figs. 62-8 to 62-10. When the defect is on the volar surface of a finger and subcutaneous fat is needed, a cross finger flap (p. 2993) may be used.

The advantages of a local flap over one from a distant part are that the involved hand is not tied to the distant donor and that in many instances finger motions may continue. When the defect is too large to be covered with a local flap, a distant flap from the abdomen (p. 2995) or a free tissue transfer (Chapter 49) is indicated.

Local Flaps

Fig. 62-7 illustrates the principles of three types of local flaps.

Local flaps usually should be avoided when treating acute hand injuries; the skin that would be used as the flap is often already contused, and this insult combined with the amount of undermining necessary for closure often causes necrosis of the flap. If skin that would be

Fig. 62-8 Angles permissible in performing Z-plasties. Angles that central limb of Z make with each of other two limbs should be between 45 and 60 degrees. When angles are less than 45 degrees, blood supply to flap is impaired; when more than 60 degrees, flaps cannot be transposed without severe tension.

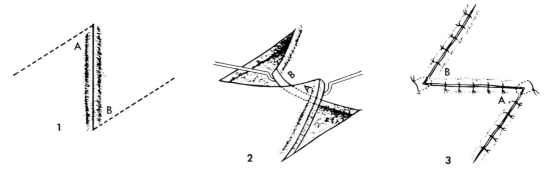

Fig. 62-9 Simple Z-plasty to release a long, narrow contracture. **1,** Central limb of Z, *solid line,* is to be made along line of contracture, and other two limbs, *broken lines,* are to be made where shown. **2,** Incisions have been made and flaps are being shifted. **3,** Flaps have been sutured in their new positions. Note special stitches at *A* and *B.*

used as a local flap is severely damaged, it should not be used in the treatment of acute hand injuries.

A variety of local flaps can be used in the hand and fingers as noted. They include local rotation flaps from the dorsum of the hand to fill defects in the web spaces, cross finger flaps, thenar flaps, "flag" flaps, Vilain and Dupuis flaps, Gibraiel flaps, lateral volar flaps, transpositional flaps, and the flap described by Lueders and Shapiro.

Local flaps are usually of the simple transposition type. This type covers vital structures but leaves a defect that must in turn be covered with a split-thickness graft (Fig. 62-11). A common error in designing a local flap is to make it too short; it must be remembered that the fixed point of pivot from which the advancement is made is at that border of the base that is opposite the defect. If the corresponding border of the flap is not long enough, tension occurs when the flap is sutured in its new bed.

Cross Finger Flaps

Cross finger flaps (Fig. 62-12) are useful for covering a defect of the skin and other soft tissues on the volar sur-

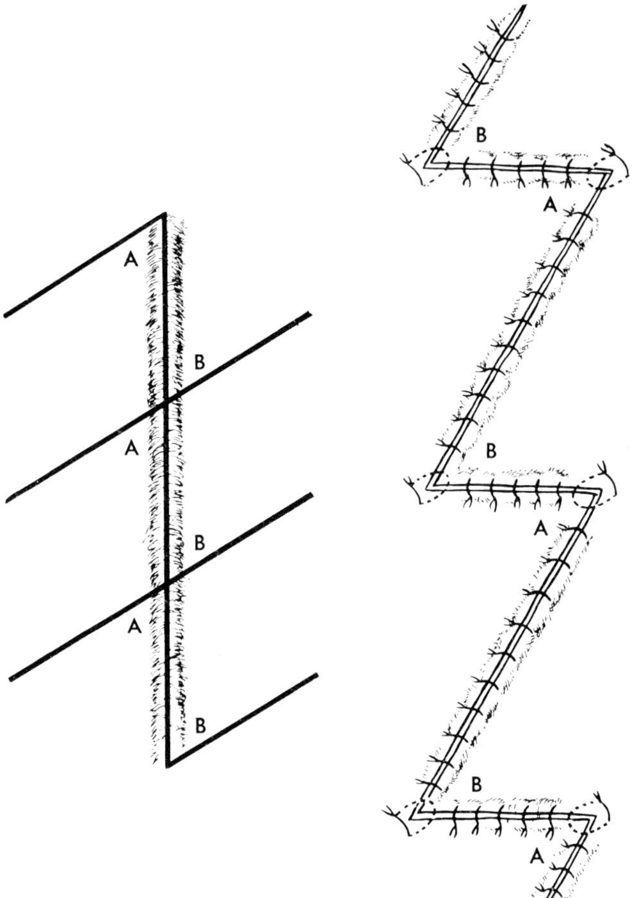

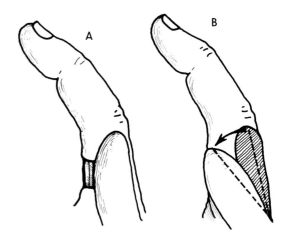

Fig. 62-11 Simple transposition type of local flap. **A,** Deep structures on anterolateral aspect of finger are exposed and must be covered by local flap; flap has been outlined. **B,** Flap has been transposed and defect thus created on posterolateral aspect of finger has been covered by split-thickness graft. Note radius, *broken lines,* of arc, *arrow,* of transposition.

Fig. 62-10 Multiple Z-plasties to release scar too long to be released by single Z-plasty.

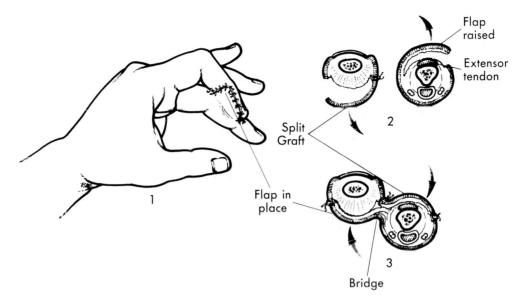

Fig. 62-12   Cross finger flap. *1,* Laterally based pedicle flap has been raised from middle finger and has been applied to distal pad of index. *2* and *3,* Cross sections of two fingers showing how cross finger flap has been applied, and how raw surfaces of donor finger and of bridge between two fingers have been covered with split-thickness skin graft (see text). (Redrawn from Hoskins HD: J Bone Joint Surg 42-A:261, 1960.)

face of the finger when tendons and neurovascular structures are exposed. They are also useful for some amputations of the thumb (Chapter 69). These grafts are best avoided in patients over 50 years of age, in hands with arthritic changes or a tendency to finger stiffness for some other reason, or when there is a local infection.

■ *TECHNIQUE.* Excise the edges of the defect so that it is rectangular, with its longer sides parallel to the long axis of the finger but not crossing skin creases. Then measure its dimensions. Place the injured finger against the donor finger and determine where to locate the base of the proposed flap. Cut the flap from the donor finger through the skin and subcutaneous tissues, leaving its base attached to the side adjacent to the recipient finger (Fig. 62-13). Make the flap 4 to 6 mm wider than the defect and long enough both to cover the defect (allowing for normal skin contraction) and to provide a bridge between the fingers. If necessary, the flap may be raised from one midlateral line of the donor finger to the other, but be careful to avoid incising the volar surface of the donor finger.

When raising the flap, make the incisions through the subcutaneous tissue but not through the paritenon of the extensor expansion (Fig. 62-14). When possible, avoid using skin distal to the distal interphalangeal joint so as not to injure the nail bed. The skin over the dorsal surface of the proximal interphalangeal joint should also be avoided unless needed for width. When necessary, the base of the flap may be further freed by cutting the oblique fibers of the deep tissue that attaches

the skin to the extensor tendon and periosteum along the side of the finger. Handle the flap with small hooks to prevent crushing and necrosis. Release the tourniquet and obtain absolute hemostasis; reinflate the tourniquet. Cut a thick split graft (up to 0.045 cm) from the forearm or thigh and suture it to the donor area and to the undersurface of the bridge. Now apply the flap to the recipient area and suture it in place with the finest suture (5-0 or 6-0 nylon); the entire recipient area should be in contact with the flap. Leave the sutures long at the edges of the free split graft, and fashion a stent dressing. Take care to avoid excessive tension on sutures transverse to the long axis of the finger to avoid vascular compromise. Cover the suture line with non-adhering gauze, then place moist cotton pledgets about the graft and apply gauze wrapping. To ensure immobility of the recipient finger, an oblique Kirschner wire through the interphalangeal joint may sometimes be used. A volar splint of plaster or fiberglass also may be used if additional support is needed.

AFTERTREATMENT. The flap may be detached after 12 to 14 days. The skin margins of the recipient finger should be trimmed so that the junction of the normal skin with the graft is at a midlateral position on the finger. Motion of both fingers can be started the day after the flap is detached.

• • •

This technique may be varied so that the base of the flap is proximal rather than lateral; such a flap is useful

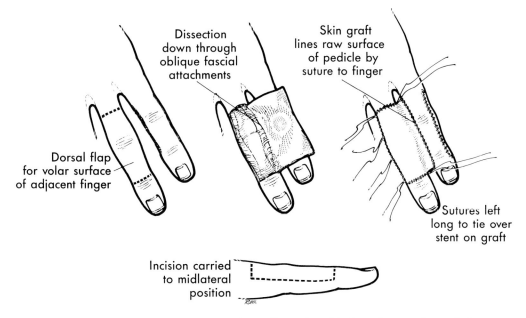

Dissection down through oblique fascial attachments

Skin graft lines raw surface of pedicle by suture to finger

Dorsal flap for volar surface of adjacent finger

Sutures left long to tie over stent on graft

Incision carried to midlateral position

Fig. 62-13   Technique of applying cross finger flap, using skin from dorsum of two phalanges (see text). (Redrawn from Curtis RM: Ann Surg 145:650, 1957.)

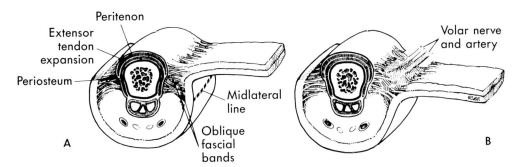

Peritenon

Extensor tendon expansion

Periosteum

Volar nerve and artery

Midlateral line

Oblique fascial bands

A

B

Fig. 62-14   Details of raising cross finger flap. **A,** Incision has been carried to but not through peritenon of extensor expansion; note oblique fascial bands. **B,** Incision has been continued to sever oblique fascial bands but avoids damage to volar digital artery and nerve. (Modified from Curtis RM: Ann Surg 145:650, 1957.)

for covering a defect near the tip of an adjacent finger or thumb (Fig. 62-15). Rotation of the flap is necessary, and care should be taken to prevent strangulation at the base and necrosis. Rotated flaps that are based proximally may be used to cover defects on the same finger (see Fig. 62-11).

Abdominal Flaps

In addition to the flaps previously discussed, the size of the defect and the thickness of the flap required may make it necessary to use a remote pedicle flap from the abdominal region. Traditionally, flaps from the abdomen have been used as *tubed pedicle flaps* or as *direct* flaps. The tubed pedicle technique requires the formation of a bipedicle tube and 6 weeks of maturation followed by detachment of one end of the tube to be applied to the hand, followed by another 3 to 6 weeks before the flap is

completely detached and "inset" into the defect. The direct abdominal flaps typically are limited in their length-to-width ratio because of the random circulation. It rarely is safe to use such a flap with a length-to-width ratio that varies significantly from 1:1. A better understanding of the skin circulation has led to the development and use of flaps with a defined arteriovenous supply — axial pattern flaps. Axial pattern flaps allow a safe length-to-width ratio of at least 3:1, the possibility of covering either the dorsal or palmar surface, and a sufficiently long pedicle to allow arm and hand movement. Because such flaps usually do not require a delay in detachment of one end, they are useful for coverage of acute hand injuries. Microvascular surgical coverage options using free flaps are discussed in Chapter 49.

RANDOM PATTERN ABDOMINAL PEDICLE FLAPS. A random pattern abdominal flap to be applied to the hand

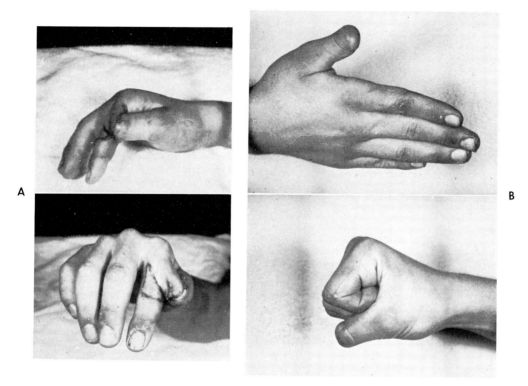

Fig. 62-15 Cross finger flap that is based proximally. **A,** Twenty days after surgery. Only radial part of flap covers defect on thumb. Triangular defect on donor finger has been covered with split-thickness graft. **B,** Six months after surgery. Flap has been detached and has healed without redundancy. Donor finger has been disfigured little. (From Hoskins HD: J Bone Joint Surg 42-A:216, 1960.)

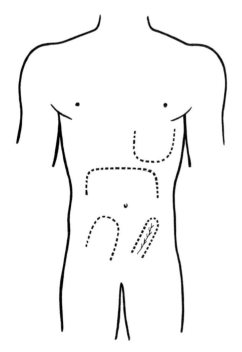

Fig. 62-16 Example of abdominal flaps (see text for details as to length and width of flaps). Lower abdominal flap may be made narrower in relation to its length if it contains superficial circumflex iliac artery and vein *(lower right)* or superficial epigastric artery and vein.

should have its base either distal, toward the superficial epigastric vessels, usually on the same side as the affected hand, or proximal, above the umbilicus toward the thoracoepigastric vessels, usually on the opposite side (Fig. 62-16). The flaps above the umbilicus should not be used in a patient with a "barrel chest" with chronic lung disease. Abdominal flaps obtained from areas above the umbilicus usually avoid the fat "storage areas." If the flap is obtained from the infra-umbilical area, the recipient grafted area usually increases in bulk, since the infra-umbilical area skin adds fat.

■ *TECHNIQUE.* On sterile paper make a pattern of the defect and outline it on the abdomen; then outline the flap making it sufficiently larger than the pattern to allow for normal skin contraction and for the pedicle "bridge" between the abdomen and the defect. As a rule the flap should be rectangular to avoid a circular outline when the flap is attached to the hand. Avoid making the flap too thick. When possible, follow the principles of appropriate hand incisions (Chapter 61) to avoid tension lines and excessive scarring. Using sharp dissection, raise the skin flap of the desired size and thickness (Figs. 62-17 and 62-18). Maintain hemostasis and handle the fat carefully to avoid necrosis. Close the donor site defect by widely undermining the skin margins

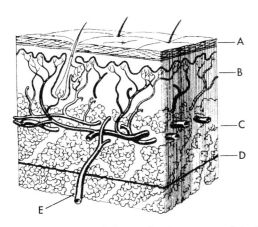

Fig. 62-17   Dissection of skin and subcutaneous fat. *A,* Epidermis; *B,* dermis; *C,* subdermal plexus of vessels; *D,* superficial fascia; *E,* arteries perforating the muscularis and deep fascia to join subdermal plexus of vessels. (From Kelleher JC, Sullivan JG, Baibak GJ, and Dean RK: J Bone Joint Surg 52-A:1552, 1970.)

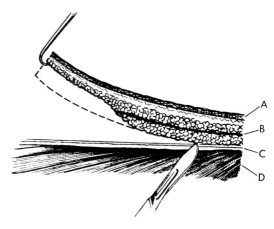

Fig. 62-18   Cross section of abdominal pedicle flap being raised. **A,** Epidermis and dermis; **B,** superficial fascia of abdomen; **C,** deep fascia of abdomen; **D,** muscularis. *Dotted line* indicates extent of defatting of portion of pedicle to be applied to hand. Base or stem should retain sufficient fat to retain its shape to prevent kinking. (From Kelleher JC, Sullivan JG, Baibak GJ, and Dean RK: J Bone Joint Surg 52-A:1552, 1970.)

and suture them together, or apply a split-thickness skin graft, or both. With a split skin graft, cover that part of the raw, exposed undersurface of the flap pedicle that will not cover the hand defect. Slightly undermine the edges of the defect on the hand and apply the flap over the entire defect. Suture the edges of the flap to those of the defect and suture the free edge of the split graft to that edge of the defect nearest to the base of the pedicle, thus covering all raw surfaces. Place strips of non-adhering gauze (Xeroform or Adaptic) over the suture line and a dry dressing on the flap; be careful to prevent kinking, tension, and rotation at its base. Using flannel cloth reinforced with either plaster or wide adhesive tape, apply a bandage around the trunk and shoulder supporting the hand. The flap should be easily accessible for inspection through the dressing. When marked pronation or supination of the forearm is necessary to prevent tension on the flap, a heavy transverse Steinmann pin through the radius and ulna just proximal to the wrist is helpful in maintaining this position.

AFTERTREATMENT. The flap should be inspected almost hourly during the first 48 hours for circulatory embarrassment produced by tension or torsion, or for the development of a hematoma. Sutures that appear to be too tight should be removed because they may apply sufficient pressure on the flap to produce ischemia.

If an area becomes necrotic, it should be excised and covered with a split skin graft. Gross infection from necrosis or hematoma usually will result in failure. The area should be redressed frequently to avoid offensive odor and decrease the chance of in-

fection. Usually the flap may be safely detached after 3 weeks. In children this can be reduced to 2 weeks.

AXIAL PATTERN FLAPS. Of the three axial pattern pedicle flaps that have been used often for hand coverage (deltopectoral, groin, and hypogastric), the groin and hypogastric flaps have been found to be the most useful. Other axial pattern flaps that have been transferred as vascularized free flaps are discussed in Chapter 49.

Groin pedicle flap. Before the 1973 description by Daniel and Taylor of its successful use as a free flap, the iliofemoral (groin) flap, popularized by McGregor, was widely used in reparative and reconstructive surgery of the upper extremity. Advantages of the groin flap include (1) its location in an area sparse in hair, (2) minimal donor site morbidity, (3) multiple arteriovenous supply, (4) potential for incorporating bone with the overlying skin flap even when used as a pedicle flap, and (5) potentially large size. Disadvantages include (1) problems with color matching, (2) possibility of damage to vessels from previous inguinal surgery, and (3) thickness of the flap in obese patients.

The groin pedicle flap usually receives its arterial supply from the superficial circumflex iliac branch of the femoral artery. Its venous drainage is via the superficial inferior epigastric and superficial circumflex iliac veins. For a discussion of the variations in the vasculature, especially as they pertain to the use of a free flap, see Chapter 49.

■ *TECHNIQUE.* Position the patient supine or turned slightly away from the affected side with sandbags or bolsters beneath the scapula and pelvis on the

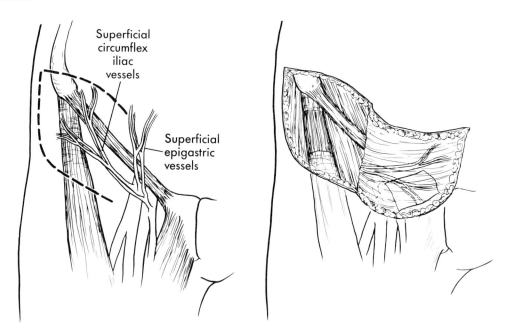

Fig. 62-19   Groin pedicle flap.

side of the flap to allow free access to the flank if a large flap is required. To help determine the central axis of the flap, identify and locate the course of the superficial circumflex iliac artery using a Doppler probe, usually about 2.5 cm distal and parallel to the inguinal ligament. After skin preparation and draping, use a suitable material such as sterile paper or plastic sheeting to outline the recipient defect with allowances for skin contraction. Place the pattern in the inguinal region, parallel with the inguinal ligament, along the course of the superficial circumflex iliac artery (Fig. 62-19).

Though somewhat unusual, a groin flap as large as 20 × 30 cm has been elevated in some situations. The usual dimensions fall within a width of about 10 cm and a length extending about 5 cm posterolateral to the anterosuperior iliac spine. Landmarks to remember and refer to include the (1) pubic tubercle, (2) anterosuperior iliac spine, (3) inguinal ligament, and (4) pulsation of the femoral artery.

Incise the skin along the outline of the pattern, tapering the margins of the flap to a narrower pedicle of skin overlying the vessels that lie about 2.5 cm distal to the inguinal ligament near the medial border of the sartorius. Incise the skin and subcutaneous tissue down to the deep fascia, and continue to elevate the flap in this plane. While dissecting along the superior margin of the flap, identify, ligate, or cauterize and divide the superficial epigastric vessels to ensure that the superficial circumflex iliac vessels are kept within the flap. Approach the lateral border of the sartorius with care because these vessels penetrate the sartorius fascia near this point. At the lateral margin of the sartorius, incise the fas-

cia and carefully elevate it to the medial border. At the medial border of the sartorius the superficial circumflex iliac artery usually has a deep branch. Dissection of the flap medial to the medial border of the sartorius requires division of this branch and might place the trunk of the artery at risk. Usually a sufficient skin flap can be elevated without extending the dissection medial to the sartorius. Dissect and handle the flap gently, maintaining hemostasis throughout the procedure. When elevation of the flap is complete, determine the best hand and forearm position for attachment of the flap. Determine also the amount of the flap required to cover the hand defect, and manage the intervening pedicle bridge of skin by either forming a tube in the pedicle or by applying a split skin graft to the raw exposed area on the pedicle. If forming a tube causes excessive pressure on the pedicle vessels, a split skin graft would provide safer coverage of this exposed tissue. While preparing the recipient area on the hand or forearm, cover the raw deep surface of the flap with moist gauze to prevent drying. Usually groin flaps will have a pale appearance after elevation. If there is any doubt regarding the axial arterial integrity after flap elevation, it may be necessary to replace the flap in its donor area, allowing a delay of 10 to 14 days.

After the recipient area has been prepared, elevate the skin at the margin of the defect to allow easier insetting of the flap. Usually after elevation of small to medium-sized flaps, close the donor site by mobilizing the skin margins, flexing the hip, and closing the subcutaneous and skin layers. Close the donor site before attaching the flap to the hand defect. Securely attach the flap skin to the skin margins of the recipient hand defect with a non-strangulating suture technique. Apply a non-adherent gauze (such as Adaptic or Xeroform) to the suture lines and pad the axilla with absorbent padding to avoid maceration of the axillary skin. With the help of assistants, elevate the patient's torso using a board or similar device to support the back while the shoulder, arm, and forearm are included in a circumferential flannel wrapping, incorporating the torso and affected extremity. Secure the cloth wrap by wrapping over it with adhesive tape. Create a small window in the bandage to allow inspection of the flap. Take care at all times while moving or assisting the patient not to pull the arm away from the body.

AFTERTREATMENT. The flap is protected by avoiding pulling on the affected arm. The flap is inspected and its circulatory status is evaluated hourly for the first 48 hours. If excessive tension, pedicle torsion, or hematoma becomes evident, the limb is repositioned, the bandage is changed, or sutures are removed to relieve ischemia. Any necrotic areas are promptly excised and hematomas are evacuated. Bandages are changed and the wound is cleaned frequently to decrease any unpleasant odor. Usually, the flap can be detached at 3 to 4 weeks. If there is any doubt concerning the axial artery or vascularity of the flap or if the pedicle bridge is to be used to cover the defect, the remainder of the flap is not detached for another 1 to 2 weeks. This will help minimize the risk of necrosis of portions of the flap.

Hypogastric (superficial epigastric) flap. Since its initial description in the 1940s by Shaw and Payne, wide application has been found for the hypogastric flap and it has been found extremely useful for coverage of the hand and forearm. Its arteriovenous pedicle consists of the superficial epigastric artery and vein (Fig. 62-20). The axis of the flap usually is oriented in a superolateral direction, with the base near the inguinal ligament centered at about the mid-point of the ligament. Flaps measuring up to 18 cm long and 7 cm wide have been used. Its advantages and disadvantages are similar to those described for the groin pedicle flap (p. 2997). Usually a bone graft cannot be incorporated into the skin flap. During preoperative planning it is important to examine the abdomen on the affected side for the presence of previous surgical or traumatic scars that might have damaged the arterial supply.

■ *TECHNIQUE.* Position the patient and elevate the affected side with a sandbag as needed. After skin preparation and draping, use a suitable material such as sterile paper to outline the recipient defect, making allowances for skin contraction. Place the pattern over the distribution of the superficial epigastric artery, arranging the base of the flap along the inguinal ligament. Arrange the axis of the flap so that it extends superiorly and slightly laterally from the inguinal ligament and is centered at about

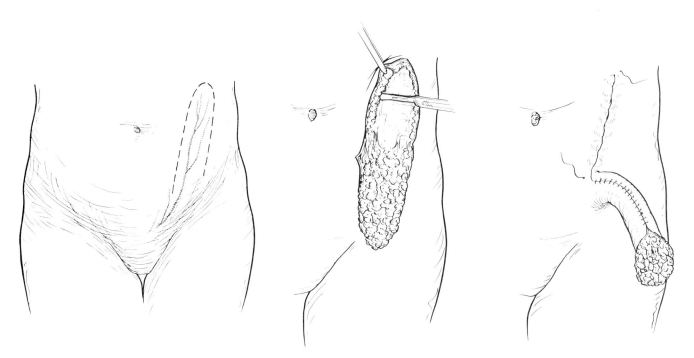

Fig. 62-20 Hypogastric (superficial epigastric) flap.

the mid-point of the ligament. Take care to avoid exceeding a length-to-width ratio of more than 3:1. Make the skin incisions along the skin markings of the pattern outline, with two parallel incisions extending superiorly and tapering toward the superiormost extreme of the flap. The distal extent of the dissection should not extend inferior to the inguinal ligament. Extend the skin incision through the subcutaneous tissue so that the plane of dissection is at the level of Scarpa's fascia. Elevate the flap inferiorly to the level of the inguinal ligament. After the flap has been elevated, cover the deep subcutaneous tissues with moistened gauze.

Prepare the recipient site on the hand, and mobilize and elevate the skin at the margins of the defect on the hand to allow ease of attachment of the flap to the hand. Close or skin graft the donor site before attaching the flap to the hand defect. After the elevation of small to medium-sized flaps, the donor site usually can be closed by mobilizing the skin margins and closing the subcutaneous and skin layers. Attach the flap skin to the skin margins of the recipient hand defect with a nonstrangulating suture technique. Apply a nonadherent gauze (such as Adaptic or Xeroform) to the suture lines. With the help of an assistant, lift the patient's torso and support it with a board or similar device while the shoulder, arm, and forearm are incorporated in a circumferential flannel wrap about the torso and affected extremity. Wrap over the cloth wrap with wide adhesive tape to secure the dressing. Arrange the bandage so that the flap can be inspected. Take care at all time while moving the patient that the flap is not disrupted by pulling on the arm.

AFTERTREATMENT. Aftertreatment is similar to that for the groin pedicle flap procedure. Pulling on the affected arm or shoulder should be avoided to prevent disruption of the suture line. The flap should be inspected hourly for the first 48 hours to evaluate its appearance and circulatory status. At any signs of excessive tension, pedicle kinking, or hematoma formation, the limb should be repositioned, the bandage changed, sutures removed, and other necessary corrections made to avoid or correct ischemic changes. Necrotic tissue is excised promptly and hematomas are evacuated. The wound is cleaned and the bandage changed frequently to minimize drainage and odor. The flap may be detached safely at 3 to 4 weeks. If the vascular status of the flap is doubtful or if the pedicle bridge will be required to cover more of the hand defect, the axial artery is divided or the pedicle is partially divided and the remainder of the flap is inset into the defect 1 to 2 weeks later.

Filleted Grafts

A filleted graft is a flap of tissue fashioned from a nearby part, usually a finger, from which the bone has been removed but in which one or more neurovascular bundles have been retained. In the hand such a graft is indicated only when deep tissues such as tendons, nerves, and joints are exposed and when a nearby damaged finger is to be sacrificed because it is not salvageable; it is *never* used at the expense of a salvageable, useful part.

A filleted graft is especially convenient when other injuries more proximal in the same extremity would interfere with positioning the hand to receive a flap from a distant part. The advantages of this graft are (1) it can be applied in a one-stage procedure at the time of injury and is obtained from within the same surgical field as the injured part, (2) its survival is almost assured because one or more of its neurovascular bundles are preserved, (3) its skin is similar to that which is to be replaced, (4) it is not attached to a distant part, and consequently after surgery the hand may be splinted in the position of function and elevated, and (5) it provides an adequate thumb web when the index finger is the donor.

■ *TECHNIQUE.* Because the main vessels course anterolaterally through the digit, it is easier to fashion a flap with its base anterior and cover a defect on the dorsum of the hand than vice versa (see Fig. 62-3). Make a midline dorsal incision along the full length of the finger and skirt it around the nail distally. Deepen the dissection to the extensor tendon. Then remove this tendon, the underlying bone, and the flexor tendons and their sheath, but preserve the fat in which the neurovascular bundles are located; take great care to avoid damaging these bundles. Spread the flap thus created and place it on the donor area. If it is too wide, trim its edges, or if it is too long, excise its end; in the latter instance ligate the digital vessels and resect the digital nerves far enough proximally to prevent their being caught in the scar. Suture the flap in place so that it lies flat; avoid strangulating its base and trim only slightly any dog-ears that may be produced at the margins of the base so as to preserve the blood supply of the flap.

REFERENCES

Aste JM: Care of the injured hand, South Med J 50:600, 1957.

Bilos ZJ and Eskestrand T: External fixator use in comminuted gunshot fractures of the proximal phalanx, J Hand Surg 4:357, 1979.

Blair WF and Marcus NA: Extrusion of the proximal interphalangeal joint: case report, J Hand Surg 6:146, 1981.

Burkhalter WE et al: Experiences with delayed primary closure of war wounds of the hand in Viet Nam, J Bone Joint Surg 50-A:945, 1968.

Daniel RK and Taylor GI: Distant transfer of an island flap by microvascular anastomoses: a clinical technique, Plast Reconstr Surg 52:111, 1973.

Flatt AE: Minor hand injuries, J Bone Joint Surg 37-B:117, 1955.

Flynn JE: Problems with trauma to the hand, J Bone Joint Surg 35-A:132, 1953.

Flynn JE: Acute trauma to the hand, Clin Orthop 13:124, 1959.

Furlong R: Injuries of the hand, Boston, 1957, Little, Brown & Co.

Gibraiel EA: A local finger flap to treat post-traumatic flexion contractures of the finger, Br J Plast Surg 30:134, 1977.

Green DP and Dominguez OJ: A transpositional skin flap for release of volar contractures of a finger at the MP joint, Plast Reconstr Surg 64:516, 1979.

Holevich J: Early skin-grafting in the treatment of traumatic avulsion injuries of the hand and fingers, J Bone Joint Surg 47-A:944, 1965.

Hoskins HD: The versatile cross-finger pedicle flap: a report of twenty-six cases, J Bone Joint Surg 42-A:261, 1960.

Kelleher JC et al: The distant pedicle flap in surgery of the hand, Orthop Clin North Am 2:227, 1970.

Kelleher JC et al: Use of a tailored abdominal pedicle flap for surgical reconstruction of the hand, J Bone Surg 52-A:1552, 1970.

Kilbourne BC and Paul EG: Do's and don'ts in the treatment of hand injuries, Surg Clin North Am 38:139, 1958.

Kleinert HE et al: Primary repair of flexor tendons, Orthop Clin North Am 4:865, 1973.

London PS: Simplicity of approach to treatment of the injured hand, J Bone Joint Surg 43-B:454, 1961.

Lueders HW and Shapiro RL: Rotation finger flaps in reconstruction of burned hands, Plast Reconstr Surg 47:176, 1971.

MacDougal B, Wray Wc Jr, and Weeks PM: Lateral-volar finger flap for the treatment of burn syndactyly, Plast Reconstr Surg 57:167, 1976.

Mason ML and Bell JL: The treatment of open injuries to the hand, Surg Clin North Am 36:1337, 1956.

Mason ML and Bell JL: The crushed hand, Clin Orthop 13:84, 1959.

Maxim ES, Webster FS, and Willander DA: The cornpicker hand, J Bone Joint Surg 36-A:21, 1954.

McCormack RM: Reconstructive surgery and the immediate care of the severely injured hand, Clin Orthop 13:75, 1959.

McCormack RM: Primary reconstruction in acute hand injuries, Surg Clin North Am 40:337, 1960.

McGregor IA: Fundamental techniques of plastic surgery, New York, 1980, Churchill Livingstone.

McGregor IA: Axial pattern flaps. In Tubiana R, editor: The hand, vol 2, Philadelphia, 1985, WB Saunders Co.

Milford L: Shotgun wounds of the hand and wrist: with a report of four cases, South Med J 52:403, 1959.

Milford L: Resurfacing hand defects by using deboned useless fingers, Am Surg 32:196, 1966.

Moberg E: The treatment of mutilating injuries of the upper limb, Surg Clin North Am 44:1107, 1964.

Nemethi CE: The primary repair of traumatic digital skeletal losses by phalangeal recession, J Bone Joint Surg 37-A:78, 1955.

Posch JL: Injuries to the hand in children, Am J Surg 89:784, 1955.

Rank BK and Wakefield AR: Surgery of repair as applied to hand injuries, Baltimore, 1960, Williams & Wilkins.

Riordan DC: Emergency treatment of compound injury of the hand, Orthopedics 1:30, 1958.

Shaw DT and Payne RL: One-staged tubed abdominal flaps: single, pedicle tubes, Surg Gynecol Obstet 83:205, 1946.

Siler VE: Primary tenorrhaphy of the flexor tendons in the hand, J Bone Joint Surg 32-A:218, 1950.

Siler VE: Combined nerve and tendon injuries in the hand and forearm, Am Surg 22:764, 1956.

Stromberg WB Jr, Mason ML, and Bell JL: The management of hand injuries, Surg Clin North Am 38:1501, 1958.

Sullivan JG et al: The primary application of an island pedicle flap in thumb and index finger injuries, Plast Reconstr Surg 39:488, 1967.

Tubiana R: Skin flaps. In Tubiana R, editor: The hand, vol 2, Philadelphia, 1985, WB Saunders Co.

Vilain R and Dupuis JF: Use of the flap for coverage of a small area on a finger of the palm: 20 years' experience, Plast Reconstr Surg 51:397, 1973.

Weeks PM and Wray RC: Skin and soft tissue replacement. In Weeks PM and Wray RC: Management of acute hand injuries: a biological approach, ed 2, St Louis, 1978, Mosby–Year Book, Inc.

CHAPTER 63

Flexor and Extensor Tendon Injuries

PHILLIP E. WRIGHT II*

This chapter considers flexor and extensor tendon injuries separately. Brief consideration is given to current concepts regarding anatomy, biomechanics, nutrition, and healing of flexor tendons and the current practice regarding repair techniques and postoperative management for both flexor and extensor tendon injuries. The reader is encouraged to refer to the excellent body of work that has developed through the efforts of many workers in the field since reports by Bunnell in the early 1900's and extending through and including the work of Boyes, Stark, and Ashworth and the more recent major contributions by Kleinert, Gelberman, Manske, Hunter, Lister, and others.

Flexor Tendons

A basic knowledge of the anatomy of the flexor tendons, especially in the forearm, wrist, and hand, is assumed, as is an understanding of the essential biomechanical aspects of flexor digitorum profundus and sublimis function in the fingers. Readers are referred to the appropriate references at the end of this chapter. Tendon nutrition is believed to be derived from two basic

*Revision of chapter by Lee W. Milford, M.D.

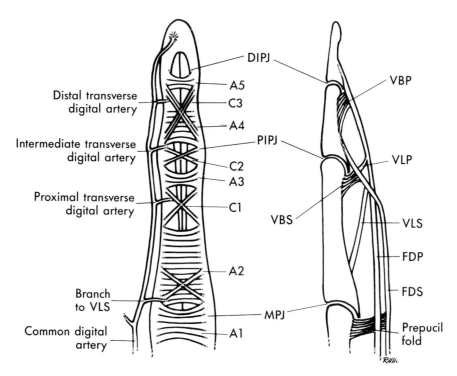

Fig. 63-1   Vascular supply to flexor tendons is by four transverse communicating branches of digital arteries. *VLS,* Vinculum longum superficialis; *VBP,* vinculum breve profundus; *VLP,* vinculum longum profundus; *VBS,* vinculum breve superficialis. (Redrawn from Hunter JM, Schneider LH, and Macklin EJ: Tendon surgery in the hand, St Louis, 1987, Mosby–Year Book, Inc.)

sources: (1) the synovial fluid produced within the tenosynovial sheath and (2) the blood supply provided through the vincular circulation (Fig. 63-1). Tendon healing is believed to occur through the activity of both extrinsic and intrinsic mechanisms. The extrinsic mechanism occurs through the activity of peripheral fibroblasts, whereas the intrinsic healing seems to occur through the activity of the fibroblasts derived from the tendon. Although tendon adhesions occur and are associated with tendon injury and healing, they are not believed to be essential to the tendon repair process itself. Experimentally, it has been shown that tendon injury alone is not sufficient to produce adhesions, whereas tendon injury accompanied by concomitant injury to the synovial sheath and combined with immobilization leads to considerable adhesions. These findings have lead to the development of postoperative mobilization techniques to diminish the formation of adhesions and enhance the end result.

EXAMINATION

Even when gross deformity is absent, the posture of the hand often provides clues as to which flexor tendons are severed (Fig. 63-2).

Traditionally, the "finger points the way" toward the injured structures. Errors are always possible when examining for flexor tendon injuries. Movements of the injured hand by the patient or the examiner may cause sufficient pain to limit motion and cause confusion. This is seen also when examining the hand after nerve injuries.

When both flexor tendons of a finger are severed, the finger lies in an unnatural position of hyperextension, especially when compared with uninjured fingers. Flexor tendon injuries may be tentatively confirmed by several passive maneuvers. First, passive extension of the wrist does not produce the normal "tenodesis" flexion of the fingers. If the wrist is flexed, even greater unopposed extension of the affected finger is produced. Gentle compression of the forearm muscle mass will at times demonstrate concomitant flexion of the joints of the uninvolved fingers, whereas the injured finger will not demonstrate this related flexion, indicating separation of the tendon ends. Gently pressing the fingertip of each digit will reveal loss of normal tension in the injured finger.

Tendon function probably is evaluated most often by voluntary active movements of the finger, usually directed by the examiner. This examination is unreliable and probably worthless when evaluating an excited, uncooperative child or an anxious, uncooperative, or intoxicated adult. At times it is best to demonstrate the maneuvers requested with the examiner's hand or the patient's uninjured hand before evaluating the injured hand. If the wound is distal to the wrist, it is helpful to

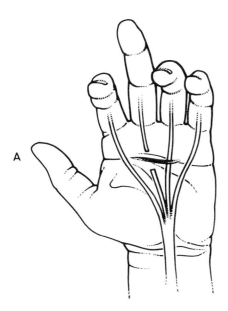
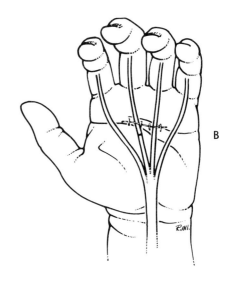

Fig. 63-2 A, If middle finger remains extended when hand is at rest, its flexor tendons have been severed. **B,** This finger becomes normally flexed after its profundus tendon or both this tendon and sublimis have been repaired.

stabilize the injured finger to obtain specific joint movements. With the proximal interphalangeal joint stabilized, the flexor digitorum profundus is presumed severed if the distal interphalangeal joint cannot be actively flexed (Fig. 63-3). If neither the proximal nor the distal interphalangeal joint can be actively flexed with the metacarpophalangeal joint stabilized, both flexor tendons probably are severed.

The method used to demonstrate the transection of a flexor digitorum sublimis tendon with an intact flexor profundus tendon involves maintaining the adjacent fingers in complete extension, anchoring the profundus tendon in the extended position, and removing its influence from the proximal interphalangeal joint. Thus, when a sublimis tendon is severed and the two adjacent fingers are held in maximum extension, flexion of the interphalangeal joint usually is not possible (Fig. 63-4). The obvious exception to this evaluation is the result of the independent function of the index finger flexor digitorum profundus; a technique advocated by Lister is helpful in evaluating an isolated injury to this tendon. In this examination, the patient is requested to pinch and pull a sheet of paper with each hand, using the index fingers. In the intact finger, this function is accomplished by the flexor sublimis with the flexor digitorum profundus relaxed, allowing hyperextension of the distal interphalangeal joint so that maximum pulp contact occurs with the paper. In the injured finger, the distal interphalangeal joint will hyperflex and the proximal interphalangeal joint will assume an extended position.

In the thumb, to check the integrity of the flexor pollicis longus tendon, the metacarpophalangeal joint of the thumb is stablized. If the flexor pollicis longus tendon is divided, flexion at the interphalangeal joint is absent.

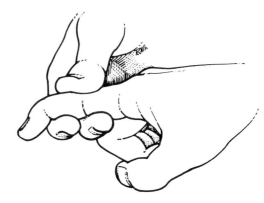

Fig. 63-3 If distal interphalangeal joint can be actively flexed while proximal interphalangeal joint is stabilized, profundus tendon has not been severed.

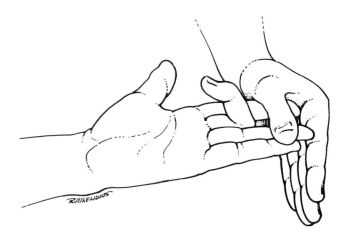

Fig. 63-4 If proximal interphalangeal joint can be actively flexed while adjacent fingers are held completely extended, sublimis tendon has not been severed (see text).

If a wound is located at the level of the wrist, the joints of a finger may be actively flexed even though the tendons to that finger are severed. This is the result of intercommunication of the flexor profundus tendons at the wrist, particularly in the little and ring fingers.

At times, a definitive diagnosis of flexor tendon transection may not be possible. These maneuvers will not detect a partially divided tendon. The partially divided tendon usually will function; however, finger motion may be limited by pain, and the examination will indicate tendon injury without allowing a definite diagnosis of tendon transection.

BASIC TENDON TECHNIQUES

The purpose of tendon suture is to approximate the ends of a tendon or to fasten one end of a tendon to adjoining tendons or to bone and to hold this position during healing. When tendons are being sutured, handling should be gentle and delicate, causing as little reaction and scarring as possible. Pinching and grasping of the uninjured surfaces should be avoided because this may contribute to the formation of adhesions.

Suture Material

A variety of satisfactory suture materials are available for tendon repair. Reports by Urbaniak et al. and Ketchum et al. are helpful in selecting appropriate suture material. Both authors found monofilament stainless steel to have the highest tensile strength; however, it is difficult to handle, tends to pull through the tendon, and makes a large knot. Although it may be used satisfactorily in the distal forearm, these disadvantages limit its use in the fingers. Absorbable sutures, both catgut and the polyglycolic acid group (Dexon; Vicryl), become weak too early after surgery to be effective in tendon repair. Although synthetic sutures of the caprolactam family (Supramid) and nylon maintain their resistance to disrupting forces longer than polypropylene (Prolene) and polyester suture, most surgeons find that the braided polyester sutures (Ticron; Mersiline) provide sufficient resistance to disrupting forces and gap formation, handle easily, and have satisfactory knot characteristics; consequently these sutures are widely used (Fig. 63-5).

Types of Sutures

The various types of suture configurations at the repair site have been studied as well. Urbaniak divided the

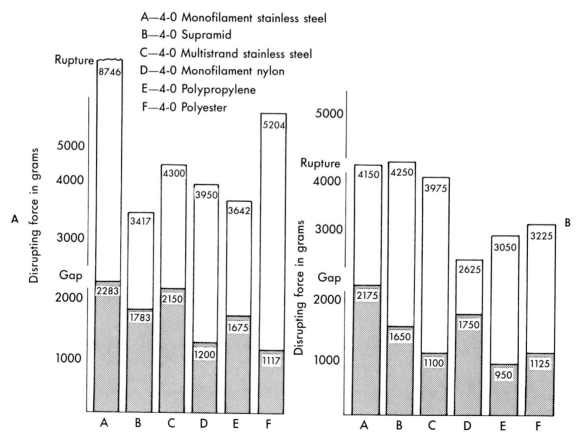

Fig. 63-5 These graphs depict ability of tendon repairs with various suture materials to withstand gap-producing and rupture-producing forces at time of tendon repair, **A,** and 3 weeks postoperatively, **B.** (Redrawn from Ketchum LD, Martin N, and Kappel D: Plast Reconstr Surg 59:708-719, 1977.)

various tendon repair types into three groups (Fig. 63-6). Group 1 is exemplified by simple sutures; the suture pull is parallel to the tendon collagen bundles, transmitting the stress of the repair directly to the opposing tendon ends. Group 2 is exemplified by the Bunnell suture; stress is transmitted directly across the juncture by the suture material and is dependent on the strength of the suture itself. Group 3 is exemplified by the Pulvertaft (fish-mouth weave); sutures are placed perpendicular to

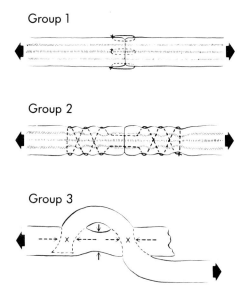

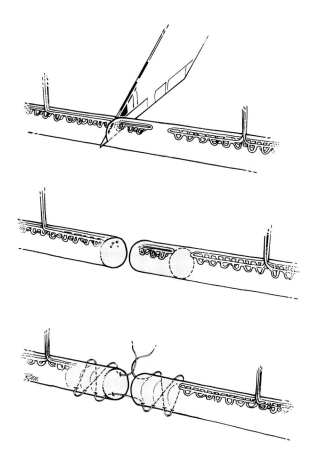

Fig. 63-6 Eight methods of tendon anastomoses could be placed into three basic groups. In group 1, suture applies shearing force to tendon ends parallel to collagen bundles and results in weak repair. In group 2, longitudinal pull of suture is converted to either oblique or transverse compressive force on tendon, and strength of repair approaches strength of suture material. In group 3, strongest union, loading of tendon applies compressive force of tendon to tendon at right angles to longitudinal shearing forces. (From American Academy of Orthopaedic Surgeons: Symposium on tendon surgery in the hand, St Louis, 1975, Mosby–Year Book, Inc.)

Fig. 63-7 Flexor tendon with segmental vascular system, each segment supplied by one dorsal vinculum vessel. A tendon is cut within one segmentally vascularized portion *(top)*. Shadowed area *(middle)* indicates area devascularized by transection of tendon. Intratendinous sutures further contribute to impaired microcirculation in tendon ends *(bottom)*. (Redrawn from Hunter JM, Schneider LH, and Macklin EJ: Tendon surgery in the hand, St Louis, 1987, Mosby–Year Book, Inc.)

Table 63-1 Tensile strength of eight different tendon suture techniques

Anastomosis	Tensile strength	Suture	
		Pulled out	Broke
Interrupted	1683 gm	20	0
Nicoladoni	2683 gm	20	0
Side-to-side	3230 gm	20	0
Bunnell	3930 gm	12	8
Kessler	3970 gm	4	16
Mason-Allen	4030 gm	4	16
Fish-mouth	4055 gm	20	0
End-weave	6430 gm	20	0

From Urbaniak J, Cahill JD, and Mortenson RA. In American Academy of Orthopaedic Surgeons: Symposium on tendon surgery of the hand, St Louis, 1975, Mosby–Year Book, Inc.

the tendon collagen bundles and the applied stress. It was found that interrupted sutures were the weakest and therefore are unsuitable in most tendon repair situations. The fish-mouth or end-weave repairs are the strongest and are most suitable for the distal forearm and palm areas, while the intermediate suture configurations (Bunnell, Kessler; Nicoladoni) did not differ significantly in strength from the bulkier repairs (Table 63-1).

Currently, it is believed that intratendinous crisscross suture techniques (Bunnell; Kleinert modification of Bunnell) tend to jeopardize the intratendinous circulation (Fig. 63-7). Wray and Weeks, using chicken flexor tendons, both compared the rupture rates and tensile strengths of the Bunnell, Kessler, Kleinert, and Tsuge (Fig. 63-8) repairs (Table 63-2). They concluded that the use of any of these techniques for flexor tendon repairs could be expected to produce about the same results. Thus, most surgeons recommend a core suture such as the Kessler technique (Fig. 63-9) or its modification (Fig. 63-10). Such techniques allow satisfactory purchase on the tendon so that satisfactory tensile strength is maintained during the early healing phase. These techniques also avoid cutting through and out of the tendon and are most dependable in the fingers. It is important to remember that no suture material or technique can be relied on to maintain tendon repairs with unlimited active movement in the early postoperative period. Most authors have found that the strength of the tendon repair diminishes considerably in the first 10 days. Thereafter the strength of the repair gradually increases, so that by the end of 10 to 12 weeks considerable active forces can be applied in the rehabilitation program.

END-TO-END SUTURES. Bunnell's "crisscross" (Fig. 63-11) is the classic technique of end-to-end suture. It is not in common use because it is believed that the intratendinous placement of the crisscross sutures tends to disturb the intratendinous circulation, rendering the ends of the tendon avascular.

The Kleinert modification of the Bunnell crisscross (Fig. 63-12) is somewhat easier to insert and probably causes less intratendinous ischemia. Because of the single crisscross, "straightening" of the suture within the tendon and gap formation are possible.

The Kessler grasping suture (Fig. 63-9) is a modification of the Mason-Allen suture. This technique is effective for tendon repair in the fingers and palm. In the fin-

Table 63-2   Strength of repair

Repair	Rupture rate (ruptured/not ruptured)	Tensile strength (mean ± 1 SE) (kg/cm²)
Bunnell	4/24	62.6 ± 9.7
Kessler	2/9	53.8 ± 8.6
Kleinert	3/9	66.8 ± 12.0
Tsuge	1/9	65.0 ± 10.4

From Wray RC and Weeks PM: J Hand Surg 5:144, 1980.

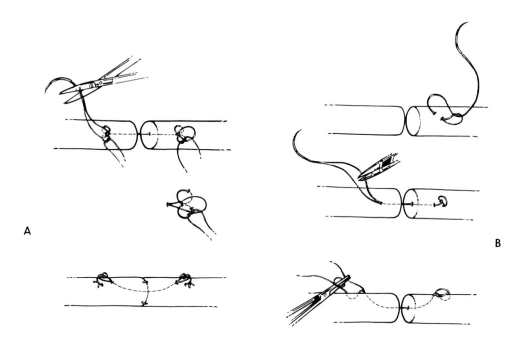

A

B

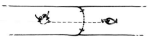

Fig. 63-8 Tsuge suture. **A,** Simplified procedure of intratendinous suture method. **B,** Another simplified procedure using only looped nylon suture. (Redrawn from Tsuge K, Ikuta Y, and Matsuishi Y.: J Hand Surg 2:436, 1977.)

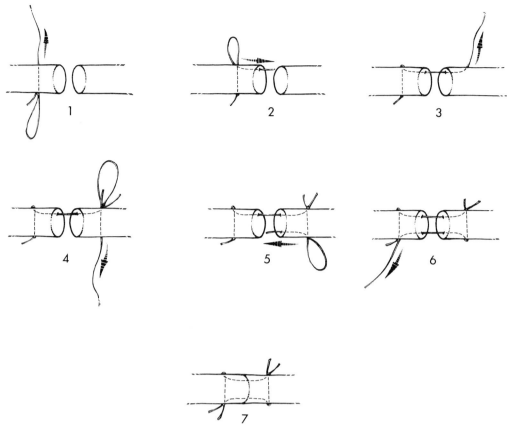

Fig. 63-9 "Grasping" technique. *1,* First knot grasps one quarter of tendon width. *2,* Needle passes longitudinally through one segment, emerging through cut surface. *3,* Thread engages second segment of tendon; half of grasping suture has been completed. *4,* Beginning of second half of suture; second needle passes transversely through other segment of tendon. *5,* Second half of suture (corresponds to *2* and *2A*). *6,* Suture is completed, but cut surfaces have not yet been approximated. *7,* End of procedure; two diagonally placed knots are tied up. (Redrawn from Hunter JM, Schneider LH, and Macklin EJ: Tendon surgery in the hand, St Louis, 1987, Mosby—Year Book, Inc.)

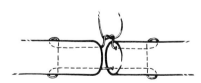

Fig. 63-10 Modified Kessler suture technique. (Redrawn from Hunter JM, Schneider LH, and Macklin EJ: Tendon surgery in the hand, St Louis, 1987, Mosby—Year Book, Inc.)

gers it has the disadvantage that the knots are left exposed on the surface of the tendon.

Kessler grasping suture

■ *TECHNIQUE (KESSLER).* Tie a knot near the end of the first suture and include one quarter of the tendon width in the first pass of the needle transversely. Then pass the needle longitudinally through this tendon segment, out through the cut surface. Next, pass the needle into the cut surface of the second segment of tendon. With a separate needle, pass another suture transversely through the second segment and lock the suture with a knot. Pass the needle from the second segment of the tendon into the first segment, through the cut surface, and exiting at the initial entry point of the first suture. Approximate the cut surfaces before tying the knots on the surface as shown in Fig. 63-9.

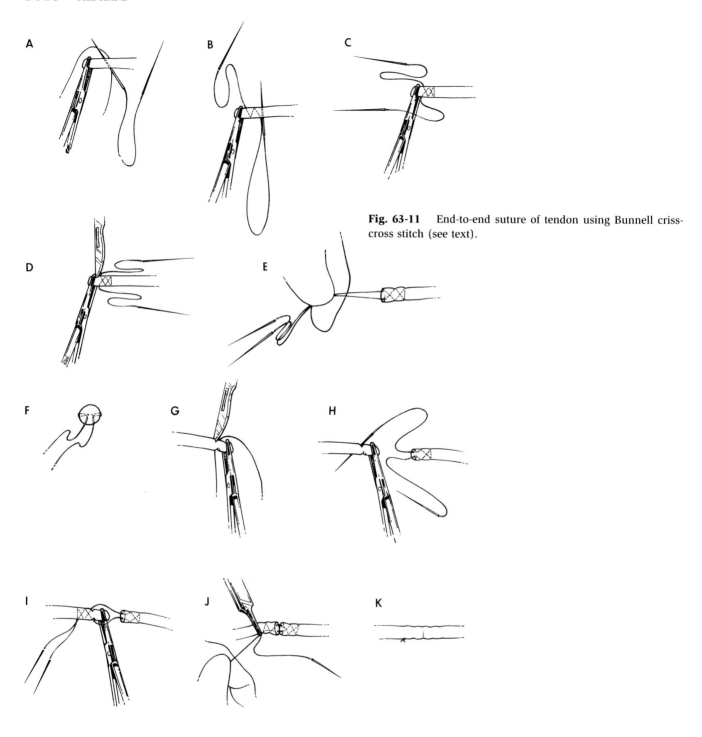

Fig. 63-11 End-to-end suture of tendon using Bunnell criss-cross stitch (see text).

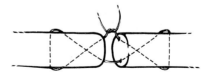

Fig. 63-12 Crisscross Bunnell suture technique. (Redrawn from Hunter JM, Schneider LH, and Macklin EJ: Tendon surgery in the hand, St Louis, 1987, Mosby–Year Book, Inc.)

"Modified" Kessler suture. This technique may be used instead of the traditional Kessler grasping suture. A single piece of suture material is used. It has the added advantage that the knot is left in the cut surface of the tendon. It may have the disadvantage that it is difficult to slide the tendon on some suture materials to achieve satisfactory approximation of the tendon ends. The needle is passed into the cut surface of one side of the cut tendon, exiting on the surface of the tendon (Fig. 63-12). The suture then is passed transversely, taking up a small portion of the surface of the tendon, and passed out on the opposite side. Next, the needle is passed through the cut surface into the other side of the cut tendon, then out and transversely again with another locking maneuver to allow passage of the suture out through the cut surface. The knot is tied after sliding the tendon on the suture to allow approximation of the cut surfaces.

The Tajima technique allows the placement of two pieces of suture material in the ends of the cut tendon (Fig. 63-13). This permits the use of the suture for traction to pass the tendon through the sheath and beneath the pulleys in difficult locations. It also has the advantage of allowing the knots to be placed within the cut surface of the tendon.

■ *TECHNIQUE (TAJIMA).* **Pass the needle into one of the cut surfaces of the tendon and then out of the tendon 5 to 10 mm from its end. Then pass the suture transversely across the tendon, exiting again. Next, pass it within the tendon and out the cut surface. Using a separate piece of suture, repeat the above steps on the opposite side of the cut tendon, and then tie the knots within the tendon, approximating the tendon ends.**

Modified Kessler-Tajima suture

■ *TECHNIQUE (STRICKLAND).* **This modification of the Kessler and Tajima techniques incorporates several advantages of each (Fig. 63-14). Separate pieces of suture are used so that the tendon ends can be passed within the flexor sheath using the free ends of the suture as traction sutures. The knots are tied within the tendon. The sutures are locked with each exit from the tendon. Use separate sutures introduced into each tendon end. Introduce a suture into one cut surface of the tendon, staying along the**

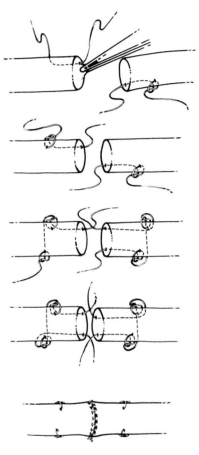

Fig. 63-14 Strickland's modification of flexor tendon repair techniques described by Kessler and Tajima is schematically depicted. Separate sutures are introduced in each tendon end at distance of 0.5 to 1.0 cm. Approximately 25% of diameter of tendon is then grasped by separate needle passage and locked on side of tendon. Suture is then passed transversely behind knot across tendon, where second-needle pass-and-lock suture is used to grasp tendon side. Finally, suture is passed behind second knot and down tendon to tendon end. Following placement of similar suture in opposite end, two tendon ends can be brought together, and repair is usually tidied up by small circumferential suture. Once in place in end of given tendon, protruding suture ends can be used to pass tendon through tendon sheath and position it for repair without need to damage tendon with further instrumentation. (Modified from Strickland JW: Orthop Clin North Am, 14:837, 1983.)

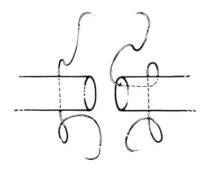

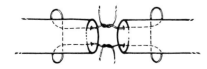

Fig. 63-13 Tajima tendon repair is shown. Double-armed needles on suture are necessary for this method. (Redrawn from Tajima T: Hand Clin 1:73, 1985.

volar portion of the tendon, and exit 5 to 10 mm from the cut edge. Grasp approximately 25% of the diameter of the tendon with passage of the needle and lock the suture on the side of the tendon with a knot. Next, pass the suture transversely behind this locked knot across the tendon and onto the tendon surface and lock the suture again. Pass the suture into the tendon behind the second knot and exit on the cut surface. Repeat this process on the opposite side of the cut tendon, locking the suture with each exit, and maintaining the suture repair on the volar third of the cut surface of the tendon. Tie the knots within the tendon. Complete the repair with circumferential running 5-0 or 6-0 nylon to invert the tendon ends to avoid adhesions.

Double right-angled suture. To suture the severed ends of a tendon together without shortening, a double right-angled stitch can be used. This suture technique is useful proximal to the palm. Although the apposition of the tendon ends is not as neat as after the other end-to-end suture techniques described, the method is easier and is more frequently used when multiple tendons are severed.

Fish-mouth end-to-end suture (Pulvertaft). A tendon of small diameter may be sutured to one of large diameter by the method shown in Fig. 63-15. This method is commonly used to suture tendons of unequal size.

END-TO-SIDE REPAIR. End-to-side repair is frequently used in tendon transfers when one motor must activate several tendons. Pierce the recipient tendon through the center with a No. 11 Bard-Parker knife blade and grasp the blade on the opposite side with a straight hemostat (Fig. 63-16). Then withdraw the blade, carrying the hemostat with it; with the latter, gently grasp the end of the tendon to be transferred and bring it through the slit. Repeat this technique with any adjacent tendons, placing the slits so that the transferred tendon approaches the recipient tendon at an acute angle to its line of pull. Suture the tendon at each passage with a vertical mattress stitch. Bury the end of the transferred tendon in the last tendon pierced.

ROLL STITCH. The roll stitch is especially useful for suturing extensor tendons over or near the metacarpophalangeal joints. Use a No. 4-0 monofilament wire or No. 4-0 monofilament nylon threaded on a small curved needle (Fig. 63-17). Pass the suture through the skin just medial or lateral to the divided tendon and through the proximal segment of the tendon near its margin from superficial to deep and then through the deep surface of the distal segment to emerge on its superficial surface. Next pass it proximally and through the opposite margin of the proximal segment and bring it out through the skin on the opposite side of the tendon from which it

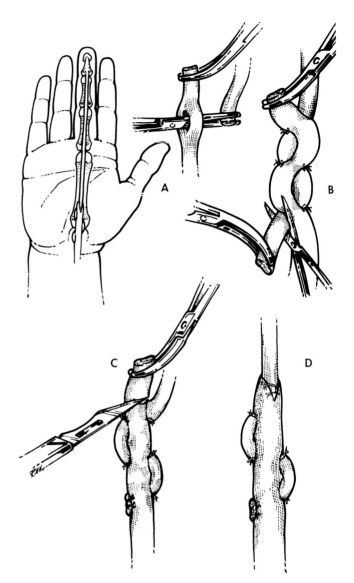

Fig. 63-15 Pulvertaft technique of suturing tendon of small diameter to one of larger diameter. **A,** Smaller tendon is brought through larger tendon and anchored with one or two sutures after tension is adjusted. **B,** Tendon is then brought through more proximal hole and is once again anchored with one or two sutures after tension is adjusted. **C,** After excess is cut flush with larger tendon, exit hole can be closed with one or two sutures. **D,** Excess of larger tendon is then trimmed as shown to permit central location of smaller tendon. This so-called fish mouth is then closed with sutures.

was introduced. Be certain that the suture slides easily in the skin and tendon. At about 4 weeks the suture can be removed by pulling on one of its ends.

TENDON-TO-BONE ATTACHMENT USING PULL-OUT SUTURE

■ *TECHNIQUE.* The attachment of tendon to bone usually requires a pull-out technique. One of several techniques may be used to arrange a pull-out wire in this situation. One involves a modification of the

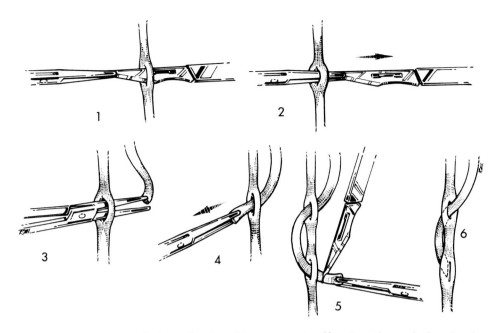

Fig. 63-16 Steps in technique of end to side anastomosis. Note in 6 that end of tendon has been buried. Sutures will be appropriately placed to fasten tendons together.

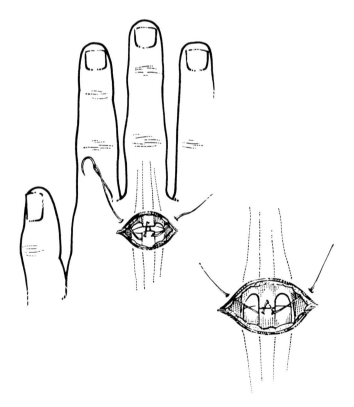

Fig. 63-17 Roll stitch using No. 4-0 wire or No. 4-0 monofilament nylon is especially useful in suturing lacerated extensor tendon over or near head of metacarpal.

Bunnell crisscross suture (see Fig. 63-11) in which the pull-out wire is looped over a straight needle that is passed transversely through the tendon approximately 10 mm from the cut end. This leaves the pull-out wire attached to a loop of the suture proximally in the tendon to be passed into the bone distally (Fig. 63-18). The modified Bunnell crisscross suture is accomplished with at least one crossing of the sutures within the tendon. The needles are brought out through the cut end of the tendon and then passed through the tunnel in the bone and out the opposite side of the bone and the skin. The needle is then passed through felt and a button and is tied over the button. The pull-out wire is passed retrograde out through the skin with a needle. At 3 to 4 weeks, to remove the wire the button is cut from the wire suture and the pull-out wire is pulled retrograde (proximally) to remove the wire. One disadvantage to this involves the retrograde traction on the tendon, which has been attached to bone. This may increase the risk of separation of the tendon from the bone.

In another technique, the suture is placed in a single loop within the tendon by passing the needle from cut surface into the tendon and then out of the tendon across the surface of the tendon and back through the tendon into the cut surface (Fig. 63-19). The loop of suture is then passed into the tunnel in bone and is secured over a piece of felt and button in the fashion previously described. At the time of suture removal, one side of the suture is cut and it is removed in an antegrade fashion, minimizing the risk of disrupting the bony attachment. As an alter-

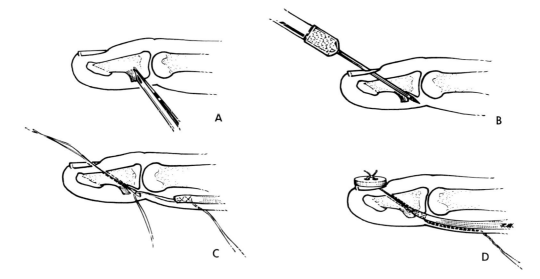

Fig. 63-18   One method of attaching a tendon to bone. **A,** Small area of cortex is being raised with osteotome. **B,** Hole is being drilled through bone with Kirschner wire in Bunnell drill. **C,** Bunnell crisscross stitch has been placed in end of tendon, and wire suture is being drawn through hole in bone. **D,** End of tendon has been drawn against bone, and suture is being tied over button.

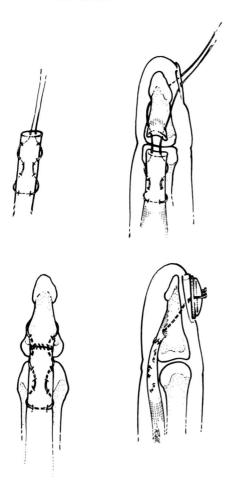

Fig. 63-19   Zone I injury: profundus tendon is advanced and reinserted into distal phalanx using pull-out wire suture and tie-over button. (Redrawn from Kleinert HE et al. In Sandzen S, editor: Current management of complications in orthopaedic surgery: the hand and wrist, Baltimore, 1985, Williams & Wilkins.)

native to passing the tendon through bone, the suture may be brought around small bones, such as the distal phalanx.

To attach a tendon to bone, use a small osteotome or dental chisel to roughen the site of insertion or raise a small area of cortex to accept the tendon (Fig. 63-18). If several tendon ends are to be fixed to bone, they are best inserted into a large hole drilled in the bone. After an area of cortex has been elevated or a large hole made, perforate the bone with a small Kirschner wire in a power drill. Then using the first needle as described for the end-to-end suture, run the suture diagonally two or three times through the end of the tendon. Loop a pull-out wire over the second needle and complete the crisscross diagonal suture. Using the needles, pass the two ends of the suture through the bone and snug the tendon against it.

TIMING OF FLEXOR TENDON REPAIR

When a wound is caused by a sharp object such as a knife and is reasonably clean, some tendons of the hand should be repaired at the time of primary wound closure. Usually a primary tendon repair is done within the first 12 hours of injury. This may be extended to within 24 hours of injury in rare situations. A so-called delayed primary repair is one that is done within 24 hours to approximately 10 days. After about 10 to 14 days, the repair is considered to be secondary, and after about 4 weeks, the secondary repair is considered to be a "late" secondary repair by Kleinert.

Primary repair may be done in those patients who

have a clean wound with either a tendon injury or a tendon injury and a neurovascular bundle injury. Primary repair may also be done if the patient has a fracture accompanying the tendon or neurovascular injury if the fracture can be satisfactorily fixed and stabilized; if this is impossible, then a secondary repair should be considered. A secondary repair is indicated when the tendon injury is associated with complicating factors that may compromise the end result. These factors include extensive crushing with bony comminution near the level of tendon injury, severe neurovascular injury, severe joint injury, and skin loss requiring a coverage procedure such as skin grafting or flap coverage.

Partial Flexor Tendon Lacerations

After partial tendon lacerations complications reported by many authors, including Kleinert; Reynolds, Wray, and Weeks; and Schlenker, Lister, and Kleinert, include rupture, triggering, and tendon entrapment. Experimental work by Dobyns, Cooney, and Wood; Wray, Holtmann, and Weeks; and McDowell and Synder suggests that a partially lacerated tendon retains varying amounts of its strength. A tendon with a 60% laceration may retain 50% or more of its strength and a tendon with a 90% laceration may retain only slightly more than 25% of its strength. In addition, it does not appear that simple suturing of partial lacerations imparts any significant additional strength to the repair. Considering these findings, a reasonable clinical approach to managing the major problems related to partial tendon lacerations would be as follows.

If a tendon is lacerated 50% or more, it is treated the same as a complete transection. A core suture is placed in the tendon, and the surface of the tendon is sutured with a continuous 6-0 nylon suture. The flexor sheath is repaired when possible. Postoperative management of a 50% or greater tendon laceration is the same as for a complete transection, with immobilization, early controlled passive motion, and restoration of forceful activities at 10 to 12 weeks.

If the laceration is less than 50%, especially in the 30% range, the flap of tendon is smoothly debrided and the flexor sheath is repaired to help avoid entrapment of the flap or triggering of the flap in the defect in the flexor sheath. Postoperatively, the part is protected with dorsal block splinting for 6 to 8 weeks and gradually more forceful activities are resumed after approximately 8 weeks.

PRIMARY FLEXOR TENDON REPAIR

Certain anatomic differences in the flexor surface of the hand influence the method and outcome of tendon repair. These differences allow the division of the flexor surface into five zones as proposed by Verdan (Fig. 63-

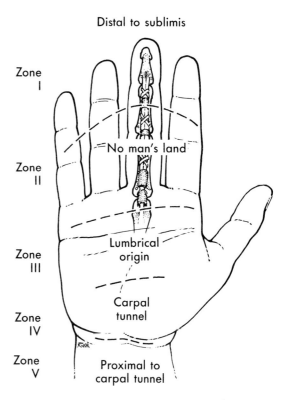

Distal to sublimis

Fig. 63-20 Flexor zones of hand. Designated zones on flexor surface of hand are helpful since treatment of tendon injuries may vary according to level of severance.

20). *Zone I* extends from just distal to the insertion of the sublimis tendon to the site of insertion of the profundus tendon. *Zone II* is in the critical area of pulleys (Bunnell's "no man's land") between the distal palmar crease and the insertion of the sublimis tendon. *Zone III* comprises the area of the lumbrical origin between the distal margin of the transverse carpal ligament and the beginning of the critical area of pulleys or first annulus. *Zone IV* is the zone covered by the transverse carpal ligament. *Zone V* is the zone proximal to the transverse carpal ligament and includes the forearm.

As a general rule, all flexor tendons should be repaired at whatever level they are severed. Because of the vincular system of the profundus tendon, when both have been severed, some surgeons believe the results are better when both are repaired than when the profundus tendon alone is repaired. When possible, especially with sharp injuries, it is better to stabilize fractures and suture digital nerves and tendons at the time of initial repair than to delay and do a secondary procedure for tendon repair. Indeed, later it may be necessary to do a tendon graft. The principle of maintaining maximum coverage of tendons with the flexor sheath has been well established; in many instances the entire sheath can be repaired after a tendon repair. Furthermore, it is essential that the A2 and A4 pulley areas of the flexor sheath be preserved; otherwise, tendon bowstringing and flexion deformity of the finger may develop and excursion of the tendon will be impaired (Figs. 63-21 and 63-22).

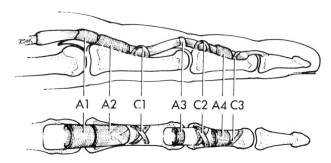

Fig. 63-21   This anatomic diagram of various parts of flexor sheath is helpful in understanding gliding of tendon. Maintenance of second annulus (A2) and fourth annulus (A4) is essential to retain appropriate angle of approach and prevent "bowstringing" of flexor tendons or tendon graft.. (Redrawn from Doyle JR and Blythe W. In American Academy of Orthopaedic Surgeons: Symposium on tendon surgery in the hand, St Louis, 1975, Mosby–Year Book, Inc.)

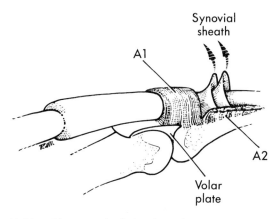

Fig. 63-22   Diagram of relationship of synovial layers (there are two) and annulus. (Redrawn from Doyle JR and Blythe W. In American Academy of Orthopaedic Surgeons: Symposium on tendon surgery in the hand, St Louis, 1975, Mosby–Year Book, Inc.)

Zone I

The flexor digitorum profundus tendon may be repaired primarily by direct suture to its distal stump or by advancement and direct insertion into the distal phalanx when the distance is 1 cm or less. Extreme care should be exercised when advancing a flexor profundus tendon. The 1 cm rule regarding advancement includes the amount of tendon that is excised, the "kinking" or bunching up that may occur, and the length of tendon inserted into bone. If the trimming of the tendon and advancement are excessive, this may result in a finger that is held in a flexed position when compared with other fingers (the finger "cascade"). Even though the finger may function reasonably well, uneven tension may be applied to the common muscle belly of the flexor profundus tendons and may lead to limited flexion of the remaining profundus tendons (the "quadriga effect" described by Verdan). In such a situation, lengthening of the tendon at the wrist should be considered, or if exces-

sive shortening has occurred tendon grafting may be considered.

A pull-out wire technique may be used to attach the proximal tendon end to its distal stump (Fig. 63-19) or directly to the bone after advancement (Fig. 63-20). When the diagnosis of interruption of this tendon is delayed and the tendon has retracted into the palm, then its vinculum has been disrupted and a decision must be made regarding repair. The recommendations of Leddy, and Leddy and Packer, especially as they pertain to flexor tendon ruptures, are helpful in this regard (see discussion of flexor tendon ruptures, p. 3026). They describe three types of flexor tendon ruptures, depending on the level to which the tendon has retracted. In type 1 the tendon is found retracted into the palm. If it is within 7 to 10 days of the injury, the tendon should be threaded back into the finger and reattached with a pull-out wire into the distal phalanx. In type 2 ruptures the tendon has retracted to the level of the proximal interphalangeal joint. At times, despite the passage of a few months, these tendons may be reattached as well. In type 3 the tendon has retracted only to the level of the distal interphalangeal joint and usually has a bony fragment attached to it. These can usually be treated by reattachment as well.

Old, untreated injuries to the flexor profundus in zone I may be treated by tendon grafting, tenodesis, or arthrodesis of the distal joint, depending on the finger involved, the age of the patient, and the needs of the patient. Flexor tendon grafting in such situations in the presence of an intact and functioning sublimis tendon has been recommended for the index and middle fingers in specific situations.

Careful patient selection has been recommended by all authors. Stark et al. concluded that highly motivated patients between the ages of 10 and 21 years can be considered as grafting candidates. The flexor profundus of the ring finger may be grafted following tendon injuries in zone I for specific needs (skilled technicians, musicians). Because of the risk of damaging the intact flexor sublimis and the additional potential complications of flexor tendon grafting, patients who are older, who have a tendency toward joint stiffness, who are noncompliant, and who do not understand the difficulty in achieving a successful result should not be considered for flexor tendon grafting.

Some, including McClinton and Curtis, pass their tendon graft around the sublimis tendon. Two-stage tendon grafting has also been advocated. In those patients who are not candidates for tendon grafting, tenodesis or arthrodesis of the distal joint should be considered, depending on the need for stability of the distal joint.

Zone II

Primary repair of flexor tendons in the fibro-osseous sheath (Bunnell's "no-man's-land"), controversial until the major contributions of Verdan and of Kleinert, is now widely accepted. If repair is done under satisfactory conditions by an experienced surgeon, satisfactory function can be expected in as high as 80% of patients. Generally the results of flexor tendon repair are better in younger patients than in those over 40 years old. Also, it seems that given appropriate circumstances the results of primary flexor tendon repair are better than secondary repair or staged reconstruction with a graft. Here especially, the primary surgeon has the greatest influence on the final result. To be qualified to make the decision and perform a primary repair, a surgeon should be sufficiently skilled to perform a tendon graft or tenolysis later, should the primary repair fail.

Primary repairs at this level frequently fail as a result of adhesions in the area of the pulleys. Exacting wound care is critical. When there is doubt as to the timing of tendon repair, the wound should be cleaned and the repair done later by an experienced surgeon.

Technical concerns during the repair procedure include the management of lacerations of both the profundus and sublimis tendons, the appropriate orientation of the profundus with the sublimis slips, the attachment of the sublimis slips in the thin flat area, the management of the flexor sheath including the annular thickening (pulleys), the postoperative management, and the timing and technique for tenolysis. Most surgeons recommend repair of both the flexor profundus and sublimis tendons in zone II. The excellent work of Doyle and Blythe, as well as of Hunter and Schneider et al., confirms that most of the annular pulley component of the fibro-osseous sheath, especially the A2 and A4 pulleys, should be preserved (Figs. 63-21 and 63-22). For the most part, repair of defects in the sheath is recommended as well. Care should be taken when the flexor sublimis has been injured in the area just proximal to the proximal interphalangeal joint and distally where the orientation of the proximal and distal portions of the tendon can be misinterpreted and repairs may be incorrectly done with the sublimis slips malrotated (Fig. 63-23). Care also should be taken to deliver the flexor profundus tendon through the split portion of the flexor sublimis when the profundus tendon has retracted proximally (Fig. 63-24).

As indicated previously, many suture configurations have been advocated. In zone II, a core suture with locking components and buried knots is recommended. The intratendinous configuration of the core sutures should remain in the volar third of the tendon and should not strangulate the intratendinous circulation. A running, circumferential 5-0 or 6-0 nylon is used by most surgeons to complete a smooth repair and to minimize adhesion formation to the sheath. The choice of suture material depends on the experience and preference of the individual surgeon; however, most authors indicate a preference for a synthetic braided suture, usually of polyester material (Mersiline, Tycron, Tevdek), while others have had success with monofilament nylon and

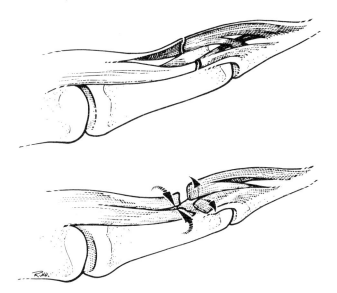

Fig. 63-23 FDS spiral. Flexor digitorum sublimis (FDS) separates just distal to level of metacarpophalangeal joint with finger in extension. It winds around profundus tendon to chiasm of Camper, where it decussates to insert in middle phalanx. Thus superficial portion of proximal sublimis tendon becomes deep at level of chiasm of Camper. If laceration is sustained in sublimis at midpoint of this spiral arrangement of both slips, proximal and distal ends both rotate through 90 degrees, but in different directions. Thus unwary surgeon will be presented with two ends that do match, that appear to lie in good relationship, and that can be so sutured. If this is done, channel for profundus tendon is obliterated. Effect, if error is not noted and corrected, will be to block excursion of tendon and eliminate satisfactory motion. (Redrawn from Lister G: Hand Clin 1:140, 1985.)

wire suture. Usually 3-0 or 4-0 sutures are required. Generally, a pull-out suture technique is unnecessary in zone II.

The postoperative management is all important, as discussed subsequently in this chapter (see discussion of primary suture of flexor tendons).

Tenolysis may be required in 18% to 25% of patients after flexor tendon repair. Usually tenolysis is considered when the patient has reached a plateau in his postoperative rehabilitation and when all wounds are supple and flexible and the skin is soft with minimal or no induration about the scars. It is hoped that fracture and joint injuries have healed and there are no or minimal residual joint contractures. A near-normal passive range of motion is preferred. Normal sensation is preferred; however, if digital nerves have been repaired progress toward return of sensation should be observed. For these criteria to be met usually requires 5 to 6 months following the tendon repair. Flexor tenolysis is a technically demanding procedure and should be undertaken by someone who has training and experience in this type of surgery. Strickland has found that function in the finger may be improved by as much as 50% by tenolysis.

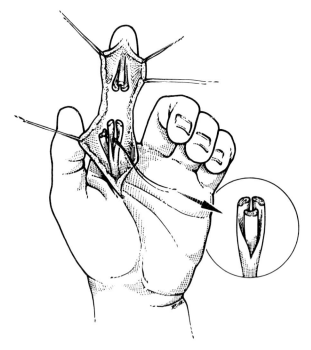

Fig. 63-24 Separated position of two tendon ends in distal palm after flexor tendon interruption and proximal retraction. Correctly position profundus in sublimis hiatus before passing tendons distally into digit. Reestablish anatomic relationship of profundus and sublimis tendon stumps so they may be correctly repaired to corresponding distal tendon stumps. In some cases, profundus will have to be passed back through hiatus created by sublimis slips to lie palmar to Camper's chiasm and re-create position of tendons that was present at level of tendon laceration. (Redrawn from Strickland JW: Hand Clin 1:55, 1985.)

Zone III

At the zone III level the muscle bellies of the lumbricals as well as the tendons are frequently interrupted. Additional incisions are often needed to further expose this area. All tendons may be repaired primarily when wound conditions are satisfactory or delayed only a few days. If conditions permit, primary repair of sharply severed nerves is extremely important since delaying the repair even a few weeks results in the development of significant gaps between the nerve ends. If wound conditions preclude tendon and nerve repair, the ends of the tendons and nerves are sutured to adjacent fascia to prevent undue retraction. Lumbrical muscle bellies usually are not sutured because this may increase the tension of these muscles and result in a "lumbrical plus" finger.

Zone IV

All tendons and nerves in zone IV may be repaired primarily when wound conditions are satisfactory; however, for exposure it may be necessary to partially or completely release the transverse carpal ligament. Should complete release be necessary, the wrist should not be placed in flexion past neutral position but the fingers should be brought into slightly more flexion than usual to permit relaxation of the musculotendinous units. Flexion of the wrist beyond neutral may permit subluxation of the repaired tendons out of their normal bed and bowstring them just under the sutured skin. When it is technically possible to accomplish tendon repair and retain part of the transverse carpal ligament, this problem is eliminated. Alternatively, the transverse carpal ligament may be released in a Z-lengthening configuration, allowing its repair after tendon repair and providing a pulley for the tendons. Remember that the flexor digitorum profundus tendons at this level may not be distinctly separated and there may be frequent interdigitations.

Zone V

Since zone V is proximal to the transverse carpal ligament, tendon gliding after repair usually is better here than in more distal zones. All tendons and nerves lacerated in this area should be repaired primarily when wound conditions are satisfactory, as advised earlier in this section. The chief difficulty of repair here usually is one of exposure, which requires a proximal extension and possibly a distal extension of the typical transverse laceration. Blood clots within the tenosynovium usually serve as clues to locating severed tendons. At this level the profundus tendons are not completely separated into individual tendon units. The sublimis tendons are usually distinctly separated and the severed ends are usually more easily matched. When the necessary expertise is not available, primary repair may be delayed and the wound cleaned. Results probably are not compromised by a brief delay of several days when required. At this level excision of some of the tenosynovial covering is necessary to identify and remove the hematoma; however, a total synovectomy usually is not indicated. An isolated laceration of the palmaris longus tendon does not absolutely require repair.

Delayed Repair of Acute Injuries

Delayed repair in any zone may be necessary in the face of severe wound contamination, crushing or avulsing injuries, soft tissue loss, multiple comminuted fractures, or lack of available surgical skill. Delayed repairs of tendons are reasonable also when other injuries require immediate surgery. In such circumstances, the patient's condition might not permit definitive management of tendons and nerves, and it is appropriate to clean the limb as well as possible and loosely close the wound or leave it open but covered with a sterile bandage and splint. Plans should then be made for definitive management of the wound and injured structures. Undue complications usually are not encountered when the repair of tendons is delayed for 2 to 3 days, providing the wound has been thoroughly cleaned. Prolonged delay may permit unacceptable retraction of tendons and nerves. If it appears that definitive management of the tendons and nerves will be delayed, an attempt should be made to secure the ends of the tendons and nerves to the adjacent soft tissues to prevent retraction before achieving satisfactory wound closure.

Primary Suture of Flexor Tendons

The preparations and techniques for primary and delayed primary suture of flexor tendons vary somewhat from zone to zone. The techniques are discussed according to requirements of each zone. Generally, further exposure of the tendon to be sutured may be necessary. Additional incisions (Fig. 63-25) should be made without crossing flexion creases at a right angle. Usually, less exposure is needed distally than proximally because the distal segment of the tendon may be delivered into the wound by flexing the distal joints. Also, the distal segment is not subject to retraction by muscle as are the proximal segments. Regardless of the zone in which the tendon is injured, careful attention should be given to the anatomic location of the respective tendons and their relationships to each other and other structures. Meticulous, gentle, and atraumatic technique should be used in the handling of the tendons. Each tendon is delivered by grasping it with a small tipped forceps with teeth. Crushing of the cut surface of the tendon should be avoided by instruments such as Allis forceps, Kocher clamps, and hemostats. Although the tip of the tendon may be held with a small hemostat, the crushed portion should be excised before the suture is tied. In certain situations, this may shorten the tendon needlessly. Suturing techniques should be exact so that the tendon ends are held together accurately and distraction, gap formation, and exposure of raw surfaces at the junction are avoided. Techniques of tendon suture are discussed on p. 3006.

REPAIR IN ZONES I AND II

■ *TECHNIQUE*

Zone I. When the flexor profundus tendon has been injured in zone I at or near its insertion, approach the distal end of the finger by extending the laceration with an oblique incision into the central portion of the pulp or through a midradial or midulnar incision. Take care to avoid injury to the terminal branches of the digital nerve and avoid devascularizing any skin flaps that are elevated. Usually the insertion of the flexor profundus is easily seen. At times the proximal stump of the tendon will have retracted very minimally. Extend the incision proximally, using a volar zigzag (Bruner), midradial, midulnar, or midline oblique (Fig. 63-25) incision. Avoid injury to the neurovascular bundles. Elevate the skin flap either by going dorsal or volar to the

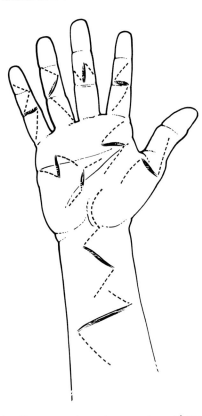

Fig. 63-25 Exposures for primary suture of tendons. Examples of skin lacerations are indicated by solid lines and direction in which they may be enlarged to obtain additional exposure by broken lines (see text).

neurovascular bundle. Expose the fibro-osseous flexor sheath. If the proximal end of the tendon can be seen, attempt to deliver it into the wound by grasping it with a small forceps, such as an Adson or a finer tissue forceps. Deliver the tendon into the wound. If the tendon has retracted more proximally, extend the incision as needed, either in a midradial or a midulnar incision or by extending the skin incision in a volar zigzag or midline oblique incision, taking care to avoid injury to the neurovascular bundle. Open the thin cruciform portion of the sheath to assist in delivering the tendon. Open the sheath by an L-shaped incision or with a trapdoor with a Z-plasty arrangement to allow easier closure if needed. If the tendon has retracted, place a grasping suture in its end, using one of the techniques previously described. When opening the flexor sheath over the middle phalanx, it is important to preserve the A4 pulley. If the flexor tendon cannot be maintained in such a way that it can be repaired easily, use a small gauge (25 or 26) hypodermic needle, Keith needle, or Bunnell needle through the skin, through the tendon, and out the skin on the opposite side of the finger as a temporary tendon retention device. These needles are removed when the tendon repair has been accomplished.

Although a pull-out wire of the Bunnell type may

be attached in such an arrangement, it is not always necessary, especially if the antegrade pull-out wire technique is used as opposed to the Bunnell retrograde pull-out technique (see Figs. 63-18 and 63-19). Using straight needles, pass the suture out through the distal pulp of the finger, usually exiting just palmar to the hyponychium. As an alternative, the proximal end of the tendon can be attached distally, using a pull-out technique in which a tunnel is drilled in bone and the needles are passed through the tunnel and out through the fingernail. Regardless of the suture material selected, usually 4-0 suture is used. If the pull-out suture is brought through the nail, a nail deformity may ensue although this does not always occur. After ascertaining satisfactory rotation and attachment of the tendon, close the wound with fine 4-0 or 5-0 monofilament nylon sutures.

Zone II. In zone II, the wound usually must be extended with proximal and distal incisions (Fig. 63-26). Regardless of which approach is used, carefully reflect the skin flaps and take care to avoid injury to neurovascular structures during the dissection. If digital nerves have been transected, gently dissect them and delay their repair until after the tendons are repaired to avoid disruption. Expose the flexor sheath in the area of injury, as well as sufficiently proximal and distal to allow location of the tendon ends. As indicated previously, the distal tendon end can usually be identified easily with passive flexion of the distal interphalangeal joint. Take care to avoid injury to the pulleys, particularly the A2 and A4 pulleys.

If opening of the flexor sheath is required, this is best done in the filamentous cruciate areas of the sheath. Small openings in the sheath can be made in the C4-A5, C2 and C3, and C1 areas where the sheath is filamentous (see Fig. 63-21). These openings can be made in several configurations. An L-shaped opening allows ease of closure and facilitates passage of the tendon through the sheath (Lister). If several days have passed and the tendon sheaths are contracting, opening the sheath with a Z-lengthening configuration will help to allow partial closure of the sheath in difficult situations. Deliver the flexor tendon into the finger by milking the forearm, hand, and wrist and flexing the wrist and fingers to allow the proximal end to be delivered if possible. If it cannot be easily delivered, a transverse incision at the distal palmar crease may be necessary to locate the tendon in the palm. Once the proximal end of the tendon has been identified, place a core suture using the definitive suture material in a locking fashion so that the suture material may be used for traction in passing the suture through the sheath.

In the fresh, acute injury, passage of the tendon usually is not difficult. After several days, tendon edema and sheath contracture may require additional techniques. The proximal end of the tendon may be easily passed through the sheath and between the slips of the sublimis using a piece of pediatric feeding tubing or plastic intravenous connecting tubing, as recommended by Lister. Deliver the tubing into the flexor sheath between the slips of the sublimis. Pass the suture into the tubing. Clamp the tubing with the suture within it and "lead" the flexor tendon through the sheath following the plastic tubing and suture.

Other techniques involve the use of 20- or 22-gauge wire fashioned into a loop passed proximally in the sheath to use as a snare for the suture, which is then delivered through the sheath followed by the tendon. The tendon may also be sutured to tubing of various types and delivered following the tubing through the sheath as well.

Once the proximal end of the tendon has been delivered to the area of repair, it may be secured in the sheath using a transverse 25- or 26-gauge hypodermic needle for temporary fixation with little or no long-term harmful effects. This is used as a temporary stabilizing device. The distal end of the tendon may be stabilized in a similar way. The core suture of the surgeon's selection is then introduced, care being taken to place it in the volar third of the flexor tendon to avoid strangulation of intratendinous circulation. Care should be taken at this point to be sure that the profundus tendon is not malrotated. Reference to the vincular attachment and the relationship to the sublimis is helpful in this regard. The knots are then tied and the tendon repair is completed with circumferential 5-0 or 6-0 nylon inverting suture to minimize exposure of the cut surface of the tendon.

If the flexor sublimis has been transected just proximal to the proximal interphalangeal joint, take care as to the arrangement of its slips of the sublimis and the so-called flexor digitorum sublimis "spiral" (see Fig. 63-23). It is helpful to recall that the flexor digitorum superficialis winds around the profundus tendon after it divides at the metacarpophalangeal joint. It inserts into the volar surface of the middle phalanx after decussating. This allows the superficial portion of the sublimis tendon to become deep in the chiasm of Camper. A laceration in this area allows the proximal and distal ends of the superficialis tendons to rotate 90 degrees in opposite directions. The tendon will thus lie in satisfactory alignment; however, if it is sutured in this alignment it will cause binding of the flexor profundus tendon.

An additional technical problem may be encountered if the flexor sublimis tendon has been tran-

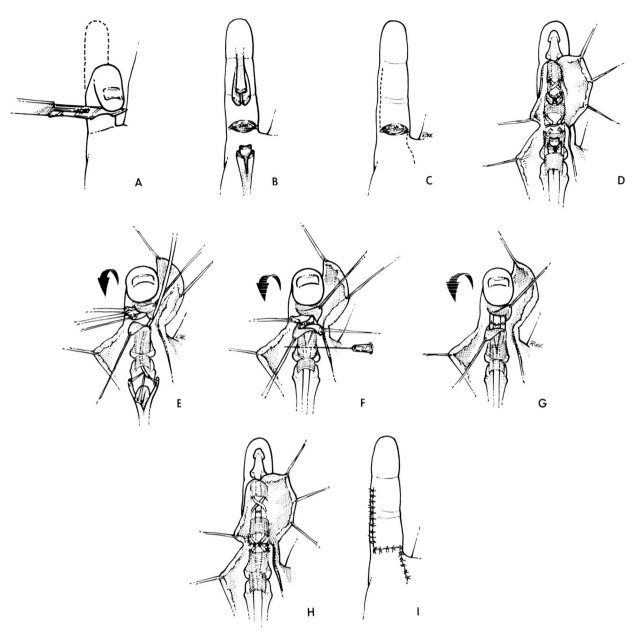

Fig. 63-26   Strickland's technique of flexor tendon repair in zone II is illustrated. **A,** Knife laceration through zone II with digit in full flexion. **B,** Level of flexor tendon retraction of same finger after digital extension. **C,** Dotted lines depict radial and ulnar incisions to allow wide exposure of flexor tendon system. **D,** Flexor tendon system of involved finger after reflection of skin flaps. In this case, laceration has occurred through C1 cruciate pulley area. Note proximal and distal position of severed flexor tendon stumps resulting from flexed attitude of finger at time of injury. Dotted lines indicate lateral incisions in cruciate-synovial portions of sheath, which will be used to provide exposure for tendon repair. **E,** Reflection of small triangular flaps at cruciate-synovial sheath allows distal flexor tendon stumps to be delivered into wound by passive flexion of distal interphalangeal joint. Profundus and sublimis stumps are retrieved proximal to A1 pulley, using small catheter or infant feeding gastrostomy tube. **F,** Proximal flexor tendon stumps are maintained at repair site by means of transversely placed small-gauge hypodermic needle, followed by repair of flexor digitorum sublimis slips. **G,** Completed repair of both tendons with the distal interphalangeal joint in full flexion. **H,** Extension of distal interphalangeal joint delivers repairs under intact distal flexor tendon sheath. Repair of cruciate (CI)–synovial pulley has been completed. **I,** Wound repair at conclusion of procedure. (Redrawn from Strickland HW: Hand Clin 1:55, 1985.)

sected more distally, near the proximal interphalangeal joint, or its insertion. Here the tendon is quite thin and it is difficult to achieve satisfactory placement of core sutures. Try to place a locked core suture in the tendon because a simple repair with 5-0 or 6-0 nylon will be insufficient to avoid rupture.

At times it may be extremely difficult to technically accomplish a flexor sublimis repair. Although most surgeons recommend against sublimis excision, if in the surgeon's judgment sublimis repair cannot be satisfactorily accomplished or its repair will compromise profundus function, excision of the superficialis in the area may be required at times.

Usually the sublimis tendon is repaired before the profundus tendon repair. Tie the knots, use the circumferential 6-0 nylon sutures as needed, and repair the sheath with 5-0 or 6-0 nylon. Close the wound with interrupted 5-0 nylon and remove the temporary retaining needle. Take care to avoid hyperextension of the finger, and immobilize the hand in a padded compression dressing with the fingers and the thumb immobilized with a dorsal splint. Splint the wrist in approximately 45 to 50 degrees of flexion; splint the fingers in flexion at the metacarpophalangeal joints to approximately 50 to 60 degrees with the proximal and distal interphalangeal joints extended.

If one or more pulleys are damaged and cannot be repaired, they should be reconstructed at the time of primary tendon repair to avoid bowstringing and restriction of motion. The flexor sheath/pulley reconstruction can be protected with orthotic thermoplastic rings during postoperative rehabilitation of the flexor tendon and while the patient is regaining motion. (See discussion of staged tendon reconstruction, p. 3036.)

AFTERTREATMENT. See p. 3023.

REPAIR IN ZONES III, IV, AND V

■ *TECHNIQUE*

Zone III. In zone III, the area between the distal edge of the transverse carpal ligament and the proximal portion of the A1 pulley, flexor tendon repair may be done in a manner similar to the zone II repair. Incisions extending the wound proximally and distally may be required. Take care to avoid crossing flexion creases at right angles. Also take care to avoid injury to neurovascular structures and devascularization of the skin flaps. Achieve proper orientation of the tendon before repair. At times if tendons have retracted into the carpal tunnel or more proximally, then partial release of the transverse carpal ligament may be required to deliver them distally into the palm. Although the flexor sheath is not involved in the palm, use a careful technique in the placement of sutures; it probably is best to use an intratendinous core suture in the palm to avoid

exposure of the suture material to adjacent structures. Satisfactory healing and functional results can be expected following repair of the tendons in the palm. The postoperative bandaging also includes a compressive bulky dressing, immobilizing the thumb and fingers and wrist. Immobilize the wrist at about 45 degrees of flexion and the fingers at about 50 to 60 degrees of flexion with the interphalangeal joints extended.

Zone IV. In zone IV, the area of the carpal tunnel, if injury occurs directly to the base of the palm it usually also involves the median nerve. If a laceration occurs just proximal to the wrist flexion crease, flexor tendon injury, especially with the fingers flexed, in zone IV should be suspected. Extend the laceration distally into the palm and proximally into the forearm with care being taken to cross flexion creases obliquely. If the laceration occurs beneath the transverse carpal ligament, partial or complete release of the transverse carpal ligament may be required. Preserve, if possible, a portion of the transverse carpal ligament to avoid bowstringing postoperatively. If it cannot be preserved, release it in a Z-lengthening configuration so it can be repaired to help minimize the risk of postoperative bowstringing. Repair the flexor profundus and sublimis tendons in the carpal tunnel; the suture configuration again probably is best an intratendinous one with a locking core suture to hold the tendons with minimal exposure of cut surface and suture material. In the carpal tunnel again take care to ensure proper orientation and location of the individual tendons. The usual arrangement of the flexor sublimis tendons in the carpal tunnel with the middle and ring finger tendons superficial to the index and small finger tendons is helpful to recall in this situation. Partial tenosynovectomy may be required to diminish the bulky and edematous tissue that may follow the repair. The skin closure usually is accomplished with 4-0 nylon, and the bandage and dorsal splint are applied to maintain the wrist in approximately 45 degrees of flexion. If the transverse carpal ligament has been completely released and repair is not possible, bring the wrist nearly to neutral and flex the fingers more acutely to diminish pressure on the volar skin and to minimize bowstringing. If the transverse carpal ligament is partially intact or has been repaired, immobilize the wrist in about 45 degrees of flexion with the fingers in about 50 to 60 degrees of flexion with the metacarpophalangeal joints in about 50 to 60 degrees of flexion and the interphalangeal joints in full extension.

Zone V. In zone V, the volar forearm proximal to the transverse carpal ligament, multiple tendons, nerves, and vessels are frequently injured by major lacerations, often from broken glass or in violent altercations with knives. In this area it is important to carefully identify the tendons accurately. Because of their common muscle origin when sublimis tendons and profundus tendons are divided, particularly at the wrist, they may be delivered into the wound as a group by finding and pulling distally on one tendon. The tendon ends can be properly matched by careful attention to their location and level in the wound, their relation to neighboring structures, their diameters, the shape of their cross sections, and the angle of the cuts through each tendon. Although it is not a disgrace to open an anatomy book in the operating room to be certain of anatomic relations, it is inexcusable to sew the median nerve to the flexor pollicis longus, the palmaris longus, or some other tendon. The proximal and distal ends of the median nerve usually can be identified easily in their appropriate anatomic location and from their more yellowish color and the presence of a volar midline vessel and the nerve fascicles, which can

usually be identified in the median nerve's severed ends.

Although 4-0 sutures are usually used in the palm and more distally, 3-0 nylon may be sufficient for suturing tendons in the distal forearm. Repairs done in the distal forearm do not absolutely require an intratendinous repair. A double right-angled or mattress suture may be satisfactory in the forearm. Repair nerves and vessels if needed after the tendon repairs in the forearm, working from the repair of deep structures to more superficial structures. Close the wounds with 4-0 nylon and immobilize the limb with the wrist flexed approximately 45 degrees and the metacarpophalangeal joints flexed 50 to 60 degrees with the interphalangeal joints in full extension.

AFTERTREATMENT. Reports based on the excellent works of Gelberman et al., Manske, Kleinert, Lister, Kutz, Duran and Houser, and Strickland and Glogovac confirm that excellent results can be achieved using one of two postoperative mobilization tech-

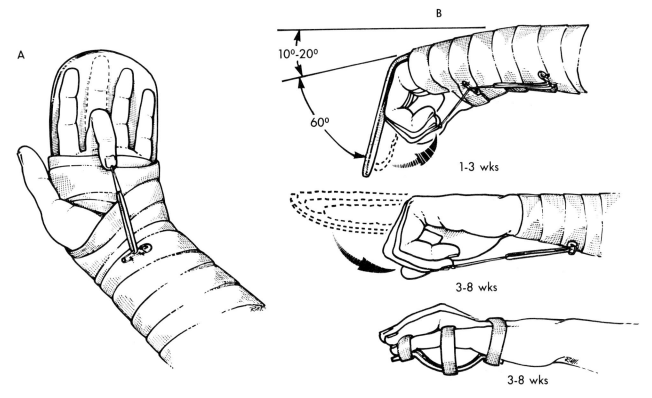

Fig. 63-27   **A,** After primary flexor tendon repair or flexor tendon graft, wrist and hand are held in a posterior plaster splint. Additionally, involved finger is held in flexion by elastic band attached at wrist level and at fingernail by wire through nail or glued-on garment hook. This permits active finger extension and protected passive flexion. **B,** Immediate controlled mobilization of repaired flexor tendon is achieved with extension block splint and proper rubber band traction, allowing PIP joint extension against traction and flexion of 40 to 60 degrees. At 3 to 8 weeks, rubber band is attached to Ace bandage cuff at wrist. After removal of rubber band traction, night splinting may be employed at 6 to 8 weeks if necessary. (**A,** Redrawn from Kleinert H: Orthop Clin North Am 4:874, 1973; **B,** redrawn from Hunter JM, Schneider LH, and Macklin EJ: Tendon surgery in the hand, St Louis, 1987, Mosby–Year Book, Inc.)

niques. In one, that advocated by Kleinert et al., active finger extension is used with passive flexion achieved using a rubber band attached to the fingernail and at the wrist. This has subsequently been modified with a roller in the palm to alter the line of force of the rubber band (Fig. 63-27). The second technique, advocated by Harmer, by Young and Harmon, and by Duran and Houser, involves a controlled passive motion technique with dorsal blocking of the fingers. It is important to understand that children younger than the age of about 10 years and noncompliant patients cannot be entrusted with understanding and following the complexities of either of these techniques and a more conservative postoperative management routine may be best selected depending on the judgment of the surgeon and the therapist. We have had success incorporating the modifications recommended by Strickland in the Duran-Houser technique and find that this is somewhat easier for patients to use and may minimize

the risk of flexion contractures at the proximal interphalangeal joint.

Although some patients can be allowed to remove a splint in the first week after surgery, we have found it safer to leave the nonremovable postoperative dorsal splint in place. Instruction in passive flexion and extension of the proximal and distal interphalangeal joints is demonstrated in the first postoperative day. The wrist is usually positioned between 20 and 45 degrees of flexion with the metacarpophalangeal joints in approximately 50 to 70 degrees of flexion and interphalangeal joints left at the neutral position. As recommended by Duran and Houser, before closure of the wound the amount of passive movement of the fingertip required to create a 3 to 5 mm excursion of the tendon is determined (Fig. 63-28). This amount of movement is started the day after surgery. According to the recommendations of Strickland and Glogovac, and of Duran and Houser, a removable splint may

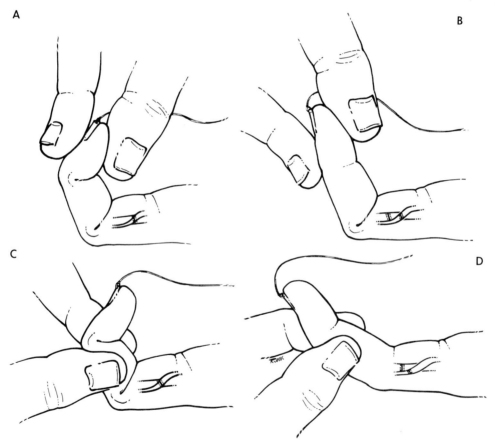

Fig. 63-28. **A,** Diagram of controlled passive motion exercise. Metacarpophalangeal joint should remain in normal balanced position. Extension of distal interphalangeal joint sufficient to move anastomosis 3 to 5 mm. Only distal interphalangeal joint moves during this exercise. **B,** Note distal migration of anastomosis of flexor digitorum profundus tendon away from that of flexor digitorum sublimis tendon. **C,** When middle phalanx is extended, both anastomoses glide distally. Only proximal interphalangeal joint moves during this exercise. **D,** Anastomoses are thus moved away from fixed structures that may have been injured. Elastic traction returns finger to original position. (Redrawn from Hunter JM, Schneider LH, and Macklin EJ: Tendon surgery in the hand, St Louis, 1987, Mosby–Year Book, Inc.)

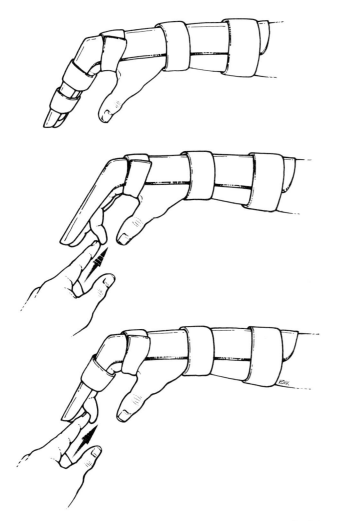

Fig. 63-29 Passive flexion of interphalangeal joints, which is done several times each day for 4 to 5 weeks. Duran and Hauser popularized early passive motion after tendon repair. (Redrawn from Strickland JW: Orthop Clin North Am 14:844, 1983.)

be used as early as 3 days after surgery in some compliant patients (Fig. 63-29). The patient is instructed in the exercise program, including eight repetitions of proximal and distal interphalangeal and composite passive flexion and extension of the joints twice daily. This is continued for at least 3 to 4 weeks, at which time a removable splint has been safe in our hands.

The controlled active motion program advocated by Kleinert et al. requires the attachment of a suture through the tip of the fingernail or a garment hook glued to the nail allowing the attachment of an elastic band (Fig. 63-27, *A*). A dorsal splint holds the wrist in 20 to 30 degrees of flexion and the metacarpophalangeal joints at 40 to 60 degrees. The interphalangeal joints are splinted in extension. The rubber band is passed beneath a roller or a safety pin in the palm and is secured to another safety pin at the level of the distal forearm (Fig. 63-27, *B*). The safety pin maintains the finger in flexion of 40 to 60 degrees at the proximal interphalangeal joint with no tension on the rubber band. The rubber band should allow full extension of the proximal interphalangeal joint against the traction of the rubber band. With this form of controlled mobilization, it is believed that the flexor tendon repair is not stretched and the movement that is allowed may enhance healing. Beginning in the first day after surgery, active extension exercises are encouraged. If it appears that the patient cannot understand and cooperate with this technique, it should be abandoned in the first week. After 3 weeks, the dorsal splint is removed and a wrist band with a hook for the rubber band is used for an additional 3 weeks. The patient actively extends the digit against the resistance of the rubber band. No passive extension or active flexion is permitted. The wrist band splint is discontinued between 6 and 8 weeks, and dynamic extension splinting is used to prevent contractures of the proximal interphalangeal joint. Between 8 and 10 weeks, strengthening exercises are permitted and the patient progresses to using his hand normally between 10 and 12 weeks following the repair.

FLEXOR TENDON INJURIES IN CHILDREN

When flexor tendons are injured in children under about the age of 10 years, the management is difficult and demanding. The same principles previously outlined apply to the management of flexor tendon injuries in the young patient. Some factors are worthy of note and emphasis.

The diagnosis of tendon and associated injuries may be more difficult in children because their examination is less reliable as a result of their anxiety, as pointed out by Entin. Because of the extremely small tolerances between the flexor sheath and flexor tendons even more attention is required to the use of meticulous technique. Finer sutures, such as 5-0 suture, may be required for repair of the tendons because of their small size; 6-0 and 7-0 sutures may be required for the circumferential repair of the surface of the tendon. Because of the inability of very young children to cooperate with the postoperative rehabilitation program their immobilization after surgery is usually more extensive and prolonged, frequently requiring the use of long arm casts extending to the axilla with the elbow and wrist flexed to nearly 90 degrees and the fingers in 50 to 60 degrees of flexion at the metacarpophalangeal joints with full interphalangeal extension. Early mobilization is not possible in the very young child because of his inability to cooperate. Should tendon grafting be required in tendon reconstruction, the sources of tendon grafts are limited. The retraining and rehabilitation of very young children are unpredictable, leading some surgeons to delay flexor tendon surgery in infants to a later age of 3 to 4 years to allow for better technical repair and to increase the chances of postoperative cooperation.

FLEXOR TENDON RUPTURES

Although rupture of flexor tendons is not as common as that of extensor tendons, it does occur and is often not diagnosed. In the athlete the most common tendon to be avulsed is the flexor digitorum profundus at its insertion in the ring finger. It may produce a small bony avulsion or articular fracture seen on the roentgenogram. Traumatic rupture usually occurs at the insertion of the tendon. Frequently the patient's initial complaint is that of a mass in the palm without awareness of any loss of finger function. The flexor tendons most frequently ruptured are the profundus tendons and more rarely the sublimis tendons or the flexor pollicis longus. These ruptures are most frequent in men during the third and fourth decades and about 20% may be associated with synovitis. (See discussion of tendon ruptures in arthritis, p. 3316.)

Treatment

The work of Leddy and of Leddy and Packer suggests a method for determining the treatment of these injuries. They have emphasized that the factors that influence the treatment and outcome of this injury are (1) the length of time between injury and treatment, (2) the extent to which the tendon retracts, (3) the blood supply to the avulsed tendon, and (4) the presence of bony fragments seen on roentgenogram. This allows the classification of these injuries into three types. In type 1 the tendon retracts completely into the palm and is held there by the lumbrical origin. In type 2 the tendon retracts to the level of the proximal interphalangeal joint with a long vinculum intact, presumably maintaining blood supply. In type 3, there is usually a bony fragment involved. The fragment may be comminuted or uncomminuted and may be nonarticular or intraarticular.

For type 1 injuries reinsertion into the distal phalanx is recommended if the injury is detected within 7 to 10 days. After this period of time, it is likely that the distal end of the tendon will become kinked and softened, prohibiting delivery into the finger and attachment to the distal phalanx. A midlateral or volar oblique incision is usually used. The sheath is opened through a transverse incision distal to the A2 pulley. Absence of the tendon end in this area indicates retraction into the palm. A transverse incision near the distal palmar crease exposes the flexor sheath proximal to the A1 pulley and allows location of the tendon end, which then can be delivered by a variety of techniques using sutures, the retrograde passage of pediatric feeding tubing or intravenous tubing, or wire loops to allow antegrade passage of the tendon without additional injury to the tendon sheath. The tendon is then attached to the distal phalanx with a pull-out wire, preferably of the antegrade type rather than the traditional retrograde Bunnell pull-out wire (see Fig. 63-19). This is left in place for 3 to 4 weeks during which time the limb is immobilized in a dorsal splint with the wrist in flexion, the metacarpophalangeal joint in 70 to 80 degrees of flexion, and the interphalangeal joints in extension. The pull-out wire is removed at 3 to 4 weeks. If a type 1 injury is seen late, consideration should be given to flexor tendon grafting in the young, cooperative patient for the index, long, or ring finger, or, as alternatives, tenodesis or arthrodesis should be considered, depending on the needs and activities of the patient.

Type 2 injuries with the tendon retracted to the level of the proximal interphalangeal joint may be repaired at a later time than those in which the tendon is retracted into the palm because the circulation is thought to be maintained. Some of these avulsions have been satisfactorily repaired several months after injury.

Type 3 injuries with a small avulsion fracture may also be treated by reattachment at a later time because of the preservation of the circulation. Early passive motion is encouraged with the finger immobilized, and if a pull-out wire technique is used, the above postoperative treatment is followed.

In many patients seen late, regardless of the level of retraction, if satisfactory reattachment is impossible, consideration should be given to arthrodesis or tenodesis. A select group of motivated patients in the 10- to 20-year age range may achieve satisfactory function following flexor tendon grafts through the intact sublimis tendon in the index and long (middle) fingers, according to Stark et al.

Postrepair Rupture

If flexor tendon rupture after a primary repair is detected promptly, satisfactory results can be achieved if the finger is explored and the ruptured tendon is located and repaired. If detection of the rupture is delayed, end-to-end repair is rarely possible and tendon graft reconstruction may be required. The flexor tendon may rupture after tenolysis. In these situations, judgment is required in making the decision regarding exploration and repair versus tendon grafting. If the tendon has ruptured in a densely scarred area, satisfactory function following reexploration and repair is unlikely and consideration should be given to delayed tendon grafting.

When a rupture of the flexor pollicis longus tendon is seen early, the tendon may be reattached to the distal phalanx; when seen late, a tendon graft may be necessary because of muscle shortening and tendon degeneration (p. 3042).

REPAIR OF FLEXOR TENDON OF THUMB

The thumb also may be arbitrarily divided into zones according to the specific anatomic structures in the zone that influence the type of repair that is chosen for the flexor pollicis longus. Zone T-1 includes the area at the interphalangeal joint and the insertion of the flexor pollicis longus. T-2 includes the fibro-osseous sheath extending just proximal to the metacarpal head and the metacarpophalangeal joint. T-3 includes the area of the metacarpal beneath the thenar muscles, T-4 corresponds to the carpal tunnel, and T-5 corresponds to the distal forearm just proximal to the wrist (Fig. 63-30).

Urbaniak has proposed an organized system of selecting repair methods for the flexor pollicis longus depending on the location of injury and the timing of repair (Table 63-3).

To locate the flexor pollicis longus, volar zigzag incisions over the thumb and linear incisions in the region of the thenar eminence and at the wrist may be required (see Fig. 63-25). Although an early mobilization routine may be used following flexor pollicis longus repair, in most situations it is not necessary. Postoperative immobilization includes splinting with the wrist flexed 30 to 45 degrees and the metacarpophalangeal and interphalangeal joints slightly extended. The splint is left intact for about 3 weeks and a removable splint is applied for an additional 3 weeks to protect the wrist and finger against excessive hyperextension. Active flexion is commenced at about 3 weeks, and passive extension and more vigorous activities may be commenced at 8 to 12 weeks.

Zone I

When the long flexor tendon of the thumb is divided in zone I within 1 cm of its insertion, it can be sutured primarily either to the distal stump or advanced and sutured directly into the bone. Some of the flexor sheath may require division. When this tendon is transected more proximally than 1 cm from its insertion, further advancement will be necessary and lengthening of the tendon by Z-plasty just proximal to the wrist should be carried out. This tendon is unique in that it may be advanced without disturbing its blood supply since it does not have a vinculum. Urbaniak and Goldner recommend advancement in preference to tendon grafting since there are fewer paratendinous adhesions after advancement than after a free tendon graft.

Zone II

In zone II, the critical pulley area at the metacarpophalangeal joint, a portion of the pulley may be excised to lessen the possibility of adherence to the pulley of the site of the tendon suture. Primary repair, however, is unpredictable and a later graft might be the better choice unless the surgeon is experienced in tendon repair. Advancement of the tendon distally to be sutured to a stump that is shortened to lie distal to the metacarpophalangeal pulley has the advantage of not placing a suture line under the pulley (Figs. 63-31 and 63-32). Lengthening of the tendon at the wrist by Z-plasty may be required for this procedure also. Urbaniak recommends an end-weave repair at the site of lengthening just proximal to the wrist.

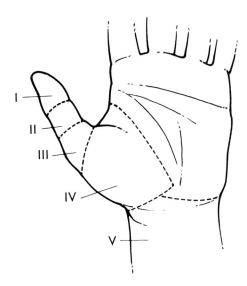

Fig. 63-30 Anatomic zones of flexor pollicis longus that influence type of repair are illustrated. (Redrawn from Urbaniak JR: Hand Clin 1:72, 1985.)

Table 63-3 Repair method for flexor pollicis longus based on zone of injury and timing of repair

	Acute injury		Chronic injury	
Zone	Sharp cut	Tendon loss	Minimal scar	Severe scar
I	Direct	Advancement	Advancement (or direct)	Advancement
II	Direct	Advancement and lengthening	Advancement and lengthening	Advancement and lengthening
III	Direct	Advancement and lengthening	Advancement and lengthening	Advancement and lengthening
IV	Direct	Free tendon graft	Free tendon graft	Two-stage free tendon graft
V	Direct	Tendon transfer (or bridge graft)	Direct	Tendon transfer

From Urbaniak JR: Hand Clin 1(1):74, 1985.

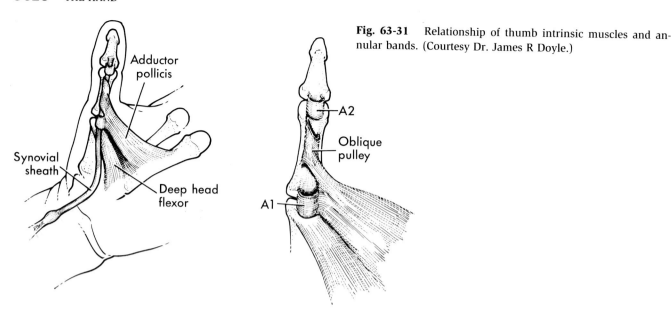

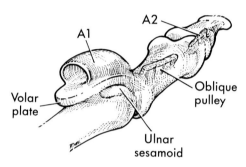

Fig. 63-32   Relationship of flexor sheath, volar plate, and metacarpophalangeal joint can be noted in this diagram of volar aspect of thumb. (Courtesy Dr. James R Doyle.)

Zone III

In zone III with a laceration of the flexor pollicis longus tendon, the proximal end frequently will retract to near the wrist level. Usually, the proximal end can be easily retrieved, and an attempt should be made to find the tendon in the thenar area. Primary repairs in this zone can be performed when the two ends are retrieved and apposed by flexing the wrist and the distal joint of the thumb. When retrieval of the proximal tendon requires an additional incision at the wrist, the tendon should be carefully rethreaded through its normal route. This may be done by inserting a 22-gauge wire loop or a tendon carrier through the sheath from the distal end, delivering a suture attached to the tendon, and threading it through from proximal to distal.

Zone IV

In zone IV the tendon is rarely cut since it is protected in part by a shelf of the radiocarpal bones. There is no contraindication to repair at this level as long as the re-

pair technique is atraumatic and the two ends are recoverable. An effort should be made to avoid the creation of a lump of suture material sufficient to cause median nerve compression within the closed space of the carpal tunnel.

Zone V

In zone V primary repair of the flexor pollicis longus tendon is indicated. Usually location of the tendon ends and end-to-end repair are not difficult.

SECONDARY REPAIR AND RECONSTRUCTION OF FLEXOR TENDONS

If flexor tendons cannot be repaired within the first 10 to 14 days (a delayed primary repair), then the repair is considered to be secondary. Kleinert et al. consider repairs done between 10 days and 4 weeks as early secondary repairs and repairs after 4 weeks as late secondary repairs. After 1 month it is extremely difficult to deliver the flexor tendon through the fibro-osseous sheath and the pulleys and in those circumstances, in the absence of extensive scarring and destruction of the tendon sheath, traditional single-stage flexor tendon grafting may be done. In the presence of extensive disturbance of the flexor sheath and pulleys, joint contractures, and nerve injury, two-stage tendon grafting should be considered.

Generally, tendons may be repaired secondarily by direct suture at the site of division, by tendon graft, or even by tendon transfer.

Before tendons are secondarily repaired, certain requirements must be met: (1) wound erythema and swelling should be minimal; (2) skin coverage must be adequate; (3) the tissues in which the tendon is expected to glide must be relatively free of scar; (4) the alignment of bones must be satisfactory, and any fractures must be healed or fixed securely; (5) joints must have a useful range of passive motion; and (6) sensation in the involved digit must be undamaged or restored, or it should be possible to repair damaged nerves directly or with nerve grafts at the time of tendon repair. Secondary repair of tendons may also be delayed for reconstruction of the flexor pulleys, especially the critical A2 and A4 pulleys. During these reconstructions a silicone rubber temporary prosthesis (Hunter) is useful to maintain the lumen of the tendon sheath while the grafted pulleys are healing. This is followed later by the insertion of the flexor tendon graft.

Flexor Tendons of Fingers

ZONE I (DISTAL HALF OF FINGER). When the profundus tendon has been lacerated or avulsed, it is best reattached within a few days, before it retracts into the palm and before avulsion of the vinculum occurs. When treated early, an avulsed or lacerated profundus tendon can be advanced 1 cm and reattached as discussed under primary repair (see discussion of flexor tendon rupture, p. 3026). After a few days the tendon end swells and it becomes difficult or impossible to thread the tendon through the bifurcation of the sublimis. Rethreading the swollen profundus may also jeopardize proximal interphalangeal joint movement. Profundus function may be restored by a tendon graft but only when indicated. It should be remembered that flexor tendon grafting through the intact sublimis tendons is somewhat unpredictable and serious discussions with the patient should be part of the preoperative planning. As noted previously, flexor tendon grafting through an intact sublimis was recommended for the index and middle fingers for children by Pulvertaft and for children and young adults by Goldner and Coonrad. Also, Stark et al. found satisfactory results in patients between the ages of 10 and 21 years, especially in the index and middle fingers, and rarely in the ring and little fingers. Honnor and Meares; Wilson; and Honnor reported satisfactory function following two-stage flexor tendon grafting after avulsion of the profundus tendon insertion.

In string musicians the motion at the distal interphalangeal joint that is provided by an intact flexor digitorum profundus is critical to enable the finger pulp to accurately fret the strings. It may also be important in technicians, artists, and others. This must be considered in those persons who have lost flexor digitorum profundus tendon function if other criteria are met that imply that tendon grafting through the intact sublimis would be worth the risk.

ZONE II (CRITICAL AREA OF PULLEYS). When the sublimis tendon alone is divided in the critical area of pulleys, it should not be repaired secondarily because the profundus tendon provides satisfactory function, and

profundus function may be jeopardized. Hyperextension deformities of the proximal interphalangeal joint occasionally occur following the laceration of a sublimis tendon in a very flexible hand. This can be dealt with by means other than sublimis tendon suture (such as tenodesis). When the profundus tendon alone is divided in this area, the sublimis tendon provides ample flexion of the proximal interphalangeal joint. In the "delayed primary" time period (10 to 14 days), meticulous repair of the flexor profundus may result in satisfactory function. During the "late secondary" time period (4 weeks), it is doubtful that a direct repair will be successful. Under these circumstances, consideration should be given to tenodesis or arthrodesis, depending on the needs of the patient. Unless the distal joint is extremely hyperextensible and "flail" it is the rare patient who will require extensive surgical treatment for this problem. Tenodesis or arthrodesis may be necessary in the index or middle finger but rarely in other digits. When both tendons are divided, if conditions do not permit primary or delayed primary repair of the tendons, flexor function may be restored with a single-stage tendon graft when all prerequisites are met in the fingers (healed and stable wound, flexible joints, and good or improving sensibility).

ZONES III, IV, AND V (FOREARM AND PALM). As late as 3 or 4 weeks after injury, flexor tendons in the forearm and palm may be repaired by direct suture because flexing the wrist usually accommodates the gap sufficiently to overcome muscle retraction. After 4 or 5 weeks the muscles become tightly contracted, and a graft is necessary at times to bring together the tendon ends. This may be in the form of a short segmental graft between the tendon ends (Fig. 63-33). When there has been destruction of tendons, profundus tendons take priority and attaching available proximal sublimis tendons to distal profundus tendons may provide satisfactory function. The tendons may be attached with a mattress suture technique, and monofilament wire may be used, especially in the distal forearm.

PROFUNDUS ADVANCEMENT

■ *TECHNIQUE (WAGNER).* Make a volar oblique, zigzag, or midateral incision over the profundus insertion (p. 2972); incise the tendon sheath at the C4 pulley area and retract it, preserving the annular pulleys. Usually the proximal end of the profundus will have retracted into the palm. This can be determined by making another opening in the sheath distal to the A2 pulley. If the tendon cannot be seen it probably is in the palm. Make a transverse incision near the distal palmar crease to recover it. Carefully thread it through the bifurcation of the sublimis and into the distal end of the finger; when this cannot be done accurately and with assurance that the relation of the sublimis to the profundus is normal two choices are available: (1) abandon the procedure be-

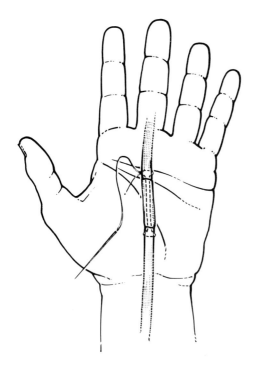

Fig. 63-33 Long-standing flexor tendon interruptions in palm may require a short segmental graft or "minigraft" to avoid too much tension.

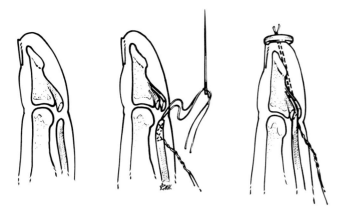

Fig. 63-34 Wagner technique of profundus advancement (see text).

cause it will end in failure not only of profundus function, but also of superficialis function, or (2) make a volar oblique incision over the proximal phalanx, open a portion of the A2 pulley, and deliver the profundus tendon into direct vision. Next, resect the distal segment of the profundus at a level just proximal to the distal interphalangeal joint and split its distal stump in a transverse plane (Fig. 63-34). Take care not to resect too much tendon, no more than 1 cm. With a Bunnell retrograde pull-out wire suture or an antegrade pull-out wire (see Figs. 63-18 and 63-19), fix the distal end of the proximal segment of tendon into the split profundus stump and tie the suture at the end of the finger through a

button. Do not disturb the capsular attachment of the profundus stump because it protects the volar plate and helps to ensure a gliding surface and mobile joint. Repair any divided digital nerves at this time. Close the wound and apply a dorsal splint with the wrist in 45 degrees of flexion, the metacarpophalangeal joints in 60 to 70 degrees of flexion, and the interphalangeal joints in full extension.

AFTERTREATMENT. See discussion of aftertreatment for primary repair (Duran-Houser, modified). Remove the pull-out suture at 3 to 4 weeks.

Reconstruction of Finger Flexors by Single-Stage Tendon Graft

When the sublimis and profundus tendons have both been divided in the critical area of pulleys, restoring flexion of the finger by grafting is indicated when several prerequisites are met: (1) the skin is pliable; (2) any wounds are well healed; (3) edema has subsided; (4) the joints allow a full passive range of motion; and (5) sensation in the finger is normal, or at least one digital nerve is intact (one divided digital nerve may be sutured at the time of grafting if the other nerve is intact). The A2 and A4 pulley systems should also be intact; otherwise, these should be reconstructed in a separate staged procedure before tendon grafting (see discussion of technique for pulley reconstruction, p. 3036). Age is a strong prognostic factor. Best results are seen in those in the 10- to 30-year age group. Worst results occur in the very young and in patients over 50 years of age.

■ *TECHNIQUE.* Make a zigzag incision on the volar aspect of the finger to expose the underlying flexor sheath up to the proximal finger crease or make a volar oblique or midlateral incision (see Fig. 61-12); carefully avoid entering the proximal interphalangeal joint, which has very thin subcutaneous fat laterally. Avoid injuring the neurovascular bundles and make the flaps wide and thick enough to prevent necrosis. Expose the flexor sheath and preserve as much of the unscarred sheath as possible. Excise no more than absolutely necessary of the A2 and A4 pulley systems; complete excision of either will result in functional failure of the grafted tendon. Free the scarred sublimis and profundus tendons and carefully preserve all of the volar plate of the proximal and distal interphalangeal joints. In the patient with hyperextensible joints, tenodesis of the sublimis will help prevent a swan neck deformity. Divide both tendons at their insertions and bring them out through a transverse palmar incision made over the midbelly of the lumbrical muscles. Then with a small chisel, raise a flap of bone just distal to the distal interphalangeal joint on the volar surface of the distal phalanx for later insertion of the profundus tendon graft (see Figs. 63-18 and 63-35). Under this bone flap, drill a small hole with a Kirschner

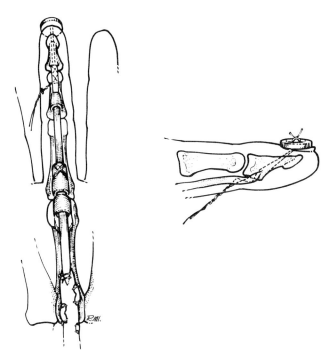

Fig. 63-35 Repair of finger flexor tendons by tendon graft. Graft has been sutured in place. Note that proximal and distal pulleys have been narrowed.

wire large enough to accommodate two No. 4-0 monofilament wire sutures.

An alternate method for distal insertion is to split the remaining distal tendon stump (see Fig. 63-34). The stump is large enough to receive and hold a suture. This method in children avoids the need for later removal of the pull-out suture. Now through the proximal palmar incision, divide the sublimis tendon as far proximally as possible and discard it; retain the profundus tendon for attachment to the graft.

In approximately 15% of people the palmaris longus tendon is absent, but when it is present, it can be taken from the same forearm and used as the graft. Expose the tendon through a transverse incision just proximal to its insertion at the wrist and through another in the upper forearm. Dissect the tendon at its musculotendinous junction proximally and detach it distally after dissecting out the various portions of its insertion; then draw the tendon out through the proximal forearm incision. Place a monofilament No. 34 pull-out wire suture in the distal end of the palmaris longus tendon before dividing it proximally. Arrange the pull-out wire either in the retrograde Bunnell technique or use a single-loop antegrade pull-out wire. This suture is much more easily placed when the proximal end of the tendon is stabilized. Thread the pull-out wire through the hole in the distal phalanx. The distal attachment may be reinforced with an absorbable mattress suture. Bring the tendon proximally

through the intact tendon sheath and into the palm by wetting the tendon and pushing it through with a probe or use a 22-gauge wire loop to pass the tendon proximally. To prevent bowstringing, determine if the pulley system is intact while bringing the tendon proximally.

A careful attempt must be made to attach the tendon to the graft under appropriate tension. Place the wrist in neutral and the finger in full extension. Now place tension on the musculotendinous junction proximally and on the graft attached to the finger distally. At the point where the tendon and graft are to be joined mark the junction with a methylene blue pen. Adjust the tension so that when the wrist is in extension, the finger will automatically be brought into about the same amount or slightly more flexion as the adjoining digits. Increase flexion a little in the more ulnar digits.

Several methods may be used to suture the proximal junction. One is a direct suture by the crisscross Bunnell method using a monofilament wire (see Fig. 63-11); another is the fish-mouth insertion described by Pulvertaft (see Fig. 63-15). Do not suture the lumbrical muscle to the tendon junction because this tends to increase the tension in the lumbrical muscle, contributing to the "lumbrical plus" finger.

Attach the tendon ends and close the wound without subcutaneous sutures. Insert a drain in the proximal palmar wound if needed, especially if the tourniquet is to be deflated after a splint is applied. Place the wrist in 40 to 45 degrees of flexion with the metacarpophalangeal joints in 60 degrees of flexion and the interphalangeal joint in full extension. The wrist should not be placed in forced flexion because this may increase postoperative pain and may cause pressure on the median nerve. Cover the wounds with a layer of nonadhesive material and then a moist molded dressing. Apply a posterior short arm splint to hold the wrist in flexion. In children, a long arm cast is applied to keep the dressing from shifting distally.

It is extremely important to prevent a postoperative hematoma. Therefore some surgeons release the tourniquet before wound closure and keep manual pressure on the wound for 5 minutes. Hemostasis is then obtained with electrocautery. As an alternative, apply a moist, conforming dressing to the volar aspect of the finger with the wrist held in flexion by a posterior splint and elevate the hand immediately following tourniquet deflation and awakening from the anesthetic.

AFTERTREATMENT. The wrist is elevated for the first 24 to 48 hours. Any drains are removed after about 24 hours or when drainage subsides. Postoperative management and rehabilitation depend on the philosophy, experience, and preferences of the surgeon and therapist. Brunelli and Brunelli report satisfactory results using an early postoperative mobilization technique. Other surgeons are more conservative, basing their rehabilitation program on the concept that the avascular tendon graft must revascularize and go through a weakened phase before commencing any significant motion. If a controlled passive motion rehabilitation program is pursued, the patient should be carefully evaluated for his ability to comply and he should be closely supervised on a nearly daily basis for at least 4 weeks. No active flexion, overextension, or passive hyperextension should be permitted. The pull-out suture is removed at 3 to 4 weeks. Protected motion is continued for at least an additional 4 weeks (total of 8 weeks). Strengthening is begun at 8 weeks after the tendon graft; however, normal forceful activity is not permitted before 12 to 14 weeks (see discussion of aftertreatment for primary repair, p. 3023)

Donor Tendons for Grafting

Donor tendons for grafting, in order of preference, are the palmaris longus, the plantaris, the long extensors of the toes, the index extensor digitorum communis, and the flexor digitorum sublimis.

PALMARIS LONGUS. The palmaris longus is the tendon of choice because it fulfills the requirements of length, diameter, and availability without producing a deformity. The presence of this tendon should be determined before any grafting procedure; its presence can be demonstrated by having the patient oppose the tips of the thumb and little finger while flexing the wrist (Fig. 63-36). The tendon is reported to be present in one arm in 85% of people and in both arms in 70%. The tendon is flat, is surrounded by paratenon, and is long enough for a graft about 15 cm in length. Excise the tendon as follows. Make a short transverse incision directly over the tendon just proximal to the flexion crease of the wrist. Divide the tendon, grasp its end with a hemostat, and apply traction so that it can be palpated easily in a proximal direction. Then make a second transverse incision over the tendon at the junction of the middle and proximal thirds of the forearm. Identify the tendon, divide it, and withdraw the segment to be used as a graft. Should paratenon be desired, a long curved incision over the forearm is necessary; this method is much more disabling, and, as an alternative, use a tendon stripper similar to that devised by Brand for the plantaris tendon (Fig. 63-37). Occasionally there is a double palmaris longus tendon, or it may have multiple insertions or an associated aberrant muscle. Any of these will make it difficult to withdraw it from only two transverse incisions.

PLANTARIS TENDON. The plantaris tendon is equally as satisfactory for a graft as the palmaris tendon, has the advantage of being almost twice as long (enough to pro-

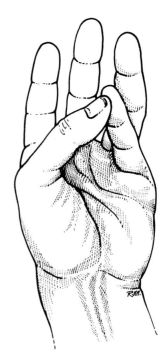

Fig. 63-36 Method of demonstrating presence of palmaris longus tendon (see text).

vide two grafts), but is not as accessible (Figs. 63-38 and 63-39). It reportedly is present in 93% of people. The tendon lies anteromedial to the tendo calcaneus proximal to the heel and may be obtained for grafting as follows. Make a small medial longitudinal incision just anterior to the insertion of the tendo calcaneus. Identify the tendon as a slip distinctly separate from the tendo calcaneus (Fig. 63-37). Divide the tendon near its insertion, and thread it through the loop of a tendon stripper made for this purpose. Keep the knee in full extension. Clamp the distal end of the tendon with a hemostat, hold it taut, and pass the stripper up the leg until the resistance of the gastrosoleus fascia is encountered; overcome this resistance with additional force on the stripper. Advance the stripper proximally for a total of about 25 cm, where resistance is again met as the loop of the stripper meets the belly of the muscle. Now palpate the loop of the stripper through the skin and over it make a longitudinal incision 5 cm long. Then free from around the plantaris tendon the gastrocnemius muscle belly, divide the tendon under direct vision, and withdraw the tendon distally. If a tendon stripper is not available, remove the tendon through multiple short transverse incisions.

LONG EXTENSORS OF TOES. Tendons of the long extensors of the toes are not as desirable as the palmaris longus or the plantaris tendons because there are many attachments between them, especially as the cruciate ligament is approached proximally. Every toe except the little one has an extensor brevis tendon to dorsiflex it after excision of the long extensor tendon. The extensor hallucis longus is much larger than the other extensors, and

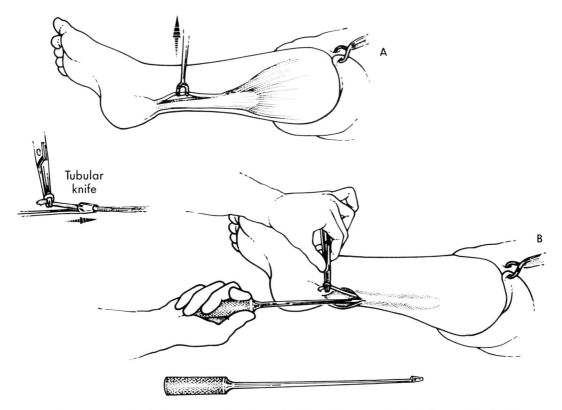

Fig. 63-37   Method of removing plantaris tendon for grafting (see text). **A,** Plantaris tendon is separated from tendo calcaneus. **B,** Brand tendon stripper. (Redrawn from White WL: Surg Clin North Am 40:403, 1960.)

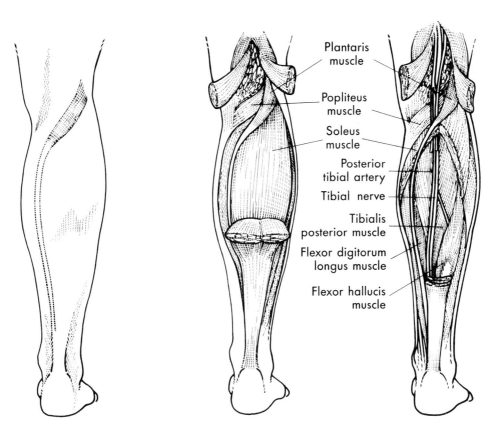

Fig. 63-38   Anatomic relations of plantaris muscle and tendon. (Modified from White WL: Surg Clin North Am 40:403, 1960.)

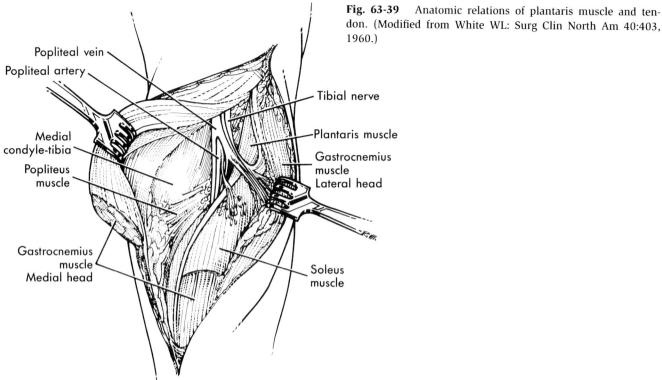

the extensor of the second toe is much more intimately related to the dorsalis pedis artery. The extensor of the third toe is probably easiest to remove and use. Make multiple short transverse incisions over the tendon and remove it by elevating the skin proximal to each incision and dissecting to a more proximal level; then make another incision at this point and repeat the procedure. Extract the divided end of the tendon through each successive incision and remove it through the proximal incision (Fig. 63-40, *A*).

A tendon may be removed much more easily through a long curved incision along the course of the tendon (Fig. 63-40, *B*), but such an incision temporarily prevents weight bearing and results in an unsightly scar.

EXTENSOR INDICIS PROPRIUS. The extensor indicis proprius tendon is usually long enough for a single flexor tendon graft but is rarely used. Divide it distally at its insertion into the extensor hood through a small transverse incision and proximally just distal to the dorsal carpal ligament through another incision. Suture the distal end of the proximal segment of tendon to the extensor digitorum communis to help maintain independent extension of the index finger.

FLEXOR DIGITORUM SUBLIMIS. A flexor digitorum sublimis tendon should not be excised simply as a graft, but at times one is available when removed in conjunction with an amputation or flexor tendon grafting. The tendon is usually too thick so that its central part may undergo necrosis when it is used as a graft; thus a local

reaction is produced that causes adhesions. The tendon may be split longitudinally to make it thinner, but this leaves a raw surface where adhesions are even more likely to develop.

Complications

"LUMBRICAL PLUS" FINGER. The "lumbrical plus" finger develops when the pull of the profundus musculotendinous unit is applied through the lumbrical muscle rather than through a flexor tendon graft distal to the lumbrical muscle origin. The pull of the profundus muscle, applied through the lumbrical muscle, creates extension of the proximal and distal interphalangeal joints. This usually occurs if the tension on a tendon graft is not appropriately set and the graft is relatively too "long" (Figs. 63-41 and 63-42). The condition may also be seen when amputations have occurred through the middle phalanx following avulsion of the insertion of the flexor digitorum profundus or division of the flexor profundus tendon. The middle finger seems to be most commonly involved. Usually with gentle flexion effort the patient can nearly make a fist with his grafted finger; however, when forceful flexion is attempted the interphalangeal joints will extend with "paradoxical extension." According to Parkes, the test for the "lumbrical plus" finger is to demonstrate first that the patient has full passive flexion of all joints of the finger. In strong gripping or active flexion of all fingers, flexion will be incomplete and partial extension of the interphalangeal joints will occur. The treatment for this condition consists of transection of

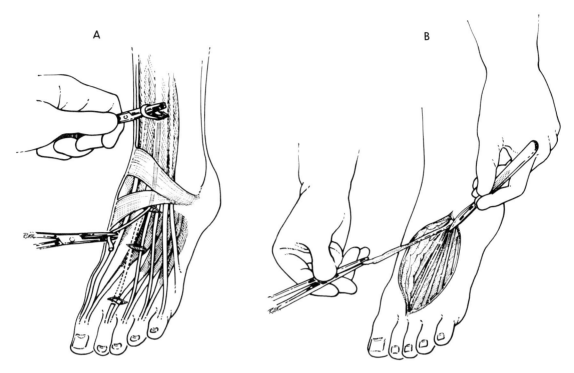

Fig. 63-40 Methods of obtaining long extensor tendon of toe for grafting (see text). **A,** Long extensor tendon of second toe is being removed through four short transverse incisions. **B,** Same tendon is being removed through one long longitudinal incision. (Redrawn from White WL: Surg Clin North Am 40:403, 1960.)

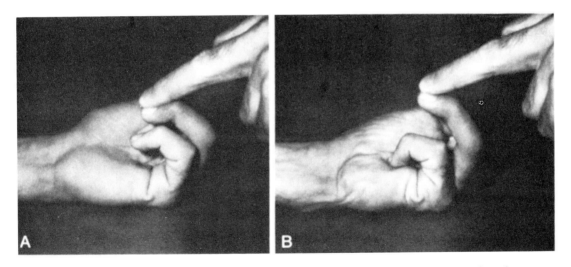

Fig. 63-41 "Lumbrical plus" finger. In this patient, a tendon graft somewhat too long has been inserted. **A,** Gentle flexion results in coordinated flexion of grafted ring finger and adjacent small finger. **B,** Powerful flexion of hand results in good flexion of small digit but paradoxical extension of interphalangeal joints of grafted ring finger against examiner's digit. (Redrawn from Lister GD: The hand: diagnosis and indications, Edinburgh, 1984, Churchill Livingstone.)

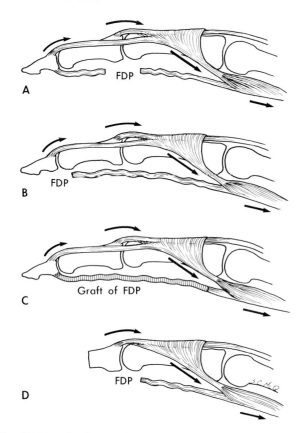

Fig. 63-42 Conditions that cause "lumbrical plus" finger. **A,** Severance of flexor digitorum profundus (FDP) (produces paradoxical extension). **B,** Avulsion of flexor digitorum profundus. **C,** Overly long flexor tendon graft. **D,** Amputation through middle phalanx. (Redrawn from Parkes A: J Bone Joint Surg 53-B:236, 1971.)

the involved lumbrical tendon through a longitudinal incision in the web space to the radial side of the involved finger, usually with the patient under a local anesthetic. If the tendon otherwise functions satisfactorily, this should cure the problem.

"QUADRIGA" EFFECT. If the tension on the tendon graft is set too tightly, when the patient attempts to flex his fingers the grafted finger will flex and reach the palm before the remaining fingers. This will block full excursion of the proximal flexor musculotendinous units and will reduce the ability to flex the uninjured digits, usually occurring in the middle, ring, and little fingers. This limitation of excursion can also occur if the flexor digitorum sublimis spiral is not corrected in the repair of any injury to the flexor profundus and sublimis, with improper repair of an oblique laceration allowing triggering or blocking of motion to occur and blocking of tendon motion because of eversion of the tendon repair. This has been emphasized by Verdan and further elucidated by Lister.

Reconstruction of Flexor Tendon Pulleys

Injury to the important annular thickenings of the fibro-osseous sheath (especially the A2 and A4 pulleys) may have occurred at the time of tendon injury, or they may have been destroyed during previous surgical procedures, either at the time of a primary repair or subsequently during tenolysis. When reconstructive procedures, including tenolyses and single-stage and two-stage graft reconstructions, are attempted without reconstruction of the pulleys the result is usually doomed. Without the presence of the pulleys, the angle of approach of the tendon to its insertion is altered, retinacular restraints are damaged, a flexion contracture frequently develops at the proximal interphalangeal joint, bowstringing of palmar skin occurs, and tendon excursion is lost. If the finger is left without the function of the A2 and A4 pulleys, it will not function satisfactorily after tenolysis and tendon graft reconstruction will be useless. Reconstruction of the A2 and A4 pulley systems is indicated when insufficient pulley remnants are left after tenolysis and as part of a single-stage or two-stage tendon graft reconstruction. In the involved digit all fractures and joint injuries should be healed, neurovascular defects should be minimal or improving, and there should be good soft tissue coverage with minimal scarring.

In two situations, flexor tenolysis and single-stage flexor tendon grafting, the pulley reconstruction may be jeopardized at the time that motion is commenced. Usually this objection can be overcome in the postoperative period using rings, taped bands, or thermoplastic material rings, as recommended by Strickland et al. to protect the pulley reconstruction.

Use of the pulley reconstruction in the two-stage tendon graft reconstruction allows the grafted material to heal satisfactorily so that by the time of the second stage of the tendon grafting procedure the pulley reconstruction has sufficiently healed. The results are usually better in young adults and adolescents because they are less likely to develop joint stiffness than are older patients. Donor grafts for pulley reconstruction include a flexor sublimis tendon that is sacrificed and split longitudinally, portions of the extensor retinaculum at the wrist or ankle as advocated by Lister, sublimis tendon, fascia lata in rare situations, and the palmaris longus if it is not needed for flexor tendon grafting (see discussion of donor sites for tendon grafts, p. 3032).

■ *TECHNIQUE.* **Make a zigzag (see Fig. 61-12, *B* and *C*), midlateral (see Fig. 61-13), or volar oblique (see Fig. 63-12, *D*) incision exposing the area of the flexor tendons. Make the exposure wide enough to show all of the flexor pulley system. Excise the scarred tendons and surrounding scar tissue. However, retain any part of the sheath that is not scarred, especially in the area of the distal joint and the A1 pulley system in the palm. Bring the tendons out through an additional palmar incision and com-**

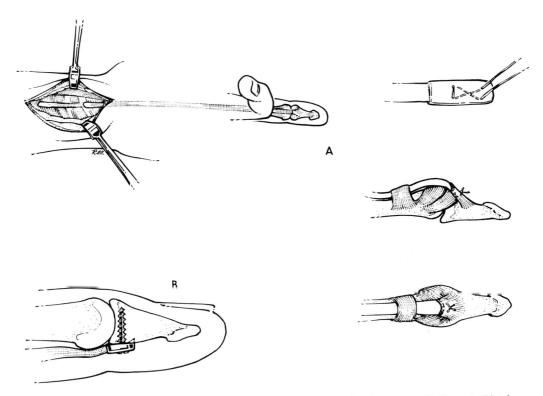

Fig. 63-43 **A,** Stage 1. Distal implant juncture; suture to profundus stump. **B,** Stage 1. Distal implant juncture; metal end plate implant model with screw fixation to distal phalanx. (**A** redrawn from Hunter JM and Salisbury RE: J Bone Joint Surg 53-A:829, 1971. **B** redrawn from Schneider LH: Hand Clin 1:113, 1985.)

plete their excision. If a two-stage tendon reconstruction is planned, insert a Silastic rod (Hunter) of appropriate size and attach it distally either to the remaining profundus tendon stump or to the bone by a small screw (Fig. 63-43) as described for the two-stage Hunter rod technique. Place the rod proximally at the forearm or palmar level in a scar-free area away from the profundus tendon. Leave the profundus tendon attached to the lumbrical muscle to maintain its length.

Several techniques are available for pulley reconstruction. If a tendon graft is to be used or a pulley substitute, a thin strip measuring at least 6 cm in length and 0.25 cm in width may be used. If the original fibro-osseous rim of the flexor sheath is satisfactory, the tendon can be woven through this rim and secured with mattress sutures. The strip is woven over the silicone rod beginning at about the A2 pulley level (Fig. 63-44). The A2 and A4 pulleys may be reconstructed individually in this method. If the fibro-osseous rim is insufficient, the tendon graft should be passed around the phalanx and sutured to itself with several mattress sutures. Over the proximal phalanx (A2 pulley reconstruction), the tendon is passed over the silicone rod and around the proximal phalanx deep to the extensor tendon. Over the middle phalanx (A4 pulley reconstruction), the tendon is passed around the middle phalanx superficial

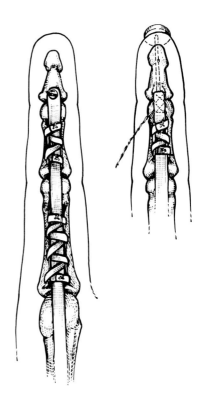

Fig. 63-44 Reconstruction of flexor tendon pulleys (see text). (Redrawn from Kleinert HE and Bennett JB: J Hand Surg 3:297, 1978.)

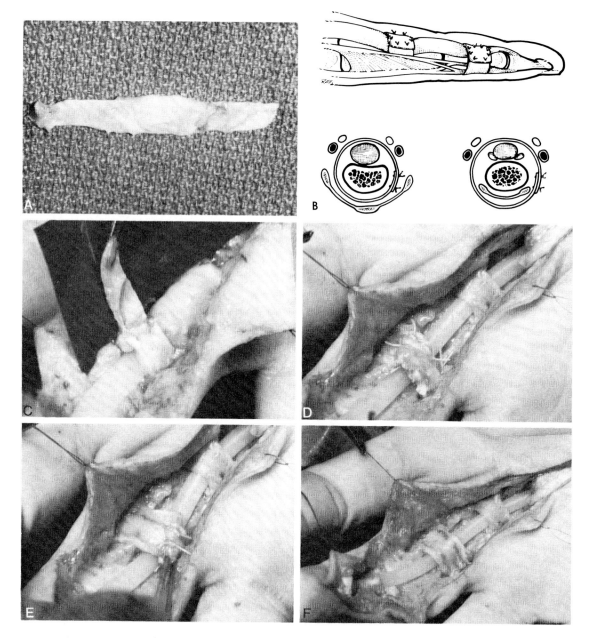

Fig. 63-45   **A,** Ideal tissue can be obtained for pulley reconstruction from extensor retinaculum of wrist or, preferably, dorsum of foot, as discussed in text. **B,** This is passed around phalanx and tendon deep to extensor tendon over proximal phalanx and superficial to it over middle. Graft is sutured securely because suture represents only weak point in this reconstruction (**C** and **D**). Overlapped repair is rotated around to side of digit, creating a strong pulley with a synovial gliding surface on its inner aspect. **E** and **F,** Intervening windows should be reconstructed with synovial tissue from dorsum of foot adjacent to retinaculum. (From Lister G: Hand Clin 1:93, 1985.)

to the extensor tendon and sutured to itself. In each case the circling pulley reconstruction is rotated so that the suture portion is to the side of the finger.

In another technique, advocated by Lister, extensor retinaculum from the wrist can be harvested and used as an encircling pulley reconstruction as well (Fig. 63-45). It is important to pass a piece of thread around the finger to estimate the amount of length of the tendon graft material that will be required for

the pulley reconstruction. Avoid reconstructing the pulley over the proximal interphalangeal joint because this may restrict motion. When pulley reconstruction is done concomitant with flexor tenolysis, plan to incorporate an orthotic protection (ring) in the rehabilitation period. Close the wound loosely and support the hand with a dorsal splint.

AFTERTREATMENT. If pulley reconstruction is part of stage 1 of a two-stage tendon reconstruction, passive motion of the finger joints is started usually at 7 to 10 days. The patient is instructed in passive finger exercises. Strapping to adjacent fingers may be helpful. For tenolyses, active motion is begun in the first 72 hours, and the therapy program progresses gradually. For staged tendon reconstruction, 3 months may be required to allow for healing and restoration of flexibility and sheath reconstitution before the second stage.

Reconstruction of Finger Flexors by Two-Stage Tendon Graft

For patients with excessive scarring, joint stiffness, and possibly nerve injury, a two-stage procedure for tendon repair may be indicated. As Schneider has emphasized, the patient who has a severely contracted, scarred digit, especially if neurovascular insufficiency is significant, may be a candidate for an arthrodesis or even amputation as reasonable alternatives to staged tendon reconstruction. The patient should clearly understand the extensive rehabilitation and effort involved in recovery following the at least two operations that will be required for such a tendon reconstruction. The first stage consists of excising the tendon and scar from the flexor tendon bed and preserving or reconstructing the flexor pulley system. A Dacron-impregnated silicone rod is inserted to maintain the tunnel in the area of the excised tendons until passive motion and sensitivity have been restored to the digit. The rod is attached distally to bone or tendon stump. It is passed proximally into the distal forearm to a level about 5 cm proximal to the wrist crease to allow proximal extension of the sheath into the forearm. The second stage consists of removal of the rod and insertion of a tendon graft (Fig. 63-46).

■ TECHNIQUE

Stage I. Make a zigzag (see Fig. 61-12, *B* and *C*) or midlateral (see Fig. 61-13) incision to expose the entire flexor sheath area. If scars are present, it is best to follow them with the incision to avoid ischemia in skin flaps. Expose the palm either by a continuation of the zigzag incision or through an additional incision at the level of the A1 pulley. Excise the profundus and sublimis tendons, but retain a stump of the profundus tendon 1 cm long at the distal phalanx. If pulley reconstruction is planned, preserve the insertion of the sublimis to reinforce the pulleys. Save excised tendon as graft material for pulley reconstruction. Retain only the unscarred portions of the flexor pulley system, but some portions of the A2 and A4 pulleys are the minimum required. Now extend the dissection into the palm; if the lumbrical muscle is scarred and contracted, excise it. Transect the profundus tendon at the level of the lumbrical.

Select a Dacron silicone rod of appropriate size and rinse it in saline to remove lint. Usually a smaller rod is selected to provide a snug fit in the sheath. Insert it into the palm and continue blunt dissection proximally so that the rod extends above the wrist level. Excising the entire sublimis tendon may be necessary to make room for the rod at the wrist. Attach the rod distally beneath the stump of the profundus with No. 32 monofilament steel wire reinforced with two 4-0 nonabsorbable sutures through the Dacron portion of the rod. As an alternative, secure the rod to the distal phalanx with a screw.

After seating the prosthesis, passively flex the fingers to observe any tendency toward buckling. Traction on the prosthesis will determine the need for possible further modification of the pulley system, either by excising more scar tissue or reconstructing a defective area in the system, especially at the A2 and A4 levels. Repair digital nerves as needed and close the wound after obtaining satisfactory hemostasis. Apply a bulky compressive dressing and a dorsal splint with the wrist at about 35 degrees of flexion, the metacarpophalangeal joints at 60 to 70 degrees of flexion, and the interphalangeal joints extended.

AFTERTREATMENT. After closing the wound, the hand is supported by a splint and gentle passive motion of the finger joints is started at 7 to 10 days. The hand should be examined regularly for synovitis or buckling of the rod. If buckling is seen, external rings are worn on the fingers to support the implant. If synovitis develops, prompt and complete immobilization is usually sufficient for resolution. The second stage is done when the finger is soft, supple, and well healed with mobile joints. The earliest time for stage 2 is about 8 weeks, but 3 months is usually required, depending on the patient's needs and the surgeon's judgment.

■ TECHNIQUE

Stage 2. Using appropriate anesthesia, open the previous incision to expose the flexor sheath over the distal portion of the middle phalanx near the distal joint, and make another incision proximally in either the palm or the forearm. Select a donor tendon, depending on the planned proximal attachment. A palmaris longus will probably suffice for a single tendon with a proximal attachment in the palm. Longer tendons will be required for attachments from the forearm to the finger. The plantaris or the extensor digitorum longus tendon to the three central toes makes a sufficiently long tendon graft. Motor tendons usually selected include the profundus mass for the long, ring, and little fingers. If suitable, the profundus to the index is used for the index finger. The sublimis muscles may also be used for motors for the tendon grafts. For the thumb flexor tendon reconstruction, the flexor pollicis lon-

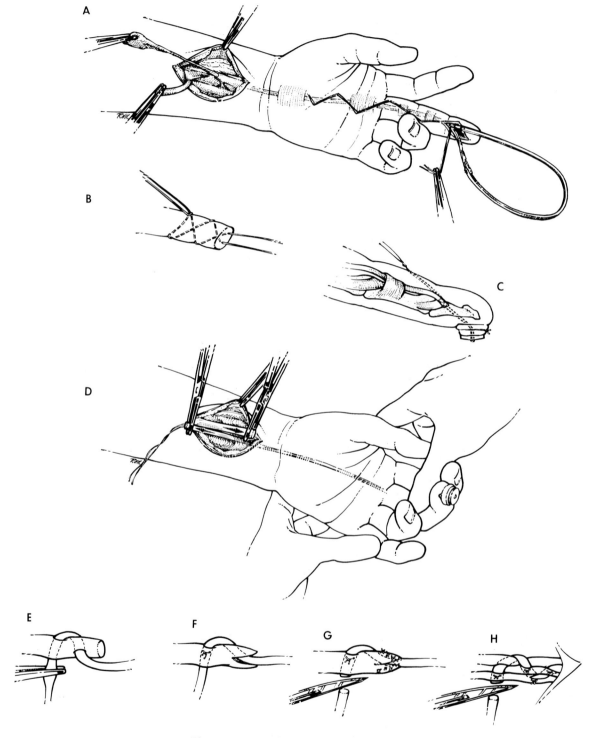

Fig. 63-46 For legend see opposite page.

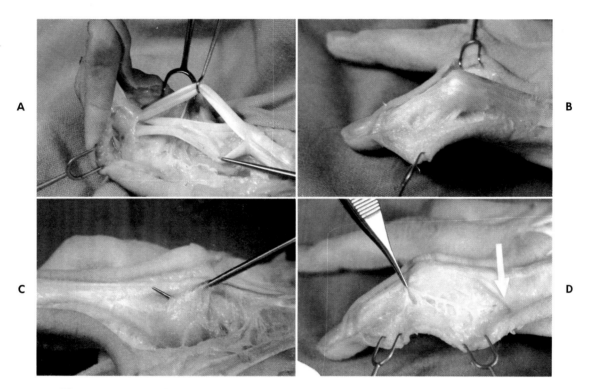

Plate 6 **A,** Injected specimen that reveals blood supply to middle area of flexor profundus digitorum tendon through its vincula longi. Note cut flexor sheaths and intact flexor sheaths distally. **B,** Cleland's ligaments as well as shorter ligaments at distal interphalangeal joint stand out in relief after dissection from proximal interphalangeal joint. **C,** Inserted probe reveals orientation of fibers of shroud ligament at level of metacarpophalangeal joint. **D,** Dorsal branch of digital nerve on radial aspect of right index finger is dissected, revealing its branches and their relationship to skin from dorsum of finger. Arrow indicates site from which nerve emerges under extensor hood.

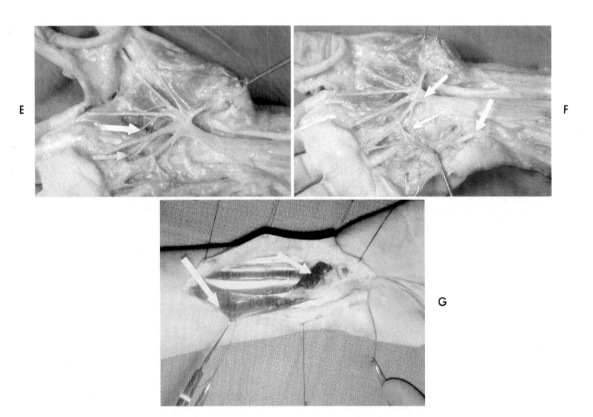

Plate 6 cont'd   **E,** Detailed dissection of median nerve reveals small branches to two radial lumbrical muscles as indicated by arrows. **F,** Arrows indicate Riche-Cannieu anastomosis. Small filament from median to ulnar nerve completes anastomosis and forms anastomotic arc. **G,** Aberrant muscle masses *(arrows)* occasionally found about palmaris longus tendon and at distal forearm on ulnar aspect.

gus or the sublimis muscles may be used. In certain selected situations, the sublimis to the ring finger may be used as both motor and tendon without the need for a free tendon graft.

While the tendon grafts are being harvested, the tourniquet is deflated and the wounds are covered with sterile bandages and compressed. After the tendon grafts have been harvested, the limb is exsanguinated and the tourniquet is reinflated. Suture the flexor graft to the proximal end of the implant and pull the implant through the sheath, trailing the tendon graft with it (Fig. 63-46, *A*). Separate the implant from the tendon graft and discard the implant. Use a pull-out technique to secure the distal attachment of the tendon graft to the distal phalanx (Fig. 64-46, *B* and *C*) or the distal end of the flexor tendon, as previously described (Fig. 63-34).

It the palm is not involved with scarring, a short graft can be used and the proximal attachment is made to the profundus tendon at the lumbrical origin with a Pulvertaft fish-mouth weave. If the profundus is not satisfactory, an adjacent sublimis may be used as a motor in the palm. If the profundus tendons of the long, ring, and little fingers are chosen for common motors, use an interweaving technique for the proximal attachment. In some circumstances, the proximal attachment is in the forearm. In the forearm the appropriate motor muscle is selected and the length of the flexor tendon graft is obtained by allowing the dorsum of the hand and wrist to lie flat on the operating table.

The "cascade of the fingers" (Schneider) is inspected with each finger somewhat more flexed than the finger to its radial side. The tendon graft is passed in an interweave method without being sutured, and traction is applied to the graft until the finger demonstrates its proper position to its adjacent fingers (Fig. 63-46, *D*); a mattress suture then is placed through the motor tendon and the tendon

graft. After testing passive movement with wrist flexion and extension, place the hand on the table and observe the finger as it assumes its position in relation to the adjacent fingers. If the position is satisfactory, complete the attachment of the graft with a Pulvertaft weave with mattress sutures (Fig. 63-46, *E* through *H*). Deflate the tourniquet, obtain satisfactory hemostasis, and close the wound using drains as needed. Apply a bulky compression dressing with a short arm dorsal splint, and maintain the wrist in about 35 degrees of flexion with the metacarpophalangeal joints in 70 degrees of flexion with full extension of the interphalangeal joints.

AFTERTREATMENT. An early protected motion program is described by Schneider. A more conservative approach may be used by surgeons concerned about rupture and disruption at the tendon attachments. If an early protected motion program is commenced, usually it begins 3 days after the operation. If a rubber band attachment to the fingernail is used as a part of the passive component of the protected motion routine, the therapist and the surgeon should closely supervise the program to avoid proximal and distal interphalangeal joint contractures. The pull-out suture is removed at 4 weeks. In a compliant patient, the dorsal splint is removed at 4 weeks also and the rubber band is attached to a wrist cuff to provide additional protection for 1 to 2 more weeks. Blocking exercises are begun at 4 to 5 weeks. Static splints are used to help avoid recurrence of flexion contractures present before stage 1. Dynamic and static splints are added as needed, possibly as early as 4 to 5 weeks in patients with poor pull-through. In those with satisfactory motion, dynamic and static splints may be added at 6 to 8 weeks. Heavy resistance should be avoided early in the program.

In those patients whose situation does not allow close supervision by the surgeon or the therapist be-

Fig. 63-46 Passive gliding technique, using Hunter tendon prosthesis. Stage 2: Removal of prosthesis and insertion of tendon graft. **A,** Graft has been sutured to proximal end of prosthesis and then pulled distally through new tendon bed. Note mesentery-like attachment of new sheath visible in forearm. **B,** Distal anastomosis. Bunnell pull-out suture in distal end of tendon graft. **C,** Distal anastomosis. Complete Bunnell suture with button over fingernail. Reinforcing sutures are usually placed through stump of profundus tendon. **D,** Proximal anastomosis. Measuring excursion of tendon graft and selecting motor. If procedure is done with patient under local anesthesia (see text) true amplitude of active muscle contraction can be measured. **E,** Proximal anastomosis graft is threaded through tendon motor muscle two or three times for added strength. **F,** Proximal anastomosis. Stump is fish-mouthed after method of Pulvertaft, tension is adjusted, and one suture is inserted as shown. Further adjustment of tension can be accomplished simply by removing and shortening or lengthening as need be. **G,** Proximal anastomosis. After appropriate tension is selected, anastomosis is completed. **H,** Proximal anastomosis. Technique when graft is anastomosed to common profundus tendon (see text). (Redrawn from Hunter JM and Salisbury RE: J Bone Joint Surg 53-A:829, 1971.)

cause of living a long distance from the physician's office or because of noncompliance, a safer routine would involve splinting of the hand without the rubberband traction for approximately 3 weeks following surgery and commencement of finger mobilization after that time. At about 3 weeks an active and passive range-of-motion exercise routine can be commenced with blocking and more active exercises commenced at 4 weeks. Protection against hyperextension should be maintained for a total of 6 to 7 weeks following surgery, and heavy resistance should not be forced for a total of 9 to 12 weeks.

Long Flexor of Thumb

The flexor pollicis longus tendon may be repaired secondarily by direct suture at any level within the thumb if the two ends can be approximated without excessive tension. Within the first few weeks after injury, tension of the muscle from contracture may be overcome by flexing the wrist. The pulley mechanism should be avoided opposite the metacarpophalangeal joint when the tendon has been divided near this level because the suture line is likely to adhere to the pulley. This can be accomplished by tendon advancement and tendon advancement with lengthening at the wrist as described under the discussion of primary repair (p. 3027). Another alternative in difficult situations is the tendon transfer of the ring finger flexor sublimis to substitute for flexor pollicis longus function. Urbaniak recommends that this tendon transfer be reserved for patients who have lost function of the flexor pollicis longus muscle belly because of anterior interosseous nerve injury, loss of blood supply, or muscle damage. As last resorts, the thumb interphalangeal joint may be stabilized by arthrodesis (p. 3190) or tenodesis (p. 3044).

FLEXOR TENDON GRAFT

■ *TECHNIQUE.* Make an incision on the radial side of the thumb from a point near the base of the nail to near the middle of the metacarpal and then angle it toward the palm to end near the middle of the thenar eminence (Fig. 61-15, *E*). Elevate the skin and subcutaneous tissue as a flap with its base toward the palm; carefully dissect the branch of the radial nerve and its corresponding vessel, and retract them with this flap. Also, dissect the digital neurovascular bundle, which lies well toward the anterior aspect of the thumb. Identify the pulley, and open the tendon sheath and the pulley sufficiently to insert the tendon graft, but leave a segment of the pulley at least 1 cm wide intact over the metacarpophalangeal joint to prevent bowstringing of the tendon. Also leave intact the oblique pulley at the proximal and middle thirds of the proximal phalanx. Free the flexor tendon, but take care not to enter the interphalangeal joint or to damage its volar plate. Now

make a transverse incision 2.5 cm long proximal to the flexor crease of the wrist and identify the flexor pollicis longus tendon and withdraw it; if possible, tag the distal end of the tendon with a suture before withdrawing it and use this suture as a guide in threading the graft into the thumb.

Now obtain a tendon graft from an appropriate site, usually the palmaris longus or toe extensor digitorum longus tendons. Anchor the graft at the point of insertion of the original tendon as described for a flexor tendon graft of a finger (p. 3030). Use the end-weave technique to suture the proximal end of the graft to the distal end of the flexor pollicis longus tendon at a level proximal to the wrist so that the juncture will not enter the carpal tunnel or encroach on the median nerve when the thumb and wrist are extended. The graft should be under enough tension to slightly flex the interphalangeal joint of the thumb when the wrist is in the neutral position. The tension on the graft may be tested by placing one mattress suture through the end weave. With the wrist in maximum extension, full flexion of the thumb is produced. With the wrist in maximum passive flexion, full extension of the thumb should be produced. When the tension is satisfactory, the additional mattress sutures are placed to secure the juncture. As an alternative method, the proximal end of the graft may be sutured to the tendon opposite the middle of the thumb metacarpal; this requires only one incision and helps avoid potential median nerve complications.

Close the wound with No. 5-0 nylon or a similar suture without subcutaneous sutures. Apply a dorsal splint to the wrist, hand, and thumb with the wrist in 45 degrees of flexion and the interphalangeal joint of the thumb in extension.

AFTERTREATMENT. At 3 weeks the pull-out suture is removed and active motion is begun. Splint protection against hyperextension is continued for 7 to 8 weeks. At 7 weeks, active flexion can be increased to approach heavy resistance by 9 to 10 weeks.

TWO-STAGE FLEXOR TENDON GRAFT FOR FLEXOR POLLICIS LONGUS. In the unusual situation in which there is extensive disruption of the flexor pollicis longus course from the carpal tunnel distally in its passage beneath the thenar muscles to the thumb and the tendon insertion, and especially if there are associated joint contractures and pulley reconstruction is required, staged tendon grafting using the silicone rod technique (Hunter) is appropriate.

■ *TECHNIQUE (HUNTER).* The incision and approach to the thumb are similar to that described for the single-stage flexor tendon graft. After the pulley has been reconstructed and the silicone rod is placed beneath the pulley reconstruction and secured distally in a manner similar to that described for the silicone rod technique in the finger (p. 3039), suture

the distal end of the silicone rod is sutured to the stump of flexor tendon with wire and nonabsorbable sutures. Pass the rod proximally through the course of the flexor pollicis longus beneath the thenar muscles and further proximally through the carpal tunnel into the distal forearm adjacent to the flexor pollicis longus tendon. After wound closure, apply a dorsal splint to maintain the wrist in slight flexion and to provide an increased length for the sheath of the flexor pollicis longus. Passive motion is commenced, and after satisfactory wound healing and motion have been achieved, the second stage is done, usually about 2 to 3 months following the first stage. Harvest a free tendon graft of sufficient length, usually the plantaris or extensor digitorum communis from a toe. Make limited incisions in the distal attachment of the thumb and proximally at the wrist for passing the tendon graft attached to the rod. Attach the graft to the proximal end of the rod and then pull it distally through the sheath. The rod is removed and discarded, and the distal attachment is accomplished with a pull-out technique similar to a single-stage tendon graft. The proximal attachment is accomplished with an end weave (Pulvertaft) using mattress sutures, and the tension is set in a manner similar to that described in the single-stage graft technique for the flexor pollicis longus.
AFTERTREATMENT. Aftertreatment for the two-stage tendon grafting is similar to that for the single-stage grafting technique.

TRANSFER OF RING FINGER FLEXOR SUBLIMIS TO FLEXOR POLLICIS LONGUS

■ *TECHNIQUE.* Expose the flexor pollicis longus insertion through a midlateral or volar zigzag incision. Take care to avoid injury to neurovascular structures and the annular thickenings of the flexor sheath of the thumb. Open only enough of the sheath to identify the flexor pollicis longus tendon insertion and leave it attached to its insertion. Make a transverse palmar incision at the level of the proximal flexion crease of the ring finger. Acutely flex the metacarpophalangeal and proximal interphalangeal joints of the ring finger to allow harvesting the greatest length of the tendon. Transect the flexor sublimis tendon and close the palmar incision with continuous 4-0 nylon sutures. Make a longitudinal incision at the wrist to the radial side of the distal forearm. Identify the transected flexor sublimis tendon to the ring finger and deliver it into the proximal wrist incision. Identify the proximal end of the transected flexor pollicis longus tendon, either at the wrist incision or by using a palmar incision over the thenar eminence (see discussion of incisions). If the flexor pollicis longus tendon is mobile in its sheath, then the distal end of the sublimis tendon can be attached to the flexor pollicis longus and the

tendon can be delivered by applying traction to the distal end of the flexor pollicis longus tendon from its insertion. If this is the case, detach the flexor pollicis longus from its insertion, deliver the sublimis tendon distally, and attach it with a pull-out technique using the retrograde Bunnell technique or the antegrade pull-out technique. If the flexor pollicis longus cannot be moved easily in its sheath, then dissect and mobilize the tendon and excise it as required by the scarred conditions in the palm and thumb; use a 22-gauge wire loop to pass retrograde down the course of the flexor pollicis longus to deliver the sublimis tendon distally through the palm and into the thumb for its insertion. Obtain adequate hemostasis and close the wound in a routine manner using 4-0 or 5-0 monofilament nylon sutures. Apply a compressive dressing and a dorsal short arm splint that immobilizes the wrist in 25 to 30 degrees of flexion, allowing the thumb metacarpophalangeal and interphalangeal joints to be in extension or only slight flexion. Drains are usually not necessary.
AFTERTREATMENT. Any drains are removed at approximately 24 hours or when drainage has ceased. Although an early postoperative mobilization program may be undertaken, it is usually unnecessary. The sutures are removed at 10 to 14 days. The initial splint is left in place for approximately 3 weeks, and then gentle active motion is commenced. The thumb is protected with an additional removable dorsal splint for another 3 to 4 weeks and then motion exercises are increased. Forceful resistance activities are not undertaken for 10 to 12 weeks.

Flexor Tenolysis After Repair and Grafting

In addition to the complications that may occur after any surgical procedure, tendon repair and grafting may be complicated by the adherence of the tendon to the sheath and its lack of gliding and consequent loss of motion. Tenolysis should not be considered until it can be documented that the patient has not made significant progress over a period of several months while cooperating with an organized progressive therapy program. Usually at least 3 months should have passed since the initial surgical procedure, and in some situations, 4 to 6 months may be required to make an accurate assessment of the patient's progress. In addition to documenting a lack of progression in the physical therapy program and motion at the distal and proximal interphalangeal joints, the following requirements should have been met: (1) all soft tissue and skin scars should be soft, pliable, and flexible and should be healed; (2) fractures and joint injuries should have healed; (3) the passive range of motion in the digital joints should be as near normal as possible; (4) the sensibility, under ideal circumstances, should be normal or there should be demonstrable recovery of nerve function following nerve repair; and (5) the patient should be demonstrating progression with strengthening exercises and should realistically understand the expectations following such a procedure; he should also understand that at the time of the procedure, if the extent of scar and adhesion is excessive, the first stage of a two-stage flexor tendon graft procedure will be a likely option. The patient should also understand that if tenolysis is successful that there is a risk of posttenolysis tendon rupture, which may approach 10% or more. After a failed graft, Boyes and others have advocated a fresh tendon graft instead of a tenolysis.

■ *TECHNIQUE.* **Make the incision through the existing skin scar. Take care when elevating the skin flaps to avoid injury to neurovascular structures and the annular portions of the fibro-osseous sheath. Using great care, dissect the scar tissue from the tendon. At times, the tendon and fibro-osseous sheath will be indistinguishable. Similarly, the tendon will at times adhere to the phalanx, particularly in areas of healed fracture callus. Use sharp dissection and periosteal elevators to free the flexor tendon from the adherent periosteum and fibro-osseous sheath. After it has been determined that complete release of the tendon has been achieved in the digit, make an incision in the distal forearm, identify the appropriate flexor tendon, and demonstrate with traction on the proximal tendon that the finger can be moved through a nearly normal full range of motion. If the tenolysis is done with the patient under a regional or local block anesthetic, the patient can voluntarily demonstrate the amount of motion in the finger. If it can be demonstrated that the annular pulleys are not present or if the remaining pulleys are insufficient for proper finger function, pulley reconstruction should be done at the time of tenolysis. If the flexor tendon cannot be salvaged because of exten-**sive injury, a silicone rod (Hunter) should be inserted beneath any pulley reconstruction as the first stage of a two-stage flexor tendon graft reconstruction. If the flexor tendon graft has ruptured or cannot be salvaged, this would also require the insertion of a silicone rod as the first stage of a two-stage flexor tendon graft. If flexion contractures are present at the proximal and distal interphalangeal joints, these should be released by capsulotomy, usually by release of the proximal extensions of the palmar plate. Usually corticosteroids are not instilled; however, this is a practice advocated by many authorities in the field. At times, especially following comminuted fractures where irregular bony surfaces are exposed, silicone sheeting has been interposed between the tendon and the bone and removed at a later date after satisfactory motion has been established. This is rarely necessary in our experience.**

AFTERTREATMENT. **A compression dressing is applied, usually with the fingers in mild flexion. Postoperative rehabilitation is begun with active motion on the first day after surgery. Indwelling catheters for pain control with local anesthetics are rarely used, although they may be helpful in controlling immediate postoperative pain.**

Tenodesis

Tenodesis is useful when the profundus is damaged, flexor tendon grafting is impossible, and the fingertip is more useful functionally when partially flexed and stabilized than when extended; this is usually true of the index finger (Fig. 63-47) and for other fingers in certain occupations as well. The operation is possible only when the distal stump of the profundus tendon is long enough to anchor proximal to the distal interphalangeal joint.

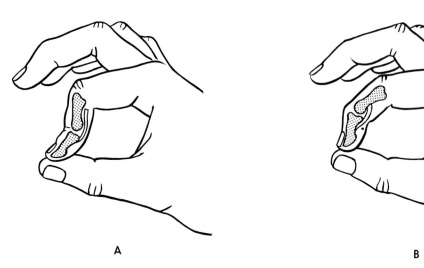

A   B

Fig. 63-47   Tenodesis for irreparable damage to profundus tendon. **A,** Before tenodesis, distal interphalangeal joint is unstable and hyperextends during pinch. **B,** After tenodesis, joint is stable and remains partially flexed during pinch.

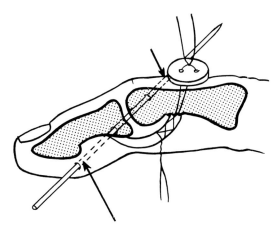

Fig. 63-48 Technique of tenodesis (see text). Kirschner wire is cut off beneath skin at points indicated by arrows.

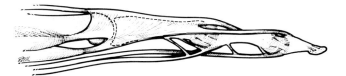

Fig. 63-49 Lateral view of entire extensor mechanism.

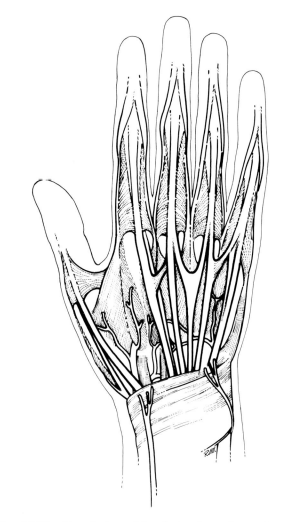

Fig. 63-50 Dorsal view of hand showing extensor tendons, accessory communicating tendons (vincular accessorium), and extensor expansions.

■ *TECHNIQUE*. Make a midlateral incision (p. 2972) and identify the stump of the tendon. Flex the distal interphalangeal joint 30 degrees and note the length of profundus tendon required for tenodesis. Insert a Bunnell pull-out wire suture in the tendon and excise any redundant tendon (Fig. 63-48). With the joint in the desired position, insert a Kirschner wire obliquely across it and cut off the wire beneath the skin. Then at the level of intended tenodesis roughen the bone of the middle phalanx with a dental chisel and drill two small holes through it from anterior to posterior. On the palmar cortex, connect the holes and make a small cortical window with a small curet. With straight needles, thread the ends of the wires through the holes leading the tendon into the cortical opening to the dorsum of the finger and tie them through a button over the middle phalanx. A pull-out technique using the Bunnell retrograde or the antegrade technique is usually required. Bring the Bunnell pull-out wire through the volar surface of the finger. Close the wound with No. 5-0 nylon. Apply a bandage. Although external splinting is usually unnecessary, a small splint is good protection from postoperative bumping and pain.

AFTERTREATMENT. The splint and sutures are removed at 10 to 14 days. The pull-out wire suture is removed at 3 weeks and the Kirschner wire at 5 or 6 weeks. Active motion of uninvolved fingers is encouraged. Heavy resistance activities are not begun for 6 to 8 weeks.

Extensor Tendons

An extensor tendon (Fig. 63-49) is presumed to be divided between the proximal and distal interphalangeal joints when active extension of the latter joint is lost; ini-

tially a gross mallet finger deformity may be absent because the surrounding capsule and other soft tissues have not yet been stretched by the strong flexor digitorum profundus. The division of the central slip of an extensor tendon between the metacarpophalangeal and proximal interphalangeal joints results in loss of extension of the latter joint only after the lateral bands prolapse anteriorly. Since the metacarpophalangeal and distal interphalangeal joints may both be actively extended, this lesion is easily overlooked during the initial examination. When the entire extensor expansion, including the lateral bands, is divided at this level, extension of the joints distal to the wound is lost; such a lesion is unlikely, however, since the expansion covers a convex surface of bone that usually blocks the injuring object before the division is complete. When the extensor tendon is divided just proximal to the metacarpophalangeal joint, the two distal finger joints can be extended by the lateral bands and their connecting transverse fibers, but extension of the metacarpophalangeal joint is incomplete. Partial or complete extension of the finger may be possible when a single extensor tendon is divided at the wrist because of the presence of accessory communicating tendons (juncturae tendinum), as shown in Fig. 63-50.

When checking the long extensor tendon of the thumb, the examiner must stabilize the metacarpophalangeal joint and must carefully test for active extension of the interphalangeal joint. Division of this tendon is often overlooked because an intact short thumb extensor can actively extend the thumb as a unit. Although the short thumb extensor will not extend the interphalangeal joint alone, the thumb intrinsic muscles assist with interphalangeal extension in some patients.

EXTENSOR TENDON REPAIR

The extensor surface of the hand may be divided into zones to conform to the different anatomic relationships of the extensor tendons and their attachments (Fig. 63-51).

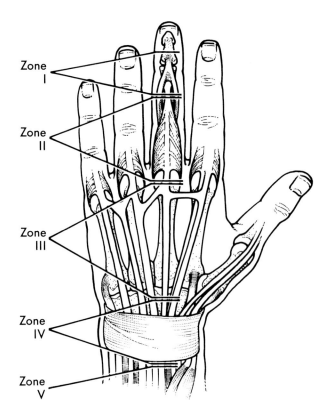

Fig. 63-51 Indications for surgery of extensor tendon lacerations vary according to level of pathologic condition; therefore various zones have been designated.

To maintain continuity of discussion and for the convenience of the reader, the acute (primary) and chronic (delayed, secondary) management of the extensor tendon injuries within each zone will be discussed together rather than separating those discussions. Similarly, extensor tendon ruptures, excluding those in rheumatoid arthritis, will be discussed within their individual zones. For additional discussion of extensor tendon ruptures, see Chapter 72.

Zone I

Zone I extends from the distal insertion of the extensor tendon to the attachment of the central slip at the proximal end of the middle phalanx. Mallet finger deformities result from an avulsion of the insertion of the tendon, sometimes including a small bone fragment, and may be treated by splinting alone (see discussion of mallet finger, below). Lateral tendons lacerated proximal to the insertion may be sutured with a very small, single-stitch suture or a roll stitch (see Fig. 63-17). An open transection of the central slip insertion at the distal phalanx is usually repaired with a roll stitch and protected with a small transarticular Kirschner wire.

EXTENSOR TENDON RUPTURE. For a closed extensor tendon rupture from its insertion into the distal phalanx, the treatment is usually nonsurgical. The distal interphalangeal joint is constantly held in hyperextension on a splint (Fig. 63-52) for 6 to 8 weeks and at night only for 1 additional week. This allows the tendon to heal, prevents stretching when the splint is removed, and usually provides a satisfactory result. The last degrees of extreme flexion of the distal joint may be lost; however, the flexion posture of the joint is usually corrected. This treatment may be successful as long as 3 months after injury

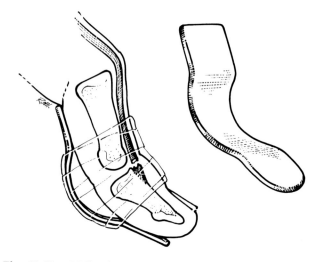

Fig. 63-52 Mallet finger uncomplicated by avulsion of large fragment of bone can be treated effectively on biconcave splint that extends distal joint alone. Plastic adhesive dressing that holds splint in place may be changed daily by patient.

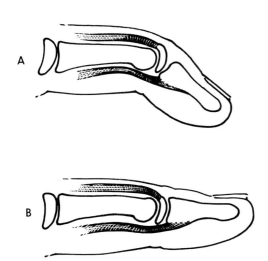

Fig. 63-53 **A,** Displacement of epiphysis of distal phalanx may cause digit to assume a mallet finger posture. **B,** Hyperextension of phalanx usually affords satisfactory reduction of displaced epiphysis.

(see discussion of treatment of chronic mallet finger below).

For a discussion of mallet finger deformities caused by fractures of the distal phalanx, see Chapter 64.

Mallet finger deformities in children may be caused by traumatic separation of the epiphysis (Fig. 63-53). These deformities can be readily recognized with radiographs. Early detection allows easy reduction with hyperextension of the distal interphalangeal joint. The finger is splinted for 3 to 4 weeks and healing is rapid when compared with the injury of the extensor tendon itself. Growth disturbance is possible but rare.

ACUTE TRANSECTION OF EXTENSOR TENDON. Treatment of an open injury of the extensor tendon insertion requires repair of the tendon. Extension of the skin laceration proximally may be required to grasp the tendon and mobilize it to its insertion where a roll suture (see Fig. 63-17) is usually sufficient to hold the insertion for healing. The repair may be protected with a transarticular Kirschner wire. The wound is closed, and the finger is temporarily splinted for comfort and to avoid additional trauma. The roll suture is removed after approximately 3 weeks, the Kirschner wire is removed at approximately 4 weeks, and the finger is splinted for an additional 4 weeks to protect the repair. Progressive motion exercises are commenced and continued until maximum function has been achieved.

CHRONIC MALLET FINGER (SECONDARY REPAIR). As late as 12 weeks after injury, a mallet finger caused by avulsion of the extensor tendon from the distal phalanx may be satisfactorily treated by splinting, as described for an acute injury (p. 3046). After 12 weeks, if

the distal phalanx droops severely but passive extension in the distal interphalangeal joint is still satisfactory, surgery may be indicated.

■ *TECHNIQUE.* Make a V-shaped incision, convex distally, with the tip 5 mm proximal to the nail base on the dorsum of the finger. Avoid injury to the germinal matrix of the nail. Develop the flap and elevate it proximally to expose the extensor tendon with its intervening scar. Attempt to identify the junction of the normal tendon with the scar, and sever the tendon transversely proximal to the joint, leaving the insertion of the tendon into bone. Resect sufficient scar or tendon to allow closure of the gap with the finger in maximum extension. To support and protect the repair, immobilize the joint with a transarticular 0.045-inch Kirschner wire. Then repair the extensor tendon with 4-0 monofilament nylon or 4-0 monofilament wire as a pull-out roll stitch (see Fig. 63-17). No additional sutures are required. Close the skin with interrupted 5-0 nylon. Maintain the finger in extension and apply a compressive dressing. Support the finger with a volar splint for postoperative comfort and to avoid reinjury in the recovery period.

AFTERTREATMENT. The sutures are removed at 10 to 14 days, and the distal joint is maintained in extension, protecting the Kirschner wire with a small metal splint for a total of 4 weeks. The Kirschner wire is removed after 4 weeks, and the repair is protected for a total of 8 weeks. Then normal activities are resumed progressively.

■ *TECHNIQUE (FOWLER).* Make a midlateral finger incision (p. 2972) from just distal to the proximal interphalangeal joint to a point level with the middle of the proximal phalanx. Open the deep tissues until the edge of the lateral band of the extensor hood is located. Then elevate this edge with a small hook (Fig. 63-54) and, with the finger in extension, continue elevating the expansion until the deep surface of the central slip is exposed at the proximal interphalangeal joint. Now elevate the entire extensor hood from the proximal phalanx. With the point of a No. 11 Bard-Parker knife blade, and beginning on the deep surface of the central slip, free the insertion of the central slip from the proximal edge of the middle phalanx. Releasing this central slip allows the entire extensor mechanism to displace proximally; thus the tension increases on the distal end and is transmitted to the avulsed tendon where the tendon has become too long after healing to the distal phalanx by scar. Close the wound with interrupted 5-0 nylon suture, apply a compressive dressing, and protect the finger with a splint for postoperative comfort.

AFTERTREATMENT. The sutures are removed at 10 to 14 days, and the splint is maintained with the proximal interphalangeal joint in no more than 30

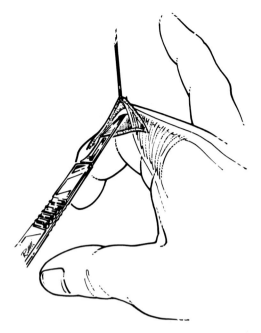

Fig. 63-54 Fowler operation to correct mallet finger (see text).

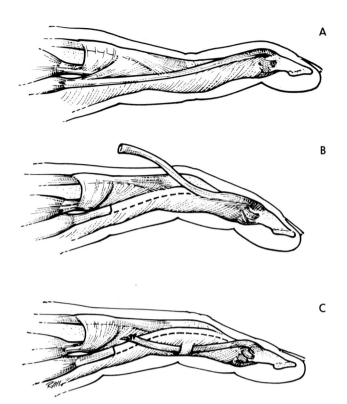

Fig. 63-55 Technique of correcting recurrent hyperextension and locking of proximal interphalangeal joint. **A,** Lateral view of extensor hood and flexor tendon sheath. **B,** One lateral band of hood has been detached proximally. **C,** Detached band has been threaded through small pulley made in flexor tendon sheath opposite proximal interphalangeal joint and has been sutured to hood under enough tension to create slight flexion contracture of joint.

degrees of flexion and the distal joint in extension. This prevention of acute flexion of the proximal interphalangeal joint will prevent the capsule of the joint from being torn following release of the central slip. The splint is removed at 3 weeks, and another splint is applied to immobilize the distal interphalangeal joint. The distal interphalangeal joint is held in extension for 4 additional weeks on a small metal splint, allowing full motion of the proximal interphalangeal and metacarpophalangeal joints.

CORRECTION OF OLD MALLET FINGER DEFORMITY BY TENDON TRANSFER OR TENDON GRAFT. The technique used for correcting hyperextension locking deformity in the proximal interphalangeal joint by transfer of a lateral band of the extensor mechanism may also be used for correction of an old mallet finger deformity when there is satisfactory passive motion and there are no more than moderate arthritic changes in the distal joint (Fig. 63-55).

Thompson, Littler, and Upton reported uniform success treating posttraumatic mallet deformities by reconstructing the oblique retinacular ligament with a palmaris tendon graft passed from the distal phalanx proximally along the path of the oblique retinacular ligament, spiraling volar to the flexor tendon sheath between the neurovascular bundle and the flexor sheath, across to the opposite side of the proximal phalanx volar to the proximal interphalangeal joint and secured to the base of the proximal phalanx through a drill hole using a pull-out technique (the spiral oblique retinacular ligament [SORL]).

■ *TECHNIQUE (MILFORD).* Make a lateral incision on the least scarred side of the digit and expose the extensor mechanism and the flexor sheath. Detach one lateral band just beyond the metacarpophalangeal joint of the finger and dissect it loose entirely to its insertion distally. Make a small pulley by opening the flexor tendon sheath with two parallel incisions opposite the proximal interphalangeal joint. Pass the lateral band tendon slip from distal to proximal through the pulley, bringing the end to be sutured to the extensor hood a bit dorsal to its original position on the lateral side of the extensor mechanism. Correct tension on this transfer is essential and will hold the proximal interphalangeal joint slightly flexed while the distal joint is fully extended. Protect this repair with a transarticular 0.045-inch Kirschner wire obliquely placed across the joint. Close the wound with interrupted 5-0 nylon suture and apply a conforming, compressing dressing, supporting the finger, hand, and wrist with a volar plaster splint over adequate padding for postoperative comfort and protection.

AFTERTREATMENT. The sutures are removed at 10 to 14 days. At approximately 3 to 4 weeks, the tran-

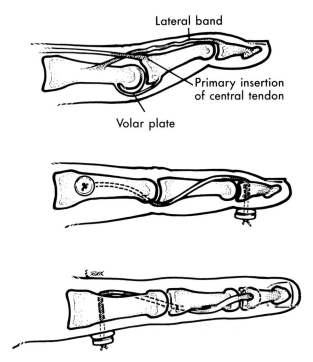

Fig. 63-56 Palmaris longus tenodesis for oblique retinacular ligament reconstruction for swan-neck deformity, called the spiral oblique retinacular ligament (SORL). Pathologic condition of swan-neck deformity involves hyperextension of PIP joint with extensor lag at distal joint, combined with laxity of volar plate, **A.** Palmaris longus can be used to provide tenodesis to correct imbalance at both joints. (See text for operative details.) (Redrawn from Thompson JS, Littler JW, and Upton J: J Hand Surg 3:482, 1978.)

sarticular Kirschner wire is removed and between exercise periods the finger is protected with a volar removable splint. The splint should be worn at night and during the day except for exercise periods. The splint may be discontinued after a total of about 8 weeks and gradual improvement in motion may progress.

■ *TECHNIQUE FOR SPIRAL OBLIQUE RETINACULAR LIGAMENT (SORL).* Make a dorsal angular incision exposing the distal phalanx and short midradial and midulnar incisions to approach the radial side of the proximal interphalangeal joint and the ulnar aspect of the proximal phalanx (Fig. 63-56). Make a vertical hole in the distal phalanx between the extensor tendon insertion and the nail germinal matrix using a small, sharp gouge. Use a hemostat for gentle blunt dissection proximally along the radial side of the middle phalanx following the lateral band, passing dorsal to Cleland's ligament to the proximal interphalangeal joint, and create a tunnel that spirals to the palmar surface between the neurovascular bundles and the volar surface of the flexor sheath, exiting through the ulnar incision at the base of the proximal phalanx. Make a transverse hole through the base of the proximal phalanx volar to the lateral

band, passing from the ulnar side to the radial side. Harvest a palmaris or plantaris tendon graft (p. 3032). Use 22-gauge or smaller stainless steel wire placed through the holes in the bone and along the tunnel that spirals from the distal phalanx along the radial side and then volar to the flexor sheath to guide the tendon graft into its appropriate position. Apply longitudinal tension to the proximal end of the graft and demonstrate that both the distal and proximal interphalangeal joints will be extended. Secure the distal bony attachment of the tendon to the distal phalanx using an antegrade pull-out wire technique over a felt-and-button gently applied to the pulp of the distal phalanx. Set the tension on the graft by adjusting it with both the proximal and the distal interphalangeal joints at neutral extension and secure the proximal free ends of the tendon graft with a button-over-felt applied to the radial side over the base of the proximal phalanx. With these attachments, passive extension of the proximal interphalangeal joint should demonstrate full passive extension of the distal interphalangeal joint with a tenodesis effect. Take care in adjusting the tension on the tendon graft to avoid excessive pull, which may cause proximal interphalangeal joint flexion and distal interphalangeal joint extension or a buttonhole posture. If necessary, transfix the proximal interphalangeal joint with a 0.045-inch Kirschner wire to protect the tenodesis. Immobilize the hand with the wrist slightly extended, the metacarpo-phalangeal joint flexed, and the proximal and distal interphalangeal joints fully extended. Apply a well-padded volar plaster splint for postoperative comfort and protection.

AFTERTREATMENT. The sutures are removed at 10 to 14 days. At about 4 weeks, any Kirschner wires are removed and the affected digit is protected with a dorsal splint holding the proximal interphalangeal joint in 20 degrees of flexion and the distal interphalangeal joint at neutral. The pull-out wires are removed at approximately 3 weeks. Active-assisted flexion exercises are begun after wire removal (approximately 4 weeks), and hyperextension is avoided beyond a position of about 20 degrees of flexion. The protective splint is gradually extended 5 to 10 degrees from 6 to 10 weeks after surgery. Stretching of the proximal interphalangeal joint beyond 5 to 10 degrees of flexion should be avoided.

Zone II

Zone II, extending from the metacarpal neck to the proximal interphalangeal joint, includes the extensor mechanism with its contoured surface encompassing the phalanx and the metacarpal head. Tendon lacerations at this level require different techniques of suture from those at other levels. Here they should be repaired with a roll stitch or some other suture technique that permits total removal of the suture later (see Fig. 63-17). Suture material and other foreign material tend to cause more inflammatory reaction over joints than over less mobile parts. No foreign material should be left permanently within this zone, especially over the metacarpophalangeal joint.

RUPTURE OR ACUTE TRANSECTION OF CENTRAL SLIP OF EXTENSOR EXPANSION (BUTTONHOLE DEFORMITY).

Rupture or laceration of the central slip of the extensor expansion at or near its insertion results in loss of active extension of the proximal interphalangeal joint and consequently persistent flexion of the joint. If left untreated, the collateral ligaments and volar plate of the proximal interphalangeal joint become contracted. The lateral bands of the extensor expansion subluxate volarward and are held there by the transverse retinacular ligaments, which also become contracted. This results in an established buttonhole deformity. The lateral bands, because they lie volar to the transverse axis of rotation of the proximal interphalangeal joint, act as flexors of the joint. The contracted oblique retinacular ligaments and the lateral bands force the distal interphalangeal joint into hyperextension, which may be increased by any attempt to passively extend the proximal interphalangeal joint.

Buttonholing also may be caused by traumatic rotation of a digit at the proximal interphalangeal joint while partially flexed. Rotation may cause a condyle of the proximal phalanx to protrude through the capsule and disrupt the triangular ligament area between the lateral band and the central tendon. This condylar herniation may cause a volar subluxation of the lateral band. A rupture of the extensor mechanism occurs, but the central tendon may not completely separate. The collateral ligament may be partially disrupted and there may be an accompanying dislocation of the proximal interphalangeal joint. After such an injury, the proximal interphalangeal joint cannot be fully extended because of hemorrhage and swelling. The joint remains in its flexed position, and the subluxated lateral band contracts, allowing the transverse retinacular ligament to also contract, securely holding the subluxated lateral band. Spinner and Choi have shown experimentally that with anterior dislocation of the proximal interphalangeal joint complete rupture of the central slip and lateral ligament may occur (Fig. 63-57).

Buttonhole deformities that are diagnosed early in closed wounds before fixed contractures occur may be treated conservatively. If the patient can demonstrate some active extension of the proximal interphalangeal joint, this suggests that an incompletely ruptured central slip may be present. The conservative treatment consists of splinting the proximal interphalangeal joint in full extension while permitting the distal interphalangeal joint to be actively flexed. Excessive pressure leading to skin necrosis over the proximal interphalangeal joint area should be avoided. Extension should be maintained around the clock for 4 to 6 weeks and continued nightly for several more weeks.

When a buttonhole deformity is traumatic and the di-

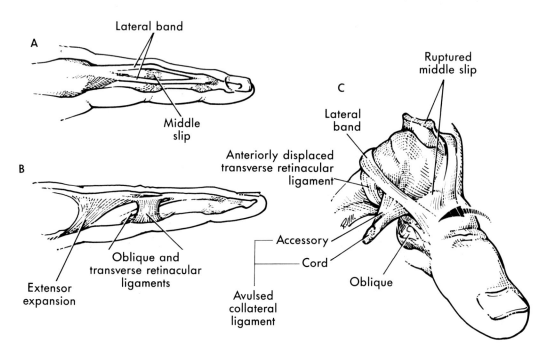

Fig. 63-57 **A,** Dorsolateral and, **B,** lateral view of extensor mechanism. **C,** Anterior dislocation of proximal interphalangeal joint with rupture of middle slip, avulsed collateral ligament, and partial tear of distal fibers of transverse retinacular ligament. Lateral band is displaced anteriorly. (Redrawn from Spinner M and Choi BY: J Bone Joint Surg 52-A:1329, 1970.)

agnosis of complete rupture, transection, or laceration of the central slip can be made, it should be exposed surgically and repaired.

■ *TECHNIQUE.* **Expose the extensor mechanism dorsally with a lazy-S or bayonet incision. Place the proximal interphalangeal joint in full extension and hold it in this position with a 0.045-inch Kirschner wire inserted obliquely across the joint. Repair the disruption of the central slip with a roll stitch of 4-0 monofilament nylon or wire. Close the wound and apply a volar splint over a gently compressing dressing.**

AFTERTREATMENT. **Remove the sutures at 10 to 14 days and the transarticular wire at 3 to 4 weeks and allow gradual protected flexion. A volar splint is worn to protect the repair for an additional 4 weeks, except for periods of exercise.**

CHRONIC BUTTONHOLE DEFORMITY (SECONDARY REPAIR AND RECONSTRUCTION). In neglected, undiagnosed, or chronic buttonhole deformity the central slip of extensor expansion has retracted and the lateral bands loosen and subluxate volarward after their dorsal transverse retaining fibers have stretched additionally. This subluxation allows the proximal interphalangeal joint to flex, the lateral bands become contracted, and a fixed flexion contracture of the proximal interphalangeal joint with hyperextension of the distal interphalangeal joint occurs. Before any surgical procedure, splinting and stretching should be done to relieve contractures of the proximal and distal interphalangeal joints. Reconstruction after rupture or laceration of the central slip of the extensor expansion is difficult and requires a precise and extensive procedure to restore the function of the damaged central slip and to release the associated contrac-

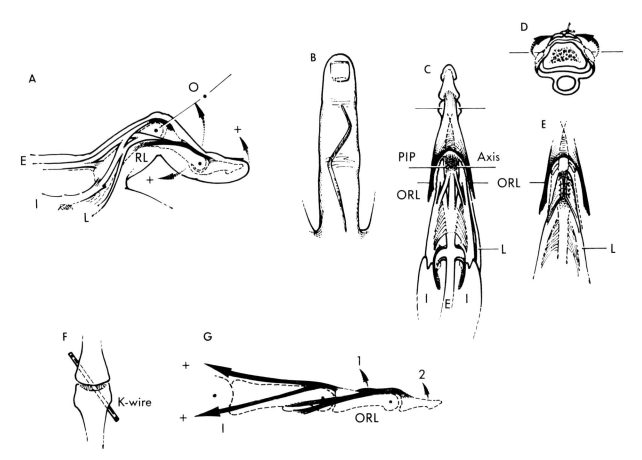

Fig. 63-58 Littler technique for repair of old buttonhole deformity. **A,** Typical deformity with flexion of proximal interphalangeal joint and extension of distal interphalangeal joint. Lateral bands have subluxated volarward. **B,** Dorsal curved longitudinal incision is made. **C,** Insertions of lateral bands are completely freed except for radialmost fibers of radial lateral band. **D** and **E,** Lateral bands are shifted dorsally and proximally and are sutured together and to soft tissues over proximal third of middle phalanx and to central tendon. **F,** Proximal interphalangeal joint is fixed in full extension by Kirschner wire. **G,** After repair, proximal interphalangeal joint is extended by extensor hood and distal interphalangeal joint by preserved lumbrical muscle and oblique retinacular ligament. (Redrawn from Littler JW and Eaton RG: J Bone Joint Surg 49-A:1267, 1967.)

THE HAND

tures. If joint contractures have developed, it is important to splint and stretch to mobilize the joints as much as possible before beginning the operative treatment.

■ *TECHNIQUE (LITTLER, MODIFIED).* Make a dorsal curved incision centered over the proximal interphalangeal joint (Fig. 63-58, *B*), exposing the lateral bands. Using the point of a probe, dissect deep to each transverse retinacular ligament from its origin near the volar plate to its insertion on the border of the lateral band. Using small scissors, divide each transverse retinacular ligament near its midportion. Free the insertions of the lateral band so that they can be replaced dorsally. On the radial side, separate with sharp dissection, leaving intact the radial fibers of the lateral band representing the contribution of the lumbrical muscles and the oblique retinacular ligament. This should preserve active extension of the distal interphalangeal joint. At this point the insertions of the lateral band should be completely free except for the radialmost fibers of the radial lateral band. Shift the bands dorsally and proximally and suture them to the soft tissue and periosteum over the proximal third of the middle phalanx (Fig. 63-58, *E*). Also, suture them to the attenuated central tendon with the proximal interphalangeal joint held in full extension. Support the repair with a transarticular 0.045-inch Kirschner wire obliquely placed across the joint. Leave the divided transverse retinacular ligaments unsutured. Close the wound with 5-0 interrupted monofilament nylon suture. Use a volar splint for immediate postoperative protection and comfort.

AFTERTREATMENT. The sutures are removed at 10 to 14 days. At 3 to 4 weeks the transarticular Kirschner wire is removed and protected motion is allowed. A volar splint is used on the finger, protecting the proximal interphalangeal joint, allowing distal interphalangeal flexion for another 4 weeks. This splint is worn during the day and night and is removed for periods of exercise three to four times daily.

Zone III

Zone III extends proximally from the metacarpal neck to the distal border of the dorsal carpal ligament. The tendons are lying free in this area without ligamentous attachment and are covered only by paratenon and fascia. Tendons may be sutured individually with a mattress suture of monofilament wire or other suture material that does not require removal since there is much less reaction to foreign materials in this area.

TRAUMATIC DISLOCATION OF EXTENSOR TENDON AT METACARPOPHALANGEAL JOINT. Traumatic dislocation of the extensor tendon toward the ulnar aspect of the metacarpophalangeal joint occurs most commonly in

the middle finger. The mechanism of dislocation is apparently a tear in the proximal portion of the shroud ligament (sagittal bands) and the more proximal fascia as the middle finger is suddenly extended against a force, as in a flicking or thumping motion. If seen within the first few days, this dislocation can be effectively treated with splinting of the metacarpophalangeal joint and wrist in extension for about 3 weeks. If the condition is undetected and has become chronic, a repair using a section of the central fibers of the extensor mechanism at the metacarpophalangeal joint may be successful.

■ *TECHNIQUE.* Make a curved incision on the radial side of the metacarpophalangeal joint to expose the joint area and the subluxating extensor tendon. Create a loop by removing a 5 cm lateral margin of the central tendon at this level, leaving the distal insertion of this segment attached. Pass the proximal segment through a small window made with vertical incisions in the capsule and through the superficial portion of the joint capsule, and suture the proximal end to the extensor tendon. Adjustment of the tension is essential to maintain the central alignment of the subluxating extensor tendon. Close the wound and apply a splint to maintain the finger in radial deviation to prevent ulnar deviation.

AFTERTREATMENT. Remove the sutures after 10 to 14 days and maintain the splint for about 3 weeks. Allow gradual improvement of motion and taping to the adjacent radial-side finger to protect the repair. Maintain protective motion for 6 to 8 weeks and allow a gradual increase in activities thereafter.

SECONDARY REPAIR OF EXTENSOR TENDONS. An extensor tendon usually can be repaired secondarily by direct suture at the level of the metacarpophalangeal joint or on the dorsum of the hand. After about 4 to 6 weeks, when the proximal segment has retracted or when a segment of tendon has been destroyed, the options for treatment include extensor indicis proprius tendon transfer to the distal segment, side-to-side suture of the distal segment to an intact adjoining extensor tendon, or segmental tendon graft. For severe injuries in which whole segments of tendon are lost, tendon grafting may be necessary. If the muscle has been damaged or denervated and has become fibrotic and scarred, transferring a suitable muscle such as the flexor carpi ulnaris or flexor carpi radialis with attachment to the distal segment will provide satisfactory function. An interposition graft may be required in such situations as well (see section on technique of tendon transfers).

Zone IV

Zone IV is the area of the wrist under the dorsal carpal ligament (extensor retinaculum). At this level the tendons have mesotenon. They are retained by the dorsal carpal ligament, which acts as a pulley, and are ensheathed in fibro-osseous canals similar to the digital flexor theca. Thus repaired tendons are likely to become stuck in their canals as they heal. Consequently primary repair of extensor tendons here may be done with a mattress or similar suture, and the sutured area should be released by excising a portion of the overlying carpal ligament. With the wrist in extension, bowstringing of the repaired tendon may occur, but it does help to avoid the adherence of the sutured tendon at this site and the loss of normal excursion. Splinting the wrist after repair in a position of moderate extension instead of full extension helps to limit the bowstring effect.

Zone V

Zone V is the zone proximal to the proximal margin of the dorsal carpal ligament. In this zone many extensor tendons are covered by their respective muscles. The tendinous portion of the musculotendinous unit may be sutured with a carefully placed stitch since sutures tend to pull out of muscle tissue. The wrist is placed in full extension postoperatively to permit maximum relaxation of the musculotendinous unit since it is quite difficult to maintain muscle-to-muscle repair by any suture technique.

AFTERTREATMENT. **Aftertreatment consists of applying a volar splint extending from just distal to the elbow to the proximal interphalangeal joints. The wrist is held in appropriate extension and the metacarpophalangeal joints in about 30 degrees of flexion with the proximal interphalangeal joints left free. This splint or some similar protection is needed for 4 to 5 weeks.**

LONG EXTENSOR OF THUMB

When an extensor pollicis longus tendon has been divided at the interphalangeal joint, its proximal segment does not retract appreciably because the adductor pollicis, abductor pollicis brevis, and extensor pollicis brevis insert into the extensor expansion; consequently the tendon can be repaired secondarily without grafting or tendon transfer. But when the tendon has been divided at the metacarpophalangeal joint or more proximally, its proximal segment retracts rapidly, and by 1 month after injury a fixed contracture of the muscle has usually developed. The contracture may often be overcome by rerouting the tendon from around Lister's tubercle and placing it in a straight line; when this maneuver does not provide enough length, the extensor indicis proprius tendon may be transferred, and in this instance only one suture line is necessary instead of the two a graft would require. When the tendon is divided at a level far enough proximal for the distal end of the palmaris longus tendon to reach the end of its distal segment, this tendon may be transferred instead of the extensor indicis proprius. A

graft is necessary to bridge a long defect when a tendon transfer is either impossible or undesirable. If a graft is selected, it should be rerouted from around Lister's tubercle to avoid adhesion and abrasion of the graft.

A splint is applied with the wrist in near full extension and the thumb extended and abducted. The splint should begin distal to the elbow but extend to the thumb tip and to the distal palmar crease. This immobilizes the thumb but releases the movement of the fingers. The splint should be maintained for 4 weeks and then the thumb is gradually permitted to move with the wrist splinted in extension for another week.

REFERENCES

Almquist EE: Nerve repair by laser, Orthop Clin North Am 19:210, 1988.
Amadio PC and Cooney WP: Current concepts of flexor tendon repair, Adv Orthop Surg 10:207, 1987.
Amis AA and Jones MM: The interior of the flexor tendon sheath of the finger: the functional significance of its structure, J Bone Joint Surg 70:583, 1988.
Araico J and Ortiz JM: Subcutaneous flexor pollicis longus tendon graft technique, Plast Reconstr Surg 45:578, 1970.
Araki S, Ohtani T, and Tanaka T: Acute dislocation of the extensor digitorum communis tendon at the metacarpophalangeal joint, J Bone Joint Surg 69:616, 1987.
Archibald SJ and Fisher TR: Micro-surgical fascicular nerve repair: a morphological study of the endoneurial bulge, J Hand Surg 12:5, 1987.
Arons MS: Purposeful delay of the primary repair of cut flexor tendons in "some-man's land" in children, Plast Reconstr Surg 53:638, 1974.
Aulicino PL, Ainsworth SR, and Parker M: The independent long extensor tendon of the fifth toe as a course of tendon grafts for the hand, J Hand Surg 14:236, 1989.
Badalamente MA, Hurst LC, Paul SB, and Stracher A: Enhancement of neuromuscular recovery after nerve repair in primates, J Hand Surg 12:211, 1987.
Bader K and Curtin JW: Clinical survey of silicone underlays and pulleys in tendon surgery in hands, Plast Reconstr Surg 47:576, 1971.
Becker H, Orak F, and Deponselle E: Early active motion following a beveled technique of flexor tendon repair: report on fifty cases, J Hand Surg 4:454, 1979.
Bell JL, Mason ML, et al: Injuries to flexor tendons of the hand in children, J Bone Joint Surg 40-A:1220, 1958.
Bennett JB: Flexor tendon laceration in Ehler-Danlos syndrome: a case report, J Bone Joint Surg 59-A:259, 1977.
Bergfield TG and Aulicino PL: Variation of the deep motor branch of the ulnar nerve at the wrist, J Hand Surg 13:368, 1988.
Bluestone L: Pin fixation technique in tendon repair, Surgery 60:506, 1966.
Bolesta MJ, Garrett WE, Ribbeck BM, et al: Immediate and delayed neurorrhaphy in a rabbit model: a functional, histologic, and biochemical comparison, J Hand Surg 13:352, 1988.
Bonnel F, Goucher G, and Saint-Andre JM: Histologic structure of the palmar digital nerves of the hand and its application to nerve grafting, J Hand Surg 14:874, 1989.
Boorman JG and Sykes PJ: Vascularised versus conventional nerve grafting: a case report, J Hand Surg 12:218, 1987.
Bora FW Jr: Profundus tendon grafting with unimpaired sublimis function in children, Clin Orthop 71:118, 1970.
Bora FW, Bednar JM, Osterman AL, et al: Prosthetic nerve grafts: a resorbable tube as an alternative to autogenous nerve grafting, J Hand Surg 12:685, 1987.

Bora FW, Osterman AL, Thomas VJ, et al: The treatment of ruptures of multiple extensor tendons at wrist level by a free tendon graft in the rheumatoid patient, J Hand Surg 12:1038, 1987.

Bourne MH, Wood MD, and Carmichael SW: Locating the lateral antebrachial cutaneous nerve, J Hand Surg 12:697, 1987.

Bowers WH, Carlson EC, Wenner SM, and Doyle JR: Nerve suture and grafting, Hand Clin 5:445, 1989.

Bowers WH and Hurst LC: Chronic mallet finger: the use of Fowler's central slip release, J Hand Surg 3:373, 1978.

Boyes JH: Flexor-tendon grafts in the fingers and thumb: an evaluation of end results, J Bone Joint Surg 32-A:489, 1950.

Boyes JH: Evaluation of results of digital flexor tendon grafts, Am J Surg 89:1116, 1955.

Boyes JH: Why tendon repair? J Bone Joint Surg 41-A:577, 1959 (editorial).

Boyes JH and Stark HH: Flexor-tendon grafts in the fingers and thumb: a study of factors influencing results in 1000 cases, J Bone Joint Surg 53-A:1332, 1971.

Boyes JH, Wilson JN, and Smith JW: Flexor-tendon ruptures in the forearm and hand, J Bone Joint Surg 42-A:637, 1960.

Brand PW: Evaluation of the hand and its function, Orthop Clin North Am 4:1127, 1973.

Brand PW, Beach RB, and Thompson DE: Relative tension and potential excursion of muscles in the forearm and hand, J Hand Surg 6:209, 1981.

Braun RM: Palmaris longus tendon transfer for augmentation of the thenar musculature in low median palsy, J Hand Surg 3:488, 1978.

Breidenbach WC: Vascularized nerve grafts: a practical approach, Orthop Clin North Am 19:81, 1988.

Broder H: Rupture of flexor tendons, associated with a malunited Colles' fracture, J Bone Joint Surg 36-A:404, 1954.

Browne EZ and Ribik CA: Early dynamic splinting for extensor tendon injuries, J Hand Surg 14:72, 1989.

Browne EZ Jr, Teague MA, and Synder CC: Prevention of extensor lag after indicis proprius tendon transfer, J Hand Surg 4:168, 1979.

Brunelli G and Brunelli F: Conventional tendon grafts: result. In Hunter JM, Schneider LH, and Mackin E, editors: Tendon surgery in the hand, St Louis, 1987, Mosby–Year Book, Inc.

Brunelli G, Vigasio A, and Brunelli F: Slip-knot flexor tendon suture in zone II allowing immediate mobilization, Hand 15:352, 1983.

Bruner JM: Surgical exposure of the flexor pollicis longus tendon, Hand 7:241, 1975.

Bunnell S: Repair of tendons in the finger and description of two new instruments, Surg Gynecol Obstet 26:103, 1918.

Bunnell S: The early treatment of hand injuries, J Bone Joint Surg 33-A:807, 1951.

Buscemi MJ and Page BJ: Flexor digitorum profundus avulsions with associated distal phalanx fractures, Am J Sports Med 15:366, 1987.

Cannon NM and Strickland JW: Therapy following flexor tendon surgery, Hand Clin 1:147, 1985.

Carter SJ and Mersheimer WL: Deferred primary tendon repair: results in 27 cases, Ann Surg 164:913, 1966.

Casscells SW and Strange TB: Intramedullary wire fixation of mallet-finger, J Bone Joint Surg 39-A:521, 1957.

Chacha P: Free autologous composite tendon grafts for division of both flexor tendons within the digital theca of the hand, J Bone Joint Surg 56-A, 960, 1974.

Chow JA, Dovelle S, Thomas LJ, et al: A comparison of results of extensor tendon repair followed by early controlled mobilisation versus static immobilisation, J Hand Surg 14:18, 1989.

Chow JA, Thomes LJ, Dovelle S, et al: Controlled motion rehabilitation after flexor tendon repair and grafting, J Bone Joint Surg 70:591, 1988.

Chow JA, Thomes LJ, Dovelle S, et al: A combined regimen of controlled motion following flexor tendon repair in "no man's land," Plast Reconstr Surg 79:447, 1987.

Christophe K: Rupture of the extensor pollicis longus tendon following Colles' fracture, J Bone Joint Surg 35-A:1003, 1953.

Chuinard RG, Dabezies EJ, and Mathews RE: Two-stage superficialis tendon reconstruction in severely damaged fingers, J Hand Surg 5:135, 1980.

Chuinard RG et al: Tendon transfers for radial nerve palsy: use of superficialis tendon for digital extension, J Hand Surg 3:560, 1978.

Clark CB: A reevaluation of selective tendon repair, Orthop Rev 4:31, July 1975.

Clark CB: Primary flexor tendon repair in the fingers, Orthop Rev 5:67, May 1976.

Crosby EB and Linsheid RL: Rupture of the flexor profundus tendon of the ring finger secondary to ancient fracture of the hook of the hamate: review of the literature and report of two cases, J Bone Joint Surg 56-A:1076, 1974.

Dellon AL, Mackinnon SE, and Crosby PM: Reliability of two-point discrimination measurements, J Hand Surg 12:693, 1987.

Dobyns RC, Cooney WP, and Wood MB: The effect of partial lacerations on canine flexor tendons, Minn Med 65:27, 1982.

Doi K, Kuwata N, Sakai K, et al: A reliable technique of free vascularized sural nerve grafting and preliminary results of clinical applications, J Hand Surg 12:677, 1987.

Dolphin JA: Extensor tenotomy for chronic boutonnière deformity of the finger: report of two cases, J Bone Joint Surg 47-A:161, 1965.

Doyle JR and Blythe WF: Anatomy of the flexor tendon sheath and pulleys of the thumb, J Hand Surg 2:149, 1977.

Doyle JR and Blythe W: The finger flexor tendon sheath and pulleys: anatomy and reconstruction. In American Academy of Orthopaedic Surgeons: Symposium on tendon surgery in the hand, St Louis, 1975, Mosby–Year Book, Inc.

Duran RJ and Houser RG: Controlled passive motion following flexor tendon repair in zones 2 and 3. In American Academy of Orthopaedic Surgeons: Symposium on tendon surgery in the hand, St Louis, 1975, Mosby–Year Book, Inc.

Duran RJ, Houser RG, Coleman CR, and Postlewaite DS: A preliminary report in the use of controlled passive motion following flexor tendon repair in zones II and III, J Hand Surg 1:79, 1976.

Elliott RA Jr: Injuries to the extensor mechanism of the hand, Orthop Clin North Am 2:335, 1970.

Entin MA: Repair of extensor mechanism of the hand, Surg Clin North Am 40:275, 1960.

Entin MA: Flexor tendon repair and grafting in children, Am J Surg 109:287, 1965.

Entin MA: Philosophy of tendon repair, Orthop Clin North Am 4:859, 1973.

Erdelyi R: Reconstruction of the flexor digitorum profundus with the aid of the flexor profundus split from an adjoining finger, Plast Reconstr Surg 37:13, 1966.

Ersek RA and Denton DR: Bovine pericardium for reconstruction and prevention of adhesions in tendon repair: a case report, Contemp Orthop 14:55, 1987.

Farkas LG: Use of interposed flap of tendon sheath to prevent adhesions after the repair of a cut flexor profundus tendon: experimental study in chickens, Plast Reconstr Surg 62:404, 1978.

Farkas L and Lindsay WK: Functional return of tendon graft protected entirely by pseudosheath — experimental study, Plast Reconstr Surg 65:188, 1980.

Fetrow KO: Tenolysis in the hand and wrist: a clinical evaluation of two hundred and twenty flexor and extensor tenolyses, J Bone Joint Surg 49-A:667, 1967.

Ford JC, Smith JR, and Carter JE: Primary tendon grafting in injuries of the thumb flexor, South Med J 64:78, 1971.

Fowler SB: The management of tendon injuries, J Bone Joint Surg 41-A:579, 1959 (editorial).

Freehafer AA, Peckham H, and Keith MW: Determination of muscle-tendon unit properties during tendon transfer, J Hand Surg 4:331, 1979.

Froehlich JA, Akelman E, and Herndon JH: Extensor tendon injuries at the proximal interphalangeal joint, Hand Clin 4:25, 1988.

Furlow LT Jr: The role of tendon tissues in tendon healing, Plast Reconstr Surg 57:39, 1976.

Gaisford JC, Hanna DC, and Richardson GS: Tendon grafting: a suggested technique, Plast Reconstr Surg 38:302, 1966.

Gama C: Results of the Matev operation for correction of boutonnière deformity, Plast Reconstr Surg 64:319, 1979.

Gattuso JM, Davies AH, Glasby MA, et al: Peripheral nerve repair using muscle autografts: recovery of transmission in primates, J Bone Joint Surg 70:524, 1988.

Gelberman RH, Amiff D, Gonsalves M, et al: The influence of protected passive mobilization on the healing of flexor tendons: a biochemical and microangiographic study, Hand 13:120, 1981.

Gelberman RH and Manske PR: Factors influencing flexor tendon adhesions, Hand Clin 1:35, 1985.

Gelberman RH, Woo SL, Lothringer K, et al: Effects of early intermittent mobilization on healing canine flexor tendons, J Hand Surg 7:170, 1982.

Goldner JL: Deformities of the hand incidental to pathological changes of the extensor and intrinsic muscle mechanisms, J Bone Joint Surg 35-A:115, 1953.

Goldner JL and Coonrad RW: Tendon grafting of the flexor profundus in the presence of a completely or partially intact flexor sublimis, J Bone Joint Surg 51-A:527, 1969.

Green WL and Niebauer JJ: Results of primary and secondary flexor-tendon repairs in no man's land, J Bone Joint Surg 56-A:1216, 1974.

Greenberg BM, Cuadros CL, Panda M, and May JW: St. Clair Strange procedure: indications, technique, and long-term evaluation, J Hand Surg 13:928, 1988.

Grundberg AB and Regan DS: Central slip tenotomy for chronic mallet finger deformity, J Hand Surg 12:545, 1987.

Grykman GK and Cally D: Interfascicular nerve grafting, Orthop Clin North Am 19:71, 1988.

Hall TD and Alves AB: Treatment of mallet finger by complete metacarpophalangeal flexion, Surg Gynecol Obstet 106:233, 1958.

Hallberg D and Lindholm A: Subcutaneous rupture of the extensor tendon of the distal phalanx of the finger: "mallet finger": brief review of the literature and report on 127 cases treated conservatively, Acta Chir Scand 119:260, 1960.

Hamas RS, Horrell ED, and Pierrett GP: Treatment of mallet finger due to intra-articular fracture of the distal phalanx, J Hand Surg 3:361, 1978.

Hamlin C and Littler JW: Restoration of the extensor pollicis longus tendon by an intercalated graft, J Bone Joint Surg 59-A:412, 1977.

Hamlin C and Littler JW: Restoration of power pinch, J Hand Surg 5:396-401, 1980.

Harmer TW: Tendon surgery, Surg Clin North Am 1:809, 1921.

Harris C Jr and Rutledge GL Jr: The functional anatomy of the extensor mechanism of the finger, J Bone Joint Surg 54-A:713, 1972.

Harvey FJ and Harvey PM: Three rare causes of extensor tendon rupture, J Hand Surg 14:957, 1989.

Hauge MF: The results of tendon suture of the hand: a review of 500 patients, Acta Orthop Scand 24:258, 1954-1955.

Henry SL and Breidenbach WC: Management of peripheral nerve injuries of the hand, Techn Orthop 1:84, 1986.

Herzog KH: Treatment of extensor tendons of the fingers (Zur Versorgung der Fingerstrecksehnenverletzungen), Arch Klin Chir 293:225, 1960. (Abstracted by Mulier JC: Int Abstr Surg 111:183, 1960.)

Hillman FE: New technique for treatment of mallet fingers and fractures of distal phalanx. JAMA 161:1135, 1956.

Hobbs RA, Magnussen PA, and Tonkin MA: Palmar cutaneous branch of the median nerve, J Hand Surg 15;38, 1990.

Hoffman S, Simon BE, and Nachamie B: Unusual flexor tendon ruptures in the hand, Arch Surg 96:259, 1968.

Holm CL and Embick RP: Anatomical considerations in the primary treatment of tendon injuries of the hand, J Bone Joint Surg 41-A:599, 1959.

Honnor R: The late management of the isolated lesion of the flexor digitorum profundus tendon, Hand 7:171, 1975.

Honnor R and Meares A: A review of 100 flexor tendon reconstructions with prosthesis, Hand 9:226, 1977.

Hunter J: Artificial tendons: early development and application, Am J Surg 109:325, 1965.

Hunter JM: Tendon salvage and the active tendon implant: a perspective, Hand Clin 1:181, 1985.

Hunter JM and Salisbury RE: Use of gliding artificial implants to produce tendon sheaths: techniques and results in children, Plast Reconstr Surg 45:564, 1970.

Hunter JM and Salisbury RE: Flexor-tendon reconstruction in severely damaged hands: a two-stage procedure using a silicone-Dacron reinforced gliding prosthesis prior to tendon grafting, J Bone Joint Surg 53-A:829, 1971.

Hunter JM, Schneider LH, and Mackin EJ, editors: Tendon surgery in the hand, St Louis, 1987, Mosby–Year Book, Inc.

Hunter JM et al: The pulley system, Orthop Trans 4:4, 1980.

Idler RS: Anatomy and biomechanics of the digital flexor tendons, Hand Clin 1:3, 1985.

Jabaley ME, Lister GD, Manske PR, et al: Flexor tendon repair, Contemp Orthop 20:421, 1990.

Jaffe S and Weckesser E: Profundus tendon grafting with the sublimis intact: an end-result study of thirty patients, J Bone Joint Surg 49-A:1298, 1967.

Jones NF and Peterson J: Epidemiologic study of the mallet finger deformity, J Hand Surg 13:334, 1988.

Kahn S: A dynamic tenodesis of the distal interphalangeal joint for use after severance of the profundus alone, Plast Reconstr Surg 51:536, 1973.

Kain CC, Russell JE, Rouse AM, and Manske PR: Regional differences in matrix formation in the healing flexor tendon, Clin Orthop 229:308, 1988.

Kaplan EB: Anatomy injuries and treatment of the extensor apparatus of the hand and the digits, Clin Orthop 13:24, 1959.

Kelly AP Jr: Primary tendon repairs: a study of 789 consecutive tendon severances, J Bone Joint Surg 41-A:581, 1959.

Kerr CD and Burczak JR: Dynamic traction after extensor tendon repair in zones 6, 7, and 8: a retrospective study, J Hand Surg 14:21, 1989.

Kessler I: The "grasping" technique for tendon repair, Hand 5:253, 1973.

Ketchum LD: Primary tendon healing: a review, J Hand Surg 2:428, 1977.

Ketchum LD: Suture materials and suture techniques used in tendon repair, Hand Clin 1:43, 1985.

Ketchum LD, Martin NL, and Kappel DA: Experimental evaluation of factors affecting the strength of tendon repairs, Plast Reconstr Surg 59:708, 1977.

Ketchum LD et al: The determination of moments for extension of the wrist generated by muscles of the forearm, J Hand Surg 3:205, 1978.

Kettelkamp DB, Flatt AE, and Moulds R: Traumatic dislocation of the long-finger extensor tendon: a clinical, anatomical, and biomechanical study, J Bone Joint Surg 53-A:229, 1971.

Kilgore ES Jr et al: Atraumatic flexor tendon retrieval, Am J Surg 122:430, 1971.

Kilgore ES Jr et al: Correction of ulnar subluxation of the extensor communis, Hand 7:272, 1975.

Kilgore ES Jr et al: The extensor plus finger, Hand 7:159, 1975.

Kleinert HE: Should an incompletely severed tendon be sutured? The voice of polite dissent, Plast Reconstr Surg 57:236, 1976.

Kleinert HE and Bennett JB: Digital pulley reconstruction employing the always present rim of the previous pulley, J Hand Surg 3:297, 1978.

Kleinert H, Kutz J, Asbell S, and Martinez E: Primary repair of lacerated flexor tendons in no-man's land, J Bone Joint Surg 49A:577, 1967.

Kleinert HE, Kutz JE, Atasoy E, and Stormo A: Primary repair of flexor tendons, Orthop Clin North Am 4:865, 1973.

Kleinert HE, Kutz JE, and Cohen MJ: Primary repair zone 2 flexor tendon lacerations. In American Academy of Orthopaedic Surgeons: Symposium of tendon surgery in the hand, St. Louis, 1975, Mosby–Year Book, Inc.

Kleinert HE and Meares A: In quest of the solution to severed flexor tendons, Clin Orthop 104:23, 1974.

Kurosawa H and Ogino T: Rupture of the extensor pollicis longus tendon after fracture of the distal end of the radius: a report of the youngest case, Ital J Orthop Traumatol 13:517, 1987.

Kutz JE: Controlled mobilization of acute flexor tendon injuries: Louisville technique. In Hunter JM, Schneider LH, and Mackin EJ, editors: Tendon surgery in the hand, St Louis, 1987, Mosby–Year Book, Inc.

Lane CS: Reconstruction of the unstable proximal interphalangeal joint: the double superficialis tenodesis, J Hand Surg 3:368, 1978.

Leddy JP: Flexor tendons — acute injuries. In Green DP, editor: Operative hand surgery, New York, 1982, Churchill Livingstone.

Leddy JP: Avulsions of the flexor digitorum profundus, Hand Clin 1:77, 1985.

Leddy JP and Packer JW: Avulsion of the profundus tendon insertion in athletes, J Hand Surg 2:66, 1977.

Leffert RD and Meister M: Patterns of neuromuscular activity following tendon transfer in the upper limb: a preliminary study, J Hand Surg 1:181, 1976.

Lindsay WK and McDougall EP: Direct digital flexor tendon repair, Plast Reconstr Surg 26:613, 1960.

Lister GD: Reconstruction of pulleys employing extensor retinaculum, J Hand Surg 4:461, 1979.

Lister G: Indications and techniques for repair of the flexor tendon sheath, Hand Clin 1:85, 1985.

Lister G: Pitfalls and complications of flexor tendon surgery, Hand Clin 1:133, 1985.

Lister GD et al: Primary flexor tendon repair followed by immediate controlled mobilization, J Hand Surg 2:441, 1977.

Littler JW: Principles of reconstructive surgery of the hand, Am J Surg 92:88, 1956.

Littler JW: The severed flexor tendon, Surg Clin North Am 39:435, 1959.

Littler JW: Basic principles of reconstructive surgery of the hand, Surg Clin North Am 40:383, 1960.

Littler JW and Eaton RG: Redistribution of forces in the correction of the boutonnière deformity, J Bone Joint Surg 49-A:1267, 1967.

Lucas GL: Fowler central slip tenotomy for old mallet deformity, Plast Reconstr Surg 80:92, 1987.

Lundborg G: Nerve regeneration and repair: a review, Acta Orthop Scand 58:145, 1987.

Lundborg G: Intraneural microcirculation, Orthop Clin North Am 19:1, 1988.

Lundborg G and Rank F: Experimental intrinsic healing of flexor tendons based upon synovial fluid nutrition, J Hand Surg 3:21, 1978.

Lundborg G et al: Superficial repair of severed flexor tendons in synovial environment: an experimental, ultrastructural study on cellular mechanisms, J Hand Surg 5:451, 1980.

Mackinnon SE and Dellon AL: A comparison of nerve regeneration across a sural nerve graft and a vascularized pseudosheath, J Hand Surg 13:935, 1988.

Mackinnon SE and Dellon AL: Evaluation of microsurgical internal neurolysis in a primate median nerve model of chronic nerve compression, J Hand Surg 13:345, 1988.

Madsen E: Delayed primary suture of flexor tendons cut in the digital sheath, J Bone Joint Surg 52-B:264, 1970.

Mahoney J, Farkas LG, and Lindsay WK: Silastic rod pseudosheaths and tendon graft healing, Plast Reconstr Surg 66:746, 1980.

Mangus DJ et al: Tendon repairs with nylon and a modified pullout technique, Plast Reconstr Surg 48:32, 1971.

Manktelow RT and McKee NH: Free muscle transplantation to provide active finger flexion, J Hand Surg 3:416, 1978.

Manske PR: The flexor tendon, Orthopedics 10:1733, 1987.

Manske PR, Bridwell K, and Lesker PA: Nutrient pathways to flexor tendons of chickens using tritiated proline, J Hand Surg 3:352, 1978.

Manske PR, Gelberman RH, and Lesker PA: Flexor tendon healing, Hand Clin 1:25, 1985.

Manske PR and Lesker PA: Flexor tendon nutrition, Hand Clin 1:13, 1985.

Manske PR, Lesker, PA, and Bridwell K: Experimental studies in chickens on the initial nutrition of tendon grafts, J Hand Surg 4:565, 1979.

Manske PR, McCarroll HR Jr, and Hale R: Biceps tendon rerouting and percutaneous osteoclasis in the treatment of supination deformity in obstetrical palsy, J Hand Surg 5:153, 1980.

Manske PR, Whiteside LA, and Lesker PA: Nutrient pathways to flexor tendons using hydrogen washout technique, J Hand Surg 3:32, 1978.

Marsh D and Barton N: Does the use of the operating microscope improve the results of peripheral nerve suture? J Bone Joint Surg 69:625, 1987.

Marshall KA, Wolfort FG, and Edlich RF: Immediate insertion of silicone rubber rods in fingers with cut flexor tendons, Plast Reconstr Surg 61:77, 1978.

Mason ML: Primary versus secondary tendon repair, Q Bull Northwestern Univ Med School 31:120, 1957.

Mason ML: Primary tendon repair, J Bone Joint Surg 41-A:575, 1959 (editorial).

Matev I, Karancheva S, Trichkova P, et al: Delayed primary suture of flexor tendons cut in the digital theca, Hand 12:158, 1980.

McClinton MA, Curtis RM, and Wilgis EFS: One hundred tendon grafts for isolated flexor digitorum profundus injuries, J Hand Surg 7:224, 1982.

McCormack RM, Demuth RJ, and Kindling PH: Flexor-tendon grafts in the less-than-optimum situation, J Bone Joint Surg 44-A:1360, 1962.

McDowell CL and Synder DM: Tendon healing: an experimental model in the dog, J Hand Surg 2:122, 1977.

McKenzie AR: Function after reconstruction of severed long flexor tendons of the hand: a review of 297 tendons, J Bone Joint Surg 49-B:424, 1967.

McNamara MJ, Garrett WE, Seaber AV, and Goldner JL: Neurorrhaphy, nerve grafting, and neurotization: a functional comparison of nerve reconstruction techniques, J Hand Surg 12:354, 1987.

Mendelaar HM: Posttraumatic ruptures of the tendon of the musculus extensor pollicis longus, Arch Chir Neerl 12:146, 1960. (Abstracted by Burnham PJ: Int Abstr Surg 111:490, 1960).

Miller H: Acute open flexor tendon injuries of the hand, Clin Orthop 13:135, 1959.

Miller RC: Flexor tendon repair over the proximal phalanx, Am J Surg 122:319, 1971.

Minami A, Ogino T, and Hamada M: Rupture of extensor tendons associated with a palmar perilunar dislocation, J Hand Surg 14:843, 1989.

Murray G: A method of tendon repair, Am J Surg 99:334, 1960.

Narakas A: The use of fibrin glue in repair of peripheral nerves, Orthop Clin North Am 19:187, 1988.

Neviaser RJ and Wilson JN: Interposition of the extensor tendon resulting in persistent subluxation of the proximal interphalangeal joint of the finger, Clin Orthop 83:118, 1972.

Neviaser RJ, Wilson JN, and Gardner MM: Abductor pollicis longus transfer for replacement of first dorsal interosseous, J Hand Surg 5:53, 1980.

Newman ED, Harrington TM, Torrett D, and Bush DC: Suppurative extensor tenosynovitis caused by *Staphylococcus aureus*, J Hand Surg 14:849, 1989.

Nichols HM: Repair of extensor-tendon insertions in the fingers, J Bone Joint Surg 33-A:836, 1951.

Norris RW, Glasby MA, Gattuso JM, and Bowden REM: Peripheral nerve repair in humans using muscle autografts: a new technique, J Bone Joint Surg 70:530, 1988.

North ER and Littler JW: Transferring the flexor superficialis tendon: technical considerations in the prevention of proximal interphalangeal joint disability, J Hand Surg 5:498, 1980.

Nunley JA, Ugino MR, Goldner RD, et al: Use of the anterior branch of the medial antebrachial cutaneous nerve as a graft for the repair of defects of the digital nerve, J Bone Joint Surg 71:563, 1989.

Ortiguela ME, Wood MB, and Cahill DR: Anatomy of the sural nerve complex, J Hand Surg 12:1119, 1987.

Parkas LG et al: An experimental study of the changes following Silastic rod preparation of a new tendon sheath and subsequent tendon grafting, J Bone Joint Surg 55-A:1149, 1973.

Parkes A: The "lumbrical plus" finger, J Bone Joint Surg 53-B:236, 1971.

Peacock EE Jr: Some technical aspects and results of flexor tendon repair, Surgery 58:330, 1965.

Peacock EE Jr and Madden JW: Human composite flexor tendon allografts, Ann Surg 166:624, 1967.

Peacock EE Jr et al: Postoperative recovery of flexor-tendon function, Am J Surg 122:686, 1971.

Pennington DG: The locking loop tendon suture, Plast Reconstr Surg 63:648, 1979.

Peterson GW and Will AD: Newer electrodiagnostic techniques in peripheral nerve injuries, Orthop Clin North Am 19:13, 1988.

Posch JL: Primary tenorrhaphies and tendon grafting procedures in hand injuries, Arch Surg 73:609, 1956.

Posch JL, Walker PJ, and Miller H: Treatment of ruptured tendons of the hand and wrist, Am J Surg 91:669, 1956.

Potenza AD: Flexor tendon injuries, Orthop Clin North Am 2:355, 1970.

Potenza AD and Melone C: Evaluation of freeze-dried flexor tendon grafts in the dog, J Hand Surg 3:157, 1978.

Pratt DR: Internal splint for closed and open treatment of injuries of the extensor tendon at the distal joint of the finger, J Bone Joint Surg 34-A:785, 1952.

Pratt DR, Bunnell S, and Howard LD Jr: Mallet finger: classification and methods of treatment, Am J Surg 93:573, 1957.

Przystawski N, McGarry JJ, Stern MB, and Edelman RD: Intratendinous ganglionic cyst, J Foot Surg 28:244, 1989.

Pulvertaft RG: Tendon grafts for flexor tendon injuries in the fingers and thumb: a study of technique and results, J Bone Joint Surg 38-B:175, 1956.

Pulvertaft RG: The treatment of profundus division by free tendon graft, J Bone Joint Surg 42-A:1363, 1960.

Pulvertaft RG: Problems of flexor-tendon surgery of the hand, J Bone Joint Surg 47-A:123, 1965.

Rath S and Bhan S: Oxytocin-induced tenosynovitis and extensor digitorum tendon rupture, J Hand Surg 14:847, 1989.

Rayan GM and Mullins PT: Skin necrosis complication mallet finger splinting and vascularity of the distal interphalangeal joint overlying skin, J Hand Surg 12:548, 1987.

Revol MP and Servant JM: Classification of main tenodesis techniques used in hand surgery, Plast Reconstr Surg 79:237, 1987.

Reynolds B, Wray RC Jr, and Weeks PM: Should an incompletely severed tendon be sutured? Plast Reconstr Surg 57:36, 1976.

Riddell DM: Spontaneous rupture of the extensor pollicis longus: the results of tendon transfer, J Bone Joint Surg 45-B:506, 1963.

Risitano G, Cavallaro G, and Lentini M: Autogenous vein and nerve grafts: a comparative study of nerve regeneration in the rat, J Hand Surg 14:102, 1989.

Rix RR: Combined nerve and tendon injury in the palm, JAMA 217:480, 1971.

Robb WAT: The results of treatment of mallet finger, J Bone Joint Surg 41-B:546, 1959.

Robertson DC: The place of flexor tendon grafts in the repair of flexor tendon injuries to the hand, Clin Orthop 15:16, 1959.

Rose EH, Kowalski TA, and Norris MS: The reversed venous arterialized nerve graft in digital nerve reconstruction across scarred beds, Plast Reconstr Surg 83:593, 1989.

Sadr B and Lalehzarian M: Traumatic avulsion of the tendon of extensor carpi radialis longus, J Hand Surg 12:1035, 1987.

Schlenker JD: Infection following pulp pull-through technique of flexor tendon grafting, J Hand Surg 6:550, 1981.

Schlenker JD, Lister GD, and Kleinert HE: Three complications of untreated partial laceration of flexor tendon, J Hand Surg 6:392, 1981.

Schmitz PW and Stromberg WB Jr: Two-stage flexor tendon reconstruction in the hand, Clin Orthop 131:185, 1978.

Schneider LH: Staged flexor tendon reconstruction using the method of Hunter, Clin Orthop 171:164, 1982.

Schneider LH: Staged tendon reconstruction, Hand Clin 1:109, 1985.

Schneider LH, Hunter JM, Norris TR, and Nadeau PO: Delayed flexor tendon repair in no man's land, J Hand Surg 2:452, 1977.

Schultz RJ: Traumatic entrapment of the extensor digiti minimi proprius resulting in progressive restriction of motion of the metacarpophalangeal joint of the little finger, J Bone Joint Surg 56-A:428, 1974.

Shibata M, Tsai TM, Firrell J, and Breidenbach WC: Experimental comparison of vascularized and nonvascularized nerve grafting, J Hand Surg 13:358, 1988.

Siegel D, Gebhardt M, and Jupiter JB: Spontaneous rupture of the extensor pollicis longus tendon, J Hand Surg 12:1106, 1987.

Smith RJ: Non-ischemic contractures of the intrinsic muscles of the hand, J Bone Joint Surg 53-A:1313, 1971.

Smith RJ and Hastings H: Principles of tendon transfers to the hand, AAOS Instr Course Lect 29:129, 1980.

Snow JW: Use of a retrograde tendon flap in repairing a severed extensor in the PIP joint area, Plast Reconstr Surg 51:555, 1973.

Snow JW: A method for reconstruction of the central slip of the extensor tendon of a finger, Plast Reconstr Surg 57:455, 1976.

Snow JW and Littler JW: A non-suture distal fixation technique for tendon grafts, Plastr Reconstr Surg 47:91, 1971.

Souter WA: The problem of boutonnière deformity, Clin Orthop 104:116, 1974.

Southmayd WW, Millender LH, and Nalebuff EA: Rupture of the flexor tendons of the index finger after Colles' fracture: case report, J Bone Joint Surg 57-A:562, 1975.

Spinner M and Choi BY: Anterior dislocation of the proximal interphalangeal joints: a cause of rupture of the central slip of the extensor mechanism, J Bone Joint Surg 52-A:1329, 1970.

Sponsel KH: Urgent surgery for finger flexor tendon and nerve lacerations: with emphasis on advancement of the divided profundus tendon distal to the level of laceration, JAMA 166:1567, 1958.

Stahl S and Wolff TW: Delayed rupture of the extensor pollicis longus tendon after nonunion of a fracture of the dorsal radial tubercle, J Hand Surg 13:338, 1988.

Stark HH, Anderson DR, Zelem NP, et al: Bridge flexor tendon grafts, Clin Orthop 242:51, 1989.

Stark HH, Zemel NP, Boyes JH, and Ashworth CR: Flexor tendon graft through intact superficialis tendon, J Hand Surg 2:456, 1977.

Stern PJ: Extensor tenotomy: a technique for correction of posttraumatic distal interphalangeal joint hyperextension deformity, J Hand Surg 14:546, 1989.

Stern PJ and Kastrup JJ: Complications and prognosis of treatment of mallet finger, J Hand Surg 13:329, 1988.

Street DM and Stambaugh HD: Finger flexor tenodesis, Clin Orthop 13:155, 1959.

Strickland JW: Management of acute flexor tendon injuries, Orthop Clin North Am 14:841, 1983.

Stickland JW: Flexor tendon repair, Hand Clin 1:55, 1985.

Strickland JW: Flexor tenolysis, Hand Clin 1:121, 1985.

Strickland JW: Opinions and preferences in flexor tendon surgery, Hand Clin 1:187, 1985.

Strickland JW: Results of flexor tendon surgery in zone II, Hand Clin 1:167, 1985.

Strickland JW: Flexor tendon injuries. III. Free tendon grafts, Orthop Rev 16:56, 1987.

Strickland JW: Flexor tendon injuries. IV. Staged flexor tendon reconstruction and restoration of the flexor pulley, Orthop Rev 16:78, 1987.

Strickland JW: Flexor tendon injuries. V. Flexor tenolysis, rehabilitation and results, Orthop Rev 16:137, 1987.

Strickland JW and Glogovac SV: Digital function following flexor tendon repair in zone II: a comparison of immobilization and controlled passive motion techniques, J Hand Surg 5:537, 1980.

Suzuki K: Reconstruction of the post-traumatic boutonnière deformity, Hand 5:145, 1973.

Suzuki K et al: Free graft of fascial tube in flexor tendon repair in the digital sheath of the hand: an attempt at a composite tissue autograft, Acta Orthop Scand 47:36, 1976.

Tajima T: History, current status, and aspects of hand surgery in Japan, Clin Orthop 184:41, 1984.

Thompson JS, Little JW, and Upton J: The spiral oblique retinacular ligament (SORL), J Hand Surg 3:482, 1978.

Thompson RV: An evaluation of flexor tendon grafting, Br J Plast Surg 20:21, 1967.

Tsuge K, Ikuta Y, and Matsuishi Y: Intra-tendinous tendon suture in the hand: a new technique, Hand 7:250, 1975.

Tubiana R: Incisions and technics in tendon grafting, Am J Surg 109:339, 1965.

Tubiana R: Results and complications of flexor tendon grafting, Orthop Clin North Am 4:877, 1973.

Tupper JW, Crick JC, and Matteck LR: Fascicular nerve repaires: a comparative study of epineurial and fascicular (perineurial) techniques, Orthop Clin North Am 19:57, 1988.

Urbaniak JR: Repair of the flexor pollicis longus, Hand Clin 1:69, 1985.

Urbaniak JR: Repair of the flexor pollicis longus. In Strickland JW, editor: Hand Clin 1:69, 1985.

Urbaniak JR, Cahill JD, and Mortenson RA: Tendon suturing methods: analysis of tensile strengths. In American Academy of Orthopedic Surgeons: Symposium on tendon surgery in the hand, St Louis, 1975, Mosby–Year Book, Inc.

Urbaniak JR and Goldner JL: Laceration of the flexor pollicis longus tendon: delayed repair by advancement, free graft or direct suture: a clinical and experimental study, J Bone Joint Surg 55-A:1123, 1973.

Urbaniak JR et al: Vascularization and the gliding mechanism of free flexor-tendon grafts inserted by the silicone-rod method, J Bone Joint Surg 56-A:473, 1974.

Van't Hof A and Heiple KG: Flexor-tendon injuries of the fingers and thumb: a comparative study, J Bone Joint Surg 40-A:256, 1958.

Verdan CE: Primary repair of flexor tendons, J Bone Joint Surg 42-A:647, 1960.

Verdan CE: Practical considerations for primary and secondary repair in flexor tendon injuries, Surg Clin North Am 44:951, 1964.

Verdan CE: Primary and secondary repair of flexor and extensor tendon injuries. In Flynn JE, editor: Hand surgery, Baltimore, 1966, Williams & Wilkins.

Verdan CE: Half a century of flexor-tendon surgery: current status and changing philosophies, J Bone Joint Surg 54-A:472, 1972.

Versaci AD: Secondary tendon grafting for isolated flexor digitorum profundus injury, Plast Reconstr Surg 46:57, 1970.

Wade PJF, Wetherell RG, and Amis AA: Flexor tendon repair: significant gain in strength from the Halsted peripheral suture technique, J Hand Surg 14:232, 1989.

Wagner CJ: Delayed advancement in the repair of lacerated flexor profundus tendons, J Bone Joint Surg 40-A:1241, 1958.

Wakefield AR: Late flexor tendon grafts, Surg Clin North Am 40:399, 1960.

Wakefield AR: The management of flexor tendon injuries, Surg Clin North Am 40:267, 1960.

Warren RA, Norris SH, and Ferguson DG: Mallet finger: a trial of two splints, J Hand Surg 13:151, 1988.

Watson AB: Some remarks on the repair of flexor tendons in the hand, with particular reference to the technique of free grafting, Br J Surg 43:35, 1955.

Weckesser EC: Tendolysis within the digit using hydrocortisone locally and early postoperative motion, Am J Surg 91:682, 1956.

Weinstein SL, Sprague BL, and Flatt AE: Evaluation of the two-stage flexor-tendon reconstruction in severely damaged digits, J Bone Joint Surg 58-A:786, 1976.

Whipple RR and Unsell RS: Treatment of painful neuromas, Orthop Clin North Am 19:175, 1988.

White WL: Secondary restoration of finger flexion by digital tendon grafts: an evaluation of seventy-six cases, Am J Surg 91:662, 1956.

White WL: Tendon grafts: a consideration of their source, procurement and suitability, Surg Clin North Am 40:403, 1960.

White WL: The unique, accessible and useful plantaris tendon, Plast Reconstr Surg 25:133, 1960.

Williams SB: New dynamic concepts in the grafting of flexor tendons, Plast Reconstr Surg 36:377, 1965.

Wilson K, Moore MJ, Rayner CR, and Fenton OM: Extensor tendon repair: an animal model which allows immediate post-operative mobilisation, J Hand Surg 15:74, 1990.

Wilson RL: Flexor tendon grafting, Hand Clin 1:97, 1985.

Wilson RL, Carter MS, Holdeman VA, and Lovett WL: Flexor profundus injuries treated with delayed two-staged tendon grafting, J Hand Surg 5:74, 1980.

Winspur I, Phelps DB, and Boswick JA, Jr: Staged reconstruction of flexor tendons with a silicone rod and a "pedicled" sublimis transfer, Plast Reconstr Surg 61:756, 1978.

Wolock BS, Moore JR, and Weiland AJ: Extensor tendon repair: a reconstructive technique, Orthopedics 10:1387, 1987.

Wray RC Jr, Holtman B, and Weeks PM: Clinical treatment of partial tendon lacerations without suturing and with early motion, Plast Reconstr Surg 59:231, 1977.

Wray RC, Jabaley ME, Puckett CL, et al: Symposium: flexor tendon injuries, Contemp Orthop 15:60, 1987.

Wray RC Jr, Moucharafieh B, and Weeks PM: Experimental study of the optimal time for tenolysis, Plast Reconstr Surg 61:184, 1978.

Wray RC and Weeks PM: Experimental comparison of techniques of tendon repair, J Hand Surg 5:144, 1980.

Yoshiyasu I, Horiuchi Y, Takahashi M, et al: Extensor tendon involvement in Smith's and Galeazzi's fractures, J Hand Surg 12:535, 1987.

Young RES and Harmon JM: Repair of tendon injuries of the hand, Ann Surg 151:562, 1960.

Zimny ML and Dabezies E: Mechano-receptors in the flexor tendons of the hand, J Hand Surg 14:229, 1989.

CHAPTER 64

Fractures, Dislocations, and Ligamentous Injuries

E. JEFF JUSTIS, JR.

Although the general principles of trauma management remain the same for all regions of the body, the hand, as a specialized vital organ interacting with the environment, is especially sensitive to functional impairment. In treating fractures, for example, anatomic and especially roentgenographic perfection does not always lead to normal function. Often it is better to accept a less than anatomic position of a fracture and strive through proper splinting and early motion for good function of the hand as a whole. In general, a closed approach to the management of hand fractures and dislocations is preferred to open operation, and, when surgery is required, the least complicated procedure to accomplish the desired functional result should be chosen. With few exceptions, prolonged immobilization (beyond 3 weeks) is not indicated in treating hand injuries. Because clinical union of fractures will often precede roentgenographic evidence of union by many weeks, early motion can be encouraged when clinical stability is assured.

When an attempt is made to restore position, angulation and lack of apposition are much more obvious immediately than an error of rotation. Rotation at the fracture may become obvious only after healing when a fist can again be made; then one finger may override another or may deviate to one side (Fig. 64-1). Observing the plane of the fingernails (Fig. 64-2) at the time of fixation helps to determine rotation; passively flexing all fingers at one time also helps to verify the position after internal fixation, and incorporating one adjacent finger in the dressing may help to prevent malrotation (see also "Complications of Fractures of Long Bones," p. 3098).

The little finger has a normal tendency to overlap the ring finger. This becomes most apparent when it can only be partially flexed while the ring finger is fully flexed. This overlap is permitted by the rotation allowable at the fifth carpometacarpal joint. In fractures causing limited flexion of this finger, it is worrisome to the patient and physician until it is understood that eventually full flexion of the little finger will align it normally with the ring finger. Once full flexion of the little finger is accomplished, external rotation is not possible while further internal rotation is. Therefore at times apparent

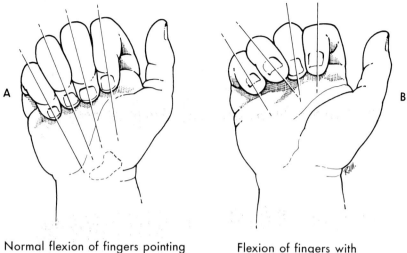

Normal flexion of fingers pointing
toward region of scaphoid

Flexion of fingers with
malrotation of ring finger

Fig. 64-1 Any malrotation of metacarpal or phalangeal fracture must be corrected. **A,** Normally all fingers point toward region of scaphoid when fist is made. **B,** Malrotation at fracture causes affected finger to deviate.

internal malrotation at the fracture may not be real (Fig. 64-3).

Exact anteroposterior and lateral roentgenograms are necessary to determine the position of the fragments before and after reduction. Even when the fracture is being reduced under direct vision, roentgenograms may prevent errors in alignment and reveal small fragments of bone not seen before reduction. When a joint cannot be completely extended, it is viewed more accurately by placing the bone segment distal to the joint parallel to the film. Cardboard cassettes are best for detail.

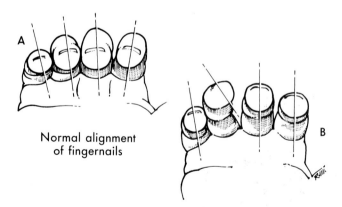

Normal alignment
of fingernails

Alignment of fingernails with
malrotation of ring finger

Fig. 64-2 Observing plane of fingernails helps to detect any malrotation at fracture; compare with opposite hand. **A,** Normal alignment of fingernails. **B,** Alignment of fingernails with malrotation of ring finger.

PRINCIPLES OF TREATMENT

For most fractures of the metacarpals and phalanges, closed manipulation, proper splinting, and protected motion will produce good functional results. There are exceptions, however, when treatment should consist of open reduction and internal fixation, or of closed manipulation and percutaneous pinning, usually with small Kirschner wires. Percutaneous pinning should be attempted before edema obliterates external landmarks. If necessary, elevate the extremity for 24 to 48 hours before reduction and pinning. Some form of fixation is most often indicated in the following instances:

1. When a displaced fracture involves a significant portion of the articular surface, exact reduction is necessary to restore smooth joint motion.
2. When a fracture is part of a major ligamentous or tendinous avulsion.
3. When a fracture is so severely displaced that interposition of tendons or other soft tissue prevents realignment by manipulation (Fig. 64-4).
4. When fractures are multiple and the hand cannot be held in the position of function without internal fixation.
5. When a fracture is open; internal fixation allows wound care after surgery without loss of reduction.

Severely comminuted closed fractures usually should not be opened since internal fixation of multiple fragments may be impossible. Limited percutaneous pinning occasionally may be indicated.

Most often dislocations are managed readily by manipulation and early function. Many are self-reduced, and protected function through "buddy taping" to an adja-

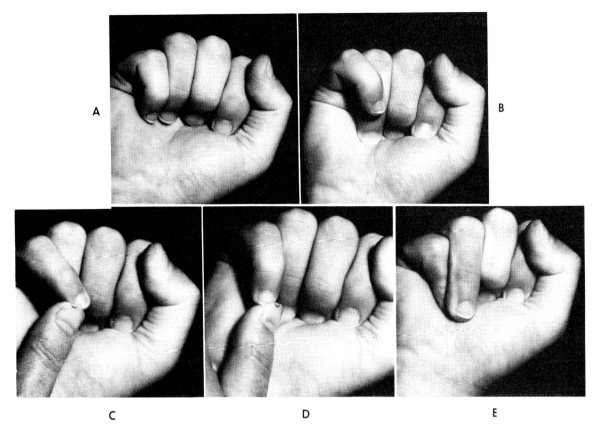

Fig. 64-3 **A**, Note normal alignment of normal little finger. **B**, Normal little finger can be made to overlap ring finger. With incomplete flexion this overlap may be perceived as rotational deformity. **C**, Rotation of little finger at carpometacarpal joint may be accentuated by passive help. **D**, From normal alignment of little finger external rotation is not possible. **E**, Incomplete flexion of ring finger may simulate rotational deformity as it tends to overlap little finger.

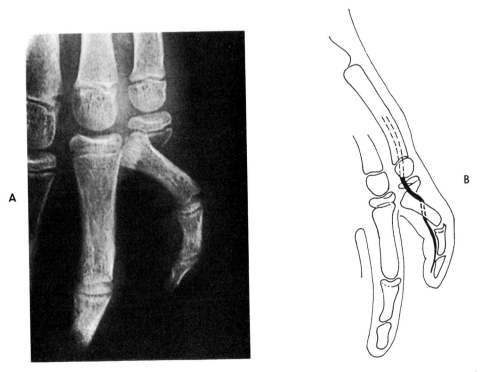

Fig. 64-4 Fracture of finger impossible to reduce by closed methods because of entrapment of tendons. **A**, Fracture of base of proximal phalanx in boy 7 years old. **B**, Flexor tendons lay on dorsum of phalangeal shaft and were trapped, making closed reduction impossible. (From von Raffler W: J Bone Joint Surg 46-B:229, 1964.)

cent finger generally will provide a good result. It is important, however, to examine carefully for associated ligamentous injury or tendon avulsion. Surgery is required most often for the following conditions:

1. Unstable dislocations of the carpometacarpal joints of the thumbs or fingers
2. Dislocations of the metacarpophalangeal joint of the thumb with complete rupture of the ulnar collateral ligament, which renders pinch weak and unstable
3. Dislocations in which a tendon is trapped, preventing manipulative reduction
4. Old, undiagnosed dislocations
5. "Buttonhole" dislocations

FRACTURES AND DISLOCATIONS WITH OPEN WOUNDS

After cleaning and examining the wound and after plans are made for its closure, fractures, if present, should be considered next. Usually fractures should be reduced and, if necessary, stabilized with small Kirschner wires to allow finger motion as soon as soft tissue healing permits; this type of fixation also permits the wound to be inspected or dressed without losing alignment of the fractures.

When the hand is severely traumatized, additional incisions are usually unnecessary to expose the fractures. The fractures should be fixed with Kirschner wires under direct vision or percutaneously to maintain the normal architectural position. In segmental defects of tubular bones, spacers made of wire bent in the shape of a U may help prevent collapse while the wound is healing. Judgment is required to determine whether the wound is sufficiently clean to permit primary closure or whether it should be only debrided and cleaned; when in doubt, do not close. Further, closure with tension on the traumatized and compromised skin edges may cause necrosis, since increased edema within the first 48 hours will create even more tension. At 48 hours the wound may be reevaluated in the operating room, and plans made at that time for closure. The target is to close the wound within the first 4 to 5 days before granulation tissues form and contractures develop. Exposed tendons without their paratenon or sheath will soon necrose without appropriate coverage (see p. 2988 for a discussion of methods of and indications for skin closure). Cultures of wound tissue are indicated, and appropriate prophylactic antibiotics should be given initially.

BASIC BONE TECHNIQUES

Many devices are available today for internal and external fixation of fractures, and considerable judgment is required to select those that provide the best opportunity for restoration of normal function. Ill-advised plating of the tubular bones of the phalanges may result in skin sloughs, tendon ruptures, or other complications. External fixators may impinge upon tendons or ligaments and interfere with function. Even with percutaneous or closed pinning, nerves may be wound around a rotating pin or tendons or ligaments may be pinned to the bone.

Rarely is more fixation needed than that afforded by Kirschner wires and external splinting, although the addition of tension band wiring techniques and 90/90 wiring of tubular bones offers the surgeon greater flexibility.

Except for the minifragment plate and screw sets and external fixator sets, little equipment is usually required in managing hand fractures. The same instruments used in handling the soft tissues are used to manipulate the bones; a straight Kocher clamp or towel clip is sufficient for a metacarpal shaft and a hemostat for smaller fragments. Because the bones of the hand are so small, dental chisels, a small rasp, and small bone cutters are useful.

Kirschner wires should be sharpened on both ends so that after being drilled in one direction they can if necessary be drilled retrograde. A small hand-held power driver or a battery-driven drill without a cumbersome air supply line is needed for accurate placement of the wire. A trocar pointed wire has been shown by Namba, Kabo, and Meals to have a greater initial holding power than either the diamond or diagonally cut wire; in addition, placement at an acute angle is easier with a trocar pointed wire. A slow insertion speed is recommended.

The wire is never allowed to project from the drill more than 5 cm to prevent bending during insertion; when more than 5 cm is needed, the first 5 cm is inserted first, and the drill is then moved on the wire. After insertion the wires should be cut off flat, and the ends should be worked well beneath the skin; end-cutting wire nippers are useful here. Kirschner wires can usually be removed in the office with the patient under local anesthesia, using a pointed extractor with grooved, corrugated, and parallel jaws. A diamond (carbide) tipped needle holder is useful in gripping and removing small Kirschner wires.

In treatment of fractures one oblique Kirschner wire is usually preferable to two wires crossed because one alone will allow some impaction at the fracture, whereas two may tend to hold the fragments apart. But sometimes a second wire is needed to control rotation. Two parallel longitudinal Kirschner wires may be used to control rotation yet avoid the distraction possible with crossed Kirschner wires.

THUMB

The integrity of the carpometacarpal joint of the thumb is far more important than that of any other joint in the function of the thumb and thus of the whole hand

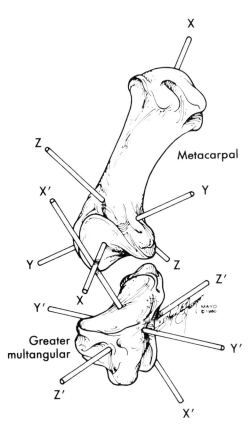

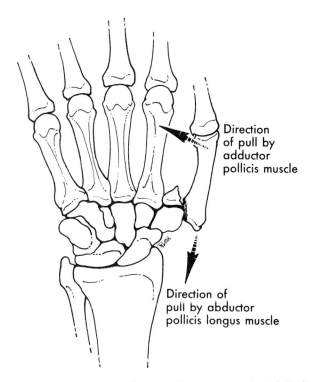

Fig. 64-6   In Bennett's fracture, first metacarpal shaft is displaced by divergent pull of muscles.

Fig. 64-5   Anatomic locations of X′, Y′, and Z′ axes of greater multangular and X, Y, and Z axes of thumb metacarpal, indicating multiple possibilities of motion between these two bones. Greater multangular is central reference for thumb metacarpal about which these movements take place. (From Cooney WP III et al: J Bone Joint Surg 63-A:1371, 1981.)

(Fig. 64-5). Unless accurately reduced, persistent dislocation or metacarpal fractures involving this joint may cause limitation of motion, pain, and weakness of pinch and of grip.

Bennett's Fracture

Edward H. Bennett, an Irish surgeon, described Bennett's fracture in 1881. It is an intraarticular fracture through the base of the first metacarpal. The shaft is laterally dislocated by the unopposed pull of the abductor pollicis longus (Fig. 64-6), but the medial projection or "hook" remains in place or slightly rotated because of its capsular attachment. Reduction by traction is easy but is difficult to maintain. Rubber band traction through a transverse pin in the proximal phalanx is not dependable: immobilization is incomplete, and verification of alignment by roentgenograms through the overlying cast is difficult. The use of a cast that maintains reduction by pressure on the base of the metacarpal is also unsatisfactory: too much pressure causes skin necrosis, and too little allows loss of reduction.

The technique of closed pinning described by Wagner

(Figs. 64-7 to 64-9) is preferred, but should reduction be unsatisfactory, open reduction is indicated.

CLOSED PINNING

■ *TECHNIQUE (WAGNER).* **Maintaining reduction of the fracture by manual traction and pressure, drill a Kirschner wire into the base of the metacarpal across the joint and into the greater multangular. Check the reduction by roentgenograms; if it is accurate, cut the wire near the skin. Then apply a forearm cast, holding the wrist in extension and the thumb in abduction; leave the distal thumb joint free.**

OPEN REDUCTION

■ *TECHNIQUE (WAGNER).* **Begin a curved incision on the dorsoradial aspect of the first metacarpal and curve it volarward at the wrist crease (Fig. 64-10). To expose the fracture, partially strip the soft tissue from the proximal end of the metacarpal shaft and incise the carpometacarpal joint. Align the articular surface of the larger fragment with that of the smaller, and under direct vision drill a wire across the joint, maintaining the reduction. If fixation by a single wire is insecure, a second wire may be added (Fig. 64-11). After closing the wound, apply a forearm cast as described previously.**

■ *TECHNIQUE (MOBERG AND GEDDA).* **Expose the joint by an incision similar to that just described or by the incision shown in Figs. 64-12 and 64-13. Pass**

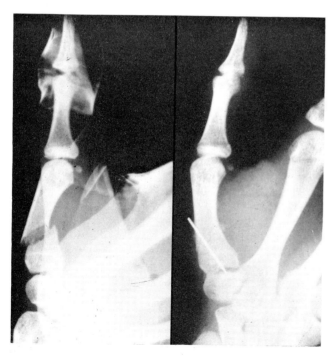

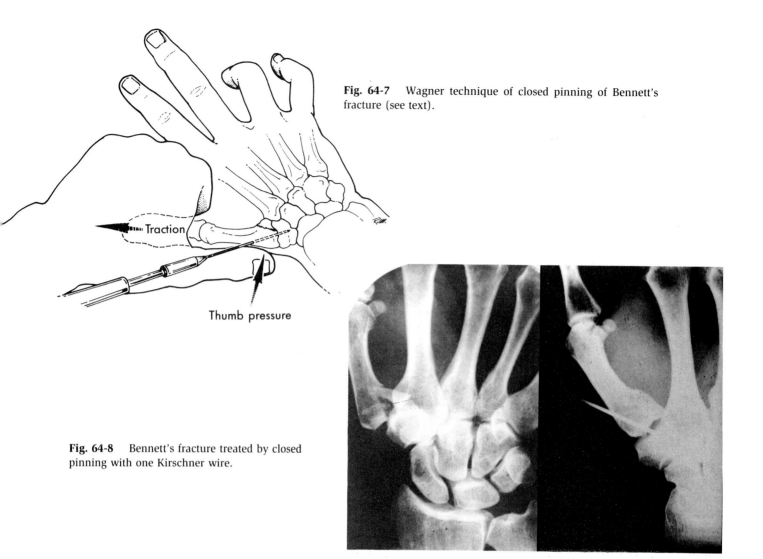

Fig. 64-7 Wagner technique of closed pinning of Bennett's fracture (see text).

Traction

Thumb pressure

Fig. 64-8 Bennett's fracture treated by closed pinning with one Kirschner wire.

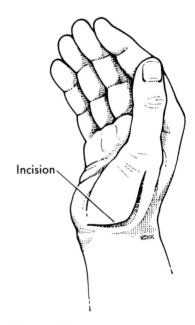

Incision

Fig. 64-9 Fracture of proximal shaft of first metacarpal treated by closed pinning as for Bennett's fracture.

Fig. 64-10 Wagner skin incision used in approaching carpometacarpal joint of thumb.

the transfixing wire through the skin of the palm into the smaller fragment until the tip of the wire is visible at the fracture. Place around the Kirschner wire tip a small loop of fine steel wire and use it to guide the fragment into accurate position. Then drill the Kirschner wire across the fracture. Remove the wire loop and complete the pinning. Close the wound and apply a cast as described previously. *AFTERTREATMENT.* The cast is removed for wound inspection at 2 to 3 weeks but is replaced and worn until 4 weeks after surgery. The wire can then be removed, but immobilization may be necessary for 2 to 4 more weeks.

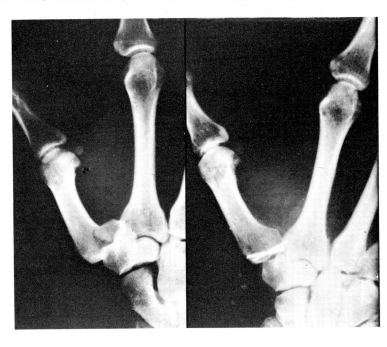

Fig. 64-11 Comminuted Bennett's fracture treated by open reduction. Two Kirschner wires were necessary to keep articular fragments reduced.

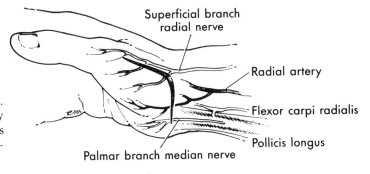

Fig. 64-12 Incision for exposure of carpometacarpal joint. Preserve branches of superficial radial nerve and radial artery and extend incision only to flexor carpi radialis tendon as shown. (From Eaton RG and Littler JW: J Bone Joint Surg 55-A:1655, 1973.)

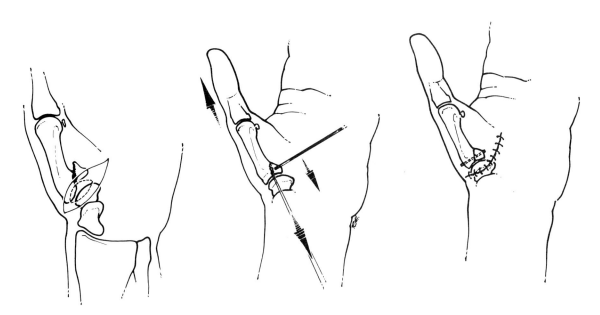

Fig. 64-13 Moberg and Gedda technique of open reduction of Bennett's fracture (see text). (From Gedda KO: Acta Chir Scand [Suppl] 193, 1954.)

Rolando's Fracture (Comminuted First Metacarpal Base) and Other Fractures Involving First Carpometacarpal Joint

Rolando in 1910 described a Y-shaped fracture involving the base of the thumb metacarpal that does not result in diaphyseal displacement as in Bennett's fracture (Fig. 64-14). Because of the likelihood of posttraumatic arthritis after these fractures or after vertical intraarticular multangular fractures, accurate reduction is important. Many may be reduced by traction and held by open or closed pinning. Some authors recommend open reduction and plate fixation with a minifragment T-plate.

OPEN REDUCTION AND INTERNAL FIXATION

■ *TECHNIQUE (FOSTER AND HASTINGS).* Make a palmar radial incision similar to the approach to a Bennett's fracture (p. 3063). Extend the radial end of the incision distally along the diaphyseal portion of the thumb metacarpal. Protect branches of the radial nerve to avoid development of a painful neuroma. Reduce the two large basilar fragments (Fig. 64-15, *A* and *B*) and provisionally fix them with a Kirschner wire (Fig. 64-15, *C*). Use a small T- or L-plate, which accepts 2.7 mm screws, on the thumb metacarpal. Place the transverse portion of the T-plate on the basilar fragments of the metacarpal (Fig. 64-15, *D*). The previously placed Kirschner wire should slide through one of the two holes in the transverse portion of the plate. If not, place a

second Kirschner wire in line with one of the two holes of the transverse portion of the plate and remove the first wire. With a 2 mm drill bit, drill through the free hole in the transverse portion of the plate and through the dorsal and palmar fragments (Fig. 64-15, *E*). Tap the hole with a 2.7 mm tap. Overdrill the hole in the dorsal fragment using a 2.7 mm drill bit for a lag screw effect. Insert a 2.7 mm cortical screw of appropriate length to compress the palmar articular fragment against the dorsal articular fragment (Fig. 64-15, *F*). Repeat the same technique with the second proximal plate hole. The exact fracture pattern may vary and require use of a lag screw separate from the plate holes or two screws placed off-center through the two proximal plate holes to compress the articular fragments together. Reduce the metacarpal to the stabilized intraarticular fragments and attach to the long portion of the T- or L-plate with 2.7 mm screws (Fig. 64-15, *G*). Close the incision appropriately and apply a soft compressive dressing and thumb spica splint.

AFTERTREATMENT. Begin active range of motion within 5 to 7 days.

• • •

Howard, on the other hand, believes the use of a combined tension band wiring technique and an external fixator to restore length will result in a serviceable articula-

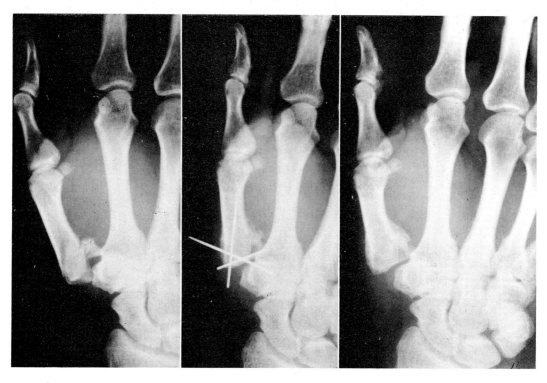

Fig. 64-14   Rolando's fracture treated by open reduction and fixation with three Kirschner wires. Early result has been excellent, but arthritic changes later may impair function.

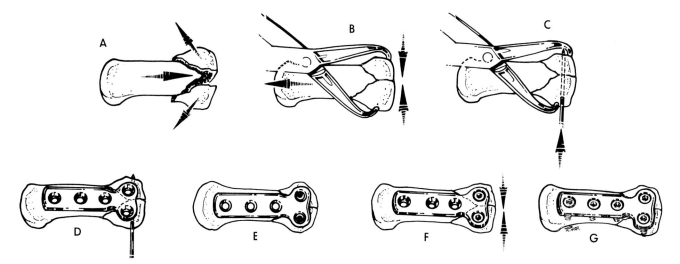

Fig. 64-15 Technique of reduction and internal fixation of T-type Rolando's fracture with miniplate and screws. **A**, Fracture. **B**, Reduction and traction. **C**, Provisional fixation with Kirschner wire. **D**, Positioning of plate. **E**, Offset drilling of two proximal holes. **F**, Tightening of two proximal screws compresses proximal fragments. **G**, Fixing rest of metacarpal to proximal fragments. (Redrawn from Foster RJ and Hastings H II: Clin Orthop 214:121, 1987.)

tion. An external fixator is used to align the comminuted fragments and to restore length; tension band wiring is then used to provide stability (Fig. 64-16). If the fracture is stable, the external fixator may be removed; if not, it should be continued for 8 weeks.

Carpometacarpal Joint Dislocation of Thumb

When this injury occurs without fracture and is recognized early, the dislocation should be reduced and the joint should be immobilized for 4 to 6 weeks to prevent recurrent dislocation. Open reduction and repair of the dorsal and radial ligaments ensure better joint stability. Immobilization for 6 weeks is still indicated after the repair.

In recurrent dislocation or subluxation of the carpometacarpal joint of the thumb, either idiopathic or traumatic, construction of a ligament to reinforce the deep capsule of the joint may be indicated. The operation is most helpful, of course, when the joint is unstable and painful and when degeneration of its articular surfaces is minimal. This procedure should not be done to relieve symptoms or subluxations of this joint from osteoarthritis.

LIGAMENT RECONSTRUCTION FOR RECURRENT DISLOCATION

■ *TECHNIQUE (EATON AND LITTLER)*. Make a dorsoradial incision along the proximal half of the first metacarpal and curve its proximal end ulnarward around the base of the thenar eminence parallel with the distal flexor crease of the wrist. Next expose the carpometacarpal joint of the thumb subpe-

riosteally and the volar aspect of the greater multangular extraperiosteally. Isolate the distal part of the flexor carpi radialis tendon from its position on the ulnar aspect of the crest of the greater multangular. Now in the distal forearm expose the same tendon through a longitudinal incision and split from its radial side a strip of tendon 6 cm long; free the strip proximally, continue the split distally, and leave the strip attached to the base of the second metacarpal (Fig. 64-17).

Before proceeding further, reduce the first metacarpal on the greater multangular and pass a Kirschner wire through this joint while holding it in appropriate orientation. Care should be taken in placing the wire so as not to interfere with the site where the transverse hole will be drilled through the first metacarpal and through which the tendon transfer will eventually pass.

Now reroute the strip of tendon previously raised from behind the crest of the greater multangular and pass it directly from the base of the second metacarpal to that of the first. Then beginning at the normal site of attachment of the deep capsule of the carpometacarpal joint of the thumb, drill a hole dorsally through the base of the first metacarpal to emerge on the ulnar side of the extensor pollicis brevis tendon. Now pass the strip of tendon through this hole, loop it back deep to the abductor pollicis longus tendon, draw it tight, and suture it to the periosteum near its exit. Finally, loop the tendon strip around the flexor carpi radialis near its insertion and suture it to the base of the first metacarpal. *AFTERTREATMENT*. The thumb is immobilized for 4 weeks in extension and abduction.

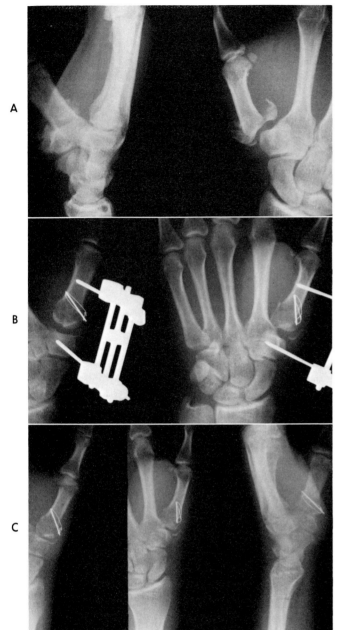

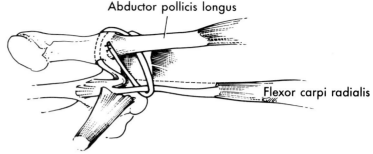

Fig. 64-17 Volar and radial ligament reconstruction with a strip from tendon of flexor carpi radialis, which is left attached at its insertion at base of second metacarpal. Course of tendon strip creates a reinforcement of volar, dorsal, and radial aspects of joint. (Redrawn from Eaton RG and Littler JW: J Bone Joint Surg 55-A:1655, 1973.)

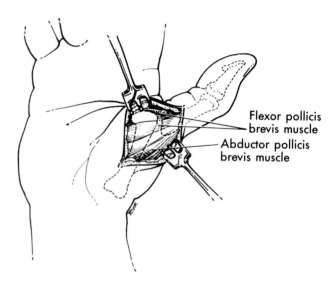

Fig. 64-18 Dislocation of metacarpophalangeal joint of thumb. Metacarpal head has penetrated joint capsule in such a way that were traction applied to thumb, metacarpal neck would be caught by capsule, and reduction would be impossible. Traction should not be applied; rather, metacarpal should be adducted and dislocated joint should be hyperextended while proximal end of proximal phalanx is pushed against and then over metacarpal head.

Fig. 64-16 **A**, Rolando's fracture treated by external fixation distractor, **B**, and tension band wiring, **C**. The distractor remained in place 8 weeks because fracture was unstable; excellent carpometacarpal and metacarpophalangeal function was obtained. (Courtesy Dr. Robert Belsole and Dr. Thomas Greene.)

Metacarpophalangeal Dislocation of Thumb

Dislocation of any of the metacarpophalangeal joints is possible from hyperextension injuries, but dorsal dislocation of the metacarpophalangeal joint of the thumb is the most common (Fig. 64-18). Early closed reduction may be easy, provided the thumb is maintained in adduction to relax its intrinsic muscles. One method is to use minimal if any tension, hyperextend the metacarpophalangeal joint, and then with the examiner's thumb push forward the proximal end of the proximal phalanx over the end of the metacarpal head. This tends to diminish the buttonhole effect on the metacarpal neck that traction accentuates. If this method is not successful, repeated attempts are contraindicated; open reduction should be done to disengage the head of the metacarpal from a buttonhole slit in the anterior capsule and from the flexor pollicis brevis muscle.

OPEN REDUCTION

■ *TECHNIQUE*. Make a transverse curved incision over the radial and volar aspects of the joint, exposing the articular surfaces of the phalanx and metacarpal. The base of the phalanx lies on the dorsal aspect of the head and neck of the metacarpal, and the head protrudes through the anterior capsule. Disengage the flexor pollicis brevis muscle, releasing the head of the metacarpal. Flex the thumb and push the head through the rent in the capsule to complete the reduction.

AFTERTREATMENT. The thumb is held in moderate flexion by a plaster splint. After 3 weeks the splint is removed and active motion is begun.

• • •

Farabeuf in 1876 recommended a dorsal surgical approach in irreducible dislocation of the metacarpophalangeal joint of the thumb. The main obstacle to reduction is the dorsally displaced volar plate, and the dorsal approach provides access to the plate, which is tethered tightly over the metacarpal head and neck. The plate is a fibrocartilaginous structure similar in appearance to articular cartilage; it is split in the midline of the thumb so that it will slip around the metacarpal head and permit reduction of the phalanx. Motion is started within a few days after surgery.

Palmar dislocation of the proximal phalanx of the thumb is rare, but sometimes it may be irreducible.

Gunther and Zielinski reported a case requiring an open reduction (Figs. 64-19 to 64-21) in which the metacarpal head was trapped between the extensor pollicis longus and extensor pollicis brevis tendons. This required opening the dorsal aponeurosis to relocate the extensor tendon. A rupture of the ulnar collateral ligament was also present and apparently the extensor pollicis longus tendon was trapped at the proximal ligamentous stump on the metacarpal head. This ligament was also repaired after reduction was accomplished.

Complete Rupture of Ulnar Collateral Ligament of Metacarpophalangeal Joint of Thumb

Incomplete rupture of the ulnar collateral ligament of the thumb is common and needs only proper rest for restoration of function, although pain and swelling may persist for several weeks. A thumb spica cast may be indicated.

Complete rupture of the ulnar collateral ligament is more common than that of the radial ligament and of course is more disabling because it renders pinch unstable. It may be suspected clinically by comparing the stability of the joint with that of the opposite thumb. Pathologic rotation of the thumb is also evident. The rupture can be demonstrated by an anteroposterior roentgenogram of the joint while under lateral stress as compared with a similar view of the opposite normal joint. Morgan

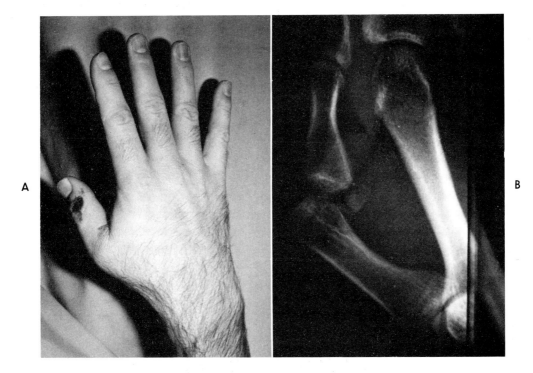

Fig. 64-19   **A**, Skin abrasion and metacarpophalangeal joint dislocation. **B**, Roentgenogram reveals palmar dislocation of proximal phalanx and widened joint space. (From Gunther SF and Zielinski CJ: J Hand Surg 7:515, 1982.)

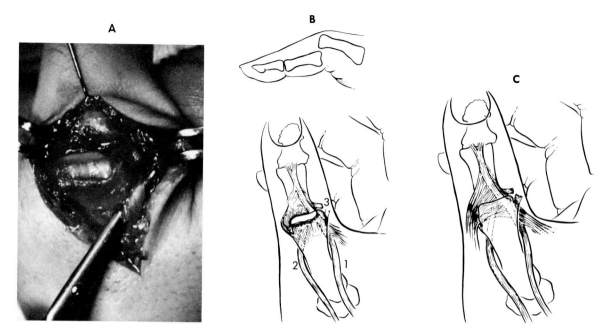

Fig. 64-20   Same patient as in Fig. 64-19. **A,** Surgical findings after incision of skin and sub-cutaneous fat. Dorsal aspect of metacarpal head is visible through rent in capsule. Whole exten-sor mechanism is trapped beneath metacarpal head. Hemostat is delivering, but cannot reduce, portion of extensor pollicis longus tendon. **B,** Visible findings: *1,* extensor pollicis longus ten-don; *2,* extensor pollicis brevis tendon; and *3,* ruptured ulnar collateral ligament. **C,** Invisible anatomy that is hidden beneath metacarpal head. Bone has buttonholed proximal and dorsal to aponeurotic expansion that connects abductor pollicis brevis to extensor pollicis longus tendon. (From Gunther SF and Zielinski CJ: J Hand Surg 7:515, 1982.)

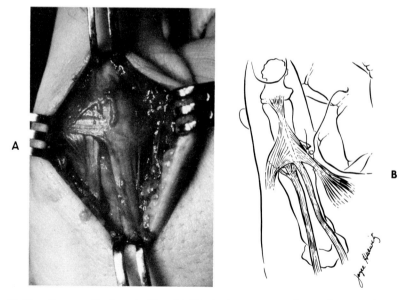

Fig. 64-21   Same patient as in Fig. 64-19. **A,** Appearance after reduction showing normal anatomy of extensor mechanism. **B,** Same patient showing single suture in ulnar collateral lig-ament. (From Gunther SF and Zielinski CJ: J Hand Surg 7:515, 1982.)

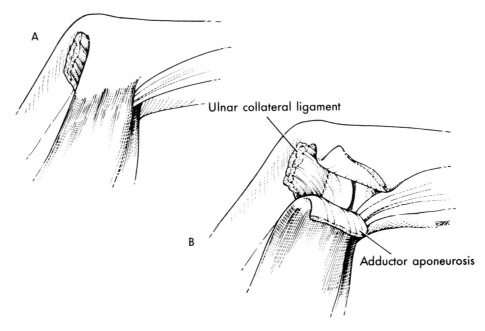

Fig. 64-22   Complete rupture of ulnar collateral ligament of metacarpophalangeal joint of thumb. **A,** Ligament is ruptured distally and is folded back so that its distal end points proximally. **B,** Adductor aponeurosis has been divided, exposing ligament and joint. (From Stener B: J Bone Joint Surg 44-B:869, 1962.)

and Lavalette suggest arthrography of the metacarpophalangeal joint to delineate the "Stener lesion" from incomplete tears that may heal conservatively.

The ligament may avulse a bony fragment from the phalanx. When this fragment is not widely displaced, the injury may be treated by applying a thumb spica cast for 6 weeks.

If a complete rupture is acute, the ligament should be repaired (Fig. 64-22), but when the diagnosis is delayed for a month or longer, fibrosis makes identification and repair of the ligament more difficult but still possible at times. Then a repair might be done by dissecting out the ligament from within the fibrotic mass and reattaching it appropriately. At that time the detached tendinous insertion of the adductor muscle might be advanced and reattached to furnish a dynamic reinforcement. When the repair is done several months after the injury, a graft may be used to replace the ligament. This may be either a boxlike graft with a strip of fascia or palmaris longus tendon passed through both the proximal and distal attachments of the ligament or a graft from the extensor pollicis brevis tendon, either split or in total, threaded through bone and attached by pull-out sutures to reconstruct the ligament. Arthrodesis of the metacarpophalangeal joint may be indicated when there are arthritic changes within the joint or gross disruption of the joint.

REPAIR BY SUTURE

■ *TECHNIQUE.* To repair an acute rupture of the ulnar collateral ligament, make a slightly curved longitudinal incision convex dorsally over the dorsoulnar aspect of the metacarpophalangeal joint or a bayonet-shaped incision with the transverse segment at the joint level. Protect the terminal branches of the superficial radial nerve, which innervate the lateral margins of the thumb pulp. Identify them as they pass distally on each side at the dorsolateral aspect of the metacarpophalangeal joint deep to the subcutaneous fat. Identify the ligament, and at the site of the avulsion drill a small hole through the proximal

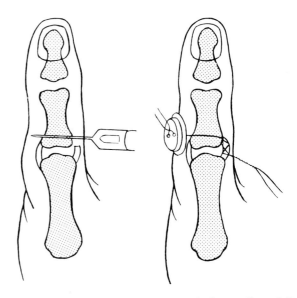

Fig. 64-23   Repair of acute rupture of ulnar collateral ligament of metacarpophalangeal joint of thumb (see text).

end of the proximal phalanx, using a Kirschner wire of the smallest diameter as a drill point (Fig. 64-23). Place a Bunnell pull-out suture through the avulsed end of the ligament, pass the ends of the suture through the phalanx, and while holding the joint in slight flexion, tie them over a padded button on the radial side. Pass the twisted pull-out wire loop through the skin near the incision before closure. The same technique is used when a small bone fragment is avulsed by the ligament if the tear is complete and the bone fragment is displaced.

AFTERTREATMENT. A thumb spica brace or splint is worn for 5 to 6 weeks. The pull-out wire is removed at 4 to 6 weeks, and normal activities are permitted.

• • •

Tension band wiring (Fig. 64-24), as suggested by Jupiter and Sheppard, offers the advantage of avoiding a pull-out wire and may provide better biomechanical fixation of an avulsion fracture.

REPAIR OF OLD ULNAR COLLATERAL LIGAMENT RUPTURE

■ *TECHNIQUE USING EXTENSOR POLLICIS BREVIS TENDON (SAKELLARIDES AND DEWEESE; Fig. 64-25).* Make a curved incision over the metacarpophalangeal joint (Fig. 64-25, *A*), so as to expose the dorsal as well as the ulnar side of this joint (Fig. 64-25, *B*). Isolate the extensor pollicis brevis tendon and detach it approximately 5 cm proximal to its insertion into the base of the proximal phalanx (Fig. 64-25, *C*). Open the expansion of the adductor tendon and inspect the joint, excising the fibrosed area of the torn ligament so as to expose adequately the ulnar aspect of the joint (Fig. 64-25, *D*). Now drill a hole beginning radial to the insertion of the exten-

sor pollicis brevis and exiting on the volar ulnar aspect of the proximal phalanx at the site of the normal ligamentous attachment (Fig. 64-25, *D*). Pass the tendon through this hole and then drill another hole transversely across the neck of the metacarpal at the site of attachment of the collateral ligament. Now pass the tendon proximally across the joint into this hole and attach it to the bone with a wire pull-out suture over a button on the radial side (Fig. 64-25, *E*). Carefully measure the tendon length and attach the pull-out suture before inserting it in the hole. Insert a Kirschner wire across the joint. Close the capsule and the expansion of the adductor muscle, close the wound (Fig. 64-25, *F*), and maintain the thumb in a cast for 4 weeks.

AFTERTREATMENT. Following cast and pin removal, protect the thumb for another 5 weeks in a soft protective dressing or a removable splint.

• • •

The following procedure is applicable when the rupture is at least a month old and when difficulty in identifying the torn ligament is expected because of scar tissue. An arthrodesis is indicated in the presence of crepitus or pain on a grinding type of manipulation of the joint.

■ *TECHNIQUE (NEVIASER ET AL.).* Make a **V**-shaped or chevron incision over the ulnar aspect of the thumb (Fig. 64-26, *A*). Take care to protect the dorsal and volar sensory nerves. Reflect the adductor aponeurosis. The original tear in the capsule and the ulnar collateral ligament may be obliterated by scar (Fig. 64-26, *B*). Detach the tendon of the adductor pollicis from the sesamoid; shape a flap of the collateral ligament in the form of a **U** based proximally to be used to reef the scarred ligament when the joint is reduced. Drill a hole through the ulnar cortex of the

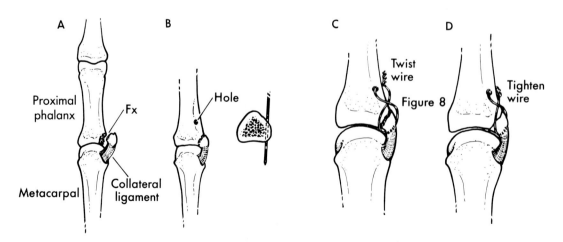

Fig. 64-24   Tension wire fixation of collateral ligament avulsion. **A,** Displaced, rotated type 2 avulsion fracture. **B,** Hole is drilled vertically approximately 1 cm distal to fracture. **C,** Wire is passed through hole and insertion of ligament on fragment. **D,** Wire is tightened, cut, and bent along palmar aspect of proximal phalanx. (Redrawn from Jupiter JB and Sheppard JE: Clin Orthop 214:113, 1987.)

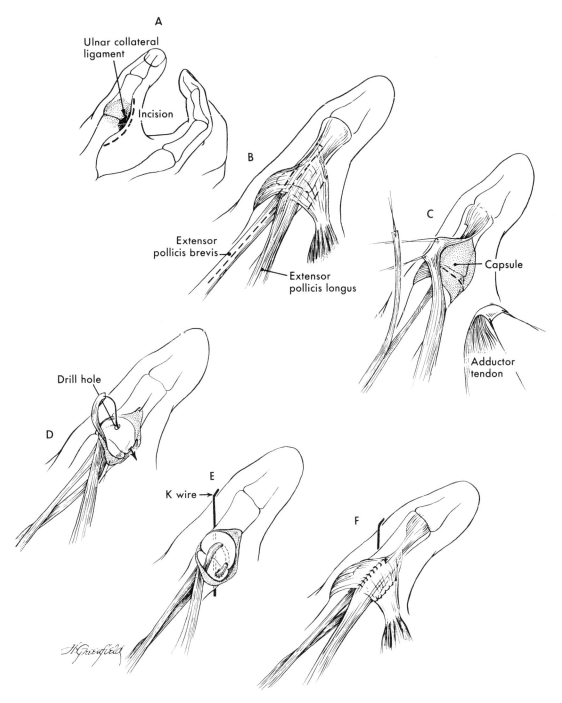

Fig. 64-25   Steps in procedure to reconstruct ulnar collateral ligament using one half of tendon of extensor pollicis brevis. (From Sakellarides HT and DeWeese JW: J Bone Joint Surg 58-A:106, 1976.)

proximal phalanx, approximately 1 cm distal to the metacarpophalangeal joint. After attaching the tightened capsule, advance and reinsert the adductor tendon distally through the hole using a pull-out wire technique (Fig. 64-26, *C*). Close the wound and immobilize the hand in plaster for a minimum of 4 weeks.

AFTERTREATMENT. Start progressive exercise when the plaster is removed.

• • •

In the series of R.J. Smith, the ulnar collateral ligament was ruptured 77% of the time and the radial collateral ligament 23% of the time. In 3 of the 21 cases, the ulnar collateral ligament was found to be superficial and proximal to the adductor apparatus as described previously by Stener. Because of a volar attachment of the ulnar collateral ligament to the proximal phalanx, Smith notes that there is also a factor of volar instability permitting subluxation of the proximal phalanx. Early surgical

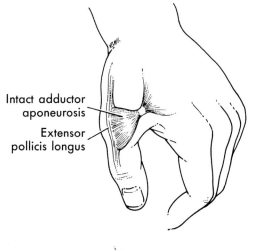

Intact adductor
aponeurosis

Extensor
pollicis longus

Fig. 64-26   Repair of old rupture of ulnar collateral ligament of thumb (see text). (Redrawn from Neviaser RJ et al: J Bone Joint Surg 53-A:1357, 1971).

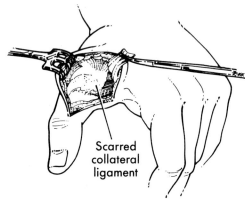

Scarred
collateral
ligament

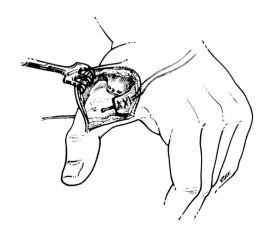

treatment is, of course, preferable, but 3 weeks after injury or longer, a tendon graft by his technique described below is recommended.

■ *TECHNIQUE* (*SMITH*). Make a midlateral incision, 3 cm long, centered over the ulnar side of the metacarpophalangeal joint of the thumb (Fig. 64-27, *A*); identify the sensory branches of the radial nerve and retract them dorsally. Expose the dorsal expansion of the extensor mechanism and transect it in the midlateral line to expose the joint capsule (Fig. 64-27, *B* and *C*). A remnant of the ruptured ulnar collateral ligament is frequently found attached to the metacarpal neck. Make a 2.8 mm hole transversely across the base of the proximal phalanx, taking care to exit on the volar ulnar side of the phalanx (Fig. 64-27, *D*). Obtain a tendon graft from the palmaris longus, attach a figure-of-eight suture to one end, pass the suture through the hole in the phalanx (Fig. 64-27, *E*), and fix it so that the end of the tendon is fastened in the hole and the other end is free on the ulnar side. Pull the free end of the graft to the area of the metacarpal head (Fig. 64-27, *F*), make parallel incisions longitudinally in the remnant of the ulnar collateral ligament, weave the graft through the portion of the ligament between the incisions, and suture it securely (Fig. 64-27, *G*).

When the collateral ligament remnant is not firm, attach the graft proximally through two adjacent drill holes connected by a tunnel in the metacarpal head. Pass the remaining free portion of the graft back distally on itself volar to the first strand and suture the parallel segments of the graft to each other (Fig. 64-27, *G*). The volar attachment of the graft helps to counteract the tendency of the phalanx to subluxate volarward. Repair the capsule by overlapping and suturing, using the double-breasted technique (Fig. 64-27, *H*). Suture the adductor expansion.

AFTERTREATMENT. Hold the thumb in plaster for 4 weeks and follow with a removable splint for an additional 5 weeks.

FOUR MEDIAL METACARPALS
Carpometacarpal Fracture-dislocation of Finger Rays

Fracture-dislocation of the proximal ends of the metacarpals is often not recognized because of swelling. All four metacarpals may be dislocated either dorsally or volarly, but the fourth and fifth are the most commonly involved and are usually displaced dorsally. A true lat-

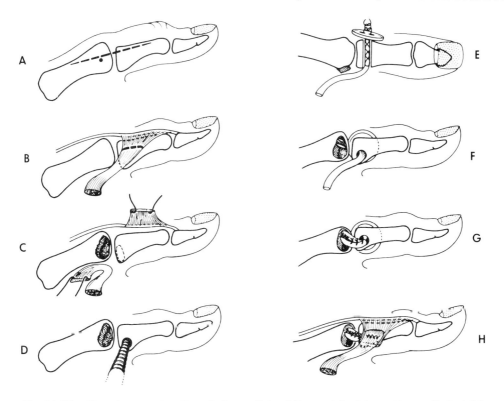

Fig. 64-27 Steps in reconstruction of ulnar collateral ligament for late posttraumatic instability. (From Smith RJ: J Bone Joint Surg 59-A:13, 1977).

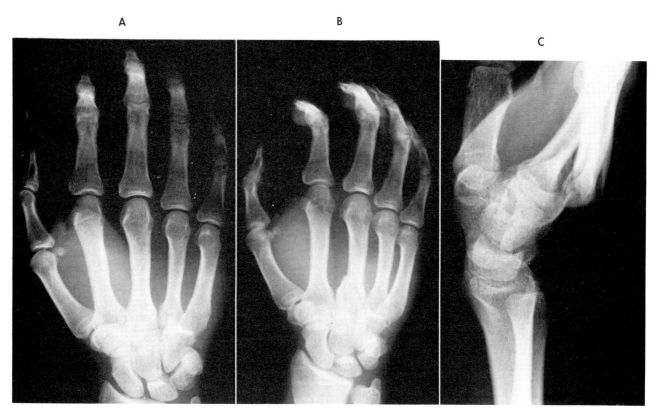

Fig. 64-28 Dislocation of fourth and fifth carpometacarpal joints and fracture of base of third metacarpal. **A**, Posteroanterior view. **B**, Oblique view. **C**, Lateral view. (From Henderson JJ and Arafa MAM: J Bone Joint Surg 69-B:212, 1987.)

eral roentgenogram is needed for accurate diagnosis since swelling may obscure the deformity. The loss of parallel joint surfaces at the carpometacarpal articulations in a posteroanterior roentgenogram should make one suspect this injury (Fig. 64-28). When the injury is seen early, manual reduction is easy, but Kirschner wire fixation is usually necessary to prevent redislocation. When seen late, the injury requires open reduction, and sometimes the proximal end of the metacarpal must be resected and the carpometacarpal joint must be fused.

Intraarticular Fracture of Base of Fifth Metacarpal

Bora and Didizian have called attention to the potentially disabling intraarticular fracture at the base of the fifth metacarpal (Fig. 64-29). When the injury is not reduced properly and malunion results, weakness of grip as well as a painful joint results. The joint consists of the base of the fifth metacarpal articulating with the hamate and the adjoining fourth metacarpal. The extensor carpi ulnaris tendon attaches to the dorsum of the proximal portion of the fifth metacarpal. The joint permits approximately 30 degrees of normal flexion and extension and the rotation necessary in grasp and in palmar cupping. This displaced intraarticular fracture might be compared with Bennett's fracture since the tendency is great for the pull of the extensor carpi ulnaris to displace proximally the metacarpal shaft, similar to the thumb metacarpal displacement in Bennett's fracture. In addition to the routine anteroposterior and lateral views, a roentgenogram should be made with 30 degrees of pronation to give a better view of the articular surface for accurate diagnosis. This fracture often may be reduced by traction

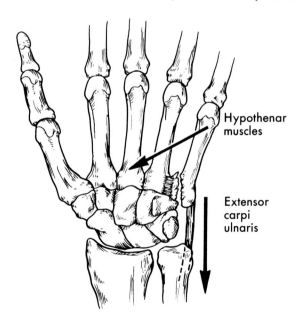

Fig. 64-29 Unstable fracture of base of fifth metacarpal may permit proximal displacement of shaft similar to Bennett's fracture (see text).

and percutaneous pinning and is then protected by a cast. However, those fractures that are not recognized early and are healing in a displaced position should have either correction by osteotomy of the malunion or resection arthroplasty (Fig. 64-30).

Metacarpophalangeal Dislocation of Fingers

Metacarpophalangeal dislocations are less common than interphalangeal dislocations. They occur most often in the index finger, and Kaplan's description of them in this finger is vivid (see Fig. 64-31).

The fibrocartilaginous plate breaks away in the region of its weakest attachment, at the neck of the volar aspect of the second metacarpal; and the flexor tendons in the vaginal ligament and the pretendinous band or the midpalmar fascia, which adheres to the vaginal ligament, are violently displaced to the ulnar side of the metacarpal head. Following this, the fibrocartilaginous plate of the joint is displaced over the head of the metacarpal, landing on the dorsum of this bone, where it becomes wedged between the base of the proximal phalanx and the head. The lateral collateral ligaments, which are now abnormally displaced, lock the phalanx in the abnormal position typical of this dislocation. At the same time the two groups of transverse fibers of the palmar fascia hold the head of the metacarpal, the distal group (the natatory ligament, which moves with the phalanx) applying pressure to the dorsum of the metacarpal head, while the proximal group (the superficial transverse ligament, which extends across the volar aspect of the metacarpal neck) applies pressure to the volar aspect.[*]

Thus the dislocated metacarpal head lies between the natatory ligament and the superficial transverse ligament of the palmar fascia. The flexor tendons are on one side and the lumbrical muscle on the other.

When the dislocation is incomplete, reduction by manipulation is easy. When complete, with the head of the metacarpal displaced volarward and the base of the phalanx dorsalward, open reduction is often required. The major obstruction preventing reduction of the metacarpophalangeal joint is the displaced volar fibrocartilaginous plate lying dorsal to the metacarpal head. Sometimes, however, manipulation alone is successful. We find that 50% can be reduced closed. The joint is hyperextended, the articular surface of the proximal phalanx is forced firmly against the metacarpal neck, and, while this force is maintained, the joint is flexed. Sometimes this maneuver will trap the displaced fibrocartilaginous plate and carry it to its normal position anterior to the metacarpal head. The following is Kaplan's technique for open reduction.

OPEN REDUCTION

■ *TECHNIQUE (KAPLAN).* "In open reduction the incision is started in the thenar crease of the hand at

---

[*]From Kaplan EB: Dorsal dislocation of the metacarpophalangeal joint of the index finger, J Bone Joint Surg 39-A:1081, 1957.

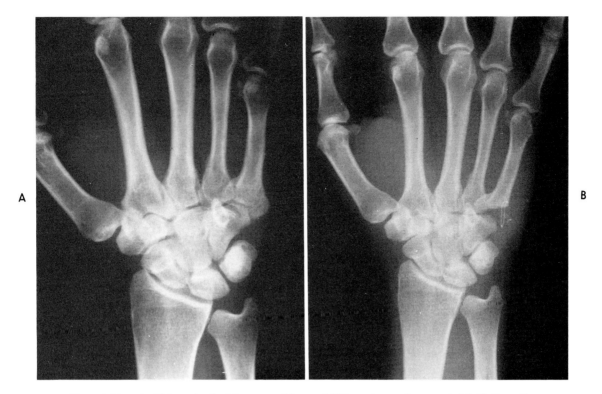

Fig. 64-30 **A,** This malunited fracture of base of fifth metacarpal was painful. **B,** Resection arthroplasty is preferred over osteotomy. Tendon of extensor carpi ulnaris must be reattached.

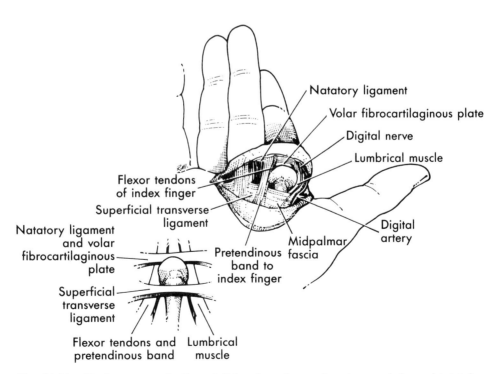

Fig. 64-31 Kaplan open reduction of dislocation of second metacarpophalangeal joint (see text). *Inset,* Diagram of four structures that surround and constrict metacarpal head. (Modified from Kaplan EB: J Bone Joint Surg 39-A:1081, 1957.)

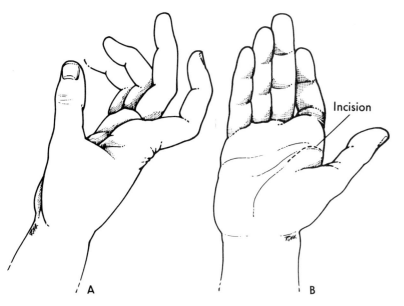

Fig. 64-32 Dislocation of second metacarpophalangeal joint. **A**, Deformity as seen from lateral side. **B**, Skin incision *(broken line)*, used in open reduction. (From Kaplan EB: J Bone Joint Surg 39-A:1081, 1957.)

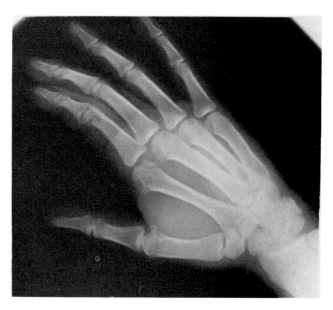

Fig. 64-33 Fracture of metacarpal head with irreducible dislocation. This fracture-dislocation of metacarpophalangeal joint of index finger is ideal for dorsal approach described by Becton et al. since direct access to fracture area is provided.

the radial base of the index finger and is continued into the proximal crease of the hand [Fig. 64-32]. . . . To reduce the dislocation following exposure, it is necessary to divide all the constricting bands. The first incision is made to free the constriction of the cartilaginous plate [Fig. 64-31]. This incision is placed parallel and radial to the vaginal ligament and extends from the free edge of the torn ligament to the junction of the periosteum with the proximal phalanx. The incision must penetrate the entire thickness of the plate. Division of the plate alone is not sufficient, however. The transverse fibers of the taut natatory ligament must also be completely divided, and following this, another longitudinal incision should be made through the transverse fibers of the superficial transverse metacarpal ligament. This third incision, which should extend to the ulnar side of the first lumbrical muscle, releases the constriction below the metacarpal head."

This triple incision "frees the base of the proximal phalanx, which then returns to its normal place over the metacarpal head. This, in turn, permits the immediate replacement of the second metacarpal head in line with the other metacarpal heads, following which the flexor tendons, the vaginal ligament, and the nerves and vessels are restored to their normal positions. The wound is then closed in the accepted manner, and the finger is immobilized in functional position for about one week."*

---

*From Kaplan EB: Dorsal dislocation of the metacarpophalangeal joint of the index finger, J Bone Joint Surg 39-A:1081, 1957.

■ *TECHNIQUE (BECTON ET AL.).* Becton et al. believe the dorsal approach has several advantages over the volar approach. The dorsal approach provides full exposure of the fibrocartilaginous volar ligament, which is the structure blocking reduction. The digital nerves are not as likely to be cut, and should there be an occult fracture of the metacarpal head, this can be reduced and fixed more easily (Fig. 64-33).

Over the metacarpophalangeal joint, make a 4 cm midline incision cutting the underlying extensor tendon and joint capsule as well. The fibrocartilaginous ligament may be difficult to identify because it has the same color as the articular cartilage, and its torn margin may not be visible. Make a small incision to ensure the tissue is in fact the fibrocartilaginous ligament; then complete the longitudinal incision (Fig. 64-34). Flex the wrist volarward to release the tension on the flexor tendons; then place traction on the finger and flex the metacarpophalangeal joint, reducing the dislocation. Observe to see if any free cartilage is missing from the metacarpal head. This may be lodged in the joint. Suture the extensor tendon and skin and splint the finger for 3 weeks.

Fracture of Metacarpal Shaft or Neck

Fracture of a metacarpal shaft is usually best treated by closed methods, but when several metacarpals are fractured and there is open soft tissue trauma, internal fixation is indicated (Fig. 64-35). Correct rotational alignment is the most important factor in reduction. Introduce the Kirschner wire at the fracture site and drill it out

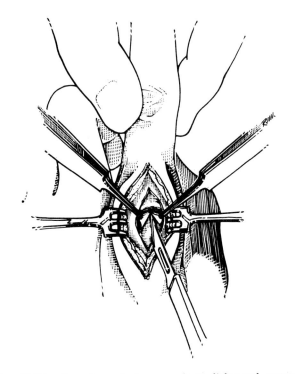

Fig. 64-34 Dorsal surgical approach to dislocated metacarpophalangeal joint. Volar plate that is caught over dorsal area of metacarpal head is incised longitudinally, and reduction is easily achieved. (Redrawn from Becton JL, Christian JD Jr, Goodwin HN, and Jackson JG: J Bone Joint Surg 57-A:698, 1975.)

through the skin at the metacarpal base; while drilling, force a bow in the wire convex toward the palm and hold the wrist in flexion so that the wire emerges on the dorsum of the wrist. Then reduce the fracture and drill the wire in the opposite direction into the distal fragment, stopping just proximal to the metacarpophalangeal joint. Cut off the proximal end under the skin (Figs. 64-36 and 64-37). Apply a splint holding the wrist in extension. A fracture of the metacarpal neck can be treated similarly if open reduction is necessary (Fig. 64-37, *B*).

An alternate method applicable in a few metacarpal shaft fractures is percutaneous pinning. With the metacarpophalangeal joint acutely flexed, introduce a 0.062-inch (0.155 cm) Kirschner wire into the metacarpal head and drill it to the level of the fracture. By manual pressure and manipulation of the wire and with the aid of an image intensifier, reduce the fracture and drill the wire out the dorsum of the wrist as just described. Withdraw the wire until the distal tip is just proximal to the metacarpophalangeal joint.

Metacarpal Head Fractures

Intraarticular metacarpal head fractures, especially of the fourth and fifth metacarpals, are often caused by the patient striking an opponent's teeth in a fist fight. Compound injuries here are almost always caused by human

bites (see section on human bite treatment in Chapter 78 for care of wound and antibiotics). Many intraarticular head fractures require open reduction and internal fixation, particularly if the articular surface is displaced so that an incongruous joint would result. These should be fixed with Kirschner wires. Occasionally these fractures result in avascular necrosis of the displaced fragment (Figs. 64-38 and 64-39).

Although the use of screws and plates has limited application in acute metacarpal fractures, the surgeon should have knowledge of the techniques and equipment now available in order to make a proper judgment in treatment of the individual patient. However, complications of this method of treatment have been reported to be as high as 42%.

OPEN REDUCTION AND PLATE FIXATION. According to Hastings, the indications for plate fixation of the metacarpals are (1) multiple fractures with gross displacement or additional soft tissue injury; (2) displaced diaphyseal transverse, short oblique, or short spiral fractures (Fig. 64-40); (3) comminuted intraarticular and periarticular fractures; (4) comminuted fractures with shortening and/or malrotation; and (5) fractures with substance loss or segmental defects.

■ *TECHNIQUE (HASTINGS).* **Plate fixation requires reduction, provisional stabilization by Kirschner wires or reduction clamps, and plate application. Expose the fracture surfaces to allow anatomic reduction. Provisional fixation with reduction forceps is more difficult in the central metacarpals than the more accessible border index and small metacarpals. In most instances, reduction forceps currently available are inadequate for clamping the plate to bone proximally and distally for provisional fixation. Instead, reduction is held by an assistant and the chosen plate contoured to the dorsal metacarpal. Fix the plate through one screw hole adjacent to the fracture. Maintain reduction and fix the first hole on the opposite side of the fracture.**

For transverse fractures when an adequate palmar cortical buttress is restored, the plate is ideally applied as a dorsal tension band plate. Compression across the fracture can best be achieved by using a 2.7 mm dynamic compression plate (DCP), but in stable situations the less bulky one-fourth tubular plate is preferred and some compression is still achievable by eccentric placement of the screws. Both screws are terminally tightened using the force of three digits on the screwdriver. Insert the remaining screws.

To function as a tension band the plate must be contoured exactly to or slightly beyond the dorsal metacarpal bow in order to restore the anterior cortical buttress. Without anterior buttressing, the plate will bend and fatigue. When an anterior buttress is properly restored, the plate is protected from

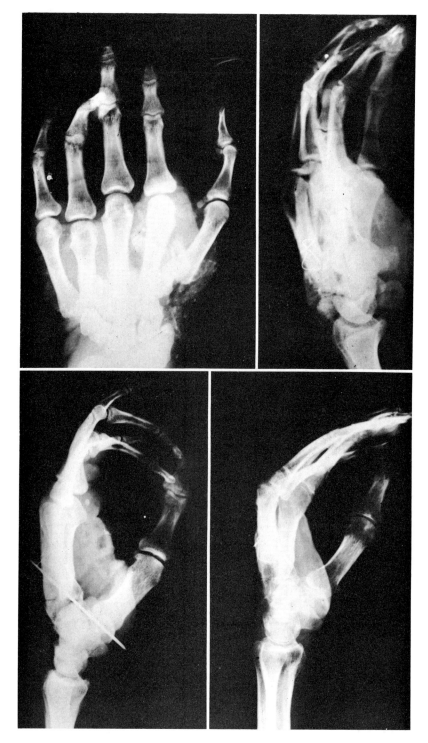

Fig. 64-35   Severely comminuted fractures of metacarpals complicated by severe injuries of soft structures require reduction and internal fixation to restore both longitudinal and transverse metacarpal arches.

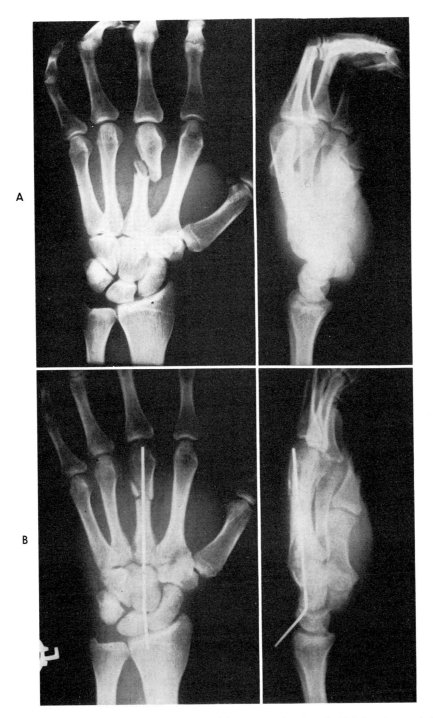

Fig. 64-36   Metacarpal shaft fracture treated by open reduction. **A**, Third metacarpal shaft is comminuted and is angulated radially and dorsally. **B**, After open reduction and medullary fixation.

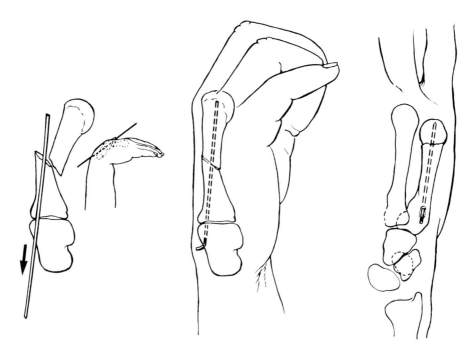

Fig. 64-37 Open reduction and medullary fixation of fracture of metacarpal shaft and neck (see text).

bending stress and is subjected mainly to tensile stress. Short oblique and spiral fractures may be stabilized by an interfragmentary screw followed by a dorsal plate to neutralize rotational stresses. When a T-shaped plate or oblique L-plate is used, apply the side arm(s) first since a rotational deformity may occur as the screws in the side arm(s) draw the underlying bone fragment up to the plate. For intraarticular fractures, the two articular fragments can be lagged together with a screw separate from the plate and perpendicular to the fracture. Alternatively, the two screws in the T or L portion of the plate can be eccentrically placed away from the fracture to compress the two fragments on terminal screw tightening. With distal metaphyseal metacarpal fractures, dorsal plating may interfere with the extensor mechanism. The interference is best avoided by use of the 2 mm condylar plate, applied dorsoradially and dorsoulnarly through the dorsal tubercle of origin of the collateral ligament.

Plate fixation for metacarpal fractures should include screw purchase in at least four cortices, both distal and proximal to the fracture. The choice of plates must be tailored to the individual situation. Short oblique or spiral fractures requiring neutralization plating are stabilized with a one-fourth tubular plate and 2.7 mm dynamic compression plate or a one-third tubular plate, which requires 3.5 mm screws. Such a strut plate will require protection from loading and early bone grafting.

OPEN REDUCTION AND SCREW FIXATION. Screw fixation alone may be indicated in long oblique or spiral fractures and displaced intraarticular fractures with greater than 25% articular surface involvement (Fig. 64-41).

■ *TECHNIQUE (HASTINGS).* Fracture reduction follows local debridement of hematoma and soft tissue. Limit periosteal stripping to 1 or 2 mm, only enough to ensure anatomic reduction. Reduction forceps or 0.028 mm Kirschner wires provide temporary fixation. Plan screw placement according to the fracture anatomy.

The compressive forces, which act to deform and shorten the metacarpals, are best resisted by a screw placed at 90 degrees to the bone's long axis. Torsional stress is best resisted by screws placed at 90 degrees to the fracture. The best compromise for resistance against axial as well as torsional loading is a bisected angle, compromising the angles 90 degrees to the fracture and 90 degrees to the bone's long axis. Screw placement near the fracture spikes must be accurate to ensure cortical purchase and avoid splintering.

The 2 mm screws are useful for shaft fractures and the 2.7 mm screws are better for metaphyses. Countersinking the screw head not only allows for better load distribution but also removes the screw head prominence. With proper screw thread grasp of the distal cortex and gliding through the overdrilled proximal cortex, the torsional load of the

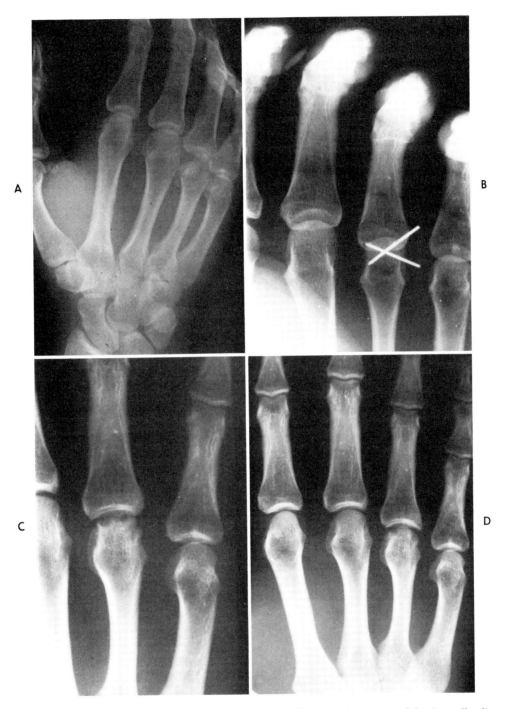

Fig. 64-38   **A,** Roentgenogram of hand of 20-year-old man who sustained horizontally directed fracture of fourth metacarpal head with palmar fragment displaced proximally. **B,** Fracture was reduced and held in place with Kirschner wires. **C,** At 4 months roentgenograms showed early avascular necrosis of metacarpal head. **D,** At 2½ years roentgenograms showed some remodeling but definite incongruities of metacarpal head. (From McElfresh EC and Dobyns JH: J Hand Surg 8:383, 1983.)

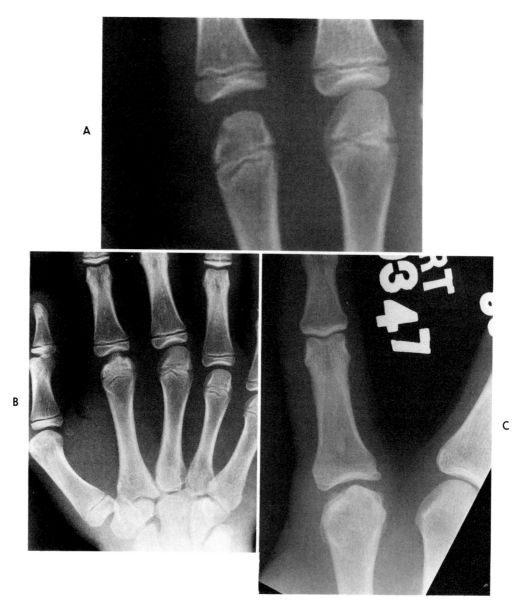

Fig. 64-39 **A**, Roentgenogram of hand of 14-year-old boy who injured his index finger metacarpophalangeal joint while playing baseball. **B**, At 9 months roentgenograms showed avascular necrosis of metacarpal head. **C**, At 8 years roentgenograms showed deformity of metacarpal head with early osteoarthritic changes. (From McElfresh EC and Dobyns JH: J Hand Surg 8:383, 1983.)

screw is converted to an axial load, which compresses the two fracture surfaces together. Metacarpal head fractures can usually be fixed with a single screw; those of the metaphysis and diaphysis require a minimum of two screws. Stable fixation by screws alone is possible for fractures with a length twice the bone diameter and fixed with two or more screws. Screw fixation alone does not provide adequate rotational stability across short fracture lines, so here a neutralization plate or external protection should be added.

MINICONDYLAR PLATE FIXATION. Buchler and Fis-

cher recommend the use of a minicondylar plate for metacarpal and phalangeal periarticular injuries. Their five indications are (1) acute fractures associated with partial or complete flexor tendon disruption treated with primary tenorrhaphy and early motion, partial or complete extensor tendon injuries that are functionally competent or repaired so as to withstand early tensile loading, and periarticular injuries in which the risk of joint stiffness is great because of the severity and location of associated soft tissue injury; (2) replantation of digits; (3) metaphyseal osteotomies of phalanges or metacarpals, especially in conjunction with capsulotomy and/or tenolysis; (4) digit reconstruction (osteoplastic, pedicle

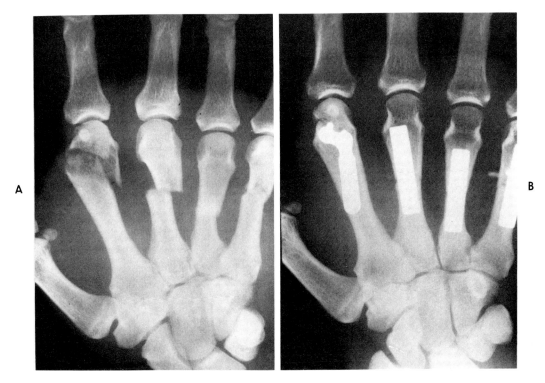

Fig. 64-40 **A**, Displaced, closed fractures of metaphyseal shafts of right middle, ring, and small digits and comminuted intraarticular fracture of head and distal metaphysis of index finger. **B**, Tubular plate fixation of index, middle, ring, and small metacarpals. (From Hastings H II: Clin Orthop 214:37, 1987.)

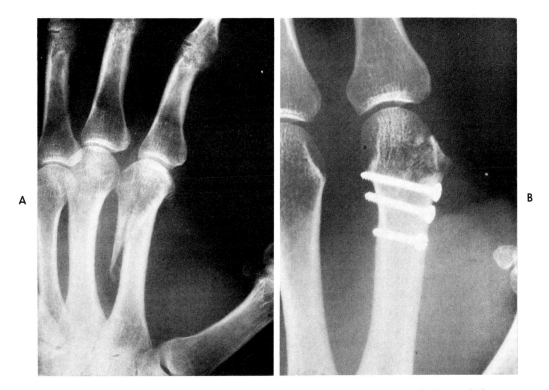

Fig. 64-41 **A**, Displaced metaphyseal fracture of left index metacarpal with dorsoradial comminution and extension into metacarpophalangeal joint. **B**, Fixation with three 2 mm interfragmentary compression screws. (From Hastings H II: Clin Orthop 214:37, 1987.)

graft, free composite tissue transfer) with need for stable fixation of skeleton; and (5) arthrodesis.

The three contraindications are (1) use in the vicinity of open epiphyses, (2) joint fragments narrower than 6 mm for the 2 mm plate or 5 mm for the 1.5 mm plate, and (3) condylar blade and screw intraarticular insertion, with the exception of the dorsal recess of the metacarpal head.

It is suggested that the surgeon review the appropriate literature on this specialized implant system.

Wiring Techniques Applicable to Long Bone Fractures

Cerclage techniques using wire or bands may result in osteonecrosis and are not recommended. However, tension band wiring and 90/90 wiring (Fig. 64-42) may increase the surgeon's choices for managing unstable fractures. Greene et al. have suggested improvements in standard tension band wiring techniques (Fig. 64-43).

PHALANGES
Fracture of Middle or Proximal Phalanx

A direct blow on the dorsum of the fingers is often the cause of fractures of the middle and proximal phalanges. Angulation is toward the palm, and the fingers may assume a claw position (Fig. 64-44). When multiple or

open, these fractures should be treated with longitudinal or oblique Kirschner wires. They may be approached through a longitudinal dorsolateral incision or, for a proximal phalangeal fracture, through one placed dorsally over the phalanx (Fig. 64-45). The latter extends from the metacarpophalangeal joint to the proximal interphalangeal joint in an S curve.

OPEN REDUCTION

■ *TECHNIQUE (PRATT).* **Expose the extensor tendon and incise it longitudinally in its center; retract it to each side to expose the fracture site. Drill a Kirschner wire into the distal fragment under direct vision, and then, after reducing the fracture, drill it retrograde. Care should be taken to correct any rotational deformity, although some shortening may be accepted. With a running suture of No. 34 monofilament wire, repair the extensor tendon. Support the finger in the position of function and the wrist in extension.**

• • •

Sometimes an unstable oblique fracture of a middle or proximal phalanx can be treated by closed reduction and percutaneous pinning with a Kirschner wire inserted across the fracture. Then the finger is splinted for 2 to 3 weeks and the wire is removed at 3 to 4 weeks.

Open or severely comminuted fractures of the phalanges, especially the proximal phalanx, may not be suitable

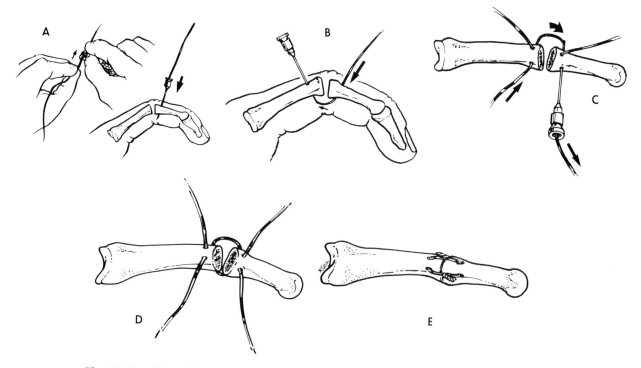

Fig. 64-42 Ninety/ninety intraosseous wiring of metacarpophalangeal joints. **A,** Wire is inserted through distal fragment with hypodermic needle. **B,** Needle is passed through proximal fragment and wire is pulled through fragment. **C,** Second wire is inserted in similar manner. **D,** Both wires in place. **E,** Wires are twisted until they begin to demonstrate color change. (Modified from Zimmerman NB and Weiland AJ: Orthopedics 12:99, 1989.)

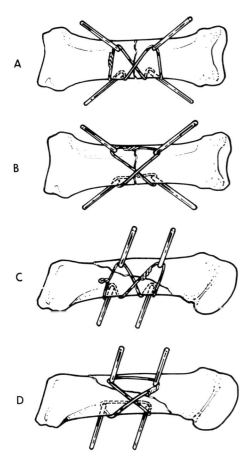

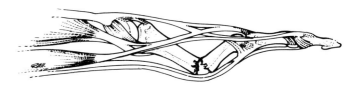

Fig. 64-44 Full flexion of metacarpophalangeal joint is required to relax deforming forces and maintain reduction. (Redrawn from Green TL, Noellert RC, and Belsole RJ: Clin Orthop 214:78, 1987.)

Fig. 64-43 Tension band wiring of hand fractures. **A** and **B**, Technique for transverse or short oblique fracture with crossed Kirschner wires and tension band in conventional figure-of-eight loop, **A**, and recommended technique, **B**. **C** and **D**, Technique for long oblique or spiral fracture with parallel Kirschner wires perpendicular to fracture in recommended pattern, **C**, and conventional figure-of-eight loop, **D**. (Redrawn from Green TL, Noellert RC, and Belsole RJ: Clin Orthop 214:78, 1987.)

for internal fixation using traditional methods. In this instance, external fixation using a mini–external fixator or, as suggested by Milford, percutaneous transverse Kirschner wires joined by a segment of polymethylmethacrylate may be appropriate. Final alignment of the bone is permitted while the plastic sets (Fig. 64-46).

Fracture-dislocation of Proximal Interphalangeal Joint

Fracture-dislocations at the proximal interphalangeal joint as a rule result in an unstable dorsal displacement of the middle phalanx caused by disruption of the attachment of the volar fibrocartilaginous plate. When there is a large single volar fragment involving more than 50% of the joint surface, open reduction and internal fixation can be carried out with one or more Kirschner wires or a wire loop pull-out. When the fragment or fragments include less than 50% of the articular surface, the technique described by McElfresh, Dobyns, and O'Brien, allowing active motion of the proximal interphalangeal joint while maintaining the finger in an extension block

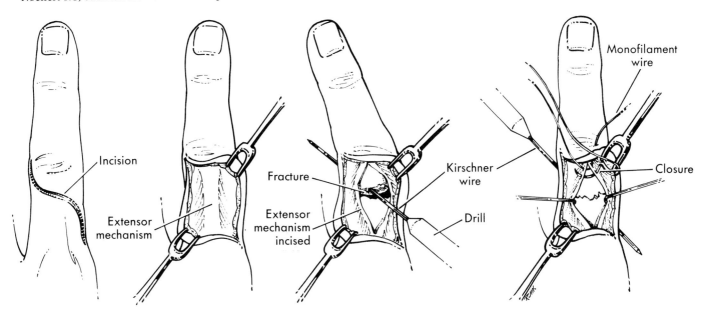

Fig. 64-45 For rare phalangeal shaft fractures that require open reduction, technique of Pratt is useful (see text).

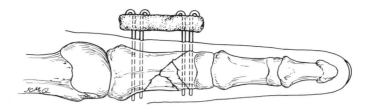

Fig. 64-46   Method for maintaining reduction of comminuted fractures of middle or proximal phalanx by using two or more percutaneous wires. These are externally stabilized by segment of polymethylmethacrylate.

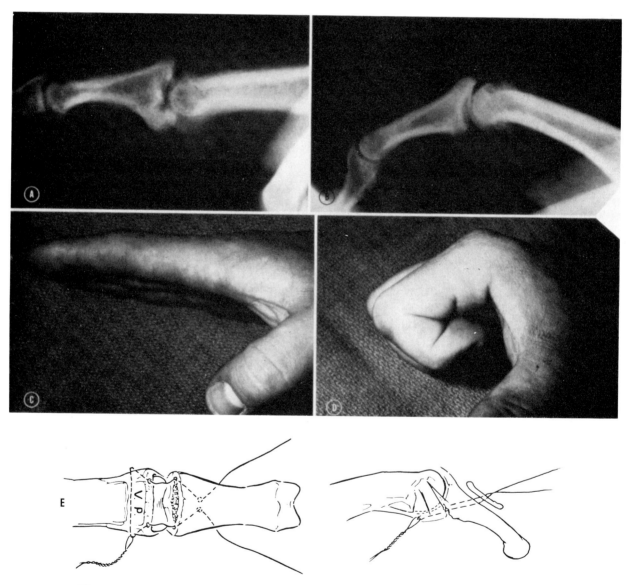

Fig. 64-47   **A,** Roentgenogram 1 year following fracture-dislocation. Patient had pain and only 20 degrees of motion. **B,** Roentgenogram 14 months following arthroplasty. Note smooth, congruous articular arc. **C,** Active extension 14 months after arthroplasty of proximal interphalangeal joint. **D,** Active flexion 14 months after arthroplasty of proximal interphalangeal joint. **E,** Schema of volar plate advancement. (**A** to **D,** From Eaton RG and Malerich MM: J Hand Surg 5:260, 1980.)

splint, gives satisfactory results especially in those without gross displacement. In proximal interphalangeal fracture-dislocations that have a comminuted surface of the proximal phalanx of 40% or less with displacement of fragments (as in persistent dorsal fracture-dislocation with preserved condyles of the proximal phalanx), the method of Eaton and Malerich is recommended. They have used this technique in old healed displaced fractures up to 2 years after injury (Fig. 64-47, *A* to *D*).

CLOSED REDUCTION

■ *TECHNIQUE (McELFRESH, DOBYNS, AND O'BRIEN).* A malleable metal dorsal splint is incorporated in a forearm gauntlet plaster cast so that the involved finger is maintained in flexion at the proximal interphalangeal joint and the metacarpophalangeal joint (Fig. 64-48). Since instability occurs when the proximal interphalangeal joint is extended, the angle at which it occurs can be determined before application of the plaster. The proximal interphalangeal joint should be blocked in flexion 15 degrees short of this demonstrated position of instability. The proximal phalanx must be held securely against the dorsal splint to avoid extension at the proximal interphalangeal joint caused by further flexion of the metacarpophalangeal joint.

AFTERTREATMENT. Immediate flexion motion of the proximal interphalangeal joint is permitted. Full extension is not permitted for 6 to 12 weeks; however, an increased amount of extension may be permitted each week and encouragement is given to increase flexion.

OPEN REDUCTION

■ *TECHNIQUE (EATON AND MALERICH).* Make a volar incision using an elongated **V** with the flap based radially. Excise the flexor tendon sheath from the proximal phalanx sufficiently to allow the tendons to be retracted to one side so as to view the entire joint. Hyperextend the joint to identify the fracture in fresh injuries. The volar plate will still be attached to the bone fragments of the middle phalanx. Detach the accessory collateral ligament from both sides, thus freeing the volar plate. Also detach the bone fragments by sharp dissection at the distal margin of the volar plate. In acute injuries the collateral ligaments and joint capsule need not be incised. Drill two small holes at the extreme margin of a trough created at the middle phalanx by the bone deficit, and possibly by some small carpentry. Place the pull-out wire through each corner of the volar plate and then through the drill holes to emerge dorsally. Place traction on these wires to snug the volar plate into the articular defect, thus effectively resurfacing the joint. Reduction can be maintained by flexing the joint no more than 35 degrees (see Fig. 64-47, *E*). Congruity of reduction should be checked by a roentgenogram. A Kirschner wire is inserted across the joint to maintain reduction. Place the hand and finger in a plaster of Paris cast for 2 weeks.

In old injuries in which the fractures have malunited, the volar plate is divided as far distally as possible. It may be necessary to excise both collateral ligaments. A transverse trough at the proximal edge of the middle phalanx must be created and extended completely across the bone to avoid an angular deformity when attaching the volar plate. The passive motion at the proximal interphalangeal joint should be 110 degrees, so as to easily touch the distal palmar crease with the fingertip. If passive motion is not 110 degrees, perform a dorsal capsular release. Then attach the volar plate as described above.

AFTERTREATMENT. After 2 weeks, the Kirschner wire is removed and active guarded flexion is started with a dorsal block splint (see Fig. 64-48). At 5 weeks, full extension should be accomplished, and

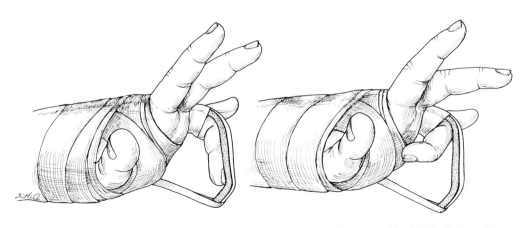

Fig. 64-48 Extension-block splinting (see text). (Redrawn from McElfresh EC, Dobyns JH, and O'Brien ET: J Bone Joint Surg 54-A:1705, 1972.)

if not, a dynamic splint should be used. The pull-out wires can be removed at 3 weeks.

• • •

The following technique is appropriate when the fracture is not comminuted and the fragment is large enough (50% of the articular surface) to be fixed in place by a Kirschner wire.

■ *TECHNIQUE.* Make a midlateral incision (p. 2971) on the proximal interphalangeal joint and divide the transverse retinacular ligament, exposing the collateral ligament and joint capsule. Detach the accessory collateral ligament at its distal insertion and expose the fibrocartilaginous volar plate. Locate the avulsed osseous fragment but preserve its periosteal attachment. Replace the fragment anatomically and fix it in position with the smallest available Kirschner wire inserted in a dorsal direction; draw the wire dorsally until its volar end lies just beneath the articular surface of the fragment and will not interfere with flexion of the joint. Cut off the wire even with the dorsal surface of the phalanx. Then place the joint in functional position and fix it with an obliquely inserted Kirschner wire. Now suture the accessory collateral and transverse retinacular ligaments and close the wound.

When the fracture is a month old or older, osteotomy may be necessary to free the small fragment; then any resulting osseous defect is filled with bone from either the proximal ulna or the volar side of the proximal phalanx. If necessary for reduction of the dislocation, both collateral ligaments may be detached.

AFTERTREATMENT. A pressed-out wet cotton cast is applied and held in place with a Kling bandage. At 3 weeks the transarticular Kirschner wire is removed, and motion is begun slowly.

FORCE-COUPLE SPLINT REDUCTION. Agee has devised an ingenious method for managing unstable fracture-dislocations of the proximal interphalangeal joint using force-couple principles.

■ *TECHNIQUE (AGEE).* The technique depicted in Fig. 64-49, *A* to *L*, was developed on fresh cadaver hands. After inserting and forming the Kirschner wires into a mechanical linkage, a small rubber band is placed with tension adequate to maintain reduction; excessive tension must be avoided. When closed reduction is possible, the force-couple splint may be applied percutaneously, preferably with the patient under digital block anesthesia, thereby allowing the patient to demonstrate the joint's active range of motion. Determine the quality of joint reduction with anteroposterior and lateral roentgenograms of the joint in the flexed position. Examine the flexion and extension lateral roentgenograms closely to assure that the intact dorsal base of the middle phalanx is concentrically reduced as evidenced by its parallel gliding motion with respect to the head of the proximal phalanx. A rocking motion of the middle phalanx on the proximal phalanx is to be avoided because it predisposes to high joint surface pressures and secondary traumatic arthritis as well as recurrent joint subluxation. Unfortunately, a "crisp and clean" gliding action is only possible with acute injuries. The force-couple splint maintains joint reduction during bone and soft tissue healing, thereby minimizing joint stiffness by allowing active range-of-motion exercises. A soft dressing is used for a day or two; then all restricting dressings are removed in favor of an antibiotic ointment that is applied daily to the pins at their exit from the skin.

Adjust the smooth Kirschner wire limbs of the device as needed to keep them centered on the finger, thereby avoiding pressure on the skin. The device is maintained for a minimum of 5 weeks, with advancing degrees of comminution and instability requiring 6 to 8 weeks. Interval roentgenograms are obtained until bone and soft tissue healing is judged to be adequate. The effect of the force couple is then removed by detaching the rubber band; flexion-extension lateral roentgenograms are repeated to confirm joint stability before removal of the force-couple splint. In chronic injuries, perform open reduction with the patient under axillary block anesthesia through a midlateral incision; divide the lateral retinacular ligament along with the dorsal part of the collateral ligament and adjacent joint capsule. Frequently the dorsal side of the opposite collateral lig-

Fig. 64-49   Force-couple splint technique for unstable fracture-dislocation of proximal interphalangeal joint (see text). **A,** Typical unstable fracture-dislocation. **B,** Manual reduction. **C,** Joint line is identified with needle. **D,** Distal Kirschner wire is inserted. **E,** Proximal Kirschner wire is inserted parallel to distal wire. **F,** Threaded Kirschner wire inserted dorsal to palmar cortex in middle phalanx. **G,** Distal wire is bent 90 degrees on each side. **H,** Second 90-degree bend is made in distal wire; hook is bent into end of wire. **I,** Proximal wire is bent 90 degrees palmarly on each side. **J,** Rubber band connects vertical arms of distal wire with threaded pin to create force couple that reduced dislocation. **K,** Completed splint. **L,** Almost full range of active motion of proximal interphalangeal joint is possible. (Redrawn from Agee JM: Clin Orthop 214:101, 1987.)

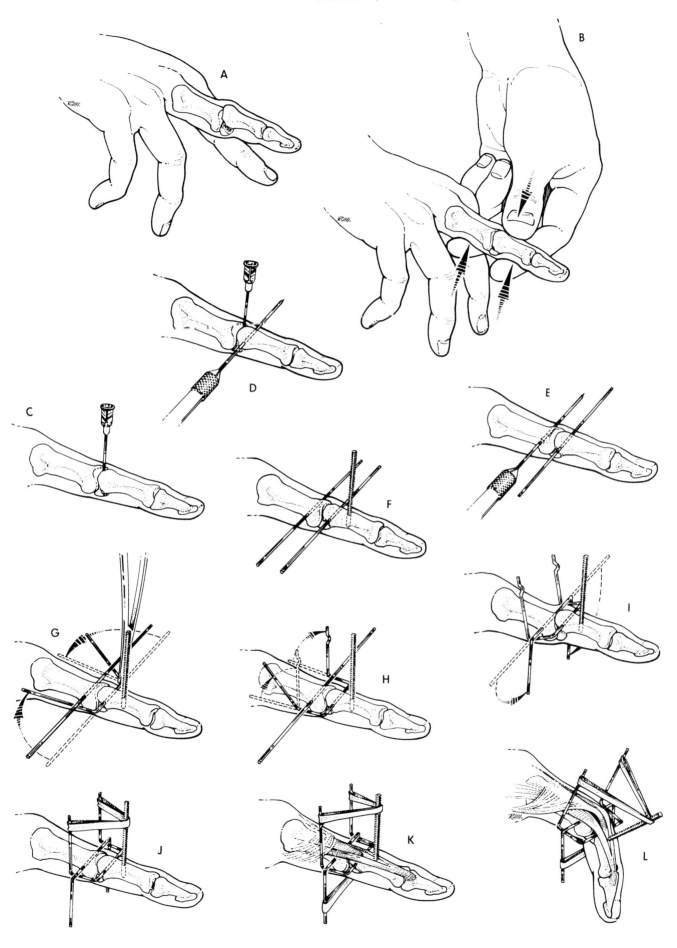

ament must be divided through a separate midlateral incision. Use a probe to free the palmar side of the joint, and a small sharp osteotome to mobilize the avulsed fragment from the palmar base of the middle phalanx; take care to preserve its blood supply. If portions of the collateral ligaments necessary for adequate stability cannot be maintained, the splint cannot be used since it will convert the dorsal dislocation to a palmar one. With adequate reduction of the intact dorsal base of the middle phalanx with respect to the condyles of the proximal phalanx, apply the force-couple splint as depicted in Fig. 64-49, allowing the smooth transverse Kirschner wires to exit through the surgical incision. When possible, repair the soft tissues and, following hemostasis, repair the skin appropriately. Obtain roentgenograms in anteroposterior view, lateral extension, and lateral flexion to evaluate the adequacy of joint reduction. Apply a soft dressing to the finger for several days.

AFTERTREATMENT. To permit active range-of-motion exercises use no dressing and an antibiotic ointment.

Interphalangeal Dislocations

Most interphalangeal dislocations are reduced immediately by the patient or by a bystander (Fig. 64-50). If a collateral ligament is not completely ruptured, joint motion can be reestablished when pain and swelling sub-

side. In a young adult if one or both of the collateral ligaments are completely ruptured, they should be repaired, especially if the ligament is ruptured on the radial side of the index finger. Dorsal dislocations of the proximal interphalangeal joint may usually be reduced manually and closed. Bony or soft tissue obstructions may be a cause of unsuccessful reduction (Fig. 64-51).

UNSTABLE PROXIMAL INTERPHALANGEAL JOINT SECONDARY TO OLD COLLATERAL LIGAMENT RUPTURE. In rare instances the proximal interphalangeal joint may be grossly unstable laterally (floppy), restoration of stability is desired, and arthrodesis is unaccept-

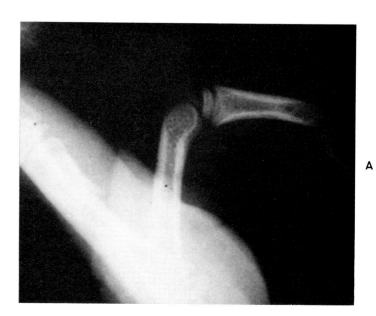

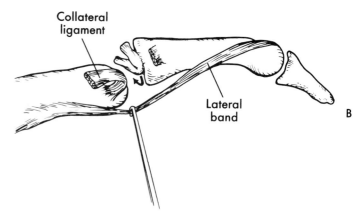

Fig. 64-50 **A** and **B,** Anteroposterior and lateral roentgenograms of fracture-dislocation after patient's self-reduction. **C,** Lateral roentgenogram after operation. (From Baugher WH and McCue FC III: J Bone Joint Surg 61-A:779, 1979.)

Fig. 64-51 **A,** Lateral roentgenogram reveals incongruous articular surface of proximal interphalangeal joint with interposed osseous tissue. **B,** Open reduction revealed rupture of proximal attachment of volar plate, but this is not displaced. Volar half of articular cartilage of middle phalanx was folded on its dorsal half, and dorsal third was detached from subchondral bone. Cartilaginous flap was restored to its anatomic position, permitting full range of passive motion immediately. (From Whipple TL, Evans JP, and Urbaniak JP: J Bone Joint Surg 62-A:832, 1980.)

able. A tendon graft may be used to replace the collateral ligament; stability and a normal range of motion may result. In several of these we have obtained satisfactory results with no loss of motion (Fig. 64-52).

Tendon graft to replace ruptured collateral ligament

■ *TECHNIQUE.* Make a midlateral incision over the proximal interphalangeal joint at the site of the origin and insertion of the cord fibers of the collateral ligament. Incise the transverse retinacular ligament and reflect the extensor mechanism dorsally. Excise any scar tissue from about the origin and insertion of the cord fibers. Drill a hole completely through the bone on each side of the joint (Fig. 64-53). Next obtain the necessary graft material, such as the palmaris longus tendon. Tie a No. 4-0 or 34-gauge wire loop around each end of the graft and bring one end out through one of the holes on the side opposite the injury. Pass the other end of the graft across the joint and through the hole in the other bone in the appropriate direction. Pass each wire loop on the ends of the graft through a piece of felt and then through separate holes in a single button. Pull the graft snug and tie the two wires together over the button. A pull-out suture is not feasible because there is insufficient tendinous material to hold this much suture. Additionally, an accessory collateral ligament may be created if necessary. Section a portion of the tendon sheath on the side opposite the

defect; maintain its insertion into the bone on the side of the involved collateral ligament and fold this fascialike sheath over the grafted tendon. Suture it to the graft with the finger in extension. Now transfix the joint with an oblique Kirschner wire.

AFTERTREATMENT. At 3 weeks remove the Kirschner wire and start motion. Remove the button and wire loop at 4 to 6 weeks.

Repair of ruptured collateral ligament of interphalangeal joint

■ *TECHNIQUE.* Make a lateral incision over the interphalangeal joint and dissect the skin and subcutaneous tissue down to the transverse retinacular ligament. Here dissect carefully underneath the transverse retinacular ligament, cut it longitudinally, and maintain the integrity of its edges for later repair. Now look at the underlying collateral ligament to determine the site of rupture. Inspect the joint for bone fragments or fragments of ligamentous material. Insert a 4-0 monofilament nylon suture proximal to the incision through the skin and into the proximal segment of the collateral ligament. Continue on into the distal segment, make a loop in the distal segment, and then proceed proximally, paralleling the first suture line. Do the same at the distal segment. Tie each of these loop sutures over a felt-padded button outside the skin (Fig. 64-54). Repair

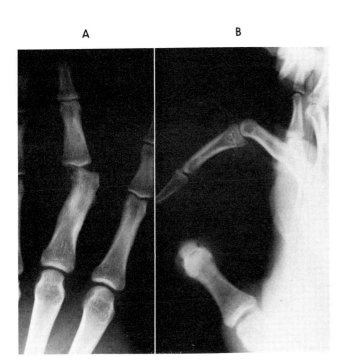

Fig. 64-52   A, Chronically unstable proximal interphalangeal joint permitted tilting and produced pain on pinch. **B,** Alignment by segmental graft from palmaris longus tendon attached through bone.

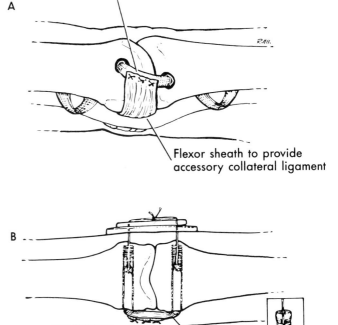

Flexor sheath to provide accessory collateral ligament

Graft

Fig. 64-53   Reconstruction of collateral ligament of proximal interphalangeal joint with tendon graft (see text).

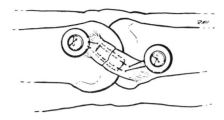

Fig. 64-54 One technique of placing removable 4-0 monofilament nylon sutures in repair of collateral ligament.

the transverse retinacular ligament with a running 4-0 monofilament nylon suture, close the skin, and maintain the finger in a blanket of wet cotton wrapped with gauze in the position of full extension. During the procedure observe whether the volar plate and accessory collateral ligament also are torn; if so, repair them.
AFTERTREATMENT. Begin motion in 2 weeks.

• • •

Rarely a dislocation of the proximal interphalangeal joint is irreducible because a lateral band of the extensor hood becomes trapped within the joint (Fig. 64-55).

UNDIAGNOSED INTERPHALANGEAL DISLOCATIONS. Failure to diagnose interphalangeal dislocations is rare but does occur because swelling soon obscures the landmarks that make early diagnosis easy. If the dislocation is not diagnosed within the first week, joint cartilage may be eroded by pressure from the articular edge of the dislocated phalanx. Open reduction is then usually necessary (Figs. 64-56 to 64-58).

Open reduction and fixation with Kirschner wire

■ *TECHNIQUE.* Make a classic midlateral incision (p. 2971) at the level of the affected interphalangeal joint. Expose the joint, remove the granulation tissue and the remaining hematoma, and reduce the joint under direct vision. Often the volar plate lies between the joint surfaces, and it and both collateral ligaments must be excised. Hold the joint with an oblique Kirschner wire and place the finger in a splint. If at surgery the joint is found to be completely destroyed, it should be arthrodesed immediately.
AFTERTREATMENT. In 2 weeks the wire can be removed and active motion is begun.

FRACTURE OF DISTAL PHALANX. Fractures of the distal phalanx are usually caused by crushing injuries and thus are usually comminuted; they require only splinting. When a circular wound is present that nearly amputates the fingertip, a Kirschner wire is of value in supporting the bone while the soft tissues heal (Fig. 64-59). Prolonged tenderness and hypesthesia of the fingertip after the fracture are results of the injury to the soft tissue, not to the bone.

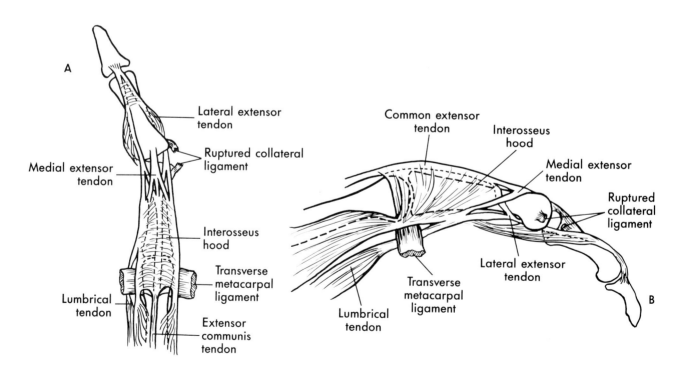

Fig. 64-55 Irreducible dislocation of proximal interphalangeal joint. Collateral ligament has been torn and lateral band of extensor hood has been trapped within joint. **A,** Dorsal view. **B,** Lateral view. (Modified from Johnson FG and Green MH: J Bone Joint Surg 48-A:542, 1966.)

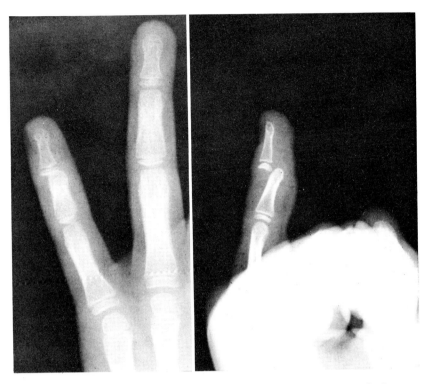

Fig. 64-56 Roentgenograms of interphalangeal dislocation in child. Injury had gone undiagnosed for 1 month because externally the deformity appeared slight. After open reduction, flexion of 30 degrees was eventually possible.

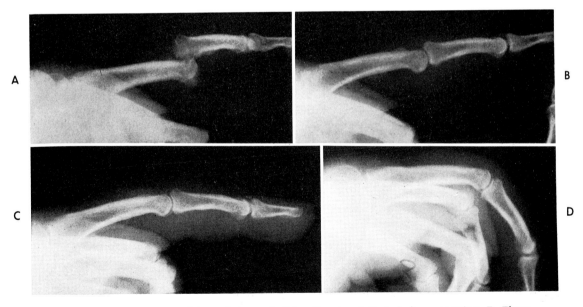

Fig. 64-57 Undiagnosed interphalangeal dislocation in adult **A**, before operation. **B**, Three weeks after open reduction. **C** and **D**, Range of extension and flexion of joint 2 months after surgery.

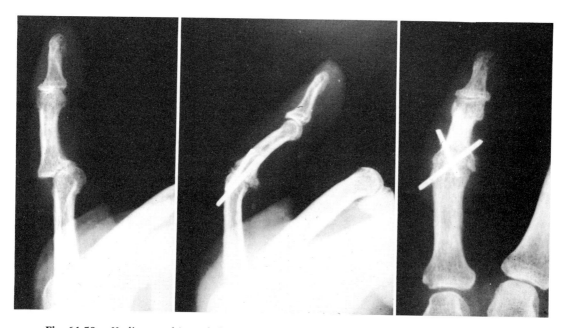

Fig. 64-58   Undiagnosed interphalangeal dislocation in adult complicated by infected wound. Note that bone has been eroded. At 6 weeks after injury, infection had been controlled, and joint was arthrodesed.

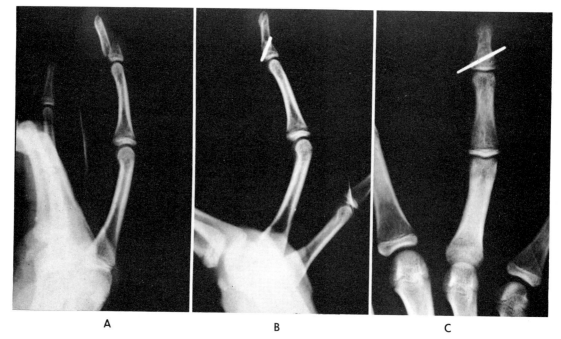

A   B   C

Fig. 64-59   **A**, Compound fracture of a distal phalanx in which fingertip has been almost amputated. **B** and **C**, Fracture has been fixed with a Kirschner wire.

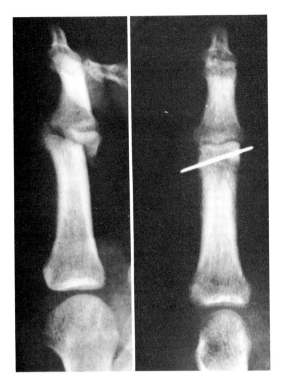

Fig. 64-60 Intraarticular fracture treated by open reduction and fixation with Kirschner wire (see text).

INTRAARTICULAR FRACTURES

See also the discussion of complications of fractures (p. 1470).

Intraarticular fractures with a single fragment involving one third or more of the joint surface usually are accompanied by subluxation and require reduction and fixation with a suture or a Kirschner wire (see "Fracture-dislocation of Proximal Interphalangeal Joint," p. 1459). Closed reduction is sometimes accomplished by flexing the finger and thus apposing the larger fragment to the smaller; the joint is then transfixed with a Kirschner wire. Another closed method is three-point skeletal traction using a vertical traction ring. Open reduction, however, usually is preferred (Fig. 64-60). Drill a Kirschner wire into the smaller fragment, reduce the fracture, and bring the wire out through the larger fragment. Then attach the drill to the opposite end of the wire and extract it until its tip is just beneath the articular cartilage of the smaller fragment. Motion usually can be started at 2 weeks, and the wire can be removed at 4 weeks (Fig. 64-61).

Intraarticular fractures include avulsion fractures at the insertions of tendons and ligaments. The fragments usually are displaced widely by the pull of the tendon or ligament and should be reduced and fixed internally to restore tendon or ligament function as well as joint integrity (Fig. 64-62). When the fragment is small (less

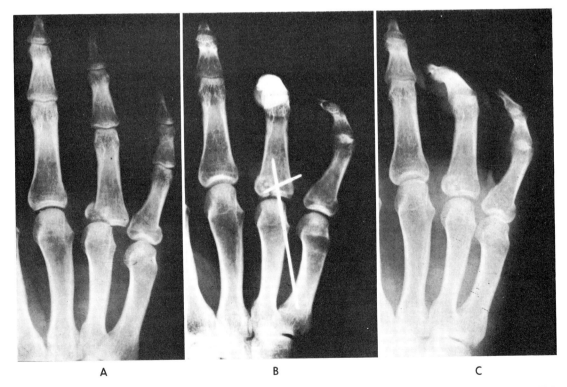

A   B   C

Fig. 64-61 **A,** Impacted intraarticular fracture. **B,** Fracture treated by open reduction and fixation with Kirschner wires. **C,** Result at 4 weeks when wires were removed. Eventually motion only 20 degrees less than normal was restored.

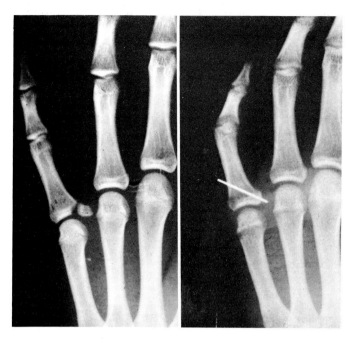

Fig. 64-62 Avulsion fracture of proximal phalanx treated by open reduction and fixation with Kirschner wire.

than one fourth of the joint surface), treatment is directed toward the soft tissue avulsion and may consist of open reduction and splinting or splinting alone in the position of function.

Hemicondylar fractures produced by lateral stress (usually at the proximal interphalangeal joint) require internal fixation if displaced. Open reduction often is necessary, but closed reduction and percutaneous pinning (Fig. 64-63) may be attempted.

COMPLICATIONS OF FRACTURES OF LONG BONES

Complications of fractures include malunion, nonunion, adhesions of tendons to the fracture site, infection (Chapter 78), and limitation of joint motion (see also discussion of reconstruction, Chapter 68).

When multiple tissues must be reconstructed, the repair of bones and joints is third in the order of priority. When good skin coverage is absent, repair will fail, and when the hand is insensitive, repair is futile. Therefore bone and joint reconstruction is indicated only after good skin coverage has been obtained and when at least protective sensation is present or is forthcoming.

Malunion

When fractures of one or more bones of the hand unite in poor position, the resulting disturbance of muscle balance causes weakness of grasp and pinch, especially when the metacarpals and proximal phalanges are involved. The kinesthetic sense also seems to be disturbed. Rotational deformity and angulation cause deviation of the digits that flexion usually increases.

Not every malunited fracture should be treated. It is the function of the fingers and the hand, not the roentgenographic appearance, that determines whether treatment is necessary. Ill-advised treatment usually fails to improve function and sometimes makes it worse. Unless a deformity is gross, it should usually be accepted when motion in the surrounding joints is satisfactory, for treatment by osteotomy may lead not only to nonunion but also to difficulty in reestablishing satisfactory joint motion. This is especially true in patients beyond middle age.

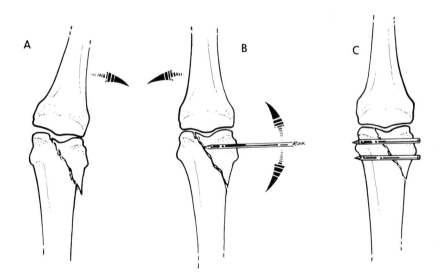

Fig. 64-63 **A,** Displaced unstable condylar fracture usually requires open reduction and fixation. **B,** Manipulation of fracture using intact collateral ligament may permit Kirschner wire insertion to hold reduction. **C,** Two wires may be necessary to avoid rotation of reduced fragment.

Most malunited fractures of the *metacarpal neck* should not be treated, particularly those of the neck of the fifth metacarpal. Flexion deformity of the neck of this bone of 40 degrees can easily be accepted with good function. When the fifth metacarpal head is displaced volarward, the carpometacarpal joint allows dorsal displacement of the distal end of the bone so that the palm can yield when a hard object is grasped; this is also true to a lesser extent of the ring finger. For the second and third metacarpals, however, there is little or no motion in the carpometacarpal joints, and when the head of one of these bones is displaced volarward, it remains as a hard unyielding mass in the palm and may be painful when a firm object is grasped; then treatment is usually indicated. When a metacarpal head is markedly displaced, hyperextension of the metacarpophalangeal joint and secondary contracture of the collateral ligaments often occur; a capsulotomy (Chapter 68) as well as an osteotomy may then be necessary.

CORRECTING MALUNION OF METACARPAL NECK

■ *TECHNIQUE.* Make a longitudinal dorsal incision just proximal and lateral to the metacarpal head; expose the extensor hood and free it on one side of the metacarpal neck with a sharp knife. Dissect the interosseus muscle from the lateral side of the neck and the extensor tendon and expansion from its dorsum as necessary for sufficient exposure. If the callus is hard, drill across the old fracture site transversely; otherwise cut across it with an osteotome. Drill the medullary canal proximally and distally so that it will accept a medullary cortical bone peg a little larger than a matchstick. The peg may be obtained from the proximal ulna or proximal tibia. Insert it proximally into the medullary canal of the shaft; then cap it with the metacarpal head. Carefully check rotational alignment and then impact the fragments. Pack cancellous bone chips about their juncture as needed. When the osteotomy is unstable despite the bone peg, insert a Kirschner wire obliquely across it (Fig. 64-64). Next examine the metacarpophalangeal joint for passive flexion; when the collateral ligaments are contracted and allow little or no motion, capsulotomy (Chapter 68) may be indicated. Now suture the lateral expansion of the extensor hood in place with fine suture. Hold the finger in moderate flexion at all joints and apply a volar splint.

AFTERTREATMENT. A dorsal splint is worn for 2 weeks to maintain the metacarpophalangeal joints in 70 degrees of flexion and the interphalangeal joints in moderate flexion, allowing some flexion of the interphalangeal joints but preventing extension of the metacarpophalangeal joints. Sutures are removed at 2 weeks, and a lighter splint is applied to prevent extension of the metacarpophalangeal joint but allow flexion and extension of the interphalangeal joints. This splint is worn an additional 1 or

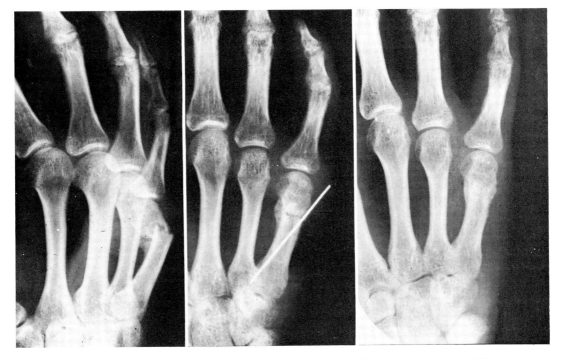

Fig. 64-64   Malunited fracture of fifth metacarpal neck treated by open reduction and fixation with one Kirschner wire inserted obliquely. This is rarely necessary because the normal motion of the fifth carpometacarpal joint permits tolerance of up to 30 degrees of angulation at fracture site.

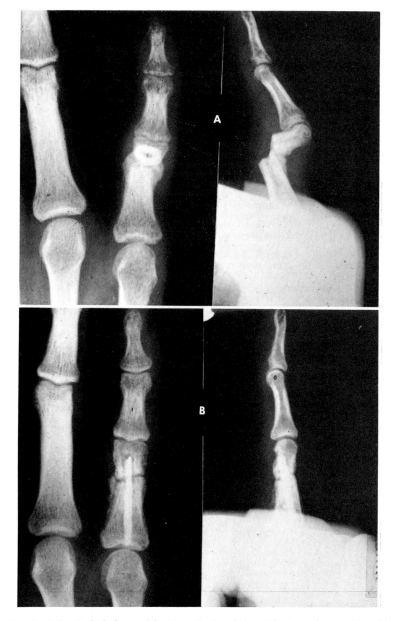

Fig. 64-65 **A,** Malunited phalangeal fracture. **B,** Result is satifactory after treatment by osteotomy and fixation with medullary bone peg.

2 weeks or until postoperative reaction has subsided.

• • •

Malunion of a metacarpal shaft or of a phalanx also may be treated with a medullary cortical bone peg; the peg must be shaped carefully to fit snugly (Fig. 64-65). Figs. 64-66 and 64-67 illustrate malunited phalangeal fractures treated by osteotomy and fixation with Kirschner wires.

Malrotation of a proximal phalanx at any level should be treated by osteotomy at the base of the phalanx. The base of the phalanx heals quite well and is cut with less difficulty than the hard cortical bone in the middle third.

It is important to make an orientation mark on each side of the proposed osteotomy line so that these reference points can be used to determine when rotation is corrected.

Nonunion

Nonunion in the *phalanges* is caused most often by distraction of the fragments by traction (Fig. 64-68); other causes are infection, lack of fixation, and bone loss. When the nonunion is associated with nerve and tendon injuries that severely impair function, amputation must be considered; this is true especially when only one finger is involved. Nonunions of comminuted

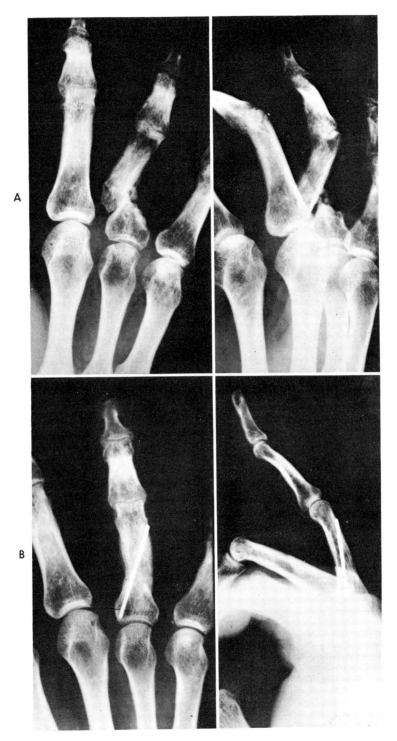

Fig. 64-66   **A**, Malunited phalangeal fracture in which fragments are severely displaced. **B**, After treatment by osteotomy and fixation with Kirschner wire.

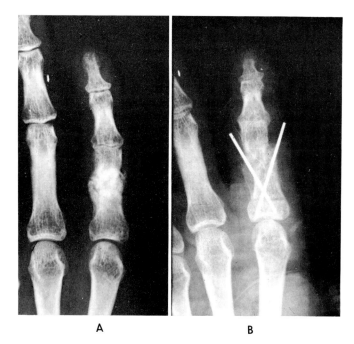

A   B

Fig. 64-67 **A**, Malunited phalangeal fracture with rotational deformity. **B**, After treatment by osteotomy through proximal end of bone and fixation with two Kirschner wires. Healing is usually more rapid after osteotomy at this level than after one at old fracture.

fractures of the tuft of the distal phalanx usually require no treatment; the fragments commonly unite or finally are absorbed. (These fractures are often the result of a crushing injury, and any local pain is evoked by the soft tissue injury, not by the presence of small bone fragments.)

Nonunions of transverse fractures of the distal phalanx, however, may require surgical treatment to obtain union when they are painful. The differentiation between pain from the nonunion and pain from scar tissue about nerve endings obviously is important. Lateral bending stress on the nonunion site should cause pain

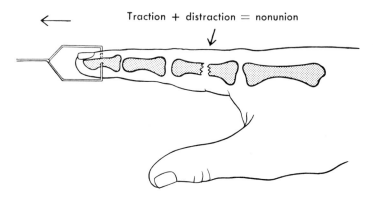

Traction + distraction = nonunion

Fig. 64-68 Nonunion of phalanx is most often caused by distraction of fragments by traction.

from a symptomatic nonunion. Simple tapping of the finger tuft when the nerve endings are tightly bound with dense scar tissue should cause pain similar to that of a neuroma.

Nonunion in the *metacarpals* is most often produced by bone loss. For a nonunion in which no bone substance is lost, the technique of repair is the same as that just described for malunion. For one in which bone substance is lost, Littler's method is recommended (Fig. 64-69).

CORRECTING NONUNION OF METACARPALS

■ *TECHNIQUE (LITTLER)*. Success of bone grafting to replace a metacarpal defect and thus to restore normal architecture and function depends on two precautions. First, the dorsum of the hand must be well covered by skin and subcutaneous tissue, even if an abdominal pedicle flap is required (p. 1443). Second, the fine details of what Bunnell called "bone carpentry" must be exact for the recipient bone is too small for ordinary plates and screws and fixation of the graft depends on exactitude of size and fit. Very small plates and screws such as the AO minifragment set are available. They may serve adequately for internal fixation. Expose the defective metacarpal with a longitudinal or curved dorsal incision, depending on location of existing scars. Dissect all scar tissue from the extensor tendons, but preserve the paratenon intact. Dissect the fibrous tissue en bloc from between the fragments so that traction can restore normal finger length. Usually the proximal fragment must be sacrificed as far as its base; resect it with an osteotome at an angle of 30 degrees (Fig. 64-70) that makes a recess in the bone. Cut the end of the distal fragment transversely with a circular saw or rongeur and open the medullary canal to receive the doweled end of the graft.

With traction on the finger, measure exactly the defect between the fragments and take from the tibia a graft at least 1.3 cm longer than the estimated defect. Fashion a dowel at one end of the graft and cut the other end obliquely at 30 degrees. Insert the doweled end into the medullary canal of the distal fragment and press the proximal end into the prepared metacarpal or carpal recess. Compression of the graft between the two fragments will hold it in place. If necessary, stabilize the graft by passing one or more Kirschner wires through it and into adjacent uninvolved metacarpals. Close the periosteal sheath, if present, and the soft tissues over the graft with fine sutures.

AFTERTREATMENT. With the hand in the position of function, a plaster cast is applied that extends to the proximal interphalangeal joints. This cast is then immediately split to allow for postoperative swelling. On about the twelfth day a new cast is applied that immobilizes only the grafted metacarpal and

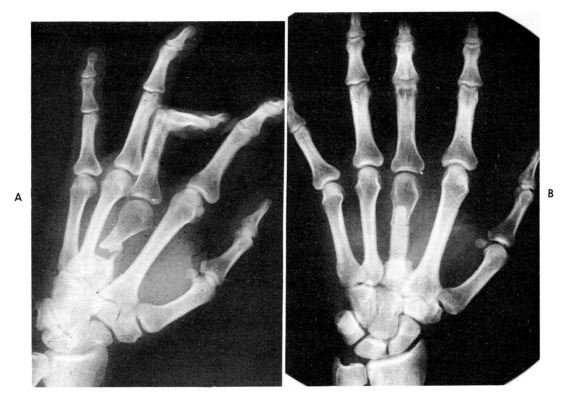

Fig. 64-69   **A**, Metacarpal nonunion in which bone substance has been lost. **B**, After grafting by Littler technique. (From Littler JW: J Bone Joint Surg 29:723, 1947.)

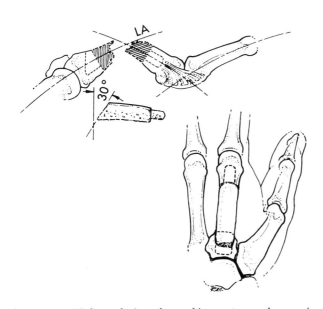

Fig. 64-70   Littler technique for grafting metacarpal nonunion in which bone substance has been lost (see text). (Courtesy Dr. JW Littler.)

the proximal phalanx; it is left in place for 2 months. Administration of prophylactic antibiotics just before or during surgery should be considered, and an antibiotic should be given for several days after surgery since the injury producing the bone defect is always open. Thus the region is potentially infected even though the original wound has healed.

REFERENCES

General

Barton N: Internal fixation of hand fractures, J Hand Surg 14-B:139, 1989 (editorial).

Friedmann E: Rupture of collateral ligaments of the hands, Orthop Rev 5:51, May 1976.

Harvey FJ and Hume KF: Spontaneous recurrent ulnar dislocation of the long extensor tendons of the fingers, J Hand Surg 5:492, 1980.

McCue FC III, Baugher WH, Kulund DN, and Gieck JH: Hand and wrist injuries in the athlete, Am J Sports Med 7:275, 1979.

Wheeldon FT: Recurrent dislocation of extensor tendons in the hand, J Bone Joint Surg 36-B:612, 1954.

Wiley AM and Dommisse I: Disabilities following basal fractures and dislocations of the ulnar border of the hand, Orthop Rev 5:43, May 1976.

Thumb

Ahmad I and DePalma AF: Treatment of game-keeper's thumb by a new operation, Clin Orthop 103:167, 1974.

Bennett EH: Fractures of the metacarpal bones, Dublin J Med Sci 73:72, 1882.

Bowers WH and Hurst LC: Gamekeeper's thumb: evaluation by arthrography and stress roentgenography, J Bone Joint Surg 59-A:519, 1977.

Camp RA, Weatherwax RJ, and Miller EB: Chronic posttraumatic radial instability of the thumb metacarpophalangeal joint, J Hand Surg 5:221, 1980.

Cho KO: Translocation of the abductor pollicis longus tendon: a treatment for chronic subluxation of the thumb carpometacarpal joint, J Bone Joint Surg 52-A:1166, 1970.

Dunn EJ: Gamekeeper's thumb, Orthop Rev 2:52, November 1973.

Dutton RO and Meals RA: Complex dorsal dislocation of the thumb metacarpophalangeal joint, Clin Orthop 164:160, 1982.

Eaton RG and Littler JW: Ligament reconstruction for the painful thumb carpometacarpal joint, J Bone Joint Surg 55-A:1655, 1973.

Farabeuf LHF: De la luxation du ponce en arriere, Bull Soc Chir 11:21, 1876.

Foster RJ and Hastings H II: Treatment of Bennett, Rolando, and vertical intraarticular trapezial fractures, Clin Orthop 214:121, 1987.

Gedda KO: Studies on Bennett's fracture: anatomy, roentgenology, and therapy, Acta Chir Scand [Suppl] 193:1, 1954.

Greenfield GQ Jr: Dislocation of the interphalangeal joint of the thumb, J Trauma 21:901, 1981.

Gunther SF and Zielinski CJ: Irreducible palmar dislocation of the proximal phalanx of the thumb: case report, J Hand Surg 7:515, 1982.

Howard FM: Fractures of the basal joint of the thumb, Clin Orthop 220:46, 1987.

Kaplan EB: The pathology and treatment of radial subluxation of the thumb with ulnar displacement of the head of the first metacarpal, J Bone Joint Surg 43-A:541, 1961.

Kessler I: A simplified technique to correct hyperextension deformity of the metacarpophalangeal joint of the thumb, J Bone Joint Surg 61-A:903, 1979.

Levy IM and Liberty S: Simultaneous dislocation of the interphalangeal and metacarpophalangeal joints of the thumb: a case report, J Hand Surg 4:489, 1979.

McCue FC III et al: The coach's finger, J Sports Med 2:270, 1974.

McCue FC III et al: Ulnar collateral ligament injuries of the thumb in athletes, J Sports Med 2:70, 1974.

Moberg E: The use of traction treatment for fractures of phalanges and metacarpals, Acta Chir Scand 99:341, 1949-50.

Moberg E: Fractures and ligamentous injuries of the thumb and fingers, Surg Clin North Am 40:297, 1960.

Moore JR, Webb CA Jr, and Thompson RC: A complete dislocation of the thumb metacarpal, J Hand Surg 3:547, 1978.

Morgan JV and Lavalette R: Arthrography for MCP joint injuries of the thumb, Techn Orthopaed 1:27, 1986.

Neviaser RJ et al: Rupture of the ulnar collateral ligament of the thumb (gamekeeper's thumb): correction by dynamic repair, J Bone Joint Surg 53-A:1357, 1971.

Osterman AL, Hayken GD, and Bora FW Jr: A quantitative evaluation of thumb function after ulnar collateral repair and reconstruction, J Trauma 21:854, 1981.

Resnick D and Danzig LA: Arthographic evauation of injuries of the first metacarpophalangeal joint: gamekeeper's thumb, Am J Roentgenol Radium Ther Nucl Med 126:1046, 1976.

Rolando S: Fracture de la base du premier metacarpien, et principalement sur une variete non encore decrite, Presse Med 33:303, 1910.

Rovere GD et al: Treatment of "gamekeeper's thumb" in hockey players, J Sports Med 3:147, 1975.

Sakellarides HT and DeWeese JW: Instability of the metacarpophalangeal joint of the thumb: reconstruction of the collateral ligaments using the extensor pollicis brevis tendon, J Bone Joint Surg 58-A:106, 1976.

Salamon PB and Gelberman RH: Irreducible dislocation of the interphalangeal joint of the thumb: report of three cases, J Bone Joint Surg 60-A:400, 1978.

Schultz RJ: Fracture eponym of the month: Rolando's fracture, Surg Rounds Orthop, p 32, November 1988.

Smith RJ: Posttraumatic instability of the metacarpophalangeal joint of the thumb, J Bone Joint Surg 59-A:14, 1977.

Solonen KA: Rupture of the ulnar collateral ligament of the metacarpophalangeal joint of the thumb, Int Surg 45:669, 1966.

Stener B: Displacement of the ruptured ulnar collateral ligament of the metacarpophalangeal joint of the thumb: a clinical and anatomical study, J Bone Joint Surg 44-B:869, 1962.

Stener B: Hyperextension injuries to the metacarpophalangeal joint of the thumb: rupture of ligaments, fracture of sesamoid bones, rupture of flexor pollicis brevis: an anatomical and clinical study, Acta Chir Scand 125:275, 1963.

Stener B: Skeletal injuries associated with rupture of the ulnar collateral ligament of the metacarpophalangeal joint of the thumb: a clinical anatomical study, Acta Chir Scand 125:583, 1963.

Strandell G: Total rupture of the ulnar collateral ligament of the metacarpophalangeal joint of the thumb: results of surgery in 35 cases, Acta Chir Scand 118:72, 1959.

Wagner CJ: Methods of treatment of Bennett's fracture-dislocation, Am J Surg 80:230, 1950.

Wagner CJ: Trans-articular fixation of fracture-dislocations of the first metacarpal joint, West J Surg Obstet Gynecol 59:362, 1951.

Zilberman Z, Rotschild E, and Krauss L: Rupture of the ulnar collateral ligament of the thumb, J Trauma 5:477, 1965.

Metacarpals and phalangeals (excluding thumb)

Adler GA and Light TR: Simultaneous complex dislocation of the metacarpophalangeal joints of the long and index fingers, J Bone Joint Surg 63-A:1007, 1981.

Agee JM: Unstable fracture dislocations of the proximal interphalangeal joint of the fingers: a preliminary report of a new treatment technique, J Hand Surg 3:386, 1978.

Agee JM: Unstable fracture dislocations of the proximal interphalangeal joint: treatment with the force couple splint, Clin Orthop 214:101, 1987.

Baldwin LW et al: Metacarpophalangeal-joint dislocations of the fingers, J Bone Joint Surg 49-A:1587, 1967.

Barash HL: An unusual case of dorsal dislocation of the metacarpophalangeal joint of the index finger, Clin Orthop 83:121, 1972.

Barenfeld PA and Weseley MS: Dorsal dislocation of the metacarpophalangeal joint of the index finger treated by late open reduction: a case report, J Bone Joint Surg 54-A:1311, 1972.

Baugher WH and McCue FC III: Anterior fracture-dislocation of the proximal interphalangeal joint: a case report, J Bone Joint Surg 61-A:779, 1979.

Becton JL et al: A simplified technique for treating the complex dislocation of the index metacarpophalangeal joint, J Bone Joint Surg 57-A:698, 1975.

Belsole RJ and Greene TL: The configuration of tension-band wires in hand fractures: the "sidewinder technique," Techniques Orthopaed 1:5, 1986.

Bohart PG, Gelberman RH, Vandell RF, and Salamon PB: Complex dislocations of the metacarpophalangeal joint, Clin Orthop 164:208, 1982.

Bora FW Jr and Didizian NH: The treatment of injuries to the carpometacarpal joint of the little finger, J Bone Joint Surg 56-A:1459, 1974.

Bowers WH: The proximal interphalangeal joint volar plate. II. A clinical study of hyperextension injury, J Hand Surg 6:77, 1981.

Bowers WH and Fajgenbaum DM: Closed rupture of the volar plate of the distal interphalangeal joint, J Bone Joint Surg 61-A:146, 1979.

Büchler U and Fischer T: Use of a minicondylar plate for metacarpal and phalangeal periarticular injuries, Clin Orthop 214:53, 1987.

Charendoff MD: Locking of the metacarpophalangeal joint: a case report, J Hand Surg 4:173, 1979.

Clendenin MB and Smith RJ: Fifth metacarpal/hamate arthrodesis for posttraumatic osteoarthritis, J Hand Surg 9-A:374, 1984.

Cunningham DM and Schwarz G: Dorsal dislocation of the index metacarpophalangeal joint, Plast Reconstr Surg 56:654, 1975.

Donaldson WR and Millender LH: Chronic fracture-subluxation of the proximal interphalangeal joint, J Hand Surg 3:149, 1978.

Dray G, Millender LH, and Nalebuff EA: Rupture of the radial collateral ligament of a metacarpophalangeal joint to one of the ulnar three fingers, J Hand Surg 4:346, 1978.

Eaton RG and Malerich MM: Volar plate arthroplasty for the proximal interphalangeal joint: a ten year review, J Hand Surg 5:260, 1980.

Espinosa RH and Renart IP: Simultaneous dislocation of the interphalangeal joints in a finger, J Hand Surg 5:617, 1980.

Giannikas AC et al: Dorsal dislocation of the first metatarso-phalangeal joint: report of four cases, J Bone Joint Surg 57-B:384, 1975.

Green DP and Terry GC: Complex dislocation of the metacarpophalangeal joint: correlative pathological anatomy, J Bone Joint Surg 55-A:1480, 1973.

Greene TL, Noellert RC, and Belsole RJ: Treatment of unstable metacarpal and phalangeal fractures with tension band wiring techniques, Clin Orthop 214:78, 1987.

Harwin SF, Fox JM, and Sedlin ED: Volar dislocation of the bases of the second and third metacarpals: a case report, J Bone Joint Surg 57-A:849, 1975.

Hastings H II: Unstable metacarpal and phalangeal fracture treatment with screws and plates, Clin Orthop 214:37, 1987.

Henderson JJ and Arafa MAM: Carpometacarpal dislocation: an easily missed diagnosis, J Bone Joint Surg 69-B:212, 1987.

Hsu JD and Curtis RM: Carpometacarpal dislocations on the ulnar side of the hand, J Bone Joint Surg 52-A:927, 1970.

Iftikhar TB: Long flexor tendon entrapment causing open irreducible dorsoradial dislocation of distal interphalangeal joint of the finger, Orthop Rev 11:117, 1982.

Iftikhar TB and Kaminski RS: Simultaneous dorsal dislocation of MP joints of long and ring fingers, Orthop Rev 10:71, 1981.

Imbriglia JE: Chronic dorsal carpometacarpal dislocation of the index, middle, ring, and little fingers: a case report, J Hand Surg 4:343, 1979.

Johnson FG and Greene MH: Another cause of irreducible dislocation of the proximal interphalangeal joint of a finger: a case report, J Bone Joint Surg 48-A:542, 1966.

Joseph RB et al: Chronic sprains of the carpometacarpal joints, J Hand Surg 6:172, 1981.

Jupiter JB and Sheppard JE: Tension wire fixation of avulsion fractures in the hand, Clin Orthop 214:113, 1987.

Kaplan EB: Dorsal dislocation of the metacarpophalangeal joint of the index finger, J Bone Joint Surg 39-A:1081, 1957.

Kleinman WB and Grantham SA: Multiple volar carpometacarpal joint dislocation: case report of traumatic volar dislocation of the medial four carpometacarpal joints in a child and review of the literature, J Hand Surg 3:377, 1978.

Krishnan SG: Double dislocation of a finger: case report, Am J Sports Med 7:204, 1979.

Lewis HH: Dislocation of the second metacarpal: report of a case, Clin Orthop 93:253, 1973.

Littler JW: Metacarpal reconstruction, J Bone Joint Surg 29:723, 1947.

McCarthy LJ: Open metacarpophalangeal dislocations of the index, middle, ring, and little fingers, J Trauma 20:183, 1980.

McCue FC III, Honner R, Johnson MC Jr, and Gieck JH: Athletic injuries of the proximal interphalangeal joint requiring surgical treatment, J Bone Joint Surg 52-A:937, 1970.

McElfresh EC, Dobyns JH, and O'Brien ET: Management of fracture-dislocation of the proximal interphalangeal joint, Clin Orthop 158:215, 1981.

Milford L: The hand: fractures and dislocations. In Crenshaw AH, editor: Campbell's operative orthopaedics, ed 7, St Louis, 1987, Mosby–Year Book, Inc.

Miller PR, Evans BW, and Glazer DA: Locked dislocation of the metacarpophalangeal joint of the index finger, JAMA 203:300, 1968.

Moneim MS: Volar dislocation of the metacarpophalangeal joint, Clin Orthop 176:186, 1983.

Murphy AF and Stark HH: Closed dislocation of the metacarpophalangeal joint of the index finger, J Bone Joint Surg 49-A:1579, 1967.

Namba RS, Kabo JM, and Meals RA: Biomechanical effects of point configuration in Kirschner-wire fixation, Clin Orthop 214:19, 1987.

North ER and Eaton RG: Volar dislocation of the fifth metacarpal: report of two cases, J Bone Joint Surg 62-A:657, 1980.

Palmer AK and Linscheid RL: Irreducible dorsal dislocation of the distal interphalangeal joint of the finger, J Hand Surg 2:406, 1977.

Palmer AK and Linscheid RL: Chronic recurrent dislocation of the proximal interphalangeal joint of the finger, J Hand Surg 3:95, 1978.

Phillips JH: Irreducible dislocation of a distal interphalangeal joint: case report and review of literature, Clin Orthop 154:188, 1981.

Portis RB: Hyperextensibility of the proximal interphalangeal joint of the finger following trauma, J Bone Joint Surg 36-A:1141, 1954.

Posner MA and Wilenski M: Irreducible volar dislocation of the proximal interphalangeal joint of a finger caused by interposition of an intact central slip: a case report, J Bone Joint Surg 60-A:133, 1978.

Pratt DR: Exposing fractures of the proximal phalanx of the finger longitudinally through the dorsal extensor apparatus, Clin Orthop 15:22, 1959.

Rayan GM and Elias LS: Irreducible dislocation of the distal interphalangeal joint caused by long flexor tendon entrapment, Orthopedics 4:37, 1981.

Rayan GM and Grana WA: Angular deformity of the middle fingers in a young athlete: case report, Am J Sports Med 10:51, 1982.

Ron D, Alkalay D, and Torok G: Simultaneous closed dislocation of both interphalangeal joints in one finger, J Trauma 23:66, 1982.

Schutt RC, Boswick JA Jr, and Scott FA: Volar fracture-dislocation of the carpometacarpal joint of the index finger treated by delayed open reduction, J Trauma 21:986, 1981.

Selig S and Schein A: Irreducible buttonhole dislocations of the fingers, J Bone Joint Surg 22:436, 1940.

Smith RS, Alonso J, and Horowitz M: External fixation of open comminuted fractures of the proximal phalanx, Orthop Rev 16:937, 1987.

Stern PJ, Wieser MJ, and Reilly DG: Complications of plate fixation in the hand skeleton, Clin Orthop 214:59, 1987.

Watson FM Jr: Simultaneous interphalangeal dislocation in one finger, J Trauma 23:65, 1982.

Waugh RL and Yancey AG: Carpometacarpal dislocations: with particular reference to simultaneous dislocation of the bases of the fourth and fifth metacarpals, J Bone Joint Surg 30-A:397, 1948.

Weeks PM: Volar approach for metacarpophalangeal joint capsulotomy, Plast Reconstr Surg 46:473, 1970.

Whipple TL, Evans JP, and Urbaniak JR: Irreducible dislocation of a finger joint in a child, J Bone Joint Surg 62-A:832, 1980.

Wiggins HE, Bundens WD Jr, and Park BJ: A method of treatment of fracture-dislocation of the first metacarpal bone, J Bone Joint Surg 36-A:810, 1954.

Wilson JN and Rowland SA: Fracture-dislocation of the proximal interphalangeal joint of the finger: treatment by open reduction and internal fixation, J Bone Joint Surg 48-A:493, 1966.

Wood MB and Dobyns JH: Chronic, complex volar dislocations of the metacarpophalangeal joint, J Hand Surg 6:73, 1981.

Zielinski CJ: Irreducible fracture-dislocation of the distal interphalangeal joint, J Bone Joint Surg 65-A:109, 1983.

Zimmerman NB and Weiland AJ: Ninety-ninety intraosseous wiring for internal fixation of the digital skeleton, Orthopedics 12:99, 1989.

Nerve Injuries

PHILLIP E. WRIGHT II*

This chapter includes the essentials of treatment of nerve injuries in the digits, palm, and wrist. Although many of the principles discussed in this chapter may be applied to injuries in the forearm and arm, more detailed discussions of more proximal nerve injuries may be found in the chapter on peripheral nerve injuries (Chapter 45). Nerve entrapments and compression neuropathies also are discussed in detail in Chapter 45. Reconstructive procedures including tendon transfers are discussed in Chapter 70 and an expansion of the discussion of microsurgical technique can be found in Chapter 49.

EVALUATION
Preoperative Assessment

At times it is difficult to evaluate the extent of nerve injury in the hand. Factors that interfere with the examination of the nerves in the hand include other injuries that may be life- or limb-threatening, patient intoxication, anxiety or lack of cooperation of the patient, and the presence of the injury in a child. These factors and others, including an extensive injury to the hand, may cause nerve injuries to be overlooked during the initial or preliminary examination. If the conditions are not satisfactory for a thorough examination during the initial evaluation, the hand should be reexamined within a reasonable period to determine the extent of nerve and other injuries to the hand. An injury to the digital nerves frequently is overlooked; however, it is worthwhile re-

membering that if a flexor tendon function deficit is present after a finger laceration, then at least one digital nerve probably has been injured as well; a high index of suspicion is necessary in the evaluation of patients with hand injuries. At least four areas of consideration are important when evaluating a patient with an injury to a nerve in the hand. These include (1) type of injury, (2) sensibility evaluation, (3) motor testing, and (4) sudomotor function evaluation (sweating).

TYPE OF INJURY. Nerve injuries seen in a civilian practice commonly are caused by one of several mechanisms, including direct trauma (blow to the limb, fracture, missile wound), laceration, traction or stretching, and entrapment or compression. To help determine the type of treatment and to arrive at tentative prognostic projections, it is helpful to recall the classification of nerve injuries according to Seddon and Sunderland (Table 65-1). Whereas common injuries such as bumping the "funny bone" (ulnar nerve at the elbow) fall easily into neurapraxia, or type I, injuries, and lacerations fall easily into type V, or neurotmesis, injuries, closed injuries with partial nerve deficits are not classified as easily and the prognosis may not be as well defined. The extent to which the nature of the injuring agent determines primary and secondary repair is discussed under those respective headings (p. 3111). Additional discussion of extent of injury may be found in Chapter 45.

SENSIBILITY. When evaluating the injured hand for sensibility, in addition to an awareness of the classic sensory distribution of the median, radial, and ulnar nerves

---

*Revision of chapter by Lee W. Milford, M.D.

Table 65-1 Classification of nerve injury

Seddon	Sunderland (degree)	
Neuropraxia	I	VI
Axonotomesis	II	(combination
	III	of any of
	IV	Sunderland
Neurotemesis	V	(I - V))

From MacKinnon SF and Dellon AL: Surgery of the peripheral nerve, New York, 1988, Thieme Medical Publishers, Inc.

(Fig. 65-1), it is helpful to recall the autonomous sensory distributions of the median, radial, and ulnar nerves in the volar pulp of the index finger, the volar pulp of the little finger, and thumb-index web space, respectively. If the injury is a laceration and the nerve has been transected, the examination usually is more definitive than in closed injuries or in lacerations the depth of which may not be fully known. Even if a wound is to be explored to determine the extent of the nerve injury, it is helpful to document the clinical deficit before surgical exploration. Careful evaluation, especially in the presence of a closed injury, will define the initial deficit, allowing for assessment of progress if observation of the injury is elected rather than exploration of the nerve. The use of a sharp pin to assess pain, a cotton-tipped applicator or a finger eraser to assess light touch, and the tips of a paper clip or commercially prepared tool to assess two-point discrimination are the customary methods used to evaluate damaged sensory nerves. The normal two-point discrimination usually is 6 mm or less. If the nerve is transected the patient will not feel light touch, he will not appreciate the pin as a sharp stimulus, and he will be unable to discriminate between one and two points. Patients with closed injuries or partial injuries to nerves may demonstrate spotty appreciation of light touch and pain and will have markedly widened two-point discrimination (Fig. 65-2).

MOTOR. Although the function in the hand served by the underlying *median nerve* includes the proximally innervated pronater teres, flexor carpi radialis, palmaris longus, flexor digitorum sublimis, flexor digitorum profundus, flexor pollicis longus, and pronator quadratus, the usual median-innervated muscles of concern in the hand include the lumbricals to the index and long fingers, the opponens pollicis, the abductor pollicis brevis, and the superficial portion of the flexor pollicis brevis. The single median-nerve–mediated motor function that usually is checked is apposition of the tip of the thumb to the pulp of the ring finger or little finger with palpation of active contraction of the abductor pollicis brevis muscle belly to supplement the visual inspection. Anatomic variations that cause cross-innervation of the mus-

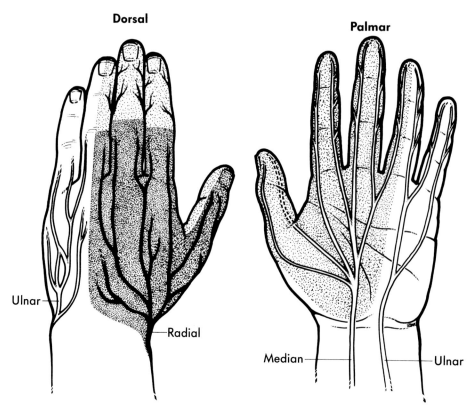

Fig. 65-1 Distribution of major nerves innervating hand for sensory function. (From American Society for Surgery of the Hand: The hand: examination and diagnosis, New York, 1983, Churchill Livingstone.)

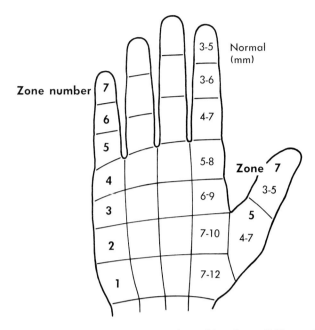

Fig. 65-2   Two-point discrimination of hand sensibility, palmar surface. Dorsal surface averages from 7 mm distally to 12 mm proximally.

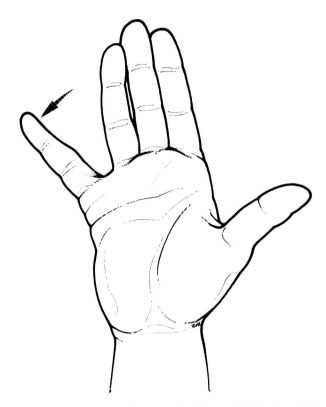

Fig. 65-3   Testing of function of abductor digiti minimi. Patient abducts little finger against resistance, while muscle belly is palpated. (From American Society for Surgery of the Hand: The hand: examination and diagnosis, New York, 1983, Churchill Livingstone.)

cles usually innervated by the median nerve should be kept in mind.

The muscles proximally innervated by the *ulnar nerve* include the flexor carpi ulnaris and flexor digitorum profundus tendons to the ring and little fingers. In the hand, the ulnar-innervated muscles of interest include the flexor pollicis brevis, adductor pollicis, adductor digiti minimi, flexor digiti minimi, opponens digiti minimi, and all of the interosseus muscles. When testing for motor function of the ulnar nerve in the hand, the usual motions mediated by the ulnar intrinsic muscles include active abduction of the middle finger from the ulnar to the radial side with the palm resting on a flat surface. This motion should be observed carefully to exclude the function of the long flexor tendons, which will tend to converge the digits and confuse accurate interpretation of the function of the volar interosseus muscles, and the long extensor tendons, which will tend to diverge the fingers and confuse accurate interpretation of the dorsal interosseus muscles. Additionally, thumb adduction usually is tested by having the patient maintain a piece of paper tightly in the thumb-index web, squeezing the paper between the thumb interphalangeal joint and the base of the index finger proximal phalanx. If the adductor is weak or paralyzed, the patient will be unable to hold the piece of paper against resistance. The function of the abductor digiti minimi also may be tested by having the patient abduct the little finger against resistance and by palpating the muscle belly of the abductor digiti minimi (Fig. 65-3). Although clawing of the little and ring fingers may not be seen at the time of an acute injury, at times it is present and careful observation of the

hand will reveal this finding. The first dorsal interosseus muscle may receive an anomalous innervation from the median nerve in about 10% of hands. The posterior interosseus or superficial branches of the radial nerve also may supply the first dorsal and the second and third dorsal interosseus muscles in some hands, as well.

Proximal muscles innervated by the *radial nerve* include the triceps, brachioradialis, supinator, and anconeus. The radially innervated muscles having influence on the hand include the extensor carpi radialis longus and brevis, the extensor carpi ulnaris, the extensor digitorum communis, the extensor indicis proprius, the extensor digiti minimi, the abductor pollicis longus, the extensor pollicis longus, and the extensor pollicis brevis. The motions that can be examined and that are mediated by the radial nerve in the hand and wrist include wrist dorsiflexion and radial and ulnar deviation, as well as thumb abduction and extension. Metacarpophalangeal extension, mediated by the radial nerve, should be evaluated carefully so that the examiner is not confused by extension of the proximal and distal interphalangeal joints of the fingers, controlled by the intrinsic muscles.

SUDOMOTOR ACTIVITY. Usually a denervated area will show no sweating within about 30 mintues after a nerve injury. It is helpful to compare the normal and suspected injured areas by palpation with a dry fingertip.

Postoperative Assessment

In 1984 the Clinical Assessment Committee of the American Society for Surgery of the Hand recommended four areas of importance in evaluating the progress of peripheral nerve injury and repair: (1) sensiblity testing, (2) motor testing, (3) subjective evaluation, and (4) sudomotor function.

SENSIBILITY EVALUATION. The basic minimum tests recommended for sensibility evaluation are the stationary two-point discrimination and moving two-point discrimination tests.

■ *TECHNIQUE.* **The hand should be warm and the instrument at room temperature. Rest the hand on a flat surface, palm up. Apply a blunt, two-pointed caliper or paper clip distally over the distal pulp in the longitudinal axis on the radial or ulnar side (Fig. 65-4). The pressure applied should be just slightly less than blanching pressure. Test each area three times. Start at a width of 10 mm and gradually decrease the distance. Do the moving two-point discrimination test in a similar fashion. Apply the caliper in an axial direction and move it from proximal to distal along the digital pad. Two out of three correct answers are considered proof of perception with either test.**

MOTOR TESTING. Three basic minimum tests are recommended for motor function: grip strength, key pinch, and tip pinch strength. The squeeze grip dynamometer should be used and the results recorded at all five positions with three successive determinations. This reflects the overall integrated function of the hand, in addition to areas of extrinsic and intrinsic muscle dificits,

Pinch strength is measured using a pinch dynamometer. Applying the thumb tip to the radial aspect of the middle phalanx of the index finger measures key pinch. Three successive determinations should be made and the opposite hand should be measured as well. Pinching with the index tip to the ulnar side of the tip of the

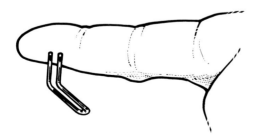

Fig. 65-4   Two-point discrimination testing. (From American Society for Surgery of the Hand: The hand: examination and diagnosis, New York, 1983, Churchill Livingstone.)

thumb allows measurement of tip pinch values. Three measurements should be made.

SUBJECTIVE EVALUATION. This is the patient's evaluation of his current status and includes symptoms such as the presence of pain, cold intolerance, dysesthesias, and functional disabilities.

SUDOMOTOR FUNCTION. The loss of sweating is an indicator of nerve disruption and loss of sympathetic function. Sweating may return without a return of two-point discrimination; however, usually it returns with the return of two-point discrimination.

A statement relative to sweating should be included in the evaluation.

NERVE REGENERATION

After a nerve injury the response in the proximal elements of the peripheral nerve include an increased rate of metabolic activity and proliferation from the nerve cell bodies distally, resulting in the sprouting of axonal processes at the injury site within the first 1 to 3 weeks. The response distally consists of the elements of wallerian degeneration, including disruption of the myelin sheath and phagocytosis, and preparation of the distal segment to receive the regenerating elements of the proximal axons. More detailed discussion of this response is found in Chapter 45.

Usually, after repair of a sensory nerve (digital, pure sensory, mixed motor, and sensory), the area of anesthesia decreases in size as regeneration progresses and the quality of sensation changes. In 2 to 3 months the entire area supplied by the nerve may become paresthetic. It then becomes hyperesthetic to light touch or cold. Firm pressure is usually less painful. With the passage of time and the use of various physical and occupational therapy modalities, the hyperesthesia resolves. Patients usually have less objectionable sensation after the period of hyperesthesia.

With progression of regeneration, the quality of sensation improves significantly within the first 1.5 to 2 years with additional gradual improvement thereafter. Rarely in adults is fully normal sensation with appreciation of functional two-point discrimination expected. Although the functional result after digital nerve regeneration is usually better than that seen for injuries to nerves more proximally and to mixed motor and sensory nerves (such as the ulnar nerve), age seems to have an influence on the final functional result after peripheral nerve repair. The reports of Omer and of Onne, as well the work of Kankaanpaa and Bakalim, suggest that patients under the age of 20 can be expected to have a better prognosis for return of functional two-point discrimination than can older patients. Although exceptions may be encountered, it is rare for patients over the age of 50 years to experience much better function than protective sensation.

In considering the repair of multiple digital nerves in the injured hand, the location of the injured nerves should be considered. Although it is general practice to repair all digital nerves, it is important to remember that the most important areas of sensory innervation of the digits include the ulnar side of the thumb, the radial side of the index and middle fingers, and the ulnar side of the little finger. These areas are important for pinch and for ulnar border contact of the hand. These nerves should be given priority if there are limiting factors such as prolonged operative time in a multiply-injured patient, multiple soft-tissue problems on the various fingers, or segmental nerve loss.

PRIMARY AND DELAYED PRIMARY NERVE REPAIR
Timing of Repair

The controversy regarding the timing of nerve repairs in general remains unresolved. The terms applied to the timing of the nerve repair include primary repair (immediately after injury, or within 6 to 12 hours), delayed primary repair (usually within the first 2 to 2.5 weeks), and secondary repair (after 2.5 to 3 weeks). The advocates of primary repair are supported by experimental work, especially the work of Grabb, Müller and Grubel, and Grabb et al., that suggests that the results may be somewhat better after primary suture. Those advocating a delay in repair are supported by the clinical observations following nerve injuries that occurred during wars. In general, the longer the delay in repair the poorer is the return of motor function that can be expected. The reinnervation of denervated muscle may occur after up to 12 months according to Sunderland; however, after that period irreversible changes occur in the muscle cells and there is little hope of recovery of motor function after reinnervation. The return of sensation has been observed when nerve repair has been peformed as long as 2 years after injury. The work of Kleinert and Griffin and Omer and Spinner suggests that satisfactory function can occur after nerve repairs done within 3 months of injury. It should be remembered that delay in nerve repair assumes the following: (1) muscle atrophy occurs, (2) contraction in the endoneural tubules of the distal segment progresses, (3) retraction of the nerve ends may occur, (4) joint contractures may develop, (5) a second operation is involved, and (6) intraneural alignment of fascicles may be more difficult. Additional factors to consider in the timing of peripheral nerve repairs include the condition of the patient and the state of preparedness of the surgeon and the institution, including the availability of instruments and personnel to allow a satisfactory primary repair.

Regardless of the timing of repair, tension should be avoided at the site of nerve repair. The work of Millesi and Meissl suggests that nerve grafts accomplished without tension heal and function better than nerve repairs performed with tension, despite the need for regeneration to occur across two suture lines with a nerve graft.

Indications

In general, a nerve repair may be done immediately after injury or within the first 2 to 2.5 weeks in the presence of a clean, sharp injury. A delay of 2 to 2.5 weeks may be caused by a variety of factors, including the condition of the patient and the availability of the appropriate personnel including the surgeon to treat the wound. It is our practice to repair injured nerves, if the wound is clean and sharp, either on the day of injury or in the first 5 to 7 days.

SECONDARY NERVE REPAIR
Indications

Several conditions should influence the surgeon to delay the repair of injured peripheral nerves. These include (1) the existence of extensive soft-tissue injury and loss with extensive trauma to the nerve, (2) the presence of extensive wound contamination, (3) the presence of multiple limb injuries requiring aggressive and expeditious management in preference to the nerve injury, (4) the existence of extensive crush injury, (5) the presence of an extensive traction injury, and (6) a nerve injury that has been treated by another surgeon, in which the extent and nature of the nerve repair are unknown to the second treating surgeon.

When multiple tissue injuries have occurred, especially in the presence of soft-tissue loss, the nerve repair is secondary and is indicated only after good skin coverage has been obtained. Following satisfactory and complete healing of all wounds and the establishment of satisfactory nutrition to the skin and other tissues of the hand, common and proper digital nerves usually can be sutured as a secondary procedure 3 weeks or more after injury. Although most reports suggest that the results following secondary repair are similar to, if not better than, those following primary repair, best results seem to occur if repairs are done within the first 3 months of injury. The reports of patients treated after World War II suggest that useful sensation can occur following repairs as late as 2 years after injury. This is not the normal expectation. Return of motor function following excessive delays is even more unpredictable.

With a severe soft tissue injury skin coverage is a priority. The extent of intraneural injury is unknown and it is best to wait 3 to 6 weeks to allow clear demarcation of intraneural scar to have a better chance at more precise nerve apposition at the time of repair.

An extensively contaminated wound may require a delay in nerve repair because infection may supervene and not only delay definitive treatment of the nerve but the wound closure itself. Although initial debridement may remove significant wound contamination and allow delayed primary repair, if wound contamination and necrotic material persist, additional debridements of necessity interpose a delay until definitive nerve repair at a later time.

Multiple limb injuries may create priorities of wound cleansing, bone stabilization, vascular repair, and soft tissue coverage. Segmental injury to nerves also might dictate secondary repair. Crush and traction injuries cause intraneural damage that cannot be assessed accurately at the time of primary wound evaluation. When the nerve has sustained extensive intraneural or extensive segmental intraneural injury or loss due to crush or traction, it is best to wait 3 to 6 weeks to allow clear demarcation between scar and normal nerve to become established. If the extent of intraneural injury is not clear or if extensive segmental loss of nerve requires grafting, primary repair should not be done and secondary repair or nerve reconstruction by graft should be considered.

A special situation occurs when the patient's initial and primary care have been accomplished by another surgeon. Frequently one does not know the extent of the initial injury and has no awareness of the nature of the repair. At times, it may be necessary to consider exploration of the nerve, possibly considering secondary repair. Exploration of the nerve may reveal that secondary repair is unnecessary. The exploration of a nerve injury in such a situation may help assure that a skillful nerve repair has been done, which is one important determinant of outcome.

SUTURING OF NERVES

For additional discussion of surgical techniques, see the chapter on peripheral nerve injuries (Chapter 45) and the chapter on microsurgery (Chapter 49).

Generally, the principles that apply to the suture of other peripheral nerves also apply to those of the hand. Important considerations include (1) mixed versus pure motor or sensory nerves, (2) internal arrangement of the nerves, (3) incisions to be used, (4) amount of mobilization and limb positioning required for tension-free apposition, (5) suture materials to be used, (6) nature of the suture arrangement, (7) magnification, and (8) postoperative management.

Careful technique is extremely important to provide the best restoration and repair of the anatomy. The internal arrangement of the nerve in the palm and digits is usually oligofascicular as described by Millesi (Fig. 65-5). In the median and ulnar nerves at the wrist an intraneural polyfascicular or group arrangement is found. The outlook is better following repair of common digital and proper digital nerves because of their internal arrangement, their pure sensory function, and the short distance from the injury to the end organ.

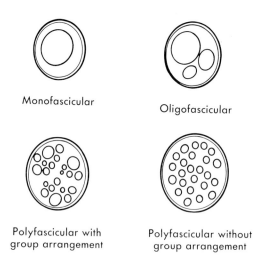

Fig. 65-5 Typical intraneural fascicular patterns in peripheral nerves.

Incisions to expose the nerve and mobilize the nerve proximally and distally should be made in accordance with proven principles of skin incisions in the palm. They should not cross flexion creases at right angles and skin flaps should not be devascularized, nor should additional neurovascular injury be created in extending the skin incisions. The exact extent to which a nerve can be mobilized without creating ischemia is unknown. Generally, within the digits, palm, and wrist, extensive mobilization of the nerve from its surrounding tissues is not sufficient to cause harm. Magnification is extremely helpful to permit the most precise and accurate restoration of the anatomy. In the palm and fingers, the magnification achieved by 3.5 to 4.5 × magnifying loupes is usually sufficient to allow accurate repair. More proximally, magnification achieved with an operating microscope is more helpful in allowing satisfactory anatomic repair. The operating microscope also may be extremely helpful in repair of the terminal branches of the proper digital nerves distal to the distal flexion crease of the finger. Suture materials reflect the amount of tension to be applied to the nerve repair. Generally in the forearm, wrist, and proximal palm 8-0 and 9-0 monofilament nylon sutures are used. In the distal palm and proximal digits 10-0 nylon suture is satisfactory, and when the digital nerve is repaired distal to the distal volar flexion crease in the finger, 11-0 nylon may be required. Usually in the palm and digits a repair using either a pure perineurial neurorrhaphy (fascicular) (Fig. 65-6) or a combination epiperineurial-perineurial neurorrhaphy (Fig. 65-7) is sufficient for satisfactory anatomic repair.

NERVE GRAFTS
Indications

At times, as a result of extensive destruction, a segmental nerve defect is created that cannot be overcome

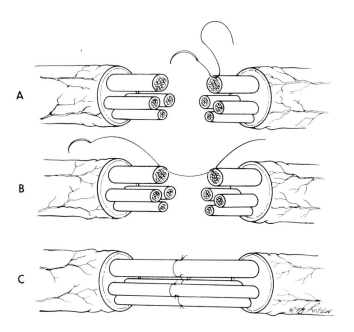

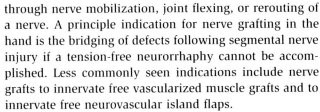

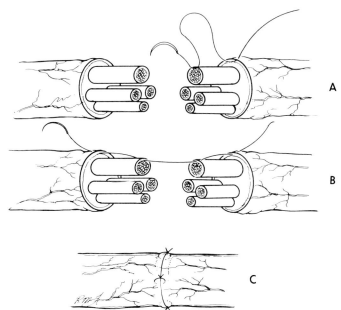

Fig. 65-6 Perineurial (fascicular) neurorrhaphy. **A,** Epineurium has been excised and fascicles exposed. **B,** Suture passed through corresponding fascicles on either side of cut surface of nerve. **C,** Neurorrhaphy completed, usually with two 10-0 nylon sutures in each fascicle.

Fig. 65-7 Epineurial-perineurial neurorrhaphy. **A,** Epineurium excised and retracted. Suture placed through epineurium, near large fascicle at periphery of nerve then through perineurium of fascicle. **B,** Suture passed through epineurium of matching fascicle on opposite side of cut surface of nerve then out through epineurium. **C,** Repair completed, after suturing other suitably matched fascicles.

through nerve mobilization, joint flexing, or rerouting of a nerve. A principle indication for nerve grafting in the hand is the bridging of defects following segmental nerve injury if a tension-free neurorrhaphy cannot be accomplished. Less commonly seen indications include nerve grafts to innervate free vascularized muscle grafts and to innervate free neurovascular island flaps.

Before performing a nerve graft, other techniques for closing the small gaps between nerve endings should be considered, since they will frequently solve the problem of closing small gaps in nerves. These techniques include mobilization of the nerve ends over a distance of a few centimeters proximally and distally, positioning of the joints near the nerve injury in less-than-awkward positions, and transposing or changing the course of nerve endings.

Sources of Nerve Grafts

Donor nerves for nerve grafts in the upper extremities include the sural, lateral antebrachial cutaneous, and medial antebrachial cutaneous, as well as digital nerves from an amputated finger, and a segment of a severed nerve from the opposite, but less critical, side of a single digit to repair the digital nerve on the opposite side (for example, for lacerations of both nerves of the long finger requiring grafting, the ulnar digital nerve may be used to graft the radial digital nerve gap.)

Tension-free Nerve Graft

The experimental and clinical observations in reports of Millesi and Millesi and Meissl suggest that a nerve repaired with a tension-free nerve graft has a better outlook than end-to-end nerve repair done under excessive tension. In general, we have had satisfactory results with nerve grafts, particularly regarding sensory return, using the technique of Millesi. It is a technique that requires microsurgical experience. Nerve gaps of greater than 20 cm have been bridged using this technique.

■ *TECHNIQUE (MILLESI, MODIFIED).* **In the digits, hand, and distal forearm use a pneumatic tourniquet to allow dissection of the injured nerve in a bloodless field. Make appropriate extensile skin incisions to locate and expose the distal glioma and the proximal neuroma on the injured nerve. Open the epineurium proximal to the neuroma in near-normal tissue on the proximal stump and in the distal segment dissect proximally toward the scarred distal stump. At the wrist and in the distal forearm, identify the major fascicle groups within the nerve and using sharp dissection with microscissors or a diamond knife for thicker scar, transect the fascicle groups so that a "step-cut" results (Fig. 65-8). Such fascicular dissection is not necessary in the common and proper digital nerves because of their pure sensory and oligofascicular nature. In a polyfascicular nerve, such as the median and ulnar nerves at the wrist, individual fascicle groups of different lengths**

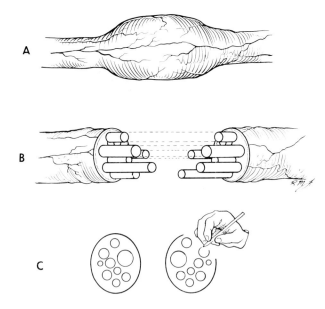

Fig. 65-8   "Step-cut" technique of Millesi.

will protrude from the nerve stump after completion of the interfascicular dissection. Carry out similar dissection on the proximal and distal stumps. In a polyfascicular nerve it is helpful to sketch the ends of the two nerve stumps with their fascicular patterns to allow matching of the respective fascicles, depending on the size, number of fascicles, and their arrangement within the proximal and distal stumps of the nerve. This clinical estimation is easier over short distances, and more difficult over longer defects.

Select a donor site that is appropriate for the size of the nerve and the gap to be filled. Generally, for common and proper digital nerves, the antebrachial cutaneous nerves are satisfactory. If a great deal of nerve tissue is required, the sural nerve is best in our experience. After the nerve graft has been harvested, place it between the proximal and distal nerve stumps. In the polyfascicular nerves, such as the median and ulnar nerves at the wrist, attempt to use the sketch of the fascicle groups to allow appropriate placement of the graft. Once coaptation of the graft has been achieved, suture the graft with 10-0 monofilament nylon through the epineurium of the graft and the perineurium of one of the fascicles in the group or in the interfascicular connective tissue. Multiple sutures may not be required with satisfactory coaptation of the graft to the nerve stump ends. Insert Silastic drains as needed. Avoid the use of suction drainage. Close the skin so that the graft is not displaced during wound closure by shearing forces. Immobilize the extremity in a padded dorsal splint in as near an anatomic position as possible.

AFTERTREATMENT. The part is immobilized for about 10 days, then the splint is removed and free

movement of the joints is allowed. Hematomas that develop early in the postoperative period are removed, unsatisfactory or necrotic skin is debrided, and local flaps or skin grafts are used to cover a nerve graft that may have become exposed as a result of wound necrosis. At about 2 weeks, physical therapy is begun with supervised active and active-assisted range-of-motion exercises. The progress of regeneration is followed using the Tinel sign. If the Tinel sign stops with no further progression for 3 to 4 months at the distal end of the graft, the nerve graft should be explored with resection of the distal suture line and another end-to-end repair.

MANAGEMENT OF SPECIFIC NERVE INJURIES
Digital Nerves

Distal to the wrist the digital nerves are the most frequently severed. It is important to repair the digital nerves, particularly the thumb ulnar digital nerve; the radial digital nerve to the index, long, ring, and little fingers; and the ulnar digital nerve to the little finger. Knowledge of the anatomy of the cutaneous sensory branches of the nerves on the dorsum of the hand will allow repair of these nerves, as well.

Digital nerves may be repaired distal to the distal volar flexion crease of the fingers in the region of the terminal branches of the nerves. If digital nerves are repaired secondarily, the suture line should lie in a well-vascularized bed free of scar. Before secondary repair the proximal end of the nerve often may be located by passing a firm object, such as a paper clip, gently distally along the course of the nerve. Upon reaching the terminal neuroma, the patient will indicate exquisite tenderness.

SUTURE OF DIGITAL NERVES

■ *TECHNIQUE.* The digital nerves lie to the radial and ulnar sides of the volar aspect of the finger and thus can be exposed through the same midradial or midulnar incision when necessary. Begin proximally and dissect a normal segment of the nerve from its investing fascia (part of Cleland's ligament) (Fig. 65-9); then proceed distally to the scar at the site of injury. Next, begin distal to the site of injury and dissect proximally to the scar. With scissors or a diamond knife, remove the neuroma from the proximal end of the nerve and the glioma from the distal end. Use loupe magnification for dissection and repair.

Approximate the nerve ends without tension; flex the finger joints minimally if necessary. If a large gap requires extreme flexion, consider a nerve graft. Use an 8-0 or 9-0 monofilament nylon suture on an atraumatic curved needle (Fig. 65-10). Use 10-0 or 11-0 nylon to repair the terminal branches distal to

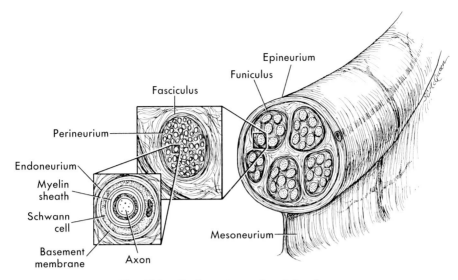

Fig. 65-9 Basic anatomy of peripheral nerves.

the distal interphalangeal joint. When necessary, the nerve ends may be held in place temporarily by passing the smallest straight Bunnell needle transversely through them into the adjoining soft tissue to avoid tension while the sutures are placed and tied. Now pass a suture through the epineurium of the nerve about 1 mm from its edge and again in a similar manner through the epineurium of the other end of the nerve; tie the knot with at least five loops to prevent its slipping or untying. Place a second suture on the exact opposite side of the nerve. Leave these first two sutures long so that they can be used as traction sutures to rotate the nerve 180 degrees, making accessible all of its surfaces. Place a total of four sutures. After the repair, slowly extend the joints and observe the suture line for tension; note the optimum position of the joints for this purpose and maintain it by splinting after closure. Always suture divided tendons before suturing any nerve to avoid disrupting the delicate repair.

AFTERTREATMENT. After 3 weeks the finger joints are allowed gradual active extension beyond the optimum position noted at surgery; when the defect in the nerve is large, active extension cannot be permitted before 4 weeks. Even though the suture line must be protected, active finger motion must be started as soon as possible to avoid stiffness.

While major nerves are regenerating after repair, the hand may assume an unnatural posture because of change in muscle balance. Even when the nerve lesion is above the wrist, the hand suffers most and may incur fixed contractures before nerve function returns. Proper splinting (p. 2979) is therefore necessary to prevent contractures during this period. The patient should be warned that until sensation returns, the anesthetic skin may become infected after even minor trauma or may be burned, frostbitten, cut, or blistered by friction unless properly protected. He should be instructed to inspect the insensitive areas routinely and to avoid extremes of heat, cold, and friction.

Fig. 65-10 Basic suture technique for laceration of peripheral nerves should result in no tension at suture line, and each small fascicle should be aligned to match opposing, mirror image.

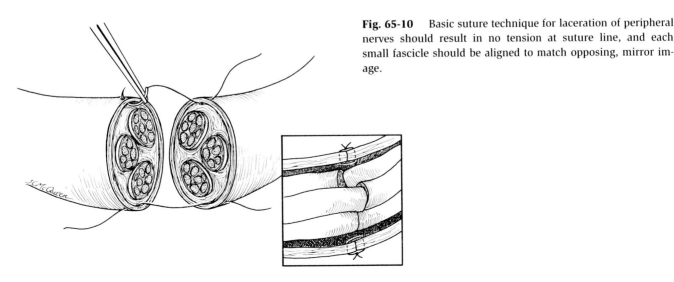

Ulnar Nerve at Wrist

When the ulnar artery and the tendon of the flexor carpi ulnaris are severed at the wrist, the ulnar nerve usually is severed too. At this level it is both motor and sensory, and therefore proper rotational alignment of the ends is important at the time of suture.

■ *TECHNIQUE.* With the pneumatic tourniquet inflated, make proximal and distal extensile skin incisions. Expose the proximal and distal segments of the nerve but do not yet remove them from their normal beds. With a suture through the epineurium, mark exactly the most anterior aspect of each segment some distance from the scarred area. Now free each segment from the surrounding soft tissues. Use loupe magnification for dissection and the operating microscope for repair. With the microscissors or a diamond knife, make clean transverse cuts and excise the neuroma from the proximal segment and the glioma from the distal segment. Inspect each cut end for a pattern of large and small bundles. By matching these patterns and using the two epineurial sutures just described, proper rotational alignment should be possible. When further length is needed for suture without tension, dissect and mobilize the nerve more proximally or, if necessary, transplant it anteriorly from behind the medial epicondyle of the humerus. Extensive freeing of a nerve may damage its blood supply. When advancing the nerve distally take care not to divide its branches to the muscles in the proximal forearm. Careful intraneural dissection of the branches may allow mobilization of the nerve. Flex the elbow as necessary to avoid tension, but avoid excessive flexion of the elbow. Use the operating microscope to help align major groups of fascicles. Although four-quadrant traction sutures may be sufficient, it is sometimes easier to start with the deep surface and close the cut surface like a book, using a combination of 8-0 or 9-0 nylon epiperineurial and 10-0 perineurial (fascicular) suture to complete the repair.

When the ulnar nerve is severed near but just distal to its division into its volar (palmar) superficial sensory branch and its deep motor branch, identify the two small proximal segments and dissect them apart in a proximal direction for ease of mobilization; suture each branch separately.

Deep Branch of Ulnar Nerve

Boyes has noted the feasibility of repairing the important deep branch of the ulnar nerve, which supplies those intrinsic muscles of the hand not supplied by the median nerve: the medial two lumbricals, all interossei, the hypothenar muscles, and the adductor pollicis. These are among those most responsible for the quick and skillful movements of the fingers. Many tendon transfers have been devised to restore motor function lost by inter-

ruption of the ulnar nerve, but when possible, direct repair of the nerve is desirable.

■ *TECHNIQUE (BOYES, MODIFIED).* Use loupe magnification for dissection and the operating microscope for repair. Expose the nerve from its origin as a branch of the main trunk at the wrist to its midpalmar part through a curved incision distal and parallel to the thenar crease; extend it over the hook of the hamate to the flexion crease of the wrist, proceed proximally and medially, crossing the crease obliquely, and proceed to the ulnar aspect of the distal forearm. Reflect the skin, divide the palmaris brevis muscle at its insertion and reflect it ulnarward so as not to disturb its nerve supply. Retract the ulnar vessels toward the thumb and divide the origins of the abductor digiti quinti, flexor digiti quinti, and opponens digiti quinti muscles. Retract the tendons of the flexor digitorum. The course of the nerve is now exposed from the pisiform to the midpalm (Fig. 65-11, *A*). When necessary, the nerve may be further exposed distally by extending the incision to the index metacarpal and by retracting the flexor tendons with the lumbrical muscles. When these are displaced ulnarward, the nerve can be identified and followed where it passes through the transverse fibers of the adductor pollicis.

When the nerve has been divided by a sharp instrument, gently free it from proximally and distally to the point of damage. This usually allows enough length for suture without tension. If a gap exists as a result of gunshot wounds or other severe injuries in which nerve substance has been lost, consider a nerve graft or reroute the nerve as follows (Fig. 65-11, *C* and *D*). Dissect its motor component from the trunk well into the distal forearm. Then divide the volar carpal ligament and free from the ulnar side of the carpus the ulnar bursa that lines the carpal tunnel; displace the proximal end of the nerve into the tunnel. Bring the proximal end to the midpalm by flexing the wrist. In some instances when branches to the hypothenar muscles are still intact, gentle dissection and mobilization of the bundles will allow branches to be saved and yet permit the nerve to be rerouted. Use microscissors or the diamond knife to freshen the ends of the nerve (Fig. 65-11, *B*). Repair the nerve using an epiperineurial or combination of epiperineurial and perineurial repairs with 8-0 or 9-0 nylon externally and 10-0 nylon within the nerves as needed. Suture the volar carpal ligament, replace the insertion of the palmaris brevis, and close the wound.

According to Boyes, the results are proportional to the accuracy of the approximation and inversely proportional to the scarring and fibrosis. Regeneration takes place in an orderly way; the recovery of nerve function may be tested by noting voluntary activity of the first dorsal interosseus muscle (Fig. 65-12).

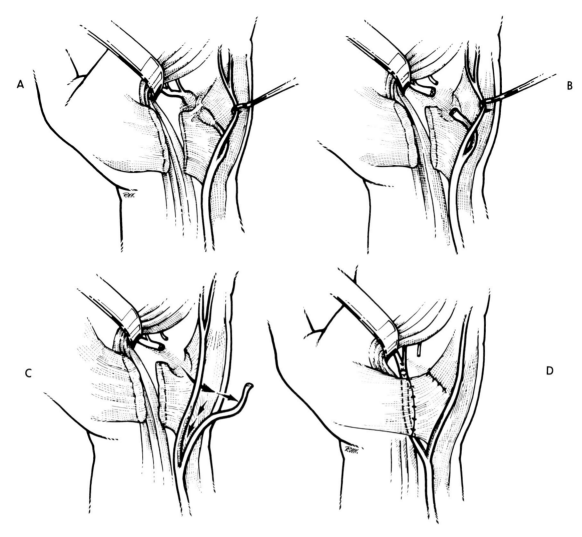

Fig. 65-11 Boyes technique of repairing deep branch of ulnar nerve. **A,** Main trunk and deep branch of ulnar nerve have both been exposed, and volar carpal ligament has been divided. **B,** Ends of deep branch have been freshened. **C,** Deep branch has been split intraneurally into distal forearm. **D,** Deep branch has been rerouted through carpal tunnel, and its ends have been sutured. (Redrawn from Boyes JH: J Bone Joint Surg 37-A:920, 1955.)

Dorsal Branch of Ulnar Nerve

This nerve is large enough at the wrist and just distal to it to be repaired like a digital nerve. It crosses the ulnar styloid superficially, even though it may have branched from the trunk 5 cm or more proximal to the wrist. If extra length is needed to appose the ends, it may be made to branch from the main trunk more proximally by intraneural dissection and is then routed more directly to the dorsum of the hand. The wrist should then be held in extension for 3 to 4 weeks after surgery, following which gradual protected motion is begun and a progressive exercise program is followed.

Median Nerve at Wrist

Division of the median nerve at the wrist is not unusual, and the vital sensory function of the hand depends on its successful repair. It is important to emphasize that (1) the neuroma must be carefully excised from the proximal end and the glioma must be excised from the distal end; (2) surrounding scar must be excised to provide a vascular bed; (3) the repair must be accurate, with the ends in proper rotation, for the nerve contains motor as well as sensory fibers; and (4) tension on the repair must be avoided.

■ *TECHNIQUE.* **Expose the median nerve at the wrist using a palmar incision parallel to the thenar crease, extending proximally and crossing the wrist flexion crease obliquely and medially. Extend the incision proximal to the nerve transection in the volar midline of the forearm. The following points are helpful. A vessel usually lies on the anterior surface of the median nerve parallel with its long axis; this vessel may be of help in securing proper rota-**

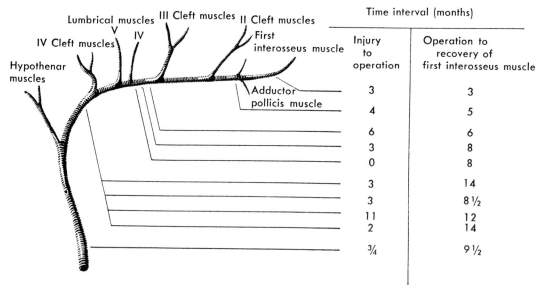

Fig. 65-12 Rate of recovery of voluntary function of first dorsal interosseus muscle after repair of deep branch of ulnar nerve in 10 patients. (Modified from Boyes JH: J Bone Joint Surg 37-A:920, 1955.)

tional alignment, or it may be obliterated by scar when the repair is late. An epineurial suture in each segment as described for the ulnar nerve at the wrist (p. 3116) may aid in obtaining proper rotation. Tension may be reduced by dissecting and mobilizing the nerve proximally in the forearm and by flexing the wrist and elbow. Use magnifying loupes and the operating microscope as needed for dissection and repair. Use 8-0, 9-0, and 10-0 nylon on an atraumatic curved needle to place epiperineurial and perineurial (fascicular) sutures as needed to complete the repair.

When a flexor tendon and the median nerve are both sutured secondarily, release of the transverse carpal ligament may be needed to help prevent scar adhesions.

Median Nerve in Palm

When the median nerve is divided where it branches in the palm, it may sometimes be repaired with a bundle suture (Fig. 65-13). This suture gathers the several branches of the nerve into a single trunk so that it in turn can be sutured to the proximal segment of the nerve.

Every effort should be made to repair the recurrent branch of the median nerve. It may be hard to find because of surrounding fascia and scar tissue, but once it is seen it can be identified readily by its yellow fibers running transversely toward the base of the thumb. This branch usually projects from the main trunk radially and superficially, passing just over the distal margin of the transverse carpal ligament. It courses slightly posteriorly and laterally to innervate the thenar muscles. There are

several important anatomic variations so that this recurrent branch may be represented by two branches instead of one; it may come off the ulnar side of the trunk, and it may perforate the distal portion of the transverse carpal ligament. It is repaired with the technique described for digital nerves (p. 3114); the prognosis is good if careful attention is given to anatomic detail.

When the median nerve cannot be repaired, a neurovascular island free graft may be indicated.

Superficial Radial Nerve

Disability after interruption of the superficial radial nerve at the wrist is less than that after interruption of sensory nerves on the volar surface of the hand; there is anesthesia over a variable area on the dorsum of the thumb and index finger. Sometimes the ulnar side of the area of pinch of the thumb receives its major innervation from this nerve. Neuromas caught in dorsal scars are particularly painful because they are stimulated not only by direct touch but also by stretching of the surrounding skin, nerve, and scar when the wrist and fingers are flexed.

Unless there is some unusual reason for repairing the nerve or one of its branches, it should be resected proximal to its site of severance to permit it to lie in an area of minimal scar. It is so common to have a painful and at times disabling neuroma after repair that the small area of lost sensibility is a small disability in comparison.

■ *TECHNIQUE.* The suture technique is as described for digital nerves. Locate the nerve proximally and dissect it distally to the scar; a consistent anatomic landmark proximally is the exit of the nerve from beneath the tendon of the brachioradialis muscle,

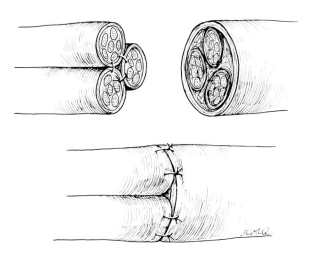

Fig. 65-13   Bundle suture for segmental gap (see text).

usually about 5 cm proximal to its insertion into the radial styloid. Then locate the nerve distally and dissect it proximally toward the scar. At the base of the thumb the nerve has usually already divided into two major branches; each is larger than a digital nerve and when severed can be repaired (for the technique of suture, see p. 3114). If the wrist must be extended to appose the nerve ends, it should be maintained in this position for 4 or 5 weeks to prevent tension on the repair. When the distal branch or branches cannot be found, take care to release the nerve proximally from the scar to relieve pain; resect some of it if necessary.

TRAUMATIC NEUROMAS

The treatment of traumatic neuromas is discussed in Chapter 77.

NEUROVASCULAR ISLAND GRAFTS

It is clear that any digit deprived of sensibility is selectively and unconsciously avoided during use of the hand. Therefore restoration of sensibility to a selected area of a given digit by transfer of a neurovascular island graft is useful at times. In permanent nerve damage, sensibility can be restored to critical areas, especially on the thumb or index finger. Transfer of a neurovascular island graft is essential to innervate an osteoplastic reconstruction of the thumb (Chapter 69). However, sensibility in the graft is never normal after transfer. In grafts critically examined some time after surgery, sensibility usually is abnormal in all. More than half of patients will have persistently hyperesthetic skin. All patients will lack precise sensory reorientation. Reorientation, although it need not be normal for a good functional result, seems to improve with time and with use of the part.

Transfer of a neurovascular island graft may be indicated to treat permanent sensory deficits on the radial side of an otherwise normal index finger or on the area

of pinch on the distal ulnar aspect of the thumb. Before the decision for surgery is made, the following factors must be considered: (1) the dominance of the involved hand, (2) the presence of any scarring in the palm through which an incision must be made for channeling of the neurovascular bundle, (3) the status of the ipsilateral ulnar nerve, (4) the condition of the opposite hand, (5) the age of the patient, and (6) the experience of the surgeon.

Early descriptions of the operation suggested transfer of skin from just the ulnar side of the distal phalanx of the ring finger. However, experience has shown that most of the skin from an entire side of the donor finger should be included in the transfer. This larger transfer increases the area of sensitive skin on the recipient digit and causes no wider sensory loss on the donor digit; usually the larger free graft required to cover the donor area is of little consequence.

In the usual case, death of the transferred neurovascular island pedicle graft is not likely; yet even temporary impairment of the circulation may cause permanent sensory deficit in the graft and thus a partial failure of the operation. Therefore in handling the neurovascular bundle, several points in technique must be emphasized: (1) the bundle, including all veins, should be dissected from proximally to distally so that any anomalies of the vessels may be properly treated; (2) the bundle should not be completely freed from the surrounding fatty tissue, especially at the base of the finger, but should be transferred along with some attached tissue; and (3) the bundle should be channeled through an incision large enough to show the entire bundle to prevent kinking, twisting, or stretching of the nerve or vessels.

■ *TECHNIQUE*. Using a skin pencil, accurately outline the area of sensory deficit on the thumb and prepare to remove skin from a similar area on the ulnar side of the ring finger. Alternate donor sites include the radial side of the little finger or, in the absence of median nerve damage, the ulnar side of the middle finger. If the entire palmar surface of the thumb is insensitive, outline on the ring finger the maximum donor area for transfer. Shape the donor area to include most of the ulnar side of the finger, with darts to near the midline on the palmar and dorsal surfaces between the finger joints. The area thus outlined will include skin supplied by the dorsal branch of the proper digital nerve and will be shaped to prevent tension on the resulting scars during finger movements.

Exsanguinate the limb by wrapping or elevation and inflate a pneumatic tourniquet on the arm. Then beginning proximally near the base of the palm, make a zigzag incision distally to the fourth web (Fig. 65-14). Identify and dissect free, along with some surrounding tissue, the common volar digital artery and nerve to the ring and little fingers and the proper digital artery and nerve to the ulnar side of the ring finger. Loupe magnification is help-

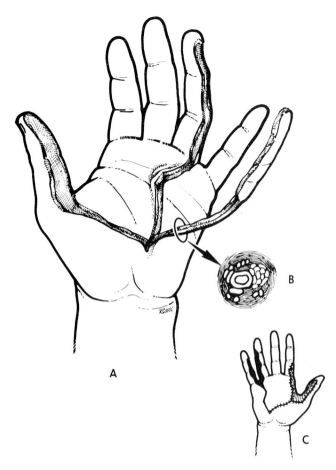

Fig. 65-14 Technique of transferring neurovascular island graft. **A,** Palmar incision has been made, neurovascular island graft has been excised from ulnar surface of ring finger and its bundle has been freed proximally, and insensitive skin has been excised from palmar surface of thumb (see text). **B,** Cross section of neurovascular bundle. **C,** Alternative technique in which neurovascular island graft includes adjacent surfaces of ring and little fingers and area covered by it is larger as shown.

ful in this dissection. Ligate and divide the proper digital artery to the radial side of the little finger. Next carefully dissect and split proximally from the common volar digital nerve the proper digital nerve to the ulnar side of the ring finger. Continue the dissection distally and excise, with this attached neurovascular bundle, the previously outlined area of skin from the ulnar side of the ring finger; take special care not to damage the artery and to preserve as many veins as possible.

Use the bipolar cautery and divide any small branches of the artery as necessary. Now free the composite graft and carry the island graft across the palm to the recipient area on the thumb; be sure the neurovascular bundle is long enough to permit the transfer without causing tension on the bundle. The island graft should cover most of the pulp area on the palmar aspect of the thumb and should extend to the ulnar aspect of the digit but not to the distal edge of the nail. Now beginning at the proximal end

of the original incision and proceeding to the thumb, make a second zigzag incision across the palm conforming to the skin creases. Excise from the thumb the previously outlined area of skin, and if large enough, save it to be used later as a free skin graft on the donor finger. Now suture the island graft in place on the thumb. Carefully check the entire neurovascular bundle for stretching, kinking, or twisting and close the palmar incisions. Next, cover the donor area of the finger with a full-thickness graft from the recipient thumb, free of fat, or with a thick split graft obtained elsewhere; cover this graft with a stent dressing. Now release the tourniquet and hold the wrist in slight flexion and the thumb in the best position to eliminate tension on the transferred bundle. Carefully observe the island graft for evidence of return of circulation. Remember that vascular spasm may cause ischemia of the graft for a few minutes. The graft eventually should become pink; if it does not, check again the positions of the wrist and thumb and, if necessary, reopen part of the palmar incision and explore the transferred neurovascular bundle for kinking.

This procedure may be altered as necessary to meet other given requirements. For instance, in complete median nerve paralysis, if sensibility on the ulnar edge of the thumb pulp is reasonably good as a result of overlap of innervation from the radial nerve, transfer of the island graft to the radial side of the proximal and middle phalanges of the index finger may be desirable. This area of the finger is used especially in strong pinch.

AFTERTREATMENT. A bulky dressing and a dorsal plaster splint are applied holding the wrist, thumb, and fingers in flexion. The hand is elevated constantly for 4 or 5 days after surgery. After suture removal at 10 to 14 days, gentle protected motion exercises are begun. The splint may be discontinued at about 3 to 4 weeks, depending on the needs of the thumb and donor finger.

REFERENCES

Anatomy, physiology, basic research

Bergfield TG and Aulicino PL: Variation of the deep motor branch of the ulnar nerve at the wrist, J Hand Surg 13-A:380, 1988.

Cabaud HE, Rodkey WG, and McCarroll HR Jr: Peripheral nerve injuries: studies in higher nonhuman primates, J Hand Surg 5:201, 1980.

Chacha PB, Krishramurti A, and Soin K: Experimental sensory reinnervation of the median nerve by nerve transfer in monkeys, J Bone Joint Surg 59-A:386, 1977.

Dellon AL: Reinnervation of denervated Meissner corpuscles: a sequential histologic study in the monkey following fascicular nerve repair, J Hand Surg 1:98, 1976.

Doyle JR, Semenza J, and Gilling B: The effect of succinylocholine on denervated skeletal muscle, J Hand Surg 6:40, 1981.

Gordon L and Buncke HJ: Heterotopic free skeletal muscle autotransplantation with utilization of a long nerve graft and microsurgical techniques: a study in the primate, J Hand Surg 4:103, 1979.

Gordon L et al: Predegenerated nerve autografts as compared with fresh nerve autografts in freshly cut and precut motor nerve defects in the rat, J Hand Surg 4:42, 1979.

Hobbs RA, Magnussen PA, and Tonkin MA: Palmar cutaneous branch of the median nerve, J Hand Surg 15-A:38, 1990.

Lundborg G: Nerve regeneration and repair: a review, Acta Orthop Scand 58:145, 1987.

Lundborg G: Intraneural microcirculation, Orthop Clin North Am 19:1, 1988.

Lundborg G and Hansson HA: Nerve regeneration through preformed synovial tubes, J Hand Surg 5:35, 1980.

Orgel MG and Terzis JK: Epineural versus perineural repair: an ultrastructural and electrophysiological study of nerve regeneration, Plast Reconstr Surg 60:80, 1977.

Rydevik B, Lundborg G, and Bagge U: Effects of graded compression on intraneural blood flow, J Hand Surg 6:3, 1981.

Seddon H: Surgical disorders of the peripheral nerves, Baltimore, 1972, Williams & Wilkins.

Starkweather RJ et al: The effect of devascularization on the regeneration of lacerated peripheral nerves: an experimental study, J Hand Surg 3:163, 1978.

Sunderland S: Nerves and nerve injuries, New York, 1978, Churchill Livingstone.

Diagnostic aids, management plan, results

Aschan W and Moberg E: The Ninhydrin finger printing test used to map out partial lesions to hand nerves, Acta Chir Scand 123:365, 1962.

Bralliar F: Electromyography: its use and misuse in peripheral nerve injuries, Orthop Clin North Am 12:229, 1981.

Dellon AL: The moving two-point discrimination test: clinical evaluation of the quickly adapting fiber/receptor system, J Hand Surg 3:474, 1978.

Dellon AL: Clinical use of vibratory stimuli to evaluate peripheral nerve injury and compression neuropathy, Plast Reconstr Surg 65:466, 1980.

Dellon AL, Mackinnon SE, and Crosby PM: Reliability of two-point discrimination measurements, J Hand Surg 12-A:693, 1987.

Eisen AA: Electromyography and nerve conduction as a diagnostic aid, Orthop Clin North Am 4:885, 1973.

Flynn JE and Flynn WF: Median and ulnar nerve injuries: a long-range study with evaluation of the Ninhydrin test, sensory and motor returns, Ann Surg 156:1002, 1962.

Frykman GK, Wolf A, and Coyle T: An algorithm for management of peripheral nerve injuries, Orthop Clin North Am 12:239, 1981.

Gellis M and Pool R: Two-point discrimination distances in the normal hand and forearm: application to various methods of fingertip reconstruction, Plast Reconstr Surg 59:57, 1977.

Henry SL and Breidenbach WC: Management of peripheral nerve injuries in the hand, Techniques Orthopaed 1:84, 1986.

Kankaanpaa U and Bakalim G: Peripheral nerve injuries of the upper extremity: sensory return of 137 neurorrhaphies, Acta Orthop Scand 47:41, 1976.

Laing PG: The timing of definitive nerve repair, Surg Clin North Am 40:363, 1960.

Levin S, Pearsall G, and Ruderman RJ: Von Frey's method of measuring pressure sensibility in the hand: an engineering analysis of Weinstein-Semmes pressure aesthesiometer, J Hand Surg 3:211, 1978.

Louis DS: Nerve function evaluation, Am Soc Surg Hand News 3(Suppl B):1, 1984.

Moberg E: Evaluation of sensibility in the hand, Surg Clin North Am 40:357, 1960.

Moberg E: Aspects of sensation in reconstructive surgery of the upper extremity, J Bone Joint Surg 46-A:817, 1964.

Moberg E: Evaluation and management of nerve injuries in the hand, Surg Clin North Am 44:1019, 1964.

Nahai F and Wolf SL: Percutaneous recordings from peripheral nerves (preliminary communication), J Hand Surg 3:168, 1978.

Nicolle FV, Chir B, and Woolhouse FM: Restoration of sensory function in severe degloving injuries of the hand, J Bone Joint Surg 48-A:1511, 1966.

Omer GE Jr: Injuries to nerves of the upper extremity, J Bone Joint Surg 56-A:1615, 1974.

Omer GE Jr: Sensation and sensibility in the upper extremity, Clin Orthop 104:30, 1974.

Omer GE Jr: Physical diagnosis of peripheral nerve injuries, Orthop Clin North Am 12:207, 1981.

Onne L: Recovery of sensibility an sudomotor activity in the hand after nerve suture, Acta Chir Scand (Suppl) 300:1, 1962.

Peacock EE Jr: Restoration of sensation in hands with extensive median nerve defects, Surgery 54:576, 1963.

Peterson GW and Will AD: Newer electrodiagnostic techniques in peripheral nerve injuries, Orthop Clin North Am 19:13, 1988.

Poppen NK et al: Recovery of sensibility after suture of digital nerves, J Hand Surg 4:212, 1979.

Stromberg WB Jr et al: Injury of the median and ulnar nerves: one hundred and fifty cases with an evaluation of Moberg's Ninhydrin test, J Bone Joint Surg 43-A:717, 1961.

Terzis JK, Dykes RW, and Hakstian RW: Electrophysiological recordings in peripheral nerve injury: a review, J Hand Surg 1:52, 1976.

Techniques of repair

Almquist EE: Nerve repair by laser, Orthop Clin North Am 19:201, 1988.

Archibald SJ and Fisher TR: Micro-surgical fascicular nerve repair: a morphological study of the endoneurial bulge, J Hand Surg 12-B:5, 1987.

Badalamente MA, Hurst LC, Paul SB, and Stracher A: Enhancement of neuromuscular recovery after nerve repair in primates, J Hand Surg 12-B:211, 1987.

Bolesta MJ, Garrett WE Jr, Ribbeck BM, et al: Immediate and delayed neurorrhaphy in a rabbit model: a functional, histologic, and biochemical comparison, J Hand Surg 13-A:364, 1988.

Bora WF, Pleasure DE, and Didizian NA: A study of nerve regeneration and neuroma formation after nerve suture by various techniques, J Hand Surg 1:138, 1976.

Bowers WH, Carlson EC, Wenner SM, and Doyle JR: Nerve suture and grafting, Hand Clin 5:445, 1989.

Cabaud HE et al: Epineurial and perineurial fascicular nerve repairs: a critical comparison, J Hand Surg 1:131, 1976.

Grabb WC: Management of nerve injuries in the forearm and hand, Orthop Clin North Am 2:419, 1970.

Grabb WC, Bement SL, Koepke GH, et al: Comparison of methods of peripheral nerve suturing in monkeys, J Plast Reconstr Surg 46:31, 1970.

Hakstian RW: Perineural neurorrhaphy, Orthop Clin North Am 4:945, 1973.

Jabaley ME et al: Comparison of histologic and functional recovery after peripheral nerve repair, J Hand Surg 1:119, 1976.

Kleinert HE and Griffin JM: Technique of nerve anastomosis, Orthop Clin North Am 4:907, 1973.

Kutz JE, Shealy G, and Lubbers L: Interfascicular nerve repair, Orthop Clin North Am 12:277, 1981.

Lewin ML: Repair of digital nerves in lacerations of the hand and the fingers, Clin Orthop 16:227, 1960.

Mackenzie IG: Causes of failure after repair of the median nerve, J Bone Joint Surg 43-B:465, 1961.

Mackinnon SE and Dellon AL: Evaluation of microsurgical internal neurolysis in a primate median nerve model of chronic nerve compression, J Hand Surg 13-A:357, 1988.

Marsh D and Barton N: Does the use of the operating microscope improve the results of peripheral nerve suture? J Bone Joint Surg 69-B:625, 1987.

McNamara MJ, Garrett WE Jr, Seaber AV, and Goldner JL: Neurorrhaphy, nerve grafting, and neurotization: a functional comparison of nerve reconstruction techniques, J Hand Surg 12-A:354, 1987.

Millesi H and Meissl G: Consequences of tension at the suture line. In Gorio A, Millesi H, and Mingrino S, editors: Posttraumatic peripheral nerve regeneration: experimental basis and clinical implications, New York, 1981, Raven Press.

Müller H and Grubel G: Long-term results of peripheral nerve sutures: a comparison of micro-macrosurgical technique, Adv Neurosurgery 9:381, 1981.

Narakas A: The use of fibrin glue in repair of peripheral nerves, Orthop Clin North Am 19:187, 1988.

Omer GE Jr and Spinner M: Peripheral nerve testing and suture techniques, AAOS Instr Course Lect 24:122, 1975.

Snyder CC: Epineurial repair, Orthop Clin North Am 12:267, 1981.

Sunderland S: The anatomic foundation of peripheral nerve repair techniques, Orthop Clin North Am 12:245, 1981.

Sunderland S: The pros and cons of funicular nerve repair, J Hand Surg 4:20, 1979.

Taylor GI: Nerve grafting with simultaneous microvascular reconstruction, Clin Orthop 133:56, 1978.

Terzis JK and Strauch B: Microsurgery of the peripheral nerve: a physiological approach, Clin Orthop 133:39, 1978.

Tupper JW, Crick JC, and Matteck LR: Fascicular nerve repairs: a comparative study of epineurial and fascicular (perineurial) techniques, Orthop Clin North Am 19:57, 1988.

Nerve grafts

Berger A and Millesi H: Nerve grafting, Clin Orthop 133:49, 1978.

Bonnel F, Foucher G, and Saint-Andre J-M: Histologic structure of the palmar digital nerves of the hand and its application to nerve grafting, J Hand Surg 14-A:874, 1989.

Boorman JG and Sykes PJ: Vascularized versus conventional nerve grafting: a case report, J Hand Surg 12-B:218, 1987.

Bora FW Jr, Bednar JM, Osterman AL, et al: Prosthetic nerve grafts: a resorbable tube as an alternative to autogenous nerve grafting, J Hand Surg 12-A:685, 1987.

Bourne MH, Wood MB, and Carmichael SW: Locating the lateral antebrachial cutaneous nerve, J Hand Surg 12-A:697, 1987.

Boyes JH: Repair of the motor branch of the ulnar nerve in the palm, J Bone Joint Surg 37-A:920, 1955.

Breidenbach WC: Vascularized nerve grafts: a practical approach, Orthop Clin North Am 19:81, 1988.

Doi K, Kuwata N, Sakai K, et al: A reliable technique of free vascularized sural nerve grafting and preliminary results of clinical applications, J Hand Surg 12-A:677, 1987.

Finseth F, Constable JD, and Cannon B: Interfascicular nerve grafting: early experiences at the Massachusetts General Hospital, Plast Reconstr Surg 56:492, 1975.

Frykman GK and Cally D: Interfascicular nerve grafting, Orthop Clin North Am 19:71, 1988.

Gattuso JM, Davies AH, Glasby MA, et al: Peripheral nerve repair using muscle autografts: recovery of transmission in primates, J Bone Joint Surg 70-B:524, 1988.

Greenberg BM, Caudros CL, Panda M, and May JW Jr: St. Clair Strange procedure: indications, technique, and long-term evaluation, J Hand Surg 13-A:928, 1988.

Hill HL, Vasconez LO, and Jurkiewicz MJ: Method for obtaining a sural nerve graft, Plast Reconstr Surg 61:177, 1978.

Mackinnon SE and Dellon AL: A comparison of nerve regeneration across a sural nerve graft and a vascularized pseudosheath, J Hand Surg 13-A:935, 1988.

McFarlane RM and Mayer JR: Digital nerve grafts with the lateral antebrachial cutaneous nerve, J Hand Surg 1:169, 1976.

Millesi H: Interfascicular nerve grafting, Orthop Clin North Am 12:287, 1981.

Norris RW, Glasby MA, Gattuso JM, and Bowden REM: Peripheral nerve repair in humans using muscle autografts: a new technique, J Bone Joint Surg 70-B:530, 1988.

Nunley JA, Ugino MR, Goldner RD, et al: Use of the anterior branch of the medial antebrachial cutaneous nerve as a graft for the repair of defects in the digital nerve, J Bone Joint Surg 71-A:563, 1989.

Ortigüela ME, Wood MB, and Cahill DR: Anatomy of the sural nerve complex, J Hand Surg 12-A:1119, 1987.

Risitano G, Cavallaro G, and Lentini M: Autogenous vein and nerve grafts: a comparative study of nerve regeneration in the rat, J Hand Surg 14-B:102, 1989.

Rodkey WG, Cabaud HE, and McCarroll HR Jr: Neurorrhaphy after loss of a nerve segment: comparison of epineurial suture under tension versus multiple nerve grafts, J Hand Surg 5:366, 1980.

Rose EH, Kowalski TA, and Norris MS: The reversed venous arterialized nerve graft in digital nerve reconstruction across scarred beds, Plast Reconstr Surg 83:593, 1989.

Shibata M, Tsai T-M, Firrell J, and Breidenbach WC: Experimental comparison of vascularized and nonvascularized nerve grafting, J Hand Surg 13-A:370, 1988.

Stromberg BV, Vlastou C, and Earle AS: Effect of nerve graft polarity on nerve regeneration and function, J Hand Surg 4:444, 1979.

Sunderland S: The restoration of median nerve function after destructive lesions which preclude end-to-end repair, Brain 97:1, 1974.

Wilgis EFS and Maxwell GP: Distal digital nerve grafts: clinical and anatomical studies, J Hand Surg 4:439, 1979.

Flaps to restore sensation

Dolich BM, Olshansky KJ, and Babar AH: Use of a cross-forearm neurocutaneous flap to provide sensation and coverage in hand reconstruction, Plast Reconstr Surg 62:550, 1978.

Edgerton MT: Cross-arm nerve pedicle flap for reconstruction of major defects of the median nerve, Surgery 64:248, 1968.

Holevich J: A new method of restoring sensibility to the thumb, J Bone Joint Surg 45-B:496, 1963.

Krag C and Rasmussen KB: The neurovascular island flap for defective sensibility of the thumb, J Bone Joint Surg 57-B:495, 1975.

Markley JM Jr: The preservation of close two-point discrimination in the interdigital transfer of neurovascular island flaps, Plast Reconstr Surg 59:812, 1977.

Morrison WA et al: Neurovascular free flaps from the foot for innervation of the hand, J Hand Surg 3:235, 1978.

Omer GE Jr et al: Neurovascular cutaneous island pedicles for deficient median-nerve sensibility: new technique and results of serial functional tests, J Bone Joint Surg 52-A:1181, 1970.

Winsten J: Island flap to restore stereognosis in hand injuries, N Engl J Med 268:124, 1963.

Rehabilitation

Adamson JE, Horton CE, and Crawford HH: Sensory rehabilitation of the injured thumb, Plast Reconstr Surg 40:53, 1967.

Frykman GK and Waylett J: Rehabilitation of peripheral nerve injuries, Orthop Clin North Am 12:361, 1981.

Leonard MH: Return of skin sensation in children without repair of nerves, Clin Orthop 95:273, 1973.

Neurolysis, neuromas, pain control

Bromage PR: Nerve physiology and control of pain, Orthop Clin North Am 4:897, 1973.

Dobyns JH et al: Bowler's thumb: diagnosis and treatment: a review of seventeen cases, J Bone Joint Surg 54-A:751, 1972.

Dunham W, Haines G, and Spring JM: Bowler's thumb (ulnovolar neuroma of the thumb), Clin Orthop 83:99, 1972.

Frykman GK, Adams J, and Bowen WW: Neurolysis, Orthop Clin North Am 12:325, 1981.

Howell AE and Leach RE: Bowler's thumb: perineural fibrosis of the digital nerve, J Bone Joint Surg 52-A:379, 1970.

Kleinert HE et al: Post-traumatic sympathetic dystrophy, Orthop Clin North Am 4:917, 1973.

Minkow FV and Bassett FH III: Bowler's thumb, Clin Orthop 83:115, 1972.

Omer GE Jr and Thomas SR: The management of chronic pain syndromes in the upper extremity, Clin Orthop 104:37, 1974.

Schuler FA III and Adamson JR: Pacinian neuroma, an unusual cause of finger pain, Plast Reconstr Surg 62:576, 1978.

Whipple RR and Unsell RS: Treatment of painful neuromas, Orthop Clin North Am 19:175, 1988.

Wilson RL: Management of pain following peripheral nerve injuries, Orthop Clin North Am 12:343, 1981.

CHAPTER 66

Wrist

PHILLIP E. WRIGHT II

This chapter discusses the anatomic, biomechanical, and kinematic aspects of wrist function, as well as diagnostic methods, treatment options, and management procedures for various wrist conditions. No attempt is made to resolve all controversies or to narrowly define the place of new procedures or technologies. In addition to the discussion of fractures and dislocations included here, also see Chapter 64. Similarly, compression neuropathies, various tendon lesions, tenosynovitis, and soft tissue aspects of rheumatoid arthritis are discussed in Chapters 76 and 72, respectively.

ANATOMY

The wrist, generally considered to be the region connecting the forearm to the hand, has indistinct boundaries especially regarding where the "wrist" ends and the "hand" begins. For the purposes of this discussion, we will consider the wrist to include the distal radioulnar, radiocarpal, and ulnocarpal joints, as well as the eight carpal bones and their articulations and attached ligaments.

The eight carpal bones include the scaphoid, lunate, triquetrum, and pisiform in the proximal row and the

trapezium, trapezoid, capitate, and hamate in the distal row (Fig. 66-1). They vary in size from the smaller pisiform and trapezoid to the largest, the capitate, and in the amount of articular cartilage allowing for articulation, with one bone by the pisiform (the triquetrum) to seven bones by the capitate.

The radiocarpal joints are formed by the articulation of the distal radius with the scaphoid and lunate through their respective concave facets on the distal radius and the triquetrum on the triangular fibrocartilage. The distal concave articular surfaces of the proximal carpal row form the mid-carpal articulations with the distal row. The distal row articulates with the metacarpals, allowing mobility in the thumb, stability in the index and long finger metacarpals, and increased mobility in the ring and little finger metacarpals.

The distal ulnar convexity articulates at the lesser sigmoid notch of the distal radius. The articular surface accommodates the ulnar head through two thirds of its arc. There is about a 20-degree inclination of the distal ulna at its articulation with the radius. The ulnar styloid lies dorsal to the ulnar head and extends distally. Separating the cartilage-covered head from the styloid is the attachment at the base of the styloid of the triangular fibrocartilage (Fig. 66-2).

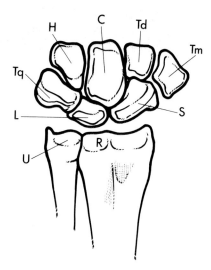

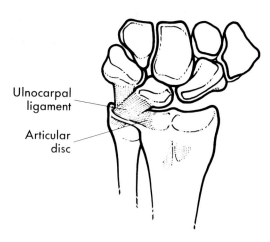

Fig. 66-1 Radiocarpal joint. *R,* radius; *U,* ulna; *S,* scaphoid; *L,* lunate; *Tm,* trapezium; *Td,* trapezoid; *C,* capitate; *H,* hamate; and *Tq,* triquetrum. (Redrawn from Poehling GG: An illustrated guide to small joint arthroscopy, Andover, Mass, 1989, Dyonics, Inc.)

Fig. 66-2 Triangular fibrocartilage complex: articular disc and ulnocarpal ligament. (Redrawn from Poehling GG: An illustrated guide to small joint arthroscopy, Andover, Mass, 1989, Dyonics, Inc.)

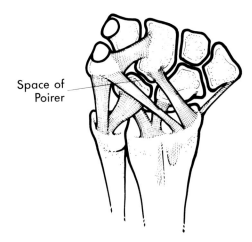

Fig. 66-3 Space of Poirier overlying palmar surface of lunate. (Redrawn from Poehling GG: An illustrated guide to small joint arthroscopy, Andover, Mass, 1989, Dyonics, Inc.)

Palmer and Werner have described the chondroligamentous supports attaching the distal radius and ulnar side of the carpus to the distal ulna, designating it the triangular fibrocartilage complex (TFCC). This structure, attached to the ulnar margin of the lunate fossa of the radius, includes the ulnar collateral ligament, the dorsal and volar radioulnar ligaments, the articular disc, the meniscal homologue, the extensor carpi ulnaris sheath, and the ulnolunate and ulnotriquetral ligament. Remaining ligaments are found in two locations: 1) between the carpal bones (interosseous intrinsic ligaments) connecting the carpal bones in the proximal and distal carpal rows and 2) extending from the radius and ulna distally across the carpal rows (extrinsic ligaments). The interosseous ligaments include the scapholunate and lunotriquetral interosseous ligaments connecting the proximal carpal row and the ligaments connecting the trapezium to the trapezoid, the trapezoid to the capitate, and the capitate to the hamate in the distal carpal row. The extrinsic or crossing ligaments include the radial collateral ligament from the radial styloid to the scaphoid waist, the ulnar collateral ligament from the base of the ulnar styloid attaching to the pisiform, and the transverse carpal ligament. The volar extrinsic or crossing ligaments also include the radioscaphocapitate ligament, the radiolunotriquetral ligament, and the radioscapholunate ligament on the radial side and the ulnolunate and ulnotriquetral components of the triangular fibrocartilage complex on the ulnar side. On the palmar side of the carpus, between the radiolunotriquetral ligament and the radioscaphocapitate ligament, is a relatively thin area, the space of Poirer, overlying the palmar surface of the lunate (Fig. 66-3).

Dorsally, there is an area of thickening in the ligaments known as the dorsal radiocarpal ligament, extending from the dorsum of the radius near Lister's tubercle ulnarward attaching to the triquetrum.

CIRCULATION

According to reports by Gelberman et al. and others, the carpus receives its extraosseous blood supply through three dorsal and three palmar transverse arterial arches. The dorsal arches are (1) the dorsal radiocarpal at the radiocarpal joint, supplying the lunate and triquetrum; (2) the dorsal intercarpal (the largest) between the proximal and distal carpal rows, supplying the distal carpal row and, through anastomoses with the radiocarpal arch, the lunate and triquetrum; and (3) the basal metacarpal arch at the base of the metacarpals (the most variable) to supply the distal carpal row. The palmar arches are (1) the palmar radiocarpal at the level of the radiocarpal joint to the palmar surfaces of the lunate and triquetrum; (2) the intercarpal arch between the proximal and distal carpal rows, which is the most variable and does not contribute to nutrient vessels in the carpus; and (3) the deep palmar arch at the level of the metacarpal bases, which is consistent and communicates with the dorsal basal metacarpal arch and the palmar metacarpal arteries. Additional descriptions of the intraosseous circulation of specific carpal bones (such as the scaphoid and lunate) are found with the discussions of afflictions of those bones in the references cited at the end of the chapter.

BIOMECHANICS AND KINEMATICS

Recent important contributions by Linscheid; Mayfield, Johnson, and Kilcoyne; Palmer et al.; Kauser; and others have led to our current understanding of wrist kinematics and biomechanics. The following summarizes what seem to be the current concepts about the functioning of the wrist.

The stability of the wrist during motion and interrelated motions depends on capsuloligamentous integrity and contact surface contours of the carpal bones. The center of rotation for most wrist motions is located in the proximal capitate. During flexion and extension, the majority of motion occurs at the radiocapitate joint, with some occurring through the midcarpal area. During radial to ulnar deviation, the proximal carpal row rotates

dorsally and the proximal row translocates or shifts radially at both the midcarpal and radiocarpal joints, with motion occurring at both the radiocarpal and intercarpal joints. During ulnar to radial deviation, the proximal carpal row tends toward palmar rotation, with most of the motion occurring in the intercarpal joints. The proximal carpal row is considered to be an intercalated segment in the forearm-to-hand connection, with the scaphoid functioning to stabilize the wrist. For purposes of understanding the ways in which forces are transmitted and motions and positions of the carpal bones are controlled by ligaments and contact surface contours, the concept of a wrist consisting of three columns has become popular. These columns generally are described as the central (force-bearing) column, the radial column, and the ulnar (control) column. The central column includes the distal articular surface of the radius, the lunate and capitate, and some would add the proximal two thirds of the scaphoid, the trapezoid, and the articulations with the second and third metacarpal bases. The radial column includes the radius, scaphoid, trapezium, trapezoid, and the thumb carpometacarpal joint. The ulnar column includes the triangular fibrocartilage (articular disc), hamate, triquetrum, and the articulations of the carpometacarpal joints of the ring and little fingers. Taleisnik has proposed that the central column includes the entire distal row and the lunate. In his concept, the scaphoid is included as the lateral column and the triquetrum as a rotatory medial column (Fig. 66-4, *A*). Lichtman proposed a ring concept of wrist kinematics (Fig.

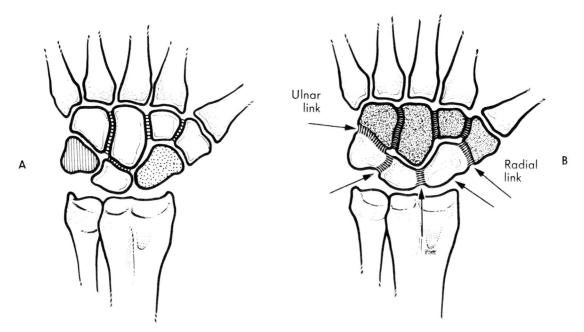

Fig. 66-4 **A,** Taleisnik's concept of central (flexion-extension) column involves entire distal row and lunate: scaphoid is lateral (mobile) column and triquetrum is rotatory medial column. **B,** Lichtman's ring concept of carpal kinematics: proximal and distal rows are semirigid posts stabilized by interosseous ligaments; normal controlled mobility occurs at scaphotrapezial and triquetrohamate joints. Any break in ring, either bony or ligamentous (*arrows*) can produce DISI or VISI deformity. (Redrawn from Lichtman DM et al: J Hand Surg 6:515, 1981.)

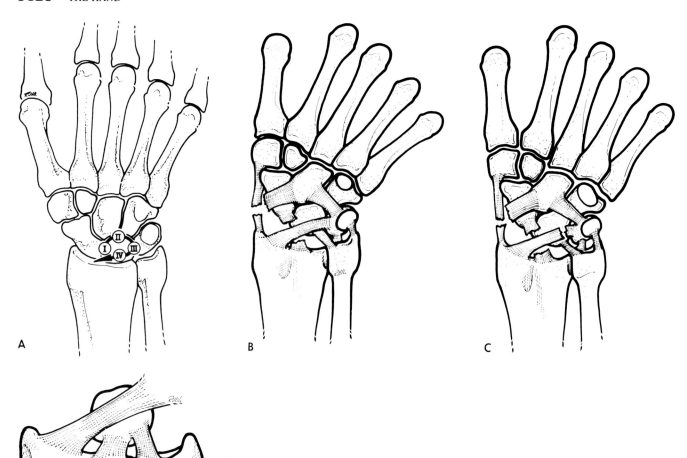

Fig. 66-5   A, Stages of perilunar instability. **B,** Volar ligamentous injury in stage II. **C,** Volar ligamentous injury in stage III. **D,** Remaining volar ligament attachments to lunate in stage IV. (Redrawn from Mayfield JK: Clin Orthop 187:36, 1984.)

66-4, *B*). According to this concept, the interosseous ligaments stabilize the semirigid proximal and distal carpal rows. Limited mobility occurs between the scaphotrapezial joints and the triquetrohamate joints. Bone or ligament disruption of the ring creates instability deformities, with the lunate tilting either dorsally (dorsal intercalated segmental instability [DISI]) or toward the volar aspect (volar intercalated segmental instability [VISI]).

DIAGNOSIS OF WRIST CONDITIONS
History

When obtaining the history of traumatic conditions, the mechanism of injury frequently is unknown. Mayfield, Johnson, and Kilcoyne have found that the various carpal injuries seem to be parts of a spectrum of injury, the extent of injury depending on (1) loading in three di-

mensions, (2) duration and amount of forces, (3) hand position at impact, and (4) mechanical properties of the ligaments and bones. A pattern can be seen in which carpal dislocations result from ulnar deviation and intercarpal supination and scaphoid fractures result from wrist extension with the dorsal articular margin of the radius serving as a fulcrum (Fig. 66-5). Flexion and pronation injuries, conversely, may contribute more to ligament injuries on the ulnar side of the wrist, especially the lunotriquetral ligament. It is therefore important to be able to document swelling, bruising, and sensations of grating, popping, crunching, and local areas of pain and point tenderness.

For long-standing problems, it is important to correlate the problem with the factors that cause worsening or improvement. The relationship to work and recreational activities; the presence and location of swelling with mechanical symptoms, such as clicking, popping, snapping, and crunching; and the response to other treatment are important. Other joint involvement and the possibility of the various arthritides in the patient or family members also should be considered.

Physical Examination

It is important to conduct a careful, detailed examination with the forearm and hand supported whether the examination is immediately following injury or for chronic problems. In addition to the usual assessment of motor, sensory, and circulatory integrity, it is important to try to correlate the patient's complaints with the underlying muscles, tendons, tendon sheaths, bones, joints, ligaments, and capsules. Old scars, bruises, and other skin findings, as well as the ranges of active and passive motion, should be documented.

The underlying anatomy may be correlated with easily identified and palpable bony structures, including the radial styloid, Lister's tubercle, the ulnar styloid, the pisiform, and the scaphoid tuberosity. It is important to differentiate overlying superficial tenosynovitis such as that seen in the first dorsal compartment (deQuervain's) from conditions related to deeper structures (e.g., thumb carpometacarpal arthritis, radial and ulnar wrist extensor tenosynovitis, masses such as ganglions, and underlying compression neuropathies of the median and ulnar nerves in their respective tunnels) from the problems related to ligamentous and bony structures.

Roentgenographic Techniques

After the history and physical, roentgenographic evaluation in a standardized and organized way is helpful in determining the diagnosis, future course, and management of wrist problems. Gilula et al. proposed a useful algorithm detailing one approach to the roentgenographic assessment of the painful wrist (Fig. 66-6).

Various roentgenographic techniques useful in assessing the painful wrist include (1) routine roentgenographic series consisting of four views (posteroanterior, lateral, oblique, and scaphoid); (2) spot views of the carpal bones for detail (carpal tunnel view; Fig. 66-7); (3) fluoroscopic spot views of the wrist (Fig. 66-8); (4) series of views for instability (anteroposterior clenched fist; posteroanterior in neutral, radial, and ulnar deviation; lateral in neutral, full flexion, and extension; semipronated oblique 30 degrees from the posteroanterior; and semisupinated oblique 30 degrees from the lateral); (5) cine or video fluoroscopy; (6) bone scan; (7) tomography; (8) arthrography of the wrist (triple injection when indicated; Fig. 66-9); (9) computed tomography; and (10) magnetic resonance imaging.

Other Diagnostic Techniques

Other clinical methods for determining the specific anatomic location of a problem include (1) differential local anesthetic injection, (2) wrist arthroscopy, and (3) various other operative procedures. If the specific structure causing the pain cannot be precisely identified (for example, extensor carpi ulnaris versus underlying ulnocarpal joint), it is sometime useful to inject a small amount (less than 3 ml) of local anesthetic into the most likely site. This helps in the localization of the pain. Sterile technique is used, and the patient is always advised of the benefits, risks, and hazards.

Wrist arthroscopy and a variety of operative procedures are available for the treatment of wrist conditions and are described in the subsequent sections.

Fig. 66-6 Roentgenographic approach to painful wrist. (From Gilula LA et al: Clin Orthop 187:52, 1984.)

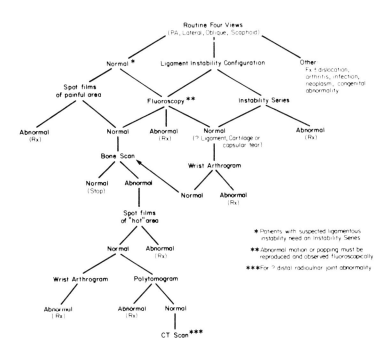

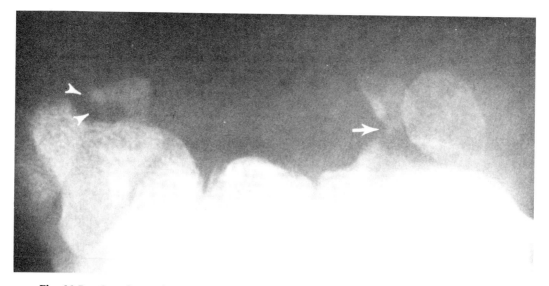

Fig. 66-7   Carpal tunnel view shows avulsion fracture of hamate hook (*arrow*) and trapezium (*arrowhead*). (From Gilula LA et al: Clin Orthop 187:52, 1984.)

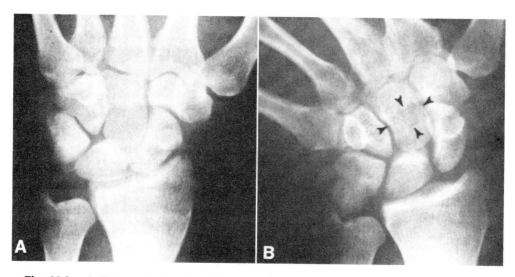

Fig. 66-8   **A,** Posteroanterior view of capitate shows no definite abnormality. **B,** On angled view, cystic defect with fracture is seen in capitate waist. (From Gilula LA et al: Clin Orthop 187:52, 1984.)

FRACTURES AND DISLOCATIONS OF CARPAL BONES, INCLUDING KIENBÖCK'S DISEASE

The diagnosis of fractures and dislocations of the carpal bones may be difficult for several reasons. The outlines of the eight tightly packed bones inevitably superimpose in most roentgenographic views. Even in the anteroposterior view at least one bone overlies another. All views must be interpreted with a thorough understanding of the normal bone contours and the relationships between the bones. Further, the carpal bones normally shift in their relationship to one another during the various arcs of wrist motion.

Because of the difficulty in recognizing fractures in acute injuries, many fractures in this region are missed until later. Articular damage and ligamentous injuries are even more difficult to evaluate. The latter may permit abnormal rotations and subluxations of the various bones. Special roentgenographic techniques are helpful, but even with their use, a precise diagnosis may be difficult to make. Often prognosis is uncertain because of the peculiarities of the blood supply of these bones, especially of the scaphoid and lunate.

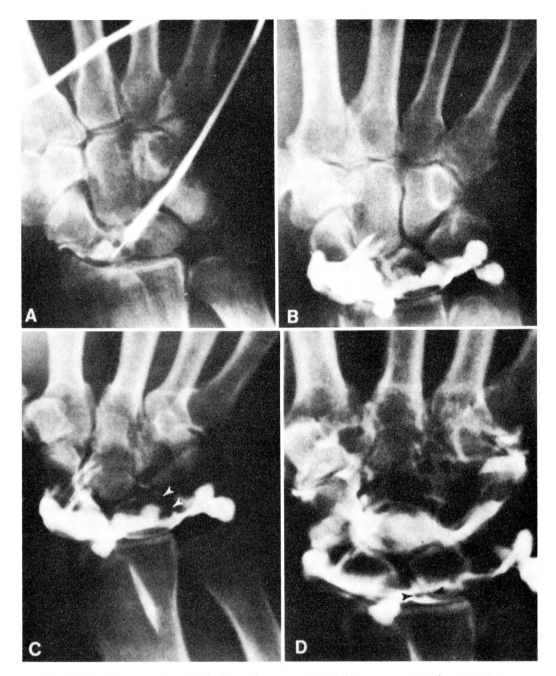

Fig. 66-9 Fluoroscopic spots during arthrogram. **A,** Needle in place, start of contrast injection. **B,** end of contrast injection, at point of slight patient discomfort: contrast is confined to radiocarpal joint. **C,** With ulnar deviation, contrast passes into midcarpal joint between lunate and triquetrum (*arrowheads*), indicating lunotriquetral ligament tear. **D,** On follow-up overhead view, contrast fills the midcarpal joints, including scapholunate joint from its distal aspect, making it difficult to see whether scapholunate or lunotriquetral ligament is torn. A small defect (*arrowheads*) between contrast in scapholunate space and radiocarpal space indicates intact scapholunate ligament. (Reprinted with permission from Gilula LA, Totty WG, and Weeks PM: Wrist arthrography: the value of fluoroscopic spot viewing, Radiology 146:555, 1983.)

Fractures of Scaphoid

Fracture of the carpal scaphoid bone is the most common fracture of the carpus, and frequently diagnosis is delayed. A delay in diagnosis and treatment of this fracture may alter the prognosis for union. A wrist sprain that is sufficiently severe to require roentgenographic examination initially should be treated as a possible frac-

ture of the scaphoid, and the roentgenograms should be repeated in 2 weeks even though initial roentgenograms may be negative.

ETIOLOGY. This fracture has been reported in people from 10 to 70 years of age although it is most common in young adult men. It is caused by a fall on the out-

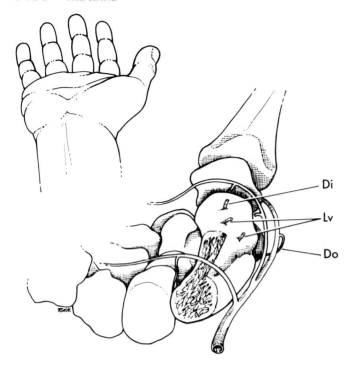

Fig. 66-10 Representation of extraosseous and intraosseous blood supply of scaphoid. *Lv,* Laterovolar vessels; *Do,* dorsal vessels; and *Di,* distal vessels. (Redrawn from Taleisnik J and Kelly PJ: J Bone Joint Surg 48-A:1125, 1966.)

stretched palm, resulting in severe hyperextension and slight radial deviation of the wrist. Seventeen percent of patients have other fractures of the carpus and forearm, including transscaphoid perilunar dislocations, fractures of the trapezium, Bennett's fractures, fractures of the radial head, dislocations of the lunate, and fractures at the distal end of the radius.

ANATOMY AND BLOOD SUPPLY OF SCAPHOID BONE. The unique anatomy of the scaphoid predisposes fracture of this carpal bone to delayed union or nonunion and to disability of the wrist. Because it articulates with the distal radius as well as with four of the remaining seven carpal bones, the scaphoid moves with nearly all carpal motions, especially volar flexion. Any alteration of its articular surface through fracture, dislocation, or subluxation or any alteration of its stability by ligamentous rupture may cause severe secondary changes throughout the entire carpus.

The blood supply of the scaphoid is precarious. Obletz and Halbstein have shown that only 67% of scaphoid bones have arterial foramina throughout their length, including the distal, middle, and proximal thirds. Of the remaining bones, 13% have blood supply predominantly in the distal third and 20% have most of the arterial foramina in the waist area of the bone with no more than a single foramen near the proximal third. This suggests that one third of the fractures occurring in the proximal third may be without adequate blood supply, and this seems to be borne out clinically; avascular necrosis occurs in 35% of fractures at this level. Taleisnik and Kelly demonstrated that vessels entered the scaphoid from the radial artery, both laterovolarly and dorsally as well as distally. The laterovolar and dorsal systems share in the

blood supply to the proximal two thirds of the scaphoid (Fig. 66-10).

TREATMENT. Treatment of scaphoid fractures is determined by displacement and stablity of the fracture. Cooney, Dobyns, and Linscheid classify scaphoid fractures as either undisplaced and stable or displaced and unstable (Fig. 66-11).

Undisplaced, stable scaphoid fractures. Prognosis is excellent in an undisplaced acute, stable fracture diagnosed early. We use a forearm cast from just below the elbow

Scaphoid nonunion associated with the location of fracture and amount of displacement		
Location	Number of fractures	Percentage of union
Distal third	2	100
Middle third	56	80
Proximal third	32	64
Displacement	Number of fractures	Percentage of union
Stable	48	85
Unstable	42	65

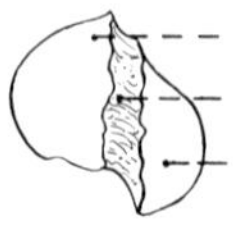

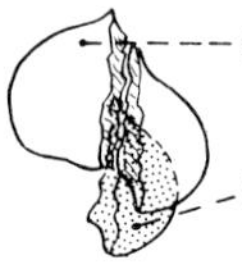

Fig. 66-11 Union of scaphoid after bone grafting is influenced significantly by both location of fracture and amount of displacement. (From Cooney WP, Dobyns JH, and Linscheid RL: J Hand Surg 5:343, 1980.)

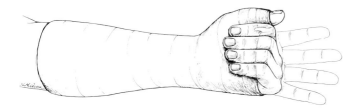

Fig. 66-12 Cast for immobilizing fractured scaphoid. It extends from base of thumbnail and proximal palmar crease distally to 1 inch distal to elbow proximally. Note that full flexion of metacarpophalangeal joints of fingers is possible.

proximally to the base of the thumbnail and the proximal palmar crease distally (thumb spica) with the wrist in slight radial deviation and in neutral flexion (Fig. 66-12). The thumb is maintained in a functional position, and the fingers are free to move from the metacarpophalangeal joints distally. The expected rate of union is 95% within 10 weeks. During this time, the fracture is observed roentgenographically for healing. If collapse of a fragment occurs, treatment is altered accordingly.

In a series of 92 patients, Terkelsen and Jepsen found that the incidence of nonunion was no greater in patients treated by a removable short arm thumb spica cast than in those treated by a long arm thumb spica cast. On the other hand, Gellman et al. found that the time to union was 3 months shorter in patients treated initially for 6 weeks in a long arm thumb spica cast.

If the fracture is displaced, the diagnosis is delayed, or the fracture is in the proximal or perhaps the middle third, the prognosis is less favorable and an initial long arm thumb spica cast for 6 weeks may be justified.

For undisplaced fracture of the scaphoid when diagnosis has been delayed for several weeks, treatment should begin with cast immobilization. Surgery should be considered only when there is no indication of new healing activity and no indication of union after a trial of cast immobilization for about 20 weeks.

When making the diagnosis of scaphoid fractures or nonunions, a bipartite scaphoid is considered so rare as to be of little or no clinical significance.

Displaced, unstable scaphoid fractures. For a displaced, unstable fracture in which the fragments are offset more than 1 mm in the anteroposterior or oblique view, or the lunocapitate angulation is greater than 15 degrees, or the scapholunate angulation is greater than 45 degrees in the lateral view (range of 30 to 60 degrees), a different course of treatment is required. Because the range of lunocapitate and scapholunate angulation can vary, comparison views of the opposite wrist may be helpful. Reduction may be attempted initially by longitudinal traction and compression of the carpus. For displaced fractures, this rarely is successful in our experience. If the reduction attempt is successful, percutaneous pinning and application of a long arm thumb spica cast may suffice. Otherwise, open reduction and internal

fixation may be required. The rate of union is reported to be 54% in these fractures. The average time for union is 16½ weeks. Cooney et al. also found that the rate of union was better when internal fixation was achieved by an inlay bone graft (Matti-Russe procedure) than by a dorsal bone peg. Regardless of the technique of bone grafting, there usually will be some loss of wrist motion even if the fracture unites, whereas with prolonged cast immobilization, once union is obtained, a more functional range of motion can be expected.

For a displaced or unstable recent fracture of the scaphoid, the best method of fixation depends on the surgeon's experience and the equipment available. In some fractures, adequate internal fixation may be obtained with Kirschner wires. The Warner compression staple, the AO cannulated screw, and the Herbert differential pitch bone screw have been used to advantage in displaced and unstable scaphoid fractures. Cannulated bone screws are useful because the screw can be accurately placed over a guide pin placed with video fluoroscopic control. The advantages of the Herbert screw, according to Sprague and Howard, are that it (1) reduces the time of external immobilization, (2) provides relatively strong internal fixation, and (3) produces compression at the fracture site. In addition, because the headless screw remains below the bone surface, removal is usually unnecessary. Screws may be used with a bone graft to correct scaphoid angulation. The disadvantages include the necessity of using a jig for insertion and the demanding surgical technique (Fig. 66-13). Contraindications include (1) avascular crumbling of the proximal pole of the scaphoid, (2) extensive trauma or osteoarthritis involving the adjacent carpals or articular surface of the radius, and (3) gross carpal collapse.

Open reduction and internal fixation of acute displaced fractures of scaphoid

■ ***TECHNIQUE.*** With the patient supine and under suitable anesthesia, prepare the hand and wrist and one iliac crest region and inflate a pneumatic tourniquet. Make a longitudinal skin incision over the palmar surface of the wrist, beginning 3 to 4 cm proximal to the wrist flexion crease over the flexor carpi radialis. Extend the incision distally to the wrist flexion crease and then curve it radially toward the scaphotrapezial and trapeziometacarpal joints. Protect cutaneous sensory nerve branches, and reflect skin flaps at the level of the forearm fascia. Open the sheath of the flexor carpi radialis, retract the tendon radially, and open the deep surface of its sheath. Expose the palmar capsule of the joint over the radioscaphoid joint. Extend the wrist in ulnar deviation and open the capsule in the longitudinal axis of the scaphoid bone, obliquely extending the incision toward the scaphotrapezial joint. With sharp dissection, expose the fracture, preserving the capsuloligamentous structures for later repair. In-

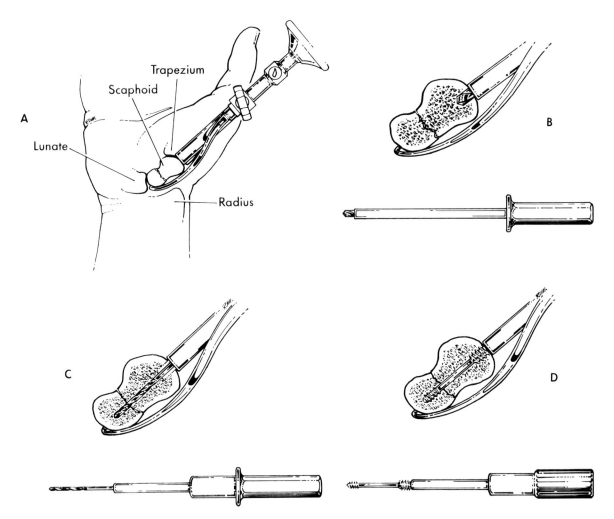

Fig. 66-13 Herbert screw fixation of scaphoid. **A**, Jig used for volar approach to scaphoid. **B**, Short drill used for making screw hole. **C**, Long drill inserted to maximum depth. **D**, Herbert screw inserted. (Redrawn from Sprague HH and Howard FM: Contemp Orthop 16:18, 1988.)

spect the fracture to determine the need for bone grafting. If comminution is absent or minimal, reduction and fixation will suffice. If comminution is extensive, especially on the palmar surface, with a tendency to flexion of the scaphoid at the fracture, obtain an iliac crest bone graft. Reduce the fracture and fix it with Kirschner wires or a stable screw technique (such as cannulated or Herbert screws), taking care that there is no rotation or angulation. For fractures through the waist and in the distal pole, inserting the fixation device through a distal portal may be easier. Placement of Kirschner wires down the long axis of the scaphoid is made easier by gentle radial deviation of the wrist, aligning the scaphoid vertically. With the wrist in this position, direct the wires almost dorsally into the scaphoid. After stable reduction and fixation are obtained, check the position and alignment of the reduction and the placement of the internal fixation with image intensification or roentgenograms. Deflate the tourniquet and obtain hemostasis. Insert a drain if needed and close the wrist capsule with nonabsorbable sutures. Close the skin and apply a dressing that includes either a sugar tong splint with a thumb spica extension or a long arm cast incorporating the thumb.

AFTERTREATMENT. The sutures are removed and the splint or cast is changed at 2 weeks. Immobilization in an elbow-thumb spica cast is continued for a total of 6 to 8 weeks. If Kirschner wires were used, they are removed at 6 to 8 weeks. Screw fixation may be left in place permanently unless tender areas develop or the screw loosens. At 6 to 8 weeks, a short arm thumb spica cast is applied; this cast is changed monthly for 6 to 8 months. If healing is progressing by roentgenographic examination, a short arm thumb spica brace is used until bone healing is assured. Finger, thumb, and shoulder motion is encouraged throughout convalescence, and after cast removal wrist motion and elbow motion are gradually increased, followed by strengthening exercises.

Nonunion of scaphoid fractures. Nonunion of scaphoid fractures is influenced by delayed diagnosis, gross displacement, associated injuries of the carpus, and impaired blood supply. Of these fractures, an estimated 40% are undiagnosed at the time of the original injury. The incidence of avascular necrosis is approximately 30% to 40%, occurring most frequently in fractures of the proximal third.

Cystic changes in the scaphoid and the adjoining bones followed by avascular necrosis may occur after untreated fractures, but this is not an absolute indication for surgery. Mazet and Hohl, and Stewart reported several patients in whom fractures of the scaphoid healed after a delay in diagnosis of 5 months when treated with cast immobilization of 8 to 12 months. Many nonunions of the scaphoid have minimal symptoms and can be tolerated well in sedentary occupations. The patient should be informed, however, that degenerative arthritis of the wrist probably is inevitable, but this may take years to develop, depending on the amount of chronic stress applied and the activity of the wrist. In old fractures with arthritis, symptoms may be decreased by excision of the radial styloid just proximal to the fracture in middle third fractures; however, other reconstructive surgery, especially for severe arthritic degeneration, may be indicated and proximal-row carpectomy or arthrodesis of the wrist joint may prove to be more dependable. When other injuries of carpal bones require open reduction, the fractured scaphoid should be accurately reduced also. Some minimally displaced fractures of the waist or middle third of the scaphoid may unite without open reduction.

We have found the following operations to be useful for nonunions of the scaphoid (not listed in order of preference): (1) styloidectomy, (2) excision of the proximal fragment, (3) proximal-row carpectomy, (4) bone grafting, and (5) partial or total arthrodesis of the wrist.

Styloidectomy. Styloidectomy alone is probably of little value in treating nonunions of the scaphoid. But when arthritic changes involve only the scaphoid fossa of the radiocarpal joint, styloidectomy is indicated in conjunction with any grafting of the scaphoid or excision of its ulnar fragment.

In older patients in whom radioscaphoid arthritis predominates and the proximal fragment is not loose, styloidectomy alone may provide pain relief. Stewart emphasized the importance of removing adequate radial styloid when the styloidectomy is performed. The distal end of the radius has two separate and distinct concave surfaces, one articulating with the scaphoid and the other with the lunate, separated by a small ridge of bone. Stewart recommends resecting enough of the styloid to remove the entire articulation with the scaphoid. It is important to preserve the palmar radiocarpal ligaments when a generous styloidectomy is done.

■ *TECHNIQUE (STEWART).* Make a bayonet-shaped incision along the radial aspect of the wrist as follows. Begin distally over the dorsum of the first metacarpal and proceed proximally to the anatomic snuffbox, then dorsally along the extensor crease of the wrist, and then proximally along the dorsoradial aspect of the distal radius. Expose and carefully protect the radial artery and the sensory branches of the radial nerve, which lie in the subcutaneous tissue. Incise the joint capsule and expose the radial styloid subperiosteally. Careful subperiosteal dissection may avoid excessive disruption of the volar radiocarpal ligaments. Locate the ridge on the radius that separates the articular fossa for the lunate from that for the scaphoid. With a sharp, thin osteotome or a thin oscillating saw blade, make the osteotomy cut perpendicular to the long axis of the radius, with its ulnar border at the ridge just located. Remove the resected styloid. Move the wrist through a full range of motion under direct vision to be sure that the irregular surfaces of the scaphoid do not impinge on the remaining radius. Close the wound in layers.

AFTERTREATMENT. An anterior plaster spint is applied with the wrist in the position of function. At 3 weeks, the splint is removed and active exercises are begun.

Excision of proximal fragment. Excising *both* fragments of the scaphoid is unwise; although the immediate result may be satisfactory, eventual derangement of the wrist is likely. Soto-Hall and Haldeman reported gradual migration of the capitate into the space previously occupied by the scaphoid, although disability was not apparent for 5 to 7 years.

When indicated, excising the proximal scaphoid fragment is usually satisfactory: the loss of one fourth or less of the scaphoid impairs wrist motion less than any other operation for nonunion, and because immobilization after surgery is brief, function usually returns rapidly. Strength in the wrist is usually decreased to some extent, although this may be difficult to detect clinically.

The indications for excising the proximal fragment of a scaphoid nonunion are as follows:

1. When the fragment consists of one fourth or less of the scaphoid: Regardless of its viability, grafting of such a small fragment frequently will fail, but not always.
2. When the fragment consists of one fourth or less of the scaphoid and is sclerotic, comminuted, or severely displaced: The comminuted fragments usually should be excised early to prevent arthritic changes; a severely displaced fragment should also be excised early when it cannot be accurately replaced by manipulation. In the past, Silastic implants have been used to act as "space fillers." Because of the possibility of silicone synovitis, we prefer to use a folded or rolled tendon graft to fill the defect.

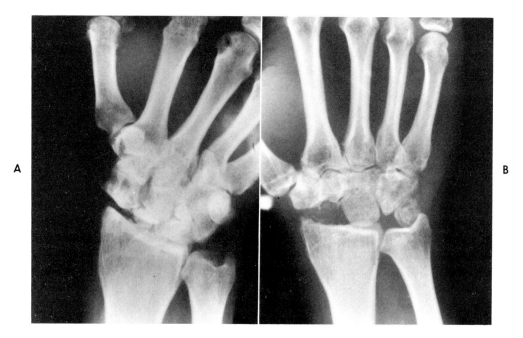

Fig. 66-14 **A,** Long-standing scaphoid nonunion with arthritis, avascular necrosis, collapse of proximal pole, and settling of capitate into proximal row. **B,** Postoperative roentgenogram of proximal-row carpectomy with radial styloidectomy. (From Neviaser RJ: J Hand Surg 8:301, 1983.)

3. When the fragment consists of one fourth or less of the scaphoid and grafting has failed.
4. When a nonviable proximal fragment consists of more than one fourth of the scaphoid, some other treatment is preferable to excision.
5. When arthritic changes are present in the region of the radial styloid, styloidectomy is indicated in conjunction with excision of the proximal fragment.

■ *TECHNIQUE.* **At the level of the styloid process of the radius, make a transverse skin incision 5 cm long on the dorsoradial aspect of the wrist. Retract the tendons of the thumb abductors in a palmar direction and the tendon of the extensor pollicis longus dorsal and ulnar. Incise the joint capsule and expose the scaphoid. To avoid excising a normal carpal bone, place a metal marker on the bone thought to be the proximal fragment of the scaphoid and identify the fragment in an anteroposterior roentgenogram. Grasp the fragment to be excised with a towel clip, apply traction, and remove the fragment by dividing its soft tissue attachments. Close the wound.**

AFTERTREATMENT. **The wrist is immobilized in a cock-up splint for 2 weeks. Active exercises are then begun and are continued until function is restored.**

Proximal-row carpectomy. Although the use of proximal-row carpectomy has been somewhat controversial, available early reports in the literature by Stamm, Crabbe, Inglis and Jones, and Jorgensen suggested that satisfactory results could be achieved. More recently, Neviaser reported satisfactory relief of pain and return of grip strength in 23 of 24 wrists treated with proximal-row carpectomy and Green reported acceptable results in 13 of 15 wrists. It generally is considered to be a satisfactory procedure in patients who are willing to accept the risk of minimal persistent pain (Figs. 66-14 and 66-15). Should it be unsuccessful, arthrodesis remains an option.

In general, manual laborers are better candidates for a wrist arthrodesis, whereas those patients requiring wrist mobility, who are willing to accept the possibility of some wrist pain, are better candidates for proximal-row carpectomy.

Proximal-row carpectomy has been used as a reconstructive procedure for posttraumatic degenerative conditions in the wrist, especially those involving the scaphoid and lunate. When proximal-row carpectomy is done for degenerative changes there should be demonstrably good articular surfaces in the lunate fossa of the radius and the distal articular surface of the capitate to allow for satisfactory articulation between these surfaces. If there are significant degenerative changes on these articular surfaces roentgenographically or to direct vision at the time of the operative procedure, consideration should be given to an alternative procedure such as arthrodesis. Primary proximal-row carpectomy may be useful in treating severe open carpal fracture dislocations in which there is significant disruption of the bony architecture, comminuted fractures of the scaphoid and lunate, and disruption of the blood supply to the lunate and scaphoid.

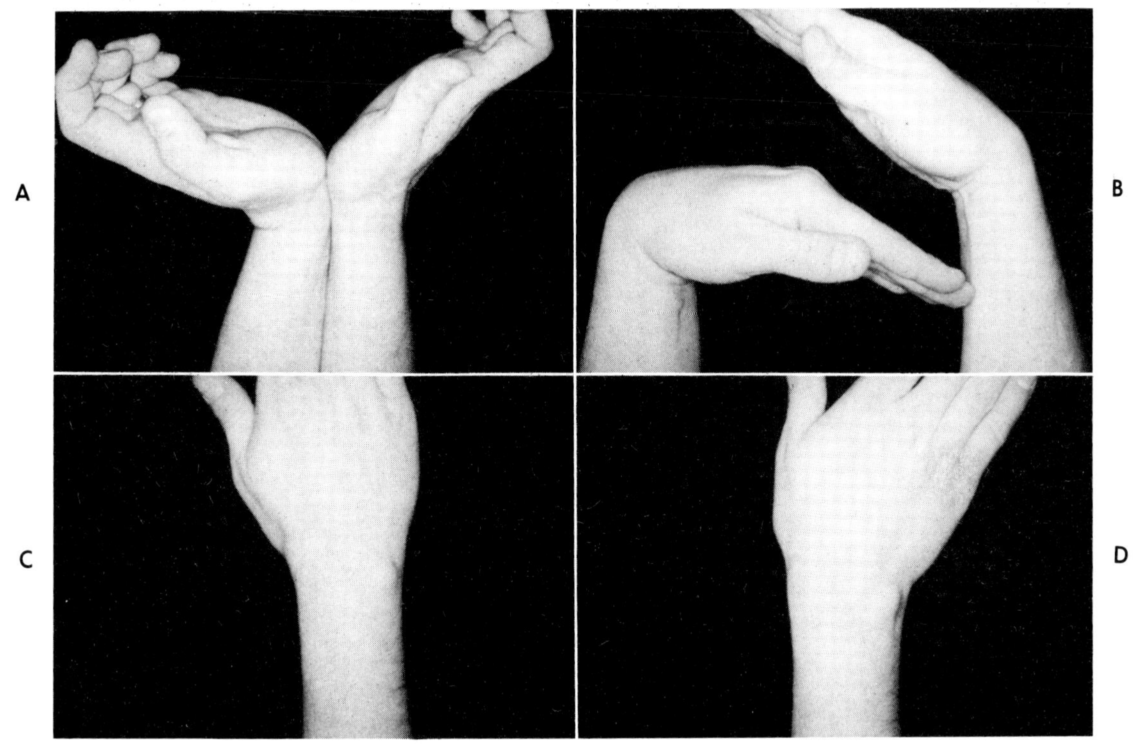

Fig. 66-15 Typical results at 6 years showing **A,** extension; **B,** flexion; **C,** radial deviation; and **D,** ulnar deviation in construction worker. (From Neviaser RJ: J Hand Surg 8:301, 1983.)

Usually excision of the triquetrum, lunate, and entire scaphoid has been recommended. However, the distal pole of the scaphoid at its articulation with the trapezium may be left to provide a more stable base for the thumb. If the distal scaphoid pole is left, radial styloidectomy should be done to avoid impingement of the distal scaphoid pole and trapezium on the radial styloid. When a radial styloidectomy is done and during proximal-row carpectomy care should be taken to avoid injury to the volar radiocapitate ligament, as stressed by Taleisnik and Green. Excision of the pisiform is unnecessary because of its location in the flexor carpi ulnaris tendon as a sesamoid. The bones usually are removed piecemeal and the use of threaded Kirschner wires or screws as "joy sticks" or handles is helpful to lever the bone out at the wrist. Two techniques are presented.

■ *TECHNIQUE.* Make a transverse incision on the dorsum of the wrist 6 mm distal to the radiocarpal joint and extending from the dorsal aspect of the ulnar styloid to that of the radial one. Deepen the incision to the extensor retinaculum, preserving the sensory branches of the radial and ulnar nerves. Ligate and divide the superficial veins. Now divide the retinaculum longitudinally both on the radial and on the ulnar sides of the extensor digitorum communis tendons; avoid damaging the extensor pollicis longus tendon that crosses the wound diagonally. Expose the dorsum of the proximal row of carpal bones through two longitudinal incisions in the capsule —

one in the interval between the extensor digitorum communis tendons and the extensor carpi ulnaris and the second between the extensor carpi radialis brevis tendon and the extensor digitorum communis. (Because the extensor pollicis longus tendon crosses this area diagonally, it can be retracted either medially or laterally as necessary.) Now expose the lunate by elevating the capsule of the wrist beneath the extensor digitorum communis tendons; insert a threaded pin into the lunate, apply traction to the bone through the pin, and excise the bone by dividing its capsular attachments with sharp pointed scissors. Carefully fragment the lunate with a small bone cutter, osteotome, or saw to facilitate removal. Next insert the pin into the triquetrum and excise it in a similar manner. (The lunate and triquetrum are excised first to provide more space for the more difficult excision of the scaphoid.) Now through the more radial of the two incisions in the capsule, first excise the ulnar fragment of the scaphoid in the manner just described above and then the radial fragment, but dissect close to this fragment to avoid injuring the radial artery. Align the capitate with the lunate fossa. Use a Steinmann pin to stabilize the capitate if needed. If the palmar radiocapitate ligament is preserved, this may not be necessary. Obtain hemostasis or drain the wound as need, and close the wound in layers. Apply a sugar tong splint with hand and wrist in a functional position.

AFTERTREATMENT. The wrist is immobilized in slight extension and with the hand in the functional position in a plaster sugar tong splint for 2 or 3 weeks. If a Steinmann pin has been used, it is removed at about 4 weeks. Active motion of the digits is encouraged soon after surgery and is continued throughout the convalescence. When the soft tissues have healed, active motion of the wrist is gradually increased. Active exercises to strengthen grip are of utmost importance.

• • •

■ *TECHNIQUE (NEVIASER).* Make a dorsal oblique or straight dorsal longitudinal incision. Preserve the extensor retinaculum by reflecting it laterally. Then make a T-shaped incision in the dorsal capsule and dissect it from the proximal carpal row, including the scaphoid, the lunate, and the triquetrum. Excise these bones piecemeal, but leave a thin shell of cortical bone adherent to the palmar capsule if necessary. Avoid injuring the proximal articular surface of the capitate and allow it to settle into the lunate fossa. If the trapezium abuts the radial styloid, thus preventing radial deviation, perform a radial styloidectomy. Cut the styloid transversely to remove the radial edge of the lunate fossa. Repair the dorsal capsule. After closure of the skin immobilize the wrist in slight extension.

AFTERTREATMENT. Immobilization is continued for 3 weeks and then progressive exercises are begun. The wrist is supported with splints for another 3 weeks.

Grafting operations. Cancellous bone grafting for scaphoid nonunion, as first described by Matti and modified by Russe, has proved to be a reliable procedure, producing bony union in from 80% to 97% of patients. Of 27 patients seen an average of 12 years after surgery, Stark et al. reported that 24 were satisfied with the result and all but one had returned to work. Mulder reported 97% bony union in 100 operations using the Matti-Russe technique.

■ *TECHNIQUE (MATTI-RUSSE).* With the patient under general anesthesia and tourniquet control, make a longitudinal incision 3 to 4 cm in length on the volar aspect of the wrist, thus avoiding the dorsal blood supply to the scaphoid. Place the incision just radial to the flexor carpi radialis tendon. Retract the tendon ulnarward and continue the incision through the wrist capsule to the scaphoid bone and expose the nonunion. It may be seen more clearly by marked dorsiflexion of the wrist. Freshen the sclerotic bone ends with a small gouge and form a cavity that extends well into each adjacent fragment. From the opposite iliac crest, obtain a piece of cancellous bone and shape it into a large lozenge-shaped peg to fit into the preformed cavity and sta-

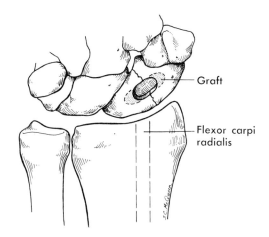

Fig. 66-16   Matti-Russe technique of bone grafting for nonunion of carpal scaphoid.

bilize the two fragments (Fig. 66-16). Place multiple small bone chips around the peg. Make a roentgenogram at surgery to assure filling of the entire cavity. After removal of the tourniquet, suture the capsule and close the skin. Apply a cast from the elbow to the tip of the thumb and to the metacarpophalangeal joints of the other digits with the wrist in neutral position. Split the cast down the palmar aspect immediately after application.

Instability found at the time of surgery and resulting in angulation of the scaphoid may require internal fixation in addition to the bone graft. Staples and more recently the Herbert screw have been used with success. According to Manske, McCarthy, and Strecker, the Herbert screw is most effective in nonunions with evidence of avascular necrosis, those involving the proximal third, or those having had previous failed bone grafts. Stark et al. recommend Kirschner wire fixation with an iliac bone graft for all nonunions because judging stability with bone grafting alone is difficult and because the technique is technically easy and adds little to the operating time. They achieved union in 97% of 151 old ununited fractures of the scaphoid.

AFTERTREATMENT. Remove the sutures at 8 to 10 days and apply a new cast. For a total of 12 to 16 weeks, check the patient every week or two and replace the cast when necessary. As an alternative, apply a well-formed sugar tong splint to include the thumb, wrap in cotton gauze, and change it at 10 days to a solid cast.

■ *TECHNIQUE (STARK ET AL.).* Expose the scaphoid through a straight or zigzag volar incision. After the wrist capsule is incised longitudinally and the wrist is dorsiflexed, both parts of the scaphoid, as well as the articular surface of the radius, can be seen readily. Remove a small, rectangular window of bone from the volar aspect of the distal fragment immediately adjacent to the fracture. Through this

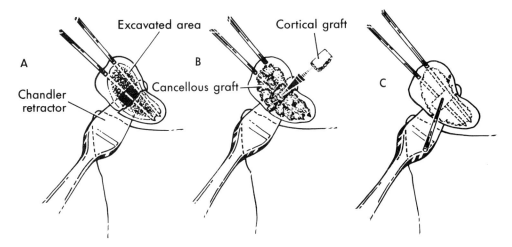

Fig. 66-17 Technique for scaphoid nonunion. **A,** Excavation of scaphoid and placement of Kirschner wires; Chandler retractor is used to protect articular cartilage of radioscaphoid joint. **B,** Cortical graft is inserted in cavity. **C,** Kirschner wire is inserted to stabilize bone graft. (Redrawn from Stark HH et al: J Bone Joint Surg 70-A:982, 1988.)

opening, clear both fragments of fibrous tissue and dead bone using a low-speed power burr or curet. As emphasized by Matti, fashion a large cavity in both the proximal and distal parts of the scaphoid. Use a Chandler retractor to protect the articular cartilage of the radioscaphoid joint (Fig. 66-17, *A*). It also helps to correct angulation, malrotation, and displacement of the fragments. The volar part of the cortex of the scaphoid is often deficient, and this deficiency permits an exaggerated volar tilt of the distal fragment, creating the so-called "humpback" deformity of the scaphoid. Realignment and reduction of the fracture and restoration of the bone to the proper length are difficult parts of the procedure. Intraoperative roentgenograms usually are necessary. Transfix the scaphoid with two 0.035-inch (0.9 mm) Kirschner wires by inserting them through the distal fragment into the proximal one; protect the articular cartilages of the scaphoid and radius with the retractor. Observe correct placement of the wires through the volar window.

Pack cancellous bone from the ilium into the cavity (Fig. 66-17, *B*). The wires can be inserted after packing the cavity with bone, but it is easier to verify their location before inserting the graft. Often a cortical bone graft can be fashioned to fit snugly into the volar window; stabilize it with one additional 0.028-inch (0.7 mm) Kirschner wire (Fig. 66-17, *C*). Cut the wires off beneath the skin. Approximate the capsule with absorbable sutures, close the skin, and immobilize the extremity in a long arm thumb spica splint with the forearm in supination, the wrist in neutral, and the thumb in abduction.

AFTERTREATMENT. The sutures are removed at 2 weeks and a long arm thumb spica cast is applied and is worn for 6 additional weeks. The Kirschner wires are removed after the fracture has united. Once immobilization is discontinued, patients are permitted to use the wrist and hand for light activities, but strenuous and forceful activity is discouraged for an additional 2 months.

• • •

Kawai and Yamamoto reported the use of a pedicle bone graft using a segment of the pronator quadratus. Their technique may be useful in difficult nonunions.

■ *TECHNIQUE (KAWAI AND YAMAMOTO).* Make a volar zigzag incision over the scaphoid tuberosity and the distal radius to expose the site of nonunion. Divide the radioscaphocapitate ligament complex, but retain it for later repair to the muscle pedicle. Excise the sclerotic bone ends and freshen them with a power burr to form an oval cavity 10 to 20 mm long and parallel to the axis of the scaphoid. Identify the pronator quadratus and outline a block of bone graft 15 to 20 mm long at its distal insertion on the distal radius close to the abductor pollicis longus tendon (Fig. 66-18). Outline the margin of the graft with Kirschner wire holes to facilitate separation with a fine osteotome. Take care that the pronator quadratus is not detached from the harvested bone graft; dissect the muscle toward the ulna to secure a pedicle 20 mm thick. The anterior interosseous vessels need not be identified. If the muscle is too tight to allow easy transfer of the pedicled bone, dissect the ulnar origin of the pronator quadratus subperiosteally from the ulna through an additional incision over the distal ulna.

Align the proximal and distal scaphoid segments carefully as a traction force is applied to the thumb. This maneuver corrects any intercalated segment instability and allows the grafted bone to be inserted

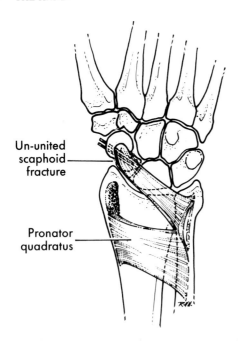

Un-united
scaphoid
fracture

Pronator
quadratus

Fig. 66-18 Pronator quadratus pedicle bone graft for scaphoid nonunion. Graft fills excavated site of nonunion and is fixed with Kirschner wires. (Redrawn from Kawai H and Yamamoto K: J Bone Joint Surg 70-B:829, 1988.)

snugly into the cavity in the scaphoid. Fix the proximal and distal scaphoid segments and the graft with two 0.047-inch (1.2 mm) Kirschner wires introduced at the scaphoid tuberosity. Do not cross the radiocarpal joint with a Kirschner wire. Close the skin and apply a long arm thumb spica cast.

AFTERTREATMENT. The long arm thumb spica cast is worn for 1 month, followed by a short arm thumb spica cast for another month. At 2 months, union is evaluated with roentgenograms and, in case of doubt, tomograms. The wrist is braced in a functional position for another 1 to 2 months, and active exercises are then begun. When stable bony union is certain, the Kirschner wires are removed, usually about 4 months after surgery.

Arthrodesis of wrist. Arthrodesis should be considered a salvage procedure for old ununited or malunited fractures of the scaphoid with associated radiocarpal traumatic arthritis. The types of wrist arthrodesis are described on pp. 3148 and 3156.

Naviculocapitate Fracture Syndrome

Although naviculocapitate fracture syndrome is rare, it should be considered among those associated injuries that can occur with a fracture of the scaphoid. Axial compression of a dorsiflexed wrist forces further dorsiflexion, and after the scaphoid fractures, the dorsal lip of the radius forcefully impacts the head of the capitate,

causing it to fracture. As the wrist continues into further dorsiflexion, after both the scaphoid and capitate are fractured, the capitate head then rotates 90 degrees. The hand, when returned to neutral position, brings the proximal fragment of the capitate into 180 degrees of rotation (Fig. 66-19). This injury can be associated with dorsal perilunate dislocation (see Fig. 66-23, *B*) or fractures of the distal end of the radius. Open reduction is necessary to derotate the capitate fragment. Some surgeons have excised this fragment, but others have replaced it, reduced both the scaphoid and capitate fractures, and maintained them with either internal fixation or cast immobilization.

Progressive Perilunar Instability

In spite of recent investigative reports, the complicated pathomechanics of carpal injuries and the link system of the carpus continue to challenge the clinician. The four stages of progressive disruption of ligamentous attachments and anatomic relations to the lunate, as described by Mayfield, Johnson, and Kilcoyne (Fig. 66-20), are the result of forced hyperextension. Stage I represents scapholunate failure; stage II, capitolunate failure; stage III, triquetrolunate failure; and stage IV, dorsal radiocarpal ligament failure allowing lunate dislocation.

ROTARY SUBLUXATION OF SCAPHOID. Rotary subluxation of the carpal scaphoid may be misdiagnosed as a wrist sprain following acute dorsiflexion of the wrist. It may be caused by and accompany fracture-dislocations of the wrist, especially transscaphoid perilunar fracture-dislocations. Tears of the scapholunate interosseous ligament (Fig. 66-21) and the volar radioscapholunate ligament allow the proximal pole of the scaphoid to rotate dorsally and become more vertical in position and permit separation of the scaphoid from the lunate. The diagnosis is made on an anteroposterior roentgenographic view when a gap is noted between the scaphoid and the lunate bones of greater than 2 mm. This gap is particularly significant when the carpus is in slight radial deviation and supinated. The affected wrist should be compared with the opposite normal wrist. The rotation of the scaphoid causes it to appear to be shortened and produces a so-called "ring sign" on the anteroposterior view. The lateral view of the wrist shows the more vertical orientation of the rotated scaphoid. The normal scapholunate angle is 30 to 60 degrees (mean of 47 degrees) and the normal capitolunate angle is less than 20 degrees (Fig. 66-22, *A*). Dorsal intercalated segment instability (DISI), in which the scapholunate angle is greater than 60 degrees and the capitolunate angle is greater than 20 degrees, is most common after a lunate or perilunate dislocation (Fig. 66-22, *B*). Conversely, volar intercalated segmental instability (VISI), in which the scapholunate angle decreases to less than 30 degrees, is often associated with triquetrolunate dissociation or midcarpal insta-

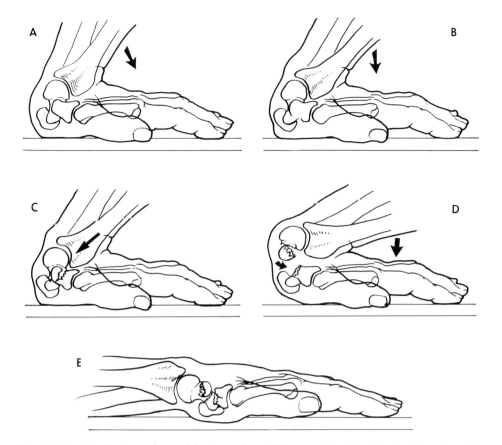

Fig. 66-19 Mechanism of carpal fractures from falls on outstretched hand with wrist going into marked dorsiflexion. **A,** Wrist in marked dorsiflexion. Note that capitate is at 90-degree angle to radius. **B,** Scaphoid fractures as result of increased dorsiflexion at midcarpal joint. **C,** Dorsal lip of radius strikes capitate, causing it to fracture. **D,** Proximal fragment of capitate is rotated 90 degrees. **E,** Return of wrist to neutral position. Note that proximal fragment of capitate is now rotated 180 degrees. (From Stein F and Siegel MW: J Bone Joint Surg 51-A:391, 1969.)

Fig. 66-20 Progressive perilunar instability: stage I — scapholunate failure, stage II — capitolunate failure, stage III — triquetrolunate failure, and stage IV — dorsal radiocarpal ligament failure allowing lunate rotation (dislocation). (Redrawn from Mayfield JK: Clin Orthop 149:45, 1980.)

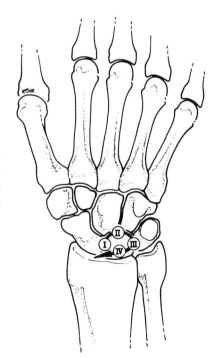

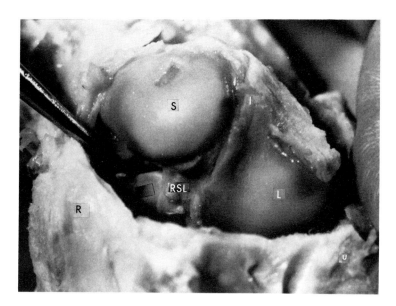

Fig. 66-21   Radioscaphoid ligament (RSL). *S,* scaphoid; *I,* scapholunate interosseous ligament; *L,* lunate; *R,* radius; *RSL,* radioscaphoid ligament. (From Mayfield J: Clin Orthop 149:45, 1980.)

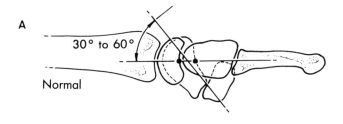

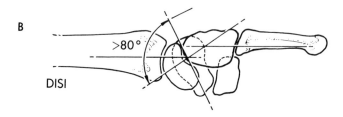

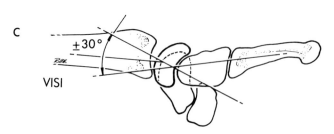

Fig. 66-22   **A,** Normal scapholunate and capitolunate angles. **B,** DISI deformity of wrist: concave surface of lunate points dorsally, scapholunate angle is greater than 60 degrees, and capitolunate angle is greater than 20 degrees. **C,** VISI deformity of wrist: concave surface of lunate points palmarly and scapholunate angle is less than 30 degrees. (Redrawn from Dobyns JH et al: AAOS Instr Course Lect 24:182, 1975.)

bility (Fig. 66-22, *C*). Occasionally the capitate migrates proximally into the gap created by the separation of the scaphoid and lunate especially when an axial force is exerted on the capitate as when making a fist.

On examination, pain and tenderness along the radiocarpal articulation, with or without edema, are usually present with some mild limitation of motion, particularly in volar flexion. Frequently the patient cannot recall the injury. Degenerative arthritic changes may eventually occur as a result of the abnormal position of these bones. A separation of 2 mm at the scapholunate articulation may not always be symptomatic. A comparative roentgenogram of the opposite wrist may be helpful. This separation may be accentuated by the patient making a clenched fist in the anteroposterior roentgenographic projection.

Closed treatment for the acute rotary subluxation of the scaphoid consists of attempting reduction by placing the wrist in neutral flexion and a few degrees of ulnar deviation. Meyer, West, and Anderson recommend percutaneous pinning with one 0.045-inch (1.16 mm) Kirschner wire placed through the scaphoid into the capitate and a second through the scaphoid into the lunate. If closed reduction is unsuccessful, then open reduction through a dorsal approach with closure of the scapholunate gap and internal fixation of the lunate and scaphoid with Kirschner wires is indicated. In addition, repair of the dorsal radiocarpal ligament is recommended, but this may be difficult. Management of an old rotary subluxation of the scaphoid may require reconstruction of the scapholunate interosseous ligament with a segment of the extensor carpi radialis brevis tendon plus a Kirschner wire for fixation after the graft has been passed through the scaphoid into the adjoining lunate. Insufficient experience with this procedure has been reported in the liter-

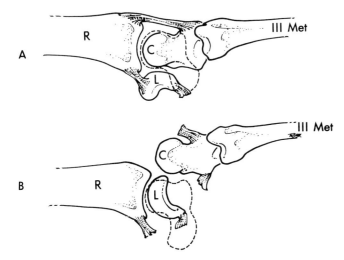

Fig. 66-23 Anterior dislocation of lunate and perilunar dislocation of carpus. **A,** Anterior dislocation of lunate. **B,** Dorsal perilunar dislocation of carpus. (Redrawn from Hill NA: Orthop Clin North Am 1(2):275, 1970.)

ature to provide data for comparing results with nontreatment. For this technique, we suggest reviewing the work of Dobyns et al., Linscheid et al., and Howard et al.

ANTERIOR DISLOCATION OF LUNATE. The most common carpal dislocation is anterior dislocation of the lunate. On a lateral roentgenographic view of the normal wrist the half-moon–shaped profile of the lunate articulates with the cup of the distal radius proximally and with the rounded proximal capitate distally. On an anteroposterior view the normal rectangular profile of the lunate when dislocated becomes triangular because of its tilt. An anteriorly dislocated lunate may cause acute compression of the median nerve (Fig. 66-23, *A*). Continued median nerve compression may result in a permanent palsy and should be relieved by reducing the lunate bone as an emergency procedure. When the injury is treated early, manipulative reduction is usually easy, and immobilization for 3 weeks with the wrist in slight flexion is required. When treated after 3 weeks, the injury may be difficult to reduce by manipulation and open reduction may be necessary. A dorsal approach to clean out the space to receive the lunate is suggested by Campbell et al. However, Hill suggests a palmar approach to decompress the median nerve as the lunate is reduced. At times, a combined dorsal and palmar approach may be required. When the lunate cannot be reduced by open reduction, a reconstructive procedure such as proximal row carpectomy or arthrodesis may be necessary.

PALMAR TRANSSCAPHOID PERILUNAR DISLOCATIONS. Palmar transscaphoid perilunar dislocations are extremely rare and are mentioned only for completeness. A report by Aitken and Nalebuff describes the mecha-

nism of injury as a fall on the dorsum of the flexed wrist. This is directly opposite the mechanism producing a dorsal perilunar dislocation (Fig. 66-23, *B*). In their patient, reduction was early, and the fracture was found to be stable with the wrist in dorsiflexion but unstable in flexion. Avascular changes were noted later in the scaphoid, and even though they eventually improved, nonunion of the scaphoid persisted.

DORSAL TRANSSCAPHOID PERILUNAR DISLOCATIONS. Like the fractured scaphoid bone alone, this entity is frequently diagnosed late. It may be associated with other injuries of the upper extremity. Early reduction by closed manipulation is best. When accurate reduction of the scaphoid fracture is not obtained, open reduction with a bone graft or other internal fixation is usually indicated. Boyes reported successful open reduction as late as 6 weeks after injury. A closed reduction can usually be carried out up to 3 weeks following injury. Later many of these injuries require open reduction. Internal fixation with Kirschner wires may be necessary for stability. After 2 months, open reduction may not be possible, and proximal-row carpectomy or arthrodesis of the wrist may be indicated.

Fracture of Hamate

A fracture of the hook of the hamate is sometimes difficult to demonstrate. Pain is elicited at the heel of the hand with firm grasp and with pressure against the bony prominence. A carpal tunnel view (Fig. 66-24, *A*) may show the fracture, but some are better demonstrated by computed tomography (Fig. 66-24, *B*). When using the latter technique, placing the patient's hands together in the praying attitude makes the diagnosis easier, because the view of both wrists rules out congenital variation of the hamate, which is usually bilateral. Occasionally, the body of the hamate is fractured, but this rarely requires surgery.

A stress fracture may develop in the hook of the hamate with some repetitive activities, such as golf. Initial diagnosis may be difficult. Transient ulnar nerve motor branch palsy may be caused by an undiagnosed stress fracture of the hook of the hamate. In most instances, unless the diagnosis is delayed, union is likely after immobilization but excision of the fragment may be necessary for nonunion, persistent pain, or ulnar nerve palsy.

Trapezium Fractures

These fractures are demonstrated roentgenographically only on the carpal tunnel view of the wrist. Palmer classified them into two types: type I is a fracture of the base of the ridge, and it may heal when treated by immobilization in plaster (Figs. 66-25 and 66-26); type II is an avulsion at the tip of the ridge, and it usually fails to heal when immobilized.

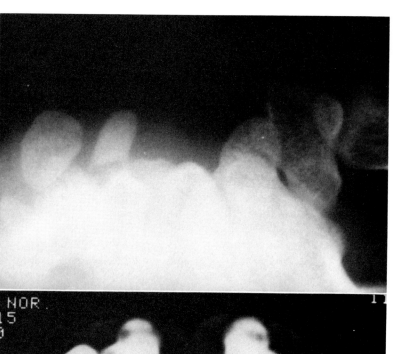

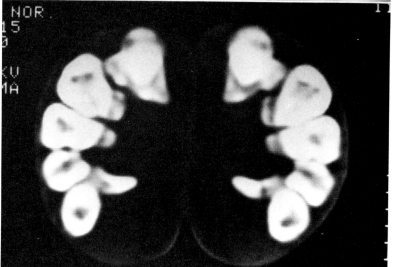

A

B

Fig. 66-24 **A,** Carpal tunnel view and **B,** CT image of patient with fracture of hook of hamate. He injured his left hand on full-swing foul ball. (From Egawa M and Asai T: J Hand Surg 8:393, 1983.)

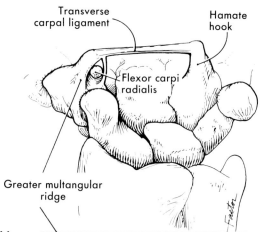

Fig. 66-25 Carpal tunnel view showing flexor carpi radialis cradled by palmar ridge of trapezium. *Inset* shows type 1 fracture at base of volar ridge of trapezium (direct loading) and type II fracture at tip (avulsion). (From Palmer AK: J Hand Surg 6:561, 1981.)

A

B

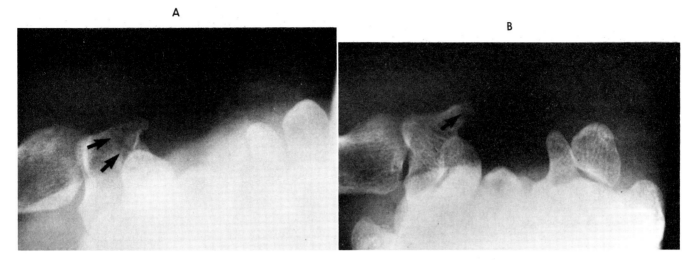

Fig. 66-26   A, Carpal tunnel view demonstrates fracture of base of palmar ridge of trapezium (*arrows*). This is designated as type I greater multangular ridge fracture. **B,** Type II fracture of tip of palmar ridge of trapezium (*arrow*) caused by fall on dorsiflexed wrist. (From Palmer AK: J Hand Surg 6:561, 1981.)

Kienböck's Disease

Kienböck's disease is a painful disorder of the wrist of unknown cause in which roentgenograms show avascular necrosis of the carpal lunate. It occurs more frequently between the ages of 15 and 40 years and in the dominant wrist of men engaged in manual labor.

In 75% of the patients the disorder is preceded by severe trauma, usually with the wrist in severe dorsiflexion. Armistead et al. demonstrated in some patients oc-

cult fractures of the lunate with computed tomography (Fig. 66-27, *A*). Untreated, the disease usually results in fragmentation of the lunate, collapse with shortening of the carpus (Fig. 66-27, *B*), and secondary arthritic changes throughout the proximal carpal area. Symptoms may develop as early as 18 months before roentgenograms show evidence of the disease. The use of magnetic resonance imaging may be helpful in the diagnosis of early avascular changes in the lunate.

Fig. 66-27   A, Common fracture pattern in Kienböck's disease is so-called anterior-pole type, isolating anterior pole of lunate from remaining portion of bone. Distraction of fracture caused by compressive force exerted by capitate diminishes likelihood of fracture healing. This detail is usually not visable on routine roentgenograms because radial styloid process is superimposed on fracture gap. As dorsal portion of lunate collapses further, anterior pole may be extruded volarly. **B,** Ratio of height of carpus to length of third metacarpal is reduced in this patient with Kienböck's disease. Youm et al. determined that this ratio in normal wrists is 0.54 ± 0.03 and that significantly reduced ratios indicate overall carpal collapse. (From Armistead RB et al: J Bone Joint Surg 64-A:170, 1982. By permission of Mayo Foundation.)

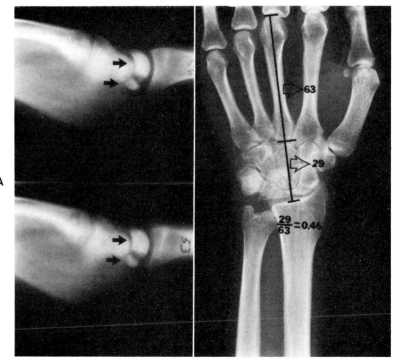

A

B

TREATMENT. Lichtman's classification of lunate changes is useful in discussing treatment.

Stage I— Normal architecture with evidence of a linear or compression fracture

Stage II— Normal outline but definite density changes within the lunate

Stage III— Collapse or fragmentation of the lunate and proximal migration of the capitate (carpal height ratio is less than 0.54 (± 0.03; Fig. 66-28)

Stage IV— Generalized degenerative changes within the carpus

The treatment of established Kienböck's disease is not standardized. Some authors recommend ulnar lengthening early in the disease (stage I or II). Hultén has described a condition known as the ulna-minus variant. He found in 78% of patients with Kienböck's disease that the ulna was shorter than the radius at their distal articulation. This was true in only 23% of normal wrists. In no patient with Kienböck's disease was the ulna longer than the radius at the distal articulation, but 16% of the control group had a so-called ulna-plus variant.

Persson in 1950 reported a series of patients in whom he lengthened the ulna for this disease. These patients were observed for several years by Moberg and Axelsson. They found 16 who had been operated on some 20 years previously, and all but one had been able to continue with manual labor after the operation. Even in one who had pain, the disease process appeared to have been halted. Because of these findings, Armistead et al. have performed the ulnar lengthening operation for Kienböck's disease, reporting 20 cases in 1982 (Fig. 66-28).

Three nonunions required a second plating and bone grafting; 18 of the 20 had pain relief. The technique is detailed below. The ulna should not be lengthened enough to impair ulnar deviation of the wrist; usually most wrist movement can be retained. Strong plate fixation of the distal ulna is recommended.

In addition to ulnar lengthening, the radius has been shortened by some to accomplish an even distal radioulnar articular surface to the lunate. Of 12 patients reported by Almquist and Burns, all but one had pain relief, and 10 of 12 showed roentgenographic revascularization of the lunate. Their indications for radial shortening include negative ulnar variance and lunate compression fracture without fragmentation or flattening (stage II). Earlier reports by Kleven, Axelsson, and Eiken and Niechajev provide similar satisfactory results. Shortening of the radius consists of making a transverse osteotomy about 3 inches (7.6 cm) proximal to the distal articular surface, shortening the radius by 2 mm, and fixing the bone with a compression plate. Edelson, Reis, and Fuchs reported development of Kienböck's disease in a patient 16 months after surgery in a lunate that appeared to have reconstituted normally. However, in a series of 35 patients, Schattenkerk, Nollen, and van Hussen reported satisfactory results in two thirds of those treated by both ulnar lengthening and radial shortening. In addition, Weiss and others reported 30 wrists with Kienböck's stages I and II treated with radial shortening of an average of 2.8 mm. At an average 3-year follow-up, 87% had decreased pain, improved motion and grip strength, and no appreciable change in the amount of lunate collapse.

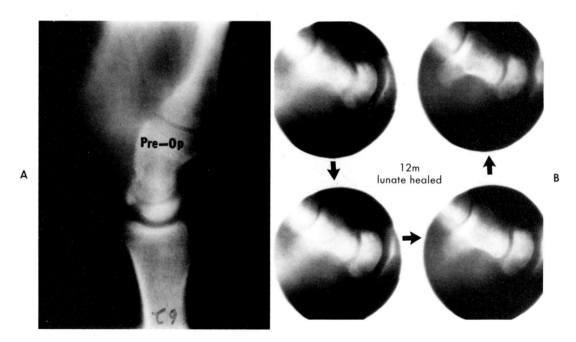

Fig. 66-28   A, Lateral tomogram of wrist, showing typical anterior-pole fracture. **B,** Lunate shows no further collapse 12 months after ulnar lengthening, and early healing is suggested. (From Armistead RB et al: J Bone Joint Surg 64-A:170, 1982. By permission of Mayo Foundation.)

Others have advised the conservative measure of simple casting if the disease is considered to be quite early (stage I or II), that is, before sclerosis, fragmentation, or collapse occurs. Conservative management includes casting of the wrist for several weeks if warranted followed by repeated roentgenograms in search of occult fracture or tardy avascular changes of the lunate or other disorders that may be more evident later, including previously undiagnosed fractures of the carpal scaphoid. However, this treatment has generally been unacceptable, since it requires 4 or more months of immobilization with an uncertain outcome. A recent study by Mikkelsen and Gelineck in which 25 wrists were observed for an average of 8 years concluded that nonoperative treatment of Kienböck's disease was ineffective.

In late cases (stage III) in which the lunate has collapsed but secondary arthritic changes are absent, the ulnar lengthening operation is still advocated by Armistead et al. Stark, Zemel, and Ashworth recommend use of a hand-carved silicone rubber spacer in the absence of significant alteration in the shape of the bone, including absence of collapse as measured by the three kinematic indices of McMurtry et al. (Fig. 66-29). The carved prosthetic device is substituted for the lunate, which is excised through a dorsal approach. Both Swanson and Lichtman and their associates advocate replacement with a previously molded lunate-shaped silicone block followed by careful repair of the capsule to avoid the potential dislocation of the block. This ligamentous and capsular reconstruction is extremely important and has been emphasized by many authors.

The patient should be warned that silicone synovitis and the formation of foreign body cysts are possible. These complications are more likely if the implant is oversized or malpositioned, if carpal instability is present, or if motion or occupational stress of the wrist is excessive. Because of this possibility, some surgeons have abandoned or limited this technique and have suggested intercarpal fusion (scaphoid-capitate, capitate-hamate, or hamate-triquetrum). Simple excision of the lunate, although controversial, has been shown in a recent study by Kawai et al., at an average follow-up of 12 years, to produce satisfactory results with continued relief of pain. In 18 patients, the carpus rearranged itself with proximal migration of the capitate, triquetrum, and palmar-flexed scaphoid, but a good range of motion was preserved and degenerative changes were less than anticipated. However, the procedure is not recommended for those who do heavy work.

When secondary arthritic changes have developed throughout the wrist (stage IV), the choice of treatment usually is between proximal carpal row resection and arthrodesis of the wrist.

Ulnar lengthening

■ *TECHNIQUE (ARMISTEAD ET AL.).* **Make a longitudinal incision over the medial border of the distal**

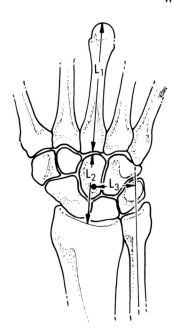

Fig. 66-29 Three kinematic indices: center of rotation, carpal height (L_2), and carpal-ulnar distance (L_3). K_1, length of third metacarpal. Carpal height ratio is L_2/L_1 and the carpal-ulnar distance ratio is L_3/L_1. (From McMurtry Y et al: J Bone Joint Surg 60-A:955, 1978.)

ulna. Reflect the extensor carpi ulnaris and flexor carpi ulnaris tendons, and expose the distal third of the ulna subperiosteally. Then make a transverse osteotomy through the medial three fourths of the ulna. Place a slotted plate with four or more holes over the bone centered at the site of the osteotomy. Insert four screws completely so that each is located at the end of the respective slotted hole nearest the center of the plate. Complete the osteotomy through the ulna with a cervical laminectomy spreader and distract the fragments without rotation. The amount of distraction needed is determined by preoperative roentgenograms. It should be 1 or 2 mm more than the negative ulnar length. Insert a cortical iliac graft of the predetermined width into the osteotomy gap. Next, loosen the two screws in the proximal fragment so that the tension of the surrounding soft tissues will compress the fragments. Now retighten all four screws. Trim any projection from the periphery of the graft. Check the new length of the ulna by roentgenograms. Finally, close the wound over suction drains and apply a padded palm-to-axilla dressing with an external plaster splint.

***AFTERTREATMENT.* The drains are removed at 24 hours. At 2 weeks the sutures are removed, and a long arm cast is applied. At 4 to 6 weeks the cast is removed, and a splint is worn until there is roentgenographic evidence of healing. The plates and screws are not removed for at least 1 year.**

Radial shortening

■ *TECHNIQUE.* With the patient under satisfactory anesthesia in the supine position and after limb exsanguination and tourniquet inflation, make an incision on the palmar aspect of the distal forearm extending distally to the wrist flexion crease. In order to protect the radial artery, incise the superficial surface of the sheath of the flexor carpi radialis. Retract the flexor carpi radialis radiolaterally and incise the dorsal surface of the sheath of the flexor carpi radialis. Carefully retract the radial artery laterally and identify the radial insertion of the pronator quadratus. Dissect proximally and identify the flexor pollicis longus. Elevate the pronator quadratus and flexor pollicis longus subperiosteally proximally so that the distal diaphysis and metaphyseal-diaphyseal junction of the radius can be easily identified. Based on preoperative roentgenograms and the amount of ulnar-minus variation, make an osteotomy in the metaphyseal-diaphyseal junction of the radius. A diaphyseal osteotomy, as recommended by Almquist and Burns, usually is required to allow enough length on the distal segment to place two or three screws. Placement of a plate in the metaphyseal-diaphyseal junction might be more difficult because of the palmar flare of the radial metaphysis, even though healing might be more predictable. Make the osteotomy proximal enough to allow placement of three screws in the distal fragment. Measure preoperative roentgenograms for the amount of shortening required. Fix the distal two screws to the distal radial fragment before osteotomy. Remove the plate and screws, perform the osteotomy with a thin-bladed oscillating saw, and shorten the radius by the appropriate amount, usually 2 to 3 mm. Reattach the plate to the distal fragment with screws. Before placing the proximal screws, compress the osteotomy and hold it with reduction forceps. Obtain image-intensifier images to check radioulnar length. Fix the radius with a compression plate technique, deflate the tourniquet, obtain satisfactory hemostasis, and drain the wound if needed. Replace the pronator quadratus over the plate and close the subcutaneous tissues and skin, leaving the forearm fascia open to minimize the chances of compartment syndrome. Immobilize the forearm in a sugar tong splint.

AFTERTREATMENT. The drain is removed after 1 or 2 days. Finger motion and wrist motion are encouraged. The sugar tong splint is removed after approximately 10 days to allow inspection of the wound, and the sutures are removed at 10 to 14 days. A solid forearm cast is applied extending above the elbow, or a solid sugar tong splint is used for 4 weeks. The cast is removed to evaluate the osteotomy with roentgenograms, and cast immobilization above the elbow is continued for another 4 weeks. After approximately 8 to 10 weeks, additional casting will depend on the roentgenographic appearance of the osteotomy. Exercise and light use of the hand are encouraged throughout convalescence.

Distal Radioulnar Joint Injuries

ANATOMY. The structures causing pain on the ulnar side of the wrist include the distal radioulnar joint and the distal ulnocarpal joint, as well as the ligamentous and cartilaginous structures attaching the distal ulna to the distal radius and ulnar side of the carpus, known as the triangular fibrocartilage complex (TFCC) of Palmer and Werner. The TFCC includes the dorsal and volar radioulnar ligaments, ulnar collateral ligament, meniscal homologue, articular disc, and extensor carpi ulnaris sheath. It begins on the ulnar side of the lunate fossa of the radius and attaches ulnarward to the head of the ulna and the ulnar styloid at its base. It is subsequently joined by the ulnar collateral ligament, and its distal insertion is the triquetrum, hamate, and base of the fifth metacarpal. During forearm rotation, the ulnar head at its articulation with the sigmoid notch moves from dorsal and distal in full pronation to proximal and palmar in full supination. Palmer et al. cite cadaver studies demonstrating that loads applied to the distal radiocarpal and ulnocarpal joints are distributed about 80% to the distal radius and 20% to the ulna.

DIAGNOSIS AND TREATMENT. When evaluating patients with painful wrists, it is important to try to localize anatomically the source of the pain and complaint. As mentioned previously, history, physical examination, roentgenograms, arthrography, and, in the case of the distal radioulnar joint, CT scans are especially helpful. In some patients, although pain complaints may persist, conservative management usually is best until a clear-cut cause for invasive treatment is seen. For the management of fractures and nonunions, see Chapter 64. Chronic distal radioulnar problems that may lend themselves to operative treatment include the subluxating distal ulna, symptomatic TFCC tears and perforations, distal radioulnar joint arthritis, and subluxation of the extensor carpi ulnaris tendon. Procedures that may be helpful in managing these problems include arthroscopy, limited ulnar head excision, ulnar shortening, and ulnar pseudarthrosis with distal radioulnar arthrodesis and distal ulnar excision (Darrach).

Most recently the works of Bowers, and Palmer et al. have contributed greatly to our understanding of the problems and treatment of distal radioulnar joint conditions. Palmer has categorized the conditions of the distal radioulnar joint, dividing them into acute and chronic problems. The acute problems include fractures of the ulnar head, styloid, radius, and carpal bones, as well as dislocations or subluxations involving the distal radioulnar joint, carpal bones, and the triangular fibrocartilage complex and extensor carpi ulnaris subluxation. The chronic conditions include bony nonunions and malunions and incongruities of the wrist joint including subluxation and dislocation of the distal radioulnar joint, the ulnocarpal region, the various carpal bones, and the triangular fibrocartilage complex, as well as localized arthritis of the pisotriquetral, lunotriquetral, and radioulnar joints and extensor carpi ulnaris subluxation related to arthritis. The management of acute fractures and dislocations as they relate to the distal radioulnar joint is discussed in Chapter 64. Procedures discussed here are indicated for the most part for chronic problems related to the distal radioulnar joint and the TFCC.

Limited ulnar head excision: hemiresection interposition arthroplasty. The TFCC provides (1) a stable radioulnar connection, (2) a stable ulnocarpal connection, (3) a mechanism for transmitting forces from the hand, (4) a suspensory ligament function for the ulnar side of the carpus from the radius, and (5) an extended dividing surface for the proximal row across the distal end of the forearm bones. A distal radioulnar joint arthroplasty involving partial ulnar head resection was developed by Bowers to maintain the triangular fibrocartilage function. This technique is indicated for (1) unreconstructable fractures of the ulnar head, (2) ulnocarpal impingement syndrome with incongruity of the distal radioulnar joint, (3) rheumatoid arthritis involving the distal radioulnar joint, (4) posttraumatic arthritis and osteoarthritis of the distal radioulnar joint, and (5) chronic painful triangular fibrocartilage tear. The procedure is contraindicated if there is no reconstructable TFCC. Without the TFCC, hemiresection interposition technique is not believed to have a significant advantage over ulnar shortening techniques.

■ *TECHNIQUE (BOWERS).* **Begin the incision 5 to 7 cm proximal to the ulnocarpal joint on the dorsal aspect of the distal ulna. Extend the incision distally and at the level of the ulnocarpal joint curve or angle palmarward for about 1 to 2 cm. Carefully protect the cutaneous nerves to the skin in the area and expose the extensor retinaculum and the distal ulnocarpal area to the fascia. Elevate retinacular flaps, raising a proximal flap based laterally and a distal flap based medially. Develop these flaps for exposure and for tissue for extensor carpi ulnaris stabilization or triangular fibrocartilage augmentation. Otherwise, reattach the flaps, use them for coverage of the arthroplasty, or excise them. If the extensor carpi ulnaris is stable, reflect it laterally with subperiosteal dissection to expose the distal ulna. If the extensor carpi ulnaris is unstable, mobilize it distally to its insertion on the retinacular fifth metacarpal. Use the proximal flap to fashion a sling, pass it around the extensor carpi ulnaris, and suture it to the fourth extensor compartment (Fig. 66-30).**

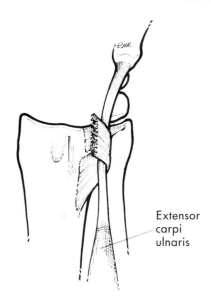

Fig. 66-30 Stabilization of extensor carpi ulnaris with retinacular sling. Flap is based on fibrous wall between compartments four and five. (Redrawn from Bowers WH: J Hand Surg 10-A:169, 1985.)

Extensor carpi ulnaris

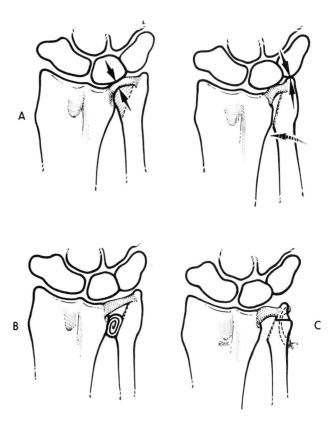

Fig. 66-31 Bowers technique of hemiresection arthroplasty. **A,** Because ulna is too long it impinges on stylocarpal ligament. This problem may be corrected by, **B,** interposition, or, **C,** shortening. (Redrawn from Bowers WH: The distal radioulnar joint. In Green DP, editor: Operative hand surgery, ed 2, New York, 1988, Churchill Livingstone.)

After the retinacular flaps have been elevated, detach the radioulnar joint capsule distally, laterally (radially), and proximally, and reflect it medially (ulnarward) to expose the articular surface. Remove the synovium, the ulnar head articular surface, and subchondral bone with osteotomes and rongeurs. Remove osteophytes around the sigmoid notch and remove all subchondral bone of the ulnar head. Leave the styloid axis and ulnar shaft resembling a tapering, 1 cm dowel (Fig. 66-31).

Carefully inspect the triangular fibrocartilage. Central perforation repairs are not necessary. With the wrist in ulnar deviation, compress and rotate the radial and ulnar shafts. If there is ulnocarpal abutment or impingement, consider ulnar shortening. If it cannot be determined preoperatively or during surgery, fill the radioulnar space with a ball of tendon or muscle and stabilize the tendon to dorsal and volar capsules with sutures. Use tendon from the palmaris longus, extensor carpi ulnaris, or flexor carpi ulnaris. This interposition helps prevent radioulnar shaft approximation and stylocarpal impingement. Close the wound by first replacing the extensor carpi ulnaris compartment or use a retinacular flap. If shortening is not required, close the wound and apply a short arm bulky dressing with dorsal and palmar splints. If ulnar shortening has been done, use a sugar tong splint to control rotation.

AFTERTREATMENT. The splint and sutures are removed at 2 weeks. A wrist splint is worn for an additional 2 weeks, and finger motion is encouraged. If ulnar shortening was done, a short arm cast is worn for another 2 weeks, and then a short arm wrist splint is worn until healing is complete. If shortening was done in the ulnar shaft, a splint or cast is worn for 8 to 12 weeks.

Ulnar shortening procedures. A number of ulnar shortening procedures have been described. They include the Darrach resection of the distal ulna (Chapter 27), and a combined distal radioulnar ankylosis (Baldwin) with formation of a pseudarthrosis of the distal ulna (Sauve and Kapandji, and Lauenstein). The formation of an ankylosis or arthrodesis of the distal radioulnar joint combined with a proximal pseudarthrosis of the distal ulna has been proposed as a solution for problems related to the distal radioulnar joint.

Although a stable distal radioulnar joint with support for the ulnocarpal area is achieved, the potential for an unstable proximal ulna remains, leaving few satisfactory solutions for the symptomatic unstable proximal ulnar stump. Ankylosis or healing of the pseudarthrosis may occur, defeating the purpose of the procedure.

Procedures to stabilize distal radioulnar joint. After undetected dislocations and surgical procedures to resect the distal ulna, a variety of techniques have been proposed to stabilize the distal radioulnar joint and the unstable distal ulna. No one procedure can be recommended to work in all situations. Bowers has emphasized the importance of repairing or reconstructing the TFCC. The difficulty of restoring the smooth carpal articulation, a flexible rotational radioulnar tether, an ulnocarpal suspension from the radius, an ulnocarpal cushion, and an ulnar shaft to the ulnar carpal connection has been emphasized by Bowers. A number of complex radioulnar tethering procedures proximal to the radioulnar joint have been described. In our experience, the simpler one keeps these procedures the better.

Arthrodesis of Wrist

Fusion of the wrist is most often done for ununited or malunited fractures of the carpal scaphoid with associated radiocarpal traumatic arthritis and for severely comminuted fractures of the distal end of the radius; it also is useful for Volkmann's ischemic paralysis, for stabilization of the wrist in poliomyelitis and cerebral palsy of the spastic type, and for tuberculosis.

The wrist should be fused in a position that will not be fatiguing and that will allow maximum grasping strength in the hand. This is usually 10 to 20 degrees of extension, with the long axis of the third metacarpal shaft being aligned with the long axis of the radial shaft. Clinically it is determined by the position that the wrist normally assumes with the fist strongly clenched.

Of the many techniques that have been described, most include the use of a bone graft. In some the graft bridges from the radius to the proximal carpal bones, but in others it extends distally to the base of the third metacarpal. The carpometacarpal joints may be preserved, retaining a small amount of "wrist" motion. However, Haddad and Riordan recommend that the second and third carpometacarpal joints always be included in the fusion to prevent development of painful motion in them. Further, the disease of the wrist frequently extends into these joints, making a complete fusion necessary.

Since the distal radial epiphysis does not close until approximately the seventeenth year of age, care should be taken not to damage it in patients under this age. After partial destruction of the plate by disease or trauma, however, the remaining part may be excised to prevent unequal growth. Fusion of the wrist in children is difficult to secure because of the amount of cartilage in the joint. When possible, operation should be postponed until the patient is 10 to 12 years of age.

In addition to many other useful procedures for rheumatoid arthritis of the upper extremity, Smith-Petersen reported a method of fusing the wrist suggested by the exposure of the wrist after resection of the distal end of the ulna. This technique should not be used unless there is disease or derangement of the distal radioulnar joint since the procedure uses the distal ulna as a bone graft

A

B

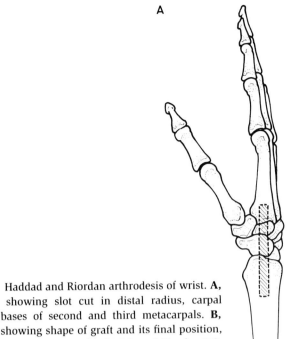

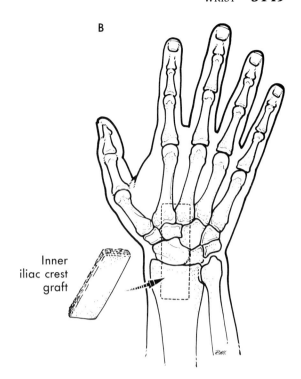

Inner
iliac crest
graft

Fig. 66-32   Haddad and Riordan arthrodesis of wrist. **A,** Radial view showing slot cut in distal radius, carpal bones, and bases of second and third metacarpals. **B,** Dorsal view showing shape of graft and its final position, *broken line,* in slot. (From Haddad RJ Jr and Riordan DC: J Bone Joint Surg 49-A:950, 1967.)

inserted between the radius and the carpus. It has the disadvantage of allowing limited access to the radiocarpal joint.

Haddad and Riordan have described a technique of arthrodesis of the wrist through a radial or lateral approach. It has these advantages: the distal radioulnar joint is not entered, the extensor tendons to the digits are not disturbed, and since dorsal thickening is avoided, the appearance of the wrist is not altered. They report only one failure in 24 wrists using this technique.

■ *TECHNIQUE (HADDAD AND RIORDAN).* **Begin a J-shaped skin incision 2.5 to 3.8 cm proximal to the radial styloid on the midlateral aspect of the forearm, extend it distally across the styloid, and then curve it dorsally to end at the base of the second metacarpal. Now mobilize and retract the superficial branch of the radial nerve. Identify the interval between the first and second dorsal compartments and incise the dorsal carpal ligament in this interval, leaving it attached to the volar aspect of the radius. Mobilize subperiosteally and retract the abductor pollicis longus, extensor pollicis brevis, and the wrist and finger extensors. Next divide the extensor carpi radialis longus tendon just proximal to its insertion on the base of the second metacarpal, leaving a stump distally so that it can be sutured later. Remove the capsule from the radiocarpal, the intercarpal, and the second carpometacarpal joints. Now locate the dorsal branch of the radial artery and ligate and divide its dorsal branch to the dorsal carpal arch. Then denude the radiocarpal joint of articular cartilage and subchondral bone. Using an os-**cillating saw and osteotomes, obtain from the inner table of the iliac crest a graft about 3.8 cm long and 2.5 cm wide. With the wrist in 15 degrees of dorsiflexion, cut a slot, using an oscillating saw, in the distal end of the radius, the carpal bones, and the bases of the second and third metacarpals. Do not cut through the medial cortex of the radius and enter the distal radioulnar joint. Then place the graft in the prepared bed (Fig. 66-32). If the wrist is unstable, insert a smooth Kirschner wire obliquely or longitudinally to engage the base of the second metacarpal and the distal radius; cut off the wire under the skin at the palm, to be removed 6 to 8 weeks later. Close the dorsal carpal ligament deep to the abductor pollicis longus and extensor pollicis brevis. Suture the extensor carpi radialis longus tendon and close the wound. Apply a sugar tong splint.**
AFTERTREATMENT. **The bandage is changed and the sutures are removed at 10 to 14 days. A solid sugar tong cast is applied and is worn for another 4 weeks, then a short-arm cast is worn until is healing is evident clinically and roentgenographically. Exercises are encouraged throughout the healing phase.**

• • •

We have used an inner table bone graft inlaid into a dorsal recess formed in the distal radius and carpus and stabilized with Kirschner wires when a dorsal approach is more appropriate than a radial or ulnar approach.

In recent years the compression plate technique has proven beneficial in providing excellent internal fixation and eliminating the need for prolonged immobilization.

■ *TECHNIQUE.* Between the third and fourth compartments, make a 10 to 15 cm longitudinal dorsal incision centered over the radiocarpal joint. Expose the extensor tendons with their retinaculum, retracting the finger extensors medially. Open the wrist capsule with an H-shaped incision to expose the radiocarpal and intercarpal joints. Denude the radiocarpal and intercarpal joint surfaces of cartilage and subchondral bone and fill the gaps with cancellous iliac bone. Place a 3.5 mm cortex lag screw through the radial styloid into the capitate to pull the carpus against the radial styloid to avoid impingement of the distal radioulnar joint. Inlay a flat rectangular corticocancellous graft from the ilium into a prepared bed between the metacarpal bases and the distal radius. Place a seven- or eight-hole 3.5 mm dynamic compression plate over the graft. Compress the radiocarpal joint with one screw in the capitate and one screw proximal to the bone graft in the radius. Attach the plate to the third metacarpal (or occasionally the second metacarpal) with two or three screws and to the radius with three or four screws (Fig. 66-33). Close the wound over drains as needed and apply a compression dressing and a sugar tong splint.

AFTERTREATMENT. The hand is kept elevated and finger motion is encouraged from the first postoperative day. The bandage is changed and the splint and sutures are removed at 10 to 14 days. Above-elbow immobilization is continued for 4 to 6 weeks; then a short arm cast is applied and is worn until healing is evident clinically and roentgenographically. Plate removal is optional, depending on the patient.

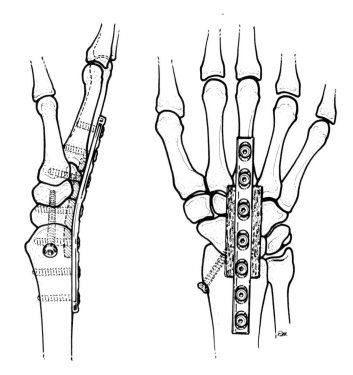

Fig. 66-33   Arthrodesis of wrist with lag screw and dynamic compression plate fixation (see text).

CARPAL LIGAMENT INJURIES AND INSTABILITY PATTERNS (TABLE 66-1)

Abnormalities in the carpal bone relationships were noted on roentgenograms obtained in the early 1900s. Subsequently reports focused on the so-called rotational instabilities of the carpal scaphoid until attention was drawn to the subject by Linscheid et al. in 1972. Describing traumatic instability of the wrist related to carpal injuries resulting in loss of alignment of the carpal bones, they were able to group the carpal instabilities into four types: (1) dorsiflexion instability, (2) palmar-flexion instability, (3) ulnar translocation, and (4) dorsal subluxation. Subsequently, it has been seen that in some instability patterns the intercarpal relationships do not change with motion and are considered to be static instability patterns, whereas in others the intercarpal relationships change with motion and manipulation and are known as dynamic. Linscheid et al. stressed the benefits of evaluating the proximal carpal row in the lateral roentgenographic projection in which the radius, lunate,

capitate, and third metacarpal should have co-linear axes within an approximately 15-degree tolerance. On this projection, the wrist-collapsed positions, which generally can be appreciated, are those in which the distal articular surface of the lunate is tilted to face dorsally (DISI collapse patterns) and those in which the distal articular surface of the lunate faces toward the palm (VISI patterns). In addition, Linscheid et al. advocated the concept of dissociative and nondissociative instabilities in the wrist. Carpal instabilities that are considered dissociative are those in which the proximal carpal row bones have lost their attachments to each other. Nondissociative instabilities are those in which the carpal bones maintain their attachments. Arthrography is helpful in delineating ligamentous injuries.

Watson and Black observed that rotatory subluxation of the scaphoid may present in four types: (1) dynamic, (2) static, (3) with degenerative arthritis, and (4) secondary to a condition such as Kienböck's osteochondrosis. Although dynamic rotatory subluxation of the scaphoid usually cannot be shown roentgenographically, the symptoms and physical findings are helpful. Typically, patients complain of pain with activity followed by aching. Watson and Black described a "scaphoid test" in which the examiner places four fingers on the dorsum of the radius with the thumb on the scaphoid tuberosity, using the right hand for the right wrist and the left hand for the left wrist. Ulnar deviation of the wrist aligns the scaphoid with the long axis of the forearm. Applying thumb pressure to the scaphoid tuberosity, the wrist is

Table 66-1   Classification of carpal instability

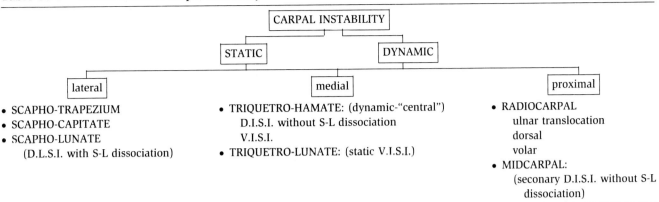

From Taleisnik J: The wrist, New York, 1985, Churchill Livingstone.

returned to radial deviation, maintaining the thumb pressure on the scaphoid tuberosity. If the scaphoid is sufficiently unstable, the proximal pole is driven dorsally and pain results.

Watson also has found the "catch-up clunk" to be helpful in evaluating rotatory instability of the scaphoid. As the wrist under load progresses from radial deviation to ulnar deviation, the scaphoid normally moves smoothly into extension, aligning with the forearm axis. If scaphoid rotatory subluxation is present, the lunate remains in a volar-flexed and dorsal position until sufficient pressure is applied so that it suddenly shifts from the volar-flexed position and "catches up" with the scaphoid with a "clunking" sensation. These maneuvers are considered to be helpful in evaluating rotatory instability of the scaphoid.

Instabilities associated with Kienböck's disease and scaphoid fractures are discussed in the section on fracture-dislocations and Kienböck's disease (p. 3128).

When the lunate becomes unstable in a position of volar displacement and dorsiflexion, it is known as dorsal intercalated segment instability (DISI) and usually is the result of injuries to the volar radioscapholunate ligaments. This pattern generally can be identified in the lateral roentgenographic projection (Fig. 66-34). Lichtman has emphasized the importance of evaluating the carpal instabilities on the ulnar side of the wrist. When assessing the wrist for triquetrolunate and midcarpal instability, Lichtman et al. reported the following findings. Patients with triquetrolunate instability usually complained of pain on the ulnar aspect of the wrist, with or without an associated wrist click in radial and ulnar deviation. Usually a traumatic event could be described. The physical examination usually reveals tenderness over the ulnar aspect of the wrist in the region of the triquetrolunate joint and a click usually can be reproduced in radial and ulnar deviation. According to Regan, Linscheid, and Dobyns, ballottement of the lunotriquetral joint can help in diagnosing this instability. The lunate is stabilized

with the thumb and index finger of one hand, and an attempt is made to displace the triquetrum and pisiform dorsally and palmarward with the opposite hand. Usually excessive laxity, pain, and crepitance constitute a positive test. If the triquetrolunate injury is a tear or sprain, the usual static roentgenograms are normal. If there is triquetrolunate dissociation, the triquetrum may be displaced proximally on the anteroposterior view. This may be exaggerated with ulnar deviation, creating overlapping of the lunate and triquetrum. Arthrography is helpful in diagnosing triquetrolunate ligament injuries.

Palmar instability in the midcarpal region (capitolunate) is thought by Lichtman et al. to be a manifestation of laxity of the ulnar arm of the arcuate ligament. This laxity allows the proximal carpal row to develop a palmar-flexed position (volar intercalated segment instability [VISI]). When dorsal midcarpal instability is present, the capitate is dorsally placed relative to the lunate and the proximal carpal row is palmarly displaced and in dorsiflexion (dorsal intercalated segment instability [DISI]). Most patients have the sensation of a painful "clunk" with ulnar deviation and pronation of the wrist. A palmar sag can be identified at the level of the midcarpal joint on physical examination. The clunk can be reproduced by passively moving the hand from the relaxed neutral position into ulnar deviation. As the wrist reaches its extreme of ulnar deviation, a palpable sensation or a "clunk" is noted. At this time the volar sag will be corrected. The roentgenographic examination usually reveals a VISI pattern, with the wrist in neutral position and unsupported. Video fluoroscopy or cineradiography may be helpful in assessing wrist instability.

Other instability patterns that have been described and may require treatment include triquetrohamate instability, ulnar translocation of the carpus, and scapholunate advanced collapsed (SLAC) wrist. According to Watson and Black, triquetrohamate instability usually is associated with other significant ligament injuries in the wrist.

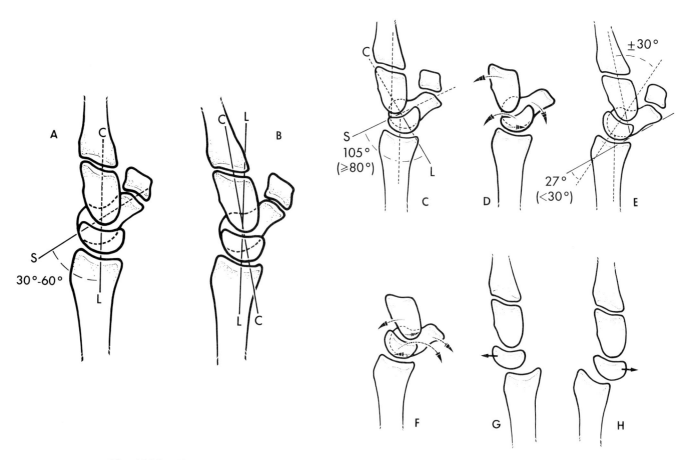

Fig. 66-34 Ligament instability patterns of wrist. **A,** Scapholunate angle is normal between 30 and 60 degrees and is sometimes normal up to 80 degrees. Although scaphoid axis (S) is shown through center of scaphoid, it is easier and also adequate to draw scaphoid axis line tangent to proximal and distal volar convexities of scaphoid. C = capitate axis, L = lunate axis. **B,** Capitolunate angle normally is less than 30 degrees. **C,** DISI is suspected with dorsal tilting of lunate and volar tilting of scaphoid causing increase in scapholunate angle, with or without increase in capitolunate angle. **D,** DISI: as lunate tilts dorsally and scaphoid tilts volarly, lunate tends to move volarly and capitate dorsally. **E,** Palmar felxion instability (VISI) is suspected with scapholunate angle of less than 30 degrees or capitolunate angle of 30 degrees or more. **F,** VISI: scaphoid and lunate both tilt volarly, and lunate tends to slide dorsally; in capitate, although distal pole tends to tilt dorsally, head (proximal end) tends to move volarly. **G,** With dorsal carpal subluxation, center of carpus is dorsal to center of midaxis of radius. **H,** With palmar carpal subluxation, central axis of carpus and lunate is volar to midaxis of radius. (From Gilula LA and Weeks PM: Radiology 129:641, 1978.)

Ulnar translocation of the carpus, usually seen in patients with rheumatoid arthritis, may also be present following major ligament disruptions in the wrist. The so-called scapholunate advanced collapse pattern usually is seen following conditions that lead to rotatory subluxation of the scaphoid resulting in loss of cartilage and degenerative changes in the radioscaphoid and capitolunate joints with sparing of the radiolunate joint.

Ligament Repair

Ligament repairs may be undertaken if closed reduction of rotatory subluxation of the scaphoid and other carpal instability patterns cannot be satisfactorily accomplished. For primary rotatory subluxation of the scaphoid and other carpal instabilities seen acutely, closed manipulation and pinning may be successful; however, because of the positioning required to reduce the subluxation or dislocation and to achieve satisfactory pinning, at times the ligaments may not be approximated as a result of positioning of the wrist in extension. Taleisnik has suggested in the case of the rotatory subluxation of the scaphoid that the scaphoid be reduced with the wrist in dorsiflexion and that the scaphoid be pinned to the capitate and lunate with three 0.045-inch (1.16 mm) Kirschner wires. After the scaphoid has been stabilized, the wrist is flexed, allowing approximation of the volar wrist ligaments.

■ *TECHNIQUE.* If open reduction is required, make an incision dorsally over the dorsoradial aspect of the wrist and on the palmar aspect paralleling the thenar crease and extending proximally to cross the volar wrist crease obliquely medially. Expose the radiovolar aspect of the wrist by retracting the digital flexor tendons to see the volar wrist capsule. Expose the dorsum of the wrist through a longitudinal or transverse incision centered in the region of the radial side of the wrist extensors. Retract the wrist extensors ulnarward and the extensor pollicis longus radially, opening the wrist dorsoradially. Take care to avoid injury to branches of the superficial radial nerve, the radial artery on the dorsal aspect, and the median nerve and flexor tendons through the palmar approach. Reduce the scapholunate disruption and fix it with three 0.045-inch (1.16 mm) Kirschner wires directed from the scaphoid into the lunate and capitate. Repair the tear in the volar capsule with interrupted nonabsorbable 3-0 or 4-0 suture. Although it is frequently difficult, attempt to repair the dorsal scapholunate interosseous ligament. This is easier if a small osteochondral fragment of bone has been avulsed. At times such a fragment can be stabilized with small Kirschner wires or with sutures placed through holes drilled in the scaphoid. Close the wound in the routine manner and immobilize the limb in a long arm thumb spica cast with mild palmar flexion and forearm pronation.

AFTERTREATMENT. Remove the sutures in 10 to 14 days and change the cast. After about 6 weeks, remove the long arm cast and apply a short arm cast for another 3 to 4 weeks. At the end of 8 to 10 weeks, remove all Kirschner wires and begin range-of-motion exercises followed by strengthening exercises in a progressive manner.

Ligament Reconstruction

Ligament reconstruction may be accomplished with free tendon grafts or tenodesis using prolonged slips of wrist flexors and extensors. Complications make ligament reconstruction, although satisfactory for some patients, unpredictable for others. Taleisnik has pointed out that satisfactory results have been achieved; however, the procedures are technically demanding, patient satisfaction is unpredictable, and the tightness required to maintain apposition of the bones limits eventual wrist motion. Palmer, Dobyns, and Linscheid reported satisfactory results using a distally attached slip of the flexor carpi radialis tendon (Fig. 66-35). They recommended that ligament reconstruction be reserved for those patients whose ligament ruptures could not be maintained with closed reduction or those who have their diagnosis made after about 1 month. Ligament reconstruction is not indicated in patients with associated degenerative

joint disease for whom other procedures, such as radial styloidectomy, wrist arthrodesis, or wrist arthroplasty, should be considered. All patients can expect to have a loss of wrist motion following most of the procedures described and advocated for these problems.

■ *TECHNIQUE (PALMER, DOBYNS, AND LINSCHEID).* After induction of anesthesia, proper application of the tourniquet, and preparation and draping of the arm with the patient in a supine position, approach the wrist through dorsal and palmar incisions, allowing sufficient exposure to identify the scapholunate articulations on the palmar and dorsal surfaces (Fig. 66-35, *A* and *B*). Dorsally, the interval between the wrist extensors and the finger extensors usually is satisfactory, although tendons might require retraction radially or ulnarward for exposure. On the palmar surface, approaching the radiovolar wrist capsule through the flexor carpi radialis sheath or to the ulnar side of the flexor carpi radialis, retract the flexor carpi radialis radially and enter the capsule at the scapholunate interval. With the scaphoid and lunate reduced, fashion drill holes in the scaphoid and lunate for tendon passage, taking care to avoid fracturing through the cortical surfaces between the scaphoid and lunate (Fig. 66-35, *B* and *C*). Start with small drill points and enlarge the holes gradually with larger drill points and curets. Incise the flexor carpi radialis, leaving its attachments distally, and split a 2 to 4 mm tendon slip from proximally to distally. Pass the flexor carpi radialis tendon slip first through the lunate from palmar to dorsal (Fig. 66-35, *C*). With the wrist reduced, stabilize the lunate with a 0.062-inch (1.59 mm) Kirschner wire drilled from proximally through the radial metaphysis into the lunate through the distal radial articular surface (Fig. 66-35, *C*). Secure the Kirschner wire stabilization after the tendon graft has been passed. Using wire loops and sutures, pass the tendon slip from dorsal to palmar through the scaphoid drill hole. Try to overreduce the carpal bones in their alignment with each other and with the radius. Stabilize the scaphoid with a 0.062-inch (1.59 mm) Kirschner wire through the radial metaphysis into the scaphoid (Fig. 66-35, *E*). Drill a hole in the distal radius at the level of the radioscapholunate ligament and pass the tendon from palmar to dorsal from within the joint on the palmar surface to extraarticular on the dorsal surface (Fig. 66-35, *F*). Suture the flexor carpi radialis back to itself dorsally.

An alternative technique described by Palmer, Dobyns, and Linscheid involves passing the flexor carpi radialis tendon slip dorsally through the scaphoid initially, then palmarward through the lunate from dorsal to palmar, and then through a drill hole in the distal radius, and then suture the flexor

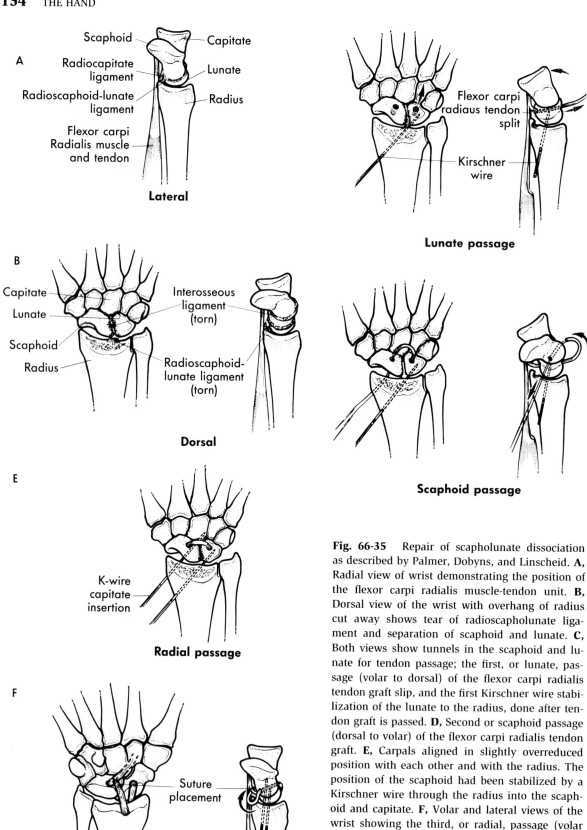

Fig. 66-35 Repair of scapholunate dissociation as described by Palmer, Dobyns, and Linscheid. **A,** Radial view of wrist demonstrating the position of the flexor carpi radialis muscle-tendon unit. **B,** Dorsal view of the wrist with overhang of radius cut away shows tear of radioscapholunate ligament and separation of scaphoid and lunate. **C,** Both views show tunnels in the scaphoid and lunate for tendon passage; the first, or lunate, passage (volar to dorsal) of the flexor carpi radialis tendon graft slip, and the first Kirschner wire stabilization of the lunate to the radius, done after tendon graft is passed. **D,** Second or scaphoid passage (dorsal to volar) of the flexor carpi radialis tendon graft. **E,** Carpals aligned in slightly overreduced position with each other and with the radius. The position of the scaphoid had been stabilized by a Kirschner wire through the radius into the scaphoid and capitate. **F,** Volar and lateral views of the wrist showing the third, or radial, passage (volar and intraarticular to volar and extraarticular) of the tendon graft, which is sutured to itself. (Redrawn from Palmer AK, Dobyns JH, and Linscheid RL: J Hand Surg 3:528, 1978.)

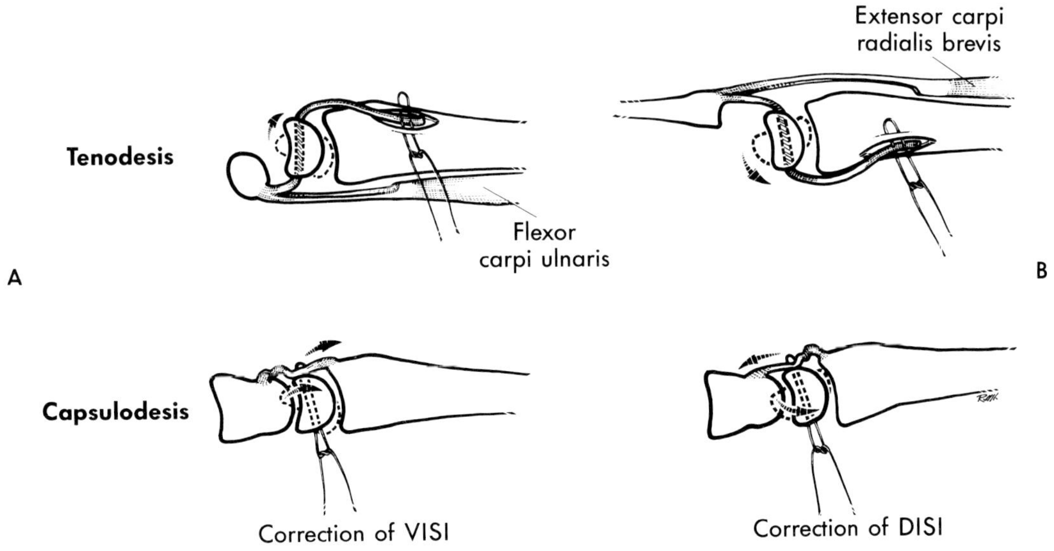

Fig. 66-36   Tenodesis and capsulodesis techniques for **A,** VISI, and **B,** DISI (see text).

carpi radialis slip to itself near its insertion. Apply a long arm thumb spica cast.

AFTERTREATMENT. The sutures are removed at 10 days to 2 weeks. The cast is changed and left in place for 6 weeks; then the cast is changed to a short arm cast, which is worn for an additional 4 weeks. The pins are removed at 8 to 10 weeks and range-of-motion and strengthening exercises are begun.

• • •

For lunate stabilization in patients with triquetrolunate instability (static VISI collapse patterns and dynamic DISI collapse patterns) in whom the instability of the lunate contributes to medial carpal instability, Taleisnik advocates for VISI deformities use of the lateral half of the flexor carpi ulnaris in a strip left attached distally and threaded from the palm through to the dorsal aspect of the lunate and secured to the dorsal surface of the distal radius (Fig. 66-36, *A*). For dynamic DISI deformities, the medial half of the extensor carpi radialis brevis is left attached distally, threaded through the lunate from dorsal to palmar, and anchored under the pronator quadratus on the anterior surface of the distal radius (Fig. 66-36, *B*).

Capsulodesis

Blatt has found that capsulodesis is useful for two conditions causing impairment of wrist function. They are scapholunate dissociation and the caput ulnae syndrome caused by distal radioulnar joint incongruity. The capsulodesis for the distal ulna is described in the section on distal radioulnar joint. Blatt has found it particularly useful in the patient with symptomatic dynamic instability

and a static deformity and has applied it to all patients with reducible scapholunate dissociations.

DORSAL CAPSULODESIS

■ *TECHNIQUE (BLATT).* Before the operative procedure, thoroughly evaluate the roentgenograms to determine the nature and extent of the scapholunate dissociation and rotatory subluxation of the scaphoid. Blatt states that "a single criterion for this procedure is the ability to anatomically reduce the scaphoid at the time of surgery." After achieving satisfactory anesthesia and appropriate skin preparation and draping of the extremity, and with the well-padded tourniquet inflated, make a longitudinal dorsoradial incision. Retract the wrist and finger extensors laterally and medially, respectively. Make a longitudinal incision through the capsule near the axis of the scaphoid. Expose the full length of the scaphoid. Preserve a 1 cm wide flap of dorsal wrist capsule and develop it from the ulnar side of the capsular incision (Fig. 66-37, *A*). This flap will be released distally, and the proximal origin on the dorsum of the distal radius will be left attached. Inspect the interosseous and dorsal scapholunate ligaments to ascertain their rupture and irreparability. Reduce the scaphoid with thumb pressure on the scaphoid tubercle on the palm side, bring the wrist into slight ulnar deviation, and transfix the scaphoid with 0.045-inch (1.16 mm) Kirschner wires placed from the distal pole of the scaphoid into the capitate and base of the third metacarpal. Make a notch in the dorsum of the distal pole of the scaphoid proximal to the distal articular surface and distal to the mid-axis of rotation of the scaphoid with a narrow osteotome or small rongeur. Trim the dorsal

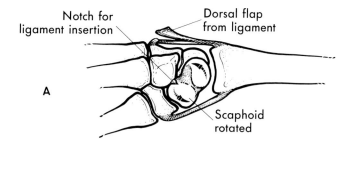

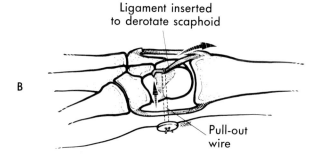

Fig. 66-37 Dorsal capsulodesis (Blatt). **A,** Proximal-based ligamentous flap is developed from dorsal wrist capsule. Notch for ligament insertion is created in dorsal cortex of distal scaphoid pole. **B,** Scaphoid has been derotated and ligament has been inserted with pull-out wire suture. (Redrawn from Blatt G: Hand Clin 3:81, 1987.)

capsuloligamentous flap to attach into the distal pole of the scaphoid with a 4-0 stainless steel pull-out wire suture. This is passed through fine drill holes to the volar tubercle of the scaphoid and the wire is tied at the level of the skin over felt and button (Fig. 66-37, *B*). Deflate the tourniquet, obtain hemostasis, and close the skin. Apply a thumb spica cast.

AFTERTREATMENT. The cast is changed at 10 to 14 days. Sutures are removed and another cast is applied and is left in place for an additional 6 weeks. After a total of 2 months, the cast is removed, as is the pull-out wire. Kirschner wires are left in place. A removable splint is provided, and progressive range-of-motion exercises are started. The Kirschner wires are removed 3 months postoperatively, and range of motion progresses with no forceful stress activities permitted for about 4 months.

Limited Wrist Arthrodesis

Limited wrist arthrodesis has been used in various forms for rotatory subluxation of the scaphoid since the 1950s. Peterson and Lipscomb in 1967 described successful fusion of the scaphoid, trapezium, and trapezoid. Subsequently, Watson and Hampton have found the "triscaphe" arthrodesis to be an effective procedure to resist the forces of movement, tending to keep the scaph-

oid in a perpendicular position relative to the forearm. Kleinman carefully reviewed the results of scaphotrapezial-trapezoid fusion for rotatory subluxation of the scaphoid and found the carpal mechanics to be disturbed by loss of the carpal shift relationship of the scaphoid and lunate. Seventy to seventy-five percent of the dorsiflexion—palmar flexion motion was preserved. Eleven of forty-one patients reviewed had major surgical complications. The development of postoperative arthrosis, on retrospective review, appeared related to imperfect reduction of the scaphoid. This procedure achieved pain relief and preserved a functional arc of motion. Other limited wrist arthrodeses have been reported on an anecdotal basis and include fusions of the capitate and lunate; scaphoid, lunate, and capitate; and capitate, hamate, lunate, and triquetrum; as well as radioscaphoid and radiolunate arthrodeses.

INDICATIONS FOR TRISCAPHE ARTHRODESIS. Watson initially considered three indications for "triscaphe" arthrodesis: (1) degenerative arthritis of the scaphotrapezial-trapezoid joint with normal thumb carpometacarpal joint, (2) radial hand dislocations, and (3) rotatory subluxation of the scaphoid. Subsequently, he has added the existence of the DISI pattern with disruption of the volar ligaments tethering the lunate, allowing the scaphoid to assume a static rotatory instability. He has also advocated this arthrodesis for resistant scaphoid nonunions, combining the triscaphe arthrodesis with bone grafts. Kleinman considered the clinical indications to be pain at the end arcs of motion, especially in radial deviation, weakness caused by instability of the proximal carpal row at the scapholunate joint, and loss of motion secondary to pain. Roentgenographic criteria included a scapholunate diastasis greater than 2 mm, scaphoid angle of greater than 60 degrees on the true lateral view of the wrist, and foreshortening of the scaphoid seen on the anteroposterior view, in which the inferior margin of the distal scaphoid pole to the proximal pole at the radioscaphoid joint is shortened to less than 7 mm.

CONTRAINDICATIONS FOR TRISCAPHE ARTHRODESIS. Scaphotrapezial-trapezoid arthrodesis probably is contraindicated in patients with radioscaphoid arthritis or early phases of degenerative changes in the wrist progressing to the scapholunate advanced collapse wrist.

SCAPHOTRAPEZIAL-TRAPEZOID FUSION

■ *TECHNIQUE (WATSON).* After the satisfactory induction of anesthesia, prepare the hand, wrist, and forearm and apply drapes in the routine manner. Make a transverse incision in the skin on the dorsum of the wrist over the area of fusion. Retract the branches of the superficial radial nerve and the veins. Open the extensor retinaculum along the tendon of the extensor pollicis longus. Approach the wrist between the tendons of the extensor carpi

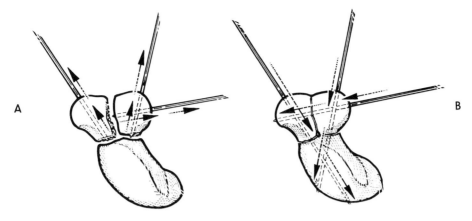

Fig. 66-38 Limited wrist (triscaphe) arthrodesis. **A,** Articular surfaces have been removed and three pins have been "preset" in retrograde fashion. **B,** Cancellous bone grafts have been packed between bones, external shape of triscaphoid unit is maintained, and pins are driven across arthrodesis sites. (Redrawn from Watson HK and Hempton RF: J Hand Surg 5:320, 1980.)

radialis longus and the extensor carpi radialis brevis or, as recommended by Kleinman, expose the wrist capsule between the first and second dorsal tendon compartments, exposing the adjacent surfaces of the scaphotrapezial-trapezoid joint and retracting the radial artery. Open the scaphotrapezial-trapezoid joint and open the capsule of the wrist to expose the proximal articular surface of the scaphoid. Triscaphe arthrodesis is contraindicated in the presence of significant radioscaphoid arthritis. If this is found, the scapholunate advanced collapse (SLAC) wrist reconstruction should be done. Observe the following principles as recommended by Watson. (1) Careful planning is essential. (2) The minimum necessary joints should be fused. (3) Packed, cancellous bone graft arthrodesis with sufficient graft should be used. (4) The external dimensions of the fused unit must equal the external dimensions of the same bones in their normal state. (5) Pin only the joints to be fused.

Careful attention to the reduction of the scaphoid is required to avoid fixing the scaphoid in an excessive longitudinal or dorsiflexed position. Kleinman recommends introducing a curved instrument palmar to the distal neck of the rotated scaphoid and dorsiflexing the distal pole with it. This allows reduction of the scaphoid to its anatomic position with the proximal pole secured in the scaphoid fossa of the radius. Insert 0.045-inch (1.16 mm) Kirschner wires through the scaphoid into the carpus to maintain this reduction and correlate the reduction by inspecting the reduced dorsal surface of the proximal pole of the scaphoid and the dorsal aspect of the lunate. The longitudinal axis attitude of the scaphoid should be 30 degrees or more to avoid excessive longitudinal orientation of the scaphoid and subsequent radioscaphoid impingement. Remove the articular surfaces of the trapezium, trapezoid, and scaphoid to cancellous bone. Kleinman's modification of removing only the dorsal two thirds of the articular surfaces allows preservation of the carpal height, maintaining the contact surfaces of the palmar one third. Obtain anteroposterior and lateral roentgenograms to confirm acceptable reduction of the scaphoid and closure of the preoperative scapholunate diastasis. Usually three 0.045-inch (1.16 mm) Kirschner wires are used to secure the scaphoid, trapezium, and trapezoid (Fig. 66-38, *A*). Two pins pass from the trapezoid toward the scaphoid and one passes across the trapezium-trapezoid joint. Remove all hyaline cartilage and subchondral bone. Bone graft can be obtained from the distal radius or from the iliac crest. If the distal radius is selected, retract the skin proximally or use a second proximal transverse incision over the distal radial metaphysis, exposing the radius between the extensor carpi radialis longus and the extensor pollicis brevis. Incise the periosteum, elevate it between these compartments, exposing the flat area of cortical bone in the distal dorsoradial metaphysis. The use of small gouges allows the removal of corticocancellous bone, and the remaining cancellous bone can be harvested with curets. Control bleeding and close the donor site wound and pack the cancellous bone into the defect left in the scaphotrapezial-trapezoid joint (Fig. 66-38, *B*).

Watson recommends placing pins by passing 0.045-inch (1.16 mm) Kirschner wires retrograde out through the raw bony surfaces. After the scaphoid, trapezium, and trapezoid are positioned for fusion, the pins are then drilled across the fusion site in an antegrade direction. To maintain the proper position of the scaphoid with the proximal pole depressed into the radial articular surface, the distal pole is elevated, as noted previously, and two pins may be used to secure the scaphoid to the capitate for temporary maintenance of reduction. Avoid passing the pins from the intercarpal arthrodesis into the radius or ulna. Ascertain that the spaces between the bones have been thoroughly packed with bone graft and that the external dimensions of the fusion unit are the same as the external dimensions of bones in the normal wrist. As an addition to the technique, a cortical bone graft may be used to bridge the fusion site on the dorsal surface and requires mortise fitting or notching into position. Pins are driven across the surfaces previously prepared. Check wrist motion to be sure that no pins obstruct radiocarpal motion and cut the pins off just beneath the skin. Deflate the tourniquet, obtain hemostasis, insert drains as needed, and close the wound. Apply a bulky compression dressing with a long arm plaster splint.

AFTERTREATMENT. The compression dressing is left in place for 7 to 10 days. After 7 to 10 days, the bandage is changed, the sutures are removed, and a long arm cast is applied. Watson has recommended a volar extension to support the index and long fingers in the intrinsic-plus position; however, Kleinman has not found this to be necessary, substituting a thumb spica cast at the time of suture removal. The second cast is left in place for another 4 to 6 weeks. Kirschner wires are removed between 6 and 8 weeks, using roentgenograms to determine healing. After about 8 weeks, roentgenograms are used to determine healing and either a short arm cast or a short arm splint may be applied for another week or two, depending on the roentgenograms and the patient's compliance. Once satisfactory healing has occurred, the hand and wrist are fully mobilized with gradual progression. Although motion usually is limited initially, it should increase within the first year after surgery. Care is taken to observe the patient closely to avoid stiffness or dystrophic complications, and intervention with physical therapy is instituted immediately if problems such as a shoulder-hand syndrome develop.

OTHER LIMITED WRIST ARTHRODESES. Arthrodesis of the scaphoid, capitate, and lunate; capitate, hamate, lunate, and triquetrum; hamate and triquetrum; radius to lunate; and radius to scaphoid can be done in a manner similar to the above through incisions centered over the respective joints to allow adequate exposure and avoid injury to neurovascular, musculoligamentous, and osteoarticular structures. Aftertreatment also is similar.

THE ARTHRITIC WRIST

Degenerative arthritis developing in the wrist (scapholunate advance collapse [SLAC] wrist) seems to be frequently related to instability about the scaphoid. The instability usually is a posttraumatic change, although primary degenerative changes are seen. The end result is a wrist with narrowing of the radioscaphoid joint, widening of the scapholunate gap, narrowing of the capitolunate joint, and remarkable preservation of the radiolunate joint. As advocated by Watson, the surgical treatment of this problem involves limited intercarpal arthrodesis of the capitohamate and triquetrolunate joints, usually with Silastic scaphoid replacement. Rheumatoid arthritis in the wrist is discussed in Chapter 72.

ARTHROSCOPY OF WRIST
Indications

According to Botte, Cooney, and Linscheid, the indications for wrist arthroscopy include the evaluation of ligamentous injuries, examination of joint articular surfaces, removal of loose bodies, biopsy of syovium, irrigation and debridement of joints, and confirmation and supplementation of wrist arthrography. Preliminary reports by Whipple et al. suggest that wrist arthroscopy may be useful in the treatment of fractures and their complications in the carpal bones and distal radius and ulna.

Equipment

1. Arthroscope
   a. Diameter: 2.5 to 3.0 mm best for routine use; 1.7 to 4 mm optional
   b. Length: 50 to 60 mm
   c. Lens-offset angle: 20 to 30 degrees best
2. Effective light source
3. Solid-state chip television camera
4. Color television monitor
5. Irrigation system: gravity feed usually satisfactory; pumps, mechanical and manual, allow better irrigation and use of suction and cutting tools
6. 18-gauge needles
7. Sterile tubing
8. Limb positioning attachments
   a. Ceiling hook or overhead pole and pulley
   b. Robotic devices, convenient and easily adjustable
   c. Finger-traps
   d. Forearm and wrist stabilizers
   e. 4 to 7 pounds of traction weights
9. Scalpel blades
10. Arthroscopy instruments
    a. Manual

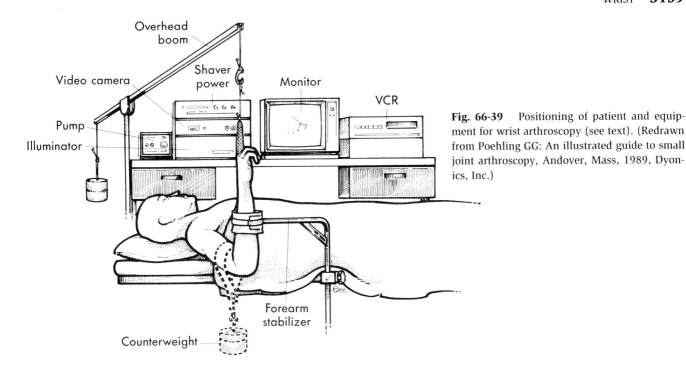

Fig. 66-39 Positioning of patient and equipment for wrist arthroscopy (see text). (Redrawn from Poehling GG: An illustrated guide to small joint arthroscopy, Andover, Mass, 1989, Dyonics, Inc.)

(1) Basket forceps 2 to 3 mm in diameter, 40 to 60 mm long
(2) Cutting tools
(3) Four-jaw, shallow probe, 40 mm long, 1.5 to 2 mm in diameter
(4) Grasping forceps with thin jaws, straight and curved
   b. Power: 2 to 3 mm in diameter usually best, full radius, efficient resector

Positioning and Preparation of Patient

Wrist arthroscopy can be done with the patient under regional block anesthesia or general anesthesia. If multiple procedures are to be done, or if the patient is uncomfortable, a general anesthetic usually is best. The use of a pneumatic tourniquet is optional but may be helpful when treating an intraarticular fracture.

■ *TECHNIQUE.* **With the patient under a suitable anesthetic, suspend the hand from the ceiling with sterile finger-traps and rope through an overhead pulley to use traction to move weight out and away from the operative field (Fig. 66-39). The thumb, index, and long fingers usually are included in the finger-traps. The elbow should be maintained in 80 to 90 degrees of flexion. The forearm is stabilized by an assistant to a mechanical well-padded forearm clamp. Before securing the arm to the clamp, if exsanguination is to be used the limb is exsanguinated and the tourniquet is inflated. Four to seven pounds of traction weight are applied through the finger-traps for distraction of the wrist.**

General Principles

The usual arthroscopic portals (Fig. 66-40) are located between the extensor compartments of the wrist. The portals are numbered according to the compartments immediately lateral to them (Fig. 66-41). Portals most often used for evaluation of the radiocarpal and ulnocarpal joints are portal 3 (between the third and fourth extensor dorsal compartments) and portal 4 (between the fourth and fifth compartments). The midcarpal joint portal lies to the radial side of the third metacarpal axis proximal to the capitate in a soft depression between the capitate and scaphoid. It is in line with Lister's tubercle (Fig. 66-42). A portal frequently used for irrigation is the portal between the fifth and sixth compartments, also known as the 6R portal, which is located on the dorsoradial aspect of the extensor carpi ulnaris.

In addition to the 3, 4, and 6 portals that are used frequently, other portals allow additional inspection of other parts of the wrist. Portal 5 permits better inspection of the TFCC and the ulnocarpal ligament on the palmar side. Portal 2, between the second and third compartments, allows inspection of the radial palmar ligaments. A probe placed through portal 1 may help to evaluate the articular surface of the distal radius. Use of needles, such as 20- and 22-gauge hypodermic needles, in the various portals before placement of the probe or other instruments helps determine which portal will work best. The use of a blunt trocar is a safer method to avoid injury to the joint surface when inserting the cannula for the arthroscope.

Although larger arthroscopes provide better fields of vision, they usually are too large and difficult to manip-

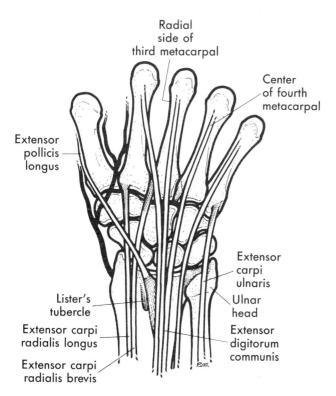

Fig. 66-40 External landmarks for wrist arthroscopy. (Redrawn from Poehling GG: An illustrated guide to small joint arthroscopy, Andover, Mass, 1989, Dyonics, Inc.)

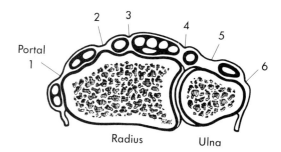

Fig. 66-41 Cross-section of wrist at level of distal radius showing compartments and portals used for examination of radiocarpal and ulnocarpal joints (Redrawn from Botte MJ, Cooney WP, and Linscheid RL: J Hand Surg 14-A(2):313, 1989.)

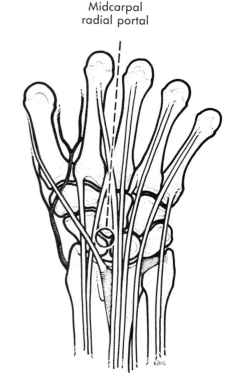

Fig. 66-42 Midcarpal radial arthroscopic portal on radial side of third metacarpal, proximal to capitate "soft spot." (Redrawn from Poehling GG: An illustrated guide to small joint arthroscopy, Andover, Mass, 1989, Dyonics, Inc.)

ulate. If continuous inflow irrigation is used, an efficient drainage system also must be used to avoid fluid extravasation and complications in the forearm. Continuous fluid infusion with positioning of the arthroscope with the camera end toward the ceiling helps avoid air bubble accumulation. The use of a probe for triangulation is helpful in examining the ligaments and cartilage surfaces.

To see in the joint satisfactorily it is important to maintain joint distraction with weight, to maintain distention with saline, and to irrigate frequently.

Radiocarpal Examination

■ *TECHNIQUE.* Distend the radiocarpal joint by locating the portal between the third and fourth extensor compartments just distal to the extensor pollicis longus and Lister's tubercle. Insert an 18-gauge needle into this portal and distend the joint with 5 to 10 ml of normal saline. Remove the needle, incise the skin over the portal, insert a cannula and blunt obturator, and establish inflow irrigation through the arthroscope. As an alternative, a continuous inflow system can be established through the ulnocarpal joint through portal 6 to the ulnar side of the exten-

sor carpi ulnaris. Outflow can occur through the arthroscope or with gravity drainage through a tube. Introduce the arthroscope into the radiocarpal joint at portal 3 through a small skin incision. Spread the subcutaneous soft tissues to retract the extensor pollicis longus tendon to the radial side. Although a sharp trocar or a No. 11 blade may be used to incise the dorsal capsule, extreme care should be taken to

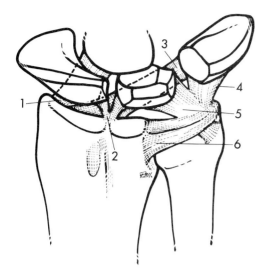

Fig. 66-43 Ligaments of radiocarpal joint: *1,* radioscaphocapitate; *2,* radioscapholunate; *3,* radiolunotriquetral; *4,* ulnotriquetral; *5,* ulnolunate; *6,* triangular fibrocartilage. (Redrawn from Poehling GG: An illustrated guide to small joint arthroscopy, Andover, Mass, 1989, Dyonics, Inc.)

avoid tendon injury. Insert the arthroscope with a palmar inclination to accommodate the palmar tilt of the distal radius. Incline the arthroscope so that the proximal end is toward the ceiling to help remove air bubbles. At this point, identify the palmar capsule of the wrist and the distal radial articular concavity. Insert a probe through portal 4 or 5 through a skin incision or through portal 6 between the ulnar margin or the extensor digitorum communis and the extensor digiti quinti or between the extensor digiti quinti and the extensor carpi ulnaris 6R portal. Follow an organized pattern of identifying structures within the wrist. Direct the arthroscope toward the distal end of the radius, follow it along the scaphoid and lunate fossas, and examine them. Move the arthroscope in the radial direction to identify the distal radius and the proximal margin of the scaphoid. Note the scapholunate articulation, which will be a small crease between the scaphoid and lunate with intimate blending of the ligament with the articular cartilage. Extend the wrist to expose the dorsal surfaces of the scaphoid and lunate and flex the wrist to examine the palmar surfaces of these bones. Identify the palmar carpal ligaments (Fig. 66-43). The radioscapholunate and radiotriquetral ligaments can be identified, as can the radiocapitate ligament. Use a probe to stress the ligaments and evaluate their integrity. Next, direct the arthroscope toward the ulnar aspect of the joint and proximally for examination of the TFCC. With a probe, palpate the TFCC to determine its integrity, especially as it leaves the ulnar margin of the radius. Moving toward the ulnar side of the wrist, identify the ulno-

carpal ligaments and the proximal articular surface of the triquetrum. Insert a probe in portal 4 or 5 to evaluate the palmar carpal ligaments, and the scapholunate and lunotriquetral interosseous ligaments. It may be necessary to move the arthroscope to a more ulnar portal to examine the TFCC and to move the probe into a more radial portal.

Midcarpal Examination

■ *TECHNIQUE.* The portal for entry into the midcarpal joint is located about 1 cm distal to the portal for the radiocarpal examination at portal 3 or 4. It is located to the radial side of the third metacarpal and proximal to the soft area between the scaphoid and capitate. Insert an 18-gauge needle into this portal and distend the joint with 5 to 7 ml of saline, incise the skin over this area, and insert a cannula and obturator, permitting inflow through the arthroscope. Another midcarpal portal is located in the center of the axis of the fourth metacarpal and proximal to the capitohamate joint. Enter this joint with an 18-gauge needle, distend the joint, and verify the position of the needle by direct vision of the needle with the arthroscope remaining in the midcarpal portal to the radial side of the extensor tendons. The scaphocapitate and capitohamate joints can be examined through these portals. The scaphotrapezial-trapezoid joint also can be examined through the midcarpal radial portal. Place the arthroscope through a skin incision into this portal to view the capitate distally and the scaphoid proximally. Moving the arthroscope toward the radial side along the scaphocapitate joint, examine the scaphotrapezial-trapezoid joint. Moving in an ulnar direction along the scaphocapitate joint, examine the scapholunate, lunotriquetral, and capitohamate joints. Traction and manipulation of the wrist allow better inspection of these joints. After the examination and operative procedures have been completed, determine that no loose objects are left within the joint and remove the arthroscope, instruments, and drainage tubing. Remove the tourniquet, obtain hemostasis, and close the portal incisions with staples or skin sutures. Infiltration of the joint with a local anesthetic agent helps minimize postoperative pain. Apply a bulky hand dressing with a splint.

AFTERTREATMENT. Depending on the nature of the procedure, the splint is removed and mobilization is commenced in the first 7 to 10 days after arthroscopy.

REFERENCES

General

Boyes JH: Bunnell's surgery of the hand, ed 5, Philadelphia, 1970, JB Lippincott Co.

Coyle MP Jr, Green DP, and Monsanto EH: Advances in carpal bone injury and disease, Hand Clin 5:471, 1989.

Lichtman DM, editor: The wrist and its disorders, Philadelphia, 1988, WB Saunders Co.

Taleisnik J: The wrist, New York, 1985, Churchill Livingstone.

Viegas SF and Ballantyne G: Attritional lesions of the wrist joint, J Hand Surg 12-A:1025, 1987.

Watson HK, Rogers WD, and Ashmead D IV: Reevaluation of the cause of the wrist ganglion, J Hand Surg 14-A:812, 1989.

Watson HK and Ryu J: Degenerative disorders of the carpus, Orthop Clin North Am 15:337, 1984.

Anatomy and biomechanics

Brumfield RH and Champoux JA: A biomechanical study of normal functional wrist motion, Clin Orthop 187:23, 1984.

Burgess RC: The effect of rotatory subluxation of the scaphoid on radio-scaphoid contact, J Hand Surg 12-A(2):771, 1987.

Gunther SF: The carpometacarpal joints, Orthop Clin North Am 15:259, 1984.

Kauer JMG and de Lange A: The carpal joint: anatomy and function, Hand Clin 3:23, 1987.

Kauer JMG: Functional anatomy of the wrist, Clin Orthop 149:9, 1980.

Mizuseki T and Ijuta Y: The dorsal carpal ligaments: their anatomy and function, J Hand Surg 14-B:91, 1989.

Palmer AK, Skahen JR, Werner FW, and Glisson RR: The extensor retinaculum of the wrist: an anatomic and biomechanical study, J Hand Surg 10-B:11, 1985.

Palmer AK and Werner FW: Triangular fibrocartilage of the wrist: anatomy and function, J Hand Surg 6:153, 1981.

Palmer AK, Werner FW, Eng MM, et al: Functional wrist motion: a biomechanical study, J Hand Surg 10-A:39, 1985.

Ruby LK, Cooney WP III, An KN, et al: Relative motion of selected carpal bones: a kinematic analysis of the normal wrist, J Hand Surg 13-A:1, 1988.

Savage R: The influence of wrist position on the minimum force required for active movement of the interphalangeal joints, J Hand Surg 13-B:262, 1988.

Seradge H, Sterbank PT, Seradge E, and Owens W: Segmental motion of the proximal carpal row: their global effect on the wrist motion, J Hand Surg 15-A:236, 1990.

Taleisnik J and Kelly PJ: The extraosseous and intraosseous blood supply of the scaphoid bone, J Bone Joint Surg 48-A:1125, 1966.

Viegas SF, Patterson R, Peterson P, et al: The effects of various load paths and different loads on the load transfer characteristics of the wrist, J Hand Surg 14-A:458, 1989.

Viegas SF, Tencer AF, Cantrell J, et al: Load transfer characteristics of the wrist. I. The normal joint, J Hand Surg 12-A:971, 1987.

Volz RG, Lieb M, and Benjamin J: Biomechanics of the wrist, Clin Orthop 149:112, 1980.

Weber ER: Wrist mechanics and its associations with ligamentous instability. In Lichtman DM, editor: The wrist and its disorders, Philadelphia, 1988, WB Saunders Co.

Youm Y and Flatt AE: Kinematics of the wrist, Clin Orthop 149:21, 1980.

Diagnosis and evaluation

Brown DE and Lichtman DM: The evaluation of chronic wrist pain, Orthop Clin North Am 15:182, 1984.

Brown DE and Lichtman DM: Physical examination of the wrist. In Lichtman DM, editor: The wrist and its disorders, Philadelphia, 1988, WB Saunders Co.

Czitrom AA and Lister GD: Measurement of grip strength in the diagnosis of wrist pain, J Hand Surg 13-A:16, 1988.

Palmer AK, Glisson RR, and Werner FW: Ulnar variance determination, J Hand Surg 7:378, 1982.

Sasaki Y and Sugioka Y: The pronator quadratus sign: its classification and diagnostic usefulness for injury and inflammation of the wrist, J Hand Surg 14-B:80, 1989.

Taleisnik J: Clinical and technologic evaluation of ulnar wrist pain, J Hand Surg 13-A:801, 1988 (editorial).

Roentgenographic techniques

Burk DL Jr, Karasick D, and Wechsler RJ: Imaging of the distal radioulnar joint, Hand Clin 7:263, 1991.

Cantor RM and Braunstein EM: Diagnosis of dorsal and palmar rotation of the lunate on a frontal radiograph, J Hand Surg 13-A:187, 1988.

Chernin MM and Pitt MJ: Radiographic disease patterns at the carpus, Clin Orthop 187:72, 1984.

Destouet JM, Gilula LA, and Reinus WR: Roentgenographic diagnosis of wrist pain and instability. In Lichtman DM, editor: The wrist and its disorders, Philadelphia, 1988, WB Saunders Co.

Gilula LA, Destouet JM, Weeks PM, et al: Roentgenographic diagnosis of the painful wrist, Clin Orthop 187:52, 1984.

Hardy DC, Totty WG, Carnes KM, et al: Arthrographic surface anatomy of the carpal triangular fibrocartilage complex, J Hand Surg 13-A:823, 1988.

Hardy DC, Totty WG, Reinus WR, and Gilula LA: Posteroanterior wrist radiography: importance of arm positioning, J Hand Surg 12-A:504, 1987.

Kricun ME: Wrist arthrography, Clin Orthop 187:65, 1984.

Manaster BJ, Mann RJ, and Rubenstein S: Wrist pain: correlation of clinical and plain film findings with arthrographic results, J Hand Surg 14-A:466, 1989.

Nakamura R, Horii E, Tanaka Y, et al: Three-dimensional CT imaging for wrist disorders, J Hand Surg 14-B:53, 1989.

Palmer AK, Levinsohn EM, and Kuzma GR: Arthrography of the wrist, J Hand Surg 8:15, 1983.

Pin PG, Semenkovich JW, Young VL, et al: Role of radionuclide imaging in the evaluation of wrist pain, J Hand Surg 13-A:810, 1988.

Posner MA and Greenspan A: Trispiral tomography for the evaluation of wrist problems, J Hand Surg 13-A:175, 1988.

Reinus WR, Hardy DC, Totty WG, and Gilula LA: Arthrographic evaluation of the carpal triangular fibrocartilage complex, J Hand Surg 12-A:495, 1987.

Zinberg EM, Palmer AK, Coren AB, and Levinsohn EM: The triple-injection wrist arthrogram, J Hand Surg 13-A:803, 1988.

Trauma (fractures and dislocations)

Aitken AP and Nalebuff EA: Volar transnavicular perilunar dislocation of the carpus J Bone Joint Surg 42-A:1051, 1960.

Allende BT: Osteoarthritis of the wrist secondary to non-union of the scaphoid, Inter Orthop (SICOT) 12:201, 1988.

Aufranc OE et al: Transnavicular perilunar carpal dislocation, JAMA 196:1146, 1966.

Botte MJ and Gelberman RH: Fractures of the carpus, excluding the scaphoid, Hand Clin 3:149, 1987.

Bryan RS and Dobyns JH: Fractures of the carpal bones other than lunate and navicular, Clin Orthop 149:107, 1980.

Bunker TD, McNamee PB, and Scott TD: The Herbert screw for scaphoid fractures: a multicentre study, J Bone Joint Surg 69-B:631, 1987.

Camp RA and Cosio MQ: Multiple percutaneous pinning of ununited scaphoid fractures, Tech Orthop 1:46, 1986.

Campbell RD Jr, Thompson TC, Lance EM, and Adler JB: Indications for open reduction of lunate and perilunate dislocation of the carpal bones, J Bone Joint Surg 47-A:915, 1965.

Carter PR, Malinin TI, Abbey PA, and Sommerkamp TG: The scaphoid allograft: a new operation for treatment of very proximal scaphoid nonunion or for the necrotic, fragmented scaphoid proximal pole, J Hand Surg 14-A:1, 1989.

Conway WF, Gilula LA, Manske PR, et al: Translunate, palmar peri-lunate fracture-subluxation of the wrist, J Hand Surg 14-A:635, 1989.

Cooney WP, Dobyns JH, and Linscheid RL: Fractures of the scaph-oid: a rational approach to management, Clin Orthop 149:90, 1980.

Cooney WP, Dobyns JH, and Linscheid RL: Nonunion of the scaph-oid: analysis of the results from bone grafting, J Hand Surg 8:343, 1980.

Cooney WP, Linscheid RL, and Dobyns JH: Scaphoid fractures: problems associated with nonunion and avascular necrosis, Or-thop Clin North Am 15:381, 1984.

Cooney WP, Bussey R, Dobyns JH, and Linscheid RL: Difficult wrist fractures: perilunate fracture-dislocations of the wrist, Clin Or-thop 214:136, 1987.

Dias JJ, Brenkel IJ, and Finlay DBL: Patterns of union in fractures of the waist of the scaphoid, J Bone Joint Surg 71-B:307, 1989.

Ferenz CC and Freundlich BD: Proximal row carpectomy for open fracture-dislocation of the carpus, J Trauma 27:85, 1987.

Fisk GR: An overview of injuries of the wrist, Clin Orthop 149:137, 1980.

Ford DJ, Khoury G, El-Hadidi S, et al: The Herbert screw for frac-tures of the scaphoid: a review of results and technical difficul-ties, J Bone Joint Surg 69-B:124, 1987.

Freund LG and Ovesen J: Isolated dorsal dislocation of the radiocar-pal joint: a case report, J Bone Joint Surg 59-A:277, 1977.

Garcia-Elias M, Dobyns JH, Cooney WP III, and Linscheid RL: Trau-matic axial dislocations of the carpus, J Hand Surg 14-A:446, 1989.

Gellman H, Caputo RJ, Carter V, et al: Comparison of short and long thumb-spica casts for non-displaced fractures of the carpal scaphoid, J Bone Joint Surg 71-A:354, 1989.

Goldberg I, Amit S, Bahar A, et al: Complete dislocation of the tra-pezium (multangulum majus), J Hand Surg 6:193, 1981.

Gordon SL: Scaphoid and lunate dislocation: report of a case in a patient with peripheral neuropathy, J Bone Joint Surg 54-A:1769, 1972.

Green DP and O'Brien ET: Open reduction of carpal dislocations: in-dications and operative techniques, J Hand Surg 3:250, 1978.

Green DP and O'Brien ET: Classification and management of carpal dislocations, Clin Orthop 149:55, 1980.

Herbert TJ: Internal fixation of the carpus with the Herbert bone screw system, J Hand Surg 14-A:397, 1989.

Herbert TJ and Fisher WE: Management of the fractured scaphoid using a new bone screw, J Bone Joint Surg 66-B:114, 1984.

Hill NA: Fractures and dislocations of the carpus, Orthop Clin North Am 1:275, 1970.

Johnson RP: The acutely injured wrist and its residuals, Clin Orthop 149:33, 1980.

Jones JA and Pellegrini VD Jr: Transverse fracture-dislocation of the trapezium, J Hand Surg 14-A:481, 1989.

Kawai H and Yamamoto K: Pronator quadratus pedicled bone graft for old scaphoid fractures, J Bone Joint Surg 70-B:829, 1988.

Korkala OL and Antti-Poika U: Late treatment of scaphoid fractures by bone grafting and compression staple osteosynthesis, J Hand Surg 14-A:491, 1989.

Manske PR, McCarthy JA, and Strecker WB: Use of the Herbert bone screw for scaphoid nonunions, Orthopedics 11:1653, 1988.

Matti H: Uber die Behandlung der Naviculare-fracture und der Re-fractura Patellae durch Plombierung mit Spongiosa, Zentralbl Chir 64:2353, 1937.

Mayfield JK: Mechanism of carpal injuries, Clin Orthop 149:45, 1980.

Mayfield JK: Patterns of injury to carpal ligaments: a spectrum, Clin Orthop 187:36, 1984.

Mayfield JK, Johnson RP, and Kilcoyne RK: Carpal dislocations: pathomechanics and progressive perilunar instability, J Hand Surg 5:226, 1980.

Mazet R and Hohl HL: Fractures of the carpal navicular: analysis of 91 cases and review of the literature, J Bone Joint Surg 45-A:82, 1963.

McCarroll HR Jr: Nerve injuries associated with wrist trauma, Or-thop Clin North Am 15:279, 1984.

McCarron RF and Coleman W: Dislocation of the pisiform treated by primary resection: a case report, Clin Orthop 241:231, 1989.

Melone CP Jr: Articular fractures of the distal radius, Orthop Clin North Am 15:217, 1984.

Meyer FN, West JL, and Anderson LD: Acute scapholunate dissoci-ation, Adv Orthop Surg 11:5, 1987.

Mulder JD: The results of 100 cases of pseudarthrosis in the scaph-oid bone treated by the Matti-Russe operation, J Bone Joint Surg 50-B:110, 1968.

Mullan GB and Lloyd GJ: Complete carpal disruption of the hand, Hand 12:39, 1980.

Neviaser RJ: Proximal row carpectomy for post-traumatic disorders of the carpus, J Hand Surg 8:301, 1983.

O'Brien ET: Acute fractures and dislocations of the carpus, Orthop Clin North Am 15:237, 1984.

Obletz BE and Halbstein BM: Non-union of fractures of the carpal navicular, J Bone Joint Surg 20:424, 1938.

Palmer AK: Scapholunate dissociation, Mimeographed, Syracuse NY, 1989.

Peltier LF: Fractures of the distal end of the radius: an historical ac-count, Clin Orthop 187:18, 1984.

Russe O: Fracture of the carpal navicular: diagnosis, nonoperative treatment, and operative treatment, J Bone Joint Surg 42-A:759, 1960.

Sarrafian SK and Breihan JH: Palmar dislocation of scaphoid and lunate as a unit, J Hand Surg 15-A:134, 1990.

Saunier J and Chamay A: Volar perilunar dislocation of the wrist, Clin Orthop 157:139, 1981.

Schwartz GB: Displaced dorsal coronal fracture of the hamate, Or-thop Rev 18:875, 1989.

Selmon LP: Compound dislocation of the trapezium: a case report, J Bone Joint Surg 54-A:1297, 1972.

Sergio G, Rosa D, DePasquali PM, and Petillo C: Treatment of non-union in fractures of the carpal navicular by the Matti-Russe op-eration, Ital J Orthop Traumatol 13:325, 1987.

Shaw JC and Wilson FC: Radial perilunar dislocation: report of a case, J Bone Joint Surg 52-A:556, 1970.

Soto-Hall R and Haldeman KO: Treatment of fractures of the carpal scaphoid, J Bone Joint Surg 16:822, 1934.

Sprague HH and Howard FM: The Herbert screw for treatment of the scaphoid fracture, Contemp Orthop 16:19, 1988.

Stark A, Broström L-A, and Svartengren G: Scaphoid nonunion treated with the Matti-Russe technique, Clin Orthop 214:175, 1987.

Stark HH, Chao E-K, Zemel NP, et al: Fracture of the hook of the hamate, J Bone Joint Surg 71-A:1201, 1989.

Stark HH, Rickard TA, Zemel NP, and Ashworth CR: Treatment of ununited fractures of the scaphoid by iliac bone grafts and Kir-schner-wire fixation, J Bone Joint Surg 70-A:982, 1988.

Stein AH Jr: Dorsal dislocation of the lesser multangular bone, J Bone Joint Surg 53-A:377, 1971.

Stewart MJ: Fractures of the carpal navicular (scaphoid): a report of 436 cases, J Bone Joint Surg 36-A:998, 1954.

Szabo RM and Manske D: Displaced fractures of the scaphoid, Clin Orthop 230:30, 1988.

Terkelsen CJ and Jepsen JM: Treatment of scaphoid fractures with a removable cast, Acta Orthop Scand 59:452, 1988.

Wagner CJ: Perilunar dislocations, J Bone Joint Surg 38-A:1198, 1956.

Walker JL, Greene TL, and Lunseth PA: Fractures of the body of the trapezium, J Orthop Trauma 2:22, 1988.

Weber ER: Biomechanical implications of scaphoid waist fractures, Clin Orthop 149:83, 1980.

Weiss C, Laskin RS, and Spinner M: Irreducible trans-scaphoid perilunate dislocation: a case report, J Bone Joint Surg 52-A:565,
1970.

Proximal row carpectomy

Crabbe WA: Excision of the proximal row of the carpus, J Bone
Joint Surg 46-B:708, 1964.

Green DP: Proximal row carpectomy, Hand Clin 3:163, 1987.

Inglis AE and Jones EC: Proximal row carpectomy for diseases of
the proximal row, J Bone Joint Surg 59-A:460, 1977.

Neviaser RJ: Proximal row carpectomy for posttraumatic disorders
of the carpus, J Hand Surg 11-A:301, 1983.

Stamm TT: Excision of the proximal row of the carpus, J Roy Soc
Med 38:74, 1944.

Stamm TT: Excision of the proximal row of the carpus, Guy's Hosp
Rep 112:6, 1963.

Wenner SM and Saperia BS: Proximal row carpectomy in arthrogry-
potic wrist deformity, J Hand Surg 12-A:523, 1987.

Kienböck's disease

Agerholm JC and Goodfellow JW: Avascular necrosis of the lunate
bone treated by excision and prosthetic replacement, J Bone Joint
Surg 45-B:110, 1963.

Alexander AH, Mack GR, and Gunther SF: Kienböck's disease: update on silicone replacement arthroplasty, J Hand Surg 7:343,
1982.

Almquist EE: Kienböck's disease, Hand Clin 3:141, 1987.

Almquist EE and Burns JF Jr: Radial shortening for the treatment of
Kienböck's disease: a 5- to 10-year follow-up, J Hand Surg 7:348,
1982.

Armistead RB, Linscheid RL, Dobyns JH, and Beckenbaugh RD: Ulnar lengthening in the treatment of Kienböck's disease, J Bone
Joint Surg 64-A:170, 1982.

Axelsson R: Behandlung av lunatomalaci, Göteborg, Sweden, 1971,
Elanders Boktrycker: Akteibolag.

Barber HM and Goodfellow JW: Acrylic lunate prostheses: a long-
term follow-up, J Bone Joint Surg 57-B:706, 1974.

Beckenbaugh RD, Shives TC, Dobyns JH, and Linscheid RL: Kienböck's disease: the natural history of Kienböck's disease and consideration of lunate fractures, Clin Orthop 149:98, 1980.

Chan KP and Huang P: Anatomic variations in radial and ulnar
lengths in the wrists of Chinese, Clin Orthop 80:17, 1971.

Crabbe WA: Excision of the proximal row of the carpus, J Bone
Joint Surg 46-B:708, 1964.

Dornan A: Results of treatment in Kienböck's disease, J Bone Joint
Surg 31-B:518, 1949.

Edelson G, Reis D, and Fuchs D: Recurrence of Kienböbock disease
in a twelve-year-old after radial shortening: report of a case, J
Bone Joint Surg 70-A:1243, 1988.

Eiken O and Niechajeu I: Radius shortening in malacia of the lunate, Scand J Plast Reconstr Surg 14:191, 1980.

Gelberman RH and Szabo RM: Kienböck's disease, Orthop Clin
North Am 15:355, 1984.

Gelberman RH et al: Ulnar variance in Kienböck's disease, J Bone
Joint Surg 57-A:674, 1975.

Gelberman RH et al: The vascularity of the lunate bone and Kienböck's disease, J Hand Surg 5:272, 1980.

Gillespie HS: Excision of the lunate bone in Kienböck's disease, J
Bone Joint Surg 43-B:245, 1961.

Graner O et al: Arthrodesis of the carpal bones in treatment of Kienböck's disease, painful ununited fractures of the navicular and lunate bones with avascular necrosis, and old fracture-dislocations
of carpal bones, J Bone Joint Surg 48-A:767, 1966.

Hultén O: Über anatomische Variationen der Handgelenkknochen,
Acta Radiol 9:155, 1928.

Inglis AE and Jones EC: Proximal row carpectomy for disease of the
proximal row, J Bone Joint Surg 51-A:460, 1977.

James JIP: A case of rupture of flexor tendons secondary to Kienböck's disease, J Bone Joint Surg 31-B:521, 1949.

Jorgensen EC: Proximal-row carpectomy: an end-result study of
twenty-two cases, J Bone Joint Surg 51:1104, 1969.

Kawai H, Yamamoto K, Yamamoto T, et al: Excision of the lunate in
Kienböbock's disease: results after long-term follow-up, J Bone
Joint Surg 70-B:287, 1988.

Kelven H: The treatment of lunatomalacia, Tidsskr Nor Laegeforen
91:1944, 1971.

Kienböck R: Uber traumatische Malazie des Mondbeins und ihre
Folgezustände, Entartungsformen und Kompressionsfrakturen,
Fortschr Geb Röntgenstr 16:77, 1910-1911.

Lichtman DM et al: Kienböck's disease: the role of silicone replacement arthroplasty, J Bone Joint Surg 59-A:899, 1977.

Linscheid RL: Ulnar lengthening and shortening, Hand Clin 3:69,
1987.

Lippman EM and McDermott LJ: Vitallium replacement of lunate in
Kienböck's disease, Milit Surg 105:482, 1949.

Lowry WE and Cord SA: Traumatic avascular necrosis of the capitate bone: case report, J Hand Surg 6:245, 1981.

Marek FM: Avascular necrosis of the carpal lunate, Clin Orthop
10:96, 1957.

Match RM: Nonspecific avascular necrosis of the pisiform bone: a
case report, J Hand Surg 5:341, 1980.

McMurtry RY, Youm Y, Flatt AE, and Gillespie TE: Kinematics of
the wrist. II. Clinical applications, J Bone Joint Surg 60-A:955,
1978.

Mikkelsen S and Gelineck J: Poor function after nonoperative treatment of Kienböck's disease, Acta Orthop Scand 58:241, 1987.

Möberg E: Treatment of Kienböck's disease by shortening of the radius. Paper presented at the joint meeting of Japanese and American hand surgeons, Hiroshima, 1974.

Mouat TB, Wilkie J, and Harding HE: Isolated fracture of the carpal
semilunar and Kienböck's disease, Br J Surg 19:577, 1932.

Nahigian SH et al: The dorsal flap arthroplasty in the treatment of
Kienböck's disease, J Bone Joint Surg 52-A:245, 1970.

Persson M: Pathogenese und Behandlung der Kienböckschen Luna-
tummalazie, die Frakturtheorie im Lichte der Erfolge operativer
Radiusverkürzung (Hultén) und einer neuen Operationsmeth-
ode — Ulnaverlängerung, Acta Chir Scand 92(suppl 98):1, 1945.

Persson M: Causal treatment of lunatomalacia: further experiences
of operative ulna lengthening, Acta Chir Scand 100:531, 1950.

Phemister DB, Brunschwig A, and Day L: Streptococcal infections of
epiphyses and short bones, their relation to Kohler's disease of
the tarsal navicular, Legg-Perthes' disease and Kienböck's disease
of the os lunatum, JAMA 95:995, 1930.

Ramakrishna B, D'Netto DC, and Sethu AU: Long-term results of
silicone rubber implants for Kienböck's disease, J Bone Joint Surg
64-B:361, 1982.

Ringsted A: Doppelseitiger Mb Kienboeck bei 2 Brüdern, Acta Chir
Scand 69:185, 1932.

Roca J et al: Treatment of Kienböck's disease using a silicone rubber implant, J Bone Joint Surg 58-A:373, 1976.

Schattenkerk ME, Nollen A, and van Hussen F: The treatment of lunatomalacia: radial shortening or ulnar lengthening? Acta Orthop
Scand 58:652, 1987.

Ståahl F: On lunatomalacia (Kienböck's disease): a clinical and
roentgenological study, especially on its pathogenesis and the
late results of immobilization treatment, Acta Chir Scand, (suppl
126), 1947.

Stark HH, Zemel NP, and Ashworth CR: Use of a hand-carved sili-
cone-rubber spacer for advanced Kienböck's disease, J Bone Joint
Surg 63-A:1359, 1981.

Sundberg SB and Linscheid RL: Kienböck's disease: results of treatment with ulnar lengthening, Clin Orthop 187:43, 1984.

Swanson AB: Silicone rubber implants for the replacement of the
carpal scaphoid and lunate bones, Orthop Clin North Am 1:299,
1970.

Swanson AB and Swanson G deG: Flexible implant resection arthroplasty: a method for reconstruction of small joints in the extremities, AAOS Instr Course Lect 27:27, 1978.

Tauma T: An investigation of the treatment of Kienböck's disease, J Bone Joint Surg 48-A:1649, 1966.

Therkelsen F and Andersen K: Lunatomalacia, Acta Chir Scand 97:503, 1949.

Viljakka T, Vastamäki M, Solonen KA, and Tallroth K: Silicone implant arthroplasty in Kienböck's disease, Acta Orthop Scand 58:410, 1987.

Werner FW, Murphy DJ, and Palmer AK: Pressures in the distal radioulnar joint: effect of surgical procedures used for Kienbock's disease, J Orthop Res 7:445, 1989.

Weiss APC, Weiland AJ, Moore JR, and Wilgis EFS: Radial shortening for Kienböck's disease, Orthop Trans 14:642, 1990.

Radioulnar joint

Aulicino PL and Siegel JL: Acute injuries of the distal radioulnar joint, Hand Clin 7:283, 1991.

Bowers WH: The distal radioulnar joint. In Green DP, editor: Operative hand surgery, ed 2, New York, 1988, Churchill Livingstone.

Bowers WH: Instability of the distal radioulnar articulation, Hand Clin 7:311, 1991.

Breen TF and Jupiter J: Tenodesis of the chronically unstable distal ulna, Hand Clin 7:355, 1991.

Chidgey LK: Histologic anatomy of the triangular fibrocartilage, Hand Clin 7:249, 1991.

Chun S and Palmer AK: Chronic ulnar wrist pain secondary to partial rupture of the extensor carpi ulnaris tendon, J Hand Surg 12-A:1032, 1987.

Darrach W: Anterior dislocation of the head of the ulna, Ann Surg 56:802, 1912.

Friedman SL and Palmer AK: The ulnar impaction syndrome, Hand Clin 7:295, 1991.

Gordon L, Levinsohn DG, Moore SV, et al: The Sauve-Kapandji procedure for the treatment of posttraumatic distal radioulnar joint problems, Hand Clin 7:397, 1991.

Hagart CG: Functional aspects of the distal radioulnar joint, J Hand Surg 4:585, 1979.

Hunter JM and Kirkpatrick WH: Dacron stabilization of the distal ulna, Hand Clin 7:365, 1991.

Imbriglia JE and Matthews D: The treatment of chronic traumatic subluxation of the distal ulna by hemiresection interposition arthroplasty, Hand Clin 7:329, 1991.

Kapandji IA: The inferior radioulnar joint and pronosupination. In Tubiana R, editor: The hand, vol 1, Philadelphia, 1981, WB Saunders Co.

Nathan R and Schneider LH: Classification of distal radioulnar joint disorders, Hand Clin 7:239, 1991.

Palmer AK: The distal radioulnar joint, Orthop Clin North Am 15:321, 1984.

Palmer AK: The distal radioulnar joint. In Lichtman DM, editor: The wrist and its disorders, Philadelphia, 1988, WB Saunders Co.

Sauve L and Kapandji M: Nouvelle technique de traitement chirurgical des luxations recidivantes isolees de l'extremite inferieure du cubitus, J Chir 47:589, 1936.

Schneider LH and Imbriglia JE: Radioulnar joint fusion for distal radioulnar joint instability, Hand Clin 7:391, 1991.

Taleisnik J: Pain on the ulnar side of the wrist, Hand Clin 3:51, 1987.

Watson HK and Brown RE: Ulnar impingement syndrome after Darrach procedure: treatment by advancement lengthening osteotomy of the ulna, J Hand Surg 14-A:302, 1989.

Webber JB and Maser SA: Stabilization of the distal ulna, Hand Clin 7:345, 1991.

Arthrodesis

Clayton ML and Ferlic DC: Arthrodesis of the arthritic wrist, Clin Orthop 187:89, 1984.

Gellman H, Kauffman D, Lenihan M, et al: An in vitro analysis of wrist motion: the effect of limited intercarpal arthrodesis and the contributions of the radiocarpal and midcarpal joints, J Hand Surg 13-A:390, 1988.

Haddad RJ and Riordan DC: Arthrodesis of the wrist: a surgical technique, J Bone Joint Surg 49-A:950, 1967.

Meyerdierks EM, Mosher JF, and Werner FW: Limited wrist arthrodesis: a laboratory study, J Hand Surg 12-A:526, 1987.

Rayan GM, Brentlinger A, Purnell D, and Garcia-Moral CA: Functional assessment of bilateral wrist arthrodeses, J Hand Surg 12-A:1020, 1987.

Rogers WD and Watson HK: Radial styloid impingement after triscaphe arthrodesis, J Hand Surg 14-A:297, 1989.

Taleisnik J: Subtotal arthrodeses of the wrist joint, Clin Orthop 187:81, 1984.

Trumble T, Bour CJ, Smith RJ, and Edwards GS: Intercarpal arthrodesis for static and dynamic volar intercalated segment instability, J Hand Surg 13-A:396, 1988.

Trumble TE, Easterling KJ, and Smith RJ: Ulnocarpal abutment after wrist arthrodesis, J Hand Surg 13-A:11, 1988.

Veigas SF, Rimoldi R, and Patterson R: Modified technique of intramedullary fixation for wrist arthrodesis, J Hand Surg 14-A:618, 1989.

Watson HK: Limited wrist arthrodesis, Clin Orthop 149:126, 1980.

Wood MB: Wrist arthrodesis using dorsal radial bone graft, J Hand Surg 12-A:208, 1987.

Instability

Alexander CE and Lichtman DM: Ulnar carpal instabilities, Orthop Clin North Am 15:307, 1984.

Armstrong GWD: Rotational subluxation of the scaphoid, Can J Surg 2:306, 1968.

Beckenbaugh RD: Accurate evaluation and management of the painful wrist following injury: an approach to carpal instability, Orthop Clin North Am 15:289, 1984.

Blatt G: Capsulodesis in reconstructive hand surgery: dorsal capsulodesis for the unstable scaphoid and volar capsulodesis following excision of the distal unla, Hand Clin 3:81, 1987.

Brown IW: Volar intercalary carpal instability following a seemingly innocent wrist fracture, J Hand Surg 12-B:54, 1987.

Dobyns JH: Current classification and treatment of carpal instabilities, Mimeographed, The Mayo Clinic, 1989.

Dobyns JH, Linscheid RL, Chao EYS, et al: Traumatic instability of the wrist, AAOS Instr Course Lect 24:182, 1975.

Goldner JL: Treatment of carpal instability without joint fusion: current assessment, J Hand Surg 7:325, 1982 (editorial).

Kleinman WB: Management of chronic rotary subluxation of the scaphoid by scapho-trapezio-trapezoid arthrodesis: rationale for the technique, postoperative changes in biomechanics, and results, Hand Clin 3:113, 1987.

Lichtman DM and Martin RA: Introduction to the carpal instabilities. In Lichtman DM, editor: The wrist and its disorders, Philadelphia, 1988 WB Saunders Co.

Linscheid RL, Dobyns JH, Beabout JW, and Bryan RS: Traumatic instability of the wrist: diagnosis, classification and pathomechanics, J Bone Joint Surg 54-A:1612, 1972.

Mayfield JK: Wrist ligamentous anatomy and pathogenesis of carpal instability, Orthop Clin North Am 15:209, 1984.

Palmer AK, Dobyns JH, and Linscheid RL: Management of posttraumatic instability of the wrist secondary to ligament rupture, J Hand Surg 3:507, 1978.

Reagan DS, Linscheid RL, and Dobyns JH: Lunotriquetral sprain, J Hand Surg 6:296, 1981.

Taleisnik J: Post-traumatic carpal instability, Clin Orthop 149:73, 1980.

Veigas SF, Tencer AF, Cantrell J, et al: Load transfer characteristics of the wrist. II. Perilunate instability, J Hand Surg 12-A:978, 1987.

Watson HK and Black DM: Instabilities of the wrist, Hand Clin 3:103, 1987.

Weber ER: Concepts governing the rotational shift of the intercalated segment of the carpus, Orthop Clin North Am 15:193, 1984.

Arthroscopy of wrist

Botte MJ, Cooney WP, and Linscheid RL: Arthroscopy of the wrist: anatomy and technique, J Hand Surg 14-A(2):313, 1989.

Cooney WP, Dobyns JH, and Linscheid RL: Arthroscopy of the wrist: anatomy and classification of carpal instability, Arthroscopy 6:133, 1990.

Kaempffe F and Peimer CA: Distraction for wrist arthroscopy, J Hand Surg 15-A:520, 1990.

Kelly EP and Stanley JK: Arthroscopy of the wrist, J Hand Surg 15-B:236, 1990.

Koman LA, Poehling GG, Toby EB, and Kammire G: Chronic wrist pain: indications for wrist arthroscopy, Arthroscopy 6:116, 1990.

North ER and Thomas S: An anatomic guide for arthroscopic visualization of the wrist capsular ligaments, J Hand Surg 13-A:815, 1988.

Osterman AL: Arthroscopy debridement of triangular fibrocartilage complex tears, Arthroscopy 6:120, 1990.

Osterman AL and Terrill RG: Arthroscopic treatment of TFCC lesions, Hand Clin 7:277, 1991.

Peterson HA and Lipscomb PR: Intercarpal arthrodesis, Arch Surg 95:127, 1967.

Poehling GG: Wrist arthroscopy: portals to progress. In An illustrated guide to small joint arthroscopy, Andover, Mass, 1989, Dyonics, Inc.

Poehling GG, Roth J, Whipple T, et al: Arthroscopic surgery of the wrist: information manual, Winston-Salem, NC, Bowman Gray School of Medicine of Wake Forest University.

Roth JH: Midcarpal arthroscopy: technique and illustrative cases, Adv Orthop Surg 12:61, 1988.

Roth JH and Poehling GG: Arthroscopic "-ectomy" surgery of the wrist, Arthroscopy 6:141, 1990.

Roth JH, Poehling GG, and Whipple TL: Arthroscopic surgery of the wrist, AAOS Instr Course Lect 37:183, 1988.

Viegas SF: Preliminary report and review of the literature: arthroscopic treatment of osteochondritis dissecans of the scaphoid, Arthroscopy 4:278, 1988.

Watson HK and Hempton RF: Limited wrist arthrodesis. I. The triscaphoid joint, J Hand Surg 6:320, 1980.

Whipple TL: Precautions for arthroscopy of the wrist, Arthroscopy 6:3, 1990.

Whipple TL, Marotta JJ, and Powell JH III: Arthroscopy 2:244, 1986.

CHAPTER 67

Special Hand Disorders

PHILLIP E. WRIGHT II*

ANEURYSM OR THROMBOSIS OF RADIAL OR ULNAR ARTERY

Sharp or blunt trauma that does not break the skin (or a small puncture wound) may cause a false aneurysm or a thrombosis of the radial or ulnar artery. Of these two vessels, the ulnar is much more frequently involved (see Fig. 76-5).

A false aneurysm of the ulnar artery results in a tender mass located at the hypothenar eminence and accompanied by a bruit and a positive Allen test (see below). Secondary spasm of the more distal vessels may suggest Raynaud's disease. A false aneurysm of the radial artery may cause few symptoms early and may be confused with a ganglion, which is so often located over this artery on the volar surface of the wrist; in this instance considerable trouble may be encountered during surgery, especially if conducted in an environment less than ideal. Treatment of these lesions usually is resection. Arteriography is helpful in preoperative planning. If the palmar arch is incomplete, excision and repair or reconstruction by vein grafting should be considered.

Thrombosis of the ulnar artery may be caused by a single injury or by repeated occupational injuries such as those that may occur when a heavy hammer is used frequently or when the hand itself is used as a hammer. Thrombosis of the ulnar artery causes persistent secondary spasm of the more distal vessels, resulting in blanching of and pain in the ulnar three digits. It may be confused with Raynaud's disease, especially since exposure to cold increases the blanching. Koman and Urbaniak reviewed 28 patients with arteriographic evidence of ulnar artery thrombosis and found that the initial diagnosis was correct in only half of the cases. Raynaud's disease was diagnosed in 6 of the 28 patients. Sometimes pain is

severe and sensibility is lost over the distribution of the ulnar nerve in the hand. There is tenderness over the artery and occasionally a feeling of fullness in the wrist and hand. The Allen test (see below) is helpful in diagnosis, but arteriography, of course, is diagnostic.

Traditionally, treatment has consisted of exploration of the artery and resection of the entire thrombotic mass. Other treatment methods include arterial reconstruction, local and regional sympathectomy, and palliation with medical and psychologic methods. A management suggested by Koman and Urbaniak individualizes treatment of ulnar artery thrombosis. The history, physical examination, and Allen test determine the initial diagnosis. If the Allen test is positive, thermography, temperature probes, Doppler studies, and pulse volume recordings are used to confirm the diagnosis. If a stellate ganglion or brachial block relieves symptoms, treatment is observation. A stellate or brachial block may block reflex vasospasm in acute thrombosis threatening digital survival. If symptoms are not relieved, arteriography is done and, at the same time, intraarterial medications (reserpine or tolazoline) usually are given. Arteriography establishes the diagnosis, identifies the extent of the thrombosis and vascular disease, and determines the probable success of surgery. Symptomatic treatment is indicated if vascular disease is generalized. If symptoms are decreased after arteriography, the patient may be observed. Surgery is indicated if symptoms persist and if digital survival is in question. After the thrombosed segment is resected, the proximal end is clamped, and the tourniquet is released. If backflow is good and pulse volume recordings of the ulnar digits are normal, the vessel is ligated and the wound is closed. If backflow is poor with no pulsative flow on digital plethysmography, vein grafting should be considered. Contraindications to vein grafting include erythrocytosis, patient refusal to modify the environment, and patient refusal to discontinue smoking. If vein

---

*Revision of chapter by Lee W. Milford, M.D.

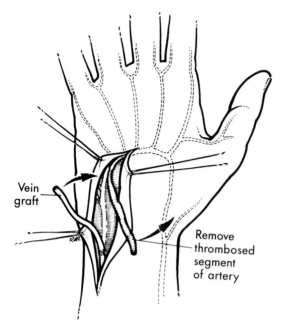

Fig. 67-1   Resection of thrombosed segment and replacement with reversed vein graft. (Redrawn from Koman LA and Urbaniak JR: Thrombosis of ulnar artery at the wrist. In American Academy of Orthopaedic Surgeons: Symposium on microsurgery: practical use in orthopaedics, St Louis, 1979, Mosby–Year Book, Inc.)

grafting is indicated, the entire thrombosed segment should be resected until normal intima is seen with the operating microscope. A reversed vein graft harvested from the forearm is inserted (Fig. 67-1). Vein grafting is contraindicated if there is inadequate peripheral "runoff" on the arteriogram. Persistent symptoms after surgery may be controlled conservatively by cessation of smoking, biofeedback techniques, and intermittent intraarterial medications. Sympathectomy may be used as a last resort.

The thrombosed mass may extend proximally in the forearm but rarely distally across the palmar arch to involve the more distal vessels; in the latter instance complete resection may be impossible. Adequate resection relieves the spasm of the distal vessels, and symptoms usually disappear; the circulation in the hand then depends entirely on the radial artery, which usually is sufficient.

Rarely thrombosis of a patent median artery may cause pain of median nerve compression within the car-

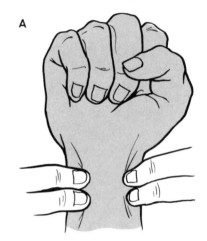

Fig. 67-2   Allen test for patency of radial and ulnar arteries. **A,** Patient elevates hand and makes fist while examiner occludes both radial and ulnar arteries. **B,** Patient extends fingers, and blanching of hand is seen. **C,** Radial artery alone is released, and color of hand returns to normal. **D,** In thrombosis of ulnar artery, test is positive (hand remains blanched) when this artery alone is released.

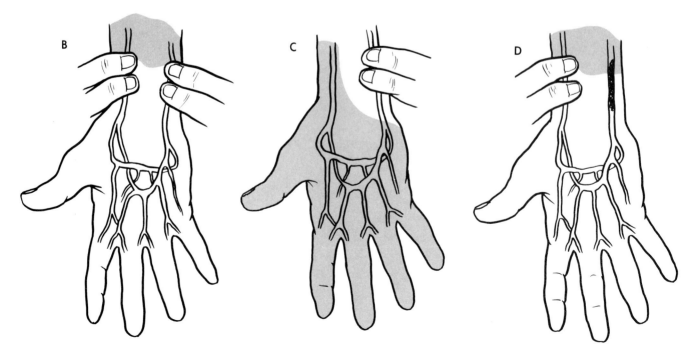

pal tunnel. It should be considered in diagnosis when acute pain in the hand is limited to the distribution of the median nerve.

Arterial lacerations in the wrist and hand are discussed in Chapter 62. (Also see Chapter 49.)

Allen Test

In 1929 Allen described maneuvers to test the patency of the radial and ulnar arteries. First the patient elevates his hand and makes a fist while the examiner occludes both the radial and ulnar arteries (Fig. 67-2, *A*). Then the patient extends his fingers, and blanching of the hand is seen (Fig. 67-2, *B*). Next, the hand is observed while the radial artery alone is released; the color of the hand should return immediately to normal (Fig. 67-2, *C*). The same maneuvers are repeated to test the ulnar artery. The test is positive when the color fails to return to normal after release of either artery alone. In thrombosis of the ulnar artery, the test is positive when the color fails to return to normal when this artery alone is released (Fig. 67-2, *D*).

The patency of the digital arteries can be tested in a similar manner (Fig. 67-3).

THERMAL BURNS

Burns from flash or flame usually involve the dorsal surface of the hand, and contact thermal and electrical burns usually involve the palmar surface. Any thermal burn of the hand must be evaluated as to depth and surface area involved and should be considered for primary debridement and skin grafting. This treatment, however, is much more urgent for third-degree burns on the dorsal surface where the skin is thin, the subcutaneous fat is scanty, and the joints and extensor tendons are poorly protected. Therefore when a burn on this surface is the main consideration in that other burns do not endanger life or require more urgent resurfacing, primary debridement and grafting may be indicated (Fig. 67-4). Accurate evaluation of the extent and depth of the full-thickness loss is essential for early replacement (Fig. 67-5). Loss of elasticity and color changes are indicative of deep burn.

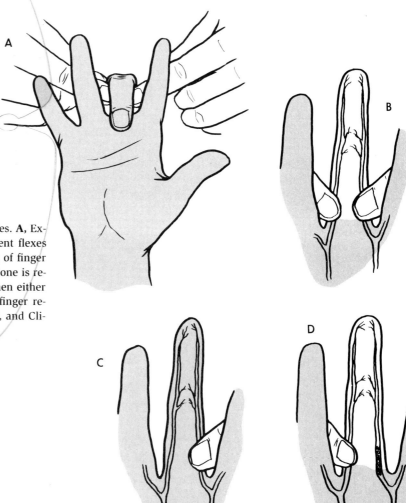

Fig. 67-3 Allen test as applied to digital arteries. **A,** Examiner occludes both digital arteries, and patient flexes finger. **B,** Patient extends finger, and blanching of finger is seen. **C,** When either artery is patent and it alone is released, color of finger returns to normal. **D,** When either artery is thrombosed and it alone is released, finger remains blanched. (From Ashbell TS, Koonce OE, and Clinard HE: Plast Reconstr Surg 39:411, 1967.)

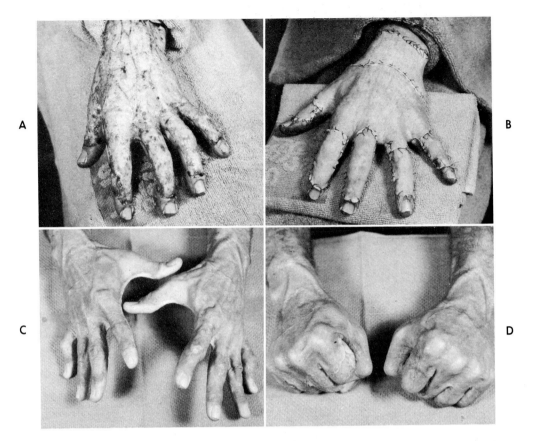

Fig. 67-4 Third-degree burn on dorsum of hand treated by primary debridement and skin grafting. **A,** Burned skin has been excised with care to preserve paratenon and venous network. Lines of excision extend into palm in all web spaces and along midlateral line of each digit with deep darts over joints. **B,** Two days after surgery. Thick split grafts have been applied and carefully anchored by fine sutures. **C** and **D,** Appearance and function of hands after recovery. (From Moncrief JA, Switzer WE, and Rose LR: Plast Reconstr Surg 33:305, 1964.)

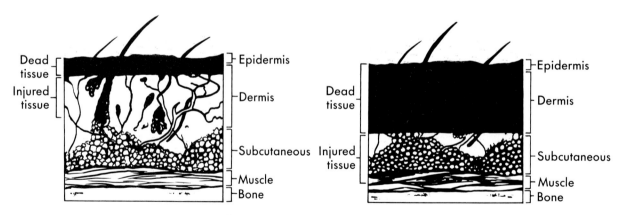

Fig. 67-5 Differential diagnosis of depth of burn. (Courtesy Dr. Hal G Bingham.)

Early coverage by debridement and grafting will help preserve the gliding mechanism of the extensor tendons. Once these tendons become adherent from scarring or from a severe fibrous reaction produced by prolonged edema or are destroyed from exposure, then later restoration of full function is almost impossible.

Immediate application of mafenide (Sulfamylon) or sulfamethazine helps prevent local infection.

Moncrief, Switzer, and Rose have had much experience in treating burns of the hand and the following remarks outline the treatment reported by them. Debridement of the burn should be delayed until about 3 days

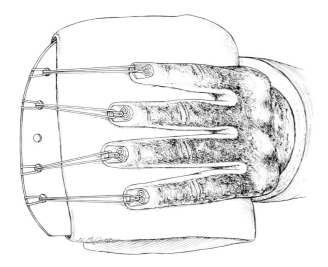

Fig. 67-6 Splinting for burned hand in antideformity position. Rubber band traction on metallic dress hooks "glued" to fingernails achieves positioning without occlusive dressing. (From Salisbury RE and Pruitt BA: Burns of the upper extremity, Philadelphia, 1976, WB Saunders Co.)

after injury; during this time the patient's general condition is evaluated, and the edema that obliterates the tissue planes and makes accurate excision of the damaged area difficult is allowed to decrease. A general anesthetic is given to the patient and a tourniquet is used. The wound and nails are cleaned, and all loose tissue is removed. The burn is inspected, its boundaries are located, and if desired, they are outlined with a skin pencil. The area to be excised should be patterned to conform to the functional skin creases as described for placing hand incisions (Chapter 61), thus avoiding tension lines and excessive scarring; this applies not only to the junction between normal skin and grafts but also to any junction between graft and graft. This proper placement of suture lines is especially important in the webs. If the webs require grafting, they should be fully covered and darts of skin should extend distally to the palm; otherwise the darts should extend distally far enough to break any suture line that crosses their proximal borders dorsally. To prevent adduction contracture of the thumb, special care must be used in locating any suture lines on the thumb web. The venous and lymphatic networks are preserved carefully to help prevent edema and to improve nutrition of the extensor tendons. Furthermore, the paratenon, so important in tendon excursion, is also preserved. After the damaged skin has been excised as necessary, small vessels are cauterized or tied with 5-0 plain catgut sutures. Then a finely woven gauze is applied to the raw surface, the hand and arm are wrapped in a bulky compression dressing, the tourniquet is released, and the extremity is elevated fully for 45 minutes to help control bleeding. This elevation is continued later in bed. After 48 hours the patient is returned to surgery and again with the patient under general anesthesia the wound is

cleaned and all bleeding is controlled. A skin graft 0.4 to 0.45 mm thick is obtained from the abdomen or medial aspect of the thigh and is sutured in place; during suture, the graft is barely stretched so that it will be elastic when finger and wrist movements are begun. A dressing is applied with the metacarpophalangeal and interphalangeal joints extended (Fig. 67-6); the wrist is supported on a volar plaster splint. The limb is elevated and the tourniquet is removed. After 72 additional hours the patient is taken to surgery a third time and is anesthetized; the grafts are inspected, any hematomas are evacuated, and any areas on which the grafting has failed are covered by new grafts. Mobilization out of bed depends on the extent of the burned area. Generally, condition permitting, the patient is encouraged to be up as soon as practical. Then the dressings are removed after about a week and active motion is begun gradually and increased as tolerated.

ELECTRICAL BURNS

Electrical burns, unfortunately, almost always involve the upper extremity. The extent of injury is determined by the characteristics of the injuring current, the duration of contact with it, and the patient's susceptibility to it. Evaluating the extent of injury is always difficult; the first assessment of the severity and depth of tissue damage is usually much too conservative because later more and more apparently normal tissue becomes necrotic.

In a large series, Hunter experienced an overall amputation rate of 43%, including the upper and lower extremities or parts thereof. Initial debridement should begin within 48 hours to help avoid the potentially lethal complication of sepsis associated with the presence of necrotic tissue.

Clinically the burn at first appears as a gray area of skin underlying blistered or charred superficial epithelium; its center is painless because of destruction of sensory nerves. Encircling the area is a line of hyperemia that later becomes edematous. At 7 to 10 days after injury the center of the damaged area begins to slough and extensive necrosis becomes apparent. Sometimes necrosis is quite deep and spreads in all directions beneath the skin. It apparently is caused by the burn and by thrombosis of vessels as well. At about 10 days the wound is invaded by bacteria, and softening of tissue and drainage result. To prevent increasing destruction by bacteria, some surgeons recommend debriding the wound early and closing it by either a split-thickness graft or a pedicle graft. This treatment may be ideal if the extent of necrosis can be reasonably determined and if no viable tissue is sacrificed, but determination is extremely difficult at times. Other surgeons are more conservative and recommend repeated debridement of obviously nonviable tissue, attempting to save all viable structures that may be useful in reconstruction later. However, the excision of nonviable tissue may uncover bones, tendons, and nerves, and unless they are soon covered they too become necrotic, probably from bacterial invasion. The wound must be closed in some manner before any reconstructive surgery. Traditional remote pedicle flaps or free tissue transfer usually suffice for this coverage. In this type of burn the danger of necrosis of major vessels is great; a large artery may rupture spontaneously during the night and consequently a tourniquet should be placed by the bed for immediate use should this complication occur.

RADIATION BURNS

In radiation burns or dermatitis caused by overexposure to roentgen rays, the skin becomes pale, dry, atrophic, and wrinkled and scattered keratoses develop; the

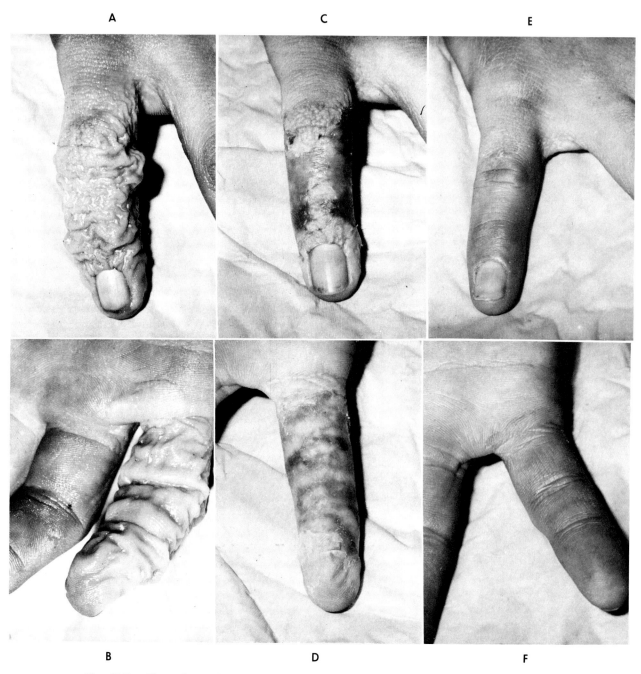

Fig. 67-7 Circumferential chemical burn. **A** and **B,** Dorsal and volar aspects of little finger showing circumferential burn from DMSO. **C,** Finger 5 days after injury. **D,** Volar aspect showing skin blanching on full extension. **E** and **F,** Dorsal and volar views of finger 3 weeks after injury. (From Walker FW and Weinstein MA: J Hand Surg 8:330, 1983.)

fingernails split longitudinally. The skin may become increasingly painful and eventually narcotics may be required. Multiple squamous cell carcinomas may develop and cause ulceration. In the past such burns have caused physicians and other medical professionals to lose digits. These burns, typically on the dorsum of the fingers of the left hand, presumably are caused in the medical profession by holding roentgen cassettes or using the fluoroscope without protection. When breakdown of tissue, pain, or malignant change make resurfacing the hand necessary, the damaged skin is excised and split-thickness grafts are applied at the same time. The area of excision should be generous, including even questionably involved skin; usually all dorsal skin from the wrist distally should be replaced.

CIRCUMFERENTIAL CHEMICAL BURNS

Chemical burns of the hand are usually splash burns. Circumferential burns of the hand are unusual. However, with the increasing availability and use of dimethyl sulfoxide (DMSO) as a "pain reliever" by some patients, circumferential burns may become more common. Walker and Weinstein reported a horse-handler and exerciser who experienced circumferential blistering of the entire small finger after wrapping it in a cloth soaked in DMSO for treatment of a minor sprain. Recovery was prompt following early debridement and a therapy program designed to prevent joint stiffness and contractures (Fig. 67-7).

FROSTBITE

In frostbite, tissue is damaged by anoxia caused early by vascular constriction and later by vascular thrombosis. In order of increasing degrees of damage the following develop: erythema, edema, vesiculation, necrosis of skin, necrosis of deeper soft tissue, and necrosis of bone. The immediate basic care of frostbite, whether the tissue is blistered or discolored, is warming in a water bath at about 40° C, and cleaning followed by minimal debridement and watchful waiting for necrosis. After warming, the hand should be washed daily. A Hubbard tank usually is satisfactory for washing. Blisters should not be debrided unless infected. Active motion should be encouraged and frequent washings continued. Amputation should be delayed until there is definite demarcation; this may require several weeks or a few months. In contrast to thermal burns, there is no place for early excision and grafting in treatment of frostbite.

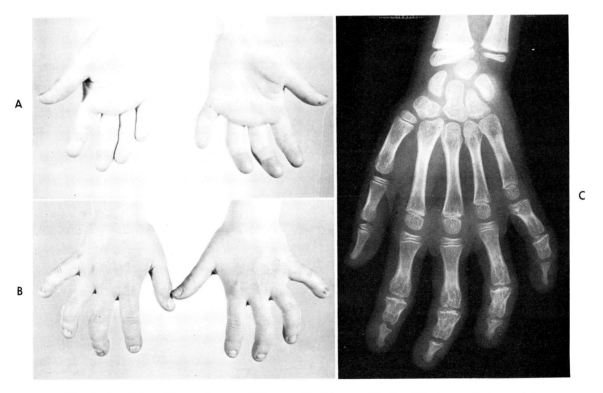

Fig. 67-8   Deformities of fingers of 12-year-old girl caused by frostbite incurred at age of 2 years. **A** and **B,** Note shortening and angulation of various fingers. **C,** Left hand. Note destruction of epiphyses of middle and distal phalanges of all fingers and deformity of epiphysis of proximal phalanx of little finger. Osseous changes in right hand were similar. (From Bigelow DR and Ritchie GW: J Bone Joint Surg 45-B:122, 1963.)

Bigelow and Ritchie reported epiphyseal arrest in several children with severe frostbite (Fig. 67-8); the index and little fingers were involved more frequently than the middle and ring fingers, and the thumb least of all. Disturbances in growth develop gradually, of course, and are probably caused by derangement of the blood supply to the involved epiphyses.

PAINT-GUN INJURIES

Paint-gun injuries usually are caused by wiping the jet opening of a high-pressure gun with the index fingertip. The stream of paint strikes the part with such pressure that it penetrates the skin and spreads widely throughout the underlying fascial planes and tendon sheaths. The resulting distention of tissues and inflammatory reaction cause marked ischemia of tissue; fever and leukocytosis follow. Stark, Ashworth, and Boyes strongly recommend immediate incision and drainage of the injured part, with the patient under general anesthesia, to relieve pressure and to remove as much of the foreign material as possible; delay in such treatment may result in loss of the part.

GREASE-GUN INJURIES

Grease-gun injuries (Figs. 67-9 and 67-10), like paint-gun injuries just described, are caused by penetration of

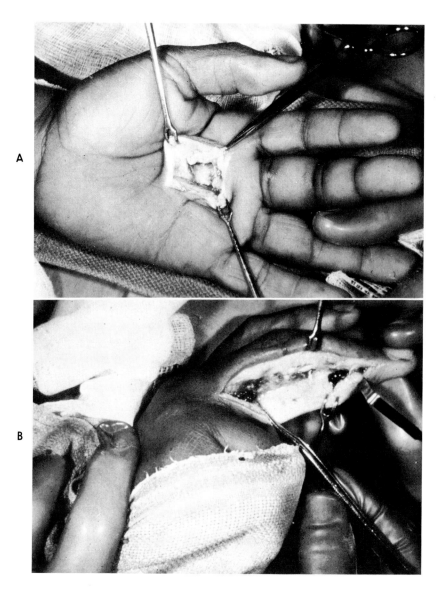

Fig. 67-9 Twelve-day-old grease-gun injury of hand. **A,** Grease had entered middle finger through a small wound on volar surface at proximal finger crease. Tendon sheath in palm was distended with grease. **B,** Tendon sheath in finger was also distended. All grease was contained within sheath. (From Stark HH, Wilson JN, and Boyes JH: J Bone Joint Surg 43-A:485, 1961.)

the tissues by grease or diesel fuel under high pressure. The grease or fuel balloons the soft tissues and follows the planes of least resistance; it causes ischemia and chemical irritation, but the inflammation is not as severe as that caused by paint. Treatment consists of relieving ischemia by decompression and, if possible, preventing infection; the distended tissues are opened immediately through bold incisions that follow the principles given for placing hand incisions (Chapter 61), and the foreign material is evacuated. The incisions are closed loosely, if at all, antibiotics are administered, and the hand is immobilized and elevated.

SHOTGUN INJURIES

Shotgun injuries are low velocity missile wounds, are multiple, and often are contaminated by such foreign material as clothing and wadding from the shotgun shell. The wadding is no longer made of horsehair, which in the past sometimes contaminated the wound by tetanus spores; it is now made of paper or plastic, but is still a dangerous contaminant. In the upper extremity such injuries usually are from close range and the clustered shots cause destruction of multiple tissues. Often the skin surrounding the wound is burned by powder.

The wound should be thoroughly debrided of foreign material, devitalized muscle, fat, and skin, but nerves, even though damaged, should not be excised. Removing every shot is unnecessary but attempts should be made to remove any lodged within joints. Any lying just beneath the skin often erode it, are painful, and require removal later. All free osseous fragments should be removed and any segmental defects in bones should be bridged by Kirschner wires to prevent collapse of the bony architecture. When the patient's condition permits and when joints, nerves, and tendons are exposed, the wound may be closed primarily on rare occasions, but a remote pedicle flap or free-tissue transfer often is necessary. A filleted finger is useful. The wound may be left open for a few days but should not be allowed to fill in slowly by granulation tissue and heal spontaneously. Certainly good coverage is necessary before any reconstructive surgery is possible.

WRINGER INJURIES

The term *wringer injury* was first used by MacCollum in 1938 to designate a crushing injury of the upper extremity caused by its passage between the rollers of the wringer on an electric washing machine. About 50% of such injuries occurred in children under the age of 5 years. Similar injuries continue to occur, more often in industrial workers. Early examination may reveal only abrasions or tears of the skin or occasionally a fracture. However, this first examination often is misleading be-

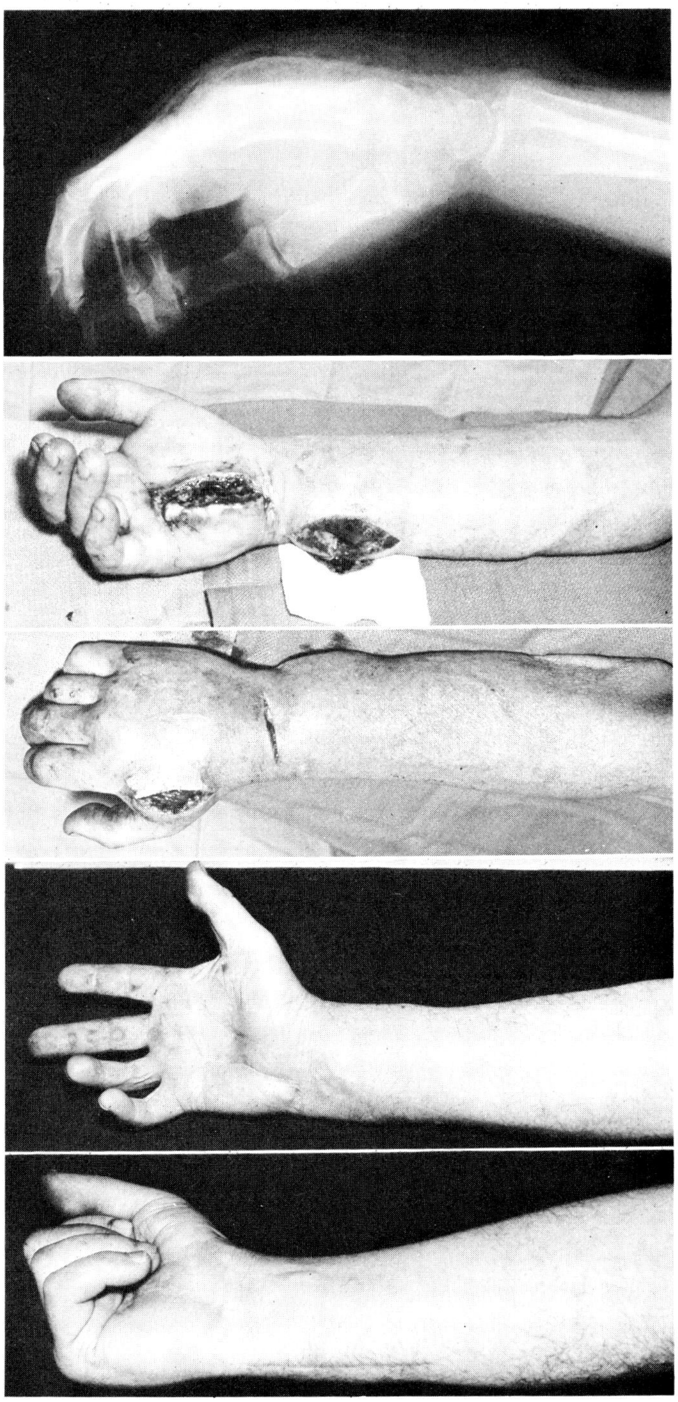

Fig. 67-10 Grease-gun injury of hand. **A,** Hand on day of injury. Air is dispersed through tissues impregnated with grease. **B** and **C,** Hand and forearm 9 days after incision and drainage. Palmar wound was incurred at time of injury, and in it ulnar nerve was found irreparably damaged. **D** and **E,** Hand and forearm 17 months after injury. Function is good. (From Tanzer RC: Surg Clin North Am 43:1277, 1963.)

cause hours later there may be severe swelling caused by hemorrhage and edema. When the injury is severe, the skin and deep tissues are burned by the rollers, often at one level where the extremity is blocked from entering farther between the rollers: usually at the base of the thumb, the antecubital fossa, or the axilla. Some of the skin avulsion may be caused by vigorous attempts of the patient to free his limb while the rollers are still in motion. These injuries typically include bursting of the skin at the thumb web with the thenar muscles protruding through the opening like toothpaste squeezed from a tube.

Some surgeons advise hospitalization for 48 hours after injury even when the skin is not broken. The limb is cleaned with soap and water and any open wounds are debrided and closed loosely, if at all. A pressure dressing that includes the entire hand is applied immediately, care being taken that pressure is evenly distributed. First the area is covered by finely woven nonadherent gauze and flat gauze pads are applied; then large masses of cotton and an elastic bandage are rolled on evenly. The extremity is elevated and is kept so throughout treatment. At 24 hours the dressing is removed, the wound is inspected for blisters, hematomas, and necrosis, and the dressing is reapplied; this is repeated every 24 hours until the injury becomes stabilized. Then if necessary, any devitalized tissue is excised and the wound is closed appropriately.

EXTRAVASATION INJURIES

Extravasation of a number of intravenously administered medications may cause deep necrosis and morbidity. Problems related to the extravasation of chemotherapeutic agents and roentgenographic contrast materials have been reported frequently over the past decade.

With an incidence of 0.5% to 6% or more, extravasation of chemotherapeutic agents is a leading cause of tissue injury. Causative agents reported by Seyfer and Solimando include doxorubicin, leteomycin, nitrogen mustards, Bacille bilié de Calmette-Guérin (BCG), and 5-fluorouracil. Lesions caused by their extravasation range from deep tissue necrosis to perivenous hyperpigmentation. Post-extravasation necrosis is determined by several factors: agent extravasated, extravasation site, host response, delay in recognition and treatment, and type of treatment. In a report of doxorubicin extravasation injuries, Linder, Upton, and Osteen found that factors causing extravasation included infusion under pressure, failure to release a proximal tourniquet, use of inadequate veins, thrombosis of proximal veins, spasm at previous venipuncture sites, active thrombophlebitis, and veins with multiple holes near the infusion site. Immediate treatment is recommended by most authors. There is no universal agreement on pharmacologic treatment. Reported antidotes include hydrocortisone, hyaluronidase, propranolol, sodium bicarbonate, isoproterenol, topical dimethyl sulfoxide (DMSO), vitamin E, and heat packs. The clinical experiences of Linder et al., Cohen, Manganaro, and Bezozo, and Seyfer and Solimando support early debridement, drainage, irrigation, repeat debridement, and delayed closure as methods consistently yielding the best results. Cohen et al. found that ultraviolet light assisted in locating and removing the fluorescent doxorubicin-containing tissue. After removing the extravasated fluid, intravenous flourescein was injected to determine the demarcation between viable and nonviable tissue for debridement. Comparing various antidotes with early surgical treatment in rats, Loth and Eversmann found early surgical debridement most effective in decreasing the size of vesicant ulcers and speeding the healing of ulcers.

While extravasation of roentgenographic contrast materials probably occurs more often than literature reports suggest, skin necrosis as a complication has been reported in 0.5% of roentgenographic contrast studies. Local inflammation may be the only response to extravasation of small amounts of contrast solutions. Large extravasations may result in skin necrosis, producing painful ulcers that are slow to heal. Loth and Jones reported that early surgical debridement, wound lavage, and delayed closure produced "excellent" functional and cosmetic results. Their management of patients with these injuries was determined by the amount of solution extravasated. Roentgenograms were used to estimate the volume and extent of extravasation. Insignificant extravasations (less than 5 ml) were treated with elevation in warm compressive dressings. Signficiant extravasations (more than 20 ml) were treated with emergency surgical drainage and wound lavage, preferably within 6 hours of extravasation. Intraoperative roentgenograms were used to assure complete removal of contrast solution. When tissue necrosis was found, closure was delayed 3 to 5 days. Treatment of extravasation of amounts between 5 and 20 ml was based on the clinical presentation; severe soft tissue reaction, swelling, and pain were indications for surgery.

PSYCHOFLEXED AND PSYCHOEXTENDED HANDS

At least two typical postures of the hand are associated with severe psychiatric depression and other mental disorders. One is the psychoflexed hand reported by Frykman et al. (Fig. 67-11). The posture is described as one in which the ulnar three digits are severely flexed and contracted, often causing maceration in the palm. It is almost uncorrectable permanently. It interferes with the hygiene of the hand and may cause an offensive odor. In addition, secondary infection can occur from pressure of the fingernails in the palm. There is no predilection for the minor or dominant hand. The psychoflexed hand

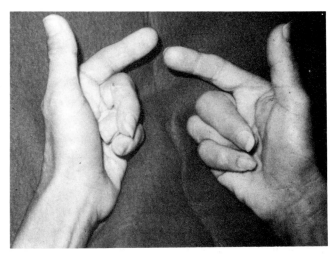

Fig. 67-11   Psychoflexed hands. Patient had flexion contractures of ulnar three fingers of both hands with palmar maceration. (From Frykman G et al: Clin Orthop 174:156, 1983.)

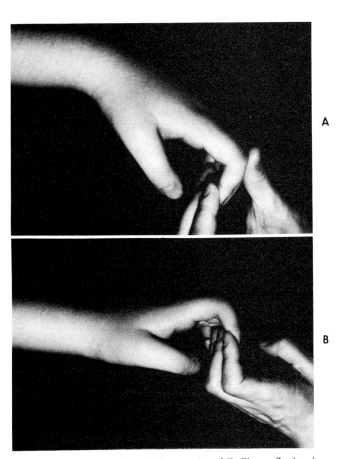

Fig. 67-12   Clenched-fist syndrome. **A** and **B,** Finger flexion is unchanged by wrist motion (paradoxical stiffness). (From Simmons BP and Vasile RG: J Hand Surg 5:420, 1980.)

should be differentiated carefully from such disorders as Dupuytren's contracture, arthrogryposis multiplex congenita, and certain spastic hand deformities secondary to stroke or cerebral palsy. These conditions usually are easily distinguished by the experienced orthopaedic surgeon.

Simmons and Vasile reported the clenched-fist syndrome (Fig. 67-12) in which the entire fist is clenched. However, the ulnar three digits are more predominantly involved.

Spiegel and Chase reported a patient who was eventually cured of severe contractures of all digits by exercises and self-hypnosis. Their method emphasizes and enhances the patient's control over the disability rather than questioning its cause.

The second posture is the psychoextended hand. It is similar to the psychoflexed hand except that the ulnar three digits are held in rigid hyperextension at the proximal interphalangeal joints and in flexion at the metacarpophalangeal joints. This seems to permit a partially functioning hand consisting of a pinch mechanism preserved between the thumb and index finger. The index finger metacarpophalangeal joint is held in flexion but active flexion and extension are preserved at the proximal interphalangeal joint, thus permitting opposition to the thumb pulp. At times these patients permit passive extension at the metacarpophalangeal joint and passive flexion at the proximal interphalangeal joint, but after release the posture quickly recurs. Increased hyperextension is eventually possible at the proximal interphalangeal joints by persistent stretching. These patients rarely are distressed by their problems and rarely demand treatment to correct the posture. However, they may permit surgery to be performed. The surgeon must be aware, however, that almost nothing is of lasting help, including casting, amputation of fingertips, or fixa-

tion of joints with Kirschner wires. Psychiatric management should be the initial treatment.

SELF-INDUCED INJURIES

Self-induced injury should be suspected when there is a history of prolonged edema, lack of wound healing, or a deformity without a plausible explanation.

Further suspicion should be aroused when the patient gives a history of having seen several competent physicians who were unable to establish an organic diagnosis after multiple diagnostic procedures such as venograms, lymphograms, and electromyograms (EMGs). Casting the edematous part or wound is not helpful because often the patient does not return or returns without the cast but with some excuse for having removed it.

Always inspect the entire extremity for evidence of some type of constricting band proximally. The edema will vary in severity depending on the length of time and the frequency with which and how recently the limb has been constricted. The constriction usually is applied when the person is alone.

3178 THE HAND

REFERENCES
Arterial injuries

Allen EV: Thromboangiitis obliterans: methods of diagnosis of chronic occlusive arterial lesions distal to the wrist with illustrative cases, Am J Med Sci 178:237, 1929.

Allen EV, Barker NW, and Hines EA Jr: Peripheral vascular diseases, ed 3, Philadelphia, 1962, WB Saunders Co.

Ashbell T, Koonce OE, and Clinard NE: The digital Allen test, Plast Reconstr Surg 39:411, 1967.

Barker NW and Hines EA Jr: Arterial occlusion in the hands and fingers associated with repeated occupational trauma, Mayo Clin Proc 19:345, 1944.

Butsch JL and Jones JM: Injuries of the superficial palmar arch, J Trauma 3:505, 1963.

Cameron BN: Occlusion of the ulnar artery with impending gangrene of the fingers: relieved by section of the volar carpal ligament, J Bone Joint Surg 36-A:406, 1964.

Caneirio RS and Mann RJ: Occlusion of the ulnar artery associated with an anomalous muscle: a case report, J Hand Surg 4:412, 1979.

Conn J Jr, Bergan JJ, and Bell JL: Hypothenar hammer syndrome: posttraumatic digital ischemia, Surgery 68:1122, 1970.

Costigan DC, Riley JN, and Coy FE: Thrombo-fibrosis of the ulnar artery in the palm, J Bone Joint Surg 41-A:702, 1959.

Diaz JE, Jones RS, and Ciceric WF: Perforation of the deep palmar arch produced by surgical wire after tenorrhaphy: a case report and review of the literature, J Bone Joint Surg 57-A:1150, 1975.

Eaton RG and Green WT: Epimysiotomy and fasciotomy in the treatment of Volkmann's ischemic contracture, Orthop Clin North Am 3:175, 1972.

Flatt AE: Tourniquet time in hand surgery, Arch Surg 104:190, 1972.

Flatt AE: Digital artery sympathectomy, J Hand Surg 5:550, 1980.

Gardner C: Traumatic vasospasm and its complications, Am J Surg 83:468, 1952.

Gelberman RH et al: Forearm arterial injuries, J Hand Surg 4:401, 1979.

Gibbon JH Jr and Landis EM: Vasodilatation in the lower extremities in response to immersing forearms in warm water, J Clin Invest 11:1019, 1932.

Goren ML: Palmar intramural thrombosis in the ulnar artery, Calif Med 89:424, 1958.

Herndon WA et al: Thrombosis of the ulnar artery in the hand: report of five cases, J Bone Joint Surg 57-A:994, 1975.

Imparato AM: Management of vascular injuries of the upper extremities, Orthop Clin North Am 2:383, 1970.

Jackson JP: Traumatic thrombosis of the ulnar artery in the palm, J Bone Joint Surg 36-B:438, 1954.

Kartchner MM and Wilcox WC: Thrombolysis of palmar and digital arterial thrombosis by intra-arterial Thrombolysin, J Hand Surg 1:67, 1976.

Kleinert HE and Volianitis GJ: Thrombosis of the palmar arterial arch and its tributaries: etiology and newer concepts in treatment, J Trauma 5:447, 1965.

Koman LA and Urbaniak JR: Thrombosis of ulnar artery at the wrist. In American Academy of Orthopaedic Surgeons: Symposium on microsurgery: practical use in orthopaedics, St Louis, 1979, Mosby–Year Book, Inc.

Koman LA and Urbaniak JR: Ulnar artery insufficiency: a guide to treatment, J Hand Surg 6:16, 1981.

Lanz U: Anatomical variations of the median nerve in the carpal tunnel, J Hand Surg 2:44, 1977.

Lawrence RR and Wilson JN: Ulnar artery thrombosis in the palm: case reports, Plast Reconstr Surg 36:604, 1965.

Leriche R, Fontaine R, and Dupertius SM: Arterectomy with follow-up studies on 78 operations, Surg Gynecol Obstet 64:149, 1937.

Lowrey CW, Chadwick RO, and Waltman EN: Digital vessel trauma from repetitive impact in baseball catchers, J Hand Surg 1:236, 1976.

Martin AF: Ulnar artery thrombosis in the palm: a case report, Clin Orthop 17:373, 1960.

McCormack LJ, Cauldwell EW, and Anson BJ: Brachial and antebrachial arterial patterns: a study of 750 extremities, Surg Gynecol Obstet 96:43, 1953.

Middleton DS: Occupational aneurysms of palmar arteries, Br J Surg 21:215, 1933.

Neviaser RJ and Adams JP: Vascular lesions in the hand: current management, Clin Orthop 100:111, 1974.

Pickering GW and Hess W: Vasodilatation of the hands and feet in response to warming the body, Clin Sci 1:213, 1934.

Poirier RA and Stansel HC Jr: Arterial aneurysms of the hand, Am J Surg 124:72, 1972.

Smith JW: True aneurysms of traumatic origin in the palm, Am J Surg 104:7, 1962.

Spittel JA Jr: Aneurysms of the hand and wrist, Med Clin North Am 42:1007, 1958.

Suzuki K, Takahashi S, and Hakagawa T: False aneurysm in a digital artery, J Hand Surg 5:402, 1980.

Teece LC: Thrombosis of the ulnar artery, Aust N Z J Surg 19:156, 1949.

Thio RT: False aneurysm of the ulnar artery after surgery employing a tourniquet, Am J Surg 123:604, 1972.

Tompkins DG: Exercise myopathy of the extensor carpi ulnaris muscle: report of a case, J Bone Joint Surg 59-A:407, 1977.

Trevaskis AE et al: Thrombosis of the ulnar artery in the hand: a case report, Plast Reconstr Surg 33:73, 1964.

Tsuge K: Treatment of established Volkmann's contracture, J Bone Joint Surg 57-A:925, 1975.

Watson HK et al: Post-traumatic interosseus-lumbrical adhesions: a cause of pain and disability in the hand, J Bone Joint Surg 56-A:79, 1974.

Wilgis EFS: Observations on the effects of tourniquet ischemia, J Bone Joint Surg 53-A:1343, 1971.

Zuckerman IC and Procter SE: Traumatic palmar aneurysm, Am J Surg 72:52, 1946.

Special hand injuries

Adams JP and Fowler FD: Wringer injuries of the upper extremity: a clinical, pathological, and experimental study, South Med J 52:798, 1959.

Adamson JE: Treatment of the stiff hand, Orthop Clin North Am 2:467, 1970.

Allen JE, Beck AR, and Jewett TC Jr: Wringer injuries in children, Arch Surg 97:194, 1968.

Ayre-Smith G: Tissue necrosis following extravasation of contrast material, J Can Assoc Radiol 33:104, 1982.

Bigelow DR and Ritchie GW: The effects of frostbite in childhood, J Bone Joint Surg 45-B:122, 1963.

Blair WF, Kilpatrick WC Jr, Saiki JH, and Alter EJ: Extravasation of chemotherapeutic agents, Clin Orthop 151:228, 1980.

Bowers D and Lynch JB: Adriamycin extravasation, Plast Reconstr Surg 61:86, 1978.

Brown H: Closed crush injuries of the hand and forearm, Orthop Clin North Am 2:253, 1970.

Browne EZ Jr, Teague MA, and Snyder CC: Burn syndactyly, Plast Reconstr Surg 62:92, 1978.

Burd DAR, Santis G, and Milward TM: Severe extravasation injury: an avoidable iatrogenic disaster? Br Med J 290:1579, 1985.

Caldwell EH and McCormack RM: Acute radiation injury of the hands: report of a case with a twenty-one year follow-up, J Hand Surg 5:568, 1980.

Cannon B and Zuidema GD: The care and the treatment of the burned hand, Clin Orthop 15:111, 1959.

Cohen FJ, Manganaro J, and Bezozo RC: Identification of involved tissue during surgical treatment of doxorubicin-induced extravasation necrosis, J Hand Surg 8:43, 1983.

Condon KC and Kaplan IJ: A method of diagnosis and management of the burned hand, Br J Plast Surg 12:129, 1959.

Crow ML and McCoy FJ: Volume increase Z-plasty to the finger skin: its application in electrical ring burns, J Hand Surg 2:402, 1977.

Drake DA et al: An unusual ring injury, J Hand Surg 2:111, 1977.

Dupertuis SM and Musgrave RH: Burns of the hand, Surg Clin North Am 40:321, 1960.

El-Adwar L and Arafa AG: A rare injury of the thumb similar to degloving, J Bone Joint Surg 57-A:998, 1975.

Elton RC and Bouzard WC: Gunshot and fragment wounds of the metacarpus, South Med J 68:833, 1975.

Flagg SV, Finseth FJ, and Krizek TJ: Ring avulsion injury, Plast Reconstr Surg 59:241, 1977.

Frykman G et al: The psychoflexed hand, Clin Orthop 174:156, 1983.

Gant TD: The early enzymatic debridement and grafting of deep dermal burns to the hand, Plast Reconstr Surg 66:185, 1980.

Gelberman RH et al: High-pressure injection injuries of the hand, J Bone Joint Surg 57-A:935, 1975.

Given KS, Puckett CL, and Kleinert HE: Ulnar artery thrombosis, Plast Reconstr Surg 61:405, 1978.

Goldner JL: Reconstructive surgery of the hand following thermal injuries, Clin Orthop 13:98, 1959.

Grace TG and Omer GE: The management of upper extremity pit viper wounds, J Hand Surg 5:168, 1980.

Hardin CA and Robinson DW: Coverage problems in the treatment of wringer injuries, J Bone Joint Surg 36-A:292, 1954.

Hawkins LG, Lischer CG, and Sweeney M: The main line accidental intra-arterial drug injection: a review of seven cases, Clin Orthop 94:268, 1973.

Horner RL, Wiedel JD, and Brailliar F: The orthopaedist and epidermolysis bullosa, Orthop Rev 1:21 August 1972.

Horner RL et al: Involvement of the hand in epidermolysis bullosa, J Bone Joint Surg 53-A:1347, 1971.

Hunter JM: Salvage of the burned hand, Surg Clin North Am 47:1059, 1967.

Iritani RI and Siler VE: Wringer injuries of the upper extremity, Surg Gynecol Obstet 113:677, 1961.

Kleinert HE and Williams DJ: Blast injuries of the hand, J Trauma 2:10, 1962.

Larmon WA: Surgical management of tophaceous gout, Clin Orthop 71:56, 1970.

Leonard LG, Munster AM, and Su CT: Adjunctive use of intravenous fluorescein in tangential excision of burns of the hand, Plast Reconstr Surg 66:30, 1980.

Leung PC and Cheng CY: Extensive local necrosis following the intravenous use of x-ray contrast medium in the upper extremity, Br J Radiol 53:361, 1980.

Lewis GK: Electrical burns on the upper extremities, J Bone Joint Surg 40-A:27, 1958.

Linder RM, Upton J, and Osteen R: Management of extensive doxorubicin hydrochloride extravasation injuries, J Hand Surg 8:32, 1983.

Loth TS and Eversmann WW Jr: Treatment methods for extravasations of chemotherapeutic agents: a comparative study, J Hand Surg 11-A:388, 1986.

Loth TS and Jones DEC: Extravasations of radiographic contrast material in the upper extremity, J Hand Surg 13-A:395, 1988.

Louis DS and Renshaw T: Injuries to the upper extremity inflicted by the mechanical cornpicker, Clin Orthop 92:231, 1973.

Lynn HB and Reed RC: Wringer injuries, JAMA 174:500, 1960.

MacCollum DW: Wringer arm: report of 26 cases, N Engl J Med 218:549, 1938.

McKay D et al: Infections and sloughs in the hands in drug addicts, J Bone Joint Surg 55-A:741, 1973.

Moncrief JA, Switzer WE, and Rose LR: Primary excision and grafting in the treatment of third-degree burns of the dorsum of the hand, Plast Reconstr Surg 33:305, 1964.

Moseley T and Hardman WW Jr: Treatment of wringer injuries in children, South Med J 58:1372, 1965.

Neviaser RJ et al: The puffy hand of drug addiction: a study of the pathogenesis, J Bone Joint Surg 54-A:629, 1972.

Peterson RA: Electrical burns on the hand: treatment by early excision, J Bone Joint Surg 48-A:407, 1966.

Posch JL and Weller CN: Mangle and severe wringer injuries of the hand in children, J Bone Joint Surg 36-A:57, 1954.

Poticha SM, Bell JL, and Mehn WH: Electrical injuries with special reference to the hand, Arch Surg 85:852, 1962.

Poulos E: The open treatment of wringer injuries in children, Am Surg 24:458, 1958.

Pulvertaft RG: Twenty-five years of hand surgery: personal reflections, J Bone Joint Surg 55-B:32, 1973.

Ramos H, Posch JL, and Lie KK: High-pressure injection injuries of the hand, Plast Reconstr Surg 45:221, 1970.

Robertson DC: The management of the burned hand, J Bone Joint Surg 40-A:625, 1958.

Robinson DW, Masters FW, and Forrest WJ: Electrical burns: a review and analysis of 33 cases, Surgery 57:385, 1965.

Robson MC and Heggers JP: Evaluation of hand frostbite blister fluid as a clue to pathogenesis, J Hand Surg 6:43, 1981.

Rudolph R: Ulcers of the hand and wrist caused by doxorubicin hydrochloride, Orthop Rev 7:93, 1978.

Salisbury RE and Pruitt BA: Burns of the upper extremity, Philadelphia, 1976, WB Saunders Co.

Sanguinetti MV: Reconstructive surgery of roller injuries of the hand, J Hand Surg 2:134, 1977.

Seyfer AE and Solimando DA: Toxic lesions of the hand associated with chemotherapy, J Hand Surg 8:39, 1983.

Simmons BP and Vasile RG: The clenched fist syndrome, J Hand Surg 5:420, 1980.

Smith JR and Gomez NH: Local injection therapy of neuromata of the hand with triamcinolone acetonide: a preliminary study of twenty-two patients, J Bone Joint Surg 52-A:71, 1970.

Spiegel D and Chase RA: The treatment of contractures of the hand using self-hypnosis, J Hand Surg 5:428, 1980.

Stark HH, Ashworth CR, and Boyes JH: Paint-gun injuries of the hand, J Bone Joint Surg 49-A:637, 1967.

Stark HH, Wilson JN, and Boyes JH: Grease-gun injuries of the hand, J Bone Joint Surg 43-A:485, 1961.

Tanzer RC: Grease-gun type injuries of the hand, Surg Clin North Am 43:1277, 1963.

Tubiana R: Hand reconstruction, Acta Orthop Scand 46:446, 1975.

Wakefield AR: Hand injuries in children, J Bone Joint Surg 46-A:1226, 1964.

Walker FW and Weinstein MA: Circumferential finger burn from dimethyl sulfoxide (DMSO), J Hand Surg 8:330, 1983.

Walton S: Injection gun injury of the hand with anticorrosive paint and paint solvent: a case report, Clin Orthop 74:141, 1971.

CHAPTER 68

Reconstruction After Injury

PHILLIP E. WRIGHT II*

Before attempting an elective procedure, the surgeon must ask himself if the expected improvement will justify the time, effort, and discomfort of the patient involved. When the answer is not clear, surgery should not be done. The patient's occupation, age, emotional maturity, and motivation all must be considered before deciding whether to undertake even a single procedure; should multiple operations be necessary to improve function, emotional maturity becomes even more important.

Each patient presents an individual problem. For example, for a laborer with a severely deformed little finger, amputation leaving a well-padded painless stump might be the wisest choice; multiple reconstructive procedures, although perhaps resulting in a more pleasing appearance, would cost him much more in time lost from work and might produce no better function. Conversely a young woman with a similar deformity might insist on almost any procedure other than amputation, no matter how long the hospitalization and convalescence involved.

Before any elective operation, the patient should be informed thoroughly of the surgeon's plans so that the patient knows not only what to expect from the operation, but also what is expected of him. He should be told the probable duration of hospitalization and disability, the discomfort involved, and the intended results. He should be advised specifically of his own responsibility for active exercises during convalescence. Unless the psychologic

preparation is painstaking and thorough, a misunderstanding may occur and may discourage not only the patient but also at times the surgeon. The plan not only should be thought out and talked out, it should be recorded. Photographs and movies are valuable parts of the record; drawings are useful for ready reference. When multiple procedures are being considered, such as skin replacement followed by tendon transfers or secondary nerve sutures, two separate examinations with complete notes are advised, the second examination being at least 2 weeks after the first and without reference to it; the conclusions from each examination should then be compared in detail and carefully considered. After a decision is reached, admitting the patient immediately to the hospital and proceeding with surgery the next day are unwise, even if the patient is willing. Instead operative arrangements should be made for several days later so that the patient has time to make personal arrangements, think over the plan, and adjust his thinking to it.

The surgeon, too, should have time to study the plan. He must see vividly what functions are impaired and determine why and how they are to be improved; he must know not only the surgical techniques required, but also the sequence in which they should be performed. For example, when multiple procedures are necessary to improve the function of the whole upper extremity, it is wise usually to begin with the hand, for if its function cannot be improved, the more proximal procedures may be futile. When multiple tissues require reconstruction, they must be treated in the proper order of precedence. Good *skin coverage* to reestablish the nutrition of the part

---

*Revision of chapter by Lee W. Milford, M.D.

is a prerequisite to any further reconstruction. Infection must not be present or threatening. Next, *nerves* must be intact or must be so repaired that return of sensation is expected. Then the *bony architecture* is restored; otherwise reconstruction may not be worthwhile. Finally, at least passive *joint motion* must be obtained before *tendon grafts* or *transfers* are indicated. Almost always, placing the wrist in extension and the metacarpophalangeal joints in flexion, either actively or passively, must be possible before a tendon is transferred or grafted. This sequence must be emphasized. First the hand is covered so that its nutrition is reestablished, then its sensation is restored or expected, next its bony architecture is restored, then joint motion is obtained, and finally tendons are repaired. This chapter is devoted to the indications and techniques involved.

For reconstruction after tendon, nerve, and bone injuries, see individual headings.

SKIN COVERAGE
Granulating Areas

A granulating area on the hand rarely should be left to heal with a scar. When a hand has not been covered completely with skin during the treatment of an acute injury, a split-thickness graft should be applied as soon as the surface is clean enough to support it; even when the entire granulating surface is not clean, any portion that is clean enough should be covered. Exposed tendons, joints, or cortical bone should be covered with flap grafts (p. 2989).

Scars

A scar is a poor substitute for skin; it is inelastic, and its sensation is abnormal. The absence of elasticity restricts the motion of otherwise unobstructed underlying joints, interferes with the nutrition of adjacent parts, and limits the motion of joints, tendons, and ligaments when the scar is adherent to them. A scar contracts during healing and will not stretch later. Attempts to stretch a scar may be beneficial only in that normal surrounding skin is stretched. When a linear scar is left spanning a joint, the intermittent stretching caused by active motion will cause it to hypertrophy. Forced passive stretching causes any scar to rupture and fissure, only to heal and become thicker. A scar not only lacks normal sensation, but it also may become painful when it adheres to nerve endings.

Scars cannot be entirely eliminated because the process of healing depends on the production of scar tissue. However, a scar can be replaced partially by tissue of better quality, and the direction or location of its lines can be changed so that they interfere less with function. A scar may be treated surgically (1) to eliminate deformity, (2) to restore joint motion, (3) to provide better skin coverage for vulnerable parts or to permit operation

on deeper structures such as tendons or nerves, (4) to relieve pain, and (5) occasionally to improve the appearance of the hand. Sometimes the excision of normal skin is necessary in moving the lines of the scar to a more desirable location.

When possible, a scar should not be replaced until it has matured, usually after a minimum of 3 months. However, it should be treated earlier when it severely limits joint motion; for example, when a metacarpophalangeal joint is held in extension or a proximal interphalangeal joint in flexion, the joint will develop a severe secondary contracture unless the offending scar is treated as soon as possible without awaiting its maturation.

For the purposes of treatment, scars may be classified as *linear* scars and *area* scars; either type, of course, may be volar or dorsal and may or may not involve the deep structures.

METHODS OF CORRECTING LINEAR SCARS. Disabling linear scars usually result from surgical incisions or traumatic lacerations that cross flexor creases. When such a scar on a finger is narrow and is surrounded by normal tissue (Fig. 68-1), it may be released by a Z-plasty (p. 2975), but a scar more than 2 mm wide on the volar surface is hard to correct in this way because the skin here is less mobile than that on the dorsum. In some instances the scar must be replaced by a full-thickness free graft (p. 2991), a cross finger flap (p. 2993), or a local flap (p. 2992). On the palm a linear scar may represent loss of skin substance, and in this instance a free thick split graft or a full-thickness graft is indicated (p. 2991); correcting a scar contracture here by Z-plasty is difficult. On the dorsum of the hand most disabling linear scars may be corrected by Z-plasty.

METHODS OF CORRECTING AREA SCARS. An area scar represents an initial skin loss greater than the area of the final scar, since it has contracted during healing; it must always therefore be replaced by a graft that is larger than the scar (Fig. 68-2). Since the skin for any graft should be as near like the lost skin as possible, a local flap (p. 2992) or cross finger flap (p. 2993) is preferable when only a small area is lost. When the area is large, when bare bone or tendon is left after excision of the scar, or when a reconstructive procedure is planned, a distant ("remote") flap, or vascularized free flap, containing both skin and subcutaneous fat is necessary. Deeper parts of the scar may be excised when the flap is applied, but tendons or nerves must not be repaired until later. They are then exposed through an incision along the edge of the flap and not through it.

An area scar on the dorsum of the hand involving only the skin may be replaced by a medium or a thick split graft of carefully planned size. The normal adult hand has about 5 cm extra skin longitudinally on the dorsum to allow flexion of the wrist and fingers and about 2.5 cm extra transversely to allow development of the metacarpal arch when making a fist. A graft here, then, must allow for some of this extra skin as well as for previous shrinkage of the scar and later shrinkage of the graft and must be placed while the hand is in the position of function. Otherwise it will be much too tight.

For an area scar on the palm, like skin cannot be used, since it is found only on the sole of the foot (palmar skin is made to withstand friction and shock and is more sensitive than dorsal skin). When the scar is superficial, a thick split graft can be used (Chapter 61); when deep vulnerable structures are involved, a full-thickness graft is preferable (Chapter 61), although it is harder to handle, is less likely to survive, and must be limited in size by the fact that it leaves a defect in the donor area that must be closed by suture after its edges are undermined.

For an insensitive large area scar on the radial side of an otherwise normal index finger or on the area of pinch of the thumb, a neurovascular island graft may be indicated (Chapter 65).

When a graft is applied to the hand, the rules that guide the location and direction of hand incisions (Chapter 61) must be followed carefully because the graft will heal to the normal skin with a linear scar (Fig. 68-3).

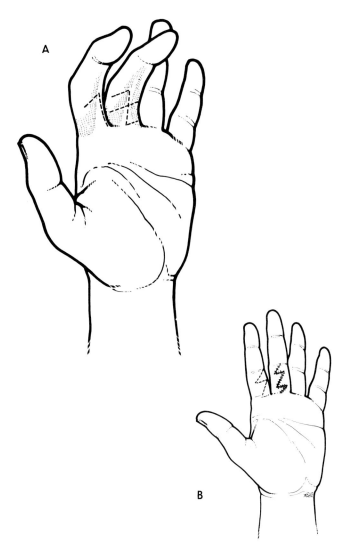

Fig. 68-1 Flexion contractures caused by linear scars may be released by Z-plasties.

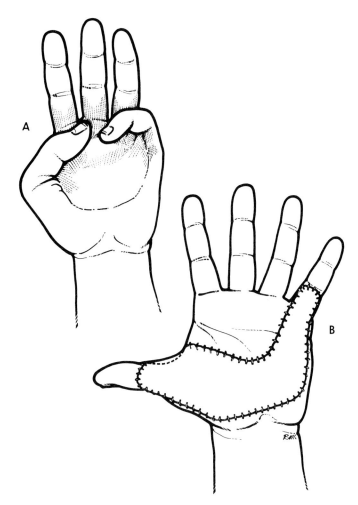

Fig. 68-3 Area scar on palm, **A,** has been replaced by graft, **B,** with margins that follow rules that guide location and direction of hand incisions.

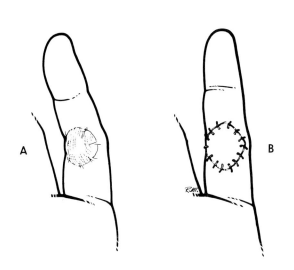

Fig. 68-2 Area scar, **A,** has been replaced by a full-thickness skin graft, **B,** which is larger than scar.

LIMITATION OF JOINT MOTION

When joint motion is limited or absent, an intelligent plan of treatment is possible only on the basis of accurate diagnosis. When there is only a single cause of limitation of motion, the diagnosis may be simple. But since a joint tends to lose motion whenever it is not actively used and since the reasons for its inactivity may be various, diagnosis of the cause of some secondary joint contractures may be complicated; the joint contracture itself may obscure the primary cause of limitation. The most frequent causes are discussed below.

Interruption of Tendons

When the continuity of a tendon is interrupted by avulsion or laceration, a specific active movement of one or more joints of the hand is lost. Passive movement in the opposite direction by the examiner will reveal complete loss of the resistance by muscle tone that is ordinarily transmitted through the tendon. The posture of the hand or fingers also may be abnormal. Some days after the injury, edema or secondary joint contracture may limit passive motion. The treatment is tendon repair or reconstruction (see Chapter 63) for basic techniques).

Adherence of Tendons

When a tendon completely adheres to bone, specific active movements of one or more joints distal to the area of adherence are lost. Specific passive movements are also limited because the adherent tendon acts as a checkrein. For example, when a profundus tendon is stuck to the shaft of the proximal phalanx, the two distal finger joints cannot be flexed actively by this tendon. However, the proximal interphalangeal joint may be actively flexed by the sublimis tendon; the metacarpophalangeal joint also may be actively flexed by the profundus and sublimis tendons along with the intrinsics. Adherence of the profundus tendon to the shaft of the proximal phalanx also checks full passive or active extension of the two distal finger joints. Active extension of the distal interphalangeal joint may be increased by passive flexion of the proximal interphalangeal joint; likewise, active extension of the proximal interphalangeal joint may be increased by passive flexion of the distal interphalangeal joint. Extension of the wrist may initiate flexion of the metacarpophalangeal joint through the adherent tendon.

Adherence of Tendon to Fracture Site

The adherence of a tendon to a fracture site is usually associated with (1) volar angulation of a phalangeal fracture after poor reduction, (2) external pressure against the tendon, forcing it against the fracture during healing, (3) crush injuries, or (4) laceration of the tendon sheath. A sublimis tendon usually adheres to the proximal phalanx, causing a flexion contracture of the proximal interphalangeal joint; a profundus tendon usually adheres to the middle phalanx, causing a flexion contracture of the distal interphalangeal joint. Although rarely involved, an extensor tendon usually adheres to the metacarpal shaft or proximal phalanx. When measurements of motion of adjacent joints demonstrate no progress in loosening the tendon by active exercise, surgery may be indicated.

■ *TECHNIQUE TO FREE ADHERENT EXTENSOR TENDON (HOWARD).* Make a longitudinal incision parallel to the lateral margin of the involved metacarpal and away from any previous scar. Free the tendon from the bone and smooth the bone with a rasp or

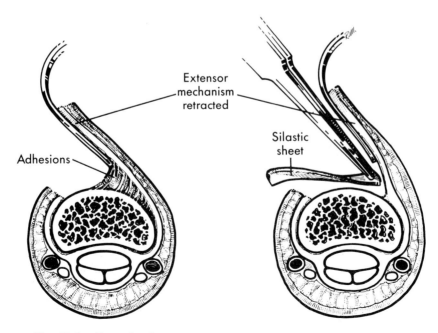

Fig. 68-4 Howard technique to free adherent extensor tendon (see text).

osteotome. Remove all scar tissue from the tendon. Place a Silastic sheet over the bone and anchor it with sutures at its corners (Fig. 68-4). Immobilize the part for 5 days and then begin voluntary motion. Improvement can be expected up to a year.

Paralysis of Muscles

Paralyzed muscles cause loss of specific active movements of joints, but passive movement usually is not limited in any direction unless the joint is secondarily contracted. The posture of the hand at rest may reveal loss of muscle tone. There will be some resistance to passive movement; however, the paralyzed muscle reveals a decrease in muscle tone. Conversely, when a tendon is severed, resistance to passive movement is absent. The treatment consists either of nerve repair or appropriate tendon transfers (see discussion of the paralytic hand, Chapter 70).

Contracture of Muscles

When muscles are contracted, as in Volkmann's ischemic contracture, active motion in the joints controlled by these muscles is limited or absent; passive motion usually is limited as well. When the finger flexors are contracted, the fingers at rest may assume a posture of flexion; passive extension is limited until a more proximal joint or joints are passively flexed. Passive flexion of the wrist may allow complete finger extension (for treatment, see Chapters 71 and 73).

Contracture of Skin

Skin contracture as a result of a scar may be an obvious cause of limitation of joint motion; when seen late, however, it may be difficult to determine whether this limitation is caused by the skin contracture, joint contracture, or both. Blanching of the skin on the extremes of passive motion is an indication of at least some skin contracture. When the contracture is on the dorsum of the hand, extension of the wrist may release the mobile skin in this area and allow an increase in passive flexion of the metacarpophalangeal joints; however, if the joints also are contracted, no increase in flexion will be gained by this maneuver. When the joint alone is contracted, the skin can be moved over the joint, at least to some extent (see Chapter 61 for methods of correcting scars).

Contracture of Joint

A joint contracture may be caused by any of the causes of limitation of motion just given, or by direct joint damage. When the limitation is produced by bone block from a malunited intraarticular fracture, motion may be equal both actively and passively but is suddenly blocked at a certain position; when the limitation is associated with ligamentous contracture, flexion is rapidly brought to a halt, but in this instance there is a springy sensation rather than a firm block. The proximal interphalangeal and metacarpophalangeal joints are more often affected by ligamentous contractures. (Correction of joint contracture by capsulotomy is discussed on p. 3193.)

Locking of Joint

The most frequent cause of locking, catching, or triggering of a finger joint (usually of the proximal interphalangeal) is stenosing tenosynovitis at the level of the proximal flexor pulley (A1) (Chapter 76). Catching or locking of the metacarpophalangeal joints may be caused by lesions other than tenosynovitis. Such lesions usually are traumatic and usually involve the fibrocartilaginous volar plate, the volar capsule, or some other structure about the metacarpophalangeal joint. The typical triggering is often absent, and flexion or extension of the joint may be firmly blocked.

The following lesions have been found responsible for locking of a metacarpophalangeal joint: (1) a tear in the volar capsule, the proximal part of which retracts and rolls up into a band caught around the metacarpal head; (2) a partial tear of the volar plate or the accessory collateral ligaments (Bruner); (3) a transverse tear of the volar plate that forms a pocket as shown in Fig. 68-5 (Yancey and Howard); (4) an osteophyte on the palmar surface of the metacarpal head that catches the fibrous cuff of the volar plate as shown in Fig. 68-6 (Goodfellow and Weaver); (5) an osteophyte on the lateral aspect of the metacarpal head that impinges on the collateral ligament as shown in Fig. 68-7 (Aston); (6) an abnormal configuration of the metacarpal head as shown in Fig. 68-8 (Flatt); (7) a large sesamoid bone that rubs against a ridge on the radial side of the palmar surface of the metacarpal head as shown in Fig. 68-9 (Flatt); (8) a trapped sesamoid and an abnormal band of tissue as shown in Fig. 68-10 (Bloom and Bryan); and (9) an irregular articular surface of the metacarpal head after an undiagnosed fracture as shown in Fig. 68-11 (Dibbell and Field).

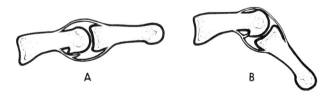

Fig. 68-5 Locking of metacarpophalangeal joint of index finger. **A,** Volar plate had been partially torn. **B,** Extension of joint was blocked when torn edge of plate became caught behind metacarpal head. Torn edge of plate and prominence of metacarpal head were excised. (Redrawn from Yancey HA Jr and Howard LD Jr: J Bone Joint Surg 44-A:380, 1962.)

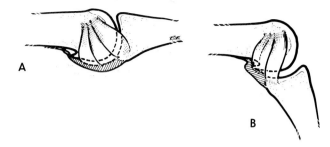

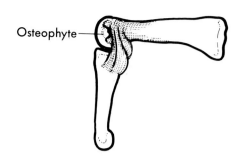

Osteophyte

Fig. 68-6 Locking of metacarpophalangeal joint of finger. **A,** Joint is extended and not locked. Note osteophyte on volar margin of metacarpal head. **B,** Osteophyte is caught in fibrous cuff of volar plate, preventing extension of joint. Treatment consisted of release over osteophyte of palmar metacarpophalangeal ligament. (Redrawn from Goodfellow JW and Weaver JPA: J Bone Joint Surg 43-B:772, 1961.)

Fig. 68-7 Locking of metacarpophalangeal joint of middle finger. Ulnar collateral ligament was caught on small osteophyte, preventing extension of joint. Treatment consisted of division of ligament. (Redrawn from Aston JN: J Bone Joint Surg 42-B:75, 1960.)

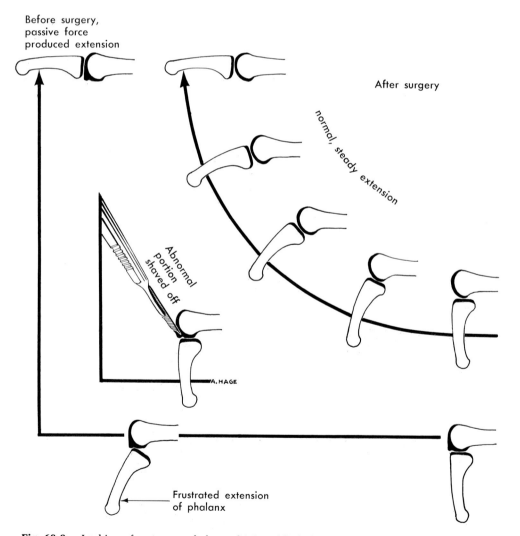

Before surgery, passive force produced extension

After surgery

normal, steady extension

Abnormal portion shaved off

Frustrated extension of phalanx

Fig. 68-8 Locking of metacarpophalangeal joint of little finger. Active extension of joint was blocked by abnormal configuration of metacarpal head. Treatment consisted of shaving off abnormal part of head. (From Flatt AE: J Bone Joint Surg 43-A:240, 1961.)

Normal   **Abnormal**

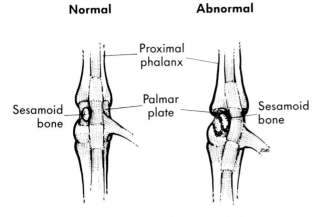

Cross sections through sesamoid bone

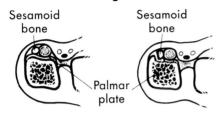

Fig. 68-9 Locking of metacarpophalangeal joint of index finger. Extension of joint was prevented by large sesamoid bone that rubbed against ridge of bone on radial side of palmar surface of metacarpal head. Tendon sheath was displaced ulnarward. Treatment consisted of excision of sesamoid and abnormal ridge of bone and repair of joint capsule. (Redrawn and modified from Flatt AE: J Bone Joint Surg 40-A:1128, 1958.)

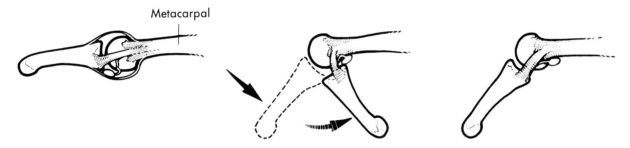

Fig. 68-10 Locking of metacarpophalangeal joint of index finger after injury. *1,* Before injury, loose abnormal band extending from sesamoid to collateral ligament caused no trouble. *2,* Direction *(arrows)* of force of injury caused abnormal flexion of joint and forced sesamoid proximal to volar margin of metacarpal head. *3,* When joint recoiled back into extension, abnormal band became tight, locking sesamoid proximal to metacarpal head and preventing full extension. Treatment consisted of excision of abnormal band and sesamoid. (Redrawn from Bloom MH and Bryan RS: J Bone Joint Surg 47-A:1383, 1965.)

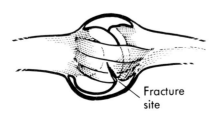

Fig. 68-11 Locking of metacarpophalangeal joint of finger caused by irregularity of metacarpal head after undiagnosed fracture. (Redrawn from Dibbell DG and Field JH: Plast Reconstr Surg 40:562, 1967.)

At the proximal interphalangeal joint other causes of triggering or catching include incomplete division of a flexor tendon, a ganglion, or other mass such as a rheumatoid nodule or giant cell tumor of the tendon sheath.

Locking or triggering of a finger joint from any cause can be corrected surgically if an accurate diagnosis is made. Release of the flexor pulley, excision of an offending osteophyte, or other surgery is then indicated.

Congenital (Infantile) Trigger Digits

Locking or triggering of a finger or thumb joint may occur in children. It usually is thought to be congenital, and may be inherited. The thumb is affected more often than the fingers. Children usually are seen at 18 to 24 months of age with inability to straighten the thumb or a finger. Attempted passive extension of the thumb causes hyperextension of the metacarpophalangeal joint, with the interphalangeal joint extending with a palpable "click." Anatomically, the inability to extend the joint usually is caused by an annular fibrous thickening in the flexor sheath, combined with a nodular enlargement of the flexor pollicis longus tendon. The report of Dinham and Meggitt of more than 130 trigger thumbs in children suggests that (1) 30% might recover between birth and 1 year of age, (2) of children presenting between 6 months and 5 years of age, about 12% might recover in another 6 months, and (3) if surgical release is done before the age of 4 years, permanent deformity is unlikely. If the interphalangeal joint is passively extensible, splinting for 3 to 4 weeks may be worthwhile. If splinting is not successful, surgical release (Chapters 74 and 76) usually relieves the problem.

Recurrent Hyperextension and Locking of Proximal Interphalangeal Joint

In this deformity the finger temporarily assumes a swan-neck posture when an attempt is made to flex it from the fully extended position. The proximal interphalangeal joint is hyperextended, the distal interphalangeal joint is flexed, and flexion of the proximal joint is impossible unless passively initiated. The lateral bands are subluxated dorsally so that they bowstring across the dorsum of the proximal interphalangeal joint, holding it extended and preventing active flexion by the flexor digitorum sublimis. The volar fibrocartilaginous plate is stretched and may even be detached, but the intrinsic muscles and joint capsule are not contracted. The deformity may be traumatic or may be caused by congenital

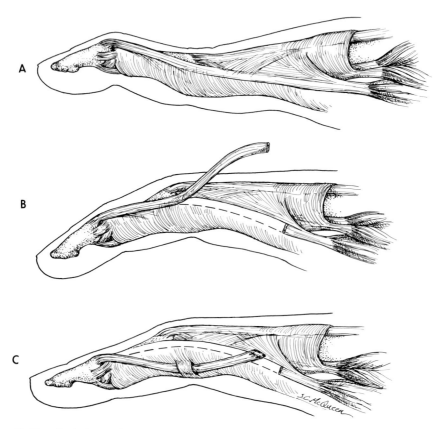

Fig. 68-12 Technique of correcting recurrent hyperextension and locking of proximal interphalangeal joint. **A,** Lateral view of extensor hood and flexor tendon sheath. **B,** One lateral band of hood has been detached proximally. **C,** Detached band has been threaded through small pulley made in flexor tendon sheath opposite proximal interphalangeal joint and has been sutured to hood under enough tension to create slight flexion contracture of joint.

hyperextensibility of joints and become worse with aging.

We have corrected the deformity and relieved the recurrent locking by transferring a lateral band of the extensor hood volarward to act as a checkrein.

■ *TECHNIQUE.* Through a curved dorsal incision centered over the proximal interphalangeal joint expose and define one lateral band of the extensor hood. Then at the junction of the proximal and middle thirds of the proximal phalanx detach the band from the extensor mechanism, leaving it attached to the distal phalanx (Fig. 68-12). Just opposite the proximal interphalangeal joint make a small pulley in the flexor tendon sheath. Then thread the detached lateral band from distal to proximal through this pulley and suture it to the extensor hood under just enough tension to create a slight flexion contracture of the joint; later the transferred lateral band will stretch and the joint will extend a few more degrees. Close the incision and apply a bulky dry dressing, incorporating a dorsal splint to avoid hyperextension.

AFTERTREATMENT. At about 2½ weeks the bandage is removed and motion is gradually begun. The repair is protected with a removable dorsal splint for about 2 more weeks. Vigorous activities are avoided for 6 to 8 weeks.

• • •

For the same deformity Curtis recommended transferring half of the flexor digitorum sublimis tendon across the volar fibrocartilaginous plate of the proximal interphalangeal joint to reinforce the plate. This gives a stronger tenodesis of the joint, such as is needed in athletes, but requires more extensive exposure about the joint.

■ *TECHNIQUE (CURTIS).* Make a midlateral incision (see Chapter 61) at the level of the proximal interphalangeal joint, incise the flexor tendon sheath, and identify the flexor tendons. Then at the proximal bifurcation of the flexor digitorum sublimis divide the ipsilateral half of the tendon (Fig. 68-13). Next, drill a hole transversely through the distal end of the proximal phalanx. Carry the freed half of the sublimis tendon deep to the flexor digitorum profundus tendon to the opposite side of the proximal phalanx, thread it through the hole in the phalanx, and anchor it with a pull-out wire suture under enough tension to cause a slight flexion contracture

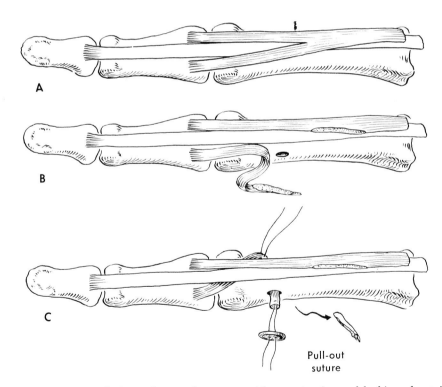

Fig. 68-13   Curtis technique of correcting recurrent hyperextension and locking of proximal interphalangeal joint. **A,** Palmar view of flexor tendons. **B,** One half of flexor digitorum sublimis tendon has been divided at bifurcation of tendon. Hole has been drilled in proximal phalanx. **C,** Freed half of tendon has been carried deep to flexor digitorum profundus tendon to opposite side of proximal phalanx, threaded through hole in bone, and anchored with pull-out suture under enough tension to cause slight flexion contracture of proximal interphalangeal joint. (From Curtis RM: In Flynn JE, editor: Hand surgery, Baltimore, 1966, The Williams & Wilkins Co.)

of the proximal interphalangeal joint. **Close the incision and splint the finger in a heavy bandage.**
AFTERTREATMENT. **At 3 weeks the bandage is removed and motion of the joint is begun.**

ARTHRODESIS

Arthrodesis of a joint of a finger or thumb may be indicated when the joint has been so damaged by injury or disease that pain, deformity, or instability makes motion a liability rather than an asset. Occasionally a joint must be arthrodesed because the muscles that control the digit are not strong enough to both stabilize and move all joints. Of the finger joints, arthrodesis is indicated most often for the proximal interphalangeal joint; it is indicated less often for the distal interphalangeal joint because sometimes stabilizing that joint by tenodesis is easier; and it is indicated least often for the metacarpophalangeal joint because motion in this joint is more valuable than in the others, and consequently when muscle power is sufficient, arthroplasty is indicated more frequently than arthrodesis. When the muscles that control the finger are weak, procedures to limit their function to the metacarpophalangeal joint are indicated. Of the joints of the thumb, arthrodesis is indicated most often for the metacarpophalangeal joint because it results in little loss of function and for the interphalangeal joint because it results in partial loss of discrete pinch only; it is indicated least often for the carpometacarpal joint because this is the most useful joint of the thumb. If the carpometacarpal joint of the thumb is to be arthrodesed, the mobility of the two distal joints should be satisfactory.

The following are the preferred positions for arthrodesis of the various joints: in the fingers, the metacarpophalangeal joints should be in flexion of 20 to 30 degrees, the proximal interphalangeal joints 40 to 50 degrees (there should be less flexion in this joint on the radial than on the ulnar side of the hand), and the distal interphalangeal joints 15 to 20 degrees; in the thumb, the interphalangeal joint should be in flexion of 20 degrees, the metacarpophalangeal joint 25 degrees, and the carpometacarpal joint with the metacarpal in opposition.

Numerous techniques for arthrodesis have been recommended, as have various methods of internal fixation, including crossed Kirschner wires, a single wire, and bone grafting techniques. Lister described a tension band wiring technique he used in 53 interphalangeal arthrodeses, with a 90.6% fusion rate. Allende and Engelem also reported good results with this technique. Büchler and Aiken reported arthrodesis of the proximal interphalangeal joint with bone grafting and plate fixation in 25 fingers with articular destruction and segmental bone loss. They used a 2 mm AO plate cut to a length that allows a minimum of two screws proximal and distal to the bone graft. All arthrodeses were successful. McGlynn, Smith, and Bogumill use one longitudinal

.035-inch or .045-inch Kirschner wire and two crossed .028-inch or .035-inch Kirscher wires for fixation, without bone grafting. They found this technique to be rapid and uncomplicated, allowing contol of the fusion position in flexion, angulation, and rotation before fixation, preserving maximal length, obtaining rapid union, and allowing early motion.

Proximal Interphalangeal Joint

■ *TECHNIQUE.* **Open the joint through either a midlateral incision (Chapter 61), a dorsal midline incision, or a dorsal incision in the form of an inverted V (see Fig. 68-15, *A*) if the extensor mechanism of the distal interphalangeal joint is destroyed. With a thin osteotome, square off the proximal end of the middle phalanx; shape the distal end of the proximal phalanx by resecting its condyles until the proper angle for arthrodesis is obtained. As an alternative, remove the articular cartilage and subchondral bone with bone-cutting instruments and a rongeur. Shape the head of the proximal phalanx into a single condyle and the base of the middle phalanx into a concave cup to allow easy changes in angulation without excessive bone removal. Do not disturb the volar cartilaginous plate; in a flexion contracture the plate may stabilize and aid in compression of the ends of the bones anteriorly as the joint is forced into extension. Stabilize the joint with parallel or crossed Kirschner wires (Fig. 68-14); be sure the bones are compressed as the wires are inserted. Use any resected bone as small grafts about the joint. Immobilize the joint with a splint until roentgenograms show solid fusion. Roentgenographic fusion may not be readily apparent for several months.**

For gross lateral instability of proximal interphalangeal joint see Chapter 64.

Distal Interphalangeal Joint

Distal interphalangeal joint arthrodesis may be performed as described for a proximal interphalangeal joint (Fig. 68-15). Herbert screw fixation of arthrodesis of the distal interphalangeal joints may prove to be an effective stabilization method.

Metacarpophalangeal Joint of Thumb

Arthrodesis of the metacarpophalangeal joint of the thumb is frequently useful in rheumatoid arthritis and is described in the discussion of the rheumatoid hand (Chapter 72).

Carpometacarpal Joint of Thumb

Arthrodesis of the carpometacarpal joint of the thumb may be indicated for degenerative arthritis after malunited Bennett's fracture, subluxation of the joint,

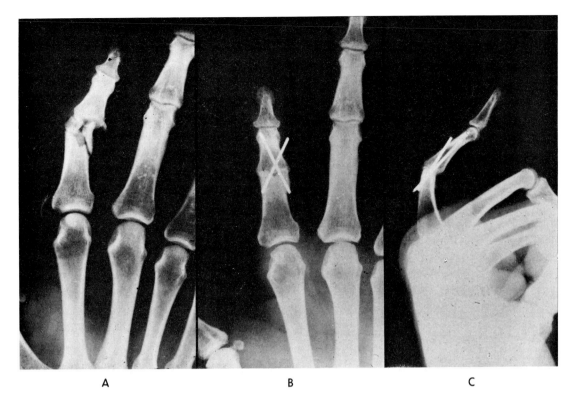

A   B   C

Fig. 68-14 Arthrodesis of proximal interphalangeal joint. **A,** Comminuted fracture involving joint. **B** and **C,** Joint has been arthrodesed. Small fragments were used as grafts, and joint was fixed with two Kirschner wires. Placing wires parallel is preferred to crossing them as shown here.

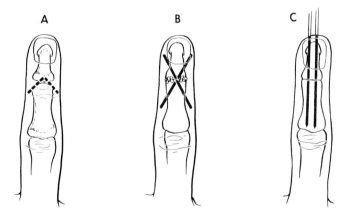

Fig. 68-15 Arthrodesis of distal interphalangeal joint. **A,** Inverted ∨ incision. **B** and **C,** Joint surfaces are resected, small chips of bone are placed about joint, and joint is fixed with two Kirschner wires, either crossed **(B)** or parallel **(C)**.

osteoarthritis, or rheumatoid arthritis. Careful consideration should be given to other causes of pain in and about the carpometacarpal area of the thumb. Signs of de Quervain's disease can be demonstrated by adduction of the thumb and ulnar deviation of the wrist (Finkelstein's test). When this maneuver produces pain, the diagnosis can be substantiated by local tenderness over the tunnel of the abductor pollicis longus and extensor pollicis brevis.

The axial compression ("grind") test, when painful, helps confirm that symptoms are mechanical and located in the carpometacarpal joint of the thumb. This test is performed by rotating the metacarpal as the joint is compressed by the metacarpal. Local tenderness is usually maximal on the radial aspect. Carpal tunnel syndrome may accompany degenerative changes at the base of the thumb joint and may worsen postoperatively; therefore careful evaluation should be made preoperatively for this cause of pain. Old fractures of the scaphoid and arthritis of adjacent joints should be ruled out by roentgenograms.

The advantages of arthrodesis versus resection arthroplasty of the joint must be considered: arthrodesis relieves pain, provides stability, and possibly increases strength; arthroplasty relieves pain, increases mobility, and probably decreases strength. Activity after resection arthroplasty usually causes sufficient pain to require protection and immobilization for several weeks after operation. When movement is started, pinch may be extremely weak and possibly painful until a buildup of heavy scar tissue takes place over several months. Activities such as opening car doors, cutting with scissors, and winding watches eventually should be possible with practice and patience but cannot be expected to be easy within the first few weeks. See Chapter 72 for discussion of resection and implant arthroplasty of this joint.

Arthrodesis requires cast immobilization for several weeks following operation with any technique; however, once fusion is accomplished, the joint is free of pain. Degenerative changes in surrounding joints do not necessarily contraindicate arthrodesis to relieve pain at the carpometacarpal joint.

Regardless of the technique used for arthrodesis of the carpometacarpal joint of the thumb, the position of the first metacarpal should be that of normal maximal abduction and opposition. This permits pulp-to-pulp pinch with the index finger and, with flexion of the thumb interphalangeal joint, with the middle finger. Extension of the thumb metacarpophalangeal joint moves the thumb to permit a full fist with unobstructed flexion of all fingers.

■ *TECHNIQUE (STARK ET AL.).* Expose the carpometacarpal joint through a curved volar incision at the base of the thumb at the level of the insertion of the abductor pollicis longus tendon, being careful to avoid the sensory branches of the superficial radial and lateral antebrachial cutaneous nerves. Divide this tendon and the origin of the opponens muscle at the base of the first metacarpal; open the joint capsule through a transverse incision. With an osteotome, bone cutting instruments, and a rongeur, remove all the articular cartilage and the subchondral cortical bone on both joint surfaces. Place the thumb as described on p. 3190 so that the index and middle finger pulps can easily reach the thumb pulp but allow sufficient room in extension to permit full finger flexion into the palm. Compress the bony surfaces in the position desired (p. 3190), and maintain this by 2 or 3 small Kirschner wires. Cannulated screws of about 4 mm also may provide satisfactory fixation. If more bony contact is needed, add an iliac bone graft. Repair the capsule and the abductor pollicis longus tendon, and suture the skin.

AFTERTREATMENT. The thumb is maintained in a thumb spica cast for 2 weeks, at which time the skin sutures are removed. The thumb spica cast is reapplied and healing is checked periodically by roentgenograms until fusion is obtained, usually at 12 weeks.

• • •

Another satisfactory method for arthrodesis of the carpometacarpal joint of the thumb consists of denuding the articular surfaces of the joint and using a bone peg for

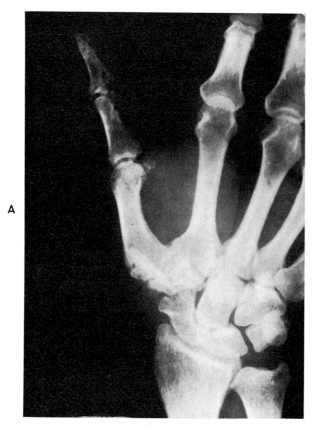
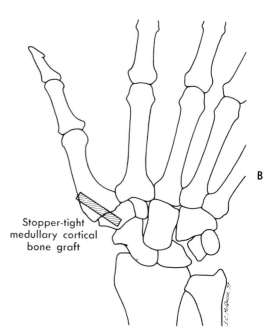

Stopper-tight
medullary cortical
bone graft

Fig. 68-16   **A,** Arthrodesis of carpometacarpal joint of thumb for osteoarthritis using square bone peg for internal fixation (see text). **B,** Drawing of roentgenogram shown in **A**. At times it is more convenient to slot graft across joint and add Kirschner wire internal fixation.

internal fixation (Fig. 68-16, *A* and *B*); thus fixation with Kirschner wires that must be removed later and the interposition of a bone graft between the osseous surfaces as required in some methods are unnecessary.

■ *TECHNIQUE.* Begin a curved incision on the dorsoradial aspect of the first metacarpal and curve it volarward at the distal wrist crease (see Fig. 64-10). Then expose the carpometacarpal joint and remove its articular cartilage. Hold the thumb in the desired position in relation to the trapezium, and starting on the base of the first metacarpal, introduce a small drill obliquely across the joint. Then check the position of both the joint and the drill by roentgenograms, remove the drill, and enlarge the hole to make it about 3 mm in diameter. Now obtain from the proximal ulna a square bone peg large enough to fit tightly in the hole (a square peg provides better fixation than a round one). Drive the peg through the hole and across the joint, taking care that its proximal end remains within the trapezium. Then place small chips of bone in any crevices about the joint and close the wound. Apply a thumb spica cast.

AFTERTREATMENT. The cast is changed as necessary but is worn until roentgenograms demonstrate osseous union, usually at 8 to 12 weeks.

ARTHROPLASTY

Of the finger joints, the metacarpophalangeal joint is treated by arthroplasty most often; the operation is indicated when traumatic, rheumatoid, or degenerative changes in the joint of an otherwise useful finger result in less than 30 degrees of motion. The muscles that control the joint must be of functional strength; otherwise the arthroplasty is of no value. Arthroplasty of the proximal interphalangeal joint is indicated only when a joint with lateral instability of 30 degrees and motion in flexion and extension of 60 degrees or more is preferable to one arthrodesed in the position of function. The two central digits are more suitable for this arthroplasty because the lateral instability is controlled somewhat by the fingers on each side. Arthroplasty of the distal interphalangeal joint of a finger and the interphalangeal joint of the thumb rarely is indicated because arthrodesis usually provides a better functioning digit.

The techniques of arthroplasty using an interpositional Silastic prosthesis for the carpometacarpal joint of the thumb and the metacarpophalangeal joints of the fingers are described in Chapter 72.

Carpometacarpal Joint of Thumb

Resecting the greater multangular may be indicated for painful degenerative arthritis of the first carpometacarpal joint or for an adduction contracture and loss of mobility of the joint caused by direct injury or contracture of the surrounding soft tissue (see discussion of the adducted thumb).

Resection of the trapezium usually is considered more strongly for a woman past middle age. If strong pinch is desired, an arthrodesis of the carpometacarpal joint should be carried out. After resection, pinch and grasp maneuvers can be accomplished with considerable force but only after several months of practice and rehabilitation. Interposition of a biological material or a Silastic prosthesis may have advantages over simple resection arthroplasty. (See p. 3324 for techniques of Burton, Stark et al., Eaton and Littler, and Swanson and Herndon); however, simple resection arthroplasty can be a satisfactory procedure. For patients older than about 70 years, Silastic arthroplasty may be the better option. For young patients, resection arthroplasty gives good stability and long-lasting results without significant functional limitations.

CAPSULOTOMY

For a stiff joint, capsulotomy is indicated more often than arthroplasty, except possibly in the rheumatoid hand. Capsulotomy may be considered for a joint in which the cartilage contours are normal and the basic cause of limited motion is contracture of the collateral ligaments from prolonged immobilization in extension. Intrinsic or long flexor muscles must be available to move the joint; otherwise, the passive motion gained by capsulotomy will be only temporary.

For capsulotomy to be successful, the surgeon must be familiar with the anatomy of the joint; otherwise the operation may result in excessive scarring and thus in further loss of motion.

Metacarpophalangeal Joint

When motion in the metacarpophalangeal joint is as much as 60 degrees, capsulotomy is contraindicated because only 60 to 70 degrees of motion usually may be expected after surgery even when the soft tissues about the joint are normal.

■ *TECHNIQUE.* Make dorsal longitudinal incisions 2.5 cm long medial and lateral to the joint. At a point 0.6 cm from the extensor tendon incise the extensor hood on the dorsolateral and dorsomedial aspects of the joint. Retract the anterior part of the extensor hood and the intrinsic tendons, expose the collateral ligaments, and excise the ligaments from each side of the joint. Now flex the joint passively, but while doing so press the proximal phalanx against the metacarpal head to keep full contact between the bones, because otherwise, if the volar plate is adherent and the pouch is obliterated, the joint will open like a book from the dorsal aspect. If the plate is adherent, strip it from the anterior part of the metacarpal head with a probe or elevator. If necessary, release the posterior part of the joint deep to the extensor hood. The same skin incision may be used to expose the extensor hood on the adjacent side of any adjacent metacarpophalangeal joint that requires capsulotomy. Close the wound with a running suture. Intraoperative injection of a long-acting local anesthetic may help reduce postoperative pain. With the joint in a little less than forced flexion, usually about 90 degrees, apply a bandage incorporating a dorsal blocking splint holding the wrist extended 15 to 20 degrees and holding the metacarpophalangeal joints in flexion.

As an alternative method, make a middorsal skin incision and split the extensor tendon longitudinally to expose the joint capsule and collateral ligaments; both ligaments may be excised through this incision. Approximate the edges of the extensor tendon with a running monofilament wire suture that is removed later by traction on an exposed end brought out through the skin. Close the skin with the same kind of suture.

AFTERTREATMENT. At 1 to 2 days active flexion exercises of the metacarpophalangeal and interphalangeal joints are started. Dynamic "knucklebender" splinting is used later to help mobilize the joint.

Proximal Interphalangeal Joint

Capsulotomy of the proximal interphalangeal joint is indicated only when the surrounding tissues are yielding, the integrity of the joint surfaces has been main-tained, and the collateral ligaments are the chief offenders. That the collateral ligaments are the cause of limited motion must be definitely established before capsulotomy is undertaken. The following is a list of causes of limited motion in this joint, as outlined by Curtis.

Flexion may be limited by the following conditions:
1. Contracture of skin on the dorsum of the finger
2. Contracture of long extensor muscle or adherence of tendon
3. Contracture of interosseus muscle or adherence of tendon
4. Contracture of capsular ligament, especially the collateral ligament
5. Bony block or exostosis

Extension may be blocked by the following conditions:
1. Scarring of skin on the volar surface of the digit
2. Contracture of the superficial fascia in the digit
3. Contracture of the flexor tendon sheath within the digit
4. Contracture of flexor muscle or adherence of tendon
5. Contracture of the volar plate of the capsular ligament
6. Adherence of the collateral ligament with the finger in the flexed position
7. Bony block or exostosis

These causes all must be considered and, except for those involving the collateral ligaments, carefully eliminated before capsulotomy.

Ideally capsulotomy is done with the patient awake and sedated so that he can move his fingers and the surgeon can observe any improvement in motion during

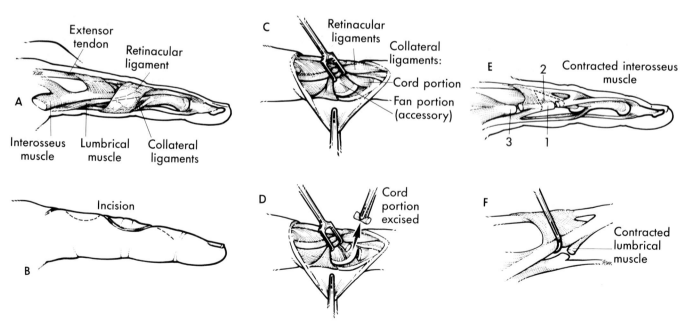

Fig. 68-17 Curtis technique for capsulotomy of proximal interphalangeal joint (see text). (From Curtis RM: Management of the stiff hand. In The practice of hand surgery, Oxford, 1981, Blackwell Scientific Publications, Inc.)

surgery. In this instance proper sedation and a regional block at the wrist or a more distal level are used. (See also discussion of anesthetics, Chapter 61.)

■ *TECHNIQUE (CURTIS).* Approach the interphalangeal joint through a midlateral incision (see Fig. 61-16) or a curved dorsal one (Fig. 68-17, *B*). On one side deepen the incision through the subcutaneous tissue to expose the tranverse retinacular ligament (Fig. 68-17, *A* and *C*). Expose the collateral ligament by approaching the joint from the base of the middle phalanx and elevating the transverse retinacular ligament; preserve this ligament for repair after capsulotomy. Starting at its distal attachment excise en bloc as much of the collateral ligament as possible (Fig. 68-17, *D*). Repeat the procedure on the opposite side of the joint.

When the contracture is of long duration, the volar synovial pouch may have been obliterated; if so, restore it with a small curved elevator or by forcing the base of the phalanx into flexion. When the interosseus muscle is contracted, lengthen its tendon by tenotomy and suture (Fig. 68-17, *E*). If necessary, free the extensor tendon over the dorsum of the finger through the same approach.

Satisfactory passive motion must be demonstrated during surgery because no further motion can be anticipated after surgery. It is also important that the flexor tendons not be adherent in the palm. This can be demonstrated by having the patient attempt to actively flex the finger. If the tendons are adherent, make a palmar incision to release them. In some situations, transarticular Kirschner wire fixation may be necessary to maintain the joint in extension.

Close the wound. Apply a dressing and palmar and dorsal splints to keep the wrist extended, the metacarpophalangeal joints flexed, and the interphalangeal joints extended.

AFTERTREATMENT. At 2 to 3 days motion is begun under supervision. The joint is splinted alternately in flexion and extension. Splinting is continued until the range of motion obtained at surgery is possible. Splinting may be necessary at least part of the time for as long as 3 or 4 months. (Also see lumbrical plus finger, Chapter 63).

• • •

At times the capsulectomy recommended by Curtis is insufficient to allow full extension of the joint. Eaton and Watson, Light, and Johnson have emphasized the importance of the "check" ligaments in maintaining persistent flexion deformities of the proximal interphalangeal joint. These are normal structures consisting of fibers from the dorsal portion of the flexor sheath and reflections of the accessory ligament inserting in the lateral margins of the volar plate. These ligaments, designated "checkreins" by Watson et al., extend from thick attachments along the

proximal edge of the volar plate, then diverge to insert separately along the volar-lateral periosteum of the proximal phalanx. These ligamentous structures may be significant in restricting proximal interphalangeal joint extension and some have recommended that their resection should be part of all middle joint releases. Careful attention to the vascular anatomy of the volar plate is necessary to avoid injury to the vascularity of the tendons.

■ *TECHNIQUE (WATSON ET AL.).* With the patient under suitable anesthesia, and with the pneumatic tourniquet inflated, approach the volar aspect of the proximal interphalangeal joint through either a midlateral or volar V-Y incision. If the flexion deformity is severe and of long standing, a longitudinal incision converted to a Z-plasty may be helpful. If a midlateral incision is selected, a second incision on the opposite side of the joint also may be required. Dissect the subcutaneous tissue, preserving the cutaneous sensory nerves. Isolate the flexor sheath and tendon, and resect portions of the flexor sheath that contribute to the flexion contracture. If possible, avoid injury to the important annular portions of the flexor sheath. Using magnification, identify

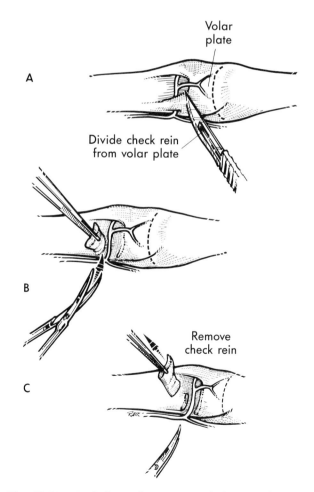

Fig. 68-18 Technique of Watson et al. for capsulotomy of proximal interphalangeal joint (see text). (Redrawn from Watson JK, Light TR, and Johnson TR: J Hand Surg 4:67, 1979.)

the vessels to the flexor tendons and retract them to avoid injury. Identify the proximal edge of the volar plate and bluntly dissect the checkreins (Fig. 68-18, *A*). Sharply excise the checkrein ligaments on either side of the volar aspect of the middle joint, taking care to avoid injury to the volar plate (Fig. 68-18, *B* and *C*). Extend the middle joint fully with a moderate amount of pressure to disrupt intraarticular adhesions and allow full passive extension. If the deformity tends to recur in a "springy" fashion, fix the joint in extension with a transarticular Kirschner wire. If pressure is excessive with the joint in full extension, avoid pinning of the joint and rely on splints for maintenance of extension of the middle joint. Obtain satisfactory hemostasis and close the wound in a routine manner. Apply a bulky dressing and splints to maintain the wrist in extension, the metacarpophalangeal joints in flexion, and the interphalangeal joints in full extension.

AFTERTREATMENT. The hand is immobilized in the bulky dressing and splint for 3 to 7 days. Then a light dressing is applied and active movement of the joint is begun. Subsequently dynamic splints are used for at least 1 hour of maximal tension while the patient is awake, with less tension throughout the night if tolerated. The sutures are removed at 12 to 14 days and special splinting is begun. Watson et al. recommend a screw-tension three-point splint with tension increased every 3 to 5 minutes and left in place overnight after the first 2 weeks. Care should be taken when using such a splint because pressure necrosis of the skin over the dorsum of the middle phalanx may occur. Night splinting is continued until full extension is obtained. Dynamic splinting may be required for as long as 4 months. At times, palmar and dorsal plaster splints may be necessary for 2 to 3 days at a time to keep the joint in full extension.

HYPEREXTENSION DEFORMITY OF METACARPOPHALANGEAL JOINT OF THUMB

Hyperextension deformity of the thumb may result from trauma, rheumatoid arthritis, or paralysis. If there is a usable joint surface with satisfactory active flexion, arthrodesis may be avoided by using the technique of Kessler, in which the extensor pollicis brevis tendon is used to tether the metacarpophalangeal joint in slight flexion. This tendon transfer reportedly does not have the disadvantage of stretching out, as may occur with the capsulorrhaphy technique.

■ *TECHNIQUE (KESSLER).* Make a 4 cm incision on each side of the metacarpophalangeal joint and slightly dorsal. Make another incision just proximal to the radial styloid to approach the extensor polli-

cis brevis tendon at its musculotendinous junction (Fig. 68-19, *A*). Sever the tendon at this point. Bring the severed segment out at the incision near the insertion of the tendon (Fig. 68-19, *B*). Thread the end of the tendon radially and volarly across the metacarpophalangeal joint obliquely and superficial to the flexor pollicis longus tendon sheath. Bring it out on

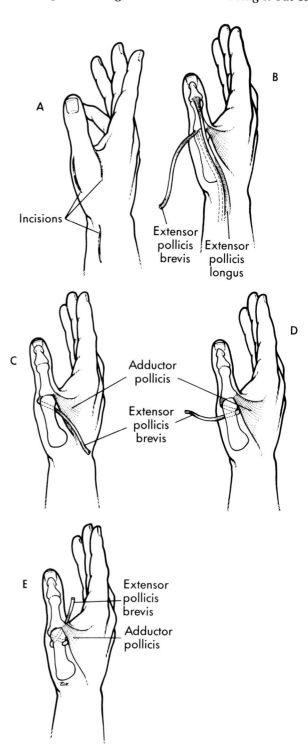

Fig. 68-19 Technique to correct hyperextension deformity of thumb at metacarpophalangeal joint. (Redrawn from Kessler I: J Bone Joint Surg 61-A:903, 1979.)

the ulnar side of the metacarpal head (Fig. 68-19, *C*). Drill a hole transversely through the neck of the metacarpal and pass the tendon through the hole to the radial side (Fig. 68-19, *D*). Place sufficient tension on the tendon to hold the metacarpophalangeal joint securely at 20 degrees of flexion. Now once again cross the tendon palmar toward the insertion of the adductor pollicis muscle. Suture it to the adductor pollicis so that the metacarpophalangeal joint is held securely in 20 degrees of flexion without permitting any further extension (Fig. 68-19, *E*). Metacarpophalangeal joint passive flexion of 30 to 40 degrees should be possible. Immobilize the thumb in a short arm-thumb spica cast for 3 weeks. A Kirschner wire also may be inserted across the metacarpophalangeal joint.

REFERENCES

Reconstruction after injury (skin coverage)

Carroll RE: Ring injuries in the hand, Clin Orthop 104:175, 1974.

Chase RA: The damaged index digit: a source of components to restore the crippled hand, J Bone Joint Surg 50-A:1152, 1968.

Chase RA: The severely injured upper limb: to amputate or reconstruct: that is the question, Arch Surg 100:382, 1970.

Chase RA: Early salvage in acute hand injuries with a primary island flap, Plast Reconstr Surg 48:521, 1971.

Chase RA and Nagel DA: Cosmetic incisions and skin, bone, and composite grafts to restore function of the hand, AAOS Instr Course Lect 23:96, 1974.

Chase RA, Hentz VR, and Apefelberg D: A dynamic myocutaneous flap for hand reconstruction, J Hand Surg 5:594, 1980.

Dabezies EJ: An advancement pedicle flap for the late coverage of pulp injuries of the digits, South Med J 67:340, 1974.

Dowden RV and McCraw JB: Muscle flap reconstruction of shoulder defects, J Hand Surg 5:382, 1980.

Eversmann WW, Burkhalter WE, and Dunn C: Transfer of the long flexor tendon of the index finger to the proximal phalanx of the long finger during index-ray amputation, J Bone Joint Surg 53-A:769, 1971.

Foucher G and Braun JB: A new island flap transfer from the dorsum of the index to the thumb, Plast Reconstr Surg 63:344, 1979.

Frackelton WH and Teasley JL: Neurovascular island pedicle-extension in usage, J Bone Joint Surg 44-A:1069, 1962.

Glanz S: Repair of contractures of the hand with pedal full-thickness skin grafts, Am J Surg 100:412, 1960.

Graham WP III: Incisions, amputations, and skin grafting in the hand, Orthop Clin North Am 2:213, 1970.

Green DP and Dominguez OJ: A transpositional skin flap for release of volar contractures of a finger at the metacarpophalangeal joint, Plast Reconstr Surg 64:516, 1979.

Hanna DC: Resurfacing the hand in acute injuries, Surg Clin North Am 40:331, 1960.

Houghland RG: Secondary index finger amputations to improve function and dexterity, Orthop Rev 4:52, July 1975.

Hurwitz DJ and White WL: Application of glove designs in resurfacing the dorsum of the hand, Plast Reconstr Surg 62:385, 1978.

Johnson RK and Iverson RE: Cross-finger pedicle flaps in the hand, J Bone Joint Surg 53-A:913, 1971.

Joshi BB: Sensory flaps for the degloved mutilated hand, Hand 6:247, 1974.

Kleinman WB and Dustman JA: Preservation of function following complete degloving injuries to the hand: use of simultaneous groin flap and partial-thickness skin graft, J Hand Surg 6:82, 1981.

Lewin ML: Digital flaps in reconstructive and traumatic surgery, Clin Orthop 15:74, 1959.

Lie KK and Posch JL: Island flap innervated by radial nerve for restoration of sensation in an index stump: case report, Plast Reconstr Surg 47:386, 1971.

Littler JW: Neurovascular skin island transfer in reconstructive hand surgery, Trans Int Soc Plast Surg 2:175, 1960.

MacDougal B, Wray RC Jr, and Weeks PM: Lateral-volar finger flap for the treatment of burn syndactyly, Plast Reconstr Surg 57:167, 1976.

Macht SD and Watson HK: The Moberg volar advancement flap for digital reconstruction, J Hand Surg 5:372, 1980.

Maquieira NO: An innervated full-thickness skin graft to restore sensibility to fingertips and heels, Plast Reconstr Surg 53:568, 1974.

May H: Plastic repair of skin defects of the hand, Clin Orthop 15:86, 1959.

May JW Jr and Barlett SP: Staged groin flap in reconstruction of the pediatric hand, J Hand Surg 6:163, 1981.

May JW Jr and Gordon L: Palm of hand free flap for forearm length preservation in nonreplantable forearm amputation: a case report, J Hand Surg 5:377, 1980.

McDonald J and Webster JP: Early covering of extensive traumatic deformities of the hand and foot, Plast Reconstr Surg 1:49, 1946.

McFarlane R and Stromberg WB: Resurfacing of the thumb following major skin loss, J Bone Joint Surg 44-A:1365, 1962.

McGarth MH, Adelbert D, and Finseth F: The intravenous fluorescein test: use in timing of groin flap division, J Hand Surg 4:19, 1979.

McGregor IA: Flap reconstruction in hand surgery: the evolution of presently used methods, J Hand Surg 4:1, 1979.

Miura T and Nakamura R: Use of paired flaps to simultaneously cover the dorsal and volar surfaces of a raw hand, Plast Reconstr Surg 54:286, 1974.

Murray JF, Ord JVR, and Gavelin GE: The neurovascular island pedicle flap: an assessment of late results in sixteen cases, J Bone Joint Surg 49-A:1285, 1967.

Pho RWH: Local composite neurovascular island flap for skin cover in pulp loss of the thumb, J Hand Surg 4:11, 1979.

Pohl AL, Larson DL, and Lewis SR: Thumb reconstruction in the severely burned hand, Plast Reconstr Surg 57:320, 1976.

Posner MA and Smith RJ: The advancement pedicle flap for thumb injuries, J Bone Joint Surg 53-A:1618, 1971.

Rose EH and Buncke HJ: Free transfer of a large sensory flap from the first web space and dorsum of the foot including the second toe for reconstruction of a mutilated hand, J Hand Surg 6:196, 1981.

Salisbury RE, McKeel DW, and Mason AD Jr: Ischemic necrosis of the intrinsic muscles of the hand after thermal injuries, J Bone Joint Surg 56-A:1701, 1974.

Schlenker JD: Transfer of a neurovascular island pedical flap based upon the metacarpal artery: a case report, J Hand Surg 4:16, 1979.

Scott JE: Amputation of the finger, Br J Surg 61:574, 1974.

Shaw DT et al: Interdigital butterfly flap in the hand (double-opposing Z-plasty), J Bone Joint Surg 55-A:1677, 1973.

Smith RC and Furnas DW: The hand sandwich: adjacent flaps from opposing body surfaces, Plast Reconstr Surg 57:351, 1976.

Thompson RVS: Closure of skin defects near the proximal interphalangeal joint — with special reference to the patterns of finger circulation, Plast Reconstr Surg 59:77, 1977.

Tubiana R and DuParc J: Restoration of sensibility in the hand by neurovascular skin island transfer, J Bone Joint Surg 43-B:474, 1961.

White WL: Flap grafts to the upper extremity, Surg Clin North Am 40:389, 1960.

Yoshimura M, Shimada T, Imura S, et al: The venous skin graft method for repairing skin defects of the fingers, Plast Reconstr Surg 80:243, 1987.

Reconstruction after injury (bone and joint)

Adams JP: Correction of chronic dorsal subluxation of the proximal interphalangeal joint by means of a criss-cross volar graft, J Bone Joint Surg 41-A:111, 1959.

Alldred A: A locked index finger, J Bone Joint Surg 36-B:102, 1954.

Alldred AJ: Rupture of the collateral ligament of the metacarpophalangeal joint of the thumb, J Bone Joint Surg 37-B:443, 1955.

Allende BT and Engelem JC: Tension-band arthrodesis in the finger joints, J Hand Surg 5:269, 1980.

Aston JN: Locked middle finger, J Bone Joint Surg 42-B:75, 1960.

Blair WF, Percival KJ, and Morecraft R: Distribution pattern of the deep branch of the ulnar nerve in the hypothenar eminence, Clin Orthop 229:194, 1988

Bloom MH and Bryan RS: Locked index finger caused by hyperflexion and entrapment of sesamoid bone, J Bone Joint Surg 47-A:1383, 1965.

Braun RM: Trephine techniques for small bone grafts, Hand 6:103, 1974.

Bruner JM: Use of single iliac-bone graft to replace multiple metacarpal loss in dorsal injuries of the hand, J Bone Joint Surg 39-A:43, 1957.

Bruner JM: Recurrent locking of the index finger due to internal derangement of the metacarpophalangeal joint, J Bone Joint Surg 43-A:450, 1961.

Buch VI: Clinical and functional assessment of the hand after metacarpophalangeal capsulotomy, Plast Reconstr Surg 53:452, 1974.

Büchler U and Aiken MA: Arthrodesis of the proximal interphalangeal joint by solid bone grafting and plate fixation in extensive injuries to the dorsal aspect of the finger, J Hand Surg 13-A:589, 1988.

Burton RI: Basal joint arthrosis of the thumb, Orthop Clin North Am 4:331, 1973.

Campbell CS: Gamekeeper's thumb, J Bone Joint Surg 37-B:148, 1955.

Camp RA and Callahan MJ: Ball-and-socket interphalangeal joint arthrodesis, Techniques Orthopaed 1:10, 1986.

Carroll RE and Hill NA: Arthrodesis of the carpo-metacarpal joint of the thumb, J Bone Joint Surg 55-B:292, 1973.

Carroll RE and Taber TH: Digital arthroplasty of the proximal interphalangeal joint, J Bone Joint Surg 36-A:912, 1954.

Coonrad RW and Goldner JL: A study of the pathological findings and treatment in soft-tissue injury of the thumb metacarpophalangeal joint: with a clinical study of the normal range of motion in one thousand thumbs and a study of post mortem findings of ligamentous structures in relation to function, J Bone Joint Surg 50-A:439, 1968.

Curtis RM: Capsulectomy of the interphalangeal joints of the fingers, J Bone Joint Surg 36-A:1219, 1954.

Curtis RM: Joints of the hand. In Flynn JE, editor: Hand surgery, Baltimore, 1966, The Williams & Wilkins Co.

Curtis RM: Management of the stiff hand. In The practice of hand surgery, Oxford, 1981, Blackwell Scientific Publications, Inc.

Dibbell DG and Field JH: Locking metacarpal phalangeal joint, Plast Reconstr Surg 40:562, 1967.

Dinham JM and Meggitt BF: Trigger thumbs in children, J Bone Joint Surg 56-B:153, 1974.

Eaton RG and Littler JW: A study of the basal joint of the thumb: treatment of its disability by fusion, J Bone Joint Surg 51-A:661, 1969.

Eaton RG and Littler JW: Ligament reconstruction for the painful thumb carpometacarpal joint, J Bone Joint Surg 55-A:1655, 1973.

Flatt AE: Recurrent locking of an index finger, J Bone Joint Surg 40-A:1128, 1958.

Flatt AE: A locking little finger, J Bone Joint Surg 43-A:240, 1961.

Fowler SB: Mobilization of metacarpophalangeal joint, J Bone Joint Surg 29:193, 1947.

Frank WE and Dobyns J: Surgical pathology of collateral ligamentous injuries of the thumb, Clin Orthop 83:102, 1972.

Froimson AI: Tendon arthroplasty of the trapeziometacarpal joint, Clin Orthop 70:191, 1970.

Gervis WH: Excision of the trapezium for osteoarthritis of the trapezio-metacarpal joint, J Bone Joint Surg 31-B:537, 1949.

Gervis WH: A review of excision of the trapezium for osteoarthritis of the trapezio-metacarpal joint after twenty-five years, J Bone Joint Surg 55-B:56, 1973.

Goldner JL and Clippinger FW: Excision of the greater multangular bone as an adjunct to mobilization of the thumb, J Bone Joint Surg 41-A:609, 1959.

Goodfellow JW and Weaver JP: Locking of the metacarpophalangeal joints, J Bone Joint Surg 43-B:772, 1961.

Gould JS and Nicholson BG: Capsulectomy of the metacarpophalangeal and proximal interphalangeal joints, J Hand Surg 4:482, 1979.

Graham WC and Riordan DC: Reconstruction of a metacarpophalangeal joint with a metatarsal transplant, J Bone Joint Surg 30-A:848, 1948.

Haraldsson S: Extirpation of the trapezium for osteoarthritis of the first carpometacarpal joint, Acta Orthop Scand 43:347, 1972.

Harrison SH: The Harrison-Nicolle intramedullary peg: follow-up study of 100 cases, Hand 6:304, 1974.

Howard LD Jr: Locking proximal finger joint (2 cases), Spectator Correspondence Club Letter, 1961 (mimeographed).

Huffaker WH, Wray RC Jr, and Weeks PM: Factors influencing final range of motion in the fingers after fractures of the hand, Plast Reconstr Surg 63:82, 1979.

Kessler I: Complete avulsion of the ulnar collateral ligament of the metacarpophalangeal joint of the thumb, Clin Orthop 29:196, 1963.

Kessler I: Silicone arthroplasty of the trapezio-metacarpal joint, J Bone Joint Surg 55-B:285, 1973.

Kessler I: A simplified technique to correct hyperextension deformity of the metacarpophalangeal joint of the thumb, J Bone Joint Surg 61-A:903, 1979.

Kleinert HE and Kasdan ML: Reconstruction of chronically subluxated proximal interphalangeal finger joint, J Bone Joint Surg 47-A:958, 1965.

Kowalski MF and Manske PR: Arthrodesis of digital joints in children, J Hand Surg 13-A:874, 1988.

Lasserre C, Pauzat D, and Derennes R: Osteoarthritis of the trapezio-metacarpal joint, J Bone Joint Surg 31-B:534, 1949.

Leach RE and Bolton PE: Arthritis of the carpometacarpal joint of the thumb: results of arthrodesis, J Bone Joint Surg 50-A:1171, 1968.

Lee BS: Degenerative arthritis of the carpometacarpal joint of the thumb, Orthop Rev 2:45, April 1973.

Light TR: Salvage of intraarticular malunions of the hand and wrist: the role of realignment osteotomy, Clin Orthop 214:130, 1987.

Lister G: Intraosseous wiring of the digital skeleton, J Hand Surg 3:427, 1978.

Mack GR, Lichtman DM, and MacDonald RI: Fibular autografts for distal defects of the radius, J Hand Surg 4:576, 1979.

Massengill JB et al: Mechanical analysis of Kirschner wire fixation in a phalangeal model, J Hand Surg 4:351, 1979.

McGarth MH and Watson HK: Late results with local bone graft donor sites in hand surgery, J Hand Surg 6:234, 1981.

McGlynn JT, Smith RA, and Bogumill GP: Arthrodesis of small joint of the hand: a rapid and effective technique, J Hand Surg 13-A:595, 1988.

Moberg E: Arthrodesis of finger joints, Surg Clin North Am 40:465, 1960.

Moberg E: Biological problems in the evolution of hand prostheses, Orthop Clin North Am 4:1161, 1973.

Moberg E and Henrikson B: Technique for digital arthrodesis: a study of 150 cases, Acta Chir Scand 118:331, 1960.

Moberg E and Stener B: Injuries to the ligaments of the thumb and fingers: diagnosis, treatment, and prognosis, Acta Chir Scand 106:166, 1953.

Morris HD: Tendon and mortise grafts for bridging metacarpal defects due to gunshot wounds, Surgery 20:364, 1946.

Müller GM: Arthrodesis of the trapezio-metacarpal joint for osteoarthritis, J Bone Joint Surg 31-B:540, 1949.

Murley AH: Excision of the trapezium in osteoarthritis of the first carpo-metacarpal joint, J Bone Joint Surg 42-B:502, 1960.

Murray RA: The injured or abnormal thumb: recommendations for treatment, South Med J 52:845, 1959.

Palmer AK and Louis DS: Assessing ulnar instability of the metacarpophalangeal joint of the thumb, J Hand Surg 3:542, 1978.

Peacock EE Jr: Reconstructive surgery of hands with injured central metacarpophalangeal joints, J Bone Joint Surg 38-A:291, 1956.

Potenza AD: A technique for arthrodesis of finger joints, J Bone Joint Surg 55-A:1534, 1973.

Pratt DR: Exposing fractures of the proximal phalanx of the finger longitudinally through the dorsal extensor apparatus, Clin Orthop 15:22, 1959.

Redler I and Williams JT: Rupture of a collateral ligament of the proximal interphalangeal joint of the fingers: analysis of eighteen cases, J Bone Joint Surg 49-A:322, 1967.

Sakellarides HT and DeWeese JW: Instability of the metacarpophalangeal joint of the thumb: reconstruction of the collateral ligaments using the extensor pollicis brevis tendon, J Bone Joint Surg 58-A:106, 1976.

Sims CD and Bentley G: Carpometacarpal osteo-arthritis of the thumb, Br J Surg 57:442, 1970.

Slocum DB: Stabilization of the articulation of the greater multangular and the first metacarpal, J Bone Joint Surg 25:626, 1943.

Smillie IS: Intermetacarpal fusion, J Bone Joint Surg 35-B:256, 1953.

Souter WA: The boutonnière deformity: a review of 101 patients with division of the central slip of the extensor expansion of the fingers, J Bone Joint Surg 49-B:710, 1967.

Stark HH et al: Fusion of the first metacarpotrapezial joint for degenerative arthritis, J Bone Joint Surg 59-A:22, 1977.

Swanson AB and Herndon JH: Flexible (silicone) implant arthroplasty of the metacarpophalangeal joint of the thumb, J Bone Joint Surg 59-A:362, 1977.

Trumble TE and Friedlaender GE: Use of allogenic bone in hand injuries, Techniques Orthopaed 1:79, 1986.

Trumble TE and Friedlaender GE: Allogenic bone in the treatment of tumors, trauma, and congenital anomalies of the hand, Orthop Clin North Am 18:301, 1987.

Turkell JH: Tenodesis as adjunct to fixation in fusion of interphalangeal joints, Bull Hosp Joint Dis 20:103, 1959.

Watson HK and Shaffer SR: Concave-convex arthrodeses in joints of the hand, Plast Reconstr Surg 46:368, 1970.

Watson HK, Light TR, and Johnson TR: Checkrein resection for flexion contracture of the middle joint, J Hand Surg 4:67, 1979.

Weckesser EC: Rotational osteotomy of the metacarpal for overlapping fingers, J Bone Joint Surg 47-A:751, 1965.

Weeks PM: The chronic boutonnière deformity: a method of repair, Plast Reconstr Surg 40:248, 1967.

Weeks PM, Wray RC Jr, and Kuxhaus M: The results of nonoperative management of stiff joints in the hand, Plast Reconstr Surg 61:58, 1978.

Wilson JN: Basal osteotomy of the first metacarpal in the treatment of arthritis of the carpometacarpal joint of the thumb, Br J Surg 60:854, 1973.

Wisnicki JL, Leathers MW, Sangalang I, and Kilgore ES Jr: Percutaneous desmotomy of digits for stiffness from fixed edema, Plast Reconstr Surg 80:88, 1987.

Yancey HA Jr and Howard LD Jr: Locking of the metacarpophalangeal joint, J Bone Joint Surg 44-A:380, 1962.

Young VL, Wray RC Jr, and Weeks PM: The surgical management of stiff joints in the hand, Plast Reconstr Surg 62:835, 1978.

Amputations

LEE W. MILFORD
MARK T. JOBE

In selected instances acute traumatic amputations may be treated primarily by vascular reanastomoses using microsurgical techniques. For these techniques and their indications, see Chapter 49.

Surgical amputation through the fingers or metacarpals is a salvage procedure (Fig. 69-1). Its object is to preserve as much function as possible in injured and uninjured parts of the hand while shortening the time required for healing, decreasing the permanent disability, and preventing continual pain; as permitted in the given instance, every effort is made to maintain the length of the osseous structures, the mobility of the joints, and the sensibility of the skin. In amputations of several digits, pinch and grasp are the chief functions to be preserved (Figs. 69-2 and 69-3).

CONSIDERATIONS FOR AMPUTATION

The only absolute indication for a primary amputation is an irreversible loss of blood supply to the part. In the absence of such an indication some other factors must be considered in deciding whether amputation is advisable.

1. The ultimate function of the part should be good enough to warrant the time and effort required of the patient if it is not amputated.
2. One should be more hesitant in amputating a finger when other fingers are also injured; immediate amputation for the same injuries might be preferred if the other fingers were normal.

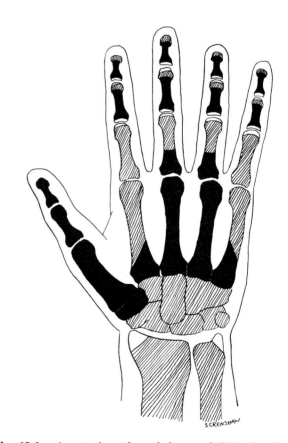

Fig. 69-1 Amputations through bones of digits, hand, and wrist. *Black parts* are most important to preserve, *oblique lines* indicate less important parts, and *white areas* are troublesome and should be amputated.

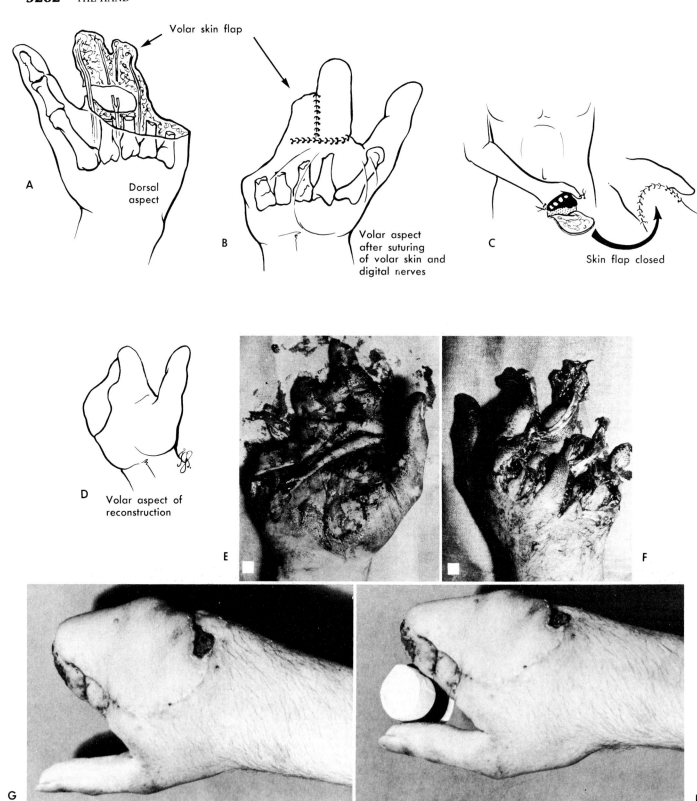

Fig. 69-2 Use of skin supported by neurovascular bundles. **A,** Dorsum of hand amputated through four ulnar metacarpals. Part of volar skin of index and middle fingers remains, is partially detached, but is viable. **B,** Volar surface after repair of severed nerves and suture of skin. **C,** Application of abdominal flap to dorsum of hand. **D,** Volar surface after application of abdominal flap. **E** and **F,** Volar and dorsal aspects of same hand soon after injury. **G** and **H,** Hand after reconstruction. Sensibility is normal in skin preserved from index finger. Bone graft to remnant of third metacarpal has provided stability for pinch and grasp. (From Entin MA: Surg Clin North Am 48:1063, 1968.)

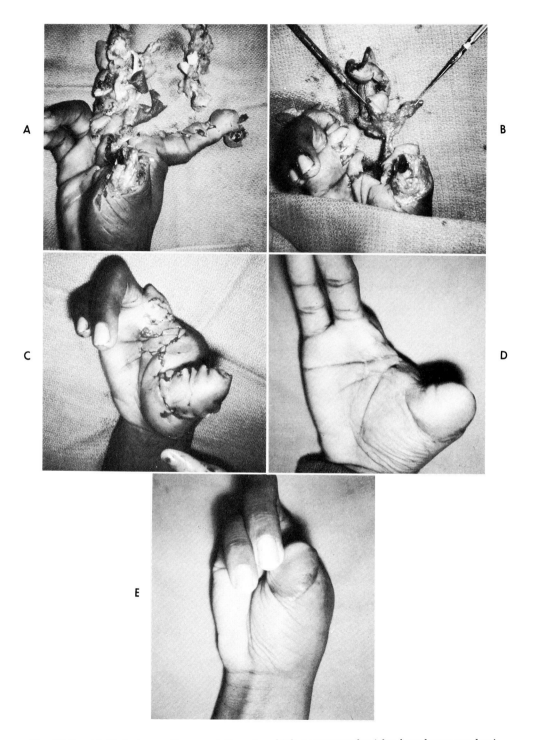

Fig. 69-3 Multiple traumatic amputations in which neurovascular island graft was used primarily. **A,** Thumb was partially amputated, including its entire area of pinch and grasp. Index and middle fingers were damaged beyond repair. **B,** Index and middle fingers were amputated, but skin of radial side of index finger and its intact neurovascular bundle were salvaged. **C,** Neurovascular island graft was sutured on thumb, providing not only immediate coverage but also sensibility. **D** and **E,** Function after healing without additional operations.

3. An analysis of the five tissue areas (skin, tendon, nerve, bone, and joint) is sometimes helpful in making the decision to amputate. When three or more of these five areas require special procedures such as grafting of skin, suture of tendon or nerve, alignment of bone, or closure of joint, then amputation should be strongly considered. In children, amputation is rarely indicated unless the part is nonviable and cannot be made viable by vascular anastomosis; however, in persons over 50 years of age, amputation of a single digit, except the thumb, may be indicated when both digital nerves and both flexor tendons are severed.

4. Even when amputation is indicated, it may be wise to delay it if parts of the finger may be useful later in a reconstructive procedure. Skin from an otherwise useless digit may be employed as a free graft. Skin and deeper soft structures may be useful as a filleted graft (p. 3000); if desired, the bone may be removed primarily and the remaining flap suitably fashioned during a secondary procedure. Skin well supported by one or more neurovascular bundles but not by bone may be saved and used as a neurovascular island graft (Chapter 65). Segments of nerves may be useful as autogenous grafts. A musculotendinous unit, especially a flexor digitorum sublimis or an extensor indicis proprius, may be saved for transfer to improve function in a surviving digit, as for example, to improve adductor power of the thumb when the third metacarpal shaft has been destroyed or to improve abduction when the recurrent branch of the median nerve has been destroyed. Tendons of the flexor digitorum sublimis of the fifth finger, the extensor digiti quinti, and the extensor indicis proprius may be useful as free grafts. Bones may be used as peg grafts or for filling osseous defects. Under certain circumstances even joints may be useful.

5. Every effort, of course, should be made to salvage the thumb.

PRINCIPLES OF AMPUTATION OF FINGERS

Whether an amputation is carried out primarily or secondarily, certain principles must be observed to obtain a painless and useful stump. The volar skin flap should be semicircular at its end and, to assure adequate coverage, almost as long as a phalanx; it must be long enough to cover the volar surface and tip of the stump and to join the dorsal flap slightly dorsally. The ends of the digital nerves should be dissected carefully from the volar flap and resected at least 6 mm proximal to its end; during this resection tension on the nerves should not be sufficient to rupture axons more proximally, since this might cause discomfort later. Neuromas at the nerve ends are inevitable but they should be allowed to develop only in

padded areas where they are less likely to be painful. The digital arteries should be cauterized. When scarring or a skin defect makes the fashioning of a classic flap impossible, one of a different shape may be improvised, but the end of the bone must be padded well. Flexor and extensor tendons should be drawn distally, divided, and allowed to retract proximally. When an amputation is through a joint, the flares of the osseous condyles should be resected to avoid clubbing of the stump. Before the wound is closed, the tourniquet should be released and any bleeding controlled because fingers are quite vascular and any hematoma is painful and delays healing. The flaps should be stitched together with small interrupted sutures; little consideration should be given to "dog-ears" at each end of the suture line because they tend to disappear and because excising them requires narrowing the base of the volar flap, which might endanger its blood supply.

The principles of handling tissues are described in the section on open hand injuries (Chapter 62).

AMPUTATIONS OF FINGERTIP

Amputations of the fingertips vary markedly depending on the amount of skin lost, the depth of the soft tissue defect, and whether the phalanx has been exposed or even partially amputated (Fig. 69-4). Proper treatment is determined by the exact type of injury and whether other digits also have been injured.

When skin alone has been lost, only it requires replacement and this is accomplished by a free graft. However, when the soft tissue defect is deep and the phalanx is exposed, deeper tissues as well as skin must be replaced. Several methods of coverage are available as follows. *Reamputation* of the finger at a more proximal level provides ample skin and other soft tissues for closure but requires shortening the finger. It may be indicated, however, when other parts of the hand are severely injured or when the entire hand would be endangered by keeping a finger in one position for a long time, as is required for a flap; this is especially true for patients with arthritis or for those over 50 years of age. For small children reamputation is not indicated because in them nature will cover the exposed bone in a remarkably short time even if the surgeon does not. A *free skin graft* may be used for coverage but normal sensibility never is restored. A split-thickness graft often is sufficient when the bone is only slightly exposed and its end is nibbled off beneath the fat. Such a graft contracts during healing and eventually becomes about half its original size. Sometimes a full-thickness graft is available from other injured parts of the hand but the fat should be removed from its deep surface. Occasionally the amputated part of the fingertip is recovered and replacing it as a free graft is tempting; although it usually survives in children, it rarely does so in adults. The medial aspect of the arm

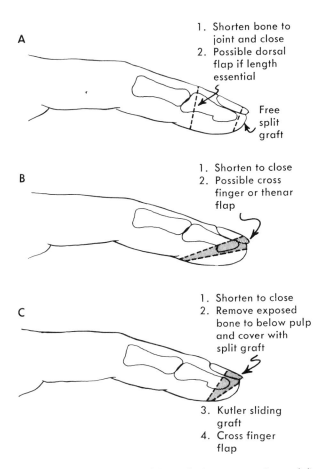

A
1. Shorten bone to joint and close
2. Possible dorsal flap if length essential

Free split graft

B
1. Shorten to close
2. Possible cross finger or thenar flap

C
1. Shorten to close
2. Remove exposed bone to below pulp and cover with split graft
3. Kutler sliding graft
4. Cross finger flap

Fig. 69-4 Techniques useful in closing amputations of fingertip. **A,** For amputations at more distal level, free split graft is applied; at more proximal level, bone is shortened to permit closure or, if length is essential, dorsal flap may be used. **B,** For amputations through *stippled area,* bone may be shortened to permit closure or cross finger or thenar flap may be used. **C,** For amputations through *stippled area,* bone may be shortened to permit closure, exposed bone may be resected and split-thickness graft applied, Kutler advancement flaps may be used, or cross finger flap may be applied. In small children, fingertip will heal without a graft nearly as fast as with a graft.

just inferior to the axilla is a convenient area from which to obtain a small full-thickness graft. Any free graft always should be secured by a stent dressing tied over the end of the finger.

When deeper tissues as well as skin must be replaced to cover exposed bone, one of several different flaps or grafts may be used. The *Kutler V-Y* or *Atasoy triangular advancement flaps* involve the injured finger alone but provide no additional skin and sometimes impair sensibility. The *bipedicle dorsal flap* is useless unless the finger has been amputated proximal to the nail bed. However, when further shortening is unacceptable, this type of flap can be raised from the dorsum of the injured finger and carried distally without involving another digit. The *cross finger flap* provides excellent coverage but may be followed by stiffness not only of the involved finger

but of the donor finger as well. This type of coverage requires operation in two stages and a split-thickness graft to cover the donor site. The *thenar flap* also requires operation in two stages. Furthermore, it usually will not cover as large a defect as will a cross finger flap and it sometimes is followed by tenderness of the donor site. It does, however, have the advantage of involving only one finger directly. A *local neurovascular island graft* shifted distally seems ideal in that a good pad with normal sensibility is provided. However, obtaining the desired result requires an experienced surgeon using almost perfect technique. A *flap from a distant area* such as the abdomen or subpectoral region should be avoided because of all the procedures mentioned, it provides the poorest coverage and is followed by the most complications. Such flaps usually are too thick and are unstable, hyperpigmented, and hypersensitive.

Reamputation of Fingertip

The technique of reamputation follows the same principles as described for amputation of a finger (see above).

Free Skin Graft

The techniques of applying free skin grafts are described on pp. 2992 to 2993.

Kutler V-Y or Atasoy Triangular Advancement Flaps

This type of fingertip coverage is appealing because it involves the injured finger alone. However, it provides only limited coverage and does not result consistently in normal sensibility.

■ *TECHNIQUE (KUTLER; FISHER).* Anesthetize the finger by digital block at the proximal phalanx and apply a rubber catheter as a tourniquet. Debride the tip of the finger of uneven edges of soft tissue and any protruding bone (Fig. 69-5). Then develop two triangular flaps, one on each side of the finger with the apex of each directed proximally and centered in the midlateral line of the digit. Avoid making the flaps too large; their sides should each measure about 6 mm and their bases about the same or slightly less. Develop the flaps farther by incising deeper toward the nail bed and volar pulp. Take care not to pinch the flaps with thumb forceps or hemostats. Rather, near the base of each insert a skin hook and apply slight traction in a distal direction. Now with a pair of small scissors and at each apex divide the pulp just enough (usually not more than half its thickness) to allow the flaps to be mobilized toward the tip of the finger. Avoid dividing any pulp distally. Round off the sharp corners of the remaining part of the distal phalanx and reshape its

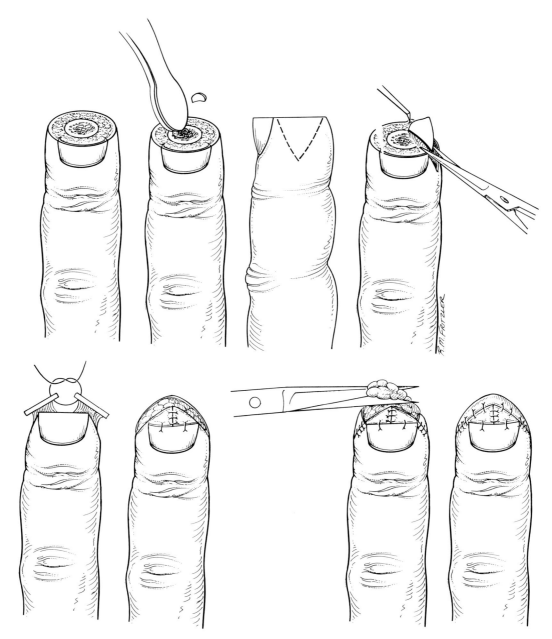

Fig. 69-5 Kutler V-Y advancement flaps (see text). (From Fisher RH: J Bone Joint Surg 49-A:317, 1967.)

end to conform with the normal tuft. Next, approximate the bases of the flaps and stitch them together with small interrupted nonabsorbable sutures; then stitch the dorsal sides of the flaps to the remaining nail or nail bed and close the defect volar to the flaps. Apply Xeroform gauze and a routine dressing.

■ *TECHNIQUE (ATASOY ET AL.)*. Under tourniquet control and using an appropriate anesthetic, cut a triangle in the remaining pulp skin area with the base of the triangle equal in width to the cut edge of the nail (Fig. 69-6). Develop a full-thickness flap with nerves and blood supply preserved. Carefully separate the fibrofatty subcutaneous tissue from the periosteum and flexor tendon sheath using sharp dissecting instruments and cutting the vertical septa that hold the flap in place. Mobilize and distally advance the flap, and suture it in place with interrupted sutures. A few millimeters of the phalanx may be removed when the bone protrudes.

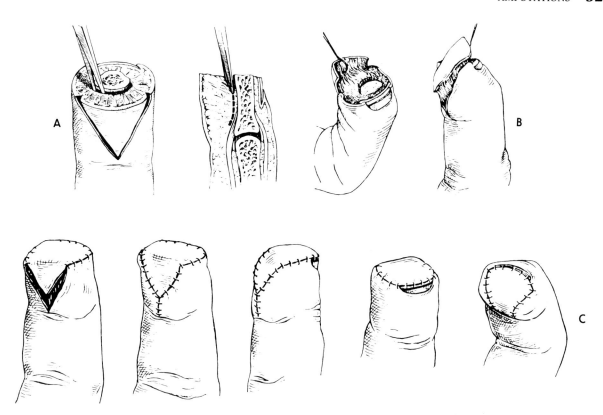

Fig. 69-6   Atasoy V-Y technique. **A,** Skin incision and mobilization of triangular flap. **B,** Advancement of triangular flap. **C,** Suturing of base of triangular flap to nail bed and closure of defect, V-Y technique. (From Atasoy E et al: J Bone Joint Surg 52-A:921, 1970.)

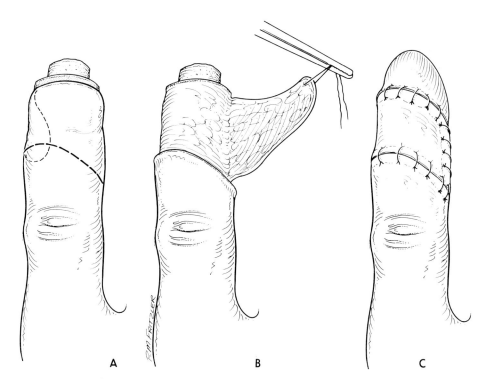

Fig. 69-7   Dorsal pedicle flap useful for amputations proximal to nail when preserving length is essential. It may have two pedicles or, as illustrated here, only one. **A,** Flap has been outlined. **B,** Flap has been elevated, leaving only single pedicle. **C,** Flap has been sutured in place over end of stump and remaining defect on dorsum of finger has been covered by split-thickness skin graft.

Bipedicle Dorsal Flaps

A bipedicle dorsal flap is useful when a finger has been amputated proximal to its nail bed and when preserving all its remaining length is essential but attaching it to another finger is undesirable. When this flap can be made wide enough in relation to its length, one of its pedicles may be divided, leaving it attached only at one side (Fig. 69-7).

■ *TECHNIQUE.* Beginning distally at the raw margin of the skin and proceeding proximally, elevate the skin and subcutaneous tissue from the dorsum of the finger. Then at a more proximal level make a transverse dorsal incision to create a bipedicle flap long enough, when drawn distally, to cover the bone and other tissues on the end of the stump. Suture the flap in place and cover the defect created on the dorsum of the finger by a split-thickness skin graft. The flap may be made more mobile by freeing one of its pedicles, but this decreases its vascularity.

Cross Finger Flaps

The technique of applying cross finger flaps is described in Chapter 62.

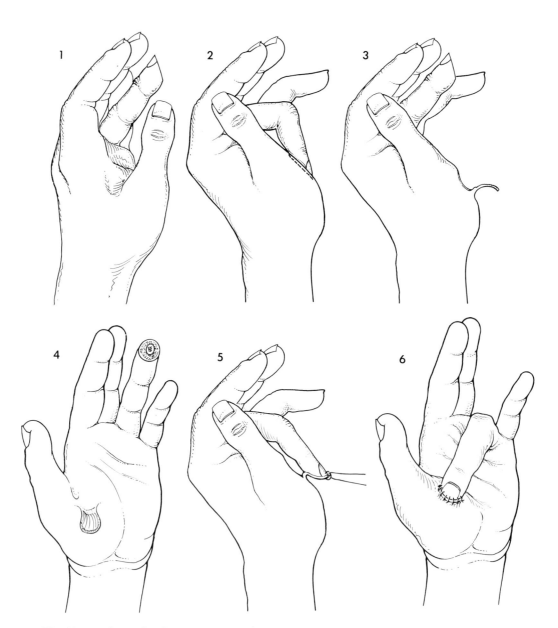

Fig. 69-8   Thenar flap for amputation of fingertip. *1*, Tip of ring finger has been amputated. *2*, Finger has been flexed so that its tip touches middle of thenar eminence, and thenar flap has been outlined. *3*, Split-thickness graft is to be sutured to donor area before flap is attached to finger. *4*, Split-thickness graft is in place. *5* and *6*, End of flap has been attached to finger by sutures passed through nail and through tissue on each side of it.

Thenar Flap

■ *TECHNIQUE.* With the thumb held in abduction, flex the injured finger so that its tip touches the middle of the thenar eminence (Fig. 69-8). Outline on the thenar eminence a flap that when raised will be large enough to cover the defect and will be properly positioned; pressing the bloody stump of the injured finger against the thenar skin will outline by bloodstain the size of the defect to be covered. With its base proximal, raise the thenar flap to include most of the underlying fat; handle the flap with skin hooks to avoid crushing it even with small forceps. Make the flap sufficiently wide that when sutured to the convex fingertip it will not be under tension. Furthermore, make its length no more than twice its width. By gentle undermining of the skin border at the donor site the defect can be closed directly without resorting to a graft. Attach the distal end of the flap to the trimmed edge of the nail by sutures passed through the nail. The lateral edges of the flap should fit the margins of the defect but, to avoid impairing circulation in the flap, suture only their most distal parts, if any, to the finger. Prevent the flap from folding back on itself and strangulating its vessels. Finally, control all bleeding, check the positions of the flap and finger, and apply wet cotton gently compressed to follow the contours of the graft and the fingertip. Now hold the finger in the proper position by gauze and adhesive tape and splint the wrist.

AFTERTREATMENT. At 4 days the graft is dressed and thereafter kept as dry as possible by dressing it every 1 or 2 days and by leaving it partially exposed. At 2 weeks the base of the flap is detached, and the free skin edges are sutured in place. The contours of the fingertip and the thenar eminence will improve with time.

Local Neurovascular Island Graft

A limited area of the touch pad may be resurfaced by a local neurovascular island graft. This graft provides satisfactory padding and normal sensibility to the most important working surface of the digit.

■ *TECHNIQUE.* Make a midlateral incision on each side of the finger (or thumb) beginning distally at the defect and extending proximally to the level of the proximal interphalangeal joint. On each side and beginning proximally, carefully dissect the neurovascular bundle distally to the level selected for the proximal margin of the graft (Fig. 69-9). Here make a transverse volar incision through the skin and subcutaneous tissues but carefully protect the neurovascular bundles. Then if necessary, make another transverse incision at the margin of the defect, thus freeing a rectangular island of the skin and underlying fat to which is attached the two neurovascular bundles. Carefully draw this island or graft distally and place it over the defect, avoiding placing too much tension on the bundles; should tension be sufficient to embarrass the circulation in the graft, then dissecting the bundles more proximally or

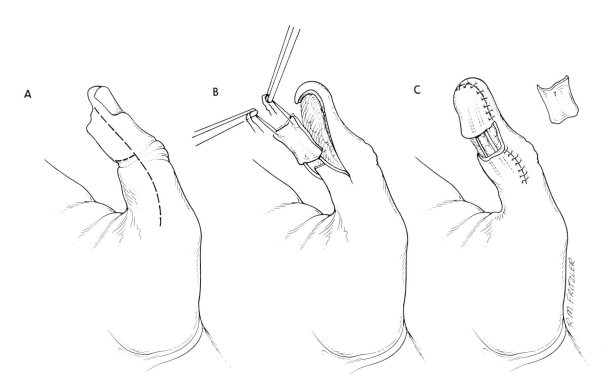

Fig. 69-9   Local neurovascular island graft (see text).

flexing the distal interphalangeal joint, or both, may be necessary. Suture the graft in place with interrupted small nonabsorbable sutures. Now cover the defect created on the volar surface of the finger with a free full-thickness graft. Place over the grafts wet cotton carefully shaped to fit the contour of the area and to prevent pressure on the neurovascular bundles. Apply a compression dressing.

AMPUTATIONS OF SINGLE FINGER
Index Finger

When the index finger is amputated at its proximal interphalangeal joint or at a more proximal level, the remaining stump is useless and may hinder pinch between the thumb and middle finger. Therefore, in most instances, when a primary amputation must be at such a proximal level, any secondary amputation should be through the base of the second metacarpal. This index ray amputation is especially desirable in women for cosmetic reasons. However, because it is a more extensive operation than amputation through the finger, it may cause stiffness of the other fingers and is contraindicated in arthritic hands and in men past middle age. Unless the surgeon's knowledge of anatomy and technique are precise, the branch of the median nerve to the second web may be accidentally damaged. Furthermore, improper technique may result in a sunken scar on the dorsum of the hand or in anchoring the first dorsal interosseus to the extensor mechanism rather than to the base of the proximal phalanx, causing intrinsic overpull.

INDEX RAY AMPUTATION

■ *TECHNIQUE.* With a skin pencil outline the incision as follows. First make a mark on the palmar edge of the second web near the base of the index finger; this is the distal point on which the skin flap will be rotated. Then outline the dorsal part of the incision that extends from this point proximally over the second metacarpal shaft and, curving radially, ends over its base. Next, from the same point on the web, outline the rest of the incision that extends first distally to the proximal interphalangeal joint of the index finger near the ulnar side of its volar surface, then radially across the volar surface of the finger, and finally proximally and ulnarward to join the dorsal part of the incision just proximal to the second metacarpophalangeal joint. Now make the incision as just outlined. Ligate and divide the dorsal veins and at a more proximal level divide the branches of the superficial radial nerve. Divide too the tendons of the extensor digitorum communis of the index finger and the extensor indicis proprius and allow them to retract. Detach the tendinous insertion of the first dorsal interosseus and dissect the muscle proximally from the second metacarpal

shaft. Then detach the volar interosseus from the same shaft and divide the transverse metacarpal ligament that connects the second and third metacarpal heads; take care not to damage the radial digital nerve of the middle finger. With bone-cutting forceps carefully divide the second metacarpal about 1.9 cm distal to its base; do not disarticulate the bone at its proximal end. Smooth any rough edges on the remaining part of the metacarpal. Divide both flexor tendons of the index finger and allow them to retract. Then divide both digital nerves of the finger proximal to the skin incision; carefully divide the ulnar digital nerve distal to the common digital nerve to prevent damaging the radial digital nerve of the middle finger. Next, anchor the tendinous insertion of the first dorsal interosseus to the base of the proximal phalanx of the middle finger; do not anchor it to the extensor tendon or its hood because this might cause intrinsic overpull. With a running suture approximate the muscle bellies in the area previously occupied by the second metacarpal shaft. Now shape the skin edges as desired, ligate or cauterize all obvious bleeders, and remove the tourniquet. Close the skin with small interrupted nonabsorbable sutures and drain the wound dorsally. Apply a well-molded wet dressing that conforms to the wide new web between the middle finger and the thumb, and support the wrist by a large bulky dressing or a plaster splint.
AFTERTREATMENT. The hand is elevated immediately after surgery for 48 hours. At 24 hours the drain is removed.

Middle or Ring Finger

In contrast to the proximal phalanx of the index finger, this phalanx of either the middle or ring finger is important functionally. Its absence in either finger makes a hole through which small objects can drop when the hand is used as a cup or in a scooping maneuver; furthermore, its absence makes the remaining fingers tend to deviate toward the midline of the hand. In multiple amputations the length of either the middle or ring finger becomes even more important. The third and fourth metacarpal heads are important too because they help stabilize the metacarpal arch by providing attachments for the transverse metacarpal ligament.

In a child or woman, when the middle finger has been amputated proximal to the proximal interphalangeal joint and especially when it has been amputated proximal to the metacarpal head, transposing the index ray ulnarward to replace the third ray may be indicated. This operation results in more natural symmetry, removes any conspicuous stump, and makes the presence of only three fingers less obvious. It must be remembered, however, that excising the third metacarpal shaft removes the origin of the adductor pollicis and thus weakens pinch. Therefore the index ray should not be transposed unless this adductor can be reattached elsewhere; furthermore, the operation is contraindicated when the hand is needed for heavy manual labor.

In the same circumstances when the ring finger has been similarly amputated, transposing the fifth ray radialward to replace the fourth rarely is indicated. Resection of the fourth metacarpal at its base or at the carpometacarpal joint and closure of the skin so as to create a common web will permit a "folding-in" of the fifth digit to close the gap without actually transposing the fifth metacarpal.

TRANSPOSING INDEX RAY

■ *TECHNIQUE (PEACOCK)*. Plan the incision so that a wedge of skin will be removed from both the dorsal and volar surfaces of the hand (Fig. 69-10). Plot in the region of the transverse metacarpal arch the exact points that must be brought together to form a smooth arch across the dorsum of the hand when the second and fourth metacarpal heads are approximated. Curve the proximal end of the dorsal incision slightly toward the second metacarpal base so that the base can be easily exposed. Fashion the distal end of the incision so that a small triangle of skin will be excised from the ring finger to receive a similar triangle of skin from the stump or the area between the fingers; transferring this triangle is important to prevent the suture line from passing through the depths of the reconstructed web. After the dorsal and volar wedges of skin have been removed and the flaps elevated, expose the third metacarpal through a longitudinal incision in its perios-

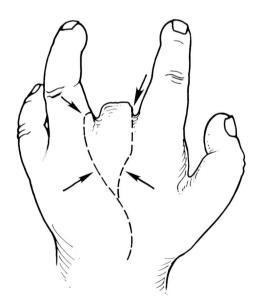

Fig. 69-10 Peacock technique of transposing index ray. Dorsal incision is shown; *arrows* indicate points along skin edges that will be brought together. Similar palmar incision is made (see text).

teum. The index ray will be the right length when its metacarpal is moved directly to the third metacarpal base. Therefore with an oscillating saw divide transversely the third metacarpal as close to its base as possible. Then excise the third metacarpal shaft and the interosseus muscles to the middle finger. Take care not to damage the interosseus muscles of the remaining fingers. Next, identify the neurovascular bundles of the middle finger; individually ligate the arteries and veins, and divide the digital nerves between the metacarpals deep within the substance of the interosseus muscle mass. While the wrist is held flexed, draw the flexor tendons distally as far as possible and divide them. Next, retract the extensor tendons of the index finger, expose the second metacarpal at its base, and divide the bone at the same level as the third metacarpal. From the radial side of the second metacarpal gently dissect the intrinsic muscles just enough to allow this metacarpal to be placed on the base of the third without placing undue tension on the muscles. Then bevel obliquely the second metacarpal base to produce a smooth contour on the side of the hand. From the excised third metacarpal fashion a key graft to extend from one fragment of the reconstructed metacarpal to the other. Then insert a Kirschner wire longitudinally through the metacarpophalangeal joint of the transposed ray and bring it out on the dorsum of the flexed wrist; draw it proximally through the metacarpal until its distal end is just proximal to the metacarpophalangeal joint. With the wrist flexed, cut off the proximal part of the wire and allow the remaining end to disappear beneath the skin. Next, flex all the fingers simultaneously to assure correct rotation of the transposed ray and insert a Kirschner wire transversely through the necks of the fourth and the transposed metacarpals. Now close the skin and insert a rubber drain. Apply a soft pressure dressing; no additional external support is needed.

AFTERTREATMENT. At 2 days the rubber drain is removed, and at 8 to 10 days the entire dressing and the sutures are removed. Then a light volar plaster splint is applied to keep the wrist in the neutral position and support the transposed ray; however, the splint is removed daily for cleaning the hand and exercising the small joints. At about 5 weeks when the metacarpal fragments have united, the Kirschner wires are removed using local anesthetic.

RING FINGER AVULSION INJURIES. The soft tissue of the left ring finger usually is forcefully avulsed at its base when a metal ring worn on that finger catches on a nail or hook. The force usually is sufficient to cause separation of the skin and nearly always damages the vascular supply to the distal tissue. Fractures and ligamentous damage may occur also, but the tendons seem to be the last to separate. Early evaluation of an incomplete avulsion may be disarming as to the severity of damage, but after 48 hours, all soft tissues usually are clearly nonviable. Attempts at salvage routinely fail unless the vascular supply can be reestablished. Amputation of the fourth ray with closure of the web is the procedure of choice in a child or woman. By resecting the fourth ray at its base or at the carpometacarpal joint, the fifth ray will close without having to be surgically transposed. Simple amputation of the finger itself should be done in the face of necrosis and infection and, if indicated, the ray amputation is done later as an elective procedure.

Little Finger

As much of the little finger as possible should be saved provided all the requirements for a painless stump are satisfied. Often this finger survives when all others have been destroyed, and then it becomes important in forming pinch with the thumb. But when the little finger alone is amputated and when the appearance of the hand is important or the amputation is at the metacarpophalangeal joint, the fifth metacarpal shaft is divided obliquely at its middle third; then the insertion of the abductor digiti quinti is transferred to the proximal phalanx of the ring finger just as the first dorsal interosseus is transferred to the middle finger in the index ray amputation already described. This smooths the ulnar border of the hand and is used most often as an elective procedure for a contracted or painful little finger.

AMPUTATIONS OF THUMB

In partial amputation of the thumb, in contrast to one of a single finger, reamputation at a more proximal level to obtain closure should not be considered because the thumb should never be shortened. Therefore the wound should be closed primarily by a free graft, an advancement pedicle flap (described later), or a local or distant flap.

When a flap is necessary, taking it from the dorsum of either the hand or the index or middle finger is preferable. A flap from one of these areas provides a touch pad that is stable but that will not regain normal sensibility.

Covering the volar surface of the thumb with an abdominal flap is contraindicated; even when thin, abdominal skin and fat provide a poor surface for pinch because they lack fibrous septa and will roll or shift under pressure. Furthermore, skin of the abdomen is dissimilar in appearance to that of the hand and its digits. When the skin and pulp, including all neural elements, have been lost from a significant area of the thumb, a neurovascular island graft (Chapter 65) may be indicated. However, the defect should be closed primarily by a split-thickness graft; then the neurovascular island graft or, if feasible, a local neurovascular island graft or advancement flap as described for fingertip amputations (p. 3206) is applied secondarily.

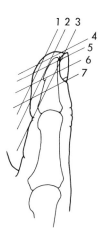

Fig. 69-11 Thumb tip amputation levels. Acceptable procedures by level are: *1*, split-thickness graft; *2*, cross finger flap or advancement flap; *3*, advancement flap, cross finger flap, or shorten thumb and close; *4*, split-thickness skin graft; *5*, shorten bone and split-thickness skin graft, advancement flap, or cross finger flap; *6*, advancement flap or cross finger flap; *7*, advancement flap and removal of nail bed remnant.

When the thumb has been amputated so that a useful segment of the proximal phalanx remains, the only surgery necessary, if any, except for primary closure of the wound, is deepening the thumb web by Z-plasty (Chapter 61). When amputation has been at the metacarpophalangeal joint or at a more proximal level, then reconstruction of the thumb may be indicated (p. 3215).

Advancement Pedicle Flap for Thumb Injuries

Advancement flaps for fingertip injuries usually will survive if the volar flap incisions are not brought proximal to the proximal interphalangeal joint. In the thumb, however, the venous drainage is not as dependent on the volar flap, and thus this technique is safer and the flap can be longer (Fig. 69-11).

Using tourniquet control and appropriate anesthesia, a midlateral incision is made on each side of the thumb from the tip to the metacarpophalangeal joint. The flap created contains both neurovascular bundles and should be elevated without disturbing the flexor tendon sheath (Fig. 69-12). Flexion of both the joints will allow the flap to be advanced and carefully sutured over the defect with interrupted sutures. The joints should be maintained in flexion postoperatively for 3 weeks. This rather large flap is used only when a large area of thumb pulp is lost.

AMPUTATIONS OF MULTIPLE DIGITS

In *partial amputations of all fingers,* preserving the remaining length of the digits is much more important than in a single finger amputation (Figs. 69-13 and 69-

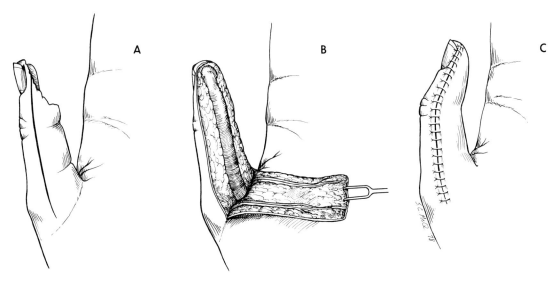

Fig. 69-12 Advancement pedicle flap for thumb injuries. **A,** Deep thumb pad defects exposing bone may be covered with advancement pedicle flap. **B,** Advancement of neurovascular pedicle. **C,** Flexion of distal joint of thumb is necessary to permit placement of flap (see text).

14). Because of the natural hinge action between the first and fifth metacarpals, any remaining stump of the little finger must play an important role in prehension with the intact thumb; this hinge action may be increased about 50% by dividing the transverse metacarpal ligament between the fourth and fifth rays.

In *complete amputation of all fingers*, if the intact thumb cannot easily reach the fifth metacarpal head, then phalangization of the fifth metacarpal is helpful. In this operation the fourth metacarpal is resected and the fifth is osteotomized, rotated, and separated from the rest of the palm. Lengthening of the fifth metacarpal is also helpful.

Phalangization of Fifth Metacarpal

■ *TECHNIQUE.* Over the fourth metacarpal make dorsal and volar longitudinal incisions that join distally. Expose and resect the transverse metacarpal ligament on each side of the fourth metacarpal head. Then divide proximally the digital nerves to the ring finger and ligate and divide the corresponding vessels. Next, resect the fourth metacarpal shaft just distal to its carpometacarpal joint. Through the same incision osteotomize the fifth metacarpal near its base. Slightly abduct and flex the distal fragment and rotate it toward the thumb. Fix the fragments with a Kirschner wire. Next, cover the raw surfaces between the third and fifth metacarpals with split-thickness grafts, creating a web at the junction of the proximal and middle thirds of the bones. Be sure the padding over the fifth metacarpal head is good and, if possible, sensation is normal at its point of maximum contact with the thumb.

• • •

In *partial amputation of all fingers and the thumb,* function may be improved by lengthening the digits relatively and by increasing their mobility. Function of the thumb may be improved by deepening its web by Z-plasty (Chapter 61) and by osteotomizing both the first and fifth metacarpals and rotating their distal fragments toward each other (Fig. 69-15) while at the same time, if helpful, tilting the fifth metacarpal toward the thumb. When the first carpometacarpal joint is functional but the first metacarpal is quite short, the second metacarpal may be transposed to the first to lengthen it and to widen and deepen the first web.

In *complete amputation of all fingers and the thumb* in which the amputation has been transversely through the metacarpal necks, phalangization of selected metacarpals may improve function. The fourth metacarpal is resected to increase the range of motion of the fifth, and function of the fifth is further improved by osteotomy of the metacarpal in which the distal fragment is rotated radialward and flexed. The second metacarpal is resected at its base but, to preserve the origin of the adductor pollicis, the third metacarpal is not. The thumb should not be lengthened by osteoplastic reconstruction (p. 3218) unless sensibility can be added to its volar surface. When the amputation has been through the middle of the metacarpal shafts, prehension probably cannot be restored, but hook can be accomplished by flexing the stump at the wrist. Furthermore, this motion at the wrist can be made even more useful by fitting an artificial platform to which the palmar surface of the stump can be actively opposed.

PAINFUL AMPUTATION STUMP

Amputation stumps are often painful enough to require revision; in fact such revision is probably the most

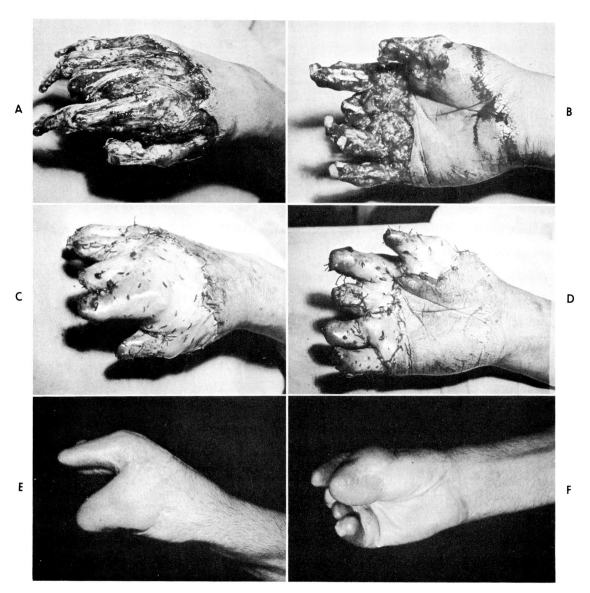

Fig. 69-13   Partial amputation of multiple digits and massive avulsion of skin and neurovascular bundles from digits and hand. **A** and **B,** Dorsal and palmar views soon after injury. **C** and **D,** Dorsal and palmar views after primary operation. Index, ring, and little fingers have been shortened as little as possible and whole area has been covered by split-thickness skin grafts. **E** and **F,** After secondary repair with pedicle graft to thumb and first web. Function is good. (From Matev I: J Bone Joint Surg 49-B:722, 1967.)

frequent elective operation in hand surgery. A neuroma located in an unpadded area near the end of the stump is the usual cause of pain. It is diagnosed by carefully pressing the stump with a small firm object such as the blunt end of a pencil; a well-localized area of extreme tenderness no more than 1 or 2 mm in diameter is found, usually in line with a digital nerve. When painful, a neuroma should be excised; it and the attached nerve are freed from the scar, and the nerve is divided at a more proximal level where its end will be covered by sufficient padding. Another neuroma will develop but should be painless when located in a padded area.

Pain in an amputation stump may also be caused by bony prominences covered only by thin skin such as a split-thickness graft or by skin made tight by scarring. In these instances excising the thin skin or scar, shortening the bone, and applying a sufficiently padded graft may be indicated. Amputation stumps that are painful because of thin skin coverage at the pulp and nail junction can be improved by using a limited advancement flap as described in the section on thumb amputations. In the finger, proximal dissection to develop these flaps should not extend proximal to the proximal interphalangeal joint.

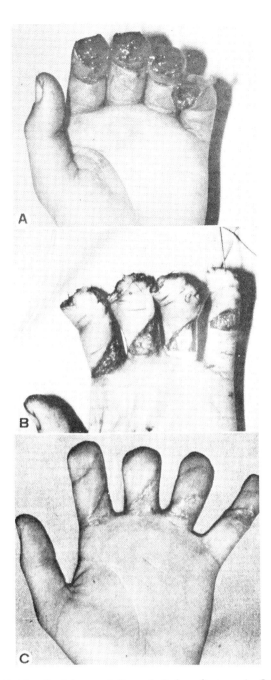

Fig 69-14   Partial amputation of all four fingers. **A,** Guillotine-type amputations of fingers. **B,** Local flaps of volar skin were transposed distally, preserving remaining length of fingers. Each flap was elevated anterior to ulnar neurovascular bundle but posterior to radial neurovascular bundle. **C,** After healing. In each finger motion was normal, and sensibility was retained in end. (From Hueston J: Plast Reconstr Surg 37:349, 1966.)

Finally, painful cramping sensations in the hand and forearm may be caused by flexion contracture of a stump resulting from overstretching of extensor tendons or adherence of flexor tendons; release of any adherent tendons is helpful.

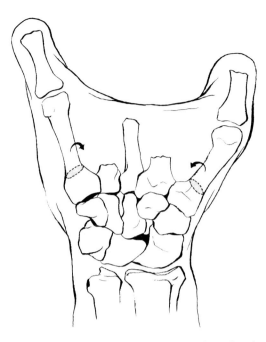

Fig. 69-15   In multiple amputations including thumb, function may be improved by osteotomizing first and fifth metacarpals and rotating their distal fragments toward each other (see text).

RECONSTRUCTIONS AFTER AMPUTATION
Reconstruction after Amputation of Hand

Amputation of both hands is, of course, extremely disabling. In selected patients the Krukenberg operation is helpful. It converts the forearm to forceps in which the radial ray acts against the ulnar ray. Swanson compares function of the reconstructed limb with the use of chopsticks. Normal sensibility between the tips of the rays is assured by proper shifting of skin during closure of the wound. The operation, because it provides not only prehension but also sensibility at the terminal parts of the limb, is especially helpful in blind patients with bilateral amputation. It is also helpful in other patients with similar amputations, especially in surroundings where modern prosthetic services are unavailable. According to Swanson, children with bilateral congenital amputation find the reconstructed limb much more useful than a mechanical prosthesis; they transfer dominance to this limb when a prosthesis is used on the opposite one (Fig. 69-16). In children the appearance of the limb after surgery has not been distressing and, furthermore, the operation does not prevent the wearing of an ordinary prosthesis when desired.

■ *TECHNIQUE (KRUKENBERG; SWANSON).* Make a longitudinal incision on the flexor surface of the forearm slightly toward the radial side (Fig. 69-17, *A*); make a similar incision on the dorsal surface slightly toward the ulnar side, but on this surface elevate a **V**-shaped flap to form a web at the junction of the rays (Fig. 69-17, *B*). Now separate the forearm muscles into two groups (Fig. 69-17, *C* and *D*): on the radial side carry the radial wrist flexors and extensors, the radial half of the flexor digitorum sublimis, the radial half of the extensor digitorum communis, the brachioradialis, the palmaris longus, and the pronator teres; on the ulnar side carry the ulnar wrist flexors and extensors, the ulnar half of the flexor digitorum sublimis, and the ulnar half of the extensor digitorum communis. If they make the stump too bulky or the wound hard to close, resect as necessary the pronator quadratus, the flexor digitorum profundus, the flexor pollicis longus, the abductor pollicis longus, and the extensor pollicis

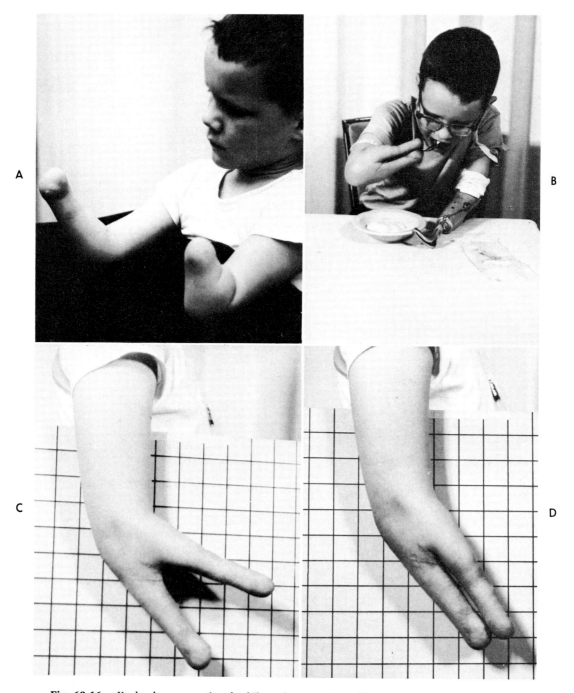

Fig. 69-16   Krukenberg operation for bilateral amputation of hand. **A,** Boy 7 years old who was born with left upper partial hemimelia and right upper archeiria. **B,** After Krukenberg operation child uses reconstructed limb as his dominant one. Secondary osteotomy of radius was necessary to improve apposition at tips of rays. **C,** Tips of rays can be separated about 7.5 cm. **D,** Pinch and grasp are excellent. (From Swanson AB: J Bone Joint Surg 46-A:1540, 1964.)

brevis; take care here not to disturb the pronator teres. Next, incise the interosseous membrane throughout its length along its ulnar attachment, taking care not to damage the interosseous vessel and nerve. The radial and ulnar rays can now be separated 6 to 12 cm at their tips depending on the size of the forearm; motion at their proximal ends occurs at the radiohumeral and proximal radioulnar joints. The opposing ends of the rays should touch; if not, osteotomize the radius or ulna as necessary.

Now the adductors of the radial ray are the pronator teres, the supinator, the flexor carpi radialis, the radial half of the flexor digitorum sublimis, and the palmaris longus; the abductors of the radial ray are the brachioradialis, the extensor carpi radialis longus, the extensor carpi radialis brevis, the radial half of the extensor digitorum communis, and the biceps. The adductors of the ulnar ray are the flexor carpi ulnaris, the ulnar half of the flexor digitorum sublimis, the brachialis, and the anconeus; the ab-

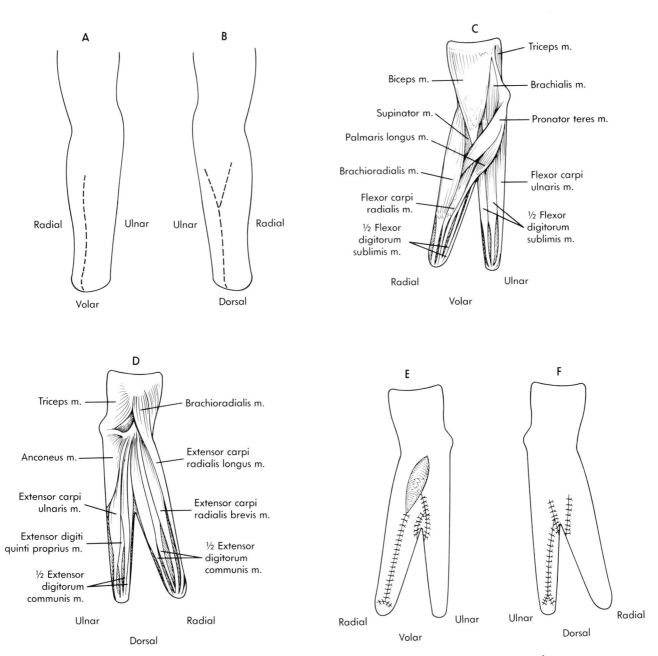

Fig. 69-17 Krukenberg operation. **A,** Incision on flexor surface of forearm. **B,** Incision on dorsal surface (see text). **C** and **D,** Forearm muscles have been separated into two groups (see text). **E,** Closure of skin on flexor surface of forearm; parallel lines indicate location of any needed split-thickness skin graft. **F,** Closure of skin on dorsal surface (see text). (Modified from Swanson AB: J Bone Joint Surg 46-A:1540, 1964.)

ductors of the ulnar ray are the extensor carpi ulnaris, the ulnar half of the extensor digitorum communis, and the triceps.

Remove the tourniquet, obtain hemostasis, and observe the circulation in the flaps. Excise any excess fat, rotate the skin around each ray, and close the skin over each so that the suture line is not on the opposing surface of either (Fig. 69-17, *E* and *F*). Excise any scarred skin at the ends of the rays and, if necessary to permit closure, shorten the bones; in children the skin is usually sufficient for closure and the bones must not be shortened because growth at the distal epiphyses will still be incomplete. Preserve any remaining rudimentary digit. Next, suture the flap in place at the junction of the rays and apply any needed split-thickness graft. Insert small rubber drains and, with the tips of the rays separated 6 cm or more, apply a compression dressing.

AFTERTREATMENT. The limb is constantly elevated for 3 to 4 days. The sutures are removed at the usual time. At 2 to 3 weeks rehabilitation to develop abduction and adduction of the rays is begun.

Reconstruction after Amputation of Multiple Digits

Several reconstructive operations are useful after amputation of multiple digits at various levels. These are discussed along with the primary treatment of these injuries (p. 3212).

Reconstruction of Thumb

Absence of the thumb, either traumatic or congenital, causes a severe deficiency in hand function; in fact, such an absence usually is considered to constitute a 40% disability of the hand as a whole. Thus when the thumb is partially or totally absent, reconstructive surgery is appealing. But before any decision for surgery is made, several factors must be considered: the length of any remaining part of the thumb, the condition of the rest of the hand, the occupational requirements and age of the patient, and the knowledge and experience of the surgeon. When the opposite thumb is normal, some surgeons question the need for reconstructing even a totally absent thumb; at least reconstruction here is not mandatory. However, function of the hand surely can be improved by a carefully planned and skillfully executed operation, especially in a young patient.

Usually the thumb should be reconstructed only when amputation has been at the metacarpophalangeal joint or at a more proximal level. When this joint and a useful segment of the proximal phalanx remain, the only surgery necessary, if any, is deepening of the thumb web by Z-plasty (Chapter 61). Furthermore, when amputation has been through the interphalangeal joint, the distal

phalanx, or the pulp of the thumb, only appropriate coverage by skin is necessary unless sensibility in the area of pinch is grossly impaired; in this latter instance, a more elaborate coverage as by a neurovascular island transfer may be indicated (Chapter 65).

A reconstructed thumb must meet five requirements. First, sensibility, although not necessarily normal, should be painless and sufficient for recognition of objects held in the position of pinch. This probably is the most important requirement. Second, the thumb should have sufficient stability so that pinch pressure does not cause the thumb joints to deviate or collapse or cause the skin pad to shift. Third, there should be sufficient mobility to enable the hand to flatten and the thumb to oppose for pinch. Fourth, the thumb should be of sufficient length to enable the opposing digital tips to touch it. Sometimes amputation or stiffness of the remaining digits may require greater than normal length of the thumb to accomplish prehension. Fifth, the thumb should be cosmetically acceptable since, if it is not, it may remain hidden and not be used.

Several reconstructive procedures are possible, and the choice depends on the length of the stump remaining and the sensibility of the remaining thumb pad (Fig. 69-18). The thumb may be lengthened by a short bone graft and transferred local skin for sensibility. The nonopposing surface then is skin grafted as in the Gillies-Millard "cocked hat" procedure. Another possibility is pollicizing a digit. A promising possibility is direct free transfer of a toe to the hand with anastomosis of both the vessels and the nerves by microsurgical technique. In this procedure, nerve restoration is never normal. The osteoplastic technique with a bone graft and tube pedicle skin graft supplemented by a neurovascular pedicle is now rarely recommended.

For congenital absence of the thumb, pollicization of the index finger is the most used technique. Congenital absence of the thumb is frequently associated with other

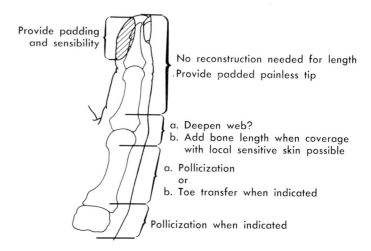

Fig. 69-18 Thumb reconstruction at various levels. Basic needs are sensibility, stability, mobility, and length.

congenital malformations such as congenital absence of the radius and occasionally metabolic disorders including blood dyscrasias. These latter conditions should be well assessed before elective procedures for thumb reconstruction are performed. These reconstructive procedures are usually done after the first year or two of life.

The so-called floating thumb, a congenital anomaly in which the distal segment of the thumb has no major attachment except a narrow soft tissue pedicle and appears to dangle from a skin thread, is not considered useful enough to attempt reconstruction. The skin of this digit may be used for a skin graft if it is needed, but as a rule it should be detached during the first few months of life.

LENGTHENING OF METACARPAL AND TRANSFER OF LOCAL FLAP. When amputation of the thumb has been at the metacarpophalangeal joint or within the condylar area of the first metacarpal, the thenar muscles are able to stabilize the digit. In these instances, lengthening of the metacarpal by bone grafting and transfer of a local skin flap may be indicated. Furthermore, the technique as described by Gillies and Millard may be completed in one stage and thus the time required for surgery and convalescence is less than in some other reconstructions. But it has disadvantages: the bone graft may resorb and

become shortened or its end, after contraction of the flap, may perforate the skin. This procedure requires that there be minimal scarring of the amputated stump.

■ *TECHNIQUE (GILLIES AND MILLARD, MODIFIED).* Make a curved incision around the dorsal, radial, and volar aspects of the base of the thumb (Fig. 69-19). Undermine the skin distally but stay superficial to the main veins to prevent congestion of the flap. Continue the undermining until a hollow flap has been elevated and slipped off the end of the stump; the blood supply to the flap is from a source around the base of the index finger in the thumb web. (If desired, complete elevation of the flap may be delayed until a second operation, as described by Gillies and Millard.) Next, attach an iliac bone graft or a phalanx excised from a toe to the distal end of the metacarpal by tapering the graft and fitting it into a hole in the end of the metacarpal. Fix the graft to the bone by a Kirschner wire and place iliac chips about its base. Be sure the graft is small enough that the flap can be easily placed over it. Now cover the raw area at the base of the thumb by a split-thickness skin graft.

AFTERTREATMENT. The newly constructed thumb is immobilized by a supportive dressing and a volar

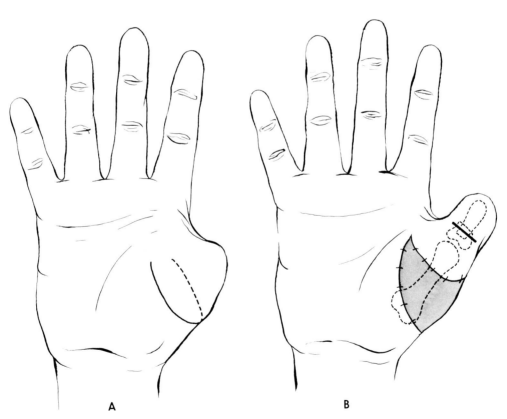

A   B

Fig. 69-19   Reconstruction of thumb by technique of Gillies and Millard, modified. **A,** Curved incision around dorsal, radial, and volar aspects of base of thumb has been outlined. **B,** Hollow flap has been undermined and elevated, iliac bone graft has been fixed (this time to base of proximal phalanx), and raw area at base of thumb has been covered by split-thickness skin graft.

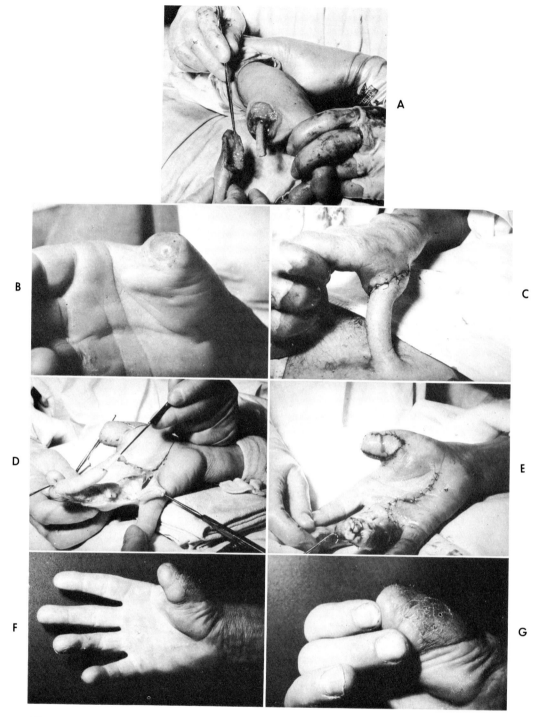

Fig. 69-20   Osteoplastic reconstruction of thumb. **A,** Large area for implantation of tubed pedicle graft has been prepared, iliac bone graft has been inserted into end of first metacarpal, and tubed pedicle graft has been prepared for suture in place over bone graft. **B** to **G,** Osteoplastic reconstruction of thumb and transfer of neurovascular island graft. **B,** Status of thumb before operation. **C,** First metacarpal has been lengthened by iliac bone graft and tubed pedicle graft has been sutured in place, enclosing bone graft. **D,** Pedicle has been freed and skin has been closed over end of newly constructed thumb; there are trophic changes in digit and sensibility is markedly deficient. Neurovascular island graft is being raised from ulnar side of ring finger. **E,** Island graft has been transferred to thumb and donor area has been covered by free skin graft. **F** and **G,** Status 3 years after surgery; trophic changes have disappeared and sensibility in skin of island graft is "normal." (From Verdan C: Surg Clin North Am 48:1033, 1968.)

plaster splint is applied to the palm and forearm. The Kirschner wire is removed when the graft has united with the metacarpal. Minor Z-plasties may be necessary later to relieve the volar and dorsal web formed by advancing the flap.

OSTEOPLASTIC RECONSTRUCTION AND TRANSFER OF NEUROVASCULAR ISLAND GRAFT. Verdan recommends osteoplastic reconstruction, especially when the first carpometacarpal joint has been spared and is functional. It is a useful method when the remaining part of the first metacarpal is short. As in the technique of Gillies and Millard, no finger is endangered and all are spared to function against the reconstructed thumb. Transfer of a neurovascular island graft supplies discrete sensibility to the new thumb but precise sensory reorientation is always lacking. For this reconstruction to be successful, the surgeon must be experienced in the use of tubed pedicle grafts and other skin grafting techniques, and the reconstructed thumb must be shorter than normal, never long enough for its end to lie opposite the proximal interphalangeal joint of the index finger.

■ *TECHNIQUE (VERDAN).* Raise from the abdomen, the subpectoral region, or some other appropriate area a tubed pedicle graft that contains only moderate subcutaneous fat. Next, excise the skin and subcutaneous tissue over the distal end of the first metacarpal; make this area for implantation of the tubed graft a long oval and as large as possible so that the graft may include many vessels and nerves and will not constrict later (Fig. 69-20, *A*). Insert into the end of the first metacarpal an iliac bone graft shaped like a palette to imitate the normal thumb. Do not place the graft in line with the first metacarpal but rather place it at an obtuse angle in the direction of opposition. Be sure the graft is not too long. Then place the end of the tubed pedicle over the bone graft and suture it to its prepared bed on the thumb (Fig. 69-20, *C*). Immobilize the hand and tubed pedicle so as to allow normal motion of the fingers and some motion of the shoulder and elbow. After 3 to 4 weeks free the tubed pedicle. Then close the skin over the distal end of the newly constructed thumb, or transfer a neurovascular island graft from an appropriate area to the volar aspect of the thumb to assist in closure and to improve sensation and circulation in the digit (Fig. 69-20, *D* to *G*). *AFTERTREATMENT.* A supportive dressing and a volar plaster splint are applied. The newly constructed thumb is protected for about 8 weeks to prevent or decrease resorption of the bone graft. If a neurovascular island graft was not included in the reconstruction (Fig. 69-21), then this transfer must be performed later.

POLLICIZATION. Because pollicization (transposition of a finger to replace an absent thumb) endangers the finger, some surgeons recommend transposition only of an already shortened or otherwise damaged finger. In this instance, full function of the new thumb hardly can be expected. In fact, full function cannot be expected even after successful transposition of a normal finger. Yet in the hands of an experienced surgeon, pollicization is worthwhile, especially in complete bilateral congenital absence of the thumb or in bilateral traumatic amputation at or near the carpometacarpal joint. When amputation has been traumatic, extensive scarring may require resurfacing by a pedicle skin graft before pollicization.

In the following techniques the index finger is transposed to replace the thumb.

■ *TECHNIQUE (LITTLER).* In congenital absence of the thumb with absence of the greater multangular or in traumatic amputation at the first carpometacarpal joint, the repositioned index finger is fixed to its own metacarpal base as described first here. In these instances, the second metacarpophalangeal joint serves as the carpometacarpal joint of the new thumb. Thus placing the new thumb in position for true opposition is impossible.

Make a racquet-shaped incision encircling the base of the index finger. Extend the handle of the racquet proximally and gently curve it first volarly and then dorsally (Fig. 69-22, *A*). Preserve the dorsal vein of the finger. Now free the neurovascular bundles and flexor mechanism of the finger by dividing the palmar fascia and septa. Next, divide the intermetacarpal ligament and interosseous fascia between the second and third metacarpals, and the proper volar digital artery to the radial side of the middle finger. Detach the insertion of the abductor indicis muscle that in the normal hand is the first dorsal interosseus (Fig. 69-22, *B*). Expose subperiosteally the metacarpal and divide it obliquely at its base at a right angle to the normal projection of the thumb. Section proximally the extensor digitorum communis tendon and separate it distally from the extensor indicis proprius and the radial lateral band to near the proximal interphalangeal joint. Next, resect the metacarpal shaft just proximal to the epiphysis, preserving a dorsal strut for better fixation of the remaining head to the metacarpal base. Thus the metacarpophalangeal joint is preserved to act as the carpometacarpal joint of the new thumb. Now fix the metacarpal head to the metacarpal base in the normal thumb projection. Next, fix the tendon of insertion of the abductor indicis at the level of the proximal interphalangeal joint by passing the extensor digitorum communis tendon twice through it, then around the ulnar lateral band, and then proximally to suture it to the abductor indicis (Fig. 69-22, *C*). Resect the redundant part of the extensor indicis proprius tendon and suture together the free ends of the tendon under proper tension.

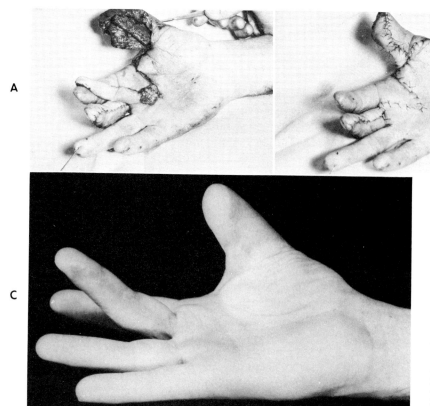

Fig. 69-21 Osteoplastic reconstruction of thumb. Thumb was traumatically amputated through metacarpophalangeal joint with loss of skin dorsally. On day of injury treatment consisted of application of tubed pedicle graft. **A,** One month after injury. Tubed pedicle has been detached from abdomen and opened, iliac bone graft has been inserted into end of first metacarpal, neurovascular island graft has been raised from ulnar side of middle finger, and donor area on finger has been covered by split-thickness skin graft. **B,** Neurovascular island graft has been sutured in place on end and palmar aspect of newly constructed thumb, and palmar incision has been closed. **C,** One year after injury. Thumb has been satisfactorily reconstructed and there is large area of sensitive skin on its end and palmar surface. (**A** and **B** courtesy Mr. JT Hueston; **C** from Hueston J: Br J Plast Surg 18:304, 1965.)

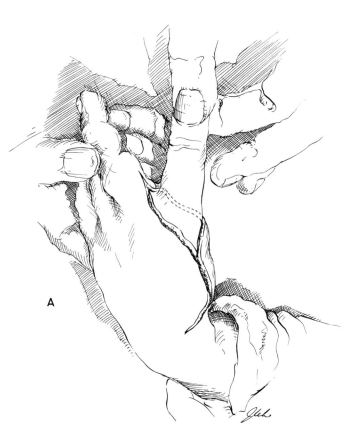

Fig. 69-22 Littler pollicization for congenital absence of thumb or amputation at carpometacarpal joint. **A,** Skin incision. **B,** Detachment of abductor indicis, resection of second metacarpal shaft, and freeing of extensor digitorum communis (see text). **C,** Readjustment of extensor mechanism and fixation of abductor indicis by extensor digitorum communis tendon (see text).

Continued.

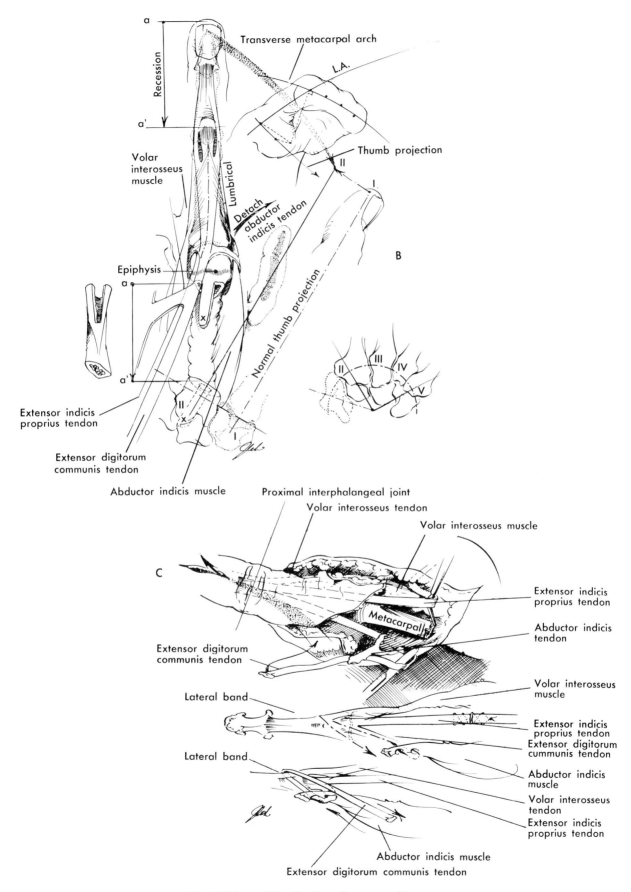

a

Recession

a'

Transverse metacarpal arch

L.A.

Volar
interosseus
muscle

Lumbrical

Detach
abductor
indicis tendon

Thumb projection

II

I

B

Epiphysis

a

Normal thumb projection

a'

x

Extensor indicis
proprius tendon

II

x

Extensor digitorum
communis tendon

I

Abductor indicis muscle

II   III   IV

V

Proximal interphalangeal joint
Volar interosseus tendon

Volar interosseus muscle

C

Metacarpal

Extensor indicis
proprius tendon

Abductor indicis
tendon

Extensor digitorum
communis tendon

Volar interosseus
muscle

Lateral band

Extensor indicis
proprius tendon
Extensor digitorum
cummunis tendon

Lateral band

Abductor indicis
muscle

Volar interosseus
tendon

Extensor indicis
proprius tendon

Abductor indicis muscle

Extensor digitorum communis tendon

Fig. 69-22, cont'd   For legend see opposite page.

Continued.

In traumatic amputation through the first metacarpal shaft, the second metacarpophalangeal joint is not needed as a substitute for the carpometacarpal joint of the thumb. Thus the index metacarpal, except for its base; the metacarpophalangeal joint; and the proximal part of the proximal phalanx are discarded, and the retained part of the proximal phalanx is rotated and fixed to the stump of the first metacarpal as described next.

Begin the incision dorsally over the junction of the middle and distal thirds of the second metacarpal, extend it distally to the web between the middle and index fingers, then laterally across the proximal flexion crease, and then proximally to the starting point; from here continue it to the end of the amputated thumb, then proximally along the dorsum of the first metacarpal, and then slightly ulnarward to permit subsequent shifting of the skin (Fig. 69-23, *A*). Be careful to protect the dorsal vein to the index finger. Next, reflect the volar flap anteriorly to expose the first dorsal interosseus, lumbrical, and adductor muscles and the radial neurovascular bundle (Fig. 69-23, *D*). Reflect distally the triangular flap from the dorsum of the finger to expose the extensor tendons and dorsal aponeurosis, the intermetacarpal ligament, and the common volar artery with its digital branches to the index and middle fingers. Then divide the juncturae tendinum and the fascia between the tendons of the extensor communis of the index and middle fingers. By further dissection at the base of the index finger carefully isolate the neurovascular pedicles. To allow radial shift of the

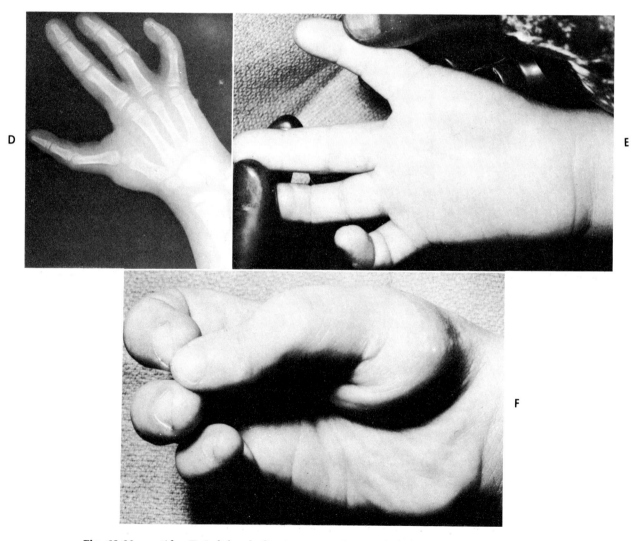

Fig. 69-22, cont'd   **D,** Left hand after treatment of congenital absence of thumb by limited repositioning of index finger. **E,** Left hand after surgery (function improved). **F,** Right hand after treatment for same anomaly by Littler technique as described in text (function is much better than in left hand; note pinch). (Modified from Littler JW: In Adams JP, editor: Current practice in orthopaedic surgery, vol 3, St Louis, 1966, Mosby–Year Book, Inc.)

nerves, vessels, and flexor tendons, section the compartmental septa of the palmar fascia. Locate the bifurcation of the common volar artery at the distal border of the intermetacarpal ligament; divide and ligate here the proper digital artery to the radial side of the middle finger (Fig. 69-23, *E*). The common volar nerve usually divides more proximally, but if necessary, separate it farther. Now section the first dorsal interosseus and volar interosseus muscles at their musculotendinous junctions. Divide as far proximally as possible the extensor tendons to the index finger and reflect them distally. Remove a

bone graft from the dorsal surface of the second metacarpal to be used for medullary fixation of the transposed finger to the first metacarpal (Fig. 69-23, *B* and *C*). Divide the index metacarpal at its base and the proximal phalanx near its base and discard the intervening bony segments; resect only enough bone from the proximal phalanx to make the new thumb of proper length. Next, place the bone graft in the medullary canal of the first metacarpal and transfix it with a Kirschner wire. Then transpose the index finger to the thumb by placing its exposed proximal phalanx over the protruding medullary

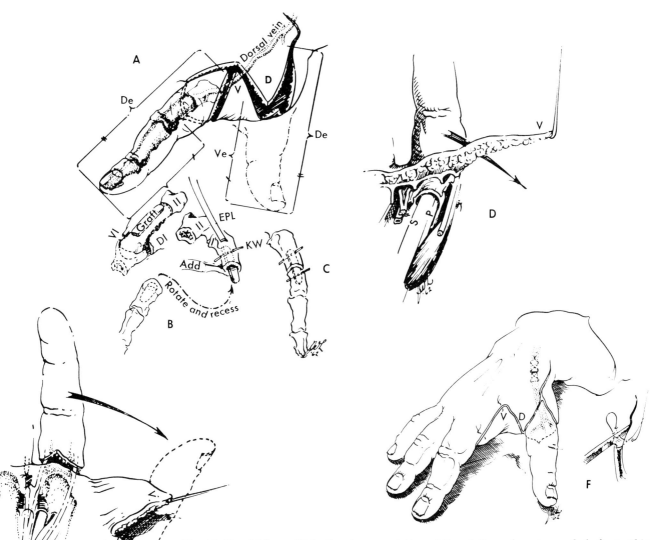

Fig. 69-23   Littler pollicization for amputation of thumb through metacarpal shaft. **A,** Skin incision. Note tenting of incision in anterior midline and preservation of dorsal vein. *Dotted line,* thumb after repositioning of index finger. Note shortening of index ray to simulate natural length of thumb. **B,** Treatment of bone: removal of graft from dorsum of second metacarpal, discard of bone between base of second metacarpal and base of proximal phalanx, and shift of index finger. **C,** Fixation of bone by graft and two Kirschner wires. **D,** Reflection anteriorly of volar flap to expose first dorsal interosseus, lumbrical, and adductor muscles and radial neurovascular bundle. **E,** Ligation of proper volar digital artery to middle finger, and division of intermetacarpal ligament and deep palmar fascia. **F,** Closure of skin flaps. Note special mattress suture used to snug tips of triangular flaps into position. Suture of extensor digitorum communis to extensor pollicis longus is shown. (Courtesy Dr. J William Littler.)

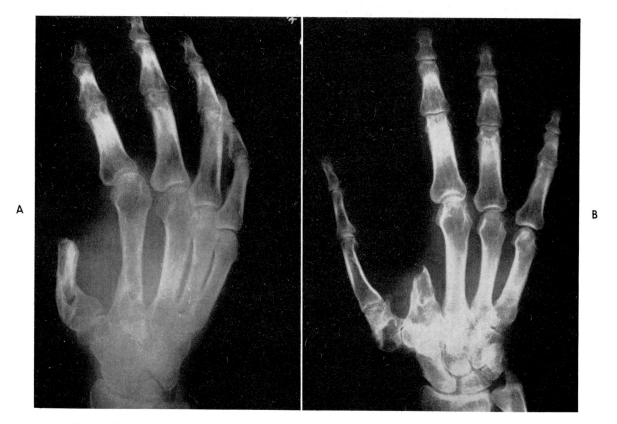

Fig. 69-24   Same as Fig. 69-23. **A,** Before surgery. **B,** After surgery. (Courtesy Dr. J William Littler.)

graft in proper pronation; transfix it also with a Kirschner wire to maintain its position after surgery. Now suture the extensor pollicis longus tendon to the extensor communis tendon of the transposed finger by the end-to-end method (Fig. 69-23, *F*). Divide the extensor indicis proprius at its junction with the common extensor, withdraw it proximal to the dorsal carpal ligament, transfer it in line with the extensor pollicis longus, and suture it to the extensor mechanism under proper tension. Now shift the volar flap ulnarward and suture it to the soft tissues at the side of the third metacarpal. Suture the dorsal flap to the margin of this flap and to the triangular flap on the dorsum of the transposed finger. Then close the remaining incisions.

AFTERTREATMENT. The hand and newly constructed thumb are immobilized in the functional position. The sutures are removed at 12 days. Function is gradually resumed 6 to 8 weeks later. The roentgenograms of a hand before and after this type of pollicization are shown in Fig. 69-24.

• • •

In the Riordan technique, again the index ray is shortened by resection of its metacarpal shaft. To simulate the greater multangular, the second metacarpal head is positioned palmar to the normal plane of the metacarpal

bases, and the metacarpophalangeal joint acts as the carpometacarpal joint of the new thumb. The first dorsal interosseus is converted to an abductor pollicis brevis and the first volar interosseus to an adductor pollicis. The technique as described is for an immature hand with congenital absence of the thumb including the greater multangular, but it can be modified appropriately for other hands.

■ *TECHNIQUE (RIORDAN).* Beginning on the proximal phalanx of the index finger make a circumferential oval incision (Fig. 69-25, *A* and *B*); on the dorsal surface place the incision level with the middle of the phalanx and on the palmar surface level with the base of the phalanx. From the radiopalmar aspect of this oval extend the incision proximally, radially, and dorsally to the radial side of the second metacarpal head, then palmarward and ulnarward to the radial side of the third metacarpal base in the midpalm, and finally again radially to end at the radial margin of the base of the palm. Dissect the skin from the proximal phalanx of the index finger, leaving the fat attached to the digit and creating a full-thickness skin flap. Next, isolate and free the insertion of the first dorsal interosseus, and strip from the radial side of the second metacarpal shaft the origin of the muscle. Then isolate and free the insertion of the first volar interosseus and strip from the

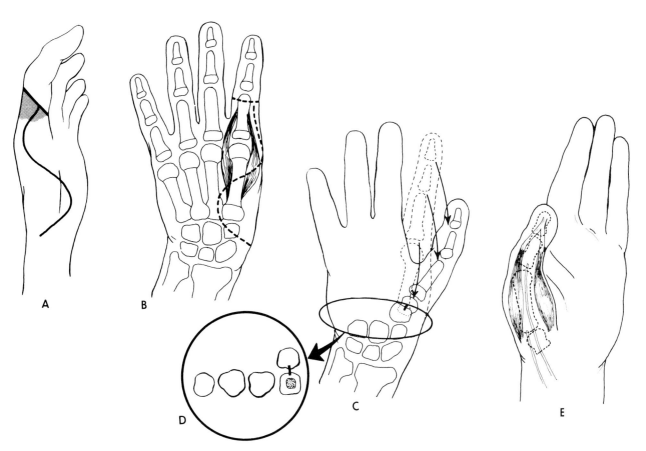

Fig. 69-25   Riordan pollicization for congenital absence of thumb, including greater multangular, in immature hand. **A** and **B,** Incision (see text). Skin of proximal phalanx, stippled area in **A,** is elevated as full-thickness skin flap. **C** and **D,** Second metacarpal has been resected by dividing base proximally and by cutting through epiphysis distally, and finger has been relocated proximally and radially. Second metacarpal head has been anchored palmar to second metacarpal base and simulates greater multangular (see text). **E,** Insertion of first dorsal interosseus has been anchored to radial lateral band of extensor mechanism of new thumb and origin to soft tissues at base of digit; insertion of first volar interosseus has been anchored to opposite lateral band and origin to soft tissues.

ulnar side of the metacarpal shaft the origin of this muscle. Take care to preserve the nerve and blood supplies to the muscle in each instance. Now separate the second metacarpal head from the metacarpal shaft by cutting through its epiphysis with a knife; preserve all of its soft tissue attachments. Then divide the second metacarpal at its base, leaving intact the insertions of the extensor carpi radialis longus and flexor carpi radialis; discard the metacarpal shaft. Next, carry the index finger proximally and radially and relocate the second metacarpal head palmar to the second metacarpal base so that it simulates a greater multangular (Fig. 69-25, *C*); take care to rotate and angulate it so that the new thumb is properly positioned. Anchor it in this position with a wire suture (Fig. 69-25, *D*). Now anchor the insertion of the first dorsal interosseus to the radial lateral band of the extensor mechanism of the new thumb and its origin to the soft tissues at

the base of the digit; this muscle now functions as an abductor pollicis brevis (Fig. 69-25, *E*). Likewise anchor the insertion of the first volar interosseus to the opposite lateral band and its origin to the soft tissues; this muscle now functions as an adductor pollicis. Shorten the extensor indicis proprius by resecting a segment of its tendon; this muscle now functions as an extensor pollicis brevis. Likewise shorten the extensor digitorum communis by resecting a segment of its tendon. Anchor the proximal segment of the tendon to the base of the proximal phalanx; this muscle now functions as an abductor pollicis longus. Trim the skin flaps appropriately; fashion the palmar flap so that when sutured it will place sufficient tension on the new thumb to hold it in opposition. Suture the flaps but avoid a circumferential closure at the base of the new thumb. Apply a pressure dressing of wet cotton and then a plaster cast.

AFTERTREATMENT. **At 3 weeks the cast is removed and motion is begun. The thumb is appropriately splinted.**

• • •

Buck-Gramcko has reported experience with 100 operations for pollicization of the index finger in children with congenital absence or marked hypoplasia of the thumb. He emphasizes a reduction in length of the pollicized digit and accomplishes this by removing the entire

second metacarpal with the exception of the head, which acts as a new greater multangular. For best results, the index finger has to be rotated initially approximately 160 degrees during the operation so that it is opposite the pulp of the ring finger. This position changes somewhat during the suturing of the muscles and the skin so that at the end of the operation there is rotation of approximately 120 degrees. In addition, the pollicized digit is angulated approximately 40 degrees into palmar abduction.

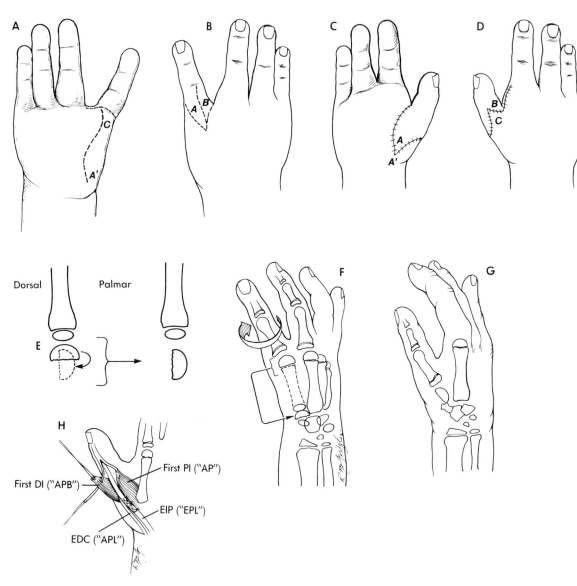

Fig. 69-26 Pollicization of index finger. **A** and **B,** Palmar and dorsal skin incisions. **C** and **D,** Appearance after wound closure. **E,** Rotation of metacarpal head into flexion to prevent postoperative hyperextension. **F,** Index finger rotated about 160 degrees along long axis to place finger pulp into position of opposition. **G,** Final position of skeleton in about 40 degrees of palmar abduction with metacarpal head secured to metacarpal base or carpus. **H,** Reattachment of tendons to provide control of new thumb. First palmar interosseous (PI) functions as adductor pollicis (AP); first dorsal interosseous (DI) functions as the abductor pollicis brevis (APB); extensor digitorum communis (EDC) functions as abductor pollicis longus (APL); and extensor indicis proprius (EIP) functions as extensor pollicis longus (EPL). (Redrawn from Buck-Gramcko D: J Bone Joint Surg 53-A:1605, 1971.)

■ *TECHNIQUE (BUCK-GRAMCKO).* Make an **S**-shaped incision down the radial side of the hand just onto the palmar surface. Begin the incision near the base of the index finger on the palmar aspect and end it just proximal to the wrist. Make a slightly curved transverse incision across the base of the index finger on the palmar surface, connecting at right angles to the distal end of the first incision. Connect both ends of the incision on the dorsum of the hand as shown in Fig. 69-26, *A*. Make a third incision on the dorsum of the proximal phalanx of the index finger from the proximal interphalangeal joint extending proximally to end at the incision around the base of the index finger (Fig. 69-26, *B*). Through the palmar incision, free the neurovascular bundle between the index and middle fingers by ligating the artery to the radial side of the middle finger. Then separate the common digital nerve carefully into its component parts for the two adjacent fingers so that no tension will be present after the index finger is rotated. Sometimes an anomalous neural ring is found around the artery; split this ring very carefully so that angulation of the artery after transposition of the finger will not occur. When the radial digital artery to the index finger is absent, it is possible to perform the pollicization on a vascular pedicle of only one artery. On the dorsal side, preserve at least one of the great veins.

Now, on the dorsum of the hand, sever the tendon of the extensor digitorum communis at the metacarpophalangeal level. Detach the interosseus muscles of the index finger from the proximal phalanx and the lateral bands of the dorsal aponeurosis. Partially strip subperiosteally the origins of the interosseus muscles from the second metacarpal, being careful to preserve the neurovascular structures.

Next, osteotomize and resect the second metacarpal as follows. If the phalanges of the index finger are of normal length, the whole metacarpal is resected with the exception of its head. When the phalanges are relatively short, the base of the metacarpal must be retained to obtain the proper length of the new thumb. When the entire metacarpal is resected except for the head, rotate the head as shown in Fig. 69-26, *E*, and attach it by sutures to the joint capsule of the carpus and to the carpal bones, which in young children can be pierced with a sharp needle. Rotate the digit 160 degrees to allow apposition (Fig. 69-26, *F*). Bony union is not essential, and fibrous fixation of the head is sufficient for good function. When the base of the metacarpal is retained, fix the metacarpal head to its base with one or two Kirschner wires, again in the previously described position. In attaching the metacarpal head, bring the proximal phalanx into complete hyperextension in relation to the metacarpal head for maximum stability of the joint. Unless this is done, hyperexten-

sion is likely at the new "carpometacarpal" joint (Fig. 69-26, *G*). Suture the proximal end of the detached extensor digitorum communis tendon to the base of the former proximal phalanx (now acting as the first metacarpal) to become the new "abductor pollicis longus." Section the extensor indicis proprius tendon, shorten it appropriately, and then suture it by end-to-end anastomosis.

Suture the tendinous insertions of the two interosseus muscles to the lateral bands of the dorsal aponeurosis by weaving the lateral bands through the distal part of the interosseus muscle and turning them back distally to form a loop that is sutured to itself. In this way, the first palmar interosseus will become an "adductor pollicis" and the first dorsal interosseus an "abductor brevis" (Fig. 69-26, *H*).

Close the wound by fashioning a dorsal skin flap to close the defect over the proximal phalanx and fashion the rest of the flaps as necessary for skin closure as in Fig. 69-26, *C* and *D*.

AFTERTREATMENT. The hand is immobilized for 3 weeks and then careful active motion is begun.

REFERENCES

Ahstrom JP Jr: Pollicization in congenital absence of the thumb, Curr Pract Orthop Surg 5:1, 1973.

Argamaso RV: Rotation-transposition method for soft tissue replacement on the distal segment of the thumb, Plast Reconstr Surg 54:366, 1974.

Atasoy E: The cross thumb to index finger pedicle, J Hand Surg 5:572, 1980.

Atasoy E et al: Reconstruction of the amputated finger tip with a triangular volar flap: a new surgical procedure, J Bone Joint Surg 52-A:921, 1970.

Bowe JJ: Thumb reconstruction by index transposition, Plast Reconstr Surg 32:414, 1963.

Brent B: Replantation of amputated distal phalangeal parts of fingers without vascular anastomoses, using subcutaneous pockets, Plast Reconstr Surg 63:1, 1979.

Broadbent TR and Woolf RM: Thumb reconstruction with contiguous skin-bone pedicle graft, Plast Reconstr Surg 26:494, 1960.

Brown H et al: Phalangizing the first metacarpal: case report, Plast Reconstr Surg 45:294, 1970.

Brown H and Getty P: Leprosy and thumb reconstruction by opponensplasty or phalangizing the first metacarpal, J Hand Surg 4:432, 1979.

Brown PW: Adduction-flexion contracture of the thumb: correction with dorsal rotation flap and release of contracture, Clin Orthop 88:161, 1972.

Brown PW: Sacrifice of the unsatisfactory hand, J Hand Surg 4:417, 1979.

Buck-Gramcko D: Pollicization of the index finger: method and results in aplasia and hypoplasia of the thumb, J Bone Joint Surg 53-A:1605, 1971.

Bunnell S: Digit transfer by neurovascular pedicle, J Bone Joint Surg 34-A:772, 1952.

Bunnell S: Reconstruction of the thumb, Am J Surg 95:168, 1958.

Butler B Jr: Ring-finger pollicization: with transplantation of nail bed and matrix on a volar flap, J Bone Joint Surg 46-A:1069, 1964.

Button M and Stone EJ: Segmental bony reconstruction of the thumb by composite groin flap: a case report, J Hand Surg 5:488, 1980.

Carroll RE: Transposition of the index finger to replace the middle finger, Clin Orthop 15:27, 1959.

Carroll RE: Ring injuries in the hand, Clin Orthop 104:175, 1974.

Clarkson P: Reconstruction of hand digits by toe transfers, J Bone Joint Surg 37-A:270, 1955.

Clarkson P: On making thumbs, Plast Reconstr Surg 29:325, 1962.

Clarkson P: Erratum (on making thumbs), Plast Reconstr Surg 30:491, 1962.

Clarkson P and Chandler R: A toe to thumb transplant with nerve graft, Am J Surg 95:315, 1958.

Clarkson P and Furlong F: Thumb reconstruction by transfer of big toe, Br Med J 2:1332, 1949.

Clayton ML: Index ray amputation, Surg Clin North Am 43:367, 1963.

Cobbett JR: Free digital transfer: report of a case of transfer of a great toe to replace an amputated thumb, J Bone Joint Surg 51-B:677, 1969.

Cook FW, Jakab E, and Pollock MA: Local neurovascular island flap, J Hand Surg 15-A:798, 1990.

Cuthbert JB: Pollicisation of the index finger, Br J Plast Surg 1:56, 1948-1949.

Davis JE: Toe to hand transfers (pedochyrodactyloplasty), Plast Reconstr Surg 33:422, 1964.

de Boer A and Robinson PH: Ray transplantation by intercarpal osteotomy after loss of the fourth digit, J Hand Surg 14-A:379, 1989.

Doi K et al: Reconstruction of an amputated thumb in one stage: case report—free neurovascular flap transfer with iliac-bone graft, J Bone Joint Surg 61-A:1254, 1979.

Entin MA: Salvaging the basic hand, Surg Clin North Am 48:1063, 1968.

Fisher RH: The Kutler method of repair of finger-tip amputation, J Bone Joint Surg 49-A:317, 1967.

Flatt AE: The thenar flap, J Bone Joint Surg 39-B:80, 1957.

Flatt AE and Wood VE: Multiple dorsal rotation flaps from the hand for thumb web contractures, Plast Reconstr Surg 45:258, 1970.

Freeman BS: Reconstruction of thumb by toe transfer, Plast Reconstr Surg 17:393, 1956.

Freiberg A and Manktelow R: The Kutler repair for fingertip amputations, Plast Reconstr Surg 50:371, 1972.

Gillies H: Autograft of amputated digit: suggested operation, Lancet 1:1002, 1940.

Gillies H and Millard RD Jr, editors: The principles and art of plastic surgery, vol 2, part V, chap 23, Boston, 1957, Little, Brown & Co.

Gordon S: Autograft of amputated thumb, Lancet 2:823, 1944.

Graham WP III: Incisions, amputations, and skin grafting in the hand, Orthop Clin North Am 2:213, 1970.

Hallock G: The simple cross-flap, technique and vascular anatomy, Orthop Rev 13:75, 1984.

Harrison SH: Restoration of muscle balance in pollicization, Plast Reconstr Surg 34:236, 1964.

Hentz V, Jackson I, and Fogarty D: Case report: false aneurysm of the hand secondary to digital amputation, J Hand Surg 3:199, 1978.

Hirshowitz B, Karev A, and Rousso M: Combined double Z-plasty and Y-V advancement for thumb web contracture, Hand 7:291, 1975.

Holm A and Zachariae L: Fingertip lesions: an evaluation of conservative treatment versus free skin grafting, Acta Orthop Scand 45:382, 1974.

Hueston J: The extended neurovascular island flap, Br J Plast Surg 18:304, 1965.

Hueston J: Local flap repair of fingertip injuries, Plast Reconstr Surg 37:349, 1966.

Hughes NC and Moore FT: A preliminary report on the use of a local flap and peg bone graft for lengthening a short thumb, Br J Plast Surg 3:34, 1950-1951.

Hung-Yin C et al: Reconstruction of the thumb, Chin Med J 79:541, 1959. (Abstracted by David E Hallstrand, Int Abstr Surg 111:177, 1960.)

Irigaray A: New fixing screw for completely amputated fingers, J Hand Surg 5:381, 1980.

Jeffery CC: A case of pollicisation of the index finger, J Bone Joint Surg 39-B:120, 1957.

Johnson HA: Formation of a functional thumb post with sensation in phocomelia, J Bone Joint Surg 49-A:327, 1967.

Joshi BB: One-stage repair for distal amputation of the thumb, Plast Reconstr Surg 45:613, 1970.

Joshi BB: A local dorsolateral island flap for restoration of sensation after avulsion injury of fingertip pulp, Plast Reconstr Surg 54:175, 1974.

Joyce JL: A new operation of the substitution of a thumb, Br J Surg 5:499, 1918.

Kaplan EB: Replacement of an amputated middle metacarpal and finger by transposition of the index finger, Bull Hosp Joint Dis 27:103, 1966.

Kaplan I: Primary pollicization of injured index finger following crush injury, Plast Reconstr Surg 37:531, 1966.

Kaplan I and Plaschkes J: One stage pollicisation of little finger, Br J Plast Surg 13:272, 1960-1961.

Keiter JE: Immediate pollicization of an amputated index finger, J Hand Surg 5:584, 1980.

Kelikian H and Bintcliffe EW: Functional restoration of the thumb, Surg Gynecol Obstet 83:807, 1946.

Kettelkamp DB and Ramsey P: Experimental and clinical autogenous distal metacarpal reconstruction, Clin Orthop 74:129, 1971.

Kleinert HE: Finger tip injuries and their management, Am Surg 25:41, 1959.

Krukenberg H: Uber Platiches Unwertung von Amputationsstumpen, Stuttgart, 1917, Ferdinand Enk.

Lassar GN: Reconstruction of a digit following loss of all fingers with preservation of the thumb, J Bone Joint Surg 41-A:519, 1959.

Leung PC and Kok LC: Use of an intramedullary bone peg in digital replantations, revascularization and toe-transfers, J Hand Surg 6:281, 1981.

Lewin ML: Partial reconstruction of thumb in a one-stage operation, J Bone Joint Surg 35-A:573, 1953.

Lewin ML: Severe compression injuries of the hand in industry: amputation versus rehabilitation, J Bone Joint Surg 41-A:71, 1959.

Lewin ML: Sensory island flap in osteoplastic reconstruction of the thumb, Am J Surg 109:226, 1965.

Littler JW: Subtotal reconstruction of thumb, Plast Reconstr Surg 10:215, 1952.

Littler JW: Neurovascular pedicle method of digital transposition for reconstruction of thumb, Plast Reconstr Surg 12:303, 1953.

Littler JW: Principles of reconstructive surgery of the hand. In Converse JM, editor: Reconstructive plastic surgery, vol 4, Philadelphia, 1964, WB Saunders Co.

Littler JW: Digital transposition. In Adams JP, editor: Current practice in orthopaedic surgery, vol 3, St Louis, 1966, Mosby–Year Book, Inc.

Littler JW: On making a thumb: one hundred years of surgical effort, J Hand Surg 1:35, 1976.

Lobay GW and Moysa GL: Primary neurovascular bundle transfer in the management of avulsed thumbs, J Hand Surg 6:31, 1981.

Ma FY, Cheng CY, Chen Y, and Leung C: Fingertip injuries: a prospective study on seven methods of treatment on 200 cases, Ann Acad Med Singapore 11:207, 1982.

Mansoor IA: Metacarpal lengthening: a case report, J Bone Joint Surg 51-A:1639, 1969.

Matev IB: First metacarpal lengthening for thumb reconstruction, Am Dig Foreign Orthop Lit 1st qtr:10, 1970.

Matev IB: Thumb reconstruction after amputation at the metacarpophalangeal joint by bone-lengthening: a preliminary report of three cases, J Bone Joint Surg 52-A:957, 1970.

Matev I: Wringer injuries of the hand, J Bone Joint Surg 49-B:722, 1967.

Mathes SJ, Buchannan R, and Weeks PM: Microvascular joint transplantation with epiphyseal growth, J Hand Surg 5:586, 1980.

Matthews D: Congenital absence of functioning thumb, Plast Reconstr Surg 26:487, 1960.

May JW Jr et al: Free neurovascular flap from the first web of the foot in hand reconstruction, J Hand Surg 2:387, 1977.

McCash C: Toe pulp-free grafts in finger-tip repair, Br J Plast Surg 11:322, 1958-1959.

McGregor IA and Simonetta C: Reconstruction of the thumb by composite bone-skin flap, Br J Plast Surg 17:37, 1964.

Metcalf W and Whalen WP: Salvage of the injured distal phalanx: plan of care and analysis of 369 cases, Clin Orthop 13:114, 1959.

Millender LH et al: Delayed volar advancement flap for thumb tip injuries, Plast Reconstr Surg 52:635, 1973.

Miller AJ: Single finger tip injuries treated by thenar flap, Hand 6:311, 1974.

Miura T: Thumb reconstruction using radial-innervated cross-finger pedicle graft, J Bone Joint Surg 55-A:563, 1973.

Miura T: An appropriate treatment for postoperative Z-formed deformity of the duplicated thumb, J Hand Surg 2:380, 1977.

Moore FT: The technique of pollicisation of the index finger, Br J Plast Surg 1:60, 1948-1949.

Morrison WA, O'Brien B McC, and MacLeod AM: Thumb reconstruction with a free neurovascular wrap-around flap from the big toe, J Hand Surg 5:575, 1980.

Murray JF, Carman W, and MacKenzie JK: Transmetacarpal amputation of the index finger: a clinical assessment of hand strength and complications, J Hand Surg 2:471, 1977.

Nemethi CE: Reconstruction of the distal part of the thumb after traumatic amputation: restoration of function and sensation using nerve, tendon, and bone from the amputated portion, J Bone Joint Surg 42-A:375, 1960.

O'Brien B McC et al: Hallux-to-hand transfer, Hand 7:128, 1975.

O'Brien B McC et al: Microvascular second toe transfer for digital reconstruction, J Hand Surg 3:123, 1978.

Ohmori K and Harii K: Transplantation of a toe to an amputated finger, Hand 7:135, 1975.

de Oliveira JC: Some aspects of thumb reconstruction, Br J Surg 57:85, 1970.

Peacock EE Jr: Metacarpal transfer following amputation of a central digit, Plast Reconstr Surg 29:345, 1962.

Pierce GW: Reconstruction of the thumb after total loss, Surg Gynecol Obstet 45:825, 1927.

Posner MA: Ray transposition for central digital loss, J Hand Surg 4:242, 1979.

Prpic I: Reconstruction of the thumb immediately after injury, Br J Plast Surg 17:49, 1964.

Reid DAC: Reconstruction of the thumb, J Bone Joint Surg 42-B:444, 1960.

Reis ND: Gillies "cocked hat" reconstruction for total loss of ulnar four fingers, Hand 5:229, 1973.

Riordan DC: Personal communication, 1969.

Robinson OG Jr: Primary reconstruction of the thumb using amputated part and tube pedicle flap, South Med J 66:1025, 1973.

Rose EH and Buncke HJ: Simultaneous transfer of the right and left second toes for reconstruction of amputated index and middle fingers in the same hand: case report, J Hand Surg 5:590, 1980.

Rose EH, Norris NS, Kowalski TA, et al: The "cap" technique: non-microsurgical reattachment of fingertip amputations, J Hand Surg 14-A:513, 1989.

Rybka FJ and Pratt FE: Thumb reconstruction with a sensory flap from the dorsum of the index finger, Plast Reconstr Surg 64:141, 1979.

Salis JG: Primary pollicisation of an injured middle finger, J Bone Joint Surg 45-B:503, 1963.

Schiller C: Nail replacement in finger tip injuries, Plast Reconstr Surg 19:521, 1957.

Schlenker JD, Kleinert HE, and Tsai T-M: Methods and results of replantation following traumatic amputation of the thumb in sixty-four patients, J Hand Surg 5:63, 1980.

Schmauk B: On the problem of thumb substitution (Zur Problematik des Daumenersatzes), Med Welt 9:482, 1960. (Abstracted by Joseph C Mulier, Int Abstr Surg 111:178, 1960.)

Scott JE: Amputation of the finger, Br J Surg 61:574, 1974.

Shaw MH and Wilson ISP: An early pollicisation, Br J Plast Surg 3:214, 1950-1951.

Smith JR and Bom AF: An evaluation of finger-tip reconstruction by cross-finger and palmar pedicle flap, Plast Reconstr Surg 35:409, 1965.

Smith RJ and Dworecka F: Treatment of the one-digit hand, J Bone Joint Surg 55-A:113, 1973.

Snow JW: The use of a volar flap for repair of fingertip amputations: a preliminary report, Plast Reconstr Surg 52:299, 1973.

Snowdy HA, Omer GE Jr, and Sherman FC: Longitudinal growth of a free toe phalanx transplant to a finger, J Hand Surg 5:71, 1980.

Soiland H: Lengthening a finger with the "on the top" method, Acta Chir Scand 122:184, 1961.

Stefani AE and Kelly AP: Reconstruction of the thumb: a one-stage procedure, Br J Plast Surg 15:289, 1962.

Stern PJ and Lister GD: Pollicization after traumatic amputation of the thumb, Clin Orthop 155:85, 1981.

Sturman MJ and Duran RJ: Late results of finger-tip injuries, J Bone Joint Surg 45-A:289, 1963.

Sullivan JG et al: The primary application of an island pedicle flap in thumb and index finger injuries, Plast Reconstr Surg 39:488, 1967.

Swanson AB: Restoration of hand function by the use of partial or total prosthetic replacement. I. The use of partial prostheses, J Bone Joint Surg 45-A:276, 1963.

Swanson AB: Restoration of hand function by the use of partial or total prosthetic replacement. II. Amputation and prosthetic fitting for treatment of the functionless, asensory hand, J Bone Joint Surg 45-A:284, 1963.

Swanson AB: The Krukenberg procedure in the juvenile amputee, J Bone Joint Surg 46-A:1540, 1964.

Swanson AB: Levels of amputation of fingers and hand: considerations for treatment, Surg Clin North Am 44:1115, 1964.

Swanson AB, Boeve NR, and Lumsden RM: The prevention and treatment of amputation neuromata by silicone capping, J Hand Surg 2:70, 1977.

Tamai S et al: Hallux-to-thumb transfer with microsurgical technique: a case report in a 45-year-old woman, J Hand Surg 2:152, 1977.

Tamai S et al: Traumatic amputation of digits: the fate of remaining blood: an experimental and clinical study, J Hand Surg 2:13, 1977.

Tanzer RC and Littler JW: Reconstruction of the thumb, Plast Reconstr Surg 3:533, 1948.

Tegtmeier RE: Thumb-to-thumb transfer following severe electrical burns to both hands, J Hand Surg 6:269, 1981.

Tubiana R and Roux JP: Phalangization of the first and fifth metacarpals: indications, operative technique, and results, J Bone Joint Surg 56-A:447, 1974.

Tubiana R, Stack H, and Hakstian RW: Restoration of prehension after severe mutilations of the hand, J Bone Joint Surg 48-B:455, 1966.

Usui M et al: An experimental study on "replantation toxemia": the effect of hypothermia on an amputated limb, J Hand Surg 3:589, 1978.

Verdan C: The reconstruction of the thumb, Surg Clin North Am 48:1033, 1968.

Watman RN and Denkewalter FR: A repair for loss of the tactile pad of the thumb, Am J Surg 97:238, 1959.

Weckesser EC: Reconstruction of a grasping mechanism following extensive loss of digits, Clin Orthop 15:60, 1959.

Weiland AJ et al: Replantation of digits and hands: analysis of surgical techniques and functional results in 71 patients with 86 replantations, J Hand Surg 2:1, 1977.

Whitaker LA et al: Retaining the articular cartilage in finger joint amputations, Plast Reconstr Surg 49:542, 1972.

White WF: Fundamental priorities in pollicisation, J Bone Joint Surg 52-B:438, 1970.

Wilkinson TS: Reconstruction of the thumb by radial nerve innervated cross-finger flap, South Med J 65:992, 1972.

Winspur I: Single-stage reconstruction of the subtotally amputated thumb: a synchronous neurovascular flap and Z-plasty, J Hand Surg 6:70, 1981.

Zancolli E: Transplantation of the index finger in congenital absence of the thumb, J Bone Joint Surg 42-A:658, 1960.

CHAPTER 70

Paralytic Hand

JAMES H. CALANDRUCCIO
MARK T. JOBE

The hand is an organ of both motion and sensibility. Motion is necessary for the highly adaptive functions of pinch, grasp, and hook; it is made possible by the many joints among the 29 bones in the hand, wrist, and forearm and by the 50 muscles that act as motors and stabilizers. To be purposeful, motion must be controlled; joints that are crossed by moving tendons but that must not themselves move during a given function must be stabilized by balanced antagonistic muscles. An outstanding example of this stabilization is that of the wrist in dorsiflexion by its extensors, which prevent the wrist from being flexed by the strong finger flexors when a fist is made; the antagonists of the wrist extensors, the wrist flexors, also contribute to stabilizing the wrist in this position.

With the wrist extended the fingers assume the position of function as a result of muscle balance (Fig. 70-1).

During use of the hand, varying joints must be stabilized at varying times for varying intervals; this dynamic stability can be provided only by the controlled balanced action of muscles. In the normal hand this transition from one stable position to another occurs in a rhythmic flow; groups of muscles act in proper phase and cooperate with other groups. The result is changing of positions by controlled balance; this is known as *coordination*. The proper timing of muscle action and the proper tension exerted by muscles are controlled at the unconscious level and by conscious effort; they are accomplishments of repetition. Some patterns of movement are used so frequently and the muscle groups involved act in coordination in such endless repetition that they are said to be *synergistic*, or working together (Fig. 70-2). The wrist extensors, finger flexors, and digital adductors act together with ease and thus are synergistic; likewise the wrist

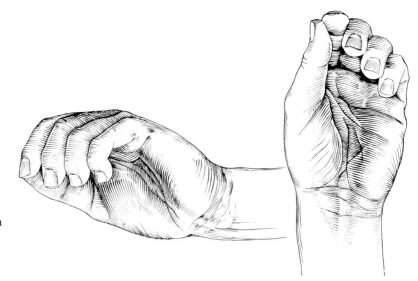

Fig. 70-1   Position of muscle balance. (From White WL: Surg Clin North Am 40:427, 1960.)

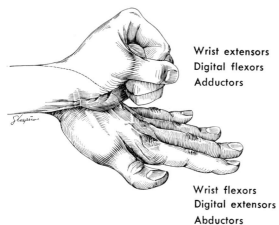

Wrist extensors
Digital flexors
Adductors

Wrist flexors
Digital extensors
Abductors

Fig. 70-2   Synergistic muscles of hand (see text). (From White WL: Surg Clin North Am 40:427, 1960.)

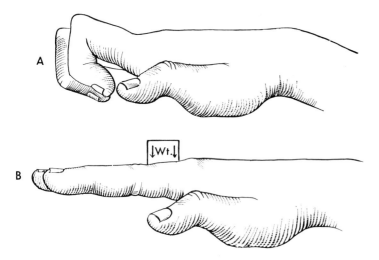

↓Wt.↓

Fig. 70-3   Clawing of hand caused by paralysis of intrinsic muscles. **A,** Long finger extensors cannot extend interphalangeal joints because metacarpophalangeal joints are hyperextended. **B,** Long finger extensors can extend interphalangeal joints because hyperextension of metacarpophalangeal joints has been prevented.

flexors, finger extensors, and digital abductors are synergistic. Beginning with the wrist flexed and the fingers extended and abducted, notice the ease with which the wrist can be extended and the fingers can be flexed and then the original position can be resumed; these positions can be exchanged with great speed. Now, beginning with both the wrist and fingers extended, flex the wrist and fingers and then resume the original position; these movements are slower and more awkward and must be directed consciously. Therefore it is obvious in treating muscle imbalance that tendons whose muscles are normally synergistic with the weakened or paralyzed ones should be first choice for transfer.

When a major muscle is paralyzed, in addition to loss of power to perform any particular function for which the muscle is directly responsible, the balance of the hand is disrupted, the various stable positions are endangered, and coordination is made difficult. Any muscle whose antagonist is paralyzed contracts unopposed and eventually develops a fixed contracture; its enveloping fascia becomes contracted, and the ligaments of any unmoved joint also contract when the joint is motionless in a position that permits shortening of the ligaments. Contractures may increase the stability of the hand, but at the same time they usually increase its disability. An imbalance resulting in contractures is demonstrated dramatically in paralysis of the intrinsic muscles which, when untreated, results in a clawhand deformity (Fig. 70-3). Because the lumbricals and other intrinsic muscles are paralyzed, the powerful long finger flexors are unopposed and flex the interphalangeal joints of the fingers; the long finger extensors, also unopposed, extend the metacarpophalangeal joints. The interphalangeal joints remain flexed even though a strong extensor force is exerted at the metacarpophalangeal joints; without stabilization of the metacarpophalangeal joints in a neutral or slightly flexed position by the intrinsics, the long extensors cannot extend the interphalangeal joints. Finally the wrist is pulled into flexion by the strong finger flexors; this causes a tenodesing effect on the long finger extensors that hyperextends the metacarpophalangeal joints even farther. In addition to deformities of the fingers, the thumb is adducted by its long extensor because this muscle is unopposed by the intrinsic muscles of opposition and abduction. This adducted position is accompanied by extension of the carpometacarpal joint, which in turn increases tension on the long thumb flexor tendon that crosses the volar side of the joint; thus the interphalangeal joint is flexed because the long flexor is unopposed by the adductor pollicis and abductor pollicis brevis muscles that normally aid in extending it. The position of the hand just described is known as the *intrinsic minus* position, and in it secondary joint contractures or even subluxations occur. Whether the loss of intrinsic function is caused by disease or by trauma, the results of dynamic muscle imbalance are the same. However, sensation in clawhand varies according to the cause of imbalance: in poliomyelitis sensation is normal, in peripheral nerve lesions the presence or absence of sensation depends on the level of the lesion and the nerve involved, in Hansen's disease sensation is absent, sometimes in a glovelike distribution, and in syringomyelia sensation is partially absent.

Spasticity of muscles can also disrupt the balance of the hand. Muscle tension may be constantly or intermittently increased and may not be controlled and balanced effectively by the opposing normal muscles. Such a situation is sometimes seen in cases of cerebral palsy and it can cause overstretching of muscles and dislocation of joints.

PRINCIPLES OF TENDON TRANSFER

Tendon transfers are useful in restoring functions of the hand lost because of paralysis produced by disease or trauma. However, some basic principles must be followed if transfers are to be successful and if an increase in imbalance and thus in deformity is to be avoided. After these principles are discussed, some frequent patterns of functional loss will be discussed, and specific tendons for transfer will be suggested for each.

Planning Tendon Transfer

Whether the original cause of imbalance has been traumatic, congenital, infectious, or vascular, the hand must be evaluated in terms of function lost and function retained. Before appropriate muscles for transfer can be selected, those available for transfer must be known; their strength, their amplitude of excursion, the synergistic group to which they belong, and the importance of their present function must all be considered. Sometimes it is helpful to list in one column functions that should be restored and in an opposite column the tendons avail-

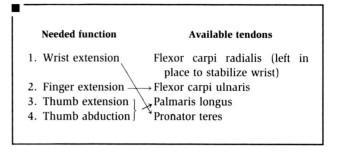

Needed function	Available tendons
1. Wrist extension	Flexor carpi radialis (left in place to stabilize wrist)
2. Finger extension	Flexor carpi ulnaris
3. Thumb extension	Palmaris longus
4. Thumb abduction	Pronator teres

able for transfer; transfers may be planned with more ease and accuracy by matching these columns, as shown in the accompanying chart of radial nerve palsy (see box above).

EVALUATING MUSCLES FOR TENDON TRANSFER. The two most important points in considering a muscle for transfer are its expendability and its strength. Restoring one major function such as finger extension is contraindicated if done at the expense of another major function such as finger flexion. The strength of a muscle is graded from 0 to 5 as follows:

0 Zero — no contraction
1 Trace — palpable contraction only
2 Poor — moves joint but not against gravity
3 Fair — moves joint against gravity
4 Good — moves joint against gravity and resistance
5 Normal — normal strength

A muscle will usually lose strength by one grade when transferred and therefore should be good or normal if the transfer is to be satisfactory. In addition to expendability and strength, the synergistic group in which the muscle acts and the amplitude of excursion of its tendon should be considered. As previously stated, rehabilitation of a muscle whose tendon has been transferred is less difficult when the transfer is synergistic (for example, a wrist flexor transfer to the finger extensors); therefore, although not essential, transferring a muscle within its own synergistic group is desirable. The amplitude of excursion of the tendon should be sufficient for satisfactory function, although it may not be as great as that of the tendon or tendons it will replace. For example, the brachioradialis, an expendable muscle for transfer, is capable of pulling its tendon through only a short excursion but can sometimes be useful, if not ideal, as a transfer to the long thumb flexor, because even limited flexion of the interphalangeal joint of the thumb is useful.

However, as pointed out by Boyes, the excursion of the brachioradialis can be increased by dissecting its tendon proximally and freeing all of its fascial attachments. The muscle is not useful as a transfer to a finger flexor because the limited motion it can produce in finger joints, even after its excursion has been increased, is of little value.

TIME OF TENDON TRANSFER. The transfer of tendons is the final step in rehabilitation of the hand. It should not be made until any scar tissue has been satisfactorily replaced because transferred tendons must be surrounded by fat to prevent their adhering to raw bone or subcutaneous scar; consequently a flap graft containing fat is necessary to replace scar. A satisfactory range of passive joint motion is also necessary *before* the transfer; proper splinting or ligamentous release is carried out as needed. Stiffness or contracture of joints cannot be corrected by tendon transfers alone; furthermore, if uncorrected, stiffness or contracture will prevent a transferred tendon from moving at the proper time after surgery so that the tendon becomes permanently adherent to the surrounding tissues. Also malalignment of bone must be corrected by osteotomy, and any necessary bone grafting must be carried out before transfer. Finally, necessary operations to restore any loss of sensibility must precede tendon transfer.

Other factors sometimes must be considered in timing tendon transfers. In poliomyelitis some recovery of muscle power may be expected until 18 months after the acute stage of the disease, and consequently this much time must pass before an accurate evaluation is possible; then any further recovery cannot be expected to improve muscle strength more than one grade, if any. During this period of waiting, parts must be properly splinted to improve available muscle function and to prevent fixed deformity. In congenital anomalies the relative muscle strength will not change. In syringomyelia weakness may increase even after transfer. Peripheral nerve injuries must be considered individually; in division of the radial nerve at the midhumerus, transfers for finger and thumb extension and for thumb abduction should be delayed for 6 months or longer after neurorrhaphy; however, early transfer to restore wrist extension should be considered. This provides an internal splint for the wrist and immediately improves the function of the hand. Transfer of the pronator teres to the extensor carpi radialis brevis is recommended. In high median nerve lesions, some function should return in the most proximal muscles in 4 months (and in 3 months in low median nerve lesions) or the nerve should be explored or tendon transfers should be considered.

Technical Considerations for Tendon Transfer

The strength of the muscle has been evaluated clinically before surgery, but its color at the time of tendon transfer provides a further check. A muscle suitable for transfer is dark pink or red, indicating satisfactory nutrition and the presence of normal muscle fibers. A weak or paralyzed muscle is pale pink and is smaller than normal, and its amplitude of excursion (Table 70-1) is less than normal when tested at surgery; such a muscle is not suitable for transfer (Fig. 70-4).

Table 70-1 Amplitude of excursion

Tendons	Amplitude (mm)
Wrist tendons	33
Flexor profundus	70
Flexor sublimis	64
Extensor digitorum communis	50
Flexor pollicis longus	52
Extensor pollicis longus	58
Extensor pollicis brevis	28
Abductor pollicis longus	28

From Curtis RM: Orthop Clin North Am 5:231, 1974.

A muscle that has been detached from its insertion some time before transfer will have developed a contracture, and consequently its tendon should be anchored under more tension than usual because it will stretch and regain some of its excursion. A muscle and its tendon should not make an acute angle between the origin of the muscle and the new attachment of the tendon — the straighter the muscle the more efficient its action. When an acute angle is necessary, a pulley must be created, but efficiency of the muscle is diminished by friction at the pulley. In freeing a muscle for transfer, care must be taken to avoid stretching or otherwise damaging the neurovascular bundle, which usually enters the proximal third of the muscle belly. A transferred tendon cannot be expected to glide properly when it crosses raw bone, passes through fascia without a sufficient opening, or is buried within scarred tissue; with a few exceptions, transferred tendons should be passed subcutaneously. Should it be necessary to split a transferred tendon and anchor it to two or more separate points, the muscle will act primarily on the slip of tendon under greatest tension and may distort function; thus great care must be taken to equalize tension on the slips at the time of attachment.

The more distal to a given joint a tendon is anchored, the more power the muscle can exert on the joint but also the more is the excursion required of the tendon to provide normal motion. Furthermore, the greater the angle of approach of a tendon to bone, the greater the force the muscle can exert on the bone and across the joint, but this creates a bowstring effect in a pulleyless system. Most muscles lie almost parallel to the bones whose joints they act on, and few approach a bone at close to a right angle; the pronator quadratus and the supinator are notable exceptions.

RESTORATION OF PINCH
Restoration of Opposition of Thumb

Opposition of the thumb is necessary for pinch — one of the three most important functions of the hand. But adduction of the thumb is necessary too (see discussion

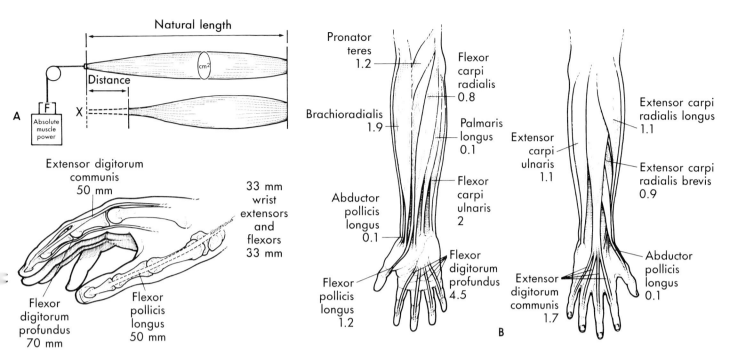

Fig. 70-4 Power of muscle transfer (**A** and **B**). **A,** Working capacity of muscle. $W = Fxd$, when F (force) = absolute muscle power, $3.65 \times cm^2$ of physiologic cross section and d (distance) = amplitude or displacement. **B,** Working capacity of muscle in mkg (meter-kilograms). **C,** Muscle amplitude in millimeters. (Redrawn from Curtis RM: Orthop Clin North Am 5:231, 1974.)

on restoration of adduction of thumb, p. 3243). Frequently opposition is either partially or totally lost in poliomyelitis or median nerve palsy. Opposition depends primarily on function of the intrinsic muscles of the thumb, especially the abductor pollicis brevis. Yet, extrinsic muscles are also necessary to stabilize dynamically the metacarpophalangeal and interphalangeal joints of the thumb, or these joints must be stabilized by arthrodesis or tenodesis. At the same time, the carpometacarpal joint of the thumb must be freely movable, unrestricted by contracture of the joint capsule or other structures of the thumb web (see discussion of the adducted thumb).

Opposition of the thumb is a complex motion made by coordination of (1) abduction of the thumb from the palmar surface of the index finger, (2) flexion of the metacarpophalangeal joint of the thumb, (3) internal rotation or pronation of the thumb, (4) radial deviation of the proximal phalanx of the thumb on the metacarpal, and finally (5) motion of the thumb toward the fingers. Although opposition is the result of coordinate function of all the long and short muscles that act on the thumb, the abductor pollicis brevis is the most important single muscle that takes part in this complex movement: it rotates internally and abducts the thumb away from the index metacarpal, internally rotates and abducts the proximal phalanx of the thumb on its metacarpal, and assists the extensor pollicis longus in extending the interphalangeal joint of the thumb. For these reasons, Littler and Riordan both recommend that in restoring opposition by

tendon transfer the transferred tendon be inserted into the tendon of the abductor pollicis brevis.

CORRECTION OF DEFORMITY OF THUMB. To restore function of the thumb properly, deformities or disabilities of the digit other than those corrected by the operation designed primarily to restore opposition frequently must be corrected either before or during such surgery. As a substitute for opposition, adduction of the thumb by the long thumb extensor may have become a habit; in these instances, adduction and extension of the thumb occur as a single function in which the flexed tip of the thumb is brought against the base of the proximal phalanx of the index finger by the pull of the long thumb extensor toward Lister's tubercle. Thus pinch occurs at the base of a finger instead of at its tip, and therefore to pick up an object, the point of contact between the thumb and finger must be rotated downward (Fig. 70-5); this is accomplished by pronating the wrist, elevating the elbow, and abducting the shoulder. As the substitution patterns become more firmly established after paralysis of the intrinsic muscles of the thumb, the long thumb extensor tendon, acting as an adductor, gradually migrates into the web space between the thumb and index finger.

Any fixed adduction and external rotational deformity of the thumb must be corrected; this usually may be accomplished by dividing the fascia in the web space between the index and thumb metacarpals and by subperiosteal stripping of the ulnar side of the first metacarpal as recommended by Goldner and Irwin. When the defor-

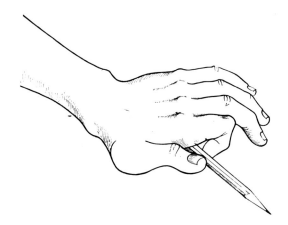

Fig. 70-5   Pattern of substitution for opposition (see text).

mity is severe, a Z-plasty of the web also may be required (see discussion of the adducted thumb, p. 3243), or if the deformity is so severe that it cannot be corrected by rotational osteotomy and release of the web space, arthrodesis of the first carpometacarpal joint may be indicated (p. 3190). A tendon transfer for opposition still may be useful after such an arthrodesis because the more proximal joints may allow some motion. However, when mobility is more desirable than stability, excising the trapezium (p. 3193) may release the soft tissues enough to make arthrodesis unnecessary.

Tendon transfers to the long thumb flexor, long thumb extensor, or long thumb abductor may be necessary to dynamically stabilize the thumb if the transfer to restore opposition is to function satisfactorily. Arthrodesis of the metacarpophalangeal joint of the thumb may be necessary when available muscle power is insufficient to stabilize it dynamically or when the joint is made unstable by relaxation of its ligaments or capsule. (Arthrodesis of this joint also may be indicated after tendon transfer to restore opposition when the tendon has been anchored in an incorrect location and hyperextends or hyperflexes the joint.) The joint is arthrodesed in 15 degrees of flexion and slight internal rotation. Arthrodesis of the interphalangeal joint of the thumb is indicated occasionally for a fixed flexion contracture; it is arthrodesed in 20 degrees of flexion (see discussion of arthrodesis, p. 3190).

TENDON TRANSFERS TO RESTORE OPPOSITION. Restoring opposition by tendon transfer has stimulated the imagination of many investigators: Steindler, Ney, Royle, Bunnell, Thompson, Irwin, Littler, Riordan, Brand, and others. Because elongated pinch is difficult to obtain in the paralytic hand but necessary to pick out objects from within a container, such as the last match from a box, new techniques of transfer still are being devised. Common to all techniques is the selection of one extrinsic, expendable, healthy muscle-tendon unit to be used as a motor and its transfer to a point on the thumb at a suitable angle to pull the thumb toward the position of oppo-

sition. The direction in which the transferred tendon approaches the thumb usually has been from the ulnar side of the wrist or palm; sometimes the tendon has been brought around a pulley to provide this direction. That a pulley is needed is now well recognized; some prefer a static pulley created by making a loop at the distal end of the flexor carpi ulnaris tendon, whereas others prefer a dynamic pulley formed by looping the transfer around this tendon.

The proper muscle for a motor is selected after carefully evaluating the strength of muscles in the rest of the hand. The flexor digitorum sublimis of the ring finger is the muscle of choice and is often used when it is strong enough to function as the transfer and when its associated flexor digitorum profundus is strong enough alone to flex the finger satisfactorily; second choice is the sublimis to the middle finger. When the preferred flexor tendons of the digits are not suitable for transfer, the extensor indicis proprius is an acceptable alternative. All other muscles require tendon grafting to reach the point of attachment on the thumb: the extensor carpi ulnaris is the next choice followed by the palmaris longus or extensor carpi radialis longus. However, a wrist extensor should be transferred only when the other wrist extensors are strong and have not been nor will be transferred elsewhere.

■ *TECHNIQUE (RIORDAN).* **Expose the sublimis tendon of the ring finger through an ulnar midlateral incision (p. 2972) over the proximal interphalangeal joint and divide the tendon at the level of the joint or just proximal to it. Divide the chiasm, thus separating the two slips of tendon at the level of the joint so they will pass around the profundus and can be withdrawn easily at the wrist. Now expose the flexor carpi ulnaris tendon through an L-shaped incision that proximally extends along the flexor carpi ulnaris tendon and distally turns radialward parallel to the flexor creases of the wrist. To make a pulley, cut halfway through the flexor carpi ulnaris tendon at a point approximately 6.3 cm proximal to the pisiform (Fig. 70-6). Then strip the radial half of the tendon distally almost to the pisiform and create a loop large enough for the sublimis tendon to pass through easily; carry the end of the radial segment of the flexor carpi ulnaris through a split in the remaining half of the tendon, loop it back, and suture it to the remaining half. Now make a wide C-shaped incision on the thumb as follows. Begin on the dorsum of the thumb just proximal to the interphalangeal joint and proceed proximally and volarward around to the radial aspect of the thumb. At a point just proximal to the metacarpophalangeal joint curve the incision dorsalward in line with the major skin creases of the thenar eminence. Preserve on the dorsoradial aspect of the thumb the fine sensory nerve from the superficial branch of the radial nerve. Expose and define the extensor pollicis lon-**

Fig. 70-6   Riordan transfer to restore opposition (see text).

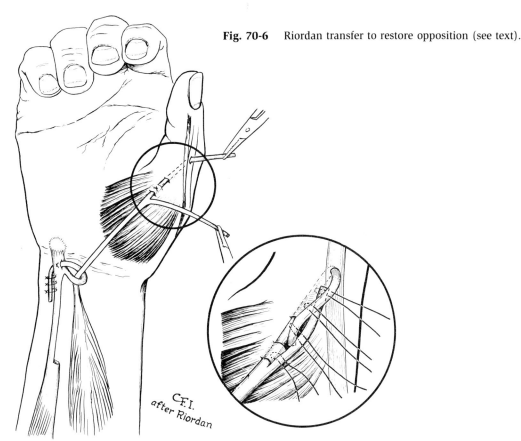

CF.I.
after Riordan

gus tendon over the proximal phalanx, the extensor aponeurosis over the metacarpophalangeal joint, and the tendon of the abductor pollicis brevis. Now at the wrist identify the sublimis tendon to the ring finger and withdraw it into the forearm incision. Pass the tendon through the loop fashioned from the flexor carpi ulnaris. Then, with a small hemostat or preferably a tendon carrier, pass the tendon subcutaneously across the thenar eminence in line with the fibers of the abductor pollicis brevis.

Now make a small tunnel for insertion of the transfer by burrowing between two small parallel incisions in the abductor pollicis brevis tendon. Split the end of the sublimis tendon for approximately 2.5 cm, or more if necessary, and pass one half of it through the tunnel. Now separate the extensor aponeurosis from the periosteum of the proximal phalanx of the thumb, make a small incision in it 6 mm distal to the first tunnel, and pass the same strip of sublimis through it. Bring the slip out from beneath the aponeurosis through a small longitudinal slit in the long extensor tendon about 3 mm proximal to the interphalangeal joint.

Next, determine the proper tension for the transfer. Grasp the two slips of sublimis with small hemostats and cross them. With the thumb in full opposition and the wrist in a straight line, place the two overlapping slips of sublimis under some tension. Releasing the thumb and passively flexing the

wrist should completely relax the transfer so that the thumb can be brought into full extension and abduction; extending the wrist 45 degrees should place enough tension on the transfer to bring the thumb into complete opposition and the tip of the thumb into complete extension. If the tension is insufficient, increase it and repeat the test. When the correct tension has been determined, suture the slips of sublimis together with the cut ends buried (Fig. 70-6). Now anchor the transfer and the tendon of the abductor pollicis brevis to the joint capsule with a single nylon or wire suture so that the transfer passes over the exact middle of the metacarpal head; this prevents later displacement of the tendon toward the palmar aspect of the joint during opposition. Close the wound with nonabsorbable sutures and immobilize the hand in a pressure dressing and a dorsal plaster splint as follows. Place the wrist in 30 degrees of flexion, the fingers in the functional position, and the thumb in full opposition with the distal phalanx extended; place a few layers of gauze between the individual fingers to prevent maceration of the skin.

AFTERTREATMENT. At 3 weeks the dressing and splint are removed and active motion is begun, but the thumb is supported with an opponens splint for an additional 6 weeks. Many patients can oppose the thumb as soon as the splint is removed. When the sublimis of the ring finger has been used for the transfer, as in the Riordan technique, training in its use may be facilitated by asking the patient to place the tip of the thumb against the ring finger; this maneuver produces flexion of the ring finger and an automatic attempt to oppose the thumb with the transferred sublimis. In patients with weak quadriceps muscles who habitually rise from a sitting position by pushing up with the flattened hands or in patients who use crutches, the transfer must be protected for 3 months or longer, or it will be overstretched and cease to function.

■ *TECHNIQUE (BRAND).* Expose and divide the sublimis tendon of the ring finger and make the incision over the thumb as just described in the Riordan technique. Withdraw the sublimis tendon through a small transverse incision about 5 cm proximal to the flexor crease of the wrist. Then make a small longitudinal incision just to the radial side of and about 6 mm distal to the pisiform. Deepen this incision until the quality of fat changes from the fibrous superficial type to a soft loose free type that bulges into the wound. This change in the fat marks the entry into a tunnel that runs proximally and contains a branch of the ulnar nerve. In this loose fat make a tunnel in the proximal direction to the forearm incision, grasp the end of the sublimis tendon, and pull it through into the palmar incision. The tunnel is superficial to the hook of the hamate, and the fibrous septa in the fat comprise the pulley. Then

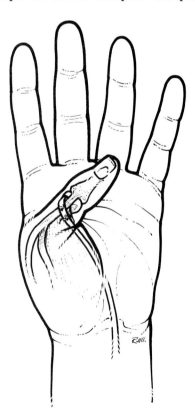

Fig. 70-7 Brand transfer to restore opposition. (Redrawn from White WL: Surg Clin North Am 40:427, 1960.)

pass the tendon to the metacarpophalangeal joint of the thumb and attach it proximal and distal to the joint after splitting its end: attach the proximal slip of the tendon to the ulnar side of the joint and the distal slip to the tendons of the abductor pollicis brevis and the extensor pollicis longus (Fig. 70-7). This dual insertion of the tendon may prevent the tendon from shifting in position as it crosses the metacarpophalangeal joint. (If an unsplit tendon shifts dorsally over the metacarpophalangeal joint, it is likely to hyperextend the joint, and if it shifts anteriorly from the radial side of the joint, it is likely to flex the joint.)

AFTERTREATMENT. Aftertreatment is similar to that described previously for the Riordan technique.

• • •

When the sublimis of the ring or middle finger is unsuitable for transfer, the extensor indicis proprius may be rerouted around the ulnar aspect of the wrist to provide opposition as described by Burkhalter et al. For high median nerve palsy or brachial plexus paralysis, a technique described by Groves and Goldner employing the flexor carpi ulnaris as a motor for a transferred sublimis tendon unit may be used.

TRANSFER OF EXTENSOR INDICIS PROPRIUS TO PROVIDE OPPOSITION OF THUMB

■ *TECHNIQUE (BURKHALTER ET AL.).* Through a short curved incision on the radial side of the dorsum of the metacarpophalangeal joint of the index finger, identify the extensor indicis proprius tendon (Fig. 70-8). Remove its insertion and a small portion of the extensor hood by sharp dissection, and then repair the hood with a single interrupted suture. If necessary, make a short incision over the midportion of the dorsum of the hand to withdraw the extensor tendon. Make a longitudinal incision about 2 cm long proximal to the wrist crease on the ulnar aspect of the forearm and through it extract the tendon. Cut the fascia as necessary to reroute the muscle. Make another small incision in the area of the pisiform bone and pass through it the tendon unit, creating a gradual curve from the dorsum of the forearm to this point. From the pisiform area, pass it subcutaneously to the tendinous portion of the abductor pollicis brevis just proximal to the metacarpophalangeal joint. Make another incision over the palmar side of the radial aspect of the metacarpophalangeal joint to expose the site of attachment. At this distal insertion, employ the technique of Riordan by splitting the tendon or simply pass it into the tendinous portion of the abductor pollicis brevis and suture it with several interrupted sutures. Suture the tendon under maximum tension with the thumb in full abduction but with the wrist in only slight volar flexion.

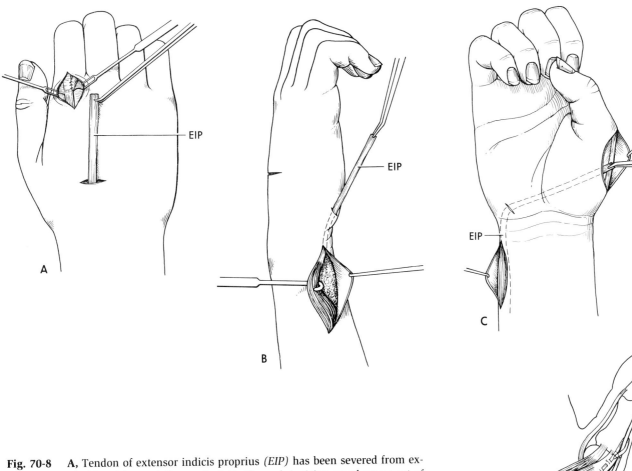

Fig. 70-8 **A,** Tendon of extensor indicis proprius *(EIP)* has been severed from extensor hood, and hood is carefully repaired. **B,** Through incision on ulnar aspect of forearm wide fascial excision is carried out and extensor indicis proprius muscle is transposed superficial to extensor carpi ulnaris through subcutaneous tissue. **C,** Tendon of extensor indicis proprius is brought out in area of pisiform and then passed again subcutaneously across palm to thumb. **D,** Method of attachment to thumb using abductor pollicis brevis tendon, metacarpophalangeal joint capsule, and extensor pollicis longus tendon over proximal phalanx. (Redrawn from Burkhalter W, Christensen RC, and Brown P: J Bone Joint Surg 55-A:725, 1973.)

AFTERTREATMENT. Aftertreatment consists of maintaining the wrist in flexion with a splint for a minimum of 3 weeks.

TRANSFER OF FLEXOR CARPI ULNARIS COMBINED WITH THE SUBLIMIS TENDON

■ *TECHNIQUE (GROVES AND GOLDNER).* Make incisions at the wrist as shown in Fig. 70-9. Remove the insertion of the sublimis tendon of the ring finger from the middle phalanx and bring it out at the wrist. Sever the flexor carpi ulnaris tendon, leaving a distal segment of this tendon sufficiently long to bring around the extensor carpi ulnaris tendon to create a pulley. Now pass the sublimis tendon through this pulley and continue it subcutaneously to the proximal end of the proximal phalanx of the thumb. Here insert one split portion of this tendon into the bone with a pull-out wire and another into the bone by direct attachment. Suture the proximal

functioning segment of the flexor carpi ulnaris and its tendon into the sublimis tendon unit under sufficient tension that dorsiflexion of the wrist provides full opposition of the thumb (Fig 70-9, *E*).

MUSCLE TRANSFER (ABDUCTOR DIGITI QUINTI) TO RESTORE OPPOSITION. When other motors are unavailable or must be transferred elsewhere, the abductor digiti quinti muscle may be transferred as first described in 1921 by Huber and more recently by Littler and Cooley (1963). This muscle, because its mass and excursion are similar to those of the abductor pollicis brevis, is an excellent substitute for it. Cosmetically the transfer is helpful, since it fills the space left by the wasted thenar muscles. It does not require a pulley.

■ *TECHNIQUE (LITTLER AND COOLEY).* Make a curved palmar incision along the radial border of the abductor digiti quinti muscle belly extending from the proximal side of the pisiform proximally to

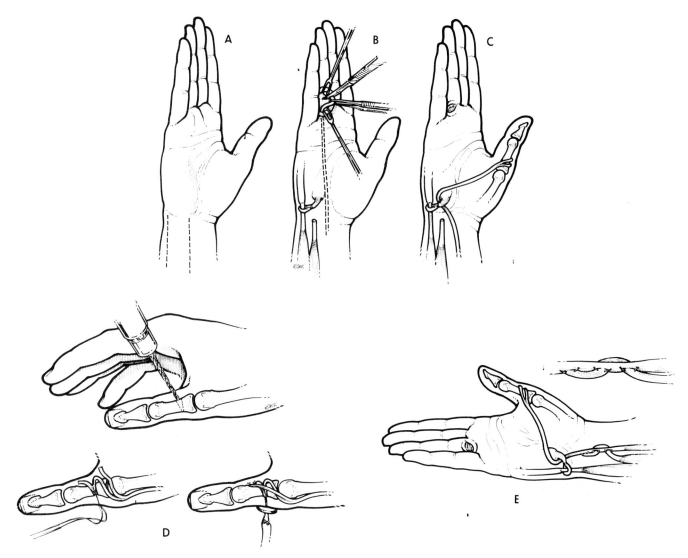

Fig. 70-9 **A,** Two incisions made at wrist. **B,** Through volar incision, flexor sublimis tendon to ring finger and flexor carpi ulnaris tendon are exposed. Through ulnar incision, extensor carpi ulnaris is exposed. Flexor carpi ulnaris tendon is divided 4 cm from its insertion, and free end of distal segment is sutured to extensor carpi ulnaris. Flexor digitorum sublimis tendon to ring finger is exposed through transverse incision at proximal flexor crease of finger, and its two slips are divided. **C,** Tendon of flexor digitorum sublimis to ring finger is drawn proximally through volar incision at wrist, threaded through pulley, and passed through subcutaneous tissue to metacarpophalangeal joint of thumb. **D,** Securing two slips of transferred tendon to base of proximal phalanx. Hole is made through proximal phalanx in ulnar-to-radial direction and is made larger on ulnar side to accept loop of one tendon slip, which is secured with pull-out suture. **E,** After transfer has been secured to thumb phalanx, tension is adjusted (see text) and proximal segment of flexor carpi ulnaris tendon is sutured to transferred tendon. (Redrawn from Groves RJ and Goldner JL: J Bone Joint Surg 57-A:112, 1975.)

the ulnar border of the little finger distally (Fig. 70-10). Free both tendinous insertions of the muscle, one from the extensor expansion and the other from the base of the proximal phalanx. Lift the muscle from its fascial compartment and carefully expose its neurovascular bundle. Isolate the bundle, taking care not to damage the veins. Next, free the origin of the muscle from the pisiform, but retain the origin on the flexor carpi ulnaris tendon; now the muscle can be mobilized enough for its insertion to reach the thumb. Make a curved incision on the radial border of the thenar eminence and create across the palm a subcutaneous pocket to receive the transfer. Now fold the abductor digiti quinti muscle over about 170 degrees (like a page of a book) and pass it subcutaneously to the thumb (Fig. 70-10, *C*). Suture its tendons of insertion to the insertion of the abductor pollicis brevis. Throughout the procedure avoid

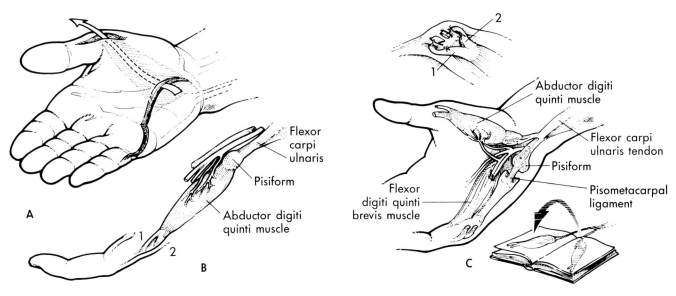

Fig. 70-10 Littler transfer of abductor digiti quinti to restore opposition. **A,** Two skin incisions. Intervening skin *(shaded area)* is undermined, creating pocket to receive transfer. **B,** Anatomy of abductor digiti quinti. Neurovascular bundle is located proximally on deep surface of muscle. Muscle inserts on both proximal phalanx, *1,* and extensor tendon, *2,* of little finger. **C,** Origin of muscle is freed from pisiform but not from flexor carpi ulnaris tendon. Muscle is folded over about 170 degrees and is passed subcutaneously to thenar area, and its two tendons of insertion, *1* and *2,* are sutured to abductor pollicis brevis tendon. (Modified from Littler JW and Cooley SGE: J Bone Joint Surg 45-A:1389, 1963.)

compression of and undue tension on the muscle and its neurovascular pedicle. Apply a carefully formed light compression dressing and then a volar plaster splint to hold the thumb in abduction and the wrist in slight flexion.

TRANSFER OF PALMARIS LONGUS TENDON TO ENHANCE OPPOSITION OF THUMB. In 1929 Camitz described a transfer of the palmaris longus tendon to enhance opposition of the thumb. Braun has recently called attention to this useful procedure. He recommends it when the abductor pollicis brevis has weakened and atrophied from a partial median nerve palsy, which happens in carpal tunnel syndrome. An advantage of the operation is its close proximity to the median nerve, which may require repair or release that can be done at the same time without much additional surgery. It does not produce true opposition, but elevates the thumb toward the flexed and abducted position.

■ *TECHNIQUE (CAMITZ).* Make a curved incision parallel to the base of the thenar crease and extend it proximally 1½ inches (3.8 cm) up the forearm. Isolate the palmaris longus tendon in the distal forearm and preserve its insertion on the deep palmar fascia. Then incise along parallel lines from the insertion to the palmaris longus into the palmar fascia, obtaining a strip of fascia distally to lengthen the tendon enough to reach the distal part of the ab-

ductor pollicis brevis tendon. Pass the lengthened tendon into a small skin incision made over the thumb metacarpal and suture it to the tendon of the abductor pollicis brevis under appropriate tension.

Restoration of Adduction of Thumb

Adduction of the thumb is as necessary for strong pinch as is opposition. Whereas opposition is the refined unique movement that places the thumb within the flexion arc of the fingers so that the tips of the thumb and fingers can oppose, adduction is the force that stabilizes the thumb in the desired position. When the adductor pollicis is paralyzed, as in ulnar nerve palsy, firm pinch between the pulps of the thumb and the flexed index and middle fingers is impossible; furthermore, the thumb cannot be brought across the palm for pinch with the ring and little fingers. Eventually the interphalangeal joint of the thumb becomes hyperflexed and the metacarpophalangeal joint becomes hyperextended. The flexor pollicis longus can provide some power of adduction when the thumb is held in slight adduction so that the muscle flexes the digit through an arc parallel to the plane of the palm.

Several transfers have been devised to restore adduction. When adduction alone is absent, the brachioradialis or one of the radial wrist extensors may be lengthened by a graft, transferred palmarward through the third interosseous space, and carried across the palm to the tendon of the adductor pollicis. Such a transfer provides adduction only and this in the direction normally provided by the adductor pollicis. It is most often indicated in ulnar nerve palsy because in this instance restoring abduction of the thumb is unnecessary; however, it should be combined with some procedure to restore abduction of the index finger. When both adduction and opposition of the thumb are absent, unless some other provision is made to restore adduction, a single tendon transfer to restore opposition should have its pulley located not near the pisiform but more distally so that some adduction also will be restored. The Royle-Thompson transfer meets this requirement. In it the flexor digitorum sublimis of the ring finger is brought out in the palm distal to the deep transverse carpal ligament that acts as a pulley. It is carried across the palm and is anchored to the tendon of the adductor pollicis. Opposition is only partially restored in that abduction and pronation of the thumb remain limited. To restore abduction of the index finger, as well as adduction of the thumb, the sublimis tendon may be split and one slip anchored to the tendon of the adductor pollicis and the other to the insertion of the first dorsal interosseus, as reported by Omer.

Several other operations are also available: the Brand transfer (Fig. 70-11) uses the sublimis of the ring finger as its motor. It traverses the palm superficial to the fascia and inserts on the radial aspect of the thumb. The sublimis is sectioned at the proximal phalanx through a short incision and is brought out at the midpalm just ulnar to the thenar crease. This tendon is passed through the natural openings of the fascia between the ring and middle fingers at the distal third of the palm. It is then passed subcutaneously to be inserted on the radial side of the thumb at the level of the metacarpophalangeal joint.

This tends to ensure pronation of the thumb as well as some restoration of power of adduction.

TRANSFER OF BRACHIORADIALIS OR A RADIAL WRIST EXTENSOR TO RESTORE THUMB ADDUCTION

■ *TECHNIQUE (BOYES)*. Transfer of the brachioradialis is preferred. Detach the insertion of the muscle and carefully free the tendon proximally of all fascial attachments, thus increasing its excursion. Then anchor a tendon graft (plantaris or palmaris longus) to the adductor tubercle of the thumb by a pull-out wire, or suture the graft to the tendon of insertion of the adductor pollicis. Pass the graft along the adductor muscle belly and through the third interosseous space to the dorsum of the hand (Fig. 70-12). Then pass it subcutaneously in a proximal and radial direction and suture it to the end of the brachioradialis tendon. When a radial wrist extensor is used, pass the tendon graft deep to the extensor digitorum communis tendons and attach it to the wrist extensor. Apply a plaster cast while holding the thumb in adduction and the wrist in extension. *AFTERTREATMENT*. At 3 weeks the cast is removed and active exercises are begun.

• • •

Smith reported 18 patients in whom he transferred the extensor carpi radialis brevis tendon to provide strong thumb adduction. To extend the tendon he used a ten-

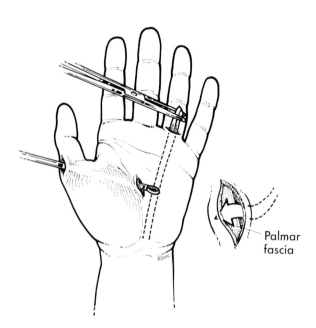

Fig. 70-11   Brand transfer (see text).

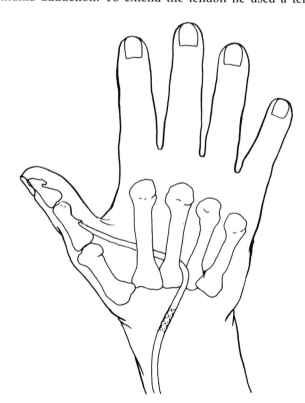

Fig. 70-12   Boyes transfer of brachioradialis or radial wrist extensor to restore thumb adduction (see text).

don graft and passed it through the second interosseous space. The operation was performed on patients in whom the power of pinch was 25% of normal or less because of paralysis of the adductor muscle. On the average, pinch was reported to have doubled in strength after the transfer (Figs. 70-13 and 70-14).

■ *TECHNIQUE (SMITH).* **Make two dorsal transverse incisions over the extensor carpi radialis brevis tendon proximal to its insertion (Fig. 70-14, *A*). Divide the tendon near its insertion on the third metacarpal base and withdraw it through the incision proximal to the dorsal retinaculum (Fig. 70-14, *B*). Now make a third incision between the second and third metacarpals and remove a window of tissue from the paralyzed interosseus muscles. Finally, make a longitudinal incision on the ulnar side of the metacarpophalangeal joint of the thumb. With a curved hemostat, tunnel deep to the adductor pollicis muscle and through the window in the second interosseous space. Secure an appropriate tendon graft (usually the palmaris longus tendon). Draw the graft through the tunnel from the thumb to the dorsum of the hand (Fig. 70-14, *C*), and suture it to the tendon of the adductor pollicis (Fig. 70-14, *D*). Now pass the proximal end of the graft subcutaneously to the most proximal incision (Fig. 70-14, *E*), and suture it to the extensor carpi radialis brevis tendon, taking up all slack, but with no tension, so that the thumb lies just palmar to the index finger with the wrist in neutral position (Fig. 70-14, *F*). Dorsiflex the wrist and note that the thumb is pulled into adduction. Then flex the wrist and note that the thumb lies firmly against the palm.**

AFTERTREATMENT. **The hand is immobilized in plaster with the thumb in neutral position and the wrist in 40 degrees of dorsiflexion. The plaster is removed in 3 weeks, and active motion is encouraged.**

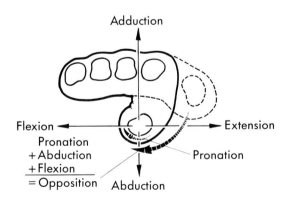

Fig. 70-13 Adduction and abduction of thumb are in plane perpendicular to palm. Flexion and extension of thumb are in palmar plane. Pronation and supination are rotation of the thumb about its longitudinal axis. Opposition is complex of abduction, flexion, and pronation of first metacarpal (as well as flexion/abduction of proximal phalanx and extension of distal phalanx). (Redrawn from Smith RC: J Hand Surg 8:4, 1983.)

ROYLE-THOMPSON TRANSFER, MODIFIED

■ *TECHNIQUE.* **Make a midlateral incision (p. 2972) over the ulnar aspect of the ring finger and free the insertion of the flexor digitorum sublimis tendon (Fig. 70-15). Then bring the tendon out of the palm through a short transverse incision and split it into two slips. Now make a curved incision on the dorsoradial aspect of the thumb as described for the Riordan transfer (p. 3238). Tunnel the slips of the sublimis tendon radially into this incision. Then suture one slip to the extensor pollicis longus tendon distal to the metacarpophalangeal joint; tunnel the other slip dorsally over the metacarpal and suture it on the ulnar side of the thumb to the tendon of insertion of the adductor pollicis (Brand's dual insertion). Close the wounds and apply a cast holding the thumb in adduction and the wrist in moderate flexion.**

AFTERTREATMENT. **At 3 weeks the cast is removed and active exercises are begun.**

RESTORATION OF ABDUCTION OF INDEX FINGER

The index is the finger against which the thumb is brought most frequently in pinch. Therefore if pinch is to be strong, this finger must be stable enough to provide the necessary resistance to the thumb; flexion, extension, abduction, and a stable metacarpophalangeal joint are required. Abduction of the index finger is also especially useful in such activities as playing a piano or using a typewriter. In poliomyelitis, abduction of the index finger is lost so frequently that its restoration is considered here separately from that of the intrinsic functions of the other fingers.

A transfer to restore abduction to this finger provides a substitute chiefly for the first dorsal interosseus muscle; therefore the transferred tendon is attached to the tendon of insertion of this muscle. The tendons most frequently transferred are those of the extensor indicis proprius, extensor pollicis brevis, and palmaris longus; any of these when transferred will abduct the index finger but will not stabilize it for strong pinch. A sublimis tendon also has been used, but this generally is contraindicated unless the hand is otherwise strong. When opposition also must be restored, the sublimis to the ring finger should be transferred to the thumb (p. 3240).

Transfer of the Extensor Indicis Proprius Tendon

■ *TECHNIQUE.* **Begin a curved incision at the midlateral point on the radial side of the proximal phalanx of the index finger; carry it proximally over the radial aspect of the metacarpophalangeal joint and then curve it dorsally to end at the middle of the in-**

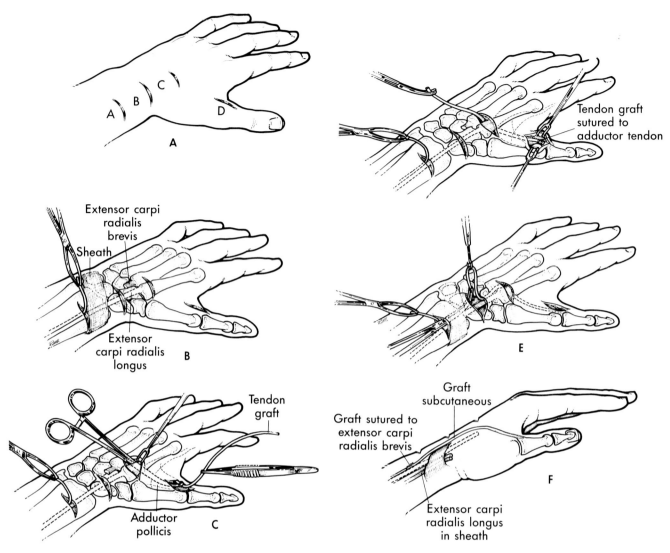

Fig. 70-14 **A** and **B,** Usual incision for detaching and withdrawing extensor carpi radialis brevis includes **C,** channeling tendon graft through second interspace, and **D,** attaching graft to tendon of adductor pollicis. **B,** Extensor carpi radialis brevis is transected distally and withdrawn proximal to dorsal retinacular ligament ("sheath"). **C,** Tendon graft (palmaris longus or plantaris) is passed deep to the adductor pollicis and between second and third metacarpals. **D,** Tendon graft is sutured to adductor tendon. **E,** Proximal end of tendon graft is passed subcutaneously to proximal incision. **F,** Tendon graft sutured proximally to extensor carpi radialis brevis with thumb adducted and wrist at zero degrees of extension. Extensor carpi radialis brevis is at resting length. Graft is made slightly longer if thenars are paralyzed. (Redrawn from Smith RC: J Hand Surg 8:4, 1983.)

dex metacarpal. To add length to the extensor indicis proprius tendon, elevate a small flap of the dorsal expansion over the metacarpophalangeal joint where it is attached to the insertion of the tendon. Withdraw the tendon proximally, free it throughout the wound, and close the defect in the expansion. Then pass the tendon radially in a gentle curve, roughen the tendon of the first dorsal interosseus muscle, and suture the transferred tendon to it with a single mattress suture.

• • •

When fusion of the metacarpophalangeal joint of the thumb is necessary because of an unacceptable hyperex-

tension deformity in ulnar nerve palsy, the extensor pollicis brevis tendon may be transferred to the first dorsal interosseus since it is no longer useful in its normal position.

Transfer of Slip of Abductor Pollicis Longus Tendon

Neviaser, Wilson, and Gardner have suggested transfer of a slip of the abductor pollicis longus tendon to replace the first dorsal interosseus muscle. In most patients the abductor pollicis longus tendon consists of two or more slips; in only 20% or less is there a single tendon here. The normal insertion is on the base of the thumb meta-

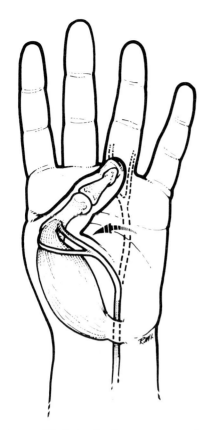

Fig. 70-15 Modified Royle-Thompson transfer to restore thumb adduction (see text).

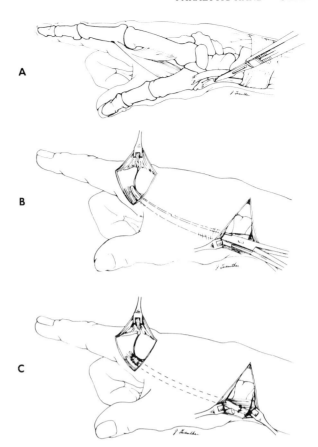

Fig. 70-16 **A,** Accessory slip inserting into trapezium is detached distal to retinaculum. Functional slip, inserting into metacarpal, is preserved. **B,** Subcutaneous tunnel is created from radial styloid to insertion of first dorsal interosseus. **C,** Tendon graft is woven into tendon of the first dorsal interosseus and sutured to the accessory slip. (From Neviaser RJ, Wilson JN, and Gardner MM: J Hand Surg 5:53, 1980.)

carpal and one or more of the extra slips insert on the trapezium or into the abductor pollicis brevis. One of these extra slips is used in this transfer. The authors reported 18 hands on which the operation was performed. They did not present comparative measurements of strength but stated that all patients had satisfactory pinch and stability and an increase in strength.

■ *TECHNIQUE (NEVIASER, WILSON, AND GARDNER).* Make a transverse incision near the insertion of the abductor pollicis longus. Identify the slips of the abductor tendon at the level of the radial styloid and note their insertions. Take care to avoid the branches of the superficial radial nerve. Apply traction to each of the slips to determine which insert on the metacarpal and which insert elsewhere. Select a slip that does not insert on the metacarpal and divide it at its insertion. Then make a second incision over the radial side of metacarpophalangeal joint of the index finger and identify the tendon of the first dorsal interosseus muscle. The authors prefer a chevron incision with its base dorsally (Fig. 70-16). Now make a subcutaneous tunnel from the radial styloid to the base of the index finger. Obtain a tendon graft from the palmaris longus or elsewhere and weave it into the first dorsal interosseus tendon distal to the metacarpophalangeal joint.

Pass the graft subcutaneously into the area of the radial styloid without disturbing the first dorsal

compartment. At the level of the radial styloid, with both the index finger and the wrist in neutral position, suture the graft to the selected slip of the abductor pollicis longus.

AFTERTREATMENT. The wrist is immobilized for 3 to 4 weeks and then active exercise is begun.

RESTORATION OF INTRINSIC FUNCTION OF FINGERS

Loss of intrinsic muscle function of the fingers may result from paralytic disease or low median and ulnar nerve lesions; low lesions of these nerves cause selective paralysis of the intrinsic muscles but spare the long extrinsics to act unopposed (Fig. 70-17) and produce a clawhand. The mechanics of development of this deformity are discussed in the introduction to this chapter.

Loss of intrinsic muscle power may cause hyperextension of the metacarpophalangeal joints in a mobile hand; however, this deformity usually is not the primary or most disabling aspect of this paralysis. It has been shown

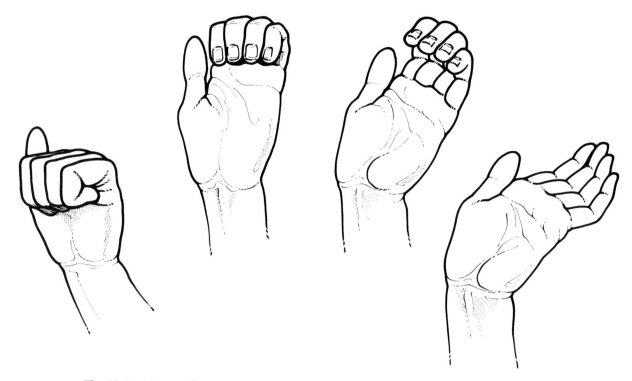

Fig. 70-17 Low median and ulnar nerve palsy. Action of extrinsic flexors of fingers when all of intrinsic muscles are paralyzed. From right to left note that these long flexors first flex distal interphalangeal joints, then flex proximal interphalangeal joints, and finally flex metacarpophalangeal joints. (Redrawn from White WL: Surg Clin North Am 40:427, 1960.)

that with intrinsic paralysis, grasp is diminished 50% or more because of the lack of power of flexion at the metacarpophalangeal joints. Additionally, there is asynchronous movement in flexion of the fingers themselves (Fig. 70-18). The roll-up maneuver of the fingers in the intrinsically paralyzed hand demonstrates this characteristic (see Fig. 70-17). The interphalangeal joints must flex first, followed next by the metacarpophalangeal joints and ultimately by full flexion of the fingers. In-phase flexion of the metacarpophalangeal joints is lost with the loss of intrinsic muscle power; thus the hand is unable to grasp a large object. As previously mentioned, it also lacks power of grasp because metacarpophalangeal flexion depends entirely on the long flexors in the absence of intrinsics. Power of pinch is also diminished in addition to the effects of paralysis of the thenar muscles since the collateral ligaments of the metacarpophalangeal joints of the fingers are lax in extension and the stabilizing intrinsic musculature that would ordinarily give lateral stability is paralyzed. Divergence of the fingers is automatic with extension produced by the long extensor tendons, and as a result of the alignment of the finger flexors, convergence of the tips on grasping is automatic. However, to stabilize the fingers in extension at the metacarpophalangeal joint, especially for the resistance of the index finger to the pinch pressure of the thumb, the intrinsics are essential.

Many procedures have been devised to block hyperextension of the metacarpophalangeal joints, but stabilizing these joints at a selected position and permitting controlled deviation from side to side requires functioning intrinsic muscles.

The restoration of grasping power should be sought when there are suitable muscles available for the reconstruction, but this will depend on individual circumstances.

In this section detailed knowledge of both the anatomy and function of the intrinsic muscles is assumed and will not be reviewed; however, it must be emphasized here that the interosseus and lumbrical muscles flex the metacarpophalangeal joints and extend the interphalangeal joints of the fingers but that the long finger extensors are capable of extending the interphalangeal joints if the metacarpophalangeal joints are stabilized and cannot hyperextend (see Fig. 70-3). This principle (that the long finger extensors can extend interphalangeal joints provided that hyperextension of the metacarpophalangeal joints is prevented) is the basis for many of the operations for intrinsic paralysis. The metacarpophalangeal joints may be stabilized by capsuloplasty (Zancolli), by tenodesis (Riordan), by bone block (Mikhail), by arthrodesis, or by tendon transfers that actively extend the interphalangeal joints as well as flex the metacarpophalangeal joints. The proper operation for

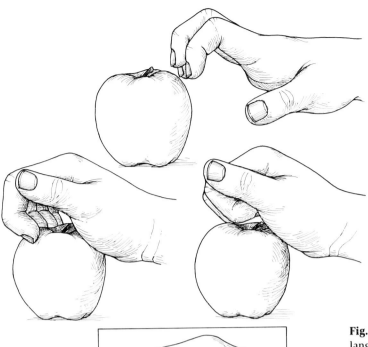

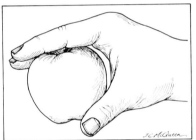

Fig. 70-18 Intrinsic muscle palsy. Flexion of metacarpophalangeal joints occurs only after interphalangeal joints are fully flexed. Fingers thus curl into the hand and push away any large object they wish to grasp. *Inset,* Object is grasped after compensatory manipulation. (Redrawn from Smith RJ: AAOS Instr Course Lect 24:200, 1975.)

a given hand depends on the muscles available for transfer, the amount of passive motion present in the finger and wrist joints, and the opinion and experience of the surgeon. Transfers to replace intrinsic function of the fingers are the most variable, complicated, and surgically difficult ones carried out in the hand. Several different transfers have been devised, but no one has been accepted universally, and rightly so, because each hand is an individual problem, even when the only concern is intrinsic paralysis.

Sir Harold Stiles in 1922 attempted to restore intrinsic function by detaching a sublimis tendon, splitting it, and transferring it to the dorsum of the fingers to the extensor tendons. He did not report on followed patients. Bunnell in 1942 modified this procedure by detaching the sublimis tendon from each finger, splitting it, and passing one slip to each side of the extensor aponeurosis of each finger by way of the lumbrical canals. This transfer removed the powerful flexor of the proximal interphalangeal joints and converted it into an extensor of the same joints. In many instances this transfer has been too strong and has pulled the proximal interphalangeal joints into extension, especially when the hand has been supple before surgery; this complication, which produces an intrinsic plus deformity, has been known to occur several months to many years after the transfer. How-

ever, a modification of this procedure in which only one sublimis is transferred to all fingers may be useful in treating clawhands with some restriction of motion in the proximal interphalangeal joints (Fig. 70-19).

Frequently, flexing the wrist in an attempt to extend the interphalangeal joints has become a necessary habit after intrinsic paralysis. Its object is to create a tenodesing effect on the long extensor tendons. If this flexion is too marked, the Bunnell transfer is rendered ineffective, but when the intrinsics are weak but not paralyzed, the transfer may be useful if the wrist extensors are strong enough to prevent flexion of the wrist. When flexing the wrist is a chronic habit and a wrist flexor can be spared, Riordan has transferred the flexor carpi radialis (see Fig. 70-26).

Fowler has split the extensor proprius tendons of the index and little fingers to form four slips and has attached one each to the extensor aponeuroses on the radial side of the index and middle fingers and on the ulnar side of the ring and little fingers. In a later modification, the tendons are split as described, but the slips are passed to the volar side of the deep transverse metacarpal ligament and are attached to the radial side of the extensor aponeurosis of each finger (Figs. 70-20 and 70-21). This is a more efficient transfer and has the advantage of a tenodesing effect when the wrist is flexed.

However, the ends of the tendon slips must be advanced about 2.5 cm to reach their destinations on the extensor aponeuroses and are therefore under considerable tension; sometimes an intrinsic overpull or intrinsic plus deformity develops. This excessive tension may be avoided as follows. The detached end of the extensor indicis proprius tendon is split into two slips, passed to the volar side of the deep transverse metacarpal ligament, and attached to the radial side of the ring and little fingers. One end of a free tendon graft is then attached to the musculotendinous junction of the extensor indicis proprius, and the other end is split into two slips that are passed distally in a similar manner and attached to the radial side of the middle and index fingers. Riordan has further

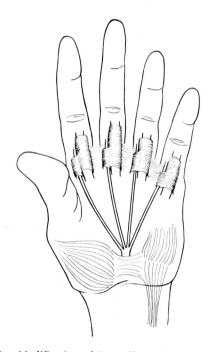

Fig. 70-19 Modification of Bunnell transfer to restore intrinsic function of fingers (see text).

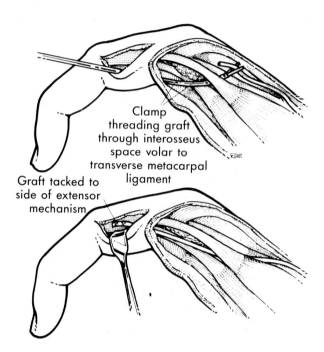

Fig. 70-20 Any tendons transferred from dorsum of hand to restore intrinsic function of fingers *must pass to volar side* of deep transverse metacarpal ligament.

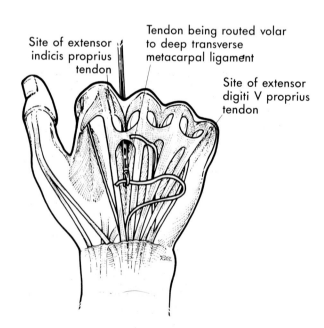

Fig. 70-21 Fowler transfer to restore intrinsic function of fingers (see text).

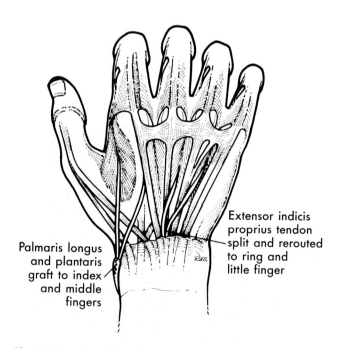

Fig. 70-22 Riordan transfer to restore intrinsic function of fingers (see text).

modified this procedure by attaching the tendon graft to the freed insertion of the palmaris longus tendon instead of to the musculotendinous junction of the extensor indicis proprius (Fig. 70-22).

Brand has had much experience in evaluating transfers for intrinsic paralysis in Hansen's disease. He devised a technique using the extensor carpi radialis brevis tendon lengthened by a free graft from the plantaris tendon (Fig. 70-23); the distal end of the graft is split into four slips or tails, and each tail is passed to the volar side of the deep transverse metacarpal ligament and is attached on the radial side of each proximal phalanx to the extensor aponeurosis, except in the index finger where it is attached on the ulnar side. In his opinion, index finger pinch can be secured more firmly when the finger is in adduction rather than in abduction (Fig. 70-24). More recently he has advised transferring the extensor carpi radialis longus or brevis to the volar side of the forearm and extending it by a four-tailed graft through the carpal tunnel and the lumbrical canals and finally to the extensor aponeuroses as before (Fig. 70-25). This transfer crowds the carpal tunnel and may cause symptoms of median nerve compression should the nerve be functioning.

For severe clawing of the hand with flexion of the wrist, Riordan advises freeing the insertion of the flexor carpi radialis and transferring it to the dorsum of the wrist; here it is prolonged with a four-tailed graft, each tail of which is passed volar to the deep transverse metacarpal ligament and is attached to the radial sides of the extensor aponeuroses (Fig. 70-26).

The procedures just described require that muscles strong enough for transfer be available. When they are not, a capsuloplasty or a tenodesing procedure to stabilize the metacarpophalangeal joints may be indicated. Zancolli described a satisfactory capsulodesis (Fig. 70-27). Riordan devised a tenodesing procedure in which the extensor carpi radialis brevis and extensor carpi ulnaris tendons are each cut halfway through at about the level of the junction of the middle and distal thirds of the forearm; a half of each tendon is then stripped distally and is left attached at its insertion on a metacarpal base. Each strand of tendon is split into two strips forming four slips; each slip is then passed through an interosseous space and along the volar side of the deep transverse metacarpal ligament to a finger and is attached to the radial side of its extensor aponeurosis. The disadvantage of this tenodesis is that it cannot be activated by motion of the wrist as can the Fowler tenodesis. Fowler uses a free tendon graft attached to the fingers as in the Riordan technique but anchored proximally in the area of the dorsal carpal ligament proximal to the wrist. Thus when the wrist is flexed the tenodesis is activated (Fig. 70-28).

When the finger flexors and the wrist flexors and extensors are strong and when there is no habitual flexion of the wrist, the operation of choice to restore function of

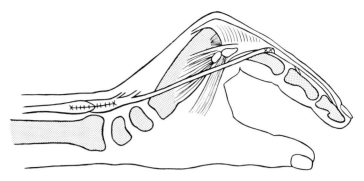

Fig. 70-23   Brand transfer of extensor carpi radialis brevis tendon prolonged with free graft to restore intrinsic function of fingers (see text).

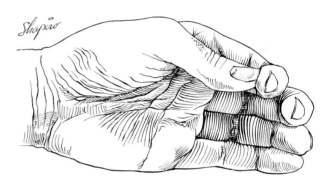

Fig. 70-24   When firm pinch will be more useful than abduction of index finger, transferred tendon is attached to ulnar lateral band of extensor hood rather than to insertion of first dorsal interosseus muscle. Note that during pinch index finger is in adduction rather than in abduction. (From White WL: Surg Clin North Am 40:427, 1960.)

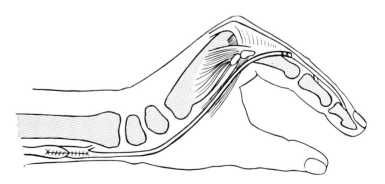

Fig. 70-25   Brand transfer of extensor carpi radialis longus or brevis, first to volar side of forearm and then, after being prolonged with free graft, to extensor aponeuroses to restore intrinsic function of fingers (see text).

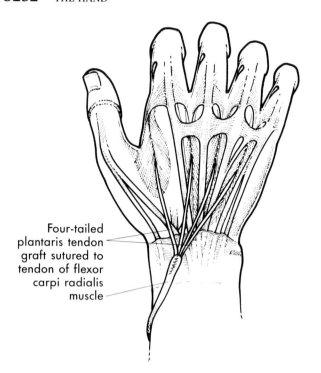

Four-tailed
plantaris tendon
graft sutured to
tendon of flexor
carpi radialis
muscle

Fig. 70-26 Riordan transfer to restore intrinsic function of fingers (see text).

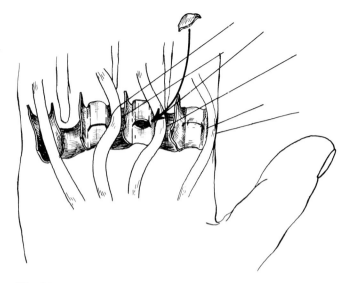

Fig. 70-27 Zancolli capsulodeses for intrinsic paralysis (see text).

the finger intrinsics is the modified Bunnell procedure in which the flexor digitorum sublimis of the ring finger is transferred (see Fig. 70-19). When flexing the wrist is habitual or there is a flexion contracture of the joint and when a wrist flexor can be spared, the Riordan transfer of the flexor carpi radialis to the dorsum of the wrist prolonged by tendon grafts (see Fig. 70-26) is a good choice; however, at least one strong wrist flexor should remain after the transfer. When the wrist extensors are strong and the flexors are weak, the Brand transfer of the extensor carpi radialis longus volarward and prolonged by a free graft through the carpal tunnel (see Fig. 70-25) may be indicated. The Brand transfer of the extensor carpi radialis brevis prolonged by a free graft carried between the metacarpals and attached to the extensor aponeuroses (see Fig. 70-23) may be complicated by difficulty in reeducation. When a flexor digitorum sublimis or a wrist flexor or extensor is not available for transfer or cannot be spared, the extensor proprius tendons of the index and little fingers may be transferred by the Fowler technique (see Figs. 70-20 and 70-21) or the Riordan modification of the Fowler technique in which the palmaris longus tendon is one of the transfers (see Fig. 70-22) that may be used. When no muscle is available for transfer and when the joints are supple, the Zancolli capsulodesis of the metacarpophalangeal joints (see Fig. 70-27), a Fowler tenodesis (see Fig. 70-28), or a Riordan tenodesis may be indicated.

The tendency to overload the extensor mechanism by routine attachment of transferred tendons to the lateral bands has been noted; this means that the desirable

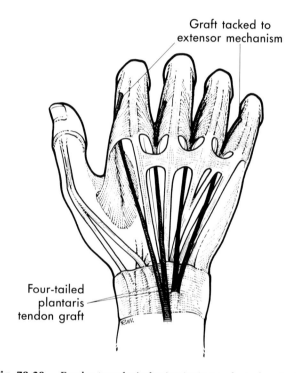

Graft tacked to
extensor mechanism

Four-tailed
plantaris
tendon graft

Fig. 70-28 Fowler tenodesis for intrinsic paralysis (see text).

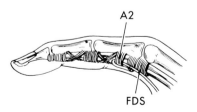

A2

FDS

Fig. 70-29 Flexor digitorum slip *(FDS)* inserted into strip of annular ligament *(A2)* at the middle of the proximal phalanx. (Redrawn from slide supplied by Brooks in Riordan DC: J Hand Surg 8:748, 1983.)

flexor power to the metacarpophalangeal joints is not obtained; therefore Brooks and Jones have suggested attaching the transfers to the flexor tendon sheath (Fig. 70-29) and, depending on the intact extensor power, extending the proximal interphalangeal joints with the metacarpophalangeal joints stabilized. Likewise, Burkhalter and others have suggested a bony attachment of the transferred tendon to the midportion of the proximal phalanx to provide leverage for flexion at the metacarpophalangeal joint and a better restoration of grip (see Fig. 70-39). However, we have found the Zancolli tendon insertion into the flexor sheath to be much less time consuming than insertion into bone. It also eliminates the tendency for hyperextension of the proximal interphalangeal joint as occurs sometimes when the tendon is inserted into the extensor mechanism.

Transfer of Flexor Digitorum Sublimis of Ring Finger

■ *TECHNIQUE (BUNNELL, MODIFIED).* Transfer the sublimis tendon of either the ring or middle finger. Make a midlateral incision (p. 2972) about 3.8 cm long on the radial side of the selected finger, beginning at the midshaft of the proximal phalanx and extending distally to beyond the proximal interphalangeal joint. Deepen the incision to the flexor tendon sheath, open the sheath laterally, and identify and divide the sublimis tendon at the level of the proximal interphalangeal joint. Separate the two slips of the tendon so that the tendon can be withdrawn into the palm. Now make a transverse incision about 3.8 cm long at the level of the proximal palmar crease. Identify the sublimis tendon, withdraw it through the palmar incision, and split it into four equal tails. Now make a longitudinal incision about 2.5 cm long on the radial side (and slightly dorsal) of the proximal phalanx of each finger, except the donor finger, and identify the extensor aponeuroses. Then with either a narrow instrument, a wire loop, or a tendon carrier, pass each tail of tendon through the lumbrical canal of a finger and over the oblique fibers of the extensor aponeurosis to its dorsum (see Fig. 70-19). Passage through the lumbrical canals should be easy; if any obstruction is met, redirect the instrument. Now with the metacarpophalangeal joint at 80 or 90 degrees of flexion, the interphalangeal joints at neutral, and the wrist at 30 degrees of flexion, suture each tail to the aponeurosis under some tension with interrupted sutures and bury its end. Usually 2.5 to 3.8 cm of redundant tendon must be excised. Close the incisions and immobilize the hand with the wrist in neutral position, the metacarpophalangeal joints in flexion, and the interphalangeal joints in extension.

Brooks recommends attaching each transfer to the flexor pulley at the level of the proximal pha-

lanx, thus preventing the development of hyperextension deformities of the proximal interphalangeal joints.

AFTERTREATMENT. At 3 weeks the cast is removed and each finger is splinted with a plaster or plastic gutter splint in a neutral position. Movement of the metacarpophalangeal joints and resisted active extension of the wrist are then encouraged. The finger splints are removed and are reapplied daily until reeducation is complete.

Transfer of the Extensor Carpi Radialis Longus or Brevis Tendon

■ *TECHNIQUE (BRAND).* Divide the extensor carpi radialis brevis tendon at the distal end of the radius through a short dorsal transverse incision (Fig. 70-30). Then make a second incision 8.9 cm proximal to the first, withdraw the tendon through it, and lay the tendon on a wet towel. Remove a plantaris tendon for a graft (p. 3032) and divide it in half or double it on itself to make two grafts. Split open the end of the motor tendon along the natural plane of cleavage, spread it out, and suture the graft to it as shown in Fig. 70-31. Then introduce a tendon-tunneling forceps at the first incision, pass it subcutaneously to the second, grasp the ends of the tendon grafts, and pull them through so that the anastomo-

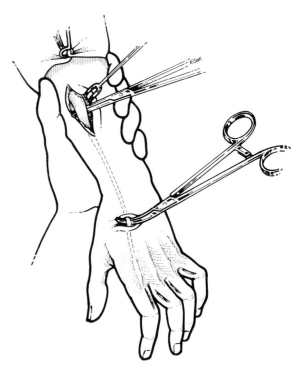

Fig. 70-30 Brand transfer of extensor carpi radialis brevis prolonged with free graft to restore intrinsic function of fingers. Tendon to be transferred has been isolated both proximally and distally. (Redrawn from White WL: Surg Clin North Am 40:427, 1960.)

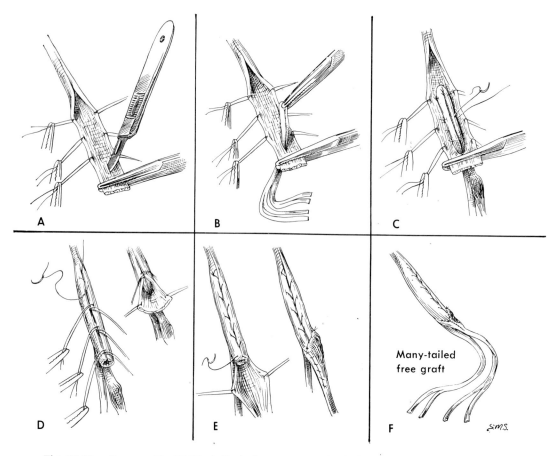

Fig. 70-31 Same as Fig. 70-30. **A,** End of extensor carpi radialis brevis tendon has been split open and spread out and is being perforated with knife. **B,** Plantaris tendon (graft) has been doubled on itself and is being pulled through perforation. **C,** Graft is being attached to tendon with interrupted sutures. **D,** Extensor carpi radialis brevis tendon is being closed over graft with running suture. **E,** On *left,* one strand of graft is being spread open to cover end of extensor carpi radialis brevis tendon. On *right,* graft has been sutured over end of tendon. **F,** Two ends of graft have been split into four slips or tails. (From White WL: Surg Clin North Am 40:427, 1960.)

sis lies under intact skin. Split the end of each graft into two parts to form a total of four slips or tails. Then make a longitudinal dorsoulnar incision over the proximal phalanx of the index finger and dorso-radial incisions over the proximal phalanx of the middle, ring, and little fingers. Identify the lumbrical tendon and lateral band of the extensor aponeurosis in each finger; tunnel from this point on each finger through the palm and appropriate interosseous space; grasp a strand of tendon graft and withdraw it into the finger. Take care to tunnel to the volar side of the deep transverse metacarpal ligament and then between the appropriate metacarpal shafts (Fig. 70-32). When all tendon grafts are in position, suture them one by one under equal tension to the lateral band of the dorsal expansion of each finger, first the index, then the little, and finally the intermediate ones (Fig. 70-33). The transfers should be relaxed completely when the wrist is dorsiflexed 45 degrees, the metacarpophalangeal joints are

flexed 70 degrees, and the interphalangeal joints are in neutral. Close the wounds and apply a light plaster cast.

As an *alternative method,* use the extensor carpi radialis longus tendon. Through a dorsal transverse incision free its insertion and withdraw it through a second incision at the middle of the forearm. Then make an incision on the anterior aspect of the forearm 7.5 cm proximal to the wrist, tunnel from the anterior incision deep to the brachioradialis to the proximal incision, and draw the tendon into the anterior incision. Suture the grafts to the motor tendon as decribed previously. Then through a midpalmar incision introduce a tunneler, pass it through the carpal tunnel into the forearm, and draw the grafts into the palm, leaving the anastomosis proximal to the carpal tunnel. Then pass each strand of the graft separately to its finger destination.

AFTERTREATMENT. Aftertreatment is as described for the modified Bunnell technique.

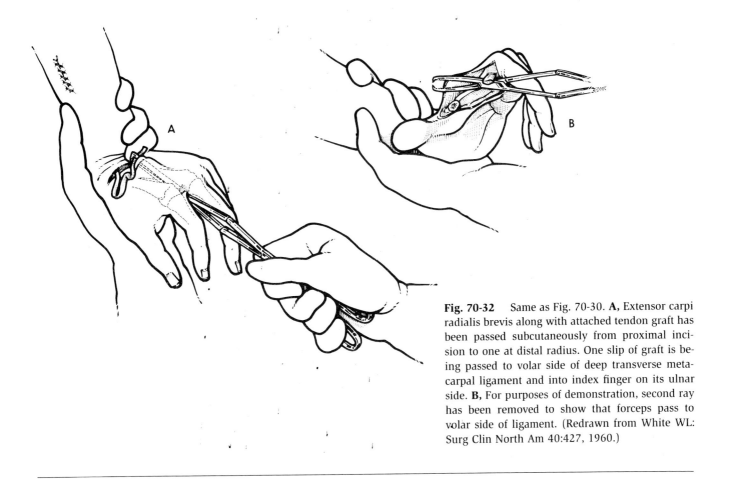

Fig. 70-32   Same as Fig. 70-30. **A,** Extensor carpi radialis brevis along with attached tendon graft has been passed subcutaneously from proximal incision to one at distal radius. One slip of graft is being passed to volar side of deep transverse metacarpal ligament and into index finger on its ulnar side. **B,** For purposes of demonstration, second ray has been removed to show that forceps pass to volar side of ligament. (Redrawn from White WL: Surg Clin North Am 40:427, 1960.)

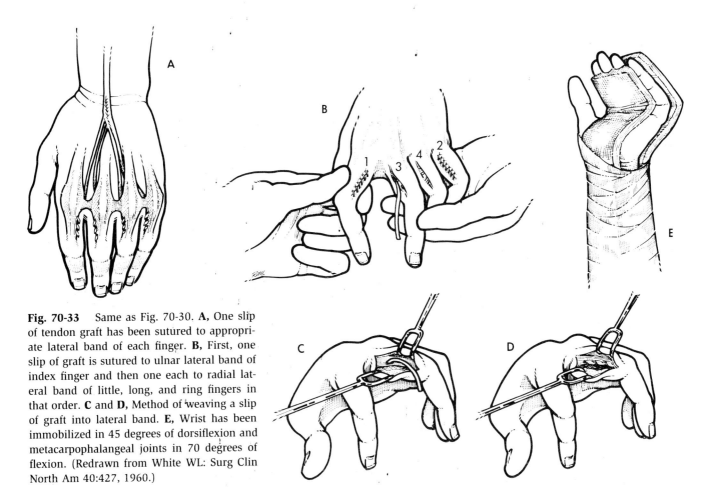

Fig. 70-33   Same as Fig. 70-30. **A,** One slip of tendon graft has been sutured to appropriate lateral band of each finger. **B,** First, one slip of graft is sutured to ulnar lateral band of index finger and then one each to radial lateral band of little, long, and ring fingers in that order. **C** and **D,** Method of weaving a slip of graft into lateral band. **E,** Wrist has been immobilized in 45 degrees of dorsiflexion and metacarpophalangeal joints in 70 degrees of flexion. (Redrawn from White WL: Surg Clin North Am 40:427, 1960.)

Transfer of the Extensor Indicis Proprius and Extensor Digiti Quinti Proprius

■ *TECHNIQUE (FOWLER)*. In this transfer, the extensor indicis proprius and the extensor digiti quinti proprius are used as motors (see Fig. 70-21). Make a dorsal incision over the radial aspect of the metacarpophalangeal joint of the index finger and identify the extensor indicis proprius tendon. Dissect the tendon from the extensor aponeurosis, obtaining as much length as possible by excising a part of the aponeurosis with it; otherwise the tendon will be too tight after transfer. Then suture the residual defect in the aponeurosis. Split the extensor indicis proprius into two equal parts, pass each volar to the deep transverse metacarpal ligament, and attach one each to the extensor aponeurosis on the radial side of the index and middle fingers, as in the Bunnell technique. Now make a dorsal incision over the little finger, identify the extensor digiti quinti proprius tendon, and free its insertion; split this tendon also into two equal parts, pass each volar to the deep transverse metacarpal ligament, and attach one each to the radial side of the ring and little fingers. Take care that this tendon is not too tight. The Riordan modification of this operation (see Fig. 70-22) does not use the extensor digiti quinti proprius. *AFTERTREATMENT*. Aftertreatment is as described for the modified Bunnell technique.

Capsulodesis

■ *TECHNIQUE (ZANCOLLI)*. Make a transverse incision in the palm at the level of the distal crease. Undermine widely the skin and fat and expose the flexor tendon sheaths; take care not to damage the neurovascular bundles. Now over each metacarpophalangeal joint make a longitudinal incision in the paratendinous fascia and tendon sheath and expose the flexor tendons. Carefully retract the tendons and expose the underlying metacarpophalangeal joint (see Fig. 70-27). Resect an elliptic segment of the volar fibrocartilaginous plate including the vertical septum and its deep origin. Resect enough tissue to produce a 10- to 30-degree flexion contracture when the plate is closed. Now close the plate by wire or heavy silk sutures placed laterally in its thickest part, this being at the insertion of the accessory collateral ligaments. If desired to maintain position of the joints, insert transarticular Kirschner wires. Close the wound and apply a dorsal plaster splint holding the metacarpophalangeal joints in flexion and the wrist in extension. *AFTERTREATMENT*. Movements of the interphalangeal joints are continued after surgery. At 3 weeks the cast and any Kirschner wires are removed and exercises of the metacarpophalangeal joints are begun.

Tenodesis

■ *TECHNIQUE (FOWLER)*. In this operation, a tendon graft is substituted for the finger intrinsics; the graft may be activated by flexing the wrist (see Fig. 70-28). Obtain a tendon graft (p. 3032) twice as long as the distance from the dorsum of the wrist to the proximal interphalangeal joints. Make a transverse incision on the dorsum of the wrist and expose the dorsal retinaculum of the wrist. Then pass the graft through the retinaculum just distal to its proximal edge. Split each end of the graft into two equal slips. Then transfer each slip to a finger, as in the Fowler transfer previously described. Suture the graft under proper tension so that when the wrist is flexed, force will be exerted on the extensor mechanism so as to extend the interphalangeal joints without hyperflexing the metacarpophalangeal joints.

PERIPHERAL NERVE PALSIES
Low Radial Nerve Palsy

In low radial nerve palsy the digital extensors, the abductor pollicis longus, and the extensor pollicis longus and brevis muscles are paralyzed. The radial wrist extensors and the brachioradialis are spared, in contrast to high radial nerve palsy in which these are also lost. Therefore the basic functions to be restored in low radial nerve palsy are extension of all digits, as well as extension and radial abduction of the thumb (Fig. 70-34). In isolated low radial nerve palsy the muscles available for

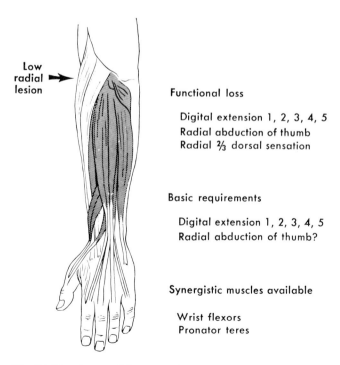

Low radial lesion →

Functional loss

Digital extension 1, 2, 3, 4, 5
Radial abduction of thumb
Radial ⅔ dorsal sensation

Basic requirements

Digital extension 1, 2, 3, 4, 5
Radial abduction of thumb?

Synergistic muscles available

Wrist flexors
Pronator teres

Fig. 70-34 Low radial nerve palsy. (Modified from White WL: Surg Clin North Am 40:427, 1960.)

transfer are essentially all those muscles left unparalyzed, resulting in numerous surgical procedures described by various authors. Low radial nerve palsy procedures are derived from the more common procedures used for high radial nerve palsy (Table 70-2). The synergistic wrist flexors, long finger flexors, palmaris longus, and pronator teres are commonly used for transfer and numerous combinations of these transfers have been described.

Jones in 1916 and 1921 published his often misquoted transfer for irreparable injury to the musculospiral (radial) nerve. He transferred the flexor carpi radialis to the extensor pollicis longus and extensor of the index finger, the flexor carpi ulnaris to the ulnar three finger extensors, and the pronator teres to the two radial wrist extensors. Thus the major wrist flexors are transferred dorsal to the extension-flexion axis of the wrist.

Zachery in a critical survey pointed out that one strong wrist flexor should be retained to prevent hyperextension of the wrist, which causes incomplete extension of the metacarpophalangeal joints. To retain one wrist flexor Starr transferred the palmaris longus to the extensor pollicis longus to provide extension of the thumb. Scuderi in 1949 modified this procedure by rerouting the extensor pollicis longus from Lister's tubercle to the region of the anatomic snuffbox so that the transferred palmaris longus provided thumb metacarpal abduction in addition to extension.

These various refinements in surgery for radial nerve paralysis have produced several commonly used series of transfers (see Table 70-2). The first set of transfers has

Table 70-2 Commonly recommended transfers for low radial nerve palsy

Needed function	Available tendons
Wrist extension (ECRB) ⟶	Pronator teres
Finger extension ⟶	Flexor carpi ulnaris
Thumb extension ⟶	Palmaris longus
Thumb abduction ⟶	

Another popular and useful set of transfers was described by Boyes

Needed function	Available tendons
Wrist extension (ECRB) ⟶	Pronator teres
Finger extension ⟷	Flexor digitorum superficialis: (Long finger — EDC Ring finger — EIP and EPL)
Thumb extension ⟶	Flexor carpi radialis
Thumb abduction ⟶	

Flexor carpi radialis transfer as advocated by Brand

Needed function	Available tendons
Wrist extension (ECRB) ⟶	Pronator teres
Finger extension ⟶	Flexor carpi radialis
Thumb extension ⟶	Palmaris longus to rerouted EPL
Thumb abduction ⟶	

From Reid RL: Hand Clinics 4(2):179, 1988.

become the most accepted surgical program. Boyes' plan is more technically difficult and adhesions often occur in the interosseous space. Conceptually, the Brand transfer may help offset the radial deviation caused by the unopposed pull of the radial wrist extensors. Furthermore, the flexor carpi ulnaris, an important wrist flexor and ulnar deviator, is not sacrificed. In low radial nerve palsy, wrist extension is maintained and pronator teres transfer is not necessary.

TRANSFER OF FLEXOR CARPI ULNARIS TO EXTENSOR DIGITORUM COMMUNIS, PALMARIS LONGUS TO EXTENSOR POLLICIS LONGUS

■ *TECHNIQUE.* Make a long, curved, radially convex incision on the volar surface of the forearm, extending proximally from the proximal wrist flexion crease over the flexor carpi ulnaris tendon (Fig. 70-35, *A*). Release the palmaris longus from the palmar fascia and dissect it free of its attachments into the proximal third of the forearm. Detach the flexor carpi ulnaris tendon near the pisiform and subperiosteally remove it from the ulna throughout the length of the incision (Fig. 70-35, *C*).

Next, make a curved incision on the dorsum of the wrist extending proximally and ulnarward from Lister's tubercle (Fig. 70-35, *B*). Isolate the extensor pollicis longus, retract it, and divide it at the musculotendinous junction.

Make a 2 cm straight incision over the thumb metacarpophalangeal joint (Fig. 70-35, *B*) and pass the extensor pollicis longus tendon to this wound. Use a tendon passer or blunt instrument to make a tunnel for the rerouted tendon. Pass the tendon along and slightly volar to the thumb metacarpal. Check that the alignment of the palmaris longus and extensor pollicis longus are reasonable. Cover the tendons in the volar wound with a saline sponge.

Expose the extensor digitorum communis tendons proximal to the extensor retinaculum and remove a portion of the retinaculum proximally. Make a tunnel for the flexor carpi ulnaris tendon around the ulnar border of the forearm into the dorsal wound. It may be necessary to remove some of the bulk of the muscle distally at this point. Make the extensor digitorum communis tendon approach the extensor digitorum communis as in line as possible and check for freedom of its excursion. Suture the extensor digitorum communis complex together with nonabsorbable sutures before weaving in the flexor carpi ulnaris tendon. Pull on the extensor digitorum communis and observe for synchronous metacarpophalangeal extension. Weave the flexor carpi ulnaris tendon through the extensor digitorum communis complex from ulnar to radial and adjust the tension so that with full passive wrist flexion the metacarpophalangeal joints extend fully and with full wrist extension the fingers can be passively

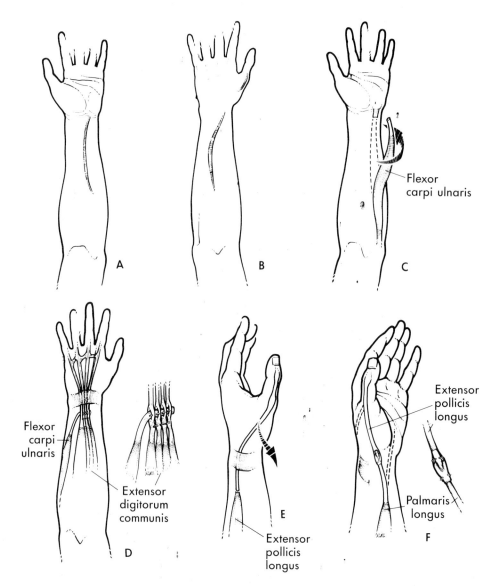

Flexor
carpi ulnaris

Flexor
carpi
ulnaris

Extensor
digitorum
communis

Extensor
pollicis
longus

Extensor
pollicis
longus

Palmaris
longus

Fig. 70-35   Transfer of flexor carpi ulnaris to extensor digitorum communis and palmaris longus to extensor pollicis longus. **A** and **B,** Incisions used in standard combination of transfers (see text). **C** and **D,** Flexor carpi ulnaris to extensor digitorum communis transfer. Flexor carpi ulnaris must be freed extensively to create direct line of pull from its origin to new insertion into extensor digitorum comunis tendons just proximal to dorsal retinaculum. End-to-side anastomosis is shown here. **E** and **F,** Palmaris longus to rerouted extensor pollicis longus transfer. By transferring extensor pollicis longus out of dorsal retinaculum, transfer creates combination of abduction and extension force on thumb. (Redrawn from Green DP: Operative hand surgery, New York, 1988, Churchill Livingstone.)

flexed. Fix the weave with multiple nonabsorbable sutures (Fig. 70-35, *D*). Next, weave the tendon of the palmaris longus into the rerouted extensor pollicis longus tendon and place it under moderate tension so that with full wrist extension the thumb can flex across the palm. Anchor the repair with multiple nonabsorbable sutures (Fig. 70-35, *E* and *F*). Obtain hemostasis and close the wounds over drains.

AFTERTREATMENT. The wrist is maintained in slight extension and the metacarpophalangeal joints are held in 40 degrees of flexion with the thumb abducted for 3 weeks. Then active exercises are begun, but the transfers are protected for 3 months.

High Radial Nerve Palsy

In high radial nerve palsy the radial wrist extensors and the brachioradialis are paralyzed in addition to those muscles paralyzed in low radial nerve palsy (Fig. 70-36). The synergistic wrist flexors, long finger flexors, and the

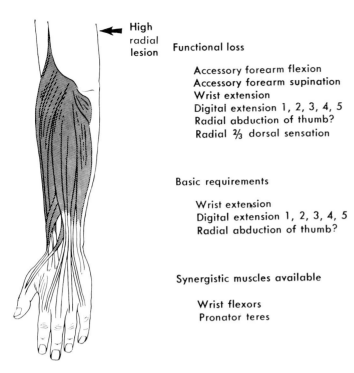

High radial lesion ←

Functional loss

Accessory forearm flexion
Accessory forearm supination
Wrist extension
Digital extension 1, 2, 3, 4, 5
Radial abduction of thumb?
Radial ⅔ dorsal sensation

Basic requirements

Wrist extension
Digital extension 1, 2, 3, 4, 5
Radial abduction of thumb?

Synergistic muscles available

Wrist flexors
Pronator teres

Fig. 70-36 High radial palsy. Boyes has added the sublimi to available synergistic muscles listed here (see text). (From White WL: Surg Clin North Am 40:427, 1960.)

pronator teres, however, are again available for transfer. A satisfactory plan is to transfer the insertion of the pronator teres to the extensor carpi radialis brevis tendon, the flexor carpi ulnaris to the long finger extensors, and the palmaris longus to the long thumb extensor. The long thumb extensor is transposed from around Lister's tubercle and is rerouted along the radial side of the wrist in line with the first metacarpal; the palmaris longus tendon can then be attached to it in a straight line. Thus both extension and abduction of the thumb are restored (Riordan), and a transfer to the long thumb abductor is not absolutely necessary. The flexor carpi radialis remains undisturbed to prevent hyperextension of the wrist. When the palmaris longus is absent, the flexor carpi ulnaris may be transferred not only to the long finger extensors but to the long thumb extensor as well. Even when the palmaris longus is present, Omer uses this transfer. He then shifts the extensor pollicis brevis tendon volarward and ulnarward and sutures the palmaris longus tendon to it; since the insertions of these tendons are not detached, some abduction of the thumb is restored and function of the palmaris longus as a flexor of the wrist is retained. However, to preserve the basic functional movements of the wrist, Boyes advises against transfer of the flexor carpi ulnaris; instead he transfers two flexor digitorum sublimis tendons (see below for the Boyes technique).

TECHNICAL CONSIDERATIONS FOR TRANSFER. The

muscle belly of the flexor carpi ulnaris extends almost to the insertion of its tendon, and all along its course the muscle takes origin from the surrounding fascia. Therefore the tendon cannot be easily withdrawn through an incision proximal to its insertion; rather, the incision should be curved and should be made over the entire distal half of the muscle; then its fibers should be dissected from the tendon proximally to the middle of the forearm so that the tendon can be transferred with gradual angulation to the long extensor tendons of the fingers. The level of suture is proximal to the dorsal carpal ligament; this ligament can be partially excised proximally if necessary, but a bowstring effect will be produced if it is completely excised.

The transferred tendons should be tunneled through subcutaneous fat without touching scar, fascia, or muscle. To prevent excessive scarring, the tunnels should be only wide enough to permit the tendons to glide without obstruction. The superficial fascia should be excised from the area in which tendons are attached. In transfers for radial nerve palsy the tendons should be sutured under a little more tension than is usual because the strong flexors tend to stretch the transferred muscles; mattress sutures of wire are preferred.

One way of adjusting tension on the transferred flexor carpi ulnaris is to maintain the wrist in a neutral position while the fingers are completely extended; place maximal pull on the transferred tendon-muscle unit, and suture the transferred tendon to the tendons of the finger extensors. The tendon is simply pulled tight, held over, and then sutured to these tendons without severing them. Through-and-through mattress sutures are used to individually attach each extensor tendon to the larger transferred tendon unit. After suture, the correct tension is verified when, on extending the wrist, full passive finger flexion is possible, and when, on flexing the wrist, there is sufficient tension on the extensors to fully extend the finger.

An additional incision on the middle third of the forearm is needed to attach the pronator teres tendon to the extensor carpi radialis brevis. The pronator teres tendon is detached from its insertion with as much periosteum as possible to make suturing easier. The tab of tendon insertion and the periosteum are inserted in the muscle belly of the extensor carpi radialis brevis and held with one untied suture. This suture is not tied until after the tension testing of the transfer to the finger extensors. An additional short incision may be made about the muscle-tendon junction of the palmaris longus to bring it out proximally for gradual angulation toward the thumb extensor. Its insertion can be reached through the dorsal incision at the wrist that extends volarward for the dissection of the flexor carpi ulnaris.

Many variations of the above are possible, including placing the palmaris longus into the abductor pollicis longus tendon or into the extensor pollicis brevis tendon; both provide some abduction of the thumb. However, if this is done, care should be taken to attach the extensor pollicis longus to the transferred flexor carpi ulnaris so that there will be an active thumb extensor with the common digital extensors.

Brand has suggested removing the insertion of the extensor carpi radialis longus and transferring it to a point between the extensor carpi radialis brevis and extensor carpi ulnaris to avoid radial deviation on extension of the wrist.

TRANSFER OF INSERTION OF PRONATOR TERES, TWO FLEXOR DIGITORUM SUBLIMIS TENDONS, AND PALMARIS LONGUS. Boyes devised an operation for high radial nerve palsy in which two sublimis tendons are included in the transfer. This operation satisfactorily restores function and preserves wrist control.

■ *TECHNIQUE (BOYES).* Make a long longitudinal incision on the volar side of the radial aspect of the forearm and free the insertion of the pronator teres. Perforate the extensor carpi radialis longus and brevis tendons, pass the insertion of the pronator teres through these tendons, and suture it under proper tension. Use stainless steel wire for all tendon attachments. Expose the sublimis tendons of the middle and ring fingers through a single incision in the distal palm over the metacarpal heads or through separate incisions at their insertions on the middle phalanges; divide each so that the free end of its distal segment lies within its sheath. Withdraw the proximal segments of the tendons through the forearm incision. Now make a dorsal transverse incision on the wrist extending from the radial styloid toward the ulnar styloid and then curving proximally. Expose the common digital extensors proximal to the dorsal carpal ligament and incise the deep fascia. Next, make a 2 cm opening in the interosseous membrane at the proximal edge of the pronator quadratus muscle. Pass the sublimis of the middle finger to the radial side of the profundus muscle mass and between it and the flexor pollicis longus muscle mass and then through the interosseous membrane. Then attach the donor tendon to the common digital extensors. Make another opening in the interosseous membrane; pass the sublimis of the ring finger to the ulnar side of the profundus muscle mass and through the opening and attach it to the extensor pollicis longus and extensor indicis proprius. Divide the flexor carpi radialis at the wrist and suture it to the extensor pollicis brevis and abductor pollicis longus at this level.

Before the transferred tendons are sutured in place, removing the tourniquet and checking the interosseous artery for bleeding is wise. If this artery has been lacerated but not properly ligated, then serious complications, including ischemic myositis, may develop after surgery.

AFTERTREATMENT. Immobilization of some type should be carried out for 5 weeks. Usually a cast is maintained on the arm for 4 weeks followed by a spring-loaded extension splint for the wrist and fingers for another week. During the cast immobilization, the metacarpophalangeal joints should not be completely extended but should be held in about 40 degrees of flexion. However, the wrist should be fully extended with the thumb in abduction and extension. The interphalangeal joints of the fingers should be in "comfortable" flexion.

Low Ulnar Nerve Palsy

The functional deficits caused by low ulnar nerve palsy are weakness of pinch resulting from paralysis of the adductor pollicis and first dorsal interosseus, weakness of grip produced by paralysis of most of the finger intrinsics, and sometimes clawing of the ring and little fingers associated with paralysis of all of their intrinsics (Fig. 70-37).

Paralysis of the adductor pollicis results in a major loss of function that should be restored when possible by appropriate tendon transfer (see discussion on restoration of adduction of thumb, p. 3243). Normal tightness of the metacarpophalangeal joints of the ring and little fingers may limit clawing of these fingers and enable the long extensors to extend their interphalangeal joints; in this instance, no treatment is indicated for clawing, but weakness of grip is still present. However, when clawing of these fingers is troublesome, function of their intrinsics should be restored by transferring the extensor indicis proprius tendon; it is split into two slips, passed volar

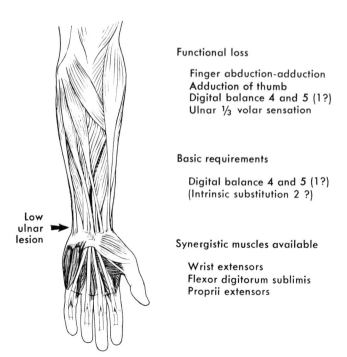

Functional loss

   Finger abduction-adduction
   Adduction of thumb
   Digital balance 4 and 5 (1?)
   Ulnar ⅓ volar sensation

Basic requirements

   Digital balance 4 and 5 (1?)
   (Intrinsic substitution 2 ?)

Synergistic muscles available

   Wrist extensors
   Flexor digitorum sublimis
   Proprii extensors

Low ulnar lesion →

Fig. 70-37 Low ulnar nerve palsy. (From White WL: Surg Clin North Am 40:427, 1960.)

to the deep transverse metacarpal ligament, and attached to the radial side of the extensor aponeurosis of each finger as in the Riordan transfer (see Fig. 70-22). Other dynamic transfers such as that of Bunnell (p. 3253) or Brand (p. 3253) may be useful. As an alternative to tendon transfer, clawing of the ring and little fingers may be corrected by Zancolli capsulodesis (p. 3256).

For low ulnar nerve palsy, Omer suggests the following procedure carried out in one stage (Fig. 70-38). The metacarpophalangeal joint of the thumb is arthrodesed. The insertion of the flexor digitorum sublimis of the middle finger is freed, and the tendon is split into two slips. One slip is carried across the palm parallel to the fibers of the adductor pollicis and is anchored to the insertion of that muscle. The other slip is split into two tails; one is carried through the appropriate lumbrical canal and is anchored to the radial side of the extensor aponeurosis of the ring finger, and the other is transferred in a similar manner to the little finger. Instead of the procedure just described, he sometimes transfers the brachioradialis tendon, prolonged with a free graft, through the third interosseous space to restore adduction of the thumb (p. 3244); to restore abduction of the index finger, he frees the radial half of the insertion of the extensor indicis proprius, splits the tendon, and anchors the freed half of the tendon to the insertion of the first dorsal interosseus.

Burkhalter has suggested several tendon transfers, all of which ultimately end by insertion directly into the diaphysis of the proximal phalanx of the involved fingers.

He believes this is a more secure attachment and also gives the advantage of a greater lever arm beyond the metacarpophalangeal joint. For motors, he has used either the brachioradialis or the extensor carpi radialis longus extended by free grafts, both of which are brought dorsally and passed through the intermetacarpal area volar to the transverse metacarpal ligament and then attached to bone (Fig. 70-39). He has also used the same bony attachment in transferring a split sublimis of the ring finger as a modification of the Stiles-Bunnell transfer. In addition, there should be a transfer to provide adduction of the thumb.

Brown has suggested several transfers for adduction of the thumb: one using the sublimis of the ring finger brought deep to the flexors of the fingers and another using the extensor indicis proprius brought into the palm through the third space of the metacarpals and then transversely across the palm, paralleling the paralyzed adductor muscle, to attach to the metacarpophalangeal joint area of the thumb. On occasion, arthrodesis of the distal thumb joint is advised to increase the power of pinch; this is accompanied at times by advancing the pulley at the metacarpophalangeal joint by sectioning it proximally to provide a greater angle of approach of the flexor pollicis longus.

High Ulnar Nerve Palsy

The functional deficits caused by high ulnar nerve palsy are the same as those described for low ulnar nerve palsy, except that functions of the flexor digitorum profundus of the ring and little fingers and of the flexor carpi ulnaris are also lost (Fig. 70-40). The transfers described for low ulnar nerve palsy may be used, except that the sublimis of the ring finger must not be trans-

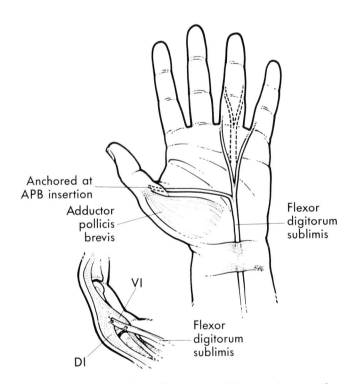

Fig. 70-38   Single flexor digitorum sublimis tendon transfer used to correct clawing and to strengthen thumb-index pinch in isolated ulnar nerve palsy. (Redrawn from Omer GE Jr: Orthop Clin North Am 5:377, 1974.)

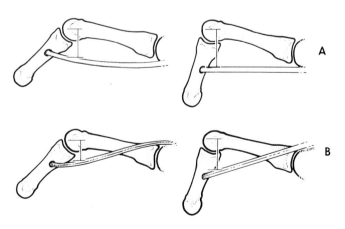

Fig. 70-39   **A,** Burkhalter modification of Stiles-Bunnell transfer increases distance of moment arm with increased flexion of metacarpophalangeal joint. Force applied distally varies with square of distance. **B,** With intermetacarpal route for this transfer, moment arm also increases with increasing flexion of metacarpophalangeal joint. (Redrawn from Burkhalter WE: Orthop Clin North Am 5:289, 1974.)

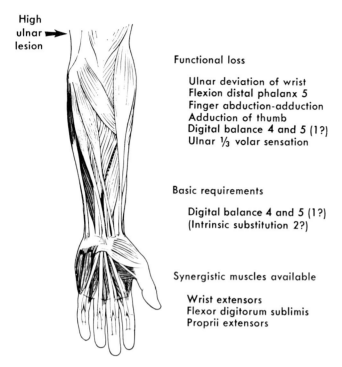

High
ulnar →
lesion

Functional loss

Ulnar deviation of wrist
Flexion distal phalanx 5
Finger abduction-adduction
Adduction of thumb
Digital balance 4 and 5 (1?)
Ulnar ⅓ volar sensation

Basic requirements

Digital balance 4 and 5 (1?)
(Intrinsic substitution 2?)

Synergistic muscles available

Wrist extensors
Flexor digitorum sublimis
Proprii extensors

Fig. 70-40 High ulnar nerve palsy. (From White WL: Surg Clin North Am 40:427, 1960.)

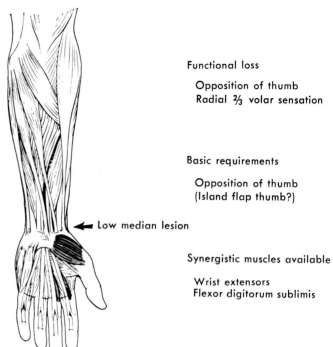

Functional loss

Opposition of thumb
Radial ⅔ volar sensation

Basic requirements

Opposition of thumb
(Island flap thumb?)

← Low median lesion

Synergistic muscles available

Wrist extensors
Flexor digitorum sublimis

Fig. 70-41 Low median nerve palsy. (From White WL: Surg Clin North Am 40:427, 1960.)

ferred because the profundus of this finger is paralyzed. Flexion of the distal interphalangeal joints of the ring and little fingers may be restored by suturing the profundus tendons of these fingers to that of the middle finger. If further power is needed, transfer of the extensor carpi radialis longus into the profundus tendons of the middle, ring, and little fingers also may be done. It should be remembered that the innervation of the profundus of the middle finger may be totally ulnar at times and frequently only partially ulnar.

Low Median Nerve Palsy

The important functional deficits caused by low median nerve palsy are loss of opposition of the thumb and loss of sensibility over the sensory distribution of the nerve; paralysis of the two radial lumbricals is of little consequence when the ulnar nerve is intact (Fig. 70-41). Restoration of thumb opposition is discussed on p. 3236. Restoration of sensibility by a neurovascular island graft is discussed on p. 3119.

High Median Nerve Palsy

The important functional deficits caused by high median nerve palsy are loss of pronation of the forearm, flexion of the wrist, flexion of the index and middle fingers, flexion of the thumb, opposition of the thumb, and sensation over the median distribution (Fig. 70-42).

Function may be restored partially as follows. The flexor digitorum profundus of the index and middle fin-

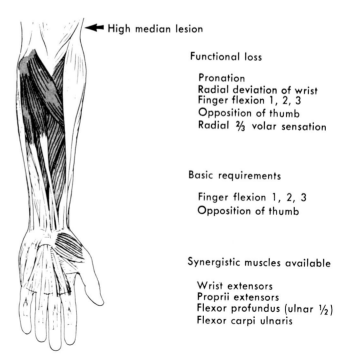

← High median lesion

Functional loss

Pronation
Radial deviation of wrist
Finger flexion 1, 2, 3
Opposition of thumb
Radial ⅔ volar sensation

Basic requirements

Finger flexion 1, 2, 3
Opposition of thumb

Synergistic muscles available

Wrist extensors
Proprii extensors
Flexor profundus (ulnar ½)
Flexor carpi ulnaris

Fig. 70-42 High median nerve palsy. (From White WL: Surg Clin North Am 40:427, 1960.)

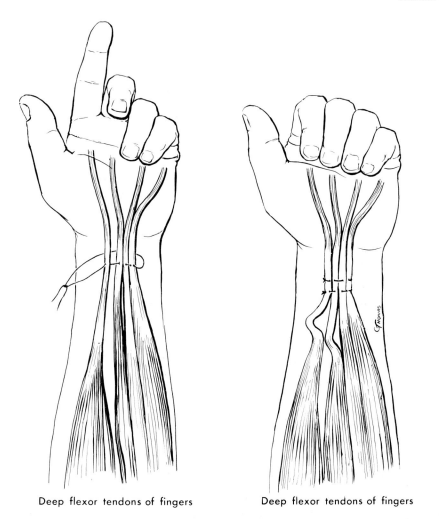

Deep flexor tendons of fingers   Deep flexor tendons of fingers

Fig. 70-43   In high median nerve palsy, distal segment of profundus tendons of index and middle fingers are tightened and tendons are sutured to profundus tendons of ring and little fingers (see text). This tendon mass may be further strengthened by transfer of extensor carpi radialis longus to insert as an additional motor. (From Omer GE Jr: J Bone Joint Surg 50-A:1454, 1968.)

gers may be attached to the ulnar-innervated flexor digitorum profundus by side-to-side suture without sectioning of any tendons (Fig. 70-43). In addition, greater power can be achieved by transferring the extensor carpi radialis longus into the profundus tendons of the index and middle fingers. Flexion of the thumb may be restored by transfer of the brachioradialis to the long thumb flexor at the wrist level. Opposition of the thumb may be restored by using the extensor indicis proprius as a transfer, bringing it around the ulnar side of the wrist so that construction of a pulley is not needed (see Burkhalter technique).

The restoration of sensibility by a neurovascular island graft is discussed on p. 3119.

Combined Low Median and Ulnar Nerve Palsy (at Wrist)

Combined median and ulnar nerve lesions at the wrist (Fig. 70-44) result in complete anesthesia of the palm and loss of function of all intrinsics of both the fingers and the thumb (see the introduction to this section). When untreated, skin and joint contractures develop, and a fixed clawhand results.

Despite the palmar anesthesia, it is possible to restore some useful function after this severe paralysis. The success of treatment depends on several factors. Often the flexor tendons have been severely injured by the same trauma that caused the paralysis; in this event, the condition of the tendons is important in planning transfers. In Hansen's disease the paralysis is not accompanied by tendon injury but at times by deformity of the skin, fingernails, and bone. For tendon transfers to be successful, any contractures of the skin or joints must be corrected first because the transfers alone cannot accomplish this. Passive extension of the interphalangeal joints and flexion of the metacarpophalangeal joints of the fingers must be possible. An attempt is made to mobilize the joints by splinting; if this fails, then arthrodesis of the proximal interphalangeal joints must be considered. Any contracture

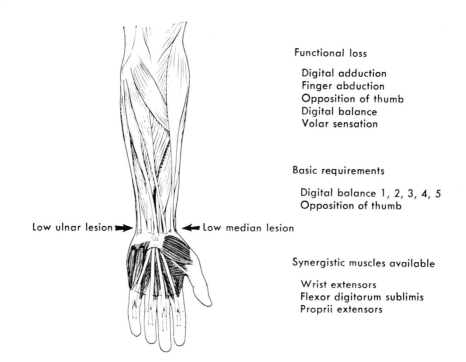

Functional loss

Digital adduction
Finger abduction
Opposition of thumb
Digital balance
Volar sensation

Basic requirements

Digital balance 1, 2, 3, 4, 5
Opposition of thumb

Low ulnar lesion ➡️   ⬅️ Low median lesion

Synergistic muscles available

Wrist extensors
Flexor digitorum sublimis
Proprii extensors

Fig. 70-44   Combined low median and low ulnar nerve palsy. (From White WL: Surg Clin North Am 40:427, 1960.)

of the thumb web, which is frequent after combined median and ulnar nerve palsy, also must be corrected (see discussion of the adducted thumb).

Function of the finger intrinsics may be restored by the Brand transfer, in which the extensor carpi radialis brevis is prolonged by tendon graft (p. 3253). Opposition of the thumb may be restored by the Riordan transfer (p. 3238) unless the sublimis tendon of the ring finger or the palmaris longus tendon has been injured by direct trauma.

For clawing, Brown suggests a transfer of the extensor carpi radialis longus tendon prolonged by a four-tailed graft to restore metacarpophalangeal flexion as Brand has described. For thumb adduction, he suggests using the extensor indicis proprius tendon passed through the third intermetacarpal space and over the paralyzed adductor muscle and attached to the adductor tendon insertion at the metacarpophalangeal joint of the thumb.

Thumb adduction also may be restored by transferring the ring flexor digitorum sublimis through the distal palmar fascia, using the vertical septum as a pulley, and then passing it across the palm superficial to the fascia, and attaching it to the radial side of the metacarpophalangeal joint of the thumb. This may cause an unsightly palmar prominence.

Omer suggests several possibilities. To restore digital balance, he uses the flexor digitorum sublimis tendon of the middle finger split into four tails or the extensor carpi radialis longus tendon prolonged by a graft. The other two possibilities are the extensor indicis proprius tendon or the extensor digiti quinti proprius tendon, each split into two tails and attached to the second and third digits and fourth and fifth digits respectively. For thumb adduction, Omer uses the middle flexor digitorum sublimis tendon or the extensor carpi radialis longus tendon brought through the third intermetacarpal space and prolonged by a graft to attach to the thumb adductor area. For opposition, he suggests using the extensor carpi ulnaris tendon prolonged by the extensor pollicis brevis tendon or a graft from the palmaris longus. Fusion is also suggested for increasing stability of the thumb.

Combined High Median and Ulnar Nerve Palsy (above Elbow)

In combined high median and ulnar nerve palsy, the entire hand is anesthetic except for its dorsal surface and the only muscles available for transfer are those innervated by the radial nerve: the brachioradialis, the extensor carpi radialis brevis, the extensor carpi radialis longus, the extensor carpi ulnaris, and the extensor indicis proprius. For this palsy Omer recommends the following treatment: arthrodesis of the metacarpophalangeal joint of the thumb; Zancolli capsulodesis of the metacarpophalangeal joints of all fingers, and release of the flexor tendon sheaths at the same time; transfer of the extensor carpi radialis longus around the radial side of the wrist to the flexor digitorum profundus; transfer of the brachioradialis to the flexor pollicis longus; and transfer of the extensor carpi ulnaris, prolonged with a free graft, around the ulnar border of the forearm to the extensor pollicis brevis.

To restore sensibility to the palm Omer has suggested amputating the index finger and its metacarpal and folding the radially innervated dorsal flap into the palm.

SEVERE PARALYSIS FROM DAMAGE TO THE CERVICAL SPINAL CORD OR OTHER CAUSES
Tetraplegia

Paralysis from spinal cord injury fortunately is not as common as paralysis caused by peripheral nerve injuries. However, improved acute management and subsequent long-term care of motor vehicular accident and sporting injury victims have placed increased emphasis on rehabilitation of patients with tetraplegia. Most patients surviving cervical spinal cord injuries are young males with 25 to 30 years of life remaining, and nearly two-thirds of all cervical cord level injury survivors have C-6 root level function remaining. Subjectively, most patients consider their lives considerably improved by upper limb surgery. Three-fourths of young tetraplegics consider the use of the hands and upper extremities to be the function which they would like most to be restored. This is considered to be more important than use of the legs, bladder and bowel function, and use and feeling of their sexual organs. Few surgeons have had vast experience in treatment of these patients, but excellent work has been published by Freehafer et al., Moberg, Lamb, Zancolli, Hentz et al., McDowell et al., House et al., Waters et al., and others.

CLASSIFICATION OF TETRAPLEGIA. McDowell, Moberg, and House, after the Second International Conference on Surgical Rehabilitation of the Upper Limb in Tetraplegia (Giens, France, 1984), provided a classification scheme on tetraplegia (Table 70-3). This classification system is a modification of that proposed from their first international meeting in Edinburgh, 1978. Forearm and hand functions are considered in terms of sensibility, motor units remaining, and the motor unit function. The sensory afferent is designated either O (ocular) or Cu (cutaneous) depending on whether visual cue or at least 10 mm two-point discrimination is preserved, respectively. The motor groupings fall into ten categories (0 through 9) depending on the lowest level of grade 4 or better motor function remaining according to the Medical Research Council (MRC) grading scale. An additional group (X) is added to accommodate those patients not falling into the ten patterned groups. The utility of this system allows patient grouping for tailoring individual surgical management and comparison of their results. The motor examination would seem to follow a predictable root level pattern (Table 70-4), but this often is not true. Asymmetric upper extremity involvement, as well as skip lesions, occur in both sensory and motor function.

PRINCIPLES OF MANAGEMENT OF TETRAPLEGIA. A surgical procedure for tetraplegia should not be stereotyped since each patient is different, even those with cord injury at the same cervical level and even each up-

Table 70-3 International classification for surgery of the hand in tetraplegia (Edinburgh 1978; Modified-Giens 1984)

Sensibility		Motor	Description
O or Cu	Group	Characteristics	Function
	0	No muscle below elbow suitable for transfer	Flexion and supination of the elbow
	1	BR	
	2	ECRL	Extension of the wrist (weak or strong)
	3*	ECRB	Extension of the wrist
	4	PT	Extension and pronation of the wrist
	5	FCR	Flexion of the wrist
	6	Finger extensors	Extrinsic extension of the fingers (partial or complete)
	7	Thumb extensor	Extrinsic extension of the thumb
	8	Partial digital flexors	Extrinsic flexion of the fingers (weak)
	9	Lacks only intrinsics	Extrinsic flexion of the fingers
	X	Exceptions	

From McDowell CL, Moberg EA, and House JH: J Hand Surg 11-A:607, 1986.
BR, brachioradialis; ECRL, extensor carpi radialis longus: ECRB, extensor carpi radialis brevis; PT, pronator teres; FCR, flexor carpi radialis.
*It is not possible to determine strength of ECRB without surgical exposure.

Table 70-4   The normal spinal segmental level of the muscles of the upper limb*

Spinal cord segment	Deltoid	Biceps	Brachio-radialis	ECRL ECRB	Pronator	Flexor carpi-radialis	Triceps	Finger extensor	Thumb extensor	Finger flexor	Intrinsics
C5											
C5 and 6											
C6											
C7											
C8											
T1											

*Modified from Lamb DW: The paralysed hand: the hand and upper limb, vol 2, Edinburgh 1987, Churchill Livingstone.

It will be seen there is a large group of muscles arising from the sixth cervical segment and that there can be a variety of muscle survival depending upon the level of the segment that the injury has occurred. The muscles are tested in an orderly sequence utilizing the MRC grading. All muscles must be tested in orderly sequence which requires knowledge of the usual spinal segmental level of supply. The shaded areas show the main segmental muscle supply.

per extremity in the same patient may require a different procedure. Careful analysis of the motor and sensory status is necessary to determine which surgical procedure is warranted, if any. Many patients are extremely hesitant to have any surgical procedure done for fear of losing what little function remains. The examiner not only must check for muscle function and grade the power but also should observe the patient going through his daily activities and try to determine what additional function would best accomplish a greater independence. According to Lamb, if there is no muscle power, not even a flicker, immediately after injury and again nothing in 1 month, then no function can be expected from this muscle. As a rule, however, surgery is begun after months of observation, usually a year or longer. In partial or incomplete quadriplegia, spasticity usually becomes a consideration since it may jeopardize the end results of surgery.

For sensibility, the two-point discrimination test with a paper clip, as described by Moberg, yields the accurate assessment of cutaneous sensation and proprioception necessary to plan treatment for improvement of grip. When sensibility is not present, then sight must substitute, and ocular substitution can be only unilateral; therefore only one upper extremity should have surgery. Furthermore, the better hand should be operated on first because rehabilitation is easier.

Following injury, it is essential to maintain joint mobility of the fingers, wrist, elbow, and shoulder, since contractures frequently develop, especially with spasticity. Elbow flexion, supination, and metacarpophalangeal extension contractures should be prevented through appropriate therapeutic modalities. Passive range-of-motion exercises and splinting as necessary of all joints of the upper extremity are necessary preoperative measures in

the post-injury period. Murphy and Chuinard (1988) developed a helpful protocol for the management of tetraplegia; they described acute, subacute, and reconstructive phases (see box, p. 3267).

Principles regarding surgical management in tetraplegia summarized by McDowell, Moberg, and House, in addition to the above, are:
1. Neurologic recovery should have ceased and at least 12 months should have passed before surgical reconstruction.
2. Uncontrolled spasticity of a muscle, despite good strength, precludes its use in transfer.
3. Painful paresthesias in a hand prohibit that hand from being reconstructed.
4. Wrist mobility and the natural tenodesis effect should be maintained.

The goal of treatment by most authors usually has been to obtain key grip or key pinch. Key pinch posture provides a stronger, broader gripping surface; is cosmetically more preferable; and is more easily achieved than the "chuckjaw" or three-fingered pinch. Grasping with all fingers is desirable, but this cannot be accomplished without more available muscles. The objective of surgery in tetraplegia, however, is not to provide complex function through complex surgery; it is to provide some degree of freedom to patients who are severely handicapped. Whenever possible a single surgical procedure for a given function should be planned. The more severe the involvement, the simpler should be the procedure.

Reconstructive surgery in tetraplegia can be simply a composite of methods necessary to provide control of a joint or a series of joints. Insufficient motor units about a joint often require arthrodesis of the joint, especially of the thumb carpometacarpal, metacarpophalangeal, and interphalangeal joints. Static and dynamic tenodeses

---

**PROTOCOL FOR MANAGEMENT OF
TETRAPLEGIA**

I. Acute phase
   A. Stabilize spine to preserve remaining neurologic function and allow early mobilization
   B. Manage associated body system problems
   C. Aggressive management of associated upper extremity injuries
   D. Occupational therapy program to prevent joint contracture and maintain joint mobility
II. Subacute phase
   A. Aggressive rehabilitation program
   B. Occupational therapy maintenance program
   C. Resolve associated problems, i.e., decubitus ulcers, bladder program
   D. Resolve psychologic problems
   E. Serial examination by the reconstruction surgeon at 3-month intervals; allow neurologic recovery to plateau
III. Reconstructive phase: upper extremity reconstruction (The patient is stable. The neurologic recovery has plateaued. The patient is psychologically well adjusted. Generally, allow at least 12 months from injury.)
   A. Reconstruction should be begun on the side with the most intact function
   B. If equal, then begin on the dominant extremity
   C. If there is no cutaneous sensibility (ocular only), reconstruction should be limited to only one extremity to allow for visual control
   D. Keep the treatment plan simple
   E. Restoration of active elbow extension by the Moberg deltoid-to-triceps should precede other upper extremity reconstruction
   F. Restoration of key grip
   G. Modify the reconstruction plan to the specific needs of the individual

(From Murphy CP and Chuinard RG: Hand Clin 4:201, 1988.)

**PATIENT EVALUATION AND MUSCLE
SELECTION GUIDELINES FOR TENDON
TRANSFERS**

PREREQUISITE CHECKS FOR TRANSFERS

Sensibility
Stability
   Bone
   Neurologic
   Psychologic
   Soft tissue
Site adequacy
   Soft tissue bed adequate
Supple joints

MUSCLE SELECTION

Strength
   Tension fraction
   Mass fraction
Excursion
Alignment
Synergy
Integrity
Expendibility

STAGING

REHABILITATION

(such as in the Moberg flexor pollicis longus tenodesis to the distal radius in group 1 tetraplegia) also are versatile, frequently used procedures. For lower level tetraplegia a variety of tendon transfers are available, often supplemented by arthrodeses and tenodeses. The continuing interest in tetraplegia has led not just to refinements in older techniques but new concepts as well.

Despite a slightly different approach to tendon transfers in spinal cord injured patients compared with those with peripheral nerve injuries, the basic checklist of prerequisites to surgery must not be overlooked (see box above right). Certainly, lower level tetraplegia with more retained motors allows the use of procedures common to peripheral nerve palsy management.

Additionally, efforts to restore sensation should follow tendon transfers, since the cortical interpretation of sensation (localization and stereognosis) seems to be enhanced by movement of the part.

High level tetraplegia without available motors for transfer is a condition that has focused attention on functional electrical stimulation. Intact neuromuscular units lacking cortical efferent control are stimulated by impulses directed along the intact neural pathways. Combinations of stimuli to different neuromuscular units allow for programming of concerted activity. Keith et al. in 1989 reported the use of an implanted stimulator in a single patient and concluded that the system provided grasp and manipulation not obtainable by other means. Freehafer et al. reported a similar implanted system, which they called a *neuroprosthesis*. They reported promising results in 30 patients with the percutaneous systems. This modality appears to be effective in patients with high level tetraplegia, but is still in the developmental stage.

ELBOW EXTENSION. Elbow extension is lost in approximately 70% of tetraplegics. Regaining this function is most appreciated by patients and should be the function achieved first or in conjunction with another procedure. Several procedures have been described for substitution for a triceps with grade 3 or less muscle power. Transfer of the biceps tendon posteriorly to the terminal insertion of the triceps may be performed only if supinator function is active (Friedenberg, Zancolli). After this procedure Zancolli reported a 24% reduction in elbow flexion.

The posterior deltoid-to-triceps transfer as described by Moberg is the most commonly used procedure to establish elbow extension. This procedure often incorporates a graft of some sort and requires relatively long periods of immobilization according to McDowell, Moberg, and Smith. However, Lacey et al. (1986) reported excellent results in 10 patients undergoing such a transfer. These authors used tibialis anterior tendon grafts instead of the toe extensor tendons as originally described by Moberg. All patients had C-6 level tetraplegia and had no voluntary triceps function before surgery. After 4 weeks of plaster immobilization at 30 degrees of flexion, active range of motion within tolerance was begun and progressed to resistive exercises at 8 weeks. Only one patient had less than grade 3 power and all were satisfied with their results. Hentz, Hamlin, and Keoshian also recommend the deltoid-to-triceps transfer. They did not interpose a graft and simply attached the deltoid to the triceps aponeurosis directly. They reserve biceps transfer for patients with significant elbow flexion contractures.

Posterior deltoid-to-triceps transfer

■ **TECHNIQUE (MOBERG, MODIFIED).** Place the patient in the lateral decubitus position and make a 10 to 13 cm incision along the posterior border of the deltoid muscle down to the insertion of the muscle. Raise flaps over the fascia of the deltoid and identify its humeral insertion. Using a periosteal elevator and sharp dissection, elevate the posterior third to half of the tendon with a strip of the periosteal insertion (Fig. 70-45, *A*). Place this portion of the deltoid under slight tension and gently split the muscle

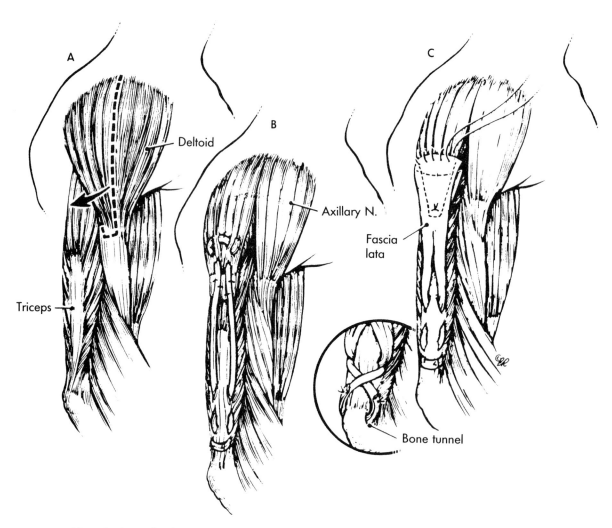

Fig. 70-45 Deltoid-to-triceps transfer (Moberg). **A,** Posterior border of muscle belly is isolated, preserving as much of tendinous insertion as possible. **B,** Tendon grafts are laced into distal end of posterior deltoid muscle belly and triceps aponeurosis. **C,** Use of fascia lata rather than tendon grafts. Direct insertion into olecranon through bone tunnel also can be done with either type of graft. (Redrawn from Green DP: Operative hand surgery, ed 2, New York, 1988, Churchill Livingstone.)

fibers in a distal-to-proximal direction, taking care to palpate and inspect for the axillary nerve and posterior circumflex humeral vessels entering the muscle on its deep surface posteriorly. End the proximal dissection when this level is identified. The triceps generally is atrophied and the posterior deltoid edge is easily palpable. Through a separate curved longitudinal incision, expose the distal triceps and its insertion on the olecranon distal to the musculotendinous junction. If there is adequate overlap of the tendinous portions of the deltoid insertion and the proximal portion of the triceps, the transfer can be accomplished without interposition grafts (Hentz et al.). However, if the overlap does not provide adequate weave fixation, a free tendon graft may be necessary (Fig. 70-45, *B*). Moberg used great toe extensors, Lacey et al. used the tibialis anterior tendon, and Hentz et al. used the fascia lata; other graft sources also have been reported (Fig. 70-45, *C*).

Adjust the tension of the attachment so that full elbow flexion can be passively obtained. Lacey et al. use intraoperative muscle stimulation to generate force-length relationships. When the length at which maximal tension is developed has been determined, hold this position and attach the transfer with the elbow in 90 degrees of flexion. As an alternative, adduct the arm, fully extend the elbow, and place the deltoid under maximal tension; preliminarily suture the transfer in place and test the passive range of motion (Lamb, 1987). Place stainless steel sutures at measured distances proximal and distal to each tendon suture for roentgenographic verification of the integrity of the attachment (Ejeskär).

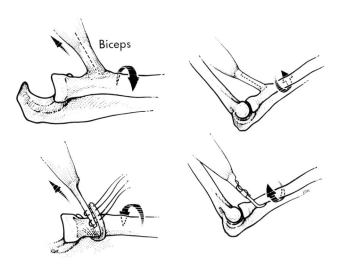

Fig. 70-46 Rerouting of distal end of biceps and release of interosseous membrane for fixed supination deformity. (Redrawn from Zancolli EA: Structural and dynamic bases of hand surgery, Philadelphia, 1978, JB Lippincott Co.)

AFTERTREATMENT. The arm is splinted in 0 to 30 degrees of elbow flexion with the arm adducted. At 4 to 6 weeks the elbow is gradually flexed at a rate of 10 to 15 degrees per week. Active and active-assisted range-of-motion exercises are then instituted, with a progressive range of motion. The elbow is maintained in an elbow extension splint at night for 3 months. The patient should refrain from wheelchair pushups and transfers for 3 months.

FOREARM PRONATION. Patients with group 3 (functioning brachioradialis, extensor carpi radialis longus and brevis) or lower function lack active forearm pronation. Resultant fixed or dynamic supination deformities prohibit the hand from being placed in a position necessary for a variety of functions. This deformity should be corrected before rehabilitation of the hand. Rerouting the biceps tendon about the lateral aspect of the proximal radius converts the biceps muscle into a pronator. Zancolli also recommends release of the interosseous membrane when the supination deformities are fixed (Fig. 70-46).

WRIST EXTENSION. Wrist extension is the goal when the only available motor is the brachioradialis, because the next most distal function is wrist extension (extensor carpi radialis longus and brevis). In group 1 patients this can be accomplished by transferring the brachioradialis into the tendon of the extensor carpi radialis brevis. Transfer into the extensor carpi radialis longus gives a more radial deviation moment and the extensor carpi ulnaris acts as a wrist extensor only when the wrist is in supination (Tubiana, Miller, and Reed). Elbow extension must be present or reconstructed to stabilize the elbow against the significant flexion moment of the brachioradialis or the transfer power will be significantly reduced. Therefore procedures for wrist extension commonly are combined with other procedures such as elbow extension and tenodesis procedures for key pinch. Only when the brachioradialis muscle has grade 4 power can it be transferred to provide wrist extension. The power of the brachioradialis can be graded by palpation over the muscle mass against resisted elbow flexion with the forearm in neutral.

Transfer of brachioradialis to extensor carpi radialis brevis

■ *TECHNIQUE.* Make a longitudinal incision approximately 8 to 10 cm long dorsally along the radial aspect of the forearm. Carefully identify the dorsal sensory branch of the radial nerve and protect it during the mobilization of the brachioradialis. Proximal mobilization of the brachioradialis allows more excursion and is safe because the nerve supply is proximal. Identify the extensor carpi radialis brevis tendon of insertion into the base of the third metacarpal and pass the tendon of the brachioradialis through this tendon several times. Place tension on

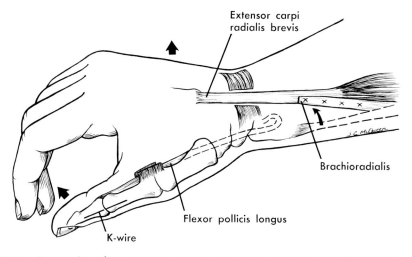

Extensor carpi
radialis brevis

Brachioradialis

Flexor pollicis longus

K-wire

Fig. 70-47 Restoration of wrist extension and key pinch when brachioradialis is only remaining functioning muscle unit, as recommended by Moberg.

the tendon and temporarily suture it to check for full wrist flexion without undue tension or laxity of the transferred unit (Fig. 70-47).

AFTERTREATMENT. A plaster splint is worn for 3 to 4 weeks and active range-of-motion exercises are then begun. Splinting is continued between exercises and at night for 8 to 12 months.

KEY PINCH. Key, or lateral pinch is more desirable and easier to achieve than chuckjaw, or three-fingered palmar pinch. This should be restored in all tetraplegics who have grade 4 or better wrist extensor motor power; however, a procedure that relies on active supination also has been described by Ejeskär. At least 75% of all tetraplegics may be candidates for a key-pinch procedure. Other prerequisites for the transfer include sufficient sensibility and thumb mobility. If ocular input is relied on, only one hand should be restored; however, if two-point discrimination is less than 12 to 15 mm, both hands should be reconstructed.

When no motors are expendable for active transfer, several well designed tenodeses are available for accomplishing key pinch.

The Moberg key-grip procedure is the precursor of and simplest of all thumb flexion tenodesis procedures. The flexor pollicis longus tendon is tenodesed to the distal radius so that on wrist extension the volar pulp of the thumb strongly contacts the radial side of the index finger. This may require stabilization procedures of the thumb interphalangeal and metacarpophalangeal joints. Moberg releases the A-1 pulley to increase the torque at the metacarpophalangeal joint by the subluxated flexor pollicis longus tendon.

Brand modified the Moberg key-grip procedure by leaving the A-1 pulley of the thumb metacarpophalangeal joint intact and routing the tendon across the palm, beneath the flexor tendons, and through Guyon's

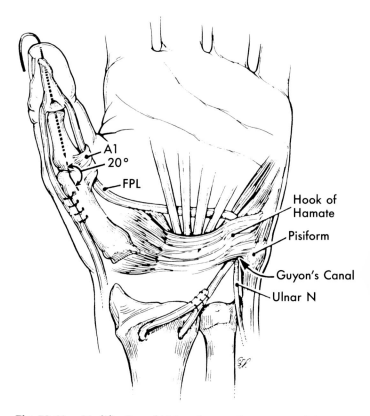

A1
20°
FPL
Hook of Hamate
Pisiform
Guyon's Canal
Ulnar N

Fig. 70-48 Modification of Moberg's operation to create "simple hand grip" (see text). (Redrawn from Green DP: Operative hand surgery, ed 2, New York, 1988, Churchill Livingstone.)

canal before tenodesing it to the distal radius. Hentz also uses this modification because the line of action is better and bowstringing of the tendon is prevented (Fig. 70-48). Bruner described a "winch" tenodesis for thumb flexion based on preservation of active forearm supination. The flexor pollicis longus tendon is routed around the distal ulna and is anchored to its dorsal aspect through a drill hole. During supination the anchored tendon flexes the thumb (Fig. 70-49).

Moberg key-grip tenodesis

■ *TECHNIQUE.* Expose the musculotendinous junction of the flexor pollicis longus through a volar approach and divide the tendon at this level. Expose the distal end of the radius by subperiosteal dissection of the pronator quadratus in a radial to ulnar direction. Drill two holes in the volar cortex of the distal radius transverse to its longitudinal axis. The holes should be large enough to allow passage of the free flexor pollicis longus tendon. Connect the drill holes with a curved curet or power burr. Carefully round the edges of the cortical bone to prevent tendon attrition. Make a 2 cm incision over the A-1 pulley and, after protecting the digital nerves, release the pulley. Deliver the flexor pollicis longus tendon into the wound. Stabilize the thumb interphalangeal

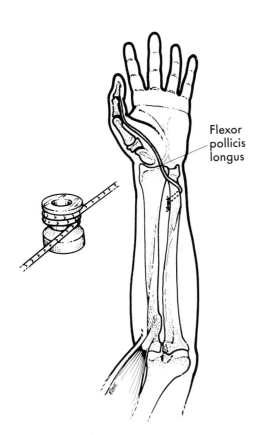

Fig. 70-49 Bruner "winch" operation: temporary arthrodesis of interphalangeal joint and tenodesis of flexor pollicis longus against dorsal aspect of ulna. (Redrawn from Ejeskär A: Hand Clin 4:585, 1988.)

joint in neutral position with a Kirschner wire (see Fig. 70-48). Make a 6 cm dorsal longitudinal incision centered over the thumb metacarpophalangeal joint. Open the hood of the dorsal apparatus in the line of the skin incision. After subperiosteal exposure, make several pairs of holes in the dorsal cortex of the thumb metacarpal. Tenodese the dorsal hood with sutures passed through them with the metacarpophalangeal joint in approximately 20 degrees of flexion. Adjust tension so that during full passive wrist extension the thumb firmly contacts the side of the index finger. Once the proper tension is obtained secure the flexor pollicis longus tendon to itself with multiple interrupted nonabsorbable sutures.

AFTERTREATMENT. The transfer is protected with a splint for 4 weeks in neutral position with the thumb tip under the index finger middle phalanx. Splint protection is continued for 8 more weeks. When transfer of the brachioradialis to the extensor carpi radialis brevis is combined with this procedure, the wrist is kept in slight extension to lessen the tension on the active transfer.

• • •

Retained active wrist extension, as in group 2 or better patients, provides active transfer potential for thumb flexion and perhaps grasp as well. Waters et al. reported transfer of the brachioradialis to the flexor pollicis longus tendon to restore lateral pinch. Before surgery their patients had no useful pinch force and at an average follow-up of 2.3 years they had a pinch force of about 4 pounds — roughly equivalent to that obtained with the Dorrance prosthetic hook. The transferred brachioradialis has been shown to have excellent excursion, muscle strength, and voluntary activation by Freehafer et al. Waters et al. also showed through electromyographic analysis that the brachioradialis muscle assumes the electrical synchrony of the paralyzed flexor pollicis longus after transfer. In normal subjects the brachioradialis is electrically silent during lateral pinch and the triceps and flexor pollicis longus have synergistic activity. Patients who had a posterior deltoid-to-triceps transfer, in addition to brachioradialis-to-flexor pollicis longus transfer, showed a pattern of synergistic electrical activity similar to normal subjects with similar tasks of thumb flexion and elbow extension. Waters et al. concluded that when wrist extensor torque is good (more than 10 foot-pounds) brachioradialis transfer for thumb flexion is preferred; when wrist torque is less, wrist extension should be augmented by the brachioradialis and thumb flexion should be augmented by tenodesis.

Patients in groups 4 and 5 comprise a large percentage of patients undergoing reconstructive efforts and systematic programs have been developed to treat these patients. The two most popular reconstructions are the House two-stage procedure and the Zancolli two-step

Table 70-5 Comparison of the Zancolli and House reconstructions*

Stage	Zancolli (1975)	House (1976)
I	Thumb CMC fusion	EDC, EPL, APL tenodesis
	Thumb MP capsuloplasty	Instrinsic tenodesis
	BR → EDC; EPL	
	MP joint stabilization (lasso)	
	PT → FCR (if FCR paralyzed)	
II	ECRL → FDP	PT → FPL
		BR → FDS (ring) → thumb (ECU & FCU)
		ECRL → FDP
	Accessory radial wrist extensor or ECRB (side-to-side)	
	Moberg key grip	

*Zancolli uses active EDC and EPL extension whereas House used tenodeses.

procedure (Table 70-5). These procedures both aim to restore grasp, key pinch, and release. They differ in that Zancolli actively restores finger extension and House adds an adduction-opposition transfer to the thumb.

House reconstruction. In 1976, House et al. described a two-stage procedure for reconstruction of digital flexion and key pinch in patients who have at least strong wrist extension and a functioning pronator teres (group 4 or better function). The procedure is divided into flexor and extensor phases; the extensor phase is performed first. Digital flexion is accomplished by transferring the extensor carpi radialis longus to the flexor digitorum profundus. Adduction and opposition of the thumb are obtained by transfer of the brachioradialis to the thumb where the flexor digitorum sublimis of the ring finger is used as an in situ graft. Key pinch and grasp strength can be enhanced by an active transfer into the flexor pollicis longus using either the pronator teres, the extensor, or flexor carpi ulnaris, or the brachioradialis. The release phase of the reconstruction consists of intrinsic and extrinsic extensor tenodeses; however, if sufficient motors are available, active extension of the thumb and fingers is possible. The thumb carpometacarpal joint is stabilized by either fusion of that joint or tenodesis of the abductor pollicis longus.

House and Shannon in 1985 compared the results of two modifications of this reconstruction. The procedures differed in the method of thumb control, intrinsic balance, and whether active extension was used. Qualitative differences between the two methods indicated that thumb carpometacarpal fusion allowed the hand better fine motor control, whereas the thumb adduction-opposition method afforded the ability to grasp larger objects.

Both methods achieved good grasp and lateral pinch. Thumb adduction-opposition transfer in the first method produced slightly greater lateral pinch and the thumb carpometacarpal arthrodesis provided slightly stronger grasp. Patients were pleased with having each hand reconstructed differently because they were able to use them for different tasks.

■ *TECHNIQUE (STAGE I, EXTENSOR PHASE).* **Make an 8 cm incision along the dorsal aspect of the distal forearm beginning just distal to Lister's tubercle on the mid-dorsum of the wrist. Curve the incision gently to the radial side of the forearm if an active transfer is chosen; otherwise make a straight incision for the tenodesis. Carefully protect the dorsal sensory branch of the radial nerve emerging beneath the brachioradialis radially and identify the extensor pollicis longus tendon ulnar and distal to Lister's tubercle and the tendons of the extensor digitorum communis in the fourth dorsal compartment. Also isolate the tendons of the abductor pollicis longus in the first dorsal compartment.**

Perform extensor tenodesis by anchoring the tendons of the abductor pollicis longus, the extensor pollicis longus, and the extensor digitorum communis to the dorsum of the distal radius through two well-rounded holes. The holes should be several cm proximal to the radiocarpal joint for the extensor digitorum communis tendons and 2 cm proximal for the abductor pollicis longus and extensor pollicis longus tendons. Make tunnels into the proximal radius with a curet to accommodate the free ends of the tendons to be tenodesed. Make two suture holes proximal to the previously prepared holes with a 0.035-inch Kirschner wire (Fig. 70-50). Remove the abductor pollicis longus tendons from the first dorsal compartment and transpose them ulnarward. Suture the extensor digitorum communis tendons together under tension so that retraction of the single sutured tendon permits synchronous extension of the fingers. Likewise, suture the abductor pollicis longus and extensor pollicis longus tendons together to form a single tendon unit to be fixed to the distal radius.

With the wrist in approximately 40 degrees of flexion place tension on the proximal end of the divided extensor digitorum communis tendon so that the metacarpophalangeal joints are in full extension. Note the position on the tendon stump that aligns with the suture holes. Weave a Bunnell heavy nonabsorbable anchor suture into the tendon so that the emerging suture ends exit at the selected site on the tendon for correct tension of the tenodesis. Introduce the free end of the extensor digitorum communis complex into the distal radius after delivering the free suture ends through the suture holes. Pull firmly on the sutures and check the tenodesis: full metacarpophalangeal extension should be

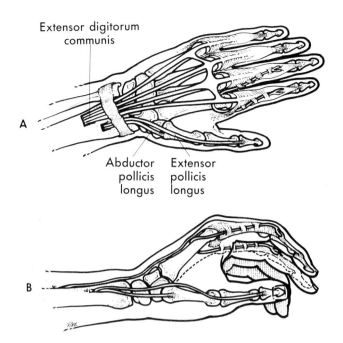

Fig. 70-50 House two-stage technique for reconstruction of digital flexion and key pinch. **A,** Stage I (extensor phase). Brachioradialis has been transferred to paralyzed flexor sublimis of ring finger as in situ graft rerouted around palmar fascial pulley to split thumb insertion. **B,** Flexor phase. Extensor carpi radialis longus has been transferred to flexor digitorum profundus and pronator teres to flexor pollicis longus. (Redrawn from House JH, Gwathmey FW, and Lundsgaard DK: J Hand Surg 1:152, 1976.)

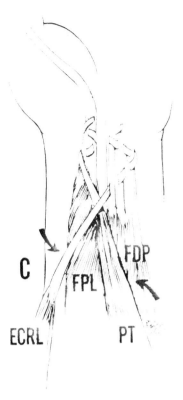

Fig. 70-51 House two-stage technique for reconstruction of digital flexion and key pinch. Stage II (flexor phase) (see text). (Redrawn from House JH, Gwathmey FW, and Lundsgaard DK: J Hand Surg 1:152, 1976.)

achieved when the wrist is flexed to 40 degrees and passive full flexion of the fingers should be obtained when the wrist is extended 40 degrees.

In the same fashion fix the rerouted abductor pollicis longus and extensor pollicis longus tendons so that with 40 degrees of wrist flexion the thumb interphalangeal joint is extended to 0 degrees and the thumb metacarpal is in the plane of the hand and radially abducted 30 to 40 degrees. After checking the tenodesis, make sure that with wrist extension the thumb has acceptable passive motion for the second stage of the transfer.

Intrinsic tenodesis may be achieved by transfer into either the A-2 pulley or the dorsal apparatus. House et al. described a procedure in which a free tendon graft is sutured into the central slip and lateral tendon of the extensor apparatus and then is taken through the lumbrical canals and around the dorsum of the metacarpal necks of the index and middle fingers. This forms in effect an "oblique retinacular ligament" so that when the proximal interphalangeal joint is flexed there is concomitant metacarpophalangeal flexion. It also prevents metacarpophalangeal hyperextension (Fig. 70-50, *B*).

AFTERTREATMENT. The wrist is held in 40 to 45 de-

grees of extension, the thumb and the metacarpophalangeal joints in 40 degrees of flexion, and the interphalangeal joints in extension for 4 weeks; then active and passive motion is begun. If thumb carpometacarpal joint arthrodesis was performed, the thumb is protected until fusion is obtained.

■ ***TECHNIQUE (STAGE II, FLEXOR PHASE) (Fig. 70-51).*** The flexor phase reconstruction is performed 2 to 6 months after the extensor phase. Access to the extensor carpi radialis longus and pronator teres for transfer into the extensor digitorum profundus and flexor pollicis longus requires three incisions. Make a volar longitudinal incision extending from the proximal wrist flexion crease just radial to the flexor carpi radialis tendon to the midshaft of the radius. Isolate the flexor pollicis longus, the pronator teres, and the flexor digitorum profundus tendons proximal to their musculotendinous junctions. Divide the extensor carpi radialis longus at its insertion into the base of the second metacarpal through a short transverse incision. Withdraw this tendon proximal to the abductor pollicis longus tendon in the mid-third of the forearm using the proximal limb of the incision from the extensor phase of the reconstruction. Free the extensor carpi radialis longus tendon from its attachments so that free excursion is possible. Remove the pronator teres tendon from the shaft of the radius with a strip of its periosteal attachment.Weave the transfers together with the pronator teres to the flexor pollicis longus and the extensor carpi radialis longus to the flexor digitorum profundus. Adjust tension so that the thumb rests against the side of the index finger when the wrist is in 30 degrees of extension. The extensor carpi radialis longus-flexor digitorum profundus tension should allow reasonable synchronous finger flexion when the wrist is in 40 degrees of extension.

The brachioradialis may be used as an opponens-adductorplasty if it was not used in the extensor phase. This procedure is essentially the same as the Royle-Thompson transfer (p. 3245). Harvest the ring finger sublimis tendon as for the Zancolli lasso procedure. Bring the sublimis tendon out through a small incision at the distal-ulnar margin of the transverse carpal ligament. Tunnel the flexor digitorum sublimis tendon with its two slips across the palm to the metacarpophalangeal region of the thumb. Suture one slip into the extensor pollicis

longus distal to the metacarpophalangeal joint and the other into the adductor tendon. Weave the free end of the brachioradialis into the intact ring flexor digitorum sublimis so that when the wrist is in neutral position the thumb rests against the side of the index finger.

AFTERTREATMENT. The wrist is immobilized in 25 degrees of dorsiflexion, the metacarpophalangeal joints in flexion, and the interphalangeal joints in extension. At 3 weeks active and passive range-of-motion exercises are begun as well as muscle reeducation. The transfers should be protected for 3 months.

Zancolli reconstruction. Zancolli in 1975 described a two-step technique for reconstruction in patients with C-6 level function. The first step provides finger and thumb extension and the second provides grasp. An accessory radial wrist extensor should be sought in the first step of the reconstruction because it may be helpful in the second step. In the first step, the thumb is stabilized by arthrodesis of the carpometacarpal joint or capsuloplasty of the metacarpophalangeal joint. The brachiorad-

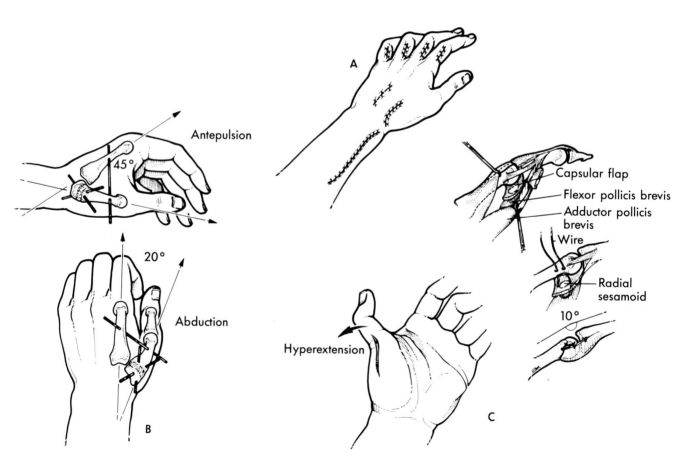

Fig. 70-52 Zancolli two-step technique for reconstruction in patients with C-6 level function (see text). **A,** Three incisions required. **B,** Thumb fusion is fixed with three Kirschner wires. **C,** For hyperextension, volar plate capsuloplasty is performed. (Redrawn from Zancolli EA: Clin Orthop 112:101, 1975.)

ialis is transferred to the extensor digitorum communis and extensor pollicis longus. If the metacarpophalangeal joints tend to hyperextend, this is corrected by the Zancolli lasso procedure. If the flexor carpi radialis is nonfunctioning, the pronator teres is transferred to obtain wrist flexion.

■ *TECHNIQUE (ZANCOLLI, FIRST STEP).* Fuse the carpometacarpal joint in 45 degrees of palmar abduction and 20 degrees of radial abduction. Fix the fusion with two crossed Kirschner wires, and with a third wire fix the relationship between the first and second metacarpals. If the metacarpophalangeal joint hyperextends, perform a volar plate capsuloplasty by suturing the volar plate and its radial sesamoid to the neck of the metacarpal (Fig. 70-52, *B* and *C*).

Transfer the brachioradialis into the extensor pollicis longus and extensor digitorum communis through a long curved radial incision (Fig. 70-52, *A*). Adhesions at the graft site may be minimized by excising a portion of the proximal aspect of the dorsal carpal ligament and by placing the sutures as far proximal as possible. Keep the elbow at 60 degrees of flexion and use slightly more tension on the extensor digitorum communis than on the extensor pollicis longus because tension is reduced on the extensor digitorum communis with elbow extension (Fig. 70-53). The tension is correct when full passive finger flexion can be obtained with maximal wrist extension and the elbow at 60 degrees of flexion. Passive wrist flexion should fully extend the metacarpophalangeal joints and the interphalangeal joint of the thumb.

The intrinsic tenodesis can be performed at this stage, but it is often combined with the second step. *AFTERTREATMENT.* The hand and elbow are immobilized for 4 weeks, after which the thumb fusion is protected with a splint for another 4 weeks. Muscle reeducation is begun by encouraging active metacarpophalangeal extension by elbow flexion. Passive finger flexion is necessary to prevent extension contractures.

• • •

Four to six months after the first step, the hand is ready for the second step of the reconstruction. This step provides finger flexion and active thumb flexion.

■ *TECHNIQUE (ZANCOLLI, SECOND STEP).* Transfer the extensor carpi radialis longus into the flexor digitorum profundus with slightly more tension applied to the more ulnar digits. The details of this are the same as in the House reconstruction (p. 3272).

The flexor pollicis longus may be activated by one of several methods. Zancolli's choice is the supernumerary radial wrist extensor (extensor carpi radialis tertius), which should be sought in the first step of the reconstruction. This is a synergistic transfer and

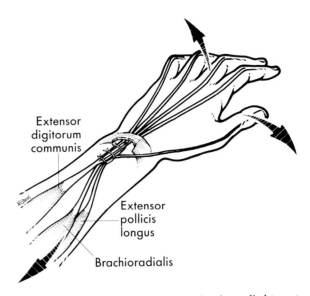

Fig. 70-53 Same as 70-52. More tension is applied to extensor digitorum communis than to extensor pollicis longus because elbow extension reduces tension on EDC. (Redrawn from Zancolli EA: Clin Orthop 112:101, 1975.)

allows independent control of thumb flexion (Fig. 70-54, *A*). When this muscle is absent, side-to-side suturing of the extensor carpi radialis brevis with the flexor pollicis longus can be performed. Thumb flexion occurs with wrist extension and conversely thumb extension occurs with wrist flexion (Fig. 70-54, *B*). Tension is set so that with complete passive wrist extension, the thumb firmly rests against the index finger. A third option is passive tenodesis to the volar aspect of the distal radius, as in the Moberg key-pinch technique (p. 3271).

The Zancolli lasso procedure for intrinsic tenodesis may be added at this step. Tenodese the paralyzed sublimis tendons through a transverse incision in the palm just proximal to the metacarpophalangeal joint flexion crease. Expose the flexor digitorum sublimis tendons and the A-1 and proximal A-2 pulleys. Retract the flexor digitorum sublimis tendons into the wound with the proximal interphalangeal joints in maximal flexion and divide them as far distally as possible. Take the two slips of each sublimis tendon out through the distal margins of the A-1 pulleys and suture them back to themselves (Fig. 70-55). Adjust tension so that with the wrist in 40 degrees of flexion the metacarpophalangeal joints extend to 0 degrees.

AFTERTREATMENT. The arm is immobilized for 4 weeks in a long arm splint, as in step one, but with the wrist in neutral, the thumb between the index and middle fingers, and the fingers gently flexed. Then active and passive exercises are begun with muscle reeducation. The transfers are protected from heavy use for 3 months.

• • •

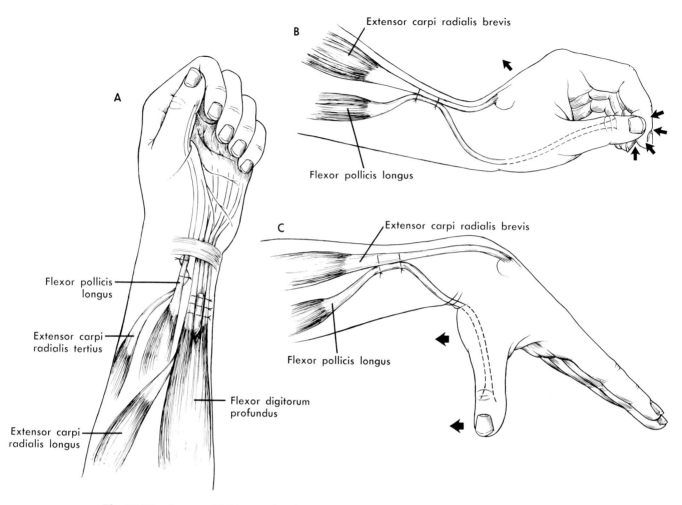

Fig. 70-54 Same as 70-52. **A,** When both radial wrist extensors are active, extensor radialis longus may be used to help provide finger flexion; thumb flexion may be benefitted by transfer of active extensor carpi radialis tertius when present (see text). **B,** Key pinch is obtained with wrist extension by active extensor carpi radialis brevis with tenodesis to flexor pollicis longus. To achieve correct tension, with wrist in complete passive extension, flexor pollicis longus tendon is sutured to extensor carpi radialis when pinching is produced. **C,** With passive wrist flexion, pinch is released. (Redrawn from Zancolli EA: Clin Orthop 112:101, 1975.)

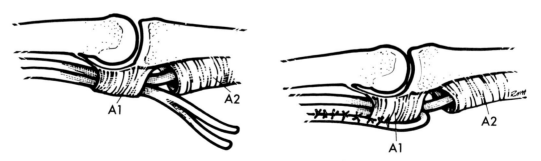

Fig. 70-55 Zancolli lasso operation. Sublimis tendon is cut distally and turned proximally and sutured to itself and to A-1 ligament with tension to prevent hyperextension of metacarpophalangeal joint. (Redrawn from Ejeskär A: Hand Clin 4:585, 1988.)

Table 70-6 Summary of surgical reconstruction options in tetraplegia according to the international classification scheme

Group	Lowest muscle grade 4 or better below elbow	Surgical reconstruction options
0	0	Elbow extension (Moberg)
1	Brachioradialis	Elbow extension, key grip
2	Extensor carpi radialis longus	Elbow extension, key grip
3	Extensor carpi radialis brevis	Zancolli two-stage Key grip BR → thumb adductor ECRL → FDP
4	Pronator teres	Zancolli two-stage
5	Flexor carpi radialis	Zancolli two-stage House two-stage
6	Finger extensors	Modified House (suture EDL to EDC side-to-side for thumb extension)
7	Thumb extensor	House two-stage
8	Partial finger flexors	Zancolli two-stage
9	Lacks only intrinsics	Opponens transfer Zancolli lasso
X	Exceptions	

Surgery in tetraplegia patients in higher groups is easier because more function is retained. The procedures outlined above can be incorporated into the management of these patients. Table 70-6 summarizes the current international classification scheme, with the surgical procedures of choice according to McDowell et al. It must be remembered that some patients do not fall neatly into groups 0 through 9, and a surgical plan must be tailored for them.

REFERENCES

Adams J and Wood VE: Tendon transfers for irreparable nerve damage in the hand, Orthop Clin North Am 12:403, 1981.

Beasley RW: Principles of tendon transfer, Orthop Clin North Am 2:433, 1970.

Beasley RW: Tendon transfers for radial nerve palsy, Orthop Clin North Am 2:439, 1970.

Belsole RJ, Lister GD, and Kleinert HE: Polyarteritis: a cause of nerve palsy in the extremity, J Hand Surg 3:320, 1978.

Blacker GJ, Lister GD, and Kleinert HE: The abducted little finger in low ulnar nerve palsy, J Hand Surg 1:190, 1976.

Boswick JA Jr: Tendon transfers for tendon injuries in the upper extremities, Orthop Clin North Am 2:253, 1974.

Boyes JH: Tendon transfers for radial palsy, Bull Hosp Joint Dis 21:97, 1960.

Boyes JH: Selection of a donor muscle for tendon transfer, Bull Hosp Joint Dis 23:1, 1962.

Boyes JH: Bunnell's surgery of the hand, ed 4, Philadelphia, 1964, JB Lippincott Co.

Boyes JH: Problems of tendon surgery, Am J Surg 109:269, 1965.

Brand PW: Paralytic claw hand: with special reference to paralysis in leprosy and treatment by the sublimis transfer of Stiles and Bunnell, J Bone Joint Surg 40-B:618, 1948.

Brand PW: Tendon grafting: illustrated by a new operation for intrinsic paralysis of the fingers, J Bone Joint Surg 43-B:444, 1961.

Brand PW: Tendon transfers for median and ulnar nerve paralysis, Orthop Clin North Am 2:447, 1970.

Brand PW: Rehabilitation of the hand with motor and sensory impairment, Orthop Clin North Am 4:1135, 1973.

Braun RM et al: Preliminary experience with superficialis-to-profundus tendon transfer in the hemiplegic upper extremity, J Bone Joint Surg 56-A:466, 1974.

Brooks AL: Personal communication, 1969.

Brooks AL and Jones DS: A new intrinsic tendon transfer for the paralytic hand, J Bone Joint Surg 57-A:730, 1975.

Brooks DM: Inter-metacarpal bone graft for thenar paralysis: technique and end-results, J Bone Joint Surg 31-B:511, 1949.

Brown PW: Zancolli capsulorrhaphy for ulnar claw hand: appraisal of forty-four cases, J Bone Joint Surg 52-A:868, 1970.

Brown PW: Reconstruction for pinch in ulnar intrinsic palsy, Orthop Clin North Am 2:323, 1974.

Bruner JM: Tendon transfer to restore abduction of the index finger using the extensor pollicis brevis, Plast Reconstr Surg 3:197, 1948.

Brys D and Waters RL: Effect of triceps function on the brachioradialis transfer in quadriplegia, J Hand Surg 12-A:237, 1987.

Buckwalter JA, Mickelson MR, and Emerson RL: Ulnar nerve palsy in Paget's disease, Clin Orthop 127:212, 1977.

Bunnell S: Surgery of the intrinsic muscles of the hand other than those producing opposition of the thumb, J Bone Joint Surg 24:1, 1942.

Bunnell S: Tendon transfers in the hand and forearm, AAOS Instr Course Lect 6:106, 1949.

Burkhalter WE: Early tendon transfer in upper extremity peripheral nerve injury, Clin Orthop 104:68, 1974.

Burkhalter WE: Restoration of power grip in ulnar nerve paralysis, Orthop Clin North Am 2:289, 1974.

Burkhalter WE: Tendon transfers in median nerve palsy, Orthop Clin North Am 2:271, 1974.

Burkhalter WE: Tendon transfers in brachial plexus injuries, Orthop Clin North Am 2:259, 1974.

Burkhalter WE and Strait JL: Metacarpophalangeal flexor replacement for intrinsic-muscle paralysis, J Bone Joint Surg 55-A:1667, 1973.

Burkhalter WE et al: Extensor indicis proprius opponensplasty, J Bone Joint Surg 55-A:725, 1973.

Camitz H: Über die behandlung der oppositionslähmung, Acta Chir Scand LXV, 77, 1929.

Carroll RE and Kleinman WB: Pectoralis major transplantation to restore elbow flexion to the paralytic limb, J Hand Surg 4:501, 1979.

Clippinger FW Jr and Irwin CE: The opponens transfer: analysis of end results, South Med J 55:33, 1962.

Cochrane RG: Leprosy in theory and practice, Bristol, 1959, John Wright & Sons, Ltd.

Curtis RM: Fundamental principles of tendon transfer, Orthop Clin North Am 2:231, 1974.

Curtis RM: Opposition of the thumb, Orthop Clin North Am 2:305, 1974.

Curtis RM: Tendon transfers in the patient with spinal cord injury, Orthop Clin North Am 2:415, 1974.

DeBenedetti M: Restoration of elbow extension power in the tetraplegic patient using the Moberg technique, J Hand Surg 4:86, 1979.

Edgerton MT and Brand PW: Restoration of abduction and adduction to the unstable thumb in median and ulnar paralysis, Plast Reconstr Surg 36:150, 1965.

Ejeskär A: Upper limb surgical rehabilitation in high-level tetraplegia, Hand Clin 4:585, 1988.

Enna CD: Use of the extensor pollicis brevis to restore abduction in the unstable thumb, Plast Reconstr Surg 46:350, 1970.

Enna CD and Riordan DC: The Fowler procedure for correction of the paralytic claw hand, Plast Reconstr Surg 52:352, 1973.

Entin MA: Restoration of function of paralyzed hand, Surg Clin North Am 44:1049, 1964.

Familla JM, Peimer CA, and Sherwin FS: Brachioradialis transfer for digital palsy, J Hand Surg 15-B:312, 1990.

Flatt AE: An indication for shortening of the thumb: description of technique and brief report of five cases, J Bone Joint Surg 46-A:1534, 1964.

Flynn JE: Reconstruction of the hand after median-nerve palsy, N Engl J Med 256:676, 1957.

Fowler SB: Mobilization of metacarpophalangeal joints, J Bone Joint Surg 29:193, 1947.

Fowler SB: Extensor apparatus of the digits, J Bone Joint Surg 31-B:447, 1949.

Freehafer AA and Mast WA: Transfer of the brachioradialis to improve wrist extension in high spinal-cord injury, J Bone Joint Surg 49-A:648, 1967.

Freehafer AA et al: Tendon transfers to improve grasp after injuries of the cervical spinal cord, J Bone Joint Surg 56-A:951, 1974.

Freehafer AA, Peckham PH, and Keith MW: New concepts on treatment of the upper limb in the tetraplegic: surgical restoration and functional neuromuscular stimulation, Hand Clin 4:563, 1988.

Freehafer AA, Peckham PH, Keith MW, and Mendelson LS: The brachioradialis: anatomy, properties, and value for tendon transfer in the tetraplegic, J Hand Surg 13-A:99, 1988.

Friedenberg ZB: Transposition of the biceps brachii for triceps weakness, J Bone Joint Surg 36-A:656, 1954.

Gansel J, Waters R, and Gellman H: Transfer of the pronator teres tendon to the tendons of the flexor digitorum profundus in tetraplegia, J Bone Joint Surg 72-A:427, 1990.

Goldner JL: Tendon transfers for irreparable peripheral nerve injuries of the upper extremity, Orthop Clin North Am 2:343, 1974.

Goldner JL and Irwin CE: An analysis of paralytic thumb deformities, J Bone Joint Surg 32-A:627, 1950.

Goldner JL and Kelly JM: Radial nerve injuries, South Med J 51:873, 1958.

Granberry WM and Lipscomb PR: Tendon transfers to the hand in brachial palsy, Am J Surg 108:840, 1964.

Groves RJ and Goldner JL: Restoration of strong opposition after median-nerve or brachial plexus paralysis, J Bone Joint Surg 57-A:112, 1975.

Hamlin C and Littler JW: Restoration of power pinch, J Hand Surg 5:396, 1980.

Henderson ED: Use of sublimis tendon transfers to extend the fingers: report of case, Mayo Clin Proc 35:438, 1960.

Henderson ED: Transfer of wrist extensors and brachioradialis to restore opposition of the thumb, J Bone Joint Surg 44-A:513, 1962.

Hentz VR, Brown M, and Keoshian LA: Upper limb reconstruction in quadriplegia: functional assessment and proposed treatment modification, J Hand Surg 8:119, 1983.

Hentz VR, Hamlin C, and Keoshian LA: Surgical reconstruction in tetraplegia, Hand Clin 4:601, 1988.

Hentz VR and Keoshian LA: Changing perspectives in surgical hand rehabilitation in quadriplegic patients, Plast Reconstr Surg 64:509, 1979.

House JH, Gwathmey FW, and Lundsgaard DK: Restoration of strong grasp and lateral pinch in tetraplegia due to cervical spinal cord injury, J Hand Surg 1:152, 1976.

House JH and Shannon MA: Restoration of strong grasp and lateral pinch in tetraplegia: a comparison of two methods of thumb control in each patient, J Hand Surg 10-A:21, 1985.

Huber E: Hilfsoperation bei Medianuslähmung, Deutsch Z Chir 162:271, 1921.

Irwin CE and Eyler DL: Surgical rehabilitation of the hand and forearm disabled by poliomyelitis, J Bone Joint Surg 33-A:825, 1951.

Irwin CE and Flinchum CE: Piedmont Orthopaedic Society Letter, October 1957 (mimeographed).

Jacobs B and Thompson TC: Opposition of the thumb and its restoration, J Bone Joint Surg 42-A:1015, 1960.

Jones R: On suture of nerves, and alternative methods of treatment by transplantation of tendon, Br Med J 1:641, 1916.

Jones R: Tendon transplantation in cases of musculospinal injuries not amenable to suture, Am J Surg 35:333, 1921.

Kaplan I, Dinner M, and Chait L: Use of extensor pollicis longus tendon as a distal extension for an opponens transfer, Plast Reconstr Surg 57:186, 1976.

Keith MW, Peckham PH, Thrope GB, et al: Implantable functional neuromuscular stimulation in the tetraplegic hand, J Hand Surg 14-A:524, 1989.

Kessler FB: Use of a pedicled tendon transfer with a silicone rod in complicated secondary flexor tendon repairs, Plast Reconstr Surg 49:439, 1972.

Lacey SH, Wilber G, Peckham PH, and Freehafer AA: The posterior deltoid to triceps transfer: a clinical and biomechanical assessment, J Hand Surg 11-A:542, 1986.

Lamb DW, editor: The paralysed hand, Edinburgh, 1987, Churchill Livingstone.

Lamb DW: Upper limb surgery in tetraplegia, J Hand Surg 14-B:143, 1989.

Lamb DW and Chan KM: Surgical reconstruction of the upper limb in traumatic tetraplegia: a review of 41 patients, J Bone Joint Surg 65-B:291, 1983.

Lamphier TA: Tendon transfer (or transplant) for paralysis of an interosseus muscle, Int Surg 27:738, 1957.

Larsen RD and Posch JL: Nerve injuries in the upper extremity, Arch Surg 77:469, 1958.

Leddy JP et al: Capsulodesis and pulley advancement for the correction of claw-finger deformity, J Bone Joint Surg 54-A:1465, 1972.

Lipscomb PR, Elkins EC, and Henderson ED: Tendon transfers to restore function of hands in tetraplegia, especially after fracture-dislocation of the sixth cervical vertebra on the seventh, J Bone Joint Surg 40-A:1071, 1958.

Littler JW: Tendon transfers and arthrodeses in combined median and ulnar nerve paralysis, J Bone Joint Surg 31-A:225, 1949.

Littler JW and Cooley SGE: Opposition of the thumb and its restoration by abductor digiti quinti transfer, J Bone Joint Surg 45-A:1389, 1963.

Makin M: Translocation of the flexor pollicis longus tendon to restore opposition, J Bone Joint Surg 49-B:458, 1967.

Mangus DJ: Flexor pollicis longus tendon transfer for restoration of opposition of the thumb, Plast Reconstr Surg 52:155, 1973.

Matev I: Functional rehabilitation of the thumb in ulnar palsy (Réhabilitation fonctionnelle du pouce dans une paralysie cubitale basse irréductible), Ann Chir Plast 5:23, 1960 (Abstracted by Joseph C Mulier, Inte Abstr Surg 111:383, 1960.)

McDowell CL, Moberg EA, and House JH: The second international conference on surgical rehabilitation of the upper limb in tetraplegia (quadriplegia), J Hand Surg 11-A:604, 1986.

McDowell CL, Moberg EA, and Smith AG: International conference on surgical rehabilitation of the upper limb in tetraplegia, J Hand Surg 4:387, 1979.

Mikhail IK: Bone block operation for clawhand, Surg Gynecol Obstet 118:1077, 1964.

Milgram JE: Tendon transplantation of biceps and triceps to paralyzed fingers through artificially created tendon sheaths, Bull Hosp Joint Dis 15:45, 1954.

Moberg E: Surgical treatment for absent single-hand grip and elbow extension in quadriplegia: principles and preliminary experience, J Bone Joint Surg 57-A:196, 1975.

Moberg E: Reconstructive hand surgery in tetraplegia, stroke, and cerebral palsy: some basic concepts in physiology and neurology, J Hand Surg 1:29, 1976.

Moberg E: The present state of upper limb surgical rehabilitation in tetraplegia, J Hand Surg 14-A (no 2 pt 2):354, 1989.

Murphy CP and Chuinard RG: Management of the upper extremity in traumatic tetraplegia, Hand Clin 4:201, 1988.

Neviaser RJ, Wilson JN, and Gardner MM: Abductor pollicis longus transfer for replacement of first dorsal interosseus, J Hand Surg 5:53, 1980.

Ney KW: A tendon transplant for intrinsic hand muscle paralysis, Surg Gynecol Obstet 33:342, 1921.

Nickel VL, Perry J, and Garrett AL: Development of useful function in the severely paralyzed hand, J Bone Joint Surg 45-A:933, 1963.

Omer GE Jr: Evaluation and reconstruction of the forearm and hand after acute traumatic peripheral nerve injuries, J Bone Joint Surg 50-A:1454, 1968.

Omer GE Jr: The technique and timing of tendon transfers, Orthop Clin North Am 2:243, 1974.

Omer GE Jr: Tendon transfers in combined nerve lesions, Orthop Clin North Am 2:377, 1974.

Omer GE Jr and Capsen DA: Proximal row carpectomy with muscle transfers for spastic paralysis, J Hand Surg 1:197, 1976.

Omer GE Jr and Elton RC: Tendon transfers for the nerve injured upper limb, Orthop Rev 1:25 July 1972.

Orticochea M: Use of the deep bundle of the flexor pollicis brevis to restore opposition in the thumb, Plast Reconstr Surg 47:220, 1971.

Palande DD: Opponensplasty in intrinsic-muscle paralysis of the thumb in leprosy, J Bone Joint Surg 57-A:489, 1975.

Palande DD: Correction of paralytic claw finger in leprosy by capsulorrhaphy and pulley advancement, J Bone Joint Surg 58-A:59, 1976.

Parkes A: Paralytic claw fingers: a graft tenodesis operation, Hand 5:192, 1973.

Peckham PH, Marsolais EB, and Mortimer JT: Restoration of key grip and release in the C6 tetraplegic patient through functional electrical stimulation, J Hand Surg 5:462, 1980.

Phalen GS and Miller RC: The transfer of wrist extensor muscles to restore or reinforce flexion power of the fingers and opposition of the thumb, J Bone Joint Surg 29:993, 1947.

Rigg BM: A simple tendon transfer for the isolated division of the flexor digitorum profundus, Hand 7:246, 1975.

Riley WB Jr, Mann RJ, and Burkhalter WE: Extensor pollicis longus opponensplasty, J Hand Surg 5:217, 1980.

Riordan DC: Tendon transplantations in median-nerve and ulnar-nerve paralysis, J Bone Joint Surg 35-A:312, 1953.

Riordan DC: Surgery of the paralytic hand, AAOS Instr Course Lect 16:79, 1959.

Riordan DC: The hand in leprosy: a seven-year clinical study. I. General aspects of leprosy, J Bone Joint Surg 42-A:661, 1960.

Riordan DC: The hand in leprosy: a seven-year clinical study. II. Orthopaedic aspects of leprosy, J Bone Joint Surg 42-A:683, 1960.

Riordan DC: Radial nerve paralysis, Orthop Clin North Am 2:283, 1974.

Riordan DC: Tendon transfers in hand surgery, J Hand Surg 8:748, 1983.

Royle ND: An operation for paralysis of the intrinsic muscles of the thumb, JAMA 111:612, 1938.

Said GZ: A modified tendon transference for radial nerve paralysis, J Bone Joint Surg 56-B:320, 1974.

Sakellarides HT: Modified pulley for opponens tendon transfer, J Bone Joint Surg 52-A:178, 1970.

Schnute WJ and Tachdjian MO: Intermetacarpal bone block for thenar paralysis following poliomyelitis: an end-result study, J Bone Joint Surg 45-A:1663, 1963.

Schottstaedt ER, Larsen LJ, and Bost FC: The surgical reconstruction of the upper extremity paralyzed by poliomyelitis, J Bone Joint Surg 40-A:633, 1958.

Scuderi C: Tendon transplants for irreparable radial nerve paralysis, Surg Gynecol Obstet 88:643, 1949.

Seddon HJ: Reconstructive surgery of the upper extremity. In Poliomyelitis, Second International Poliomyelitis Congress, Philadelphia, 1952, JB Lippincott Co.

Selvapandian AJ and Brand PW: Reconstructive surgery in leprosy hands, Indian J Surg 20:524, 1958.

Skielboe BE and Koh JY: Tendon transference for ulnar and combined ulnar-median nerve paralysis, Acta Orthop Scand 36:137, 1965-1966.

Smith RJ: Non-ischemic contractures of the intrinsic muscles of the hand, J Bone Joint Surg 53-A:1313, 1971.

Smith RJ: Intrinsic muscles of the fingers: function, dysfunction, and surgical reconstruction, AAOS Instr Course Lect 24:200, 1975.

Smith RJ: Extensor carpi radialis brevis tendon transfer for thumb abduction: a study of power pinch, J Hand Surg 8:4, 1983.

Snow JW and Fink GH: Use of a transverse carpal ligament window for the pulley in tendon transfers for median nerve palsy, Plast Reconstr Surg 48:238, 1971.

Spinner M: Reconstruction of the hand in high median nerve injuries, Bull Hosp Joint Dis 26:191, 1965.

Srinivasan H: The extensor diversion graft operation for correction of intrinsic minus fingers in leprosy, J Bone Joint Surg 55-B:58, 1973.

Starr CL: Army experience with tendon transference, J Bone Joint Surg 4:3, 1922.

Steindler A: Flexor plasty of the thumb in thenar paralysis, Surg Gynecol Obstet 50:1005, 1930.

Steindler A: Reconstruction of the poliomyelitic upper extremity, Bull Hosp Joint Dis 15:21, 1954.

Stiles HJ and Forrester-Brown MF: Treatment of injuries of the peripheral spinal nerves, Stoughton, 1922, H Frowde & Hodder.

Thompson TC: Modified operation for opponens paralysis, J Bone Joint Surg 24:632, 1942.

Tubiana R: Palliative treatment of paralytic deformities of the thumb, Orthop Clin North Am 4:1141, 1973.

Tubiana R, Miller HW IV, and Reed S: Restoration of wrist extension after paralysis, Hand Clin 5:53, 1989.

Tubiana R and Yabe Y, chairmen: Section on paralysis symposium. Paralysis including tetraplegia: plenary symposium, J Hand Surg 14-A (no 2 pt 2):353, 1989.

Versaci AD: Tendon transfers in ulnar-nerve injuries, N Engl J Med 262:801, 1960.

Versaci AD: Tendon transfers in ulnar nerve injuries, Plast Reconstr Surg 26:500, 1960.

Waters RL: Upper extremity surgery in stroke patients, Clin Orthop 131:30, 1978.

Waters R, Moore KR, Graboff SR, and Paris K: Brachioradialis to flexor pollicis longus tendon transfer for active lateral pinch in the tetraplegic, J Hand Surg 10-A:385, 1985.

Waters RL, Stark LZ, Gubernick I, et al: Electromyographic analysis of brachioradialis to flexor pollicis longus tendon transfer in quadriplegia, J Hand Surg 15-A:335, 1990.

White WL: Restoration of function and balance of the wrist and hand by tendon transfers, Surg Clin North Am 40:427, 1960.

Williams HWG: The treatment of peripheral nerve lesions of the hand in leprosy, Int Surg 46:573, 1966.

Wilson JE: Providing automatic grasp by flexor tenodesis, J Bone Joint Surg 38-A:1019, 1956.

Zachary RB: Tendon transplantation for radial paralysis, Br J Surg 33:358, 1946.

Zancolli EA: Claw-hand caused by paralysis of the intrinsic muscles: a simple surgical procedure for its correction, J Bone Joint Surg 39-A:1076, 1957.

Zancolli EA: Surgery for the quadriplegic hand with active, strong wrist extension preserved: a study of 97 cases, Clin Orthop 112:101, 1975.

Cerebral Palsied Hand

MARK T. JOBE

Cerebral palsy is a nonprogressive, nonhereditary encephelopathy that occurs in the prenatal or perinatal period and is characterized by altered motor, sensory, and often intellectual function. It occurs in the United States with an approximate annual frequency of 7 per 1000 live births. It can be classified as pyramidal, which includes spastic hemiplegia, diplegia, paraplegia, and quadriplegia, or as extrapyramidal, which includes athetoid and ataxic patterns. A mixed variety also occurs, with both spasticity and athetosis (see also Chapter 46). Hand function is impaired to some extent in all types, except possibly spastic paraplegia, with the most common deformities being shoulder adduction, and internal rotation, elbow flexion, forearm pronation, wrist and finger flexion, thumb-in-palm, and swan-neck deformities (Fig 71-1). Many surgical procedures have been performed in an attempt to correct these deformities. Earlier results were unpredictable and disappointing, primarily because of inappropriate patient selection. The extensive works of such surgeons as Green, Goldner, Swanson, Zancolli, and Hoffer have proved certain principles in the evaluation and management of the cerebral palsied hand.

PATIENT EVALUATION

Probably fewer than 4% of patients with hands disabled by cerebral palsy can be helped by surgery. Careful, repeated evaluations, often over a considerable period of time, are required before surgery can either be advised for this small group or discouraged for most other patients. Important information includes any birth or perinatal medical problems, achievement of developmental milestones, and especially the degree with which the child has previously used the hand. If the hand is completely ignored by the child, then it is doubtful that function will be restored or improved with surgery. The early development of handedness may be especially helpful, because it is uncommon before the age of 3 years and may represent some degree of particular weakness or uncoordination in the less preferred extremity. The particular cerebral lesion should be identified and characterized as either pyramidal with associated spasticity or extrapyramidal, because children with athetoid patterns will not be surgical candidates. The persistence of any infantile postural reflexes should be documented. Deformities should be classified as either static contractures (deformities that do not correct with compensatory positioning of either muscle or joint) or dynamic deformities that are spastic and slowly correctable. Most children demonstrate dynamic deformities early in life, and, if left untreated, these deformities may progress to static contractures.

Muscle examination should determine the degree of spasticity, strength, and coordination of each major muscle, with special attention given to the child's ability to pinch, grasp, and release objects. The patient also should have sufficient proximal control of the extremity to voluntarily place the hand on top of the head and then on the opposite knee within 5 to 10 seconds. If the child does not demonstrate this degree of control, it is doubtful that he will use the extremity enough to justify reconstruction.

The sensibility pattern of the hand should be determined. Even though most patients have intact epicritic sensation (the ability to discern pinprick, heat, and cold),

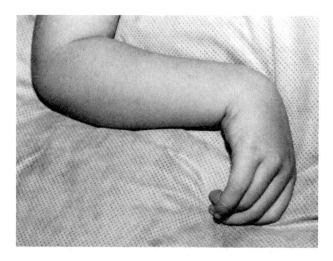

Fig. 71-1 Typical upper extremity deformities in cerebral palsy. Elbow flexion, forearm pronation, wrist and finger flexion.

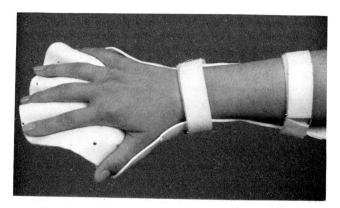

Fig. 71-2 Splint for spastic hand.

about half have impaired sensibility, with diminished two-point discrimination, stereognosis, and proprioception. Because sensibility in the hand is so important in determining prognosis after surgery, its status should be evaluated as accurately as possible before surgery. An indication may be gained by observing whether the hand is used or ignored; unless motor coordination is extremely poor, an ignored hand probably indicates the absence of sensibility. Further evaluation requires communication with the child, and this usually is impossible before the age of 4 years. A cursory examination may be carried out by asking the blindfolded child to differentiate between a sphere and a cube or to indicate the position of the hand when the palm has been placed, by the examiner, facing upward or downward. A more detailed examination testing recognition of blunt and sharp points, of familiar objects such as coins, and of differences in temperature also is valuable.

Further evaluation using dynamic electromyography, as described by Hoffer, Perry, and Melkonian, may be helpful in determining which muscles are in phase with the function to be augmented and thus allow for appropriate donor muscle selection. Neuromuscular blocking agents, such as 1% lidocaine, 0.25% bupivacaine, and 45% ethanol, are helpful in assessing weaker muscle groups without the overbearing effect of antagonist muscles and can assist in predicting surgical outcome following tendon lengthening or tenotomy.

NONOPERATIVE MANAGEMENT

Splinting is indicated early to prevent fixed contractures of the muscles and joints. A well-padded splint that avoids pressure points should hold the wrist in as much

extension as tolerated, the fingers in almost complete extension, and the thumb out of the palm (Fig. 71-2).

OPERATIVE MANAGEMENT
Goals

The goals of operative treatment in the child with cerebral palsy should be very specific and should be aimed at providing useful grasp and release and acceptable hygiene. At times, improving the appearance of the hand by correcting an unsightly contracture may be a modest goal as well. Fine manipulation rarely will be improved by surgery, and normal hand function is an unrealistic goal. Grasp and release will be possible only in children who have at least sufficient sensibility to allow an awareness of the extremity. Undercorrection rather than overcorrection of the deformity or dysfunction is always preferred.

Principles

The ideal candidate for surgery is a spastic hemiplegic who is cooperative, intelligent, and well motivated and who has a pattern of grasp and release so functional that the hand is already useful to some extent; furthermore, the hand should be reasonably sensitive. On the contrary, a poor candidate for surgery is a patient who is severely retarded mentally (IQ usually below 70) and who has definite athetosis in the extremity, a hand that has developed joint contractures and is insensitive, a wrist that passively cannot be brought to neutral, and fingers that cannot be extended even when the wrist is flexed. Children with spastic diplegia rarely have sufficient upper extremity spasticity to warrant surgery, and children with spastic quadriplegia or total body involvement have too little voluntary control to benefit from surgery aimed at improving grasp and release; however, they may benefit from surgery that improves hygiene.

Surgical options include myotomy, tenotomy, tendon lengthening, tendon transfer, tenodesis, capsulotomy, excisional arthoplasty, and arthrodesis. Tendon lengthening requires no particular compliance and can be performed in both spastic and athetoid patients. It weakens the muscle and diminishes its excursion and stretch reflex, which subsequently diminishes spasticity, thereby allowing antagonistic muscles to influence function to a greater extent. Tendon transfers require some postoperative compliance, should be synergistic, cannot overcome fixed deformity, and are not reliable in athetoid patients. Arthrodesis is useful in stabilizing the thumb metacarpophalangeal joint during reconstruction of a thumb-in-palm deformity and also in correcting fixed flexion deformities of the wrist when sacrifice of its windlass effect is believed justifiable.

As to when the various types of operations may be indicated, myotomies are likely to be effective at the earliest age, tendon transfers later, and arthrodeses even later. Soft tissue operations to correct flexion deformity of the wrist and pronation deformity of the forearm are probably indicated earliest. As a rule, indicated surgery usually is carried out between 4 and 8 years of age and ideally before significant contractures develop.

Pronation Contracture of Forearm

Pronation deformity of the forearm is common and disabling in children with cerebral palsy and is caused by spasticity of the pronator teres and at times the pronator quadratus. At times it may be aggravated by lengthening of the biceps tendon for elbow flexion contracture. It may be improved by simple tenotomy of the insertion of the pronator teres. Supination also may be improved by transfer of the extensor carpi ulnaris around the ulnar side of the forearm during augmentation of the extensor digitorum communis or the extensor carpi brevis. Sakellarides, Mitral, and Lenzi have devised an operation principally to correct pronation contracture of the forearm. According to them, transferring the pronator teres tendon will produce better correction than any other transfer. This method corrects one deforming force and at the same time provides a force for supination. The tendon is released, wrapped around the radius, and inserted into the bone. In their series of 22 patients so treated, 82% gained an average of 46 degrees of active supination.

TRANSFER OF PRONATOR TERES

- ■ *TECHNIQUE.* Make a zigzag, curvilinear, or straight longitudinal incision over the anterior and radial aspects of the midforearm (Fig. 71-3, *A*). Protect the lateral cutaneous nerve of the forearm and the superficial radial nerve. Next identify the borders of the brachioradialis muscle, and mobilize and retract it medially. Identify the oblique fibers that insert into bone at the musculotendinous insertion of the pronator teres (Fig. 71-3, *B*). Use sharp dissection to detach the insertion of the pronator teres, along with an attached strip of periosteum (Fig. 71-3, *C*).

Mobilize the muscle extraperiosteally, well proximal in the forearm. Now free the interosseous membrane from the radius as far as necessary to gain maximum passive supination. Pass the pronator teres and attached periosteum posteriorly and laterally around the radius. At the same level as the previous muscle insertion, drill an anchoring hole on the anterolateral aspect of the radial cortex (Fig. 71-3, *D*). Drill a smaller hole through the posteromedial part of the radius using a 1.6 mm Kirschner wire. Enlarge the hole in the anterolateral cortex to 2.8 mm (⁷⁄₆₄ inch). Pass a suture with the tendon attached through the two holes from anterolateral to posteromedial (Fig. 71-3, *E*). In this manner the tendon is introduced into the larger hole and is secured (Fig. 71-3, *F* and *G*). Apply further stay sutures through the tendon as indicated. Hold the forearm in approximately 45 degrees of supination and snug the tendon up to hold this position. Allow the brachioradialis to fall in place and close the incision. Apply a long arm cast, maintaining the elbow in 45 degrees of flexion and the forearm in 60 degrees of supination. Elevate the arm immediately after surgery. *AFTERTREATMENT.* After 3 weeks a new cast is applied, which may be bivalved at any time for observation. The cast is removed during the day but is reapplied at night for at least 6 months.

Flexion Deformities of Wrist and Fingers

The most frequent deformities in the upper extremity in spastic paralysis are those of flexion of the wrist and fingers. These deformities are usually accompanied by pronation of the forearm, flexion of the elbow, and the thumb-in-palm deformity. Zancolli, Goldner, and Swanson classified spastic flexion deformities of the wrist and hand into three patterns.

Pattern 1. The fingers can be actively extended with the wrist in less than 20 degrees of flexion. This is a fairly mild deformity in which grasp and release are possible. Extension of the wrist is not possible with the fingers in full extension. Consideration may be given to flexor carpi ulnaris tenotomy combined with lengthening of the finger flexors, preferably by tenotomy at the musculotendinous junction, allowing for selective fractional lengthening as required. A flexor slide may also be selected.

Pattern 2. Active finger extension is possible only with the wrist in more than 20 degrees of flexion. This pattern is further divided into two subgroups. In pattern 2A the patient has voluntary wrist extension with the fingers in flexion, indicating that the wrist extensors are active and the finger flexors are not severely spastic. In pattern 2B the patient is unable to extend the wrist with the fingers in flexion, indicating that the wrist extensors are paralyzed and will require augmentation to improve function. In pattern 2, lengthening of the finger flexors, com-

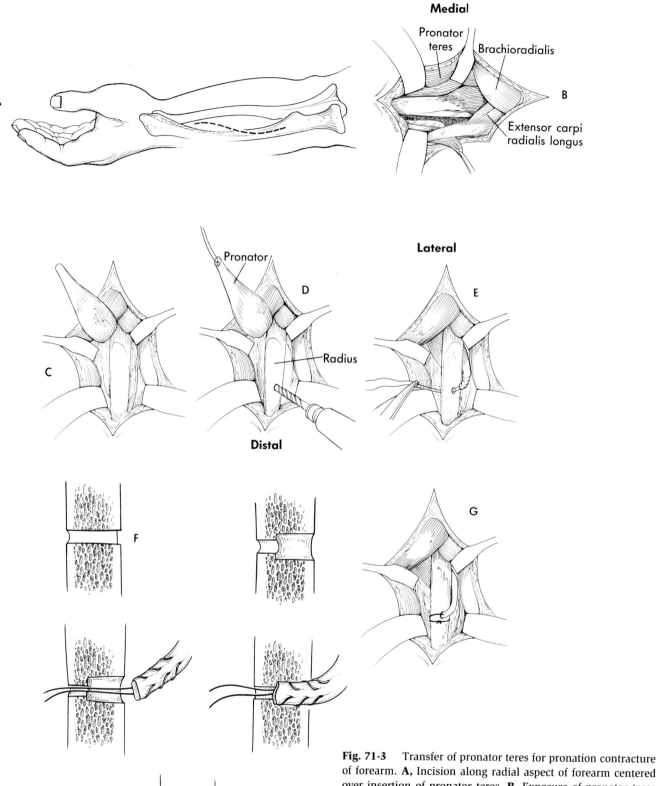

Fig. 71-3   Transfer of pronator teres for pronation contracture of forearm. **A,** Incision along radial aspect of forearm centered over insertion of pronator teres. **B,** Exposure of pronator teres insertion on radius. **C,** Elevation of pronator teres insertion with strip of periosteum from radius. **D,** Anchoring hole drilled in anterolateral part of radial cortex, with smaller hole drilled through posteromedial part. **E, F,** and **G,** Pronator teres tendon rerouted posteriorly through interosseous membrane, passed from lateral to medial through hole drilled in radius, and sutured. (Redrawn from Sakellarides MT, Mital MA, and Lenzi WD: J Bone Joint Surg 63-A:645, 1981.)

bined with a tendon transfer to augment either finger or wrist extension, should be considered. The classic transfer is of the flexor carpi ulnaris to the extensor carpi radialis brevis, which improves supination, wrist extension, and finger flexion (grasp). If weakness in finger extension (release) is considerable, then transfer into the extensor digitorum communis is preferred. Preoperative electromyography may be useful to determine in which phase the donor muscle is active: grasp or release.

Pattern 3. The patient has severe flexion deformities and is unable to actively extend the fingers or wrist even when starting from a position of maximal flexion. Hand sensibility usually is poor. Surgery will not improve function, but it may improve hygiene. Tenotomy of the wrist flexors and sublimis-to-profundus transfers as described by Braun and Vice may be considered. Wrist arthrodesis and carpectomy may improve appearance in these severe deformities.

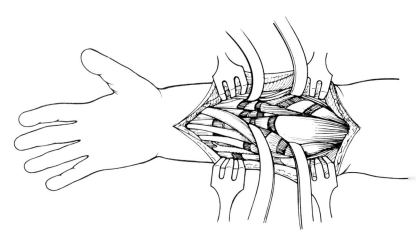

Fig. 71-4 Fractional lengthening of flexor carpi radialis muscle and finger flexors (see text).

FRACTIONAL LENGTHENING OF FLEXOR CARPI RADIALIS MUSCLE AND FINGER FLEXORS

■ *TECHNIQUE.* Begin a curved volar incision over the forearm about 3 cm proximal to the volar wrist crease and continue it proximally for 6 cm. Identify the flexor carpi radialis muscle, and follow it proximally to the musculotendinous junction and then farther proximally until the muscle belly is identified. The distal portion of the muscle belly is surrounded by an aponeurosis that thickens distally and forms the tendon of the muscle itself. Lengthen the muscle-tendon unit and leave it in continuity by making transverse cuts in the aponeurosis proximal to the musculotendinous junction. Completely identify the muscle circumferentially and make a transverse cut through the aponeurosis but not through the muscle (Fig. 71-4). It is important to divide the aponeurosis transversely and not leave any of the tendon intact; otherwise, the muscle-tendon unit will not lengthen. After the cut in the aponeurosis is made, place the wrist in dorsiflexion. The transverse cut in the aponeurosis will widen as the muscle lengthens, but the entire muscle-tendon unit will remain intact. A second cut for recession may be made if necessary.

Other musculotendinous units may be contracted in addition to the flexor carpi radialis muscle. Frequently the palmaris longus muscle also is spastic and contracted, and also may require lenthening in the same manner. Through this same incision the finger flexors may be lengthened in a similar manner. First lengthen the flexor digitorum sublimis muscles and then the flexor digitorum profundus if they contribute to the contracture.

AFTERTREATMENT. A palmar (volar) short arm splint with the wrist in neutral position or slightly extended is worn for 3 to 4 weeks. Then mobilization of the wrist is begun, and a removable splint is used for protection. A volar short arm night splint is used for an additional 4 to 6 months.

RELEASE OF FLEXOR-PRONATOR ORIGIN. Release of the flexor-pronator origin may improve appearance and function of a hand with severe flexion deformities of the wrist and fingers. It is not indicated in hands that can be corrected passively but that assume a flexed position during grasp; for these, less extensive operations such as transfer of the flexor carpi ulnaris to a wrist extensor, are more useful. Release of the flexor-pronator origin was described by Page in 1923 and more recently by Inglis and Cooper and by Williams and Haddad.

■ *TECHNIQUE (INGLIS AND COOPER).* Make an incision over the anterior part of the medial epicondyle of the humerus beginning 5 cm proximal to the epicondyle and continuing distally to the midpoint of the forearm over the ulna (Fig. 71-5, *A*). The medial antebrachial cutaneous nerve is often seen in the distal part of the incision, and the medial brachial cutaneous nerve may be seen posterior to the medial part of the epicondyle. Next identify the ulnar nerve proximal to the epicondyle, dissect and elevate it from its groove behind the epicondyle, and carefully free it distally (Fig. 71-5, *B*). Identify, free, and protect the branches of the ulnar nerve to the flexor carpi ulnaris and to the two ulnar heads of the flexor digitorum profundus. Next release the origins of the flexor carpi ulnaris and flexor digitorum profundus as follows. Begin distally at about the middle of the ulna and elevate both muscles from the bone at the subcutaneous border; the interosseous membrane is then seen around the volar surface of the bone. Then continue proximally along the ulna as far as the ulnar groove at the epicondyle. During this dissection the interosseous membrane and the fascia of the brachialis muscle are seen in the depths of the wound. Replace the ulnar nerve in

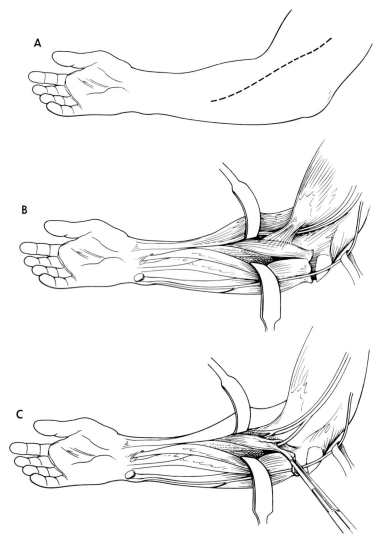

Fig. 71-5 Flexor slide (Inglis and Cooper). **A,** Incision on medial aspect of volar side of arm, beginning approximately 5 cm proximal to medial epicondyle and continuing distally to midpoint of forearm over ulna. **B,** Ulnar nerve is identified, protected, and released from cubital tunnel. Tendinous origin of muscles on medial epicondyle is cut, and flexor carpi ulnaris and flexor digitorum profundus muscles are completely released from medial epicondyle and ulna. **C,** Lacertus fibrosus is divided, along with any remaining portions of flexor muscle origin, and ulnar nerve is transposed anteriorly.

its groove and divide the entire flexor-pronator muscle mass at its origin from the medial part of the epicondyle. At this point the median nerve can be seen as it passes through the pronator teres. Now continue the dissection anteriorly over the flexor aspect of the elbow, dividing the lacertus fibrosus (Fig. 71-5, *C*) and any remaining parts of the flexor muscle origin. If a flexion contracture of the elbow persists, incise the fascia of the brachialis muscle. Then transplant the ulnar nerve anterior to the epicondyle. Now the muscle mass will have been displaced 3 to 4 cm distal to its original location. Close

the wound and apply a cast or plaster splints to hold the forearm in supination and the wrist and fingers in neutral positions.

AFTERTREATMENT. At 3 weeks the cast or splints and the sutures are removed. Then an extension hand splint is applied (Fig. 71-6, *G*); it is worn constantly for 3 months and then only at night for 3 more months or, in children, until growth is complete.

• • •

Williams and Haddad recommend a similar but more extensive release of the flexor-pronator origin than that just described. It frees completely the origins of the flexor mass almost to the wrist.

■ *TECHNIQUE (WILLIAMS AND HADDAD).* Make an incision over the medial aspect of the arm and forearm anterior to the medial epicondyle of the humerus beginning 5 cm proximal to the elbow and extending distally to about 5 cm proximal to the wrist (Fig. 71-7, *A*). Protecting the medial antebrachial cutaneous nerve and the basilic vein, dissect anteriorly a flap of skin and subcutaneous tissue to expose the lacertus fibrosus and the antecubital fossa (Fig. 71-7, *B*). Then expose the ulnar nerve as it passes between the two heads of origin of the flexor carpi ulnaris. Now, avoiding the ulnar collateral ligament and capsule of the elbow joint, divide the common tendon of origin of the superficial group of muscles just distal to the epicondyle (Fig. 71-7, *C*). Protecting the median nerve and its motor branches to the superficial group of muscles, free the ulnar origin of the pronator teres. Extend the dissection along the lateral border of the pronator teres to its insertion on the radius, but avoid injuring the radial artery. At this level divide the aponeurotic, radial origin of the flexor digitorum sublimis. Now retract anteriorly the ulnar nerve and the stump of the common flexor tendon, and free the origin of the flexor carpi ulnaris from the medial border of the olecranon. During this dissection ligate and divide the posterior ulnar recurrent artery. Avoiding the periosteum of the ulna, release the aponeurotic origin of the flexor carpi ulnaris and flexor digitorum profundus from the ulna throughout its entire length (Fig. 71-7, *D*). Next identify the common interosseous artery, its volar branch, and the anterior interosseous nerve, and release from the volar aspect of the ulna and adjacent interosseous membrane the origin of the flexor digitorum profundus as far distally as the pronator quadratus (Fig. 71-7, *E*). Release from the radius the origin of the flexor digitorum profundus to the index finger. Then release from the medial side of the coronoid process the remaining origin of the flexor digitorum sublimis proximal to the common interosseous artery (Fig. 71-7, *F*). Extend the wrist and fingers, and identify and release any remaining tight bands. If there is any tension on the ulnar nerve, transplant it anteriorly into the brachialis (Fig. 71-7, *G*) and, if any elbow contracture persists, divide the brachialis tendon. If necessary, divide or lengthen the tendon of the flexor pollicis longus through a separate incision proximal to the wrist. Splint the extremity with the wrist and fingers extended and the elbow flexed.

AFTERTREATMENT. At 3 weeks the splint and sutures are removed, and another splint is applied that keeps the wrist and fingers extended and the thumb abducted. This splint is worn for 3 months except when it is removed for exercises of the wrist and fingers. It is then worn only at night for 6 weeks. Occupational and physical therapy are continued as necessary.

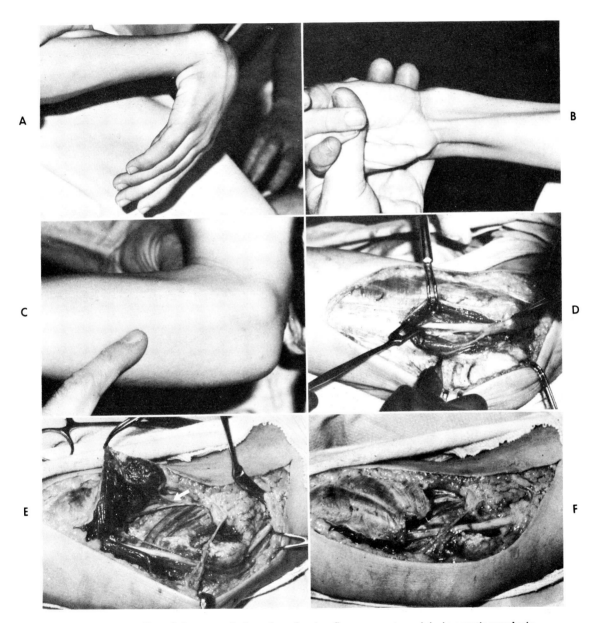

Fig. 71-6 Inglis and Cooper technique for releasing flexor-pronator origin in spastic paralysis. **A,** Posture of hand and wrist before surgery. Wrist cannot be actively extended beyond 90 degrees, and fingers cannot be actively flexed. **B,** Flexor muscles on volar surface of forearm are contracted. **C,** Contracted flexor-pronator muscle mass is attached to medial humeral epicondyle. **D,** Ulnar nerve is dissected free and elevated from behind epicondyle. Its branches to flexor carpi ulnaris and to two ulnar heads of flexor digitorum profundus are identified, freed, and protected. **E,** Entire flexor-pronator muscle mass is divided at its origin from medial part of epicondyle. Median nerve *(arrow)* is seen as it passes through pronator teres. **F,** Ulnar nerve is transplanted anterior to epicondyle (see text).

Continued.

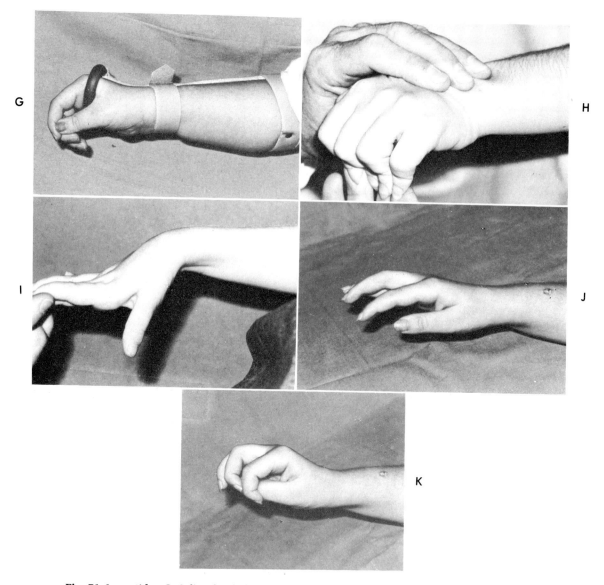

Fig. 71-6, cont'd **G,** Splint that holds wrist extended but interferes little with function of fingers is applied 3 weeks after surgery. **H** and **I,** Before release of flexor-pronator origin. Active extension of wrist and fingers is absent. When wrist is passively extended, **H,** finger flexors are tight. When fingers are passively extended, **I,** wrist flexors are tight. **J** and **K,** After surgery. While wrist is extended, fingers can be actively extended, **J,** and actively flexed, **K.** (From Inglis AE and Cooper W: J Bone Joint Surg 48-A:847, 1966.)

TRANSFER OF FLEXOR CARPI ULNARIS. Transfer of the flexor carpi ulnaris dorsally to a radial wrist extensor removes a deforming force that pulls the hand into ulnar deviation and flexion and provides a force that promotes supination of the forearm and extension of the wrist. For this operation to be effective, active finger extension, passive flexibility of the hand, wrist, and forearm, and a favorable diagnostic profile are all necessary. Any fixed deformity should be corrected before surgery either by successive casts or by any operations as indicated. If active supination is possible before surgery, the muscle may be carried through the interosseous membrane instead of around the ulnar side of the forearm and will thus be prevented from acting as a supinator. This procedure should not be performed in conjunction with a release or lengthening of the flexor carpi radialis, because it may cause a hyperextension deformity of the wrist. As emphasized by Hoffer, Leham, and Mitani (1986), a wrist flexion deformity may be accompanied by a primary weakness of the finger extensors. The child is thus able to release objects only by flexing the wrist. In this situation a transfer of the flexor carpi ulnaris to the wrist extensors will only strengthen grasp, making it even more difficult for the child to release objects. They recommend transfer of the flexor carpi ulnaris to the extensor digitorum communis if electromyography demonstrates activ-

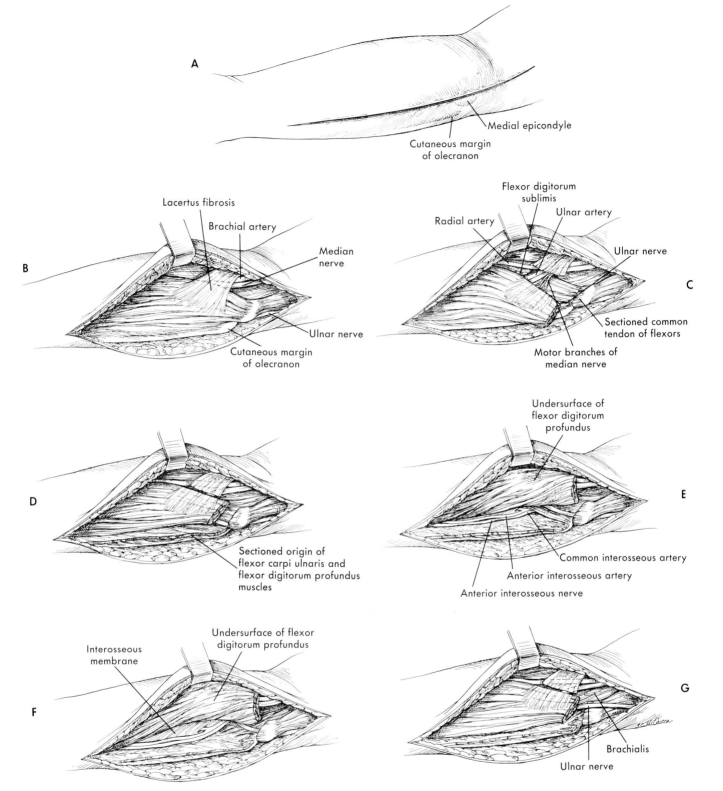

Fig. 71-7 Williams and Haddad technique for releasing flexor-pronator origin. **A,** Incision. **B,** Structures anteriorly and medially at elbow have been exposed (see text). **C,** Lacertus fibrosus has been divided, origin of superficial flexors has been released from medial epicondyle, and origin of flexor digitorum sublimis has been released from radius (see text). **D,** Origin of flexor carpi ulnaris has been released from olecranon, and common origin of flexor carpi ulnaris and flexor digitorum profundus has been released from ulna (see text). **E,** Origin of flexor digitorum profundus has been released from volar aspect of ulna and interosseous membrane (see text). **F,** Origin of flexor digitorum profundus to index finger has been released from radius, and remaining origin of flexor digitorum sublimis has been released from coronoid process (see text). **G,** Ulnar nerve has been transplanted anteriorly into brachialis muscle (see text). (Modified from Williams R and Haddad RJ: South Med J 60:1033, 1967.)

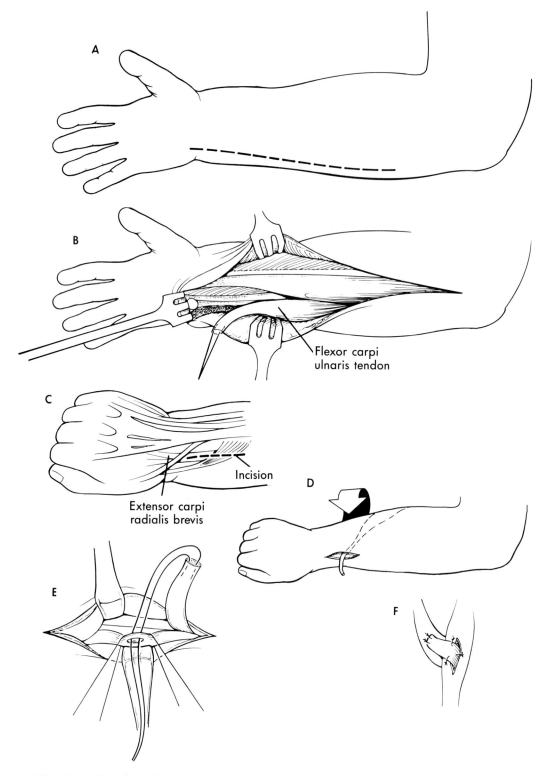

Fig. 71-8   Transfer of flexor carpi ulnaris. **A,** Anterior longitudinal incision over flexor carpi ulnaris. This may be divided into two separate incisions as described in text. **B,** Flexor carpi ulnaris tendon is detached from pisiform insertion, and muscle is dissected proximally off ulna. **C,** Small longitudinal incision on dorsum of wrist over extensor carpi radialis brevis just proximal to first extensor compartment. **D,** Flexor carpi ulnaris tendon is passed subcutaneously around ulnar border of forearm using tendon passer. **E,** Buttonhole is made in extensor carpi radialis brevis tendon. **F,** Flexor carpi ulnaris is passed through buttonhole and sutured to itself under appropriate tension.

ity of the flexor carpi ulnaris during the release phase, especially if finger extension is weak. In their series of 17 patients so treated, all had improved function without loss of grip.

■ *TECHNIQUE (GREEN AND BANKS)*. Make an anterior longitudinal incision (Fig. 71-8, *A*) extending from the flexor crease of the wrist proximally for about 3 cm to expose the insertion of the flexor carpi ulnaris on the pisiform bone. Detach the tendon from the bone and dissect it proximally (Fig. 71-8, *B*). The attachment of the muscle to the ulna often extends almost the full length of the tendon; free it by sharp dissection from the ulna, leaving the periosteum in place. The ulnar nerve now may be seen in a sheath posterior to the tendon. Next introduce a nylon suture into the distal end of the tendon and, by pulling on it gently, outline the course of the muscle proximally. Then, beginning about 5 cm distal to the medial epicondyle of the humerus, make a second incision 7 to 10 cm long over the belly of the muscle. Define the lateral margin of the muscle and make an incision there through the deep fascia to expose this margin and the deep surface of the muscle. Once the muscle belly has been defined, dissect it from its origin on the deep surface of the deep fascia and from the ulna distally. Then pull the tendon into the proximal incision. Free the muscle further until it will pass straight from its origin across the border of the ulna to the dorsal aspect of the wrist. Take care to locate and preserve branches of the ulnar nerve to the muscle; they limit the dissection proximally. Now, at a suitable level at the medial margin of the ulna, excise the intermuscular septum separating the volar and dorsal compartments of the forearm for 4 to 5 cm and expose the dorsal compartment. Then, starting just proximal to the transverse skin crease on the dorsum of the wrist and extending proximally, make a third incision (Fig. 71-8, *C*) about 3 cm long over the extensor carpi radialis brevis and longus tendons. Expose these tendons and choose either for insertion of the transferred tendon; that of the brevis gives a more central action in extension of the wrist, whereas that of the longus gives a better pull for supination of the forearm and radial deviation of the wrist. Using a tendon passer (Fig. 71-8, *D*), direct the free end of the flexor carpi ulnaris from the proximal incision into the dorsal compartment along the path of the extensor tendons to the chosen extensor radialis tendon. Make a buttonhole (Fig. 71-8, *E*) in the chosen tendon and pass through it the flexor carpi ulnaris tendon; suture the flexor carpi ulnaris tendon (Fig. 71-8, *F*) there under tension with the forearm in full supination and the wrist in at least 45 degrees of extension. If the flexor carpi ulnaris is to be transferred into the extensor digitorum communis tendons, suture it under tension such that when the wrist is in the neu-

tral position the metacarpophalangeal joints are hyperextended. Close the wounds. Now apply a cast extending from near the axilla to the tips of the fingers, holding the wrist in extension, the forearm in supination, the fingers in almost complete extension, and the thumb in abduction and opposition.

AFTERTREATMENT. The cast is bivalved soon after surgery, and exercises are started with the arm out of the cast 4 or 5 days later. These are continued daily for at least 6 weeks, with the cast remaining in place between exercise periods. Then the cast is worn at night and intermittently for several more weeks or months as necessary to keep the hand in its corrected position.

WRIST ARTHRODESIS. Wrist fusion may improve function in the cerebral palsied hand; however, most authors agree that this is unlikely, and fusion is used much less frequently now than previously. It is primarily used to control position and improve hygiene in a hand with poor motor control and sensibility. In this circumstance Hoffer and Zeitzew reported wrist arthrodesis to be fairly predictable in achieving these goals in their series of 19 patients. Because the epiphysis of the distal radius will be damaged, fusion must be delayed until the patient is at least 12 years old. The wrist should be fused in neutral flexion and ulnar deviation. Osteopenia usually precludes the use of plates and screws for fixation.

■ *TECHNIQUE*. After lengthening or releasing the flexor tendons as necessary, make a dorsal longitudinal incision over the wrist. Excise carpal bones as necessary to achieve correction. Denude all remaining cartilage from the radiocarpal and intercarpal joints, as well as from the second and third carpometacarpal joints. Use corticocancellous portions of the excised carpal bones or iliac crest grafts to supplement the fusion. Transfix the carpus with two Steinmann pins measuring $\frac{7}{64}$ to $\frac{9}{64}$ of an inch (Fig. 71-9). Apply a long arm cast with the elbow at 90 degrees of flexion and the forearm in neutral pronation and supination. If the finger flexors have been lengthened, extend the cast to include the fingers in the extended position.

AFTERTREATMENT. At 4 weeks the long arm cast may be converted to a short arm cast, and finger flexion and extension are encouraged. The wrist is protected until fusion is apparent, usually around 10 to 12 weeks. The pins may be removed once the arthrodesis is solid.

CARPECTOMY. Omer and Capen reported proximal row carpectomies to improve appearance in eight patients with cerebral palsy. At the same time transfers of the flexor carpi ulnaris tendon around the ulna to the extensor carpi radialis brevis were carried out to strengthen wrist extension and increase supination. They warn that this does not necessarily improve function. All of their

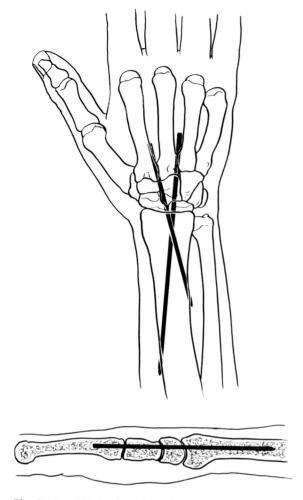

Fig. 71-9 Wrist arthrodesis using two Steinmann pins.

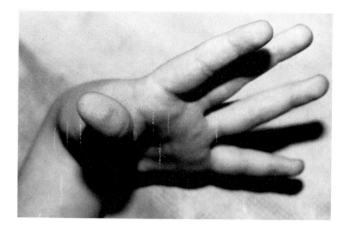

Fig. 71-10 Typical thumb-in-palm deformity.

patients were older than 11 years of age. They emphasize prolonged postoperative splinting because the procedure increases the relative length of all flexor muscle tendon units that cross the wrist and increases wrist extension and forearm supination. They further emphasize that only the proximal half of the carpal scaphoid is taken.

■ *TECHNIQUE (OMER AND CAPEN).* **Make a longitudinal incision over the dorsum of the wrist. Identify the distal edge of the dorsal carpal ligament and retract the common digital extensor tendons ulnarward. Make a T-shaped incision in the dorsal capsule to expose the carpal bones. Excise the lunate and the proximal half of the scaphoid. Leave the distal half of the scaphoid with its capsular attachments. Excise the triquetrum but leave the pisiform bone. Make a longitudinal incision over the volar aspect of the wrist, beginning at the pisiform and extending proximally over the flexor carpi ulnaris tendon. Protect the neurovascular bundle and free the flexor carpi ulnaris from the intermuscular septum. Divide the muscle near its insertion and pass its tendon through a window in the interosseous**

membrane. (To give more supination, pass the transfer around the ulna.) Insert the flexor carpi ulnaris into the extensor carpi radialis brevis and anchor it with nonabsorbable monofilament sutures. Place the wrist in maximum passive dorsiflexion and imbricate the dorsal capsule of the wrist.

AFTERTREATMENT. The arm is placed in a bulky dressing and a volar plaster splint holding the fingers and wrist in extension. On or about the fifth day, a circular long arm cast is applied, holding the elbow flexed, the forearm supinated, and the wrist and fingers extended. This position is maintained for 6 weeks. Then a circular short arm cast, incorporating outriggers for extension of the fingers, is applied. Splinting is continued for 4 months and then used only at night for an indefinite time.

Thumb-in-Palm Deformity

The second frequent and important deformity of the hand in cerebral palsy is the thumb-in-palm, adducted thumb, or clutched thumb deformity (Fig. 71-10). This deformity blocks entry of objects into the palm and, in addition, prevents the thumb from assisting fingers in grasp or pinch. Contributing to thumb-in-palm deformity are spasticity of the flexor pollicis longus, flexor pollicis brevis, adductor pollicis, and first dorsal interosseus, as well as weakness of the extensor pollicis longus, extensor pollicis brevis, and adductor pollicis longus muscles. Spasticity in the extensor pollicis longus muscle also may contribute to an adduction deformity of the thumb during the release phase (Fig. 71-11). In 1981 House, Gwathney, and Fidler classified thumb-in-palm deformities into four major types based on the clinical appearance of the thumb. A type I deformity consists of a simple metacarpal adduction contracture and is the most common pattern. A type II deformity consists of a metacarpal adduction contracture combined with a metacarpophalangeal flexion deformity. A type III deformity consists of a metacarpal adduction contracture combined

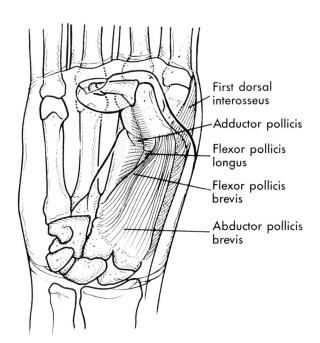

Fig. 71-11 Adducted thumb position in cerebral palsy is result of forces exerted by powerful muscles. (Redrawn from Inglis AE, Cooper W, and Bruton W: J Bone Joint Surg 52-A:253, 1970.)

First dorsal interosseus
Adductor pollicis
Flexor pollicis longus
Flexor pollicis brevis
Abductor pollicis brevis

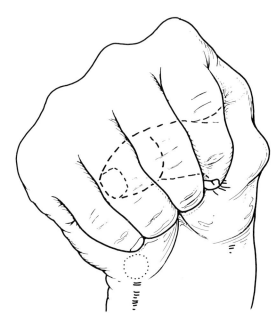

Fig. 71-12 With spastic thumb-in-palm deformity caused by tight flexor pollicis longus, thumb is flexed at interphalangeal and metacarpophalangeal joints, and carpometacarpal joint is flexed and adducted. (From Smith RJ: J Hand Surg 7:327, 1982.)

with a metacarpophalangeal hyperextension deformity or instability; this is the second most common pattern. A type IV deformity consists of a metacarpal adduction contracture combined with metacarpophalangeal and interphalangeal flexion deformities; this is believed to be the most severe deformity, being caused by spasticity in the flexor pollicis longus, as well as in the intrinsic muscles in the thumb (Fig. 71-12).

Although thumb-in-palm deformity may be caused principally by spasticity of the flexor pollicis longus muscle, it is not caused solely by this muscle. The flexor pollicis longus flexes the interphalangeal joint, the metacarpophalangeal joint, and the carpometacarpal joint, and also acts as an adductor of the thumb. To be certain that it is a principal deforming force, the patient should be able to decrease the flexion of these joints by flexing the wrist. Conversely, extending the wrist will cause an increase in deformity. The examiner should determine whether an accompanying severe adduction deformity, caused by contracture of muscle or other structures, is present. A weak adductor pollicis may be overpowered by a tendon transfer; active adduction of the thumb by the adductor pollicis should be checked with the wrist palmar flexed to determine the strength of the muscle.

TREATMENT. Treatment of thumb-in-palm deformity must be individualized after careful, repeated assessments of the overall hand function, as well as function of the specific muscles contributing to the deformity. Currently, a dynamic approach is used in the surgical cor-

rection of this deformity, as described by House et al. This involves release of contractures, augmentation of weak muscles, and skeletal stabilization, especially of the metacarpophalangeal joint when necessary. A myotomy of the adductor pollicis may be carried out through a palmar incision as described by Matev (1963) or through a Z-plasty incision placed in the first web if a skin contracture is present. Hoffer et al. (1983) found that preoperative electromyography of the adductor pollicis was useful in determining whether a partial or complete release of this muscle was necessary. If the adductor was active during grasp, the patients were said to have selective control, and release of the transverse head of the muscle only was considered because in the experience of Hoffer et al., pinch may be weak if complete myotomy is performed. Release of the origin of the first dorsal interosseus muscle also may be required. In longstanding type II deformities the origin of both the adductor and the flexor pollicis brevis may require release, as described by Matev. In type IV deformities the flexor pollicis longus may require lengthening proximal to the wrist. Augmentation of a weak adductor pollicis longus may be necessary. The most common muscles used for this augmentation are the palmaris longus, the brachioradialis, and the flexor carpi radialis. Fusion of the thumb metacarpophalangeal joint is especially useful if a hyperextension deformity of that joint is present. Arthrodesis may be performed without damage to the epiphysis if only articular cartilage is removed and a smooth Kirschner wire is used for fixation.

Smith has proposed transfer of the flexor pollicis longus tendon to the radial side of the thumb combined with tenodesis of the distal joint. He recommends the operation for patients who have some use of the affected hand, in addition to passive extension of the metacarpophalangeal joint and abduction of the carpometacarpal joint with the wrist in flexion.

If the extensor pollicis longus contributes to the thumb deformity, it may be rerouted from Lister's tubercle as recommended by Manske (1985). Significant improvement in functional activities was noted in 90% of his patients treated with this technique.

MYOTOMY

■ *TECHNIQUE.* Make an incision bordering the thenar crease in the palm, but avoid damaging the recurrent branch of the median nerve or the innervation of the adductor pollicis. After retracting the long flexors of the fingers, strip from the third metacarpal the origin of the adductor pollicis. Cut from the deep transverse carpal ligament about two thirds of the origin of the abductor pollicis brevis and all of the origins of the flexor pollicis brevis and opponens pollicis (Fig. 71-13). Also strip from the second metacarpal the origin of the first dorsal interosseus. If necessary, carry out a capsulorrhaphy of the metacarpophalangeal joint.

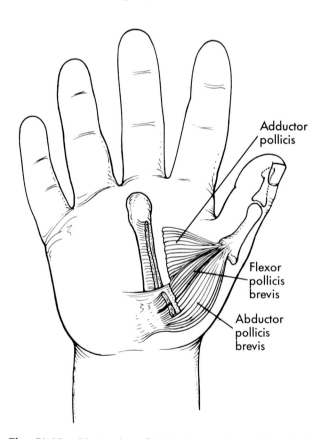

Fig. 71-13 Myotomies of intrinsic muscles of thumb for thumb-in-palm deformity (see text). (Modified from Swanson AB: Surg Clin North Am 48:1129, 1968.)

AFTERTREATMENT. A pressure dressing and a cast are applied holding the first metacarpal (not the phalanges) in wide abduction and opposition. At 3 weeks the cast and sutures are removed and a splint is applied to hold the thumb in this same position. If tendon transfers have been necessary, the cast is retained for 6 weeks. Splinting at night may be necessary for a long time if the deformity tends to recur.

RELEASE OF CONTRACTURES, AUGMENTATION OF WEAK MUSCLES, AND SKELETAL STABILIZATION

■ *TECHNIQUE (HOUSE ET AL.) Step 1 (release of contractures).* Through a Z-plasty incision located along the first web space, release the origin of the first dorsal interosseus muscle from the thumb metacarpal (Fig. 71-14, *A*). Expose the intramuscular portion of the tendon of the adductor pollicis and divide it obliquely to allow a relative lengthening of the tendon while preserving bridging muscle fibers. If a long-standing type II deformity exists with a flexion deformity of the metacarpophalangeal joint, release the origin of both the adductor and the flexor pollicis brevis if necessary. For a type IV deformity with spasticity of the flexor pollicis longus muscle and interphalangeal flexion deformity, lengthen the tendon of the flexor pollicis longus proximal to the wrist.

Step 2 (augmentation of weak muscles). If adduction of the thumb at the carpometacarpal joint is considerable, with weakness of the abductor pollicis longus, then release the abductor pollicis longus tendon from the first extensor compartment and allow the tendon to subluxate volarly. Divide the palmaris longus tendon at the level of the wrist and suture it into the abductor pollicis longus tendon in an end-to-side fashion (Fig. 71-14, *B*). The brachioradialis, as well as the flexor carpi radialis, may be used instead of the palmaris longus if desired. If there is no suitable donor for active transfer, then divide the abductor pollicis longus tendon and reroute its distal portion volarly, attaching it in an end-to-side fashion to the flexor carpi radialis tendon under sufficient tension to maintain metacarpal abduction (Fig. 71-14, *C*). This provides a dynamic abductor tenodesis. If the flexion deformity at the metacarpophalangeal joint is significant but stability of the joint is normal, then a similar tenodesis of the extensor pollicis brevis tendon may be performed. Care must be taken not to create a disabling hyperextension deformity at this joint.

Step 3 (skeletal stabilization). If there is a hyperextension deformity of the metacarpophalangeal joint (type III deformity), then carefully remove the articular cartilage of the metacarpophalangeal joint without damaging the epiphysis. Position the thumb and secure it with one centrally placed 1 mm Kirschner wire (Fig. 71-14, *D*).

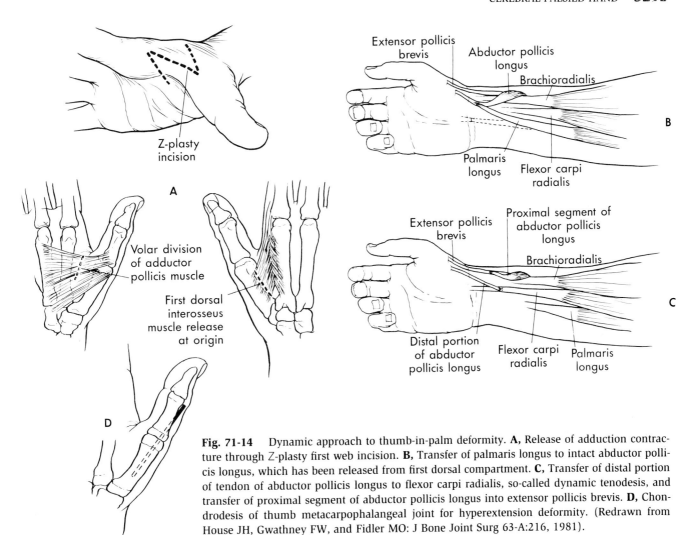

Fig. 71-14 Dynamic approach to thumb-in-palm deformity. **A,** Release of adduction contracture through Z-plasty first web incision. **B,** Transfer of palmaris longus to intact abductor pollicis longus, which has been released from first dorsal compartment. **C,** Transfer of distal portion of tendon of abductor pollicis longus to flexor carpi radialis, so-called dynamic tenodesis, and transfer of proximal segment of abductor pollicis longus into extensor pollicis brevis. **D,** Chondrodesis of thumb metacarpophalangeal joint for hyperextension deformity. (Redrawn from House JH, Gwathney FW, and Fidler MO: J Bone Joint Surg 63-A:216, 1981).

AFTERTREATMENT. The forearm and hand are immobilized for 4 weeks with the thumb held in abduction and extension by a volar plaster splint. Then active and assisted exercises of the wrist, thumb, and fingers are started. A long opponens splint modified by the addition of a **C** bar or molded plastic orthosis is worn between exercise periods for the next few weeks, after which splinting is continued at night only until growth is completed or dynamic balance is attained and stabilized.

FLEXOR POLLICIS LONGUS ABDUCTOR-PLASTY

■ *TECHNIQUE (SMITH).* Make a radial midlateral incision from the middle of the distal phalanx of the thumb to the neck of the first metacarpal (Fig. 71-15, *A*). Elevate a volar skin flap and transect the flexor pollicis longus tendon opposite the proximal phalanx (Fig. 71-15, *B*). Tenodese the flexor pollicis longus stump to the proximal phalanx or arthrodese the distal joint in 15 degrees of flexion (Fig. 71-15, *C, D,* and *E*). Now make a

longitudinal incision in the forearm just radial to the tendon of the flexor carpi radialis, curving its distal portion ulnarward. Identify the flexor pollicis longus tendon and draw it out through this incision. Tunnel subcutaneously by blunt dissection on the radial side of the thumb to the lateral side of the metacarpophalangeal joint and pass the flexor pollicis longus tendon through this tunnel. With the wrist in neutral position and the thumb at 50 degrees of abduction, suture the tendon to the dorsoradial aspect of the metacarpophalangeal joint with tension (Fig. 71-15, *F*).

AFTERTREATMENT. The hand is immobilized for 6 weeks with the thumb in abduction and the wrist in 30 degrees of flexion. The thumb is splinted with a **C**-splint in the web for an additional 6 weeks.

REDIRECTION OF EXTENSOR POLLICIS LONGUS

■ *TECHNIQUE (MANSKE).* Through a palmar incision, release the adductor pollicis and the deep head of the flexor pollicis brevis, as described by Matev and by Swanson. Release the first dorsal interosseus

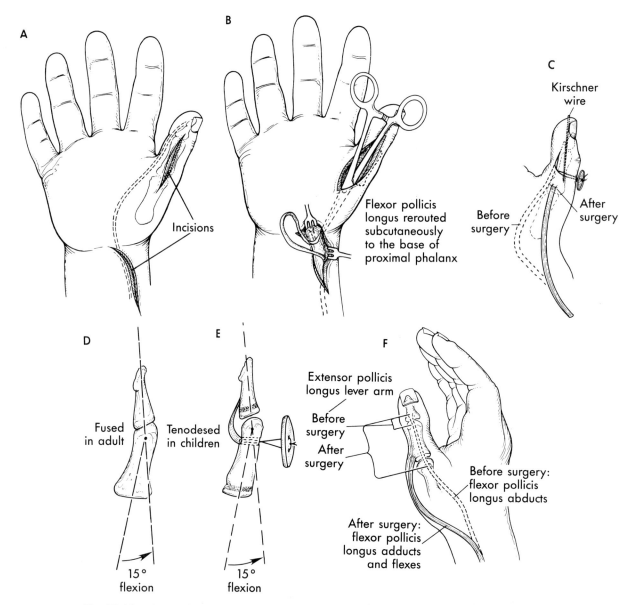

Fig. 71-15 **A,** Incision to radial side of thumb exposes insertion of flexor pollicis longus, interphalangeal joint, and base of proximal phalanx. Second curved incision to radial side of wrist exposes flexor pollicis longus near its musculotendinous juncture and permits tendon to be withdrawn from carpal canal. **B,** Flexor pollicis longus is transected at its insertion and withdrawn from carpal canal through wrist incision. It is then passed subcutaneously to radial side of base of proximal phalanx. **C, D,** and **E,** Interphalangeal joint of thumb is arthrodesed in about 15 degrees of flexion in adult. In child with open epiphysis, distal joint may be tenodesed in about 15 degrees of flexion. **F,** Transfer of flexor pollicis longus to radial side of proximal phalanx reduces adduction-flexion deformity and augments thumb abduction by transferred position of flexor pollicis longus. Interphalangeal arthrodesis improves metacarpophalangeal joint extension by increasing lever arm of extensor pollicis longus on metacarpophalangeal joint. (From Smith RJ: J Hand Surg 7:327, 1982).

muscle at its origin from the first metacarpal through a longitudinal incision on the dorsum of the thumb. Next extend the incision on the dorsum of the thumb distally to the proximal phalanx, exposing the extensor aponeurotic hood (Fig. 71-16, *A*). Identify the extensor pollicis longus at the metacarpophalangeal joint and dissect it out from the extensor aponeurosis for a distance of 10 mm distal to the joint. This leaves a longitudinal defect 4 mm wide in the extensor hood. Take care to preserve the margins of the aponeurosis sufficiently for subsequent closure. Identify the extensor pollicis longus through a longitudinal incision at the distal radius and withdraw it into the forearm (Fig. 71-16,

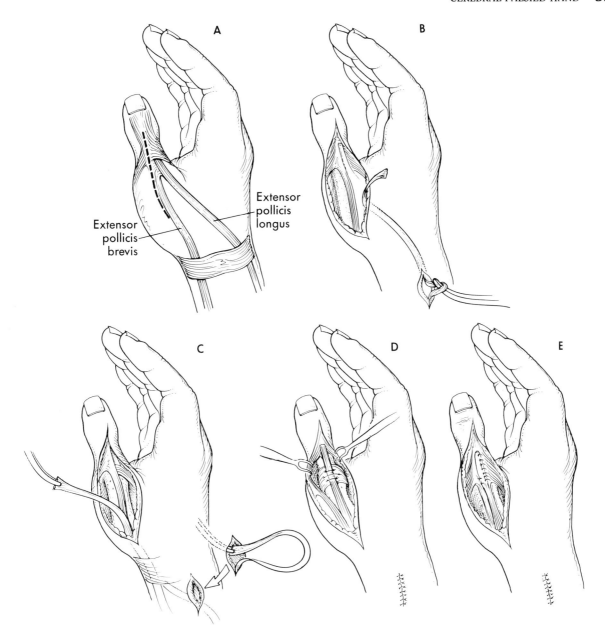

Fig. 71-16   Manske technique for redirecting extensor pollicis longus tendon to correct thumb-in-palm deformity (see text). (Redrawn from Manske PR: J Hand Surg 10-A:553, 1985).

B). Redirect the extensor pollicis longus tendon along the radial aspect of the wrist, using the first extensor retinacular compartment as a pulley to maintain its position by passing a curved hemostat or tendon passer from the dorsal incision on the thumb along the course of the extensor pollicis brevis tendon through the first extensor compartment. Grasp the extensor pollicis longus tendon with the hemostat and retract it distally through the first extensor compartment (Fig. 71-16, *C*). If redirecting the tendon through this compartment is difficult, the extensor pollicis longus can be routed around the extensor pollicis brevis and adductor pollicis longus tendons just proximal to the com-

partment and then into the dorsal incision on the thumb. Next pass the extensor pollicis longus tendon through a transverse tunnel made in the capsule of the metacarpophalangeal joint and suture it under sufficient tension to advance it 1 to 2 cm from its original position (Fig. 71-16, *D*). If the metacarpophalangeal joint is hyperextensible, this tunnel should be placed proximal to the articular surface to prevent further hyperextension. Suture the distal portion of the extensor pollicis longus tendon into the extensor aponeurosis to close the longitudinal defect and prevent flexion deformity at the interphalangeal joint (Fig. 71-16, *E*). Close the incisions in routine fashion.

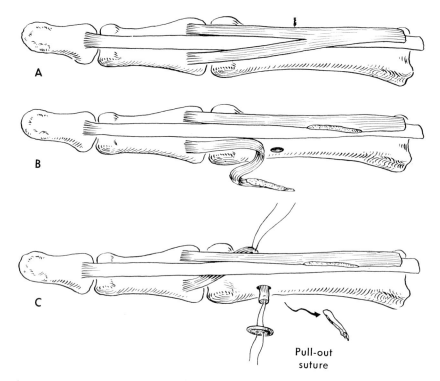

Fig. 71-17 Curtis technique for correcting recurrent hyperextension and locking of proximal interphalangeal joint. **A,** Palmar view of flexor tendons. **B,** One half of flexor digitorum sublimis tendon has been divided at bifurcation of tendon. Hole has been drilled in proximal phalanx. **C,** Freed half of tendon has been carried deep to flexor digitorum profundus tendon to opposite side of proximal phalanx, threaded through hole in bone, and anchored with pull-out suture under enough tension to cause slight flexion contracture of proximal interphalangeal joint. (Redrawn from Curtis RM: In Flynn JE, editor: Hand surgery, Baltimore, 1966, Williams & Wilkins.)

AFTERTREATMENT. The thumb is immobilized in abduction and extension in a short arm thumb spica cast for 4 weeks. Then a removable thumb spica splint is worn for 2 weeks; this splint is removed three to four times daily for controlled active motion.

Swan-Neck Deformity

Compared with other deformities of the upper extremity in cerebral palsy, swan-neck deformities of the fingers are infrequent; however, they may be quite disabling. They are caused by muscle imbalance and by secondary ligamentous and capsular relaxation at the proximal interphalangeal joints that allows these joints to hyperextend. In the involved finger the middle extensor band is relatively short as compared with the lateral bands because of tension exerted on the middle band by the long extensor and the intrinsic muscle. In this deformity the Curtis sublimis tenodesis of the proximal interphalangeal joint may improve function.

SUBLIMIS TENODESIS OF PROXIMAL INTERPHALANGEAL JOINT

■ *TECHNIQUE (CURTIS).* The Curtis technique is described in the section on hyperextension and locking of the proximal interphalangeal joint. It employs one slip of the flexor digitorum sublimis that is left at its insertion on the bone and cut free at the bifurcation. It is then brought to the opposite side of the joint under the remaining tendons and inserted into the lateral aspect of the middle phalanx with a pull-out wire suture (Fig. 71-17). The proximal interphalangeal joint is held in flexion by a traversing Kirschner wire for 6 weeks.

REFERENCES

Braun RM and Vice BT: Sublimis to profundus transfers in the hemiplegic upper extremity, J Bone Joint Surg 55-A:873, 1973.

Chait LA, Kaplan I, Stewart-Lord B, and Goodman M: Early surgical correction in the cerebral palsied hand, J Hand Surg 5:122, 1980.

Curtis RM: Treatment of injuries of proximal interphalangeal joints of fingers. In Adams JP, editor: Current practice in orthopaedic surgery, vol 2, St Louis, 1964, Mosby–Year Book, Inc.

Goldner JL: Reconstructive surgery of the hand in cerebral palsy and spastic paralysis resulting from injury to the spinal cord, J Bone Joint Surg 37-A:1141, 1955.

Goldner JL: Upper extremity reconstructive surgery in cerebral palsy or similar conditions, AAOS Instr Course Lect 18:169, 1961.

Goldner JL: Upper extremity tendon transfers in cerebral palsy, Orthop Clin North Am 2:389, 1974.

Goldner JL: Surgical reconstruction of the upper extremity in cerebral palsy, AAOS Instr Course Lect 36:207, 1987.

Goldner JL: Surgical reconstruction of the upper extremity in cerebral palsy, Hand Clin 4:223, 1988.

Goldner JL and Ferlic DC: Sensory status of the hand as related to reconstructive surgery of the upper extremity in cerebral palsy, Clin Orthop 46:87, 1966.

Green NE: Cerebral palsy. In Canale ST and Beaty JH, editors: Operative pediatric orthopaedics, St Louis, 1991, Mosby–Year Book, Inc.

Green WT and Banks HH: Flexor carpi ulnaris transplant and its use in cerebral palsy, J Bone Joint Surg 44-A:1343, 1962.

Haddad RJ Jr and Riordan DC: Arthrodesis of the wrist: a surgical technique, J Bone Joint Surg 49-A:950, 1976.

Hoffer MM, Leham M, and Mitani M: Long-term follow-up on tendon transfers to the extensors of the wrist and fingers in patients with cerebral palsy, J Hand Surg 11-A:836, 1986.

Hoffer MM, Lehman M, and Mitani M: Surgical indications in children with cerebral palsy, Hand Clin 5:69, 1989.

Hoffer MM, Perry J, Garcia M, and Bullock D: Adduction contracture of the thumb in cerebral palsy: a preoperative electromyographic study, J Bone Joint Surg 65-A:755, 1983.

Hoffer MM, Perry J, and Melkonian GJ: Dynamic electromyography and decision-making for surgery in the upper extremity of patients with cerebral palsy, J Hand Surg 4:424, 1979.

Hoffer MM and Zeitzew S: Wrist fusion in cerebral palsy, J Hand Surg 13-A:667, 1988.

House JH, Gwathney FW, and Fidler MO: A dynamic approach to the thumb-in-palm deformity in cerebral palsy: evaluation and results in fifty-six patients, J Bone Joint Surg 63-A:216, 1981.

House JH and Shannon MA: Restoration of strong grasp and lateral pinch in tetraplegia: a comparison of two methods of thumb control in each patient, J Hand Surg 10-A:21, 1985.

Inglis AE and Cooper W: Release of the flexor-pronator origin for flexion deformities of the hand and wrist in spastic paralysis: a study of eighteen cases, J Bone Joint Surg 48-A:847, 1966.

Inglis AE, Cooper W, and Bruton W: Surgical correction of thumb deformities in spastic paralysis, J Bone Joint Surg 52-A:253, 1970.

Kaplan EB: Surgical treatment of spastic hyperextension of the proximal interphalangeal joint of the fingers, accompanied by flexion of the distal phalanges: case report, Bull Hosp Jt Dis Ortho Inst 23:35, 1962.

Keats S: Surgical treatment of the hand in cerebral palsy: correction of thumb-in-palm and other deformities: report of nineteen cases, J Bone Joint Surg 47-A:274, 1965.

Kilgore ES Jr and Graham WP: Operative treatment of swan neck deformity, III, Plast Reconstr Surg 39:468, 1967.

Koman LA, Gelberman RH, Toby EB, and Poehling GG: Cerebral palsy: management of the upper extremity, Clin Orthop 253:62, 1990.

Lam SJS: A modified technique for stabilizing the spastic thumb, J Bone Joint Surg 54-B:522, 1972.

Manske PR: Redirection of extensor pollicis longus in the treatment of spastic thumb-in-palm deformity, J Hand Surg 10-A:553, 1985.

Martz C and Schaffer E: Orthopaedic management and care of the cerebral palsied. Symposium on cerebral palsy in Indiana, 1956 (mimeographed).

Matev IB: Surgical treatment of spastic "thumb-in-palm" deformity, J Bone Joint Surg 45-B:703, 1963.

Matev IB: Surgical treatment of flexion-adduction contracture of the thumb in cerebral palsy, Acta Orthop Scand 41:439, 1970.

Matev IB: Thumb reconstruction through metacarpal bone lengthening, J Hand Surg 5:482, 1980.

McCue FC, Honner R, and Chapman WC: Transfer of the brachioradialis for the hands deformed by cerebral palsy, J Bone Joint Surg 52-A:1171, 1970.

Mital MA: Lengthening of the elbow flexors in cerebral palsy, J Bone Joint Surg 61-A:515, 1979.

Mital MA and Sakellarides HT: Surgery of the upper extremity in the retarded individual with spastic cerebral palsy, Orthop Clin North Am 12:127, 1981.

Mortens J: Surgery of the hand in cerebral palsy, Acta Orthop Scand 36:441, 1965-1966.

Mowery CA, Gelberman RH, and Rhoades CE: Upper extremity tendon transfers in cerebral palsy: electromyographic and functional analysis, J Pediatr Orthop 5:69, 1985.

Omer GE and Capen DA: Proximal row carpectomy with muscle transfers for spastic paralysis, J Hand Surg 1:197, 1976.

Page CM: An operation for the relief of flexion-contracture in the forearm, J Bone Joint Surg 21:233, 1923.

Perry J and Hoffer MM: Preoperative and postoperative dynamic electromyography as an aid in planning tendon transfers in children with cerebral palsy, J Bone Joint Surg 59-A:531, 1977.

Sakellarides HT, Mital MA, and Lenzi WD: Treatment of pronation contractures of the forearm in cerebral palsy, J Bone Joint Surg 63-A:645, 1981.

Sakellarides HT, Mital MA, and Lenzi WD: Treatment of pronation contractures of the forearm in cerebral palsy by changing the insertion of the pronator radii teres, J Bone Joint Surg 63-A:645, 1982.

Samilson RL and Morris JM: Surgical improvement of the cerebral palsied upper limb: electromyographic studies and results of 128 operations, J Bone Joint Surg 46-A:1203, 1964.

Sherk HH: Treatment of severe rigid contractures of cerebral palsied upper limbs, Clin Orthop 125:151, 1977.

Skoff H and Woodbury DF: Current concepts review: management of the upper extremity in cerebral palsy, J Bone Joint Surg 67-A:500, 1985.

Smith RJ: Flexor pollicis longus abductor-plasty for spastic thumb-in-palm deformity, J Hand Surg 7:327, 1982.

Sprenger TR: Pronation deformities in the forearm in cerebral palsy. Symposium on cerebral palsy in Indiana, 1956 (mimeographed).

Stein I: Gill turnabout radial graft for wrist arthrodesis, Surg Gynecol Obstet 160:231, 1958.

Strecker WB, Emanuel JP, Dailey L, and Manske PR: Comparison of pronator tenotomy and pronator rerouting in children with spastic cerebral palsy, J Hand Surg 13-A:540, 1988.

Swanson AB: Surgery of the hand in cerebral palsy and the swan-neck deformity, J Bone Joint Surg 42-A:951, 1960.

Swanson AB: Surgery of the hand in cerebral palsy, Surg Clin North Am 44:1061, 1964.

Swanson AB: Treatment of the swan-neck deformity in the cerebral palsied hand, Clin Orthop 48:167, 1966.

Swanson AB: Surgery of the hand in cerebral palsy and muscle origin release procedures, Surg Clin North Am 48:1129, 1968.

Tachdjian MO and Minear WL: Sensory disturbances in the hands of children with cerebral palsy, J Bone Joint Surg 40-A:85, 1958.

Wenner SM and Johnson KA: Transfer of the flexor carpi ulnaris to the radial wrist extensors in cerebral palsy, J Hand Surg 13-A:231, 1988.

White WF: Flexor muscle slide in the spastic hand: the Max Page operation, J Bone Joint Surg 54-B:453, 1972.

Williams R and Haddad RJ: Release of flexor origin for spastic deformities of the wrist and hand, South Med J 60:1033, 1967.

Zancolli EA, Goldner LJ, and Swanson AB: Surgery of the spastic hand in cerebral palsy. Report of the Committee on Spastic Hand Evaluation, J Hand Surg 8(2):766, 1983.

Arthritic Hand

PHILLIP E. WRIGHT II*

Arthritic hand deformities may be caused by any of several diseases that should be identified individually. Although the surgical treatment may be similar for all, the operative indications and prognosis after surgery may differ with each disease entity. Furthermore, the systemic rheumatoid diseases have different effects on other areas of the body. In severe disorders the diagnosis may have already been established before referral. If not, a diagnosis should be determined before surgery, and the necessary medical treatment should be initiated and continued during and after surgery. Operative treatment should be considered a part of the general management of the disease.

The goals of surgery are to relieve pain, restore function, correct or prevent deformity, and inhibit progression of the disease. If pain is not the primary consideration, then the surgeon must be quite certain he can restore sufficient function to justify the surgery. On the other hand, relieving pain alone by a surgical procedure is worthwhile when adequate medical treatment has failed to do so. Although they may complain principally of pain, cosmesis is an important consideration for some, if not most, patients. If rheumatoid synovitis or tenosynovitis persists despite good medical treatment and supervision, synovectomy and tenosynovectomy are worthwhile as prophylactic procedures that may help delay further distention of the joint capsule and ligament and prevent tendon rupture.

Before surgery the surgeon should advise the patient on what the procedure entails, including (1) the insertion of pins, (2) the location of incisions, (3) the expected appearance after surgery, (4) the application of splints, (5) the expected stay in the hospital, (6) the type of anesthesia, (7) the approximate cost of the operation, (8) the alternatives to and risks of surgery, (9) the after-treatment and the rehabilitation period, and especially (10) the expected benefit from the operation. Patients with severe deformities may have developed substitution patterns that enable them to perform their daily tasks; these should not be interrupted without careful analysis of the pathologic anatomy and functional patterns. This is especially true in those who are older, who have retired, and who have no pain. The patient should be advised emphatically that surgery will not cure the disease process, but that deformities are correctible and local progression of the disease can be altered by surgical procedures.

The management of arthritic patients should be accomplished with a team approach, including an internist or rheumatologist, surgeon, therapist, and counselor. Patients with medical illnesses in addition to systemic rheumatic diseases (rheumatoid arthritis, psoriatic arthritis,

*Revision of chapter by Lee W. Milford, M.D.

or anklylosing spondylitis) may require medications that have significant side effects. Salicylates and nonsteroidal antiinflammatory drugs commonly are used. Because of their effect on platelet function, salicylates should be discontinued at least 1 week before surgery, and nonsteroidal antiinflammatory drugs should be discontinued 2 to 5 days before surgery, depending on dosage. Patients who have taken steroids for more than a 3-week period in the previous 12 months should receive supplemental corticosteroid therapy before, during, and after surgery to enhance their response to the stress of surgery. Other medications that have side effects to be considered include gold, penicillamine, hydrochloroquine, sulfasalazine, methotrexate, azathioprine, and various analgesics.

When a general anesthetic is to be used during an operation on a rheumatoid patient, the alignment and stability of the cervical spine should be investigated before surgery. If the disease has been generalized and prolonged, roentgenograms of the cervical spine are indicated to discover any subluxations. The degree of cervical spine involvement forewarns the anesthesiologist as to possible spinal cord damage that may result from hyperextension of the neck during intubation or while maintaining a free airway.

OSTEOARTHRITIS

Osteoarthritis may be unilateral, but occurs as frequently in the minor hand as in the dominant one. Although it is associated with tendon ruptures and triggering of fingers, they are not seen as frequently in osteoarthritis as in rheumatoid arthritis. It generally affects women more often than men and is frequently seen at the carpometacarpal joint of the thumb, sometimes as a single joint involvement. The distal interphalangeal joints most frequently involved are finger joints, often in association with Heberden nodes. The proximal interphalangeal joints may be affected with this form of arthritis, but their involvement is more common in rheumatoid arthritis. Spur formation, cartilage fragmentation, and limited motion without dislocation are the frequent sequelae. During the active phase pain is severe, and the joints and overlying skin may be inflamed. Direct trauma to an inflamed joint is especially painful. One of the most frequent complaints regarding the osteoarthritic hand is the painful, unstable carpometacarpal joint of the thumb.

RHEUMATOID ARTHRITIS

Rheumatoid arthritis, characterized by hypertrophic synovitis that eventually destroys the cartilage of joints, erodes and ruptures tendons, compresses adjacent nerves, and dislocates and erodes the joint itself, is one of the more painful chronic arthritic conditions. It may

cause such grotesque deformities of the hands that the patient may become so ashamed of his appearance that he may be reluctant to be seen in public.

Rheumatoid hand deformities usually are bilateral and symmetric, at times presenting a bizarre mirror imagery. Each deformity must be analyzed in detail before surgery is considered. Although combinations of deformities occur, involvement of the fingers, thumb, and wrist is typical. The metacarpophalangeal joints and the wrist are the joints most often affected early in rheumatoid arthritis, whereas the distal two joints usually are affected later. The metacarpophalangeal is the most important joint affecting finger function in rheumatoid disease. Ulnar deviation with palmar subluxation or dislocation of the finger typifies the rheumatoid hand deformity. Osteochondral and ligamentous intraarticular damage, as well as the forces applied through the intrinsic and extrinsic muscles at the metacarpophalangeal joint, affect the deformities at the metcarpophalangeal joint and at the proximal and distal interphalangeal joints. The extent of disease and deformity at the wrist also has an effect on the finger joint deformities. In addition to the typical metacarpophalangeal deformities, the proximal interphalanageal joints may develop boutonniere or swanneck deformities, and the distal interphalangeal joints usually develop a mallet or hyperflexed deformity, depending on the extent of capsular disruption.

Thumb involvement may cause a variety of deformities, depending on the joint at which synovitis begins. Nalebuff et al. noted that synovitis beginning at the metacarpophalangeal joint frequently leads to palmar subluxation and flexion of the proximal phalanx, with hyperextension of the interphalangeal joint (boutonniere deformity). When synovitis begins at the carpometacarpal joint, the deformity includes dorsal subluxation of the metacarpal base and hyperextension of the metacarpophalangeal joint (swan-neck deformity). Another thumb deformity caused by synovitic destruction of the capsuloligamentous supports on the ulnar side of the metacarpophalangeal joint is the gamekeeper's equivalent resulting from laxity of the ulnar collateral ligament of the thumb at the metacarpophalangeal joint. Involvement of the metacarpophalangeal joint also may result in laxity of the capsuloligamentous structures in the volar plate, leading to hyperextension of the metacarpophalangeal joint and interphalangeal hyperflexion but with a stable carpometacarpal joint. Other more severe deformities of the fingers and thumb may be caused by an erosive rheumatoid disease, leading to the "main en lorgnette" (opera glass hand).

Significant tenosynovitis of the flexor and extensor tendons in the digits and over the flexor and extensor surfaces of the wrist can lead to erosive and attritional changes and rupture of the tendons.

Rheumatoid wrist deformities have a significant effect on hand function, especially the position of the fingers at the metacarpophalangeal joint. Rheumatoid synovitis can result in disruption of the intercarpal ligaments, especially the radioscaphocapitate ligament, leading to rotatory instability of the carpal scaphoid and subsequent destructive changes throughout the entire wrist. The distal radioulnar joint–stabilizing ligaments are destroyed in a similar fashion, leading to dorsal dislocation of the ulnar head distally and subluxation of the extensor carpi ulnaris tendons with secondary ulnar translocation of the carpus.

SYSTEMIC LUPUS ERYTHEMATOSUS

Systemic lupus erythematosus is caused by an abnormality in the immune system. A number of autoantibodies are produced in excessive amounts and result in the formation and deposition of immune complexes in small vessels, joints, and other tissue. As a result, whole organ systems are involved, including the skin, heart, lungs, kidneys, central nervous system, and a variety of gastrointestinal system organs. Musculoskeletal involvement is characterized by stiffness, swelling, tenderness, and pain with tendons, joint capsules, and ligaments particularly involved. Joint surface destruction may occur late in the disease process. Hand involvement may be among the earliest manifestations of systemic lupus erythematosus. Usually the metacarpophalangeal and proximal interphalangeal joints are involved, as first manifested by ligamentous laxity. Raynaud's phenomenon, with tissue necrosis, ulceration, and cold intolerance, also is seen (Fig. 72-1). Although the hand deformities of systemic lupus erythematosus are similar to rheumatoid hand deformities, they result from primarily soft tissue abnormalities unrelated to proliferative synovitis, and the articular cartilage is well preserved. Procedures that may be of benefit include digital and arterial symphathectomy for the treatment of Raynaud's phenomenon abnormalities, as well as soft tissue procedures, joint replacement, and arthrodesis in the fingers.

PSORIATIC ARTHRITIS

Psoriatic arthritic deformities are similar to those in rheumatoid arthritis. An estimated 7% of patients with psoriasis have some form of inflammatory arthritis. Of patients with severe skin involvement, 40% have arthritic changes. The distal interphalangeal joints are typically affected and the disease here may produce a fusiform swelling of the entire digit. Uniquely, the nails may separate from the nail bed and have a white, flaking discoloration near their distal borders; they may also be ridged. Roentgenographic changes in psoriatic arthritis of the hand include erosion of terminal phalangeal tufts (acro-osteolysis), tapering of the phalanges and metacarpals, cupping of the proximal ends of phalanges and metacarpals ("pencil-in-cup" deformity), severe destruc-

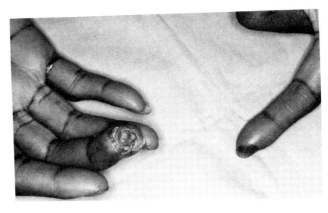

Fig. 72-1 Vasculitis associated with lupus erythematosus has resulted in necrosis of these fingertips in 33-year-old woman.

tion or ankylosis of isolated small joints, and a predilection for the interphalangeal joints with sparing of the metacarpophalangeal joints. Contractures of the proximal interphalangeal joints most often require surgical treatment, usually arthrodesis. In their report of 25 patients with psoriatic arthritis, Belsky et al. found proximal interphalangeal joint involvement in 22; seven patients had spontaneous fusion of all eight proximal interphalangeal joints, and 13 developed fixed flexion contractures of more than 90 degrees in all proximal interphalangeal joints. Although fusion or arthroplasty improved hand function, the authors warn that infection may occur more frequently after implant arthroplasty in these patients than in patients with rheumatoid disease.

REITER'S SYNDROME

Reiter's syndrome is described as a triad of conjunctivitis, urethritis, and synovitis. The synovitis usually involves asymmetrically four or fewer joints. Heel pain, back pain, and nail deformities may occur in this syndrome, sometimes making it difficult to distinguish from psoriatic arthritis. It affects the lower extremity more often than the upper, and 90% of the patients have remission of symptoms after several weeks; in about 10% the disease may become chronic. It is typically found in young males. Surgery is rarely indicated.

GOUT

Gout usually causes an erythematous, painful joint in adult males. The attack is often sudden with severe pain about a single joint. The joint is swollen, hot, and tender, suggesting a severe cellulitis or abscess. The area may be incised and drained by the unsuspecting surgeon. In chronic gout massive deposits of monosodium urate crystals may be found about the joints and tendon sheaths, causing nerve compression such as carpal tunnel syndrome. The skin may be ulcerated by pressure from within (Fig. 72-2). Amputation may be necessary because of the extreme bony disruption resulting from gout. The deposits may be visible on roentgenograms. Women rarely have gouty arthritis until after menopause; however, the patient with tophaceous gout is typ- ically an elderly woman. The presence of hyperuricemia alone does not establish the diagnosis of gout, and in fact, the uric acid level may be elevated and an acute attack of gout never occur. Conversely, during an acute attack of gout the uric acid level may be normal. Aspiration of a joint provides the only definitive diagnosis of gout: polarized microscopy usually shows negatively bi-

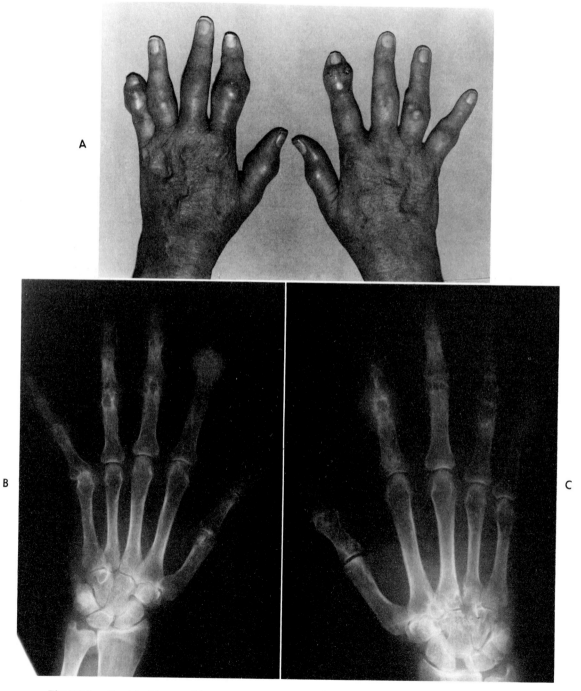

Fig. 72-2   Gout in 56-year-old woman. **A,** Heavy calcium urate deposits have caused skin erosion. **B** and **C,** Roentgenograms of hands showing destructive lesions in bones of digits.

refringent crystals in the joint fluid. Surgery for tophaceous deposits is rarely indicated unless an important structure is compressed or if the patient cannot tolerate uric acid–lowering measures.

Pseudogout, although more common in the knee, may involve the hands and can mimic septic arthritis. Deposition of calcium pyrophosphate crystals may be visible on routine roentgenograms as opaque areas in the articular cartilage or the fibrocartilaginous disc of the distal radioulnar joint. As with gout, definitive diagnosis is made by the identification of calcium pyrophosphate crystals in the joint aspirate. Treatment of pseudogout is medical.

SCLERODERMA (PROGRESSIVE SYSTEMIC SCLEROSIS)

Diffuse scleroderma, or progressive systemic sclerosis (PSS), affects both the extremities and the trunk. The disease may involve not only the skin but also the gastrointestinal tract, especially the esophagus, the heart, lungs, and kidneys. Telangiectasia may also be seen. The hand surgeon may see these patients because of calcinosis of the fingertips, ulcerations, or Raynaud's phenomenon. The age of onset is usually past 40 years.

Arthritic involvement usually causes contractures of the fingers, but synovial thickening is minimal. Involvement of tendons and tendon sheaths of the hand may cause a palpable tendon friction rub or a rather leathery crepitus as distinguished from the coarse, grittylike crepitus palpable in osteoarthritis. These rubs may also be felt in the tendons about the foot and ankle. Ulceration of the fingertips because of vascular impairment is best treated by an extremely conservative surgical approach, including waiting for the tips to amputate spontaneously since this will retain length of the digits. Surgical sympathectomies and intraarterial injection of drugs to help dilate the vessels have been recommended. Calcification about the eroded pulps of the fingers may be excised through a lateral incision, but healing may be quite slow. Local applications of medications may be helpful. Smoking should be avoided.

NONOPERATIVE TREATMENT FOR SYNOVITIS

Persistent tenosynovitis or arthritis with obvious swelling that persists for several weeks even when treated with antiinflammatory drugs may be treated by local injections of a steroid preparation and a local anesthetic. This treatment is especially applicable to trigger fingers and carpal tunnel syndrome frequently seen in rheumatoid disease or osteoarthritis of the carpometacarpal joint of the thumb. Even osteoarthritis of the distal interphalangeal joints and rheumatoid arthritis of the proximal interphalangeal joints will respond favorably to injec-

tions for a period of several weeks. However, after repeated injections the response may be less dramatic. In many instances pain may be relieved and surgery may at least be delayed by this technique.

STAGING OF OPERATIONS

When considering operative procedures for patients with rheumatoid arthritis, all aspects of the musculoskeletal involvement should be considered. Souter recommends starting with a procedure that is likely to succeed, beginning with the least involved hand. In addition, he advocates correcting significant disease and deformity in the elbow and shoulder before correcting hand deformities. According to Ferlic, Smyth, and Clayton surgical priorities are, in descending order of importance, the spine, foot, hip, knee, wrist, shoulder, thumb, elbow, and fingers. Each patient should be considered individually, and the patient's requirements, as well as the forces and demands on the extremity, should be considered.

When several operations are indicated on a single hand, their order of priority must be considered. In general, when wrist arthroplasty or arthrodesis is indicated, it should be done first since the position of the wrist determines the balance of the digital flexor and extensor tendons. However, at the time of wrist surgery it may be possible to do an additional procedure such as arthrodesis of the metacarpophalangeal joint of the thumb. But other extensive surgery should be delayed.

When multiple small-joint procedures such as metacarpophalangeal arthroplasties or proximal interphalangeal joint fusions are to be performed, plans should be made to do them all at one time to reduce the number of times operations are performed on a single hand. Frequently a rheumatoid patient will require surgery not only on the opposite hand but also on the feet, the hips, and other joints. However, surgery should be performed on only one hand at a given time because of the requirements for daily independent living and personal hygiene. If the lower extremities require external support, a platform or forearm crutch should be provided.

FINGER DEFORMITIES IN RHEUMATOID ARTHRITIS

Deformities of the finger may be caused by tightness of the intrinsic muscles, displacement of the lateral bands of the extensor hood, rupture of the central slip of the hood, or rupture of the long extensor or long flexor tendons. Here abnormal forces act on joints already weakened by the disease.

In addition, flexor tenosynovitis may produce limitation of interphalangeal joint motion so that the range of active flexion of these joints is significantly less than that obtained passively.

Intrinsic Plus Deformity

In the intrinsic plus deformity, caused by tightness of the intrinsic muscles, the proximal interphalangeal joint cannot be flexed while the metacarpophalangeal joint is fully extended; often the deformity develops in combination with ulnar deviation of the fingers. If the classical Bunnell test for tightness of the intrinsics is to be accurate, it must be performed with the proximal phalanx in line with its metacarpal. Any ulnar deviation at the metacarpophalangeal joint during the test will slacken those intrinsics on the ulnar side of the finger and confuse the findings. For instance a tight first volar interosseus will pull the extended index finger ulnarward, but if the finger is held in line with the second metacarpal during the test, tightness of this muscle can be demonstrated. It should be remembered that the first volar interosseus is a flexor as well as an adductor of the second metacarpophalangeal joint and that usually the first dorsal interosseus is only an abductor. Release of the volar intrinsics, especially of the abductor digiti quinti, once thought to reduce ulnar drift when performed early, is usually ineffective in itself because factors other than tight intrinsics also contribute to the deformity (p. 3312).

To test for intrinsic tightness, the metacarpophalangeal joint is held in extension, causing flexion of the proximal interphalangeal joint to be markedly limited; however, when the metacarpophalangeal joint is flexed, the intrinsics are relaxed and flexion of the proximal interphalangeal joint is increased. With ulnar drift of the fingers, this intrinsic tightness may be present only on the ulnar side. To test this accurately, axial alignment of the finger with the metacarpal should be maintained in checking intrinsic tightness. When indicated, intrinsic tightness may be released in conjunction with synovectomy by mobilization of the lateral band. When degeneration of the metacarpophalangeal joints requires arthroplasty, there may be sufficient resection of bone to release the intrinsic mechanism; however, it must be specifically determined at the time of surgery when a release is necessary. A specific tendon release of the intrinsics may be indicated (see Littler technique, Chapter 73).

Swan-Neck Deformity

Swan-neck deformity may be described as a flexion posture of the distal interphalangeal joint and hyperextension posture of the proximal interphalangeal joint with flexion at times of the metacarpophalangeal joint. It is caused by muscle imbalance and may be passively correctable, depending on the fixation of the original and secondary deformities.

This deformity may begin as a mallet deformity associated with a disruption of the extensor tendon with secondary overpull of the central tendon, causing hyperextension of the lax proximal interphalangeal joint. The proximal interphalangeal joint may actively flex normally.

This deformity may also begin at the proximal interphalangeal joint, as hyperplastic synovitis causes herniation of the capsule, tightening of the lateral bands and central tendon, and eventual adherence of the lateral bands in a fixed dorsal position so that they can no longer slide over the condyles when the proximal interphalangeal joint is flexed. This limits proximal interphalangeal flexion. The centrally displaced lateral bands may be ineffective in extending the distal interphalangeal joint, which may secondarily assume a mallet deformity without actual rupture of the lateral tendons. This mallet deformity, however, is usually not as severe as that produced by a rupture of the lateral tendons. A swan-neck deformity may require synovectomy of the proximal interphalangeal joint, mobilization of the lateral bands, and release of the skin distal to the proximal interphalangeal joint. Wrinkles and normal laxity of the skin are lost at the level of the proximal interphalangeal joint after several weeks (see technique for release of skin and mobilization of lateral bands, p. 3308).

Nalebuff, Feldon, and Millender categorized swan-neck deformities into four types and recommended appropriate treatment plans for each type. Type I deformities are flexible and require dermodesis, flexor tenodesis of the proximal interphalangeal joint, fusion of the distal interphalangeal joint, and reconstruction of the retinacular ligament. Type II deformities are caused by intrinsic muscle tightness and require intrinsic release in addition to one or more of the above procedures. Type III deformities are stiff and do not allow satisfactory flexion, but do not have significant joint destruction roentgenographically. These deformities require joint manipulation, mobilization of the lateral bands, and dorsal skin release. Type IV deformities are those with roentgenographic destruction of the joint surface and stiff proximal interphalangeal joints, which usually can be best treated with arthrodesis of the proximal interphalangeal joint or, in the ring and small fingers, with Swanson implant arthroplasty of the proximal interphalangeal joint.

Beckenbaugh emphasizes that flexor tenosynovitis results in ineffective support by the sublimis tendon and may be an important factor in initiating the development of swan-neck deformity in the rheumatoid hand. Every patient in his series had tenosynovitis with adherence of the sublimis tendon, the tendon being rendered ineffective in stabilizing the proximal interphalangeal joint against hyperextension. The overpull of the central tendon, combined with synovitis of the proximal interphalangeal joint and surrounding tissue that results in stretching, may cause a swan-neck or hyperextended position. Beckenbaugh treats this disorder by creating a tenodesis across the proximal interphalangeal joint with one half of the flexor sublimis tendon. He emphasizes that postoperative immobilization of the joint is unnecessary and allows immediate movement at the joint without protective splinting. The chief complication in his technique is flexion contracture of the proximal interphalangeal joint of more than 30 degrees. Some of these are corrected by releasing the tenodesis.

When there is marked hyperextension at the proximal interphalangeal joint and a normal roentgenographic appearance with maintenance of a normal joint space, tenodesis by the flexor sublimis tendon may be combined with release of the lateral bands and the distal skin. The technique of tenodesis of the sublimis tendon is the same as for the hand in cerebral palsy (see Chapter 71, Swan-Neck Deformity).

When there is marked proximal interphalangeal joint extension associated with joint destruction on roentgenograms, arthrodesis may be best if there is a near normal metacarpophalangeal joint or if metacarpophalangeal joint resection arthroplasty is anticipated. Numerous fixation techniques have been described to obtain successful proximal interphalangeal joint arthrodesis in arthritic joints, including a single Kirschner wire, crossed Kirschner wires, intraosseous wiring, bone pegs, polypropylene pegs, miniplates, compression plates, tension bands, and Herbert screws.

USE OF KIRSCHNER WIRES IN RHEUMATOID HAND

In the rheumatoid hand most Kirschner wires eventually loosen and require removal. Fortunately, however, fusion occurs rapidly in most instances after arthrodesis. Therefore we cut off Kirschner wires under the skin at a level that makes them easily recoverable, even sometimes leaving them protruding at the proximal interphalangeal joints. The dressing is then applied over the wires. Wires left embedded in the pulp of the fingers or near the metacarpophalangeal joint on the palmar side of the thumb are extremely painful. Wires in these areas should be inserted with the end nearest the skin on the dorsal surface. Most wires can then be removed in the office using a local anesthetic.

• • •

Arthroplasty of the proximal interphalangeal joints of the ring and little fingers may be performed when there are near-normal metacarpophalangeal joints proximally. Arthroplasties of both the metacarpophalangeal joint and proximal interphalangeal joint of the same finger rarely are done even in stages (see Swanson technique for implant at proximal interphalangeal joint, p. 3311). Pelligrini and Burton compared the results of arthroplasty and fusion in 43 proximal interphalangeal joints. All cemented arthroplasty devices failed at an average of 2.25 years after surgery. None of the flexible silicone interposition arthroplasties in ulnar digits required revision, but progressive bone resorption was evident roentgenographically adjacent to the implant. They concluded that no currently available cemented articulated device provides adequate lateral stability in the radial proximal in-

terphalangeal joints; arthrodesis remains their procedure of choice for the index and occasionally the long finger proximal interphalangeal joints with osteoarthritic involvement that interferes with lateral pinch. Adams, Blair, and Shurr reported long-term evaluation of the Schultz articulated, cemented metacarpophalangeal implant in 36 metacarpophalangeal joints with rheumatoid arthritis. Although they found medullary cement fixation satisfactory at long-term follow-up, the articulated portion of the implant did not consistently withstand the stresses transmitted across the joint and did not provide long-term stability.

INTRINSIC RELEASE. See Chapter 73.

CORRECTING HYPEREXTENSION DEFORMITY OF PROXIMAL INTERPHALANGEAL JOINT

■ **TECHNIQUE (BECKENBAUGH).** Make a zigzag incision over the middle and proximal phalanges (Fig. 72-3, *A*). Take care not to damage the digital nerves that may adhere to the cruciate pulley system anterior to the hyperextended proximal interphalangeal joint. Expose the cruciate pulleys by elevating medially and laterally the neurovascular bundles. Expose the A2 pulley (Fig. 72-3, *B*). Incise the central pulley centrally to expose the flexor tendons. Retract the profundus tendon and release any adhesions; then expose the sublimis tendon and its adhesions and perform a synovectomy (Fig. 72-3, *C*). Pull the sublimis tendon distally and incise the decussation, splitting the tendon into two slips. If necessary, extend the incision proximally and release the adhesions at the A1 pulley level to allow distal translocation of the tendon. Pull the divided sublimis tendon distally and incise the ulnar slip, leaving a 5 cm slip of tendon attached to the ulnar side of the middle phalanx (Fig. 72-3, *D*). Pull the slip firmly to ensure that its insertion is not weakened by synovitis. In the little finger both slips are incised because a single slip is usually too small. Puncture the A2 pulley 3 to 4 mm from its distal border (Fig. 72-3, *E*). Pass a small curved hemostat through the hole distally into the sheath and clamp the tip of the sublimis tendon slip and pull it proximally through the A-2 pulley (Fig. 72-3, *F*). Now bring the slip of tendon distally and suture it to itself with nonabsorbable 4-0 sutures (Fig. 72-3, *G* and *H*). Adjust the tension so that the digit is held at only 5 degrees of flexion at the proximal interphalangeal joint. A tenodesis is accomplished by this slip of tendon fixed across the joint. Repair the cruciate pulley if feasible. Close the skin over a small drain. Several fingers may be operated on at one sitting.

AFTERTREATMENT. Motion is begun on the third day after removal of the dressing. A static splint is worn at night for 6 weeks to hold the metacarpophalangeal joints in extension and the proximal inter-

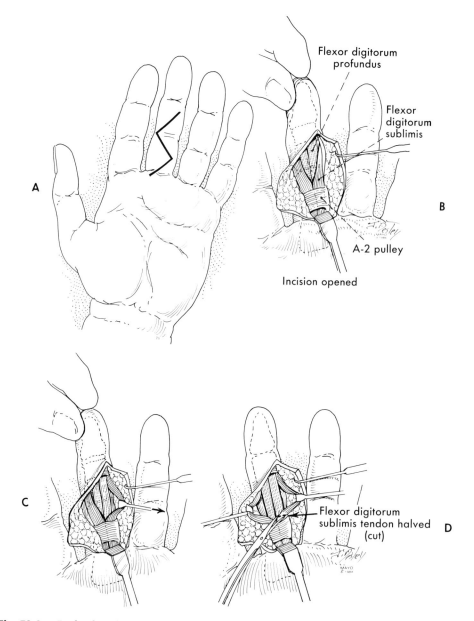

Fig. 72-3   Beckenbaugh technique for correcting hyperextension deformity of proximal interphalangeal joint (see text). (Copyright Mayo Clinic.)

phalangeal joints in slight flexion. If the distal interphalangeal joints are fixed in a flexed position, they may be manipulated and pinned in extension for 3 weeks.

LATERAL BAND MOBILIZATION AND SKIN RELEASE

■ *TECHNIQUE (NALEBUFF AND MILLENDER).* Begin a slightly curved dorsal incision at the midportion of the proximal phalanx, continue it distally from this point over the dorsolateral aspect of the proximal interphalangeal joint and over the middle of the middle phalanx, and then traverse obliquely dorsally to form the tail of a **J** (Fig. 72-4, *A*). Elevate the skin carefully, taking with it the necessary venous anastomoses. Make a longitudinal incision between each

lateral band and the central tendon, releasing them from their fixed dorsal position (Fig. 72-4, *B* and *C*). Passively flex the proximal interphalangeal joint to observe that the lateral bands will now slip volarward, sliding over the condyles of the joint (Fig. 72-4, *D*). A synovectomy may now be done, and good passive motion is usually established unless there is a bulging synovitis of the flexors. Suture the skin incision proximally. Distally suturing may not be possible; therefore the distal incision, being placed obliquely across the middle phalanx, gapes open and accomplishes a skin release. If the distal portion of the skin incision is sutured routinely, it might again contribute to hyperextension of the joint. The open portion of the incision usually will

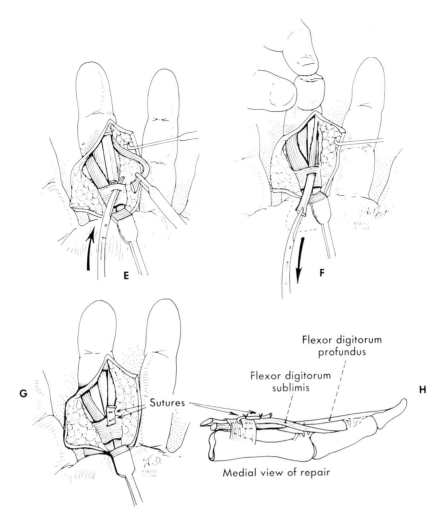

Fig. 72-3 cont'd   For legend see opposite page.

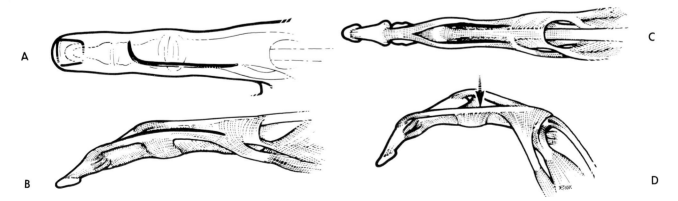

Fig. 72-4   Nalebuff and Millender technique for correction of swan-neck deformity. Skin incision is shown curved to permit release of contracted skin. Incision should not be completely sutured. Lateral tendons are then mobilized by two longitudinal releasing incisions, and joint is flexed (see text).

heal without a graft in about 2 weeks. Make certain postoperatively that active motion can be established by evaluating active flexion of the joint by the profundus and sublimis tendons. When active flexor function is not confirmed, check the tendons by making an incision in the palm and pulling on the tendons through the palm to see that they are not stuck and are not held by rheumatoid nodules.

Pass a Kirschner wire across the proximal interphalangeal joint to maintain this joint in flexion postoperatively for approximately 3 weeks. During this time, the open portion of the skin wound should close.

Buttonhole, or Boutonniere, Deformity

The so-called buttonhole deformity commonly is seen in patients with rheumatoid arthritis, although this tendon imbalance is not unique for rheumatoid disease. It is caused by synovitis of the proximal interphalangeal joint with a stretching out of the central slip, forcing the lateral bands to begin subluxating volarward. As the deformity progresses, the lateral bands are forced farther over the condyles of the proximal interphalangeal joint and therefore become tightened by their new course and by pressure from the underlying swollen joint. They finally become fixed in a subluxated position volar to the transverse axis of the joint and then act as flexors of the proximal interphalangeal joint. This tightening causes a secondary hyperextension deformity of the distal interphalangeal joint. The flexion deformity of the proximal interphalangeal joint is compensated for by an extension of the metacarpophalangeal joint. The metacarpophalangeal joint deformity does not become fixed, as do the distal two joints. Nalebuff and Millender categorized buttonhole deformities, depending on the roentgenographic appearance of the joint surface and the amount of active and passive motion. The mildest deformities, with satisfactory motion and normal-appearing roentgenograms, may be treated with repositioning of the lateral band, portion of the extensor mechanism, proximal interphalangeal joint synovectomy, and extensor tenotomy over the middle phalanx (Dolphin-Fowler procedure). For moderate deformities with a passively correctable proximal interphalangeal joint, normal flexor tendon function, and satisfactory preservation of joint space roentgenographically, a soft tissue procedure with central slip reconstruction using the lateral band or a tendon graft are options. For severe deformities with stiff joints, the long, ring, and little fingers may be treated with extensor reconstruction and silastic implant arthroplasty; in the index finger arthrodesis of the proximal interphalangeal joint may suffice.

In mild buttonhole deformities there is a flexion deformity at the proximal interphalangeal joint with lessened ability to fully flex the distal joint, but the joint is not necessarily fixed in hyperextension. The flexion defor-

mity at the proximal interphalangeal joint is passively correctable from a position of approximately 15 degrees of flexion. In these deformities treatment may consist of releasing the lateral tendons near their insertion into the distal phalanx (technique follows).

A moderate buttonhole deformity has an approximately 40-degree flexion contracture of the proximal interphalangeal joint, most of which is passively correctable. The distal joint is hyperextended, and usually the metacarpophalangeal joint is correctable to full flexion passively. The lateral bands are fixed in their subluxated position volarward by virtue of the contracted transverse retinacular ligament. To correct this deformity there must be functional restoration of the central slip and correction of the subluxation of the lateral bands (technique follows). Roentgenogenograms of these joints should show no severe joint destruction. If the metacarpophalangeal joint is destroyed and fixed but the interphalangeal joint is preserved, this deformity can be treated with metacarpophalangeal joint arthroplasty or fusion.

A fixed buttonhole deformity usually has joint changes on roentgenograms and a passively uncorrectable flexion contracture of the proximal interphalangeal joint (technique follows). Combined procedures on both joints, usually metacarpophalangeal joint arthroplasty or fusion with interphalangeal joint release or fusion, are necessary.

CORRECTION OF MILD BUTTONHOLE DEFORMITY BY EXTENSOR TENOTOMY

■ *TECHNIQUE.* Make a dorsal transverse or oblique incision over the distal third of the middle phalanx and expose the extensor tendon. Divide this tendon obliquely to enable it to lengthen and remain partially in apposition after the distal interphalangeal joint is flexed. Now carefully stretch the distal interphalangeal joint into flexion. This may uncommonly become overstretched and develop a mallet deformity that requires splinting. Do not suture the extensor tendon. Close the wound and begin motion in the next several days, making sure that active motion is carried out by the patient. Splint only if there is a mallet deformity.

CORRECTION OF MODERATE BUTTONHOLE DEFORMITY

■ *TECHNIQUE.* Make a curved, dorsal, longitudinal incision over the proximal interphalangeal joint and extend it distally to the distal interphalangeal joint. Mobilize the lateral bands by incising the transverse retinacular ligament longitudinally and dissecting underneath the displaced lateral slips. Tenotomize the two lateral tendons just proximal to the distal interphalangeal joint. When the central tendon appears to be stretched, shorten it by suture after tenotomy, taking care not to create an extension contracture at the proximal interphalangeal joint. Align the lateral bands with the central tendon at the proximal portion of the middle phalanx. Be certain of 80 degrees' passive flexion at the proximal interphalangeal joint to ensure that no extension contracture is being created. Tendon balance is critical in this operation. Perform a synovectomy after mobilizing the lateral bands. Pass a transfixing Kirschner wire of small caliber obliquely through the joint to hold it in extension. After 3 to 4 weeks, remove the wire and place the joint in a dynamic extension splint if it is indicated. Active motion should be initiated promptly so as not to lose joint flexion.

CORRECTION OF SEVERE BUTTONHOLE DEFORMITY

■ *TECHNIQUE.* When arthrodesis of the proximal interphalangeal joint is indicated, release the distal interphalangeal joint by oblique tenotomy of the lateral tendons just proximal to the joint and use the technique of arthrodesis described in Chapter 68.

The resection arthroplasty and implant technique (Swanson) may be used as an option if the flexion contracture is not so severe that it requires extreme bone shortening to accommodate the implant.

IMPLANT AT PROXIMAL INTERPHALANGEAL JOINT

■ *TECHNIQUE (SWANSON).* Swanson advises proximal interphalangeal joint resection arthroplasty and implant for the index finger when the deformity is singular and severe. If the proximal interphalangeal joints of both the index and middle fingers are involved, then arthrodesis of the joint of the index finger and resection arthroplasty of the joint of the middle finger may be indicated. This will give a more stable index finger for pinch and permit flexion of the middle finger for grasp. Resection arthroplasty for the ring and little fingers may also be done when indicated.

Make a dorsal longitudinal incision, slightly curved, over the joint. Incise the central tendon longitudinally, preserving the insertion at the middle phalanx. Maintain the collateral ligament insertions as much as possible. Resect the head of the proximal phalanx sufficiently to accommodate the implant. Ream the medullary canal if needed. Insertion of the prosthesis in the middle phalanx should be done after reaming, but the articular surface is not resected. Make a trial for size of the prosthesis with the joint in extension, noting that neither the middle nor proximal phalanx should impinge on the implant, but the implant should be well seated at the cortex of each bone. In flexion the cortices of the phalanges should not abut. Care should be taken not to have too tight a fit, which will cause buckling. Reattach the central tendon, if necessary, through a hole drilled at the dorsal cortex of the proximal phalanx.

In the swan-neck deformity (Fig. 72-5), a release

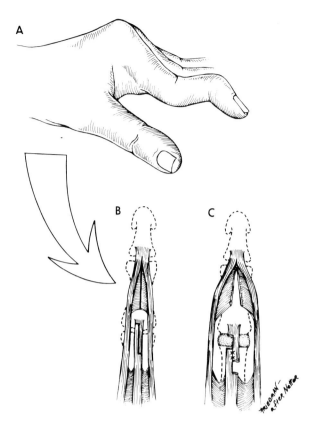

Fig. 72-5 Technique for swan-neck deformity. **A,** Swan-neck deformity of fingers. **B,** Central tendon is separated from lateral tendons by dividing connecting fibers. Central tendon is step-cut transversely and dissected proximally, thereby lengthening it. **C,** Lateral tendons relocate palmarward. After insertion of implant, cut ends of central tendon are reapproximated with interrupted sutures. Knots are buried. (Adapted from an original painting by Frank H. Netter, M.D., from Clinical Symposia, copyright by CIBA Pharmaceutical Company, Division of CIBA-GEIGY Corporation.)

of the triangular ligament may be necessary, as well as a release of the lateral tendon from the central tendon and elongation of the central tendon. In the buttonhole deformity (Fig. 72-6), release and imbrication of the triangular ligament are necessary to permit extension of the proximal interphalangeal joint. The central tendon may have to be advanced and reinserted at the dorsum of the middle phalanx. Collateral ligaments at times may require excision to permit alignment of the joint. Transfixing the joint with a pin is at times helpful to maintain alignment.

Deformities of Distal Joint

The rheumatoid deformities at the distal joint include a mallet, hyperflexed distal interphalangeal joint, which may occur in conjunction with a swan-neck deformity or as a result of attenuation of the terminal central slip of

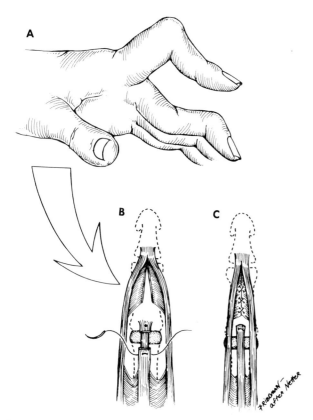

Fig. 72-6 Technique for buttonhole deformity. **A,** Buttonhole deformity of index finger with swan-neck deformity of other fingers. **B** and **C,** Lengthened central tendon is advanced, and lateral tendons are released and relocated dorsally by suturing their connecting fibers. (Adapted from an original painting by Frank H. Netter, M.D., from Clinical Symposia, copyright by CIBA Pharmaceutical Company, Division of CIBA-GEIGY Corporation.)

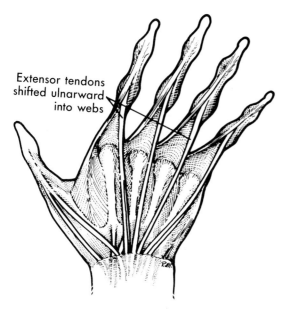

Extensor tendons shifted ulnarward into webs

Fig. 72-7 Ulnar deviation of fingers in rheumatoid arthritis (see text).

the extensor tendon, and a hyperextensible distal interphalangeal joint, which also may be related to attenuation of capsuloligamentous structures or to flexor tendon rupture. Usually either of these deformities can be treated with distal interphalangeal joint arthrodesis. In a patient who has had a proximal interphalangeal joint arthrodesis, the distal interphalangeal joint mallet deformity might be left untreated, because the small amount of mobility remaining in the distal interphalangeal joint can contribute significantly to fingertip function.

ULNAR DRIFT OR DEVIATION OF FINGERS

The deformity of ulnar drift or deviation of the fingers (Fig. 72-7) is found in conditions other than rheumatoid arthritis. Although its pathogenesis is not completely understood, its causes have been studied by many researchers (Flatt; Straub; Inglis; Smith and Kaplan; Long and Brown; Steinberg and Parry; Vainio, Reiman, and Pulkki; Kessler and Vainio; Tubiana; Hakstian; and Lipscomb). Space permits the listing of only a few of the factors that seem to cause this deformity. Those factors found in the *normal hand* are (1) the ulnar deviation of the phalanges at the metacarpophalangeal joints, especially of the index finger; (2) the small and sloping ulnar condyle of asymmetric metacarpal heads, especially those of the index and middle fingers; (3) the approach to the metacarpophalangeal joints from the ulnar direction of the long flexor and extensor tendons; (4) the greater ulnar deviation than radial deviation of the digits permitted by the radial collateral ligaments when the metacarpophalangeal joints are flexed; and (5) the greater strength of the abductor digiti quinti and flexor digiti quinti than of the third volar interosseus. Those factors found in the *rheumatoid hand* are (1) stretching of the collateral ligaments of the metacarpophalangeal joints by the volarly directed forces of the flexor tendons that permits volar displacement of the proximal phalanges; (2) stretching of the accessory collateral ligaments that permits ulnar displacement of the flexor tendons within their tunnels; (3) stretching of the flexor tunnels that permits even more ulnar displacement of the long flexor tendons; (4) ulnar displacement of the long flexor tendons caused by surgical release of their sheaths for multiple trigger fingers or for improving strength of grasp by changing their angle of approach to the fingers; (5) contracture of the interosseus muscles that causes (in addition to ulnar deviation of the digits) hyperextension of the proximal interphalangeal joints, flexion of the metacarpophalangeal joints, and eventually subluxation of these latter joints; (6) ulnar displacement of the long extensor tendons that further increases their deforming influence (this displacement is caused by ineffective radial sagittal bands); and (7) rupture of long extensor tendons at the distal edge of the dorsal carpal ligament that increases the possibility of dislocation of the metacarpophalangeal joints.

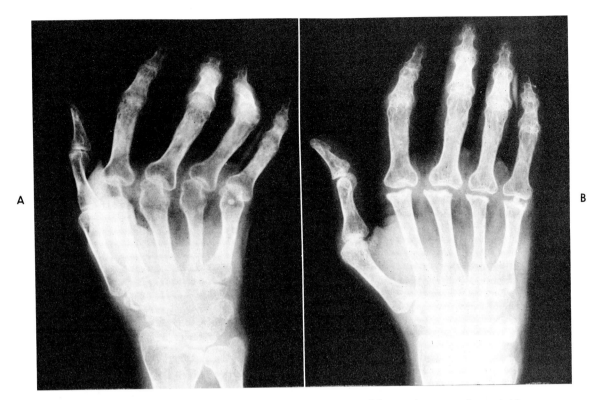

Fig. 72-8 **A,** Subluxation of metacarpophalangeal joints of fingers in severe rheumatoid arthritis. **B,** Subluxations have been treated by resecting metacarpal heads. Because at surgery articular cartilage of joints was eroded, intrinsic release would have been insufficient treatment.

Mild-to-Moderate Ulnar Drift

In the surgical treatment of mild-to-moderate ulnar drift, reasonable success is possible only when the major deforming forces have been properly evaluated. This type of ulnar drift implies the absence of severely diseased articular surfaces of dislocated joints (Fig. 72-8). Often, however, the flexor and extensor tendons are displaced ulnarward, the intrinsic muscles are imbalanced, and the joints are swollen. Surgical procedures that may be indicated are intrinsic release or transfer for balance, extensor tendon realignment, and metacarpophalangeal joint synovectomy. No operation has been devised to easily realign the ulnarly displaced flexor tendons and their sheaths.

EXTENSOR TENDON REALIGNMENT AND INTRINSIC REBALANCING

■ *TECHNIQUE.* With a skin pencil, outline on the hand the major dorsal veins so that, after their collapse on application of the tourniquet, they can be located and preserved when possible. They usually are found in the "valleys" between the metacarpal heads. Make a transverse dorsal incision over the metacarpal heads. Identify and preserve the dorsal veins. Enter each metacarpophalangeal joint through a longitudinal incision on the radial side of the extensor hood. Dissect the extensor hood from the underlying capsule to release the ulnarly displaced extensor mechanism. Make an incision in the capsule so that it will not lie directly under the tendon incision. Dissect between the synovium and joint capsule, if possible, and remove the synovium, especially that herniating out through the capsule and over the dorsal neck of the metacarpal. Usually most of the dorsal capsule must be removed in severe cases. Note the synovium usually lying under the collateral ligaments at the metacarpal head, and remove it by abrasion with two or three layers of gauze sponge wrapped over the point of a hemostat. Make another incision on the ulnar side of the central tendon, and reposition the displaced extensor mechanism, leaving the ulnar incision open. With fine interrupted sutures or a running pull-out suture of No. 4-0 monofilament nylon or No. 4-0 monofilament wire, maintain the extensor tendon over the metacarpophalangeal joint. When the index finger is markedly deviated, a transfer of the extensor indicis proprius tendon to its radial side may be of benefit (Fig. 72-9). In addition, the intrinsic tendons may be transferred from the ulnar side of the digits to the radial side of the adjacent joint, as shown in Fig. 72-10.

AFTERTREATMENT. At 2 weeks the sutures are removed and the hand is continually supported on a splint to avoid recurrence of ulnar deviation. The splint is worn for another 4 to 6 weeks.

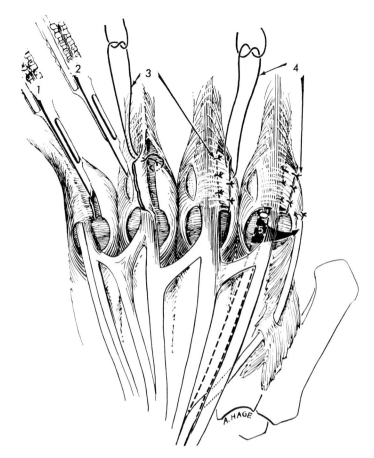

Fig. 72-9   Correction of mild-to-moderate ulnar drift. *1,* Joint is entered through incision in radial side of hood. *2,* Relaxing incision is made in ulnar side of hood to permit repositioning of extensor tendon. *3* and *4,* Incision in radial side of hood is closed after its edges are overlapped. *5,* Extensor indicis proprius tendon is transferred to first dorsal interosseus muscle to reinforce it. (From Flatt AE: In Converse JM, editor: Reconstructive plastic surgery, Philadelphia, 1964, WB Saunders Co.)

Severe Ulnar Drift and Metacarpophalangeal Dislocation

In severe ulnar drift often one or more metacarpophalangeal joints will have dislocated (Fig. 72-11); consequently, this type of drift and dislocation of these joints will be discussed together. Here the dislocation of the metacarpophalangeal joint in effect will have released the soft structures that cross the joint, and thus by decreasing tension will have protected, at least partially, the proximal interphalangeal joint. Conversely, if it is the proximal interphalangeal joint that dislocates first, then the metacarpophalangeal joint will be partially protected. Because of the deforming forces mentioned earlier in this section, the metacarpophalangeal joints will have deviated ulnarward more and more. It should be emphasized, however, that the long flexor tendons are a major deforming force. They will have shifted ulnarward either within or without their sheaths, exerting a force on the finger in the ulnar direction. In addition they exert a force on the proximal phalanx in a palmar direction that dislocates the metacarpophalangeal joint. For this type of ulnar drift, surgery is carried out mainly on the metacarpal head and its surrounding ligaments and tendons.

Function of a dislocated metacarpophalangeal joint may be improved by interposition arthroplasty in which bone is resected. Many different designs of interposition arthroplasty for the metacarpophalangeal joint are available, but we have had more experience with the Swanson implant than any other. An average expected range of motion at the metacarpophalangeal joint is about 55 degrees, and usually this occurs in the critical functional range. The incidence of complications is acceptable, with an infection rate of less than 1% and a breakage rate between 2% and 22%. With the newer high-density silicone construction, breakage has been reduced considerably. Even though obvious fractures of the prosthesis may occur and occult fractures often may be demonstrated on tomograms, the function of the joint usually is not impaired since it is not only the prosthesis but also the encapsulating scar that provides stability and permits motion. Metal sleeves have been added to diminish abrasion at the bone-prosthesis interface. The prostheses are easily removed when necessary. Interposition arthroplasty of the metacarpophalangeal joint can be depended on to relieve pain, maintain stability and alignment, and permit acceptable motion.

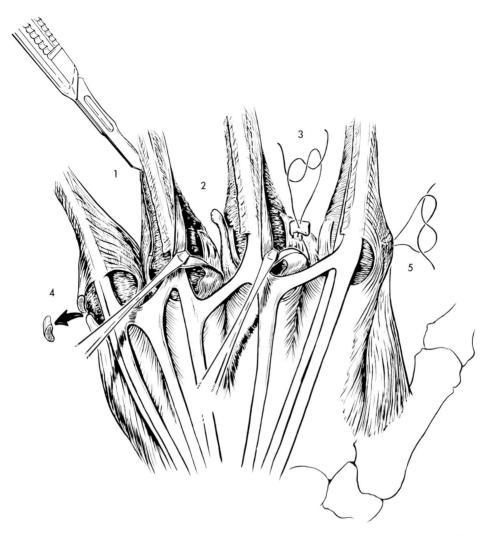

Fig. 72-10 Flatt transfer of released ulnar intrinsics to radial side of digits for ulnar drift. *1,* Incision is made on ulnar side of central tendon, releasing ulnar intrinsic insertion. *2,* Ulnar intrinsic insertion is free. *3,* Insertion is sutured to capsule on radial side of metacarpophalangeal joint of adjacent finger. *4,* Segment of abductor digiti quinti tendon is excised to relieve ulnar pull of muscle on little finger. *5,* First dorsal interosseus tendon is shortened to increase radial pull of muscle on index finger. (Courtesy Dr. AE Flatt.)

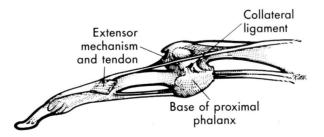

Fig. 72-11 Metacarpophalangeal dislocation in rheumatoid arthritis (see text).

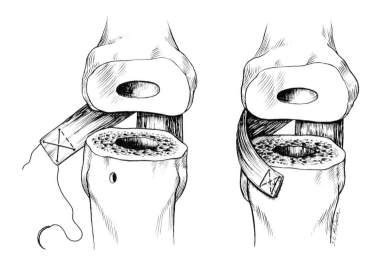

Fig. 72-12 Swanson technique for reconstruction of radial collateral ligament of index metacarpophalangeal joint by using a slip of volar plate. (Redrawn from Swanson AB: Flexible implant arthroplasty in hand and extremities, St Louis, 1973, Mosby–Year Book, Inc.)

■ *TECHNIQUE (SWANSON).* Make a transverse incision on the dorsum of the hand, beginning on the radial aspect of the second metacarpophalangeal joint, and extend it ulnarward to the ulnar aspect of the fifth metacarpophalangeal joint. Carefully observe the pattern of the superficial veins, and preserve them where possible. This incision permits a slight flap that can be dissected proximally and folded back, exposing the heads of the metacarpals. Through this, incise the shroud ligament of the extensor mechanism on the radial aspect of each joint and, if necessary, on the ulnar aspect also. This permits entry into the joint capsule, which already may be ruptured dorsally, with herniation of hypertrophied synovium. Incise the capsule longitudinally, and excise it partially as well as all the synovium that presents itself, either then or after resection of the metacarpal head. With a thin osteotome or a bone-biting instrument, resect each metacarpal head to shorten the bone sufficiently to permit easy reduction of the dislocated joint. This usually requires resection proximal to the origin of the collateral ligaments. After synovectomy, introduce into the medullary canal of the metacarpal either a square-shaped awl or, if necessary, a drilling broach to provide space for the stem of the prosthesis. The metacarpal head-neck region should be carefully cut so that it is at a 90-degree angle with the axis of the metacarpal shaft. Do not resect the concave articular surface of the proximal phalanx, but into this also insert the reaming device and ream the proximal phalanx to accept the distal stem of the prosthesis. Usually a No. 4 or No. 5 Swanson implant is used, but the largest one that can comfortably be inserted is required. Resection of bone should be sufficient to prevent buckling of the prosthesis or abutment of the metacarpal and phalanx on the palmar aspect with flexion.

To avoid pronation of the index finger, Swanson recommends that a radial slip of the volar plate be split off proximally and reattached to the radial aspect of the metacarpal to provide a mooring for the proximal phalanx (Fig. 72-12). Remove the prosthesis from the package only after a trial prosthesis has been inserted and the exact size determined. Handle the prosthesis with instruments without sharp edges to avoid scoring or other damage. Insert the prosthesis first proximally and then distally. Accomplish reduction of the joint with a comfortable seating of the prosthesis, and demonstrate passive motion of the metacarpophalangeal joint from full extension to near 90 degrees of flexion. Check all fingers carefully for alignment and for rotary deformity. Replace and realign the extensor tendon, and be sure that an intrinsic release has been accomplished by bony resection. Use a running pull-out No. 4-0 monofilament wire or nylon suture since multiple buried sutures at this level are more likely to erode and cause inflammation with movement. Insert a drain, close the wound, and apply a supportive dressing to splint the fingers in slight radial deviation. Additional surgery may be done on the same hand at the time of the insertion of the prostheses. Occasionally the fifth metacarpophalangeal joint may not require resection arthroplasty.

RUPTURE OF TENDONS
Extensor Tendon Rupture

Rupture of tendons is a major cause of deformity and disability in the rheumatoid hand. Rheumatoid tenosynovitis is the basic cause of such ruptures.

The long extensor tendons of the middle, ring, and little fingers seem to rupture as a group, and these ruptures can be easily overlooked because of more grotesque deformities elsewhere in the hand. Dorsal subluxation of the distal ulna contributes to rupture of these three tendons because the diseased end of the bone is rough and they usually glide between it and the tight, intact dorsal carpal ligament. Other extensor tendons also usually rupture at the level of this ligament (Fig. 72-13). The long extensor tendon of the thumb, because of its tortuous course, frequently ruptures at the level of Lister's tubercle where it angles through an enclosed tunnel or pulley. At surgery a white strip of connective tissue representing an effort toward regeneration of the tendon (pseudotendon) may be seen, but it is not a true tendon.

A ruptured extensor tendon may be repaired by direct suture when found within a few days if the remaining tendon is adequate. When surgery must be delayed for several days, it is well to splint the wrist in extension to relieve the constant tension on the remaining intact tendons. When the ruptured tendon is diagnosed after several weeks, a segmental tendon graft, transfer of a tendon to the distal segment of the ruptured tendon, or possibly a side-to-side suture of the proximal and distal segments of the ruptured tendon to an adjoining intact tendon are options for treatment (Fig. 72-14). A synovectomy is always indicated in the region of the rupture and the repair.

When the tendon of the ring finger or little finger alone is ruptured, repair of the ring finger tendon may be possible by suturing both its distal and proximal segments to the intact middle finger extensor tendon under appropriate tension. A transfer of the extensor indicis proprius might be used as a motor to the little finger. Another alternative, transfer of the extensor pollicis brevis as a motor, is possible when it is also necessary to arthrodese the metacarpophalangeal joint of the thumb. When three extensor tendons, those of the middle, ring, and little fingers, have been ruptured for an extended period of time, the transfer of a motor is usually indicated, and an acceptable source for this motor is the sublimis of the ring finger. This tendon has enough excursion and might be even more effective because of the tenodesing effect when the wrist is flexed. Extensor pollicis longus tendon rupture may be repaired by transfer of the extensor indicis proprius, a useful transfer when the extensor pollicis ruptures from other causes.

Flexor Tendon Rupture

Rupture in rheumatoid patients is not as common as extensor tendon rupture but is much more difficult to treat surgically. Rupture may occur within the digit as a result of infiltrative tenosynovitis or at wrist level because of bony erosion of the tendon, especially the flexor pollicis longus tendon. Rupture of one sublimis slip may cause triggering of the finger. Rupture of a profundus tendon may be easily demonstrated, but the level of rupture may be quite difficult to determine. A ruptured profundus or ruptured sublimis may cause secondary joint stiffness. Tendon grafts for rupture of flexor tendons in the digits of rheumatoid patients almost always fail. The exception is at the wrist, where a segmental graft may

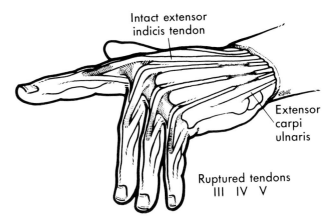

Fig. 72-13   Rupture of extensor tendons at level of dorsal carpal ligament in rheumatoid arthritis. Nearly all ruptures of common finger extensors occur at abrasive point created by dorsally dislocated distal ulna.

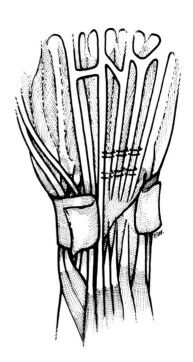

Fig. 72-14   Extensor tendon rupture under dorsal carpal ligament. Repair may be accomplished by side-to-side anastomosis with adjacent intact tendon.

occasionally be used as treatment for a ruptured flexor pollicis longus tendon. Another approach to rupture of the flexor pollicis longus is arthrodesis of the distal joint of the thumb.

PERSISTENT SYNOVITIS OF PROXIMAL INTERPHALANGEAL JOINT

Synovectomy is a useful operation for persistent synovitis of the proximal interphalangeal joint. It can be done on all four fingers of one hand at the same time and in conjunction with other synovectomies.

Synovectomy

■ *TECHNIQUE.* On one side, and occasionally on both sides, of the finger make a midlateral incision (Chapter 61) centered over the proximal interphalangeal joint, and on each side do the following procedure. Locate the transverse retinacular ligament, sever its attachment, and elevate the extensor hood. Then under the hood identify the collateral ligament. Enter the joint dorsal to this ligament and lateral to the central tendon, explore the joint, and excise as much synovium as possible. Remove the synovium from both the area behind the volar plate and the area inferior to the collateral ligament, dividing, if necessary, the accessory collateral ligament. Relocate the lateral tendon and transverse retinacular ligament. Close the incisions.

TENOSYNOVITIS OF FLEXOR TENDON SHEATHS

Savill reported that 50% of patients with chronic rheumatoid arthritis have tenosynovitis; Brewerton reported a 64% incidence. Often there is a progressive fusiform swelling of one or more flexor tendon sheaths extending from the middle of the palm to the distal interphalangeal joint. The swelling is painful and causes a gradual decrease in flexion of the fingers. On palpation the synovium is thickened, and nodules can be felt along the tendon sheath with tendon excursion; crepitus and grating usually are present. Should passive motion at the proximal interphalangeal joint be greater than active, synovitis within the proximal interphalangeal joint may be causing the major problem. Tenosynovectomies seem to have a lasting effect. Brown and Brown reported only 7 recurrences of tenosynovitis after 173 tenosynovectomies at a mean follow-up of 70 months. A tenosynovectomy may increase joint motion, but, although synovectomy of a joint may relieve pain, increased motion cannot always be expected.

Synovectomy

■ *TECHNIQUE.* Make a long zigzag incision (Chapter 61) on the palmar surface of each involved finger.

Expose the flexor tendon sheath by raising flaps on each side, but take care not to damage the neurovascular bundles that lie anterolaterally (not laterally). Now excise the sheath except for pulleys 1 cm wide or wider that are left at the middle of the proximal and middle phalanges. Excise as much synovium as possible, taking care to remove it from behind the slips of the sublimis and from between the profundus and sublimis. Close the incision with interrupted sutures, apply a compression dressing, support the wrist with a volar plaster splint, and elevate the hand. Motion of the fingers is started as soon as tolerated.

DEFORMITIES OF THUMB
Classification of Deformities

Rheumatoid thumb deformities frequently are complex and may involve the joints individually or in combination. The classification of rheumatoid thumb deformities proposed by Nalebuff is helpful in understanding the problems and developing a plan for treatment. He described four types of rheumatoid thumb deformities: type I, the most common, is a boutonniere deformity; type II, which is rare, includes metacarpophalangeal joint flexion, interphalangeal joint hyperextention, and carpometacarpal joint subluxation or dislocation; type III, the second most common, is a swan-neck deformity; and type IV, which is unusual, results from ulnar collateral ligament laxity and includes abduction of the proximal phalanx with metacarpal adduction. Type I (boutonniere) deformity results from synovitis that begins at the metacarpophalangeal joint and bulges dorsally to stretch the capsule and extensor hood, with attenuation of the extensor pollicis brevis insertion. The extensor pollicis longus migrates medially. The deformities that eventually develop are metacarpophalangeal joint flexion, palmar subluxation of the proximal phalanx on the metacarpal, and interphalangeal joint hyperextension. As the deformity begins to develop, the joints usually can be passively corrected; with progression, the deformities become fixed.

TYPE I. Treatment of type I thumb deformities depends on the passive correctability of the joints and the extent of joint destruction. If the metacarpophalangeal subluxation and interphalangeal joint hyperextension are correctable and roentgenographically the joints are normal, metacarpophalangeal synovectomy and extensor reconstruction may suffice. If the metacarpophalangeal contracture is fixed and the interphalangeal joint is correctable, but there is significant roentgenographic joint destruction, metacarpophalangeal arthrodesis provides a satisfactory thumb. In the presence of joint destruction at the interphalangeal and carpometacarpal joints, metacarpophalangeal arthroplasty may be more satisfactory, especially in older patients with fewer demands on their hands. If the deformities at the metacarpophalangeal and interphalangeal joints are fixed, with a satisfactory carpometacarpal joint but interphalangeal and metacarpophalangeal joint damage, metacarpophalangeal motion may be preserved with arthroplasty, and interphalangeal arthrodesis may provide a satisfactory thumb for patients with low demands. If both joints are severely damaged roentgenographically and if bone stock is reduced, metacarpophalangeal and interphalangeal arthrodeses usually provide a satisfactory thumb.

TYPE II. Type II thumb deformities include metacarpophalangeal joint flexion, interphalangeal joint hyperextension, and dislocation or subluxation of the carpometacarpal joint. Using combinations of interphalangeal fusion and metacarpophalangeal and carpometacarpal arthroplasty, type II deformities can be treated similar to type I and type III deformities.

TYPE III. Type III (swan-neck) thumb deformities generally are believed to begin with synovitis at the carpometacarpal joint. Eventually the carpometacarpal joint subluxates laterally because of joint destruction and capsular attenuation. An adduction contracture of the metacarpal develops, and the metacarpophalangeal joint hyperextends as a result of the extension forces on the metacarpophalangeal joint and laxity of the volar plate. The treatment of the type III deformities depends on the extent of metacarpophalangeal joint destruction, pain, the passive correctability of the metacarpophalangeal joint deformity and carpometacarpal subluxation, metacarpal adduction contractures, and metacarpophalangeal joint hyperextension. For mild type III deformities, if conservative treatment fails and pain persists, carpometacarpal hemiarthroplasty, without total excision of the trapezium, provides a satisfactory basal joint. Most authorities avoid total trapezial resection with replacement because of the instability that may result. If the metacarpophalangeal deformity is mild, carpometacarpal implant hemiarthroplasty or resection arthroplasty may provide a satisfactory joint. However, if the deformity and metacarpophalangeal joint destruction are advanced, metacarpophalangeal joint fusion may be added to the carpometacarpal hemiarthroplasty or resection arthroplasty. In advanced metacarpophalangeal deformity with carpometacarpal dislocation, a fixed thumb metacarpal adduction contracture, and a fixed hyperextension of the metacarpophalangeal joint, better results may be obtained with carpometacarpal hemiarthroplasty or resection arthroplasty, combined with metacarpophalangeal fusion. This usually relieves the adduction contracture of the thumb metacarpal without release of the first dorsal interosseus or first web space.

TYPE IV. Type IV (game keeper's) thumb deformity includes a thumb metacarpophalangeal abduction deformity and an adducted metacarpal caused by stretching of

the ulnar collateral ligament and attenuation of the capsuloligamentous structures by the chronic rheumatoid synovitis. Metacarpophalangeal synovectomy, ligament reconstruction, and adductor release may be sufficient for milder deformities. For more advanced deformities, metacarpophalangeal arthroplasty or arthrodesis may be required to stabilize the joint. Additional adduction deformity of the thumb metacarpal usually is avoided after metacarpophalangeal stabilization.

• • •

Techniques for correction of rheumatoid thumb deformities are described after the discussion of osteoarthritic deformities of the thumb. Although the pathomechanics may be somewhat different, techniques for treating the thumb, including soft tissue procedures, arthrodesis, and arthroplasty, are similar in both diseases.

Osteoarthritis

The thumb joints affected by osteoarthritis are, in descending order of frequency, the carpometacarpal, metacarpophalangeal, and distal interphalangeal joints. The carpometacarpal joint is most often affected by primary or posttraumtic arthritis, and the metacarpophalangeal joint is most often disabled by ligament instability, usually of the ulnar collateral ligament.

Correction of Arthritic Thumb Deformities

The operative techniques available for the treatment of arthritic thumb deformities include synovectomy, soft tissue reconstructions, arthroplasty, and arthrodesis. The following techniques may be used for both rheumatoid arthritis and osteoarthritis. Although most of the soft tissue procedures are used more frequently for rheumatoid arthritis, the bony procedures, including arthroplasty and arthrodesis, are used in the treatment of osteoarthritis as well.

SYNOVECTOMY. Synovectomy may prevent rheumatoid capsular distension and capsuloligamentous destruction and attenuation and is effective especially in the absence of significant roentgenographic changes or joint instability. Synovectomy is done more commonly for interphalangeal and metacarpophalangeal involvement and less often for carpometacarpal involvement.

Thumb interphalangeal joint synovectomy

■ *TECHNIQUE.* Approach the interphalangeal joint of the thumb using either a straight dorsal incision or a longitudinal curved incision. If there is a palmar bulge of synovium, approach the joint through a radial midaxial incision, releasing the collateral ligament. If the dorsal approach is used, release the extensor tendon on either the radial or ulnar side and open the joint capsule dorsally to allow removal of involved synovium. If the radial collateral ligament is released, use a curet and rongeur to remove involved synovium, reattach the collateral ligament to bone with a pull-out wire, and fix the joint with Kirschner wire for temporary stabilization. Close the wound and apply a splint with the interphalangeal joint in extension.

AFTERTREATMENT. The sutures and Kirschner wire are removed at about 10 days, and active movement is begun. The finger is splinted in extension except for exercise periods for another 10 to 14 days.

Thumb metacarpophalangeal joint synovectomy

■ *TECHNIQUE.* Approach the metacarpophalangeal joint through a dorsal curved incision. Expose the dorsal joint capsule between the extensor pollicis longus and extensor pollicis brevis tendons, retracting them to either side of the joint. Open the capsule dorsally and clean the joint using a rongeur and curet. Apply traction to the distal phalanx to open the joint and flex the joint to allow access to the more volar recesses. Clean the collateral ligament well. Close the capsule, extensor mechanism, and skin. Apply a splint to maintain the metacarpophalangeal joint in extension.

AFTERTREATMENT. The splint and sutures are removed at 10 to 14 days, and exercises are begun. Splinting of the joint is continued for another 2 weeks except for exercise periods.

Thumb carpometacarpal joint synovectomy

■ *TECHNIQUE.* Approach the thumb carpometacarpal joint through a straight dorsal incision curving toward the palm over the carpometacarpal joint. Retract the skin, taking care to avoid injury to the cutaneous nerve branches. Open the capsule to the dorsal side of the abductor pollicis longus and clean the joint as much as possible with a rongeur and curet. Close the capsule and skin and splint the thumb in extension and abduction. If extensive ligamentous laxity is noted, reconstruction of the carpometacarpal capsuloligamentous structures may be required as described in the following text.

SOFT TISSUE RECONSTRUCTION. Soft tissue reconstruction may be required for rheumatoid deformities at the thumb interphalangeal, metacarpophalangeal, and carpometacarpal joints or for joint instability related to osteoarthritic deformities, especially at the metacarpophalangeal and carpometacarpal joints.

Interphalangeal soft tissue reconstruction

■ *TECHNIQUE.* If the interphalangeal joint is passively correctable and there are no significant roentgenographic changes, release of this joint may be effective in restoring some of its flexion. Make medial and lateral incisions at the interphalangeal joint or

make a longitudinal incision over the dorsum of the joint. If there is a severe deformity and a dorsal incision is used, plan to convert it to a Z-plasty as the wound is closed. Perform a tenolysis of the extensor tendon and release the dorsal capsule by retracting the extensor tendon to the side and incising the dorsal part of the metacarpophalangeal joint capsule along with the dorsal portions of the collateral ligament. Flex the joint 20 to 30 degrees and pin it with a Kirschner wire. If a dorsal incision is required and there is insufficient skin for closure, Z-plasty may provide sufficient coverage. If there is a small portion of the wound that cannot be closed distally, leave it open and it usually will heal in 10 to 14 days. Apply a splint to protect the thumb.

AFTERTREATMENT. The splint and Kirschner wire are removed at 10 days and gentle exercises are begun. The sutures are removed at about 14 days. The thumb is splinted for another 2 to 3 weeks except for periods of exercise. If an incomplete extension (extensor lag) develops, splinting is continued for another 2 to 3 weeks. Normal motion rarely is regained.

Metacarpophalangeal synovectomy with extensor tendon reconstruction. Soft tissue reconstructions are effective for mild, easily correctable rheumatoid deformities of the metacarpophalangeal joint without significant roentgenographic changes. Metacarpophalangeal synovectomy and extensor tendon reconstruction usually will restore metacarpophalangeal joint extension. Nalebuff and Inglis both described effective procedures for improving function in the rheumatoid thumb. In patients with long-standing posttraumatic ulnar collateral ligament laxity or ligament laxity related to osteoarthritis, ulnar collateral ligament reconstruction may be required to stabilize the joint if there is no significant roentgenographic joint destruction.

■ *TECHNIQUE.* Determine the passive correctability of the metacarpophalangeal flexion. Make either a straight or curved incision over the dorsum of the metacarpophalangeal joint and retract skin flaps, taking care to avoid injury to cutaneous nerves. Identify the extensor pollicis brevis and longus tendons, which may be displaced medially, and make an incision between them. Incise along each side of the extensor pollicis longus to free it of its intrinsic muscle attachment. Transect the extensor pollicis longus over the distal third of the proximal phalanx. Dissect and release the extensor pollicis brevis from the base of the proximal phalanx and detach it from the extensor mechanism. Make a transverse incision in the capsule and mobilize a flap of capsule based distally at its attachment to the base of the proximal phalanx. Make a transverse slit incision in the base of the capsule to allow passage of the extensor pollicis longus. Remove the synovium from the joint with

a rongeur and curet. Pass the extensor pollicis longus through the transverse slit incision in the capsule and reflect it over itself. Hold the joint in full extension and suture the extensor pollicis longus tendon to itself under tension. Apply traction to the extensor pollicis brevis distally and suture it into the side of the extensor pollicis longus. Make sure that the intrinsic tendon insertions into the extensor mechanism are properly positioned to maintain active extension of the distal phalanx and that the intrinsic tendons do not subluxate toward the palm. Tighten the transverse fibers of the extensor tendons over the dorsal aspect of the distal phalanx if needed. Insert a Kirschner wire across the metacarpophalangeal joint to maintain it in extension. Apply a splint to maintain interphalangeal extension.
AFTERTREATMENT. The splint and sutures are removed at 10 to 14 days and the splint is reapplied. The Kirschner wire across the metacarpophalangeal joint is removed at 4 weeks and splinting of the metacarpophalangeal joint in extension is continued for another 2 weeks. Interphalangeal joint flexion and extension are maintained from the early postoperative period throughout the recovery.

Reconstruction of metacarpophalangeal joint of thumb for rheumatoid arthritis

■ *TECHNIQUE (INGLIS ET AL.).* Make a longitudinal incision over the dorsum of the metacarpophalangeal joint from the middle of the proximal phalanx to the midshaft of the first metacarpal. Observe the extensor pollicis brevis to determine if it has become detached from the bone of the proximal phalanx and retracted proximally (Fig. 72-15, *A*). Split the extensor hood longitudinally between the extensor pollicis longus and extensor pollicis brevis. Detach the abductor pollicis brevis from the extensor hood on the radial side, and detach the adductor pollicis from the ulnar side (Fig. 72-15, *B*). Retract the remaining tendon structures laterally to expose the capsule and synovium. Preserve the collateral ligaments, but excise all the synovium within the joint (Fig. 72-15, *C*). This may be facilitated by flexing the joint. Drill a hole for sutures on each side of the dorsum of the base of the proximal phalanx, and make a large hole just distal to and between them for insertion of the extensor pollicis brevis tendon. Attach the extensor pollicis brevis with sufficient tension to maintain extension of the metacarpophalangeal joint, and then attach the abductor pollicis brevis and adductor pollicis dorsally to preserve the balance of this joint (Fig. 72-15, *D*). Maintain the metacarpophalangeal joint in extension by two transfixing Kirschner wires for 4 weeks. Apply a splint to maintain the thumb in the desired position.
AFTERTREATMENT. The splint and sutures are removed at about 2 weeks, and the splint is reapplied.

The Kirschner wires are removed at about 4 weeks, and splinting is continued, except for exercise periods, for another 2 to 3 weeks.

• • •

Procedures for ulnar collateral ligament laxity are described in Chapter 64.

Carpometacarpal soft tissue reconstruction usually is reserved for posttraumatic ligamentous laxity related to recurrent dislocation. It rarely is indicated for laxity related to rheumatoid or osteoarthritic changes, because arthroplasty or arthrodesis usually is a better option (see Chapter 68).

ARTHROPLASTY. Arthroplasty is more useful than soft tissue reconstruction for metacarpophalangeal and carpometacarpal deformities caused by both rheumatoid arthritis and osteoarthritis. It is indicated for severe rheumatoid deformities with joint destruction, fixed metacarpophalangeal contractures, and metacarpophalangeal subluxation. In patients with rheumatoid arthritis, it is preferable to attempt to maintain metacarpophalangeal joint motion if the interphalangeal joint is sufficiently damaged to require arthrodesis. Sufficient bone stock should be present to allow stable arthroplasty, and it should be possible to obtain reasonable stability of the joint with restoration or preservation of capsuloligamentous structures. If restoration of joint stability is doubtful, arthrodesis is more predictable. Normal motion is not expected after metacarpophalangeal arthroplasty. Resection arthroplasty (Fig. 72-16), popular in the past, does not provide a stable metacarpophalangeal joint. Silicone implant arthroplasty, as advocated by Swanson and others, provides a satisfactorily functioning joint. Although implant breakage, dislocation, and particulate synovitis related to the Silastic are potential problems, implant arthroplasty is worthwhile in selected older patients with low demands on their thumbs.

Metacarpophalangeal arthroplasty

■ *TECHNIQUE.* Expose the metacarpophalangeal joint through a longitudinal dorsal oblique or curved incision. Release the extensor pollicis longus from the extensor expansions on each side of the extensor pollicis longus. Release the extensor pollicis brevis from the base of the proximal phalanx. Resect the metacarpal head perpendicular to the shaft, leaving the metaphyseal flare of the metacarpal. Preserve the collateral ligaments. If a flexion contracture persists, partially release the collateral ligament proximally. Leave the base of the proximal phalanx unless additional space is required for the prosthesis, in which case remove a portion of the cartilage and subchondral bone. Ream the medullary canal of the metacarpal and the proximal phalanx using the temporary trial prostheses to determine the largest size the metacarpal shaft will accept. Drill small holes in the dorsal base of the proximal phalanx to

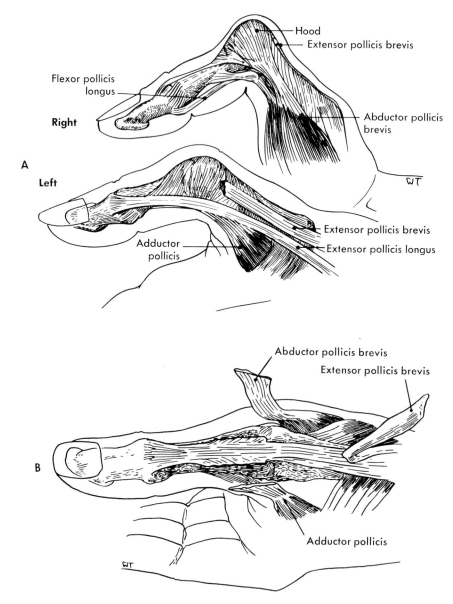

Fig. 72-15 Reconstruction of metacarpophalangeal joint of thumb in rheumatoid arthritis. **A,** Metacarpophalangeal joint of thumb with extensive tendon damage. After rupture of insertion of extensor pollicis longus tendon into base of proximal phalanx and proximal retraction, extensor hood becomes attenuated and allows abductor pollicis brevis and extensor pollicis longus to migrate volarward below center of rotation of metacarpophalangeal joint. **B,** Extensor pollicis brevis and adductor pollicis insertions are dissected free from remaining attenuated extensor tendon hood.

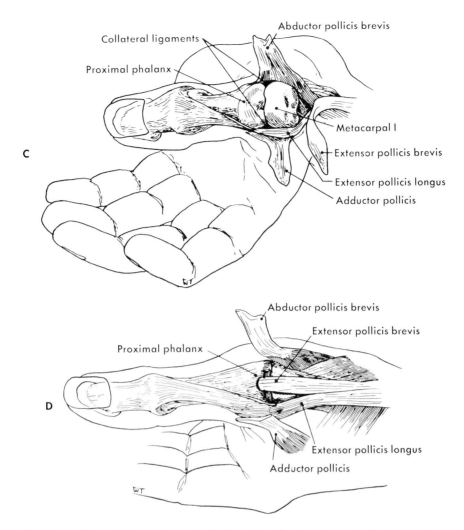

Fig. 72-15, cont'd C, Synovectomy is facilitated by flexion of proximal phalanx. Note that collateral ligaments are preserved. D, Attachment of extensor pollicis brevis tendon into base of proximal phalanx. When extensor pollicis brevis cannot be advanced, tendon of extensor indicis proprius may be transferred from index finger and inserted into base of proximal phalanx (see text). (From Inglis AE et al: J Bone Joint Surg 54-A:704, 1972.)

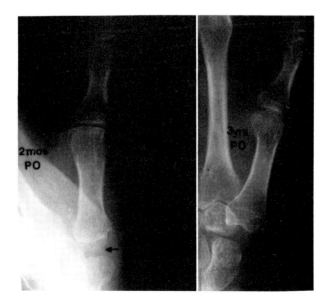

Fig. 72-16   At 2 months and at 3 years after excision of trapezium, settling of metacarpal and narrowing of the new joint is absent, but thumb is unstable.

Table 72-1 Classification systems of thumb CMC arthrosis

	Eaton (16-18)	Burton (7)	Dell (14)
Stage	No joint destruction. Joint space widened if effusion present. Less than one-third subluxation.	Ligamentous laxity. Pain, positive grind test. Dorsoradial metacarpal subluxation.	Symptoms with heavy use, positive grind test. Narrowed joint space, subchondral sclerosis.
Stage II	Slight decrease in joint space. Marginal osteophytes less than 2 mm. May be one-third of subluxation.	Crepitus, instability, chronic subluxation. Degenerative changes on radiograph.	Pain with normal use, crepitus. Ulnar osteophyte, less than one-third subluxation.
Stage III	Significant joint destruction with cysts and sclerosis. Osteophytes greater than 2 mm. Greater than one-third subluxation.	Pentrapezial degenerative changes.	CMC adduction deformity, MP joint hyperextension. May have pantrapezial arthritis and one-third subluxation.
Stage IV	Involvement of multiple joint surfaces.	Stage II or III with arthritis at the MCP joint.	Cystic changes and total loss of joint space. CMC joint may be totally immobile.

From Wolock BS, Moore JR, and Weiland AJ: J Arthroplasty 4:65, 1989.

allow reattachment of the extensor pollicis brevis. Pass a suture through these holes so that it is in place for reattachment of the extensor pollicis brevis after the prosthesis has been inserted. Insert the silicone implant. If needed, use the metal sleeve "grommets" to protect against irregular bony surfaces. Reattach the extensor pollicis brevis under sufficient tension to allow proximal phalangeal extension. Repair the extensor expansion over the insertion of the extensor pollicis brevis tendon. Advance and repair the extensor pollicis longus tendon centered over the extensor expansion. Close the skin and apply a splint to immobilize the hand and thumb with the metacarpophalangeal joint held in extension. Pin the distal joint if needed.

AFTERTREATMENT. The sutures are removed at about 7 days if the wound permits, and a splint is applied over the metacarpophalangeal joint to hold it in extension. Interphalangeal joint motion is encouraged. The metacarpophalangeal joint is splinted in extension for 3 to 4 weeks. Forceful, strenuous activities are avoided for at least 6 to 8 weeks.

Carpometacarpal arthroplasty. Arthroplasty techniques available for the thumb carpometacarpal joint include excisional arthroplasty, as advocated by Goldner and Clippinger and by Gervis; resection arthroplasty with tendon interposition, with or without ligament reconstruction; silicone implant arthroplasty or hemiarthroplasty; and total joint arthroplasty. Although patients with rheumatoid arthritis involving the carpometacarpal joint appear to benefit more from either resection arthroplasty, with or without tendon interposition or ligament reconstruction, or from hemiarthroplasty, this is related to the extent of ligament attenuation and joint disruption

as well as osteoporosis. Carpometacarpal deformities related to osteoarthritis may be more amenable to a wider option of procedures, including those mentioned above for rheumatoid arthritis as well as carpometacarpal arthrodesis in younger patients with heavy demands on their joints.

Burton, as well as Eaton and Littler, have proposed classification systems of thumb carpometacarpal arthrosis (Table 72-1). The deformities are divided into four stages, with stages III and IV involving significant joint destruction, pantrapezial changes, osteophyte formation, adduction deformities, and advanced osteoarthritic changes. These stages lend themselves to treatment with arthroplasty or arthrodesis.

Resection arthroplasty involving total trapeziectomy may relieve pain in patients with rheumatoid arthritis, but those with extreme ligamentous laxity may not have as good results. Patients with advanced osteoarthritic changes may obtain satisfactory results. Resection arthroplasty allows early mobilization of the thumb and is technically easier than other arthroplasty methods.

Excising trapezium

■ *TECHNIQUE (GOLDNER AND CLIPPINGER).* Make an incision parallel with the abductor pollicis longus tendon and extend it into the web space as far as necessary to release the soft tissues. Divide the superficial fascia and release the fascia over the abductor, the adductor insertion, and that part of the adductor origin on the third metacarpal. Reflect dorsally the dorsal branch of the radial artery and the sensory branch of the radial nerve and identify the base of the first metacarpal. Remove the periosteum and capsule to expose the first trapeziometacarpal joint and then the scaphotrapezial joint. With a small osteotome split the trapezium into three segments and remove it. Maintain the volar oblique ligaments so that the base of the thumb metacarpal retains its attachments to the index finger metacarpal. Remove small segments of bone from the base of the thumb metacarpal, and, if necessary, resect a part of the base of the index (second) metacarpal. Perform a tenolysis of the extensor pollicis longus and abductor pollicis longus if needed. Insert Gelfoam into the space left by the trapeziectomy. Hold the thumb and index metacarpals with a Kirschner wire, maintaining the thumb in a rotated, abducted position. Skin grafting of the thumb web may be necessary or adjacent soft tissues that are contracted may require rotation flaps or Z-plasties. Close the skin and apply a compression dressing combined with a plaster splint to maintain thumb abduction and rotation.

AFTERTREATMENT. The splint or cast and sutures are removed at 2 weeks. If necessary, the Kirschner wire is removed at 2 to 3 weeks and exercises are begun; the thumb is splinted between exercise sessions.

• • •

Biological interposition materials used for resection arthroplasty have included fascia lata and the flexor carpi radialis or palmaris longus tendon as advocated by Froimson and by Carroll. Ligament reconstructions have included free grafts and strips of the flexor carpi radialis tendon, as advocated by Eaton and by Burton, or of the abductor pollicis longus tendon, as advocated by Thompson. Ligament reconstruction alone appears to be suitable for posttraumatic or early osteoarthritic changes at the carpometacarpal joint.

The procedure for ligament reconstruction with tendon interposition arthroplasty is that described by Burton and Pelligrini. The technique for resection arthroplasty, ligament reconstruction, and interposition is that described by Eaton, Glickel, and Littler and by Burton and Pelligrini. These techniques are similar, may be used in patients with rheumatoid arthritis or osteoarthritis, provide a predictable and reliable method of stabilizing the thumb metacarpal base to the index metacarpal base, may be used with complete or partial excision of the trapezium, and have provided satisfactory results in our experience.

Excising trapezium

■ *TECHNIQUE (BURTON AND PELLIGRINI).* With the patient under satisfactory anesthesia and a pneumatic tourniquet inflated, expose the carpometacarpal joint of the thumb with a dorsoradial incision in line with the thumb metacarpal, extending proximally across the carpometacarpal joint and then medially toward the palm. Elevate the thenar muscles extraperiosteally and expose the trapezium by opening the capsule of the carpometacarpal joint. Reflect the abductor pollicis longus palmarward. If preoperative roentgenograms reveal only carpometacarpal arthrosis, excise the distal half of the trapzium. If there is pantrapezial involvement or if there is a severe thumb-web contracture, excise the entire trapezium. Take care to avoid damage to the flexor carpi radialis tendon during trapezial excision. Remove a portion of the trapezoid if needed to enlarge the trapezium fossa. Excise only the articular surface of the thumb metacarpal perpendicular to its long axis, including the articular surface. Make the hole in the base of the radial cortex of the thumb metacarpal with a 6 mm gouge perpendicular with the plane of the thumbnail. Split the flexor carpi radialis longitudinally and release a 10 to 12 cm portion of the radial half of the flexor carpi radialis, leaving it attached distally. Harvest the flexor carpi radialis either through a series of short transverse incisions or through a single longitudinal incision. Split the flexor carpi radialis tendon to its insertion on the index metacarpal base and then pass it into the dorsoradial wound through the trapezium fossa. Take care to avoid transecting the flexor carpi radialis at its insertion. Place two nonabsorbable sutures in the deep capsule for later use. Seat the metacarpal in a medial direction toward the index metacarpal and stabilize it in the abducted position with a longitudinal Kirschner wire. Apply traction to the metacarpal and slide it on the Kirschner wire to preserve the arthroplasty space in the trapezium fossa. Pass the free end of the flexor carpi radialis from its distal insertion proximally to the base of the metacarpal cortex, into the medullary canal, and out of the hole in the radial metacarpal cortex. Pull the tendon slip tight and suture it to the lateral periosteum and soft tissues around the metacarpal, then back onto itself to resurface the base of the metacarpal. Fold the remainder of the tendon to act as a spacer in the trapezium fossa and suture it to itself and the deep palmar capsule with one of the previously placed sutures. Use the second capsular suture to complete a two-layered lateral capsular closure over, and including, the tendon arthroplasty spacer. The distal orientation of the flexor carpi radialis tendon slip from the base of the thumb metacarpal to its insertion on the base of the index metacarpal is important, since this is the ligament reconstruction that supports the thumb metacarpal, preventing proximal migration and radial subluxation of the thumb. Transfer the extensor pollicis brevis proximally and insert it on the metacarpal shaft to augment the metacarpal abduction and remove the hyperextension-deforming force in the proximal phalanx at the metacarpophalangeal joint. Apply a thumb spica short arm splint.

AFTERTREATMENT. The sutures are removed in about 10 days. A splint is worn for an additional 3 weeks, at which time the Kirschner wire is removed and a removable thumb spica splint is applied. Range-of-motion exercises are begun at about the end of the first month. Inititally range-of-motion exercises are focused on metacarpal abduction and extension, avoiding the flexion and adduction. Splinting is continued, except for hand exercises and bathing, for 2 to 4 weeks after commencement of exercises. At about 6 weeks thenar strengthening is begun and is continued for 4 to 6 months. Pinch and grip strengthening exercises are begun at about 8 weeks. Splinting is discontinued when range of motion and thenar strengh are improved to a functional level, usually at 8 to 12 weeks.

Tendon interposition arthroplasty

■ *TECHNIQUE (EATON ET AL.).* With the patient under satisfactory anesthesia and after inflation of a pneumatic tourniquet, expose the trapeziometacarpal joint of the thumb through a radiopalmar excision extending from the thumb metacarpal proximally and then palmarward (Wagner). Elevate the thenar muscles extra-periosteally from the base of the metacarpal and the trapezium. Make a transverse incision in the trapeziometacarpal and scaphotrapezial joints. If degenerative changes are present in both joints by inspection and roentgenograms, trapezial resection is indicated, and consideration might be given to trapezial replacement arthroplasty. If only the trapeziometacarpal joint is involved, proceed with tendon interposition arthroplasty. Remove osteophytes and the prominent "posts" of the trapezial "saddle." Minimally resect the base of the thumb metacarpal, creating flat surfaces perpendicular to the functional axis of the thumb ray. With a gouge make an extraarticular hole in the sagittal plane from dorsal to palmar in the base of the thumb metacarpal, approximately 3 mm distal to the base of the thumb metacarpal. Align this hole perpendicular to the plane of the thumbnail. Pass a Kirschner wire from the center of the resected metacarpal base through the medullary canal from proximal to distal, emerging distally through the metacarpal head. Withdraw the wire distal to the gouge hole in the metacarpal to avoid entanglement in the reconstructed ligament.

Harvest the flexor carpi radialis tendon slip next. Make multiple short transverse incisions 2 to 3 cm apart over the course of the flexor carpi radialis tendon from the wrist crease to the musculotendinous junction. Split the tendon and dissect a strip consisting of about one half to two thirds of its width from distal to proximal, extending to the musculotendinous junction. Dissect the slip distally beneath the skin bridges and emerge just distal to the wrist flex-

ion crease. Dissect the distal 4 cm of the flexor carpi radialis tendon slip, leaving it attached distally, divide it from the proximal 6 to 10 cm of tendon, and set aside the free segment to use as a tendon "sandwich." Usually about 40% of the flexor carpi radialis strip is used for ligament reconstruction, and 60% for tendon interposition. Pass the distally attached segment of the flexor carpi radialis through the gouge hole in the metacarpal base from palmar to dorsal. Leave this tendon protruding dorsally to suture it to the abductor pollicis longus tendon and capsule. Fold the remaining free segment of tendon and suture the free ends together with a 3-0 catgut suture on a straight needle through the center of the folded and doubled tendon segment, passing the suture between the resected surfaces of the bone and out through the skin of the dorsal surface of the thumb web space. Pull on the suture ends to fold the tendon in half, creating a four-layered tendon "sandwich" lying between the resected base of the metacarpal and thumb trapzium. Tie the ends of the traction suture loosely on the dorsum of the thumb web, allowing the tendon "sandwich" to form a cushion between the resected bone surfaces. Reduce the trapeziometacarpal joint and maintain it in extension and abduction by passing the previously positioned Kirschner wire down the metacarpal shaft proximally into the trapezium. Pass the remaining stump of the flexor carpi radialis tendon beneath the abductor pollicis longus insertion and suture the flexor carpi radialis tendon to the abductor pollicis longus tendon and the dorsal capsule. Do not excessively tighten the reconstructed ligament. Close the arthrotomy with absorbable sutures and approximate the thenar muscles. Close the skin and apply a bandage reinforced with a plaster splint, immobilizing the carpometacarpal and metacarpophalangeal joints of the thumb.

AFTERTREATMENT. If the wound is healing satisfactorily, the sutures are removed at about 10 days. The thumb is immobilized for 4 weeks, and then the cast and Kirschner wire are removed. If capsulodesis was done at the metacarpophalangeal joint at the time of the carpometacarpal procedure, it is immobilized in a small aluminum splint for an additional week. At 4 to 5 weeks, progressive range-of-motion exercises of the thumb carpometacarpal and metacarpophalangeal joints are begun. Extension and circumduction exercises are begun first, then opposition, followed by thumb flexion toward the metacarpal heads, and then pinch strengthening. Residual stiffness of the carpometacarpal joint can be expected for at least 6 to 10 weeks, depending on the patient's ability to cooperate with rehabilitation.

Implant arthroplasty. Implant arthroplasty of the carpometacarpal joint may be indicated when pain from rheumatoid arthritis or osteoarthritis has not responded to conservative treatment. Several techniques are available that provide stability and relief of pain yet preserve some mobility and strength of pinch. We are most familiar with the technique of Swanson et al., that is, silicone implant arthroplasty that replaces the entire trapezium. Their technique is generally used in patients with a subluxated carpometacarpal joint with synovitis, joint narrowing, osteophytes, and a positive grind test. Complications include implant subluxation (5% to 20%) or dislocation (0% to 19%) and silicone synovitis (as high as 50%). The ligaments and capsule around this prosthesis must be carefully reconstructed, and its position must be maintained in a cast for 6 weeks to prevent subluxation. Relief of pain has been excellent in most instances. However, some joint motion and power of pinch are lost with various degrees of subluxation. We no longer place a transfixing wire across the prosthesis or suture the prosthesis to the surrounding bone.

Sometimes in severe rheumatoid arthritis, absorption of bone causes marked displacement of the carpometacarpal joint. This results in secondary shortening of the associated intrinsic muscles and other surrounding structures. In these instances replacement of the trapezium and realignment of the thumb may cause an unacceptable increase in tension in the surrounding musculature, resulting in secondary deformities distally. To prevent this, techniques of resurfacing arthroplasty of the joint have been devised by Swanson et al. and Ashworth et al.

■ *TECHNIQUE (SWANSON ET AL.).* **Make an incision along the radiopalmar side of the first metacarpal shaft at its proximal half. Extend it over the base of the thumb and across toward the palm (Fig. 72-17). Expose and protect the underlying superficial branches of the radial nerve and the dorsal branch of the radial artery. Then excise the joint capsule just at its insertion on the trapezium, thus preserving its distal insertion for maximum use later. If this capsule is excised from the base of the thumb, excision of the trapezium will then remove it completely. Release the insertion of the abductor pollicis longus tendon. Before releasing it, remember to retain a slip of tendon to reinforce the capsule if indicated. Next, remove the trapezium by fragmenting it with an osteotome. Usually cutting it in thirds will provide better exposure. Remove the fragments with a rongeur. Leaving small fragments of bone attached to the palmar capsule preserves its integrity and prevents the tendency of the prosthesis to subluxate in this direction. Now debride the osteophytes along the base of the thumb metacarpal. Ream the medullary canal with an awl or reamer to permit insertion of a prosthesis of appropriate size. The awl reamer is less likely to damage the cortex of the metacarpal. Seat the prosthesis into the thumb metacarpal and on the distal articular surface of the carpal scaphoid. Shake the thumb gently to confirm that the**

prosthesis is stable. If necessary, use an osteotome to remove the part of the trapezoid that faces the prosthesis. This provides better seating against a larger surface. Be certain that the stem of the prosthesis is completely seated in the medullary canal of the first metacarpal. Some trimming of the stem may be needed. Place the thumb in abduction and extension and repair the joint capsule with nonabsorbable 4-0 sutures. Capsular reinforcements may be obtained from a segment of the abductor pollicis longus as mentioned above or from the flexor carpi radialis. Be sure not to create an imbalance of the intrinsics, causing hyperextension at the metacarpophalangeal joint.

Metacarpophalangeal and interphalangeal arthrodeses may be done at the same time if needed. It is especially important to correct metacarpophalangeal joint hyperextension with volar capsulodesis, arthroplasty, or arthrodesis as needed.

Reattach the abductor pollicis longus. Suture the skin and insert a drain. Place the hand in a soft dressing and a volar plaster splint.

AFTERTREATMENT. **The bandage and sutures are removed at 10 to 14 days. A full thumb spica cast is applied and is worn for 4 weeks. Then a removable splint is applied, and rehabilitation is begun. Thumb metacarpophalangeal hyperextension is prevented by splinting for another 4 weeks.**

• • •

Ashworth et al. prefer to resect only part of the trapezium, thus permitting the insertion of a small silicone rubber prosthesis. Less bone resection and a smaller prosthesis decrease the tendency for subluxation at the carpometacarpal joint. We have had little experience with this prosthesis, but it meets the needs of resurfacing the joint and preventing the subluxation.

■ *TECHNIQUE (ASHWORTH ET AL.).* **Make a transverse or curved longitudinal incision and expose the carpometacarpal joint of the thumb. Identify and protect the superficial sensory branch of the radial nerve. Now detach the abductor pollicis longus at its insertion and retract the extensor pollicis brevis. Enter the joint capsule and remove any marginal osteophytes from the base of the metacarpal and the trapezium. Distract the joint to expose the distal surface of the trapezium, and, with either an osteotome or a power saw, resect bone to create a flat distal surface. Excise the medial osteophyte and reduce the subluxated metacarpal. Curet a crater 5 to 7 mm wide in the body of the trapezium to receive the prosthesis. Trim the peripheral portion of the disc-shaped prosthesis to fit the diameter of the distal surface of the trapezium. Now advance the abductor pollicis longus tendon distally to the base of the metacarpal and anchor it with a nonabosorbable 4-0 suture through the periosteum or a hole drilled**

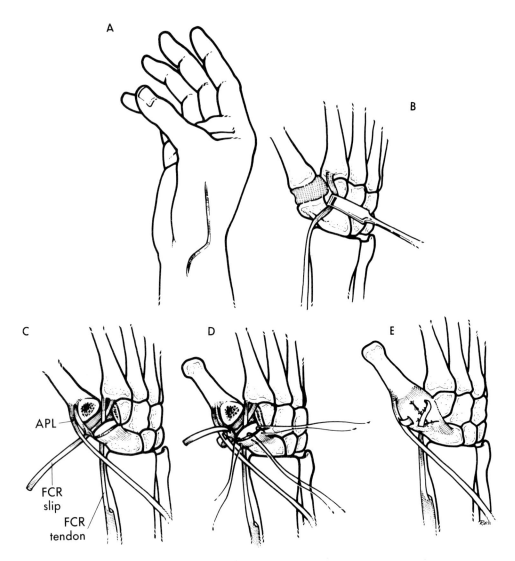

Fig. 72-17 Method of reinforcing thumb carpometacarpal capsule during implant arthroplasty. **A,** Longitudinal incision parallel to extensor pollicis brevis has short transverse and palmarward arm to continue proximally parallel to flexor carpi radialis tendon. **B,** Proper exposure and retraction of radial artery over scaphoid bone essential for proper exposure. Adequate excision of trapezium, including projection between first and second metacarpals is most important. Radial aspect of trapezoid is removed when it is necessary to improve fit of implant over scaphoid facet. **C,** Excision of bone is completed. Flexor carpi radialis tendon slip is dissected to its insertion on second metacarpal, passed under flexor carpi radialis tendon, and sutured to flexor carpi radialis tendon and palmar capsule to exit radially through abductor pollicis brevis muscle. **D,** Flexor carpi radialis slip passed anteriorly through abductor pollicis longus tendon and lateral capsule. Sutures are passed through capsular reflections off scaphoid bone to secure capsular closure. **E,** After implant insertion and temporary fixation are completed, capsule is sutured; flexor carpi radialis slip is brought over and through radial capsule and over implant to exit through ulnar capsule. Slip is then pulled, folded over and across dorsal capsule, and sutured in position. (Redrawn from Swanson AB, deGroot-Swanson G, and Watermeier JJ: J Hand Surg 6:125, 1981.)

in the bone. Close the capsule tightly and reinforce it with additional sutures along the side of the abductor pollicis longus. Also reinforce the capsule in any way necessary. Occasionally the abductor pollicis longus sends a separate tendon to the abductor pollicis brevis. If this tendon is present, use it for reinforcement. Close the wound and apply a large compression dressing and a volar plaster splint with the thumb in abduction. Occasionally the first metacarpal must be fixed by a Kirschner wire.

AFTERTREATMENT. The splint and sutures are removed at about 10 days, and a thumb spica cast is worn for an additional 5 weeks. Active motion should be started gradually at 6 weeks after surgery. Unrestricted free motion is usually present at the end of the third month, when ordinary activity can be resumed.

• • •

Eaton designed a prosthesis that is stabilized by passing a segment of tendon through a perforation in its body, thereby anchoring it to the adjacent bone. The prosthesis was designed in an effort to avoid subluxation or dislocation, which occurred in 10% of the patients in his series. He defines subluxation as a state in which the articular surfaces of the prosthesis and the adjoining bone are in less than 50% apposition. A slip of the abductor pollicis longus seems to work best. There are two sizes of prosthesis to select from.

■ *TECHNIQUE (EATON).* Expose the carpometacarpal joint of the thumb by a palmar approach. Reflect the muscles and expose the joint capsule. Avoid injury to the superficial branch of the radial artery and nerve and the palmar cutaneous branch of the median nerve. Remove the trapezium, preserving as much capsule and periosteum as possible. Avoid damage to the deep branch of the radial artery. Now resect a portion of the distal pole of the scaphoid along a line perpendicular to the anticipated positioning of the thumb metacarpal. Square off the thumb metacarpal perpendicular to its long axis. Remove all osteophytes. Next ream the medullary canal of the metacarpal to accept the round stem of the implant. Shave off the radial facet of the trapezoid down to subchondral bone and gouge a channel in the bone to receive the tendon reinforcement. This channel will emerge near one of the tendons of the radial wrist extensors. See Fig. 72-18 for the direction of the channel. Pass a 28-gauge wire loop through the channel with which to pass the strip of tendon. Through a J-shaped incision over the anatomic snuff box, isolate a strip of tendon of the abductor pollicis longus, retaining its normal insertion distally on the first metacarpal. Using the wire loop, pass this strip through the capsule, through the perforation in the body of the implant, and then through the channel previously created in the lesser multangular. Adjust the strip and suture it to the ad-

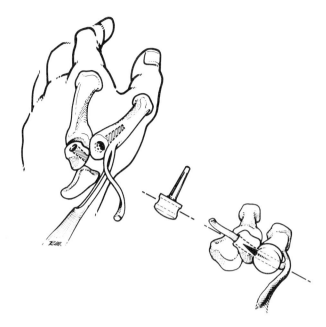

Fig. 72-18   Method for inserting Eaton trapezial prosthesis. Stabilization of implant is accomplished by passage of strip of abductor pollicis longus tendon through base of implant and into adjacent trapezium. (Redrawn from Eaton RG: J Bone Joint Surg 61-A:76, 1979.)

jacent wrist extensor tendons after the capsule has been securely reconstructed. Keep the implant seated while holding the thumb in abduction and extension. Next divide the extensor pollicis brevis at the metacarpophalangeal joint and reattach it under moderate tension to the base of the extended thumb metacarpal. The distal free end may be used to reinforce the capsule. Plicate the intact portion of the abductor pollicis longus tendon or divide and reattach it to the base of the thumb metacarpal under moderate tension while keeping the thumb abducted. Be certain that hyperextension has not developed at the metacarpophalangeal joint. If extension is more than 20 degrees, perform a volar capsulodesis and transfix the metacarpophalangeal joint in flexion with a Kirschner wire. If the metacarpophalangeal joint is hyperextended more than 40 degrees, arthrodese it in 20 to 25 degrees of flexion. Now anchor the slip of tendon of the abductor pollicis longus emerging at the dorsum of the lesser multangular while maintaining slight tension on the adjacent wrist extensors. Avoid excessive tension because this will place a stress on the base of the implant stem.

AFTERTREATMENT. The thumb is immobilized for 5 weeks in a well-padded reinforced dressing. Then the Kirschner wires are removed, and the metacarpophalangeal joint is protected with a splint for 4 more weeks while rehabilitation progresses.

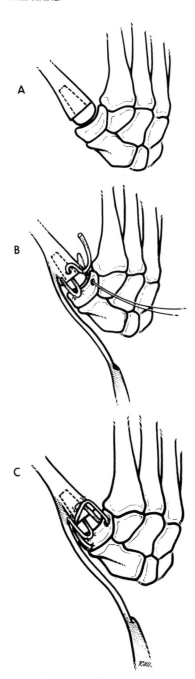

Fig. 72-19 Swanson et al. technique for convex condylar arthroplasty. (Redrawn from Swanson A, deGroot-Swanson G, and Watermeier JJ: J Hand Surg 6:125, 1981.)

Convex condylar implant arthroplasty

■ *TECHNIQUE (SWANSON ET AL.).* As in some of the previous techniques, approach the carpometacarpal joint through a palmar incision. Incise the capsule longitudinally on the radial side and resect enough of the base of the first metacarpal to allow 45 degrees of radial abduction of the bone. Ream the medullary canal of the metacarpal to receive the implant. Select the implant of appropriate size from the 11 sizes available. Align the bone, excise the ul-

nar distal projection of the trapezium, and with a burr make a slightly concave surface to receive the convex implant (Fig. 72-19, *A*). Now reconstruct the capsule and ligamentous structures with a slip of the abductor pollicis longus as described in the previous technique. As an alternative prepare an 8 cm slip of the abductor pollicis longus, preserving its insertion on the metacarpal, loop it into the medullary canal of the metacarpal, and pull it out through a hole drilled in the radiodorsal aspect of the bone (Fig. 72-19, *B*). Now pass the slip through a 3 mm hole drilled in the trapezium from inside out. Position the implant and hold the thumb in 45 degrees of abduction, tighten and interweave the slip of tendon, pass its distal end through or under the abductor pollicis longus insertion, and suture it to the radial capsular structures of the trapezium with a nonabsorbable suture (Fig. 72-19, *C*). If reduction of a severely displaced metacarpal causes a hyperextension deformity of the metacarpophalangeal joint of no more than 10 to 15 degrees, the joint may be fixed in proper position by a Kirschner wire passed through the joint. If the hyperextension is more than 20 degrees, the palmar aspect of the capsule should be fixed by a capsulodesis. Severe hyperextension and instability may require arthrodesis of the metacarpophalangeal joint. The care after surgery is similar to that described for the Swanson et al. Silastic implant at the carpometacarpal joint.

Millender et al. described a technique of arthroplasty using a Swanson T-shaped great toe Silastic prosthesis. In most instances this does not require resection of all of the greater multangular, thus preserving bone stock. In their series most patients also initially had instability and a hyperextension deformity at the metacarpophalangeal joint. This required arthrodesis of the joint is shown in Fig. 72-20. In rare instances the entire trapezium was excised.

Interpositional arthroplasty for rheumatoid carpometacarpal joint

■ *TECHNIQUE (MILLENDER ET AL.).* Make a dorsal zigzag incision over the proximal one third of the first metacarpal and extend it along the first wrist extensor compartment. Identify and free the radial artery from the underlying fascia and retract it for protection. When the joint is dislocated, the artery may be displaced deep to the metacarpal. Now incise the carpometacarpal joint vertically and release the capsule from the base of the metacarpal; carefully preserve the capsule for later closure. If the joint is loose, dislocate it completely so that the end of the metacarpal is exposed.

The palmar and ulnar surfaces of the trapezium may be eroded and may require resection or reshaping. Resect the metacarpal base perpendicular to its long axis. Shape the base to allow the insertion of a size 0 or 1 Swanson great toe prosthesis. Ream the medullary canal of the metacarpal to permit introduction of the prosthetic stem. Insert the stem and seat the base of the prosthesis on the flat surface of the reshaped trapezium. Insert a small Kirschner wire through the first metacarpal and into the carpus to ensure proper alignment. Then close the capsule and reinforce the closure with a section of the abductor pollicis longus if indicated. A secure closure is essential. Close the wound.

AFTERTREATMENT. The thumb is supported on a splint for 3 weeks. Then the Kirschner wire is removed, but splinting is continued for a total of 6 weeks, during which progressive motion exercises are begun.

Infection following insertion of Silastic thumb prosthesis. If a Silastic implant becomes infected, it should be removed. The wound is drained, and the thumb is then held in abduction and opposition in a cast or splint if necessary until the thumb is stable. Once the infection has cleared and the wound is healing, motion of the thumb can be started with what is a resection arthroplasty. In most instances the capsular scarring will stabilize the joint, and subluxation is unlikely if a night splint is used and motion is started gradually. We have salvaged several joints in this manner. However, several months may pass before maximum improvement is reached.

ARTHRODESIS OF THUMB JOINTS. Arthrodesis may be required for thumb joint deformities caused by rheumatoid arthritis or osteoarthritis. In patients with rheumatoid arthritis, soft bone, insufficient bone, and lax tissues allow easy positioning of the joints. The soft bone and small remaining bone may limit the choice of internal fixation to small Kirschner wires. In addition, insufficient bone may require bone grafting. If adequate bone is present, fixation may be obtained with combinations of Kirschner wires, plates and screws, and wire loops in a tension band configuration. The more stable and rigid the fixation, the shorter the time required for immobilization.

Interphalangeal arthrodesis

■ *TECHNIQUE.* Approach the interphalangeal joint through either a straight dorsal incision or a proximally based flap incision. Divide the extensor tendon and open the joint. Expose the articular surfaces by flexing the joint. Release the collateral ligaments and remove the articular surface and a small amount of subchondral bone from the distal and proximal phalanges. Position the interphalangeal joint in approximately 15 to 20 degrees of flexion and fix it with small Kirschner wires driven out through the distal phalanx distally and then proxi-

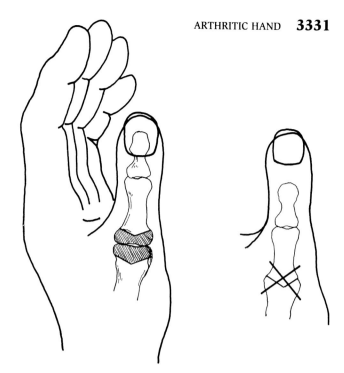

Fig. 72-20 Technique for arthrodesis of metacarpophalangeal joint of the thumb (see text).

mally into the proximal phalanx after the interphalangeal joint has been appropriately positioned. After the interphalangeal joint has been stabilized with the Kirschner wires, evaluate the thumb for appropriate position and length. If the thumb is shortened excessively, as may be seen in patients with arthritis mutilans, obtain a small corticocancellous iliac crest bone graft to restore length and transfix it with Kirschner wires.

Metacarpophalangeal joint

■ *TECHNIQUE.* If the metacarpophalangeal joint of the thumb is unstable but not subluxated, bone should be resected straight across the joint. Make a straight dorsal incision and cauterize the exposed vein. Then retract the extensor pollicis longus tendon to the ulnar side and the extensor pollicis brevis to the radial side, or detach it and suture it later to the capsule. With an osteotome, cut across the articular surface of the proximal phalanx in a straight line at 90 degrees to the long axis of the bone. After the articular surface is resected, place the phalanx at an angle of 15 degrees of flexion with the metacarpal. There is a tendency to osteotomize the distal metacarpal also at 90 degrees; rather, make the osteotomy so that the metacarpophalangeal joint is flexed 15 degrees. This requires removing more bone toward the palmar aspect. The two raw surfaces should fit flush. Remove any protruding small edges of bone to smooth the site of arthrodesis. Fix the arthrodesis with three Kirschner wires inserted longitudinally. Insert them first through the metacarpal and advance them through the phalanx. Be certain that the wires do not pierce the flexor tendon or the distal joint. Cut them off under the skin and approximate the tendons with a small absorbable suture. Finally close the wound and place the hand in a small splint to be replaced later by a cast if indicated.

When this joint is subluxated, shortening of the bone may be required. A chevron-shaped excision of bone that permits interlocking of the exposed surfaces may be used to accomplish shortening. Make a dorsal longitudinal incision over the joint and displace the extensor pollicis longus tendon to the ulnar side. On the proximal end of the proximal phalanx, shape a tongue of bone; on the distal end of the first metacarpal, create a V-shaped notch. These should fit like a tongue in a groove (see Fig. 72-20). Thus large surfaces of bone are put in contact, but the angle of fusion can be adjusted easily. Now fix the joint in the proper position by two Kirschner wires that are cut off flush with the bone. Pack small fragments of bone into any spaces about the joint margins. Close the wound and apply a volar plaster splint that includes the thumb but no other digits. In both of the techniques described here, be certain that the thumb is in appropriate pronation so that the pulp of the thumb can be placed against the other digits. Also, as already mentioned, if the first metacarpal is adducted, some of this adduction may be overcome by fusing the joint in slight abduction. This places the thumb in proper position without releasing soft tissues in the palm.

AFTERTREATMENT. At 10 to 14 days the splint and sutures are moved. The thumb is protected in a thumb spica short arm cast for another 4 weeks. T.. Kirschner wires are removed at about 6 weeks, and a splint is worn another 3 to 4 weeks. Active use of the thumb is gradually resumed, despite absence of roentgenographic evidence of fusion.

Carpometacarpal joint. Although arthroplasty of the thumb carpometacarpal joint has usually been advised instead of arthrodesis, arthrodesis usually is recommended for joints affected by osteoarthritis and in some patients when it is the only joint of the thumb affected by rheumatoid arthritis or when strong pinch is more important than motion. Arthrodesis of the carpometacarpal joint of the thumb may be indicated for posttraumatic arthritis after a malunited Bennett's fracture, unstable chronic subluxation of the joint, osteoarthritis, or rheumatoid arthritis. Arthrodesis can be expected to relieve pain and to provide a stable and strong joint at the expense of thumb mobility. It has traditionally been used for patients who require a strong, powerful, stable, and painless thumb. Although its most frequent application has been in younger patients, it may be useful for some

older patients. It also is useful in stabilizing the joint for congenital and paralytic deformities and in hands impaired by cerebral palsy. Techniques of carpometacarpal joint arthrodesis are described in Chapter 68.

DEFORMITIES OF WRIST
Synovitis of Wrist

Often the dorsum of the wrist is the location of the first painful swelling in rheumatoid arthritis. The tenosynovial swelling may contribute to de Quervain's disease, trigger finger, or carpal tunnel syndrome, whereas rheumatoid arthritis as the underlying cause may not be suspected. The swelling may begin as a small soft mass at the distal end of the ulna; then roentgenograms may reveal a small pit at the base of the ulnar styloid as the first roentgenographic evidence of the disease. The synovitis may spread and cause a massive swelling shaped like an hourglass, its middle being constricted by the dorsal carpal ligament. Eventually destruction of joints may contribute to dorsal subluxation of the distal ulna, ulnar shifting of the carpal bones, radial angulation of the metacarpals, and ulnar deviation of the fingers. Finally, the wrist may subluxate volarly. Tendons, especially those of the three ulnar finger extensors, may rupture (p. 3316).

When the synovitis is only moderate and when changes in the bones are absent but pain is significant, dorsal synovectomy of the wrist seems to be of lasting benefit. Persistent swelling at the dorsum of the wrist that continues for 6 weeks or longer despite adequate medical treatment may be an indication for a dorsal synovectomy. This may be considered a prophylactic measure to avoid rupture of the extensor tendons. Their rupture is quite disabling, and function can never be restored completely.

Any tendons ruptured at the level of the wrist may be repaired at the time of synovectomy. Options include side-to-side suture anastomosis, free tendon graft, and tendon transfers to bridge a defect in a tendon. Often when synovitis involves both the wrist and the metacarpophalangeal joints, synovectomy may be done at both levels through carefully planned incisions during the same operation, usually only on one limb at a time.

On the volar aspect of the wrist, even slight hypertrophy of the synovium undetectable clinically may cause compression of the median nerve and thus classic symptoms of carpal tunnel syndrome (Chapter 76). Synovitis is considered one of the most frequent causes of the syndrome. Compression of the nerve in rheumatoid arthritis should be relieved surgically when conservative treatment with splinting and steroid injections has been unsuccessful. When hypertrophy of the tenosynovium on the volar aspect of the wrist is obvious clinically, with or without symptoms of compression of the median nerve, a palmar (flexor) tenosynovectomy may be useful in relieving pain and in preventing rupture of tendons. The level of the deep transverse carpal ligament is a frequent site of rupture of flexor tendons. Erosion of the distal end of the radius or carpal scaphoid into the floor of the carpal tunnel may cause fraying and eventual rupture of several profundus tendons. More commonly the flexor pollicis longus or index profundus is involved. Synovitis within the carpal articulations themselves, as well as in the surrounding tendon sheaths, is common in rheumatoid arthritis.

The various options for surgical treatment depend on the pathology involved and the severity of the disease. As already mentioned, synovectomy of the dorsal compartment is a worthwhile procedure when indicated. Capsuloligamentous repairs may be required to stabilize joints. Repair of tendons on the extensor surface is often necessary but is best done by anastomosis to an adjoining tendon rather than by segmental grafting. Flexor tendon rupture at the wrist level is best repaired either by suture to adjoining tendons or by segmental grafts; however, in the thumb an arthrodesis of the distal joint is the procedure of choice. Tendon transfer or relocation also may be needed to prevent deformities.

Should bony procedures on the wrist be necessary bilaterally, arthroplasty should be strongly considered. In some cases arthroplasty may be indicated initially because eventual collapse of the opposite wrist may require reconstruction. Several types of arthroplasties are available. Resection arthroplasty does not provide stability. Albright and Chase resected the distal radius to form a shelf in cases of palmar dislocation. This was an effort to maintain some stability, increase motion, and relieve pain without the insertion of foreign material. Implant arthroplasties include those made of silicone (Swanson) and those of plastic and metal. Silicone prostheses designed by Swanson have gained widespread popularity. This procedure does not require fixation by polymethylmethacrylate, entails minimal bone resection, and usually is an easily salvaged procedure. It is the choice of many surgeons, despite an 8% to 10% prosthetic fracture rate.

DORSAL SYNOVECTOMY

■ *TECHNIQUE.* Make a dorsal longitudinal incision curved only slightly ulnarward and long enough to expose both the distal ulna and the dorsal carpal ligament; avoid curving it sharply, otherwise the circulation in a flap may be impaired. Preserve the larger veins, the dorsal branch of the ulnar nerve, and the superficial radial nerve. Detach from the radial side and reflect as a sheet the dorsal carpal ligament. Now carefully excise the synovium from around the finger and radial wrist extensor tendons. Excise any hypertrophied synovium from the distal ulna and the distal radioulnar joint. If the attachments of the distal ulna to the radius and carpus seem to be intact, do not disturb them. But if the distal ulna is

found subluxated, excise about 1 cm of it, smooth off the remaining end, and cover the end with periosteum and surrounding soft tissues.

Incise the sheath of the extensor carpi ulnaris tendon near its attachment to the base of the fifth metacarpal. If the sheath is disintegrated and the tendon is dislocated palmarward, it then has become a flexor causing palmar flexion and ulnar deviation of the wrist. In this case, remove the tendon from the sheath as needed and return it to the dorsum of the wrist. Create a pulley with a strip of the dorsal retinaculum to keep it in position. If before surgery the patient could not actively deviate and dorsiflex the wrist from a position of radial deviation, it may be necessary to transfer the insertion of the extensor carpi radialis longus tendon to the extensor carpi ulnaris tendon to correct radial deviation. While an assistant applies traction to the hand, remove the synovium from among the carpal bones. Now pass the dorsal carpal ligament deep to the long extensor tendons, and suture its detached end in place. Elevate the hand, control bleeding by manual pressure, and release the tourniquet. Close the skin with interrupted sutures and leave a rubber drain in the wound. Apply a compression dressing and then a volar plaster splint to hold the wrist in neutral position.

AFTERTREATMENT. Active motion of the finger joints is encouraged early. The wound is periodically inspected, and any hematoma beneath the skin is evacuated. At 10 to 14 days the sutures are removed, and at 3 weeks the splint.

VOLAR SYNOVECTOMY

■ *TECHNIQUE.* Make a volar longitudinal incision beginning distally at the middle of the palm and proceeding proximally to the wrist parallel to the thenar crease, then curving slightly radialward and then slightly ulnarward, and ending about 7.5 cm proximal to the wrist (Chapter 61). Open the deep fascia proximally and identify the median nerve. Stay on the ulnar side of this nerve and protect its recurrent branch and, if identified, its palmar branch. Divide the deep transverse carpal ligament to expose the flexor tendons; its distal border is more distal in the palm than is usually realized. Beginning proximally and proceeding distally and keeping constantly in mind the location of the median nerve, dissect the synovium from each flexor tendon. Do not close the deep transverse carpal ligament. Release the tourniquet, obtain hemostasis, insert a drain, and close the wound. Apply a compression dressing and a volar plaster splint from the proximal forearm to the distal palmar crease. Keep the wrist extended for a minimum of 3 weeks.

AFTERTREATMENT. The aftertreatment is the same as for dorsal synovectomy (see above).

Arthrodesis of Wrist Versus Arthroplasty

Whether arthrodesis or arthroplasty of the wrist is best in rheumatoid arthritis is controversial. Obviously retention of wrist motion is desirable. However, wrist arthroplasty usually has a higher percentage of late complications than does arthrodesis. Arthrodesis provides a painless and stable wrist once fusion has taken place. Most consider it the procedure of choice for marked flexion deformity of the wrist and fingers, for carpal dislocation, or for a painful wrist associated with multiple ruptures of tendons. This is especially true for ruptures of the extensor carpi radialis longus and brevis, since these muscles are necessary for wrist balance. Also, when wrist deformities are bilateral and require major procedures on both sides, one wrist may be arthrodesed to provide stability, especially when the use of crutches may be necessary; then an arthroplasty may be performed on the other wrist. Arthrodesis will reliably relieve pain, correct deformity, and maintain stability.

The exact position in which to fuse for maximum function is also controversial. Haddad and Riordan prefer 10 degrees of dorsiflexion, whereas Boyes prefers 30 degrees. Clayton and Ferlic prefer the neutral position with the alignment of the axis of the third metacarpal coaxial with the axis of the radius in the lateral roentgenographic projection, especially if bilateral wrist fusions are to be carried out. In bilateral fusions some prefer to place one wrist in dorsiflexion and the other in palmar flexion. Usually, both wrists should not be fused in dorsiflexion because this will make it impossible for the patient to take care of personal toilet needs. Several satisfactory techniques are available for arthrodesis. Most require some type of internal fixation, usually by a medullary pin. Mannerfelt and Malmsten have described the use of a Rush pin inserted between the second and third metacarpal shafts, through the carpus, and then through the medullary canal of the radius, with a supplementary staple to prevent rotation. Clayton and Ferlic inserted a medullary Steinmann pin and bone grafted the dorsum of the wrist. Millender and Nalebuff described a method of arthrodesing the wrist using medullary fixation with a Steinmann pin down the shaft of the third metacarpal with additional fixation by a staple or oblique pin. This permits operations to be done on the metacarpophalangeal joints at the same time. Because all of the procedures for rheumatoid wrist fusions are similar, the procedure of Millender and Nalebuff is described here.

ARTHRODESIS

■ *TECHNIQUE (MILLENDER AND NALEBUFF).* Make a dorsal, straight longitudinal incision and protect the extensor tendons of the digits and wrist. Curet the cartilage and sclerotic bone from the carpus and radius down to cancellous bone. Varying amounts of bone may require resection for reduction of a dislocated wrist. Drill a Steinmann pin of appropriate size into the carpus and out distally between the second and third metacarpals. Then drill it proximally into the medullary canal of the radius and cut off its end beneath the skin. Or as an alternative method resect the head of the third metacarpal for later insertion of a joint prosthesis. Insert the Steinmann pin through the medullary canal of the third metacarpal, then through the carpus, and finally into the radius, leaving sufficient room distally in the metacarpal to allow insertion of the proximal stem of a metacarpophalangeal prosthesis. This places the wrist in neutral position. To avoid rotational deformities, drive a staple across the radiocarpal joint or insert an oblique Kirschner wire. Insert a small plug of polymethylmethacrylate into the metacarpal shaft to prevent the Steinmann pin from shifting and protruding, or, if desired, pack bone from the resected metacarpal head around the pin to accomplish the same purpose. Close the wound loosely to permit ample drainage. Now proceed with any other operations necessary on the digits.

AFTERTREATMENT. At least for the first 2 weeks, a splint is preferred to avoid complications from swelling. The wrist is protected with a cast or splint until bony union has occurred. The extent and type of splinting depends on the activities and needs of the patient.

ARTHROPLASTY. Because patients with juvenile rheumatoid arthritis have such small bones, it is usually better to insert a Swanson silicone prosthesis. But silicone prostheses alone cannot be depended on to stabilize the wrist. The soft tissues must be released adequately, the bones must be aligned correctly, and the musculotendinous units must be balanced if possible to prevent recurrence of deformity.

Silicone wrist arthroplasty

■ *TECHNIQUE (SWANSON).* Make a slightly curved dorsal longitudinal incision, preserving the veins and sensory nerves. Avoid the S-shaped incision because it may increase the risk of skin necrosis. Split the dorsal retinaculum over the extensor digitorum tendons and reflect it to the radial side; protect it for later use to reinforce the capsule and provide a floor for the extensor tendons. Detach the dorsal capsule from the radius and reflect it distally as a widely based flap. Detach the radial collateral ligament from the radius and carefully protect the abductor pollicis longus and extensor pollicis brevis tendons. Now hyperflex the radiocarpal joint to expose the distal radius. Remove the lunate, the proximal half of the scaphoid, and the radial side of the triquetrum. Resect the radial styloid in line with the distal articular surface of the radius at 90 degrees to the long axis of the radius. Preserve as much cortical bone as possible to provide support. When the joint is dislocated, resect more of the radius as necessary. Align the wrist and prepare the capitate and the base of the third metacarpal to receive the prosthesis. To ensure proper placement of the reamer in the medullary canal of the third metacarpal, insert a Kirschner wire and check its position by roentgenograms. Then ream with an awl or if necessary with a power reamer. Do not perforate the metacarpal shaft. The size of the third metacarpal shaft will determine the size of the prosthesis. Use this shaft for size and then ream the radius to fit the opposite stem of the prosthesis. Smooth the base of the capitate and radius to eliminate any sharp bony edges that could cause a prosthetic fracture. Use metal sleeve "grommets" as needed. Now seat the prosthesis against the radius and capitate so that there is no tendency for buckling. Align the hand on the wrist, avoiding ulnar deviation or flexion. See that passive flexion and extension of about 30 degrees each are possible without blockage. Strip the volar capsule if it is too tight. Next resect the distal ulna. Close the capsule with sutures passed through holes drilled in the dorsal cortex of the distal radius. Reattach the collateral ligament of the radius and realign the dorsal retinaculum under the finger and wrist extensors. Relocate the extensor carpi ulnaris tendon dorsally to prevent it from functioning as a wrist flexor if it has shifted palmarward; pass it through a pulley created from a segment of the dorsal retinaculum if necessary. Repair any extensor tendons as indicated and close the wound loosely. Insert a suction drain and apply a bulky dressing and a plaster splint.

AFTERTREATMENT. The splint is worn for 5 to 6 weeks. At 3 weeks limited wrist motion is started, and at 4 weeks active motion is begun. A total motion of 60 degrees is considered satisfactory, and 95% of patients obtain relief from pain.

Total Joint Arthroplasty

Although total joint arthroplasty has the advantages of preserving motion, providing a fixed fulcrum, and obtaining stable fixation, problems such as distal component loosening compromise the results in as many as 50% of patients. Constrained designs, such as the Meuli and Volz wrists, allow excessive forces to be transmitted to the prosthesis, resulting in displacement of the distal portion of the prosthesis and leading to median nerve compression and flexor tendon abrasion. Beckenbaugh and Linscheid reported satisfactory preliminary results with a semi-constrained "biaxial" wrist implant. It is porous-coated to either improve cement fixation or to eliminate the need for cement. The reader is referred to the bibliography and current literature for information on the evolution of total wrist arthroplasty.

REFERENCES

Adams BD, Blair WF, and Shurr DG: Schultz metacarpophalangeal arthroplasty: a long-term follow-up study, J Hand Surg 15A:641, 1990.

Albright JA and Chase RA: Palmar-shelf arthroplasty of the wrist in rheumatoid arthritis: a report of nine cases, J Bone Joint Surg 52-A:896, 1970.

Amadio PD, Millender LH, and Smith RJ: Silicone spacer or tendon spacer for trapezium resection arthroplasty: comparison of results, J Hand Surg 7:237, 1982.

Aptekar RG and Duff IF: Metacarpophalangeal joint surgery in rheumatoid arthritis: long-term results, Clin Orthop 83:123, 1972.

Aptekar RG, Davie JM and Cattell, HS: Foreign body reaction to silicone rubber: complication of a finger joint implant, Clin Orthop 98:231, 1974.

Aro H, Ekfors T, Hakkarainen S, and Aho AJ: Osteolytinen vierasesinereaktio Silastic-proteesikomplikaationa ranteesa, Suomen Kirugiyhd 3:66, 1982.

Ashworth CA, Blatt G, Chuinard RG, and Stark H: Silicone rubber interposition arthroplasty, J Hand Surg 2:345, 1977.

Ayres JR, Goldstrohm GL, Miller GJ, and Dell PC: Proximal interphalangeal joint arthrodesis with the Herbert screw, J Hand Surg 13A:600, 1988.

Beckenbaugh RD: Total joint arthroplasty—the wrist, Mayo Clin Proc 54:513, 1979.

Beckenbaugh RD and Linscheid RL: Total wrist arthroplasty: a preliminary report, J Hand Surg 2:337, 1977.

Beckenbaugh RD and Linscheid RL: Arthroplasty in the hand and wrist In Green DP, editor: Operative hand surgery, ed 2, New York, 1988, Churchill Livingstone.

Belsky MR, Feldon P, Millender LH, et al: Hand involvement in psoriatic arthritis, J Hand Surg 7:203, 1982.

Berger RA, Blair WF, and Andrews JG: Resultant forces and angles of twist about the wrist after ECRL to ECU tendon transfer, J Orthop Res 6:443, 1988.

Bigelow DR: A surgical solution to the problem of swan-neck deformity of rheumatoid arthritis, Clin Orthop 123:89, 1977.

Black MR, Boswick JA Jr, and Wiedel J: Dislocation of the wrist in rheumatoid arthritis: the relationship to distal ulna resection, Clin Orthop 124:184, 1977.

Boland DM and Craig EV: Rheumatoid disease, Hand Clin 5:359, 1989

Bora FW, Osterman AL, Thomas VJ, et al: The treatment of ruptures of multiple extensor tendons at wrist level by a free tendon graft in the rheumatoid patient, J Hand Surg 12A:1038, 1987.

Boulas HJ and Milek MA: Ulnar shortening for tears of the triangular fibrocartilaginous complex, J Hand Surg 15A:415, 1990.

Bowers WH: Distal radioulnar joint arthroplasty: the hemiresection interposition technique, J Hand Surg 10A:169, 1985.

Boyce T et al: Clinical and experimental studies on the effect of extensor carpi radialis longus transfer in the rheumatoid hand, J Hand Surg 3:390, 1978.

Boyes JH: Bunnell's surgery of the hand, Philadelphia, 1970, JB Lippincott Co.

Brannon EW and Klein G: Experiences with a finger-joint prosthesis, J Bone Joint Surg 41-A:87, 1959.

Braun RM: Total joint replacement at the base of the thumb: preliminary report, J Hand Surg 7:245, 1982.

Braun RM and Chandler J: Quantitative results following implant arthroplasty of the proximal finger joints in the arthritic hand, Clin Orthop 83:135, 1972.

Brewerton DA: Hand deformities in rheumatoid disease, Ann Rheum Dis 16:183, 1957.

Brown FE and Brown M-L: Long-term results after tenosynovectomy to treat the rheumatoid hand, J Hand Surg 13A:704, 1988.

Brumfield RH Jr, Conaty JP, and Mayes JD: Surgery of the wrist in rheumatoid arthritis, Clin Orthop 142:159, 1979.

Brunelli G, Monini L, and Brunelli F: Stabilization of the trapezio-metacarpal joint, J Hand Surg 14-B:209, 1989.

Buch VI: Clinical and functional assessment of the hand after metacarpophalangeal capsulotomy, Plast Reconstr Surg 53:452, 1974.

Bunnell S: Surgery of the rheumatic hand, J Bone Joint Surg 37-A:759, 1955.

Burton RI: Basal joint arthrosis of the thumb, Orthop Clin North Am 4:331, 1973.

Burton RI and Pelligrini VD Jr: Surgical management of basal joint arthritis of the thumb. II. Ligament reconstruction with tendon interposition arthroplasty.

Campbell RD Jr and Straub LR: Surgical considerations for rheumatoid disease in the forearm and wrist, Am J Surg 109:361, 1965.

Carroll RE: Arthrodesis of the carpometacarpal joint of the thumb: a review of patients with a long postoperative period, Clin Orthop 220:106, 1987.

Carroll RE and Dick HM: Arthrodesis of the wrist for rheumatoid arthritis, J Bone Joint Surg 53-A:1365, 1971.

Chamay A and Gabbiani G: Digital contracture deformity after implantation of a silicone prosthesis: light and electron microscopic study, J Hand Surg 3:266, 1978.

Clawson MC and Stern PJ: The distal radioulnar joint complex in rheumatoid arthritis: an overview, Hand Clin 7:373, 1991.

Clayton ML: Surgery of the thumb in rheumatoid arthritis, J Bone Joint Surg 44-A:1376, 1962.

Clayton ML: Surgery of the rheumatoid hand, Clin Orthop 36:47, 1964.

Clayton ML: Surgical treatment at the wrist in rheumatoid arthritis: a review of thirty-seven patients, J Bone Joint Surg 47-A:741, 1965.

Clayton ML and Ferlic DC: Tendon transfer for radial rotation of the wrist in rheumatoid arthritis, Clin Orthop 100:176, 1974.

Clayton ML and Ferlic DC: The wrist in rheumatoid arthritis, Clin Orthop 106:192, 1975.

Comstock CP Louis DS, and Eckenrode JF: Silicone wrist implant: long-term follow-up study, J Hand Surg 13A:201, 1988.

Cooney WP III, Beckenbaugh RD, and Linscheid RL: Total wrist arthroplasty: problems with implant failure, Clin Orthop 187:121, 1984.

Cooney WP, Linscheid RL, and Askew LJ: Total arthroplasty of the thumb trapeziometacarpal joint, Clin Orthop 220:35, 1987. Crawford GP: Ligament augmentation with replacement arthroplasty of the CMC joint, Hand 12:91, 1980.

Cregan JCF: Indications for surgical intervention in rheumatoid arthritis of the wrist and hand, Ann Rheum Dis 18:29, 1959.

Crosby EB, Linscheid RL, and Dobyns JH: Scaphotrapezial trapezoidal arthrosis, J Hand Surg 3:223, 1978.

Culver JE and Fleegler EJ: Osteoarthritis of the distal interphalangeal joint, Hand Clin 3:385, 1987.

Dell PC: Compression of the ulnar nerve at the wrist secondary to a rheumatoid synovial cyst: case report and review of the literature, J Hand Surg 4:468, 1979.

Dell PC and Muniz RB: Interposition arthroplasty of the trapeziometacarpal joint for osteoarthritis, Clin Orthop 220:27, 1987.

Dell PC, Brushart TM, and Smith RJ: Treatment of trapeziometacarpal arthritis: results of resection arthroplasty, J Hand Surg 3:243, 1978.

Devas M and Shah V: Link arthroplasty of the metacarpophalangeal joints: a preliminary report of a new method J Bone Joint Surg 57-B:72, 1975.

Digby JM: Malignant lymphoma with intranodal silicone rubber particles following metacarpophalangeal joint replacements, Hand 14:326, 1982.

Dobyns JH and Linscheid RL: Rheumatoid hand repairs, Orthop Clin North Am 3:629, 1971.

Eaton RG: Replacement of the trapezium, J Bone Joint Surg 61-A:76, 1979.

Eaton RG, Glickel S, and Littler J: Tendon interposition arthroplasty for degenerative arthritis of the trapeziometacarpal joint of the thumb, J Hand Surg 10-A:645, 1985.

Eaton RG and Littler JW: Ligament reconstruction for the painful thumb carpometacarpal joint, J Bone Joint Surg 55-A:1665, 1973.

Ehrlich GE et al: Pathogenesis of rupture of extensor tendons at the wrist in rheumatoid arthritis, Arthritis Rheum 2:332, 1959.

Ellison MR, Kelly KJ, and Flatt AE: The results of surgical synovectomy of the digital joints in rheumatoid disease, J Bone Joint Surg 53-A:1041, 1971.

Ellison MR, Flatt AE, and Kelly KJ: Ulnar drift of the fingers in rheumatoid disease: treatment by crossed intrinsic tendon transfer, J Bone Joint Surg 53-A:1061, 1971.

Engel J, Tsur H, and Farin I: A comparison between K-wire and compression screw fixation after arthrodesis of the distal interphalangeal joint, Plast Reconstr Surg 60:611, 1977.

Ertel AN: Flexor tendon ruptures in rheumatoid arthritis, Hand Clin 5:177, 1989.

Ertel AN, Millender LH, Nalebuff E, et al: Flexor tendon ruptures in patients with rheumatoid arthritis, J Hand Surg 13A:860, 1988.

Feldon P and Belsky MR: Degenerative diseases of the metacarpophalangeal joints, Hand Clin 3:429, 1987.

Ferlic DC: Implant arthroplasty of the rheumatoid wrist, Hand Clin 3:169, 1987.

Ferlic DC: Boutonniere deformities in rheumatoid arthritis, Hand Clin 5:215, 1989.

Ferlic DC, Busbee GA, and Clayton ML: Degenerative arthritis of the carpometacarpal joint of the thumb: a clinical follow-up of eleven Niebauer prostheses, J Hand Surg 2:212, 1977.

Ferlic DC and Clayton ML: Flexor tenosynovectomy in the rheumatoid finger, J Hand Surg 3:364, 1978.

Ferlic DC, Clayton ML, and Holloway M: Complications of silicone implant surgery in the metacarpophalangeal joint, J Bone Joint Surg 57-A:991, 1975.

Ferlic DC, Smyth CJ, and Clayton ML: Medical considerations and management of rheumatoid arthritis, J Hand Surg 8:662, 1983.

Figgie MP, Inglis AE, Sobel M, et al: Metacarpal-phalangeal joint arthroplasty of the rheumatoid thumb, J Hand Surg 15A:210, 1990.

Figgie HE III, Inglis AE, Straub LR, and Ranawat CS: A critical analysis of alignment factors influencing functional results following trispherical total wrist arthroplasty, J Arthroplasty 1:149, 1986.

Figgie HE III, Ranawat CS, Inglis AE, et al: Preliminary results of total wrist arthroplasty in rheumatoid arthritis using the trispherical total wrist arthroplasty, J Arthroplasty 3:9, 1988.

Fitzgerald JP, Peimer CA, and Smith RJ: Distraction resection arthroplasty of the wrist, J Hand Surg 14A:774, 1989.

Flatt AE: Surgical rehabilitation of the arthritic hand, Arthritis Rheum 2:278, 1959.

Flatt AE: Restoration of rheumatoid finger joint function: interim report on trial of prosthetic replacement, J Bone Joint Surg 43-A:753, 1961.

Flatt AE: Salvage of the rheumatoid hand, Clin Orthop 23:207, 1962.

Flatt AE: Restoration of rheumatoid finger joint function, J Bone Joint Surg 45-A:1101, 1963.

Flatt AE: Some pathomechanics of ulnar drift, Plast Reconstr Surg 37:295, 1966.

Flatt AE: The care of the rheumatoid hand, ed 3, St Louis, 1974, Mosby–Year Book, Inc.

Flatt AE and Ellison MR: Restoration of rheumatoid finger joint function III A follow-up note after fourteen years of experience with a metallic hinge prosthesis, J Bone Joint Surg 54-A:1317, 1972.

Folmar RC, Nelson CL, and Phalen GS: Ruptures of the flexor tendons in hands of non-rheumatoid patients, J Bone Joint Surg 54-A:579, 1972.

Freiberg RA and Weinstein A: The scallop sign and spontaneous rupture of finger extensor tendons in rheumatoid arthritis, Clin Orthop 83:128, 1972.

Froimson AI: Hand reconstruction in arthritis mutilans: a case report, J Bone Joint Surg 53-A:1377, 1971.

Gervis W: Excision of the trapezium for osteoarthritis of the trapeziometacarpal joint, J Boint Joint Surg 31-B:537, 1949.

Gervis W: A review of excision of the trapezium for osteoarthritis of the trapeziometacarpal joint after twenty-five years, J Bone Joint Surg 55-B:56, 1973.

Girzadas DV and Clayton ML: Limitations of the use of metallic prosthesis in the rheumatoid hand, Clin Orthop 67:127, 1969.

Goldner JL: Tendon transfers in rheumatoid arthritis, Orthop Clin North Am 2:425, 1974.

Goldner JL and Clippinger FW: Excision of the greater multangular bone as an adjunct to mobilization of the thumb, J Bone Joint Surg 41-A:609, 1959.

Goldner JL, Gould JS, Urbaniak JR, and McCollum DE: Metacarpophalangeal joint arthroplasty with silicone-Dacron prostheses (Niebauer type): six and a half years' experience, J Hand Surg 2:200, 1977.

Goodman MJ, Millender LH, Nalebuff EA, and Phillips CA: Arthroplasty of the rheumatoid wrist with silicone rubber: an early evaluation, J Hand Surg 5:114, 1980.

Gordon M and Bullough PG: Synovial and osseous inflammation in failed silicone rubber prostheses, J Bone Joint Surg 64-A:574, 1982.

Granberry WM and Mangum GL: The hand in the child with juvenile rheumatoid arthritis, J Hand Surg 5:105, 1980.

Granowitz S and Vainio K: Proximal interphalangeal joint arthrodesis in rheumatoid arthritis: a follow-up study of 122 operations, Acta Orthop Scand 37:301, 1965-1966.

Green DP: Pisotriquetral arthritis: a case report, J Hand Surg 4:465, 1979.

Haddad RJ and Riordan DC: Arthrodesis of the wrist: a surgical technique, J Bone Joint Surg 49-A:950, 1967.

Haffajee D: Endoprosthetic replacement of the trapezium for arthrosis in the carpometacarpal joint of the thumb, J Hand Surg 2:141, 1977.

Hagan HJ and Hastings H II: Fusion of the thumb metacarpophalangeal joint to treat posttraumatic arthritis, J Hand Surg 13A:750, 1988.

Hakstian RW and Tubiana R: Ulnar deviation of the fingers: the role of joint structure and function, J Bone Joint Surg 49-A:299, 1967.

Harris C Jr and Riordan DC: Intrinsic contracture in the hand and its surgical treatment, J Bone Joint Surg 36-A:10, 1954.

Harrison SH: The importance of middle or long finger realignment in ulnar drift, J Hand Surg 1:87, 1976.

Hay EL, Bomberg BC, Burke C, and Misenheimer C: Long-term results of silicone trapezial implant arthroplasty, J Arthroplasty 3:215, 1988.

Henderson ED and Lipscomb PR: Surgical treatment of rheumatoid hand, JAMA 175:431, 1961.

Herndon JH: Trapeziometacarpal arthroplasty: a clinical review, Clin Orthop 220:99, 1987.

Howard LD Jr: Surgical treatment of rheumatic tenosynovitis, Am J Surg 89:1163, 1955.

Inglis AE: Rheumatoid arthritis in the hand, Am J Surg 109:368, 1965.

Inglis AE, Hamlin C, Sengelmann RP, and Straub LR: Reconstruction of the metacarpophalangeal joint of the thumb in rheumatoid arthritis, J Bone Joint Surg 54-A:704, 1972.

Jackson IT, Milward TM, Lee P, and Webb J: Ulnar head resection in rheumatoid arthritis, Hand 6:172, 1974.

Jennings CD and Livingstone DP: Convex condylar arthroplasty of the basal joint of the thumb: failure under load, J Hand Surg 15A:573, 1990.

Jensen JS: Operative treatment of chronic subluxation of the first carpometacarpal joint, Hand 7:269, 1975.

Jones NF, Imbriglia JE, Steen VD, and Medsger TA: Surgery for scleroderma of the hand, J Hand Surg 12A:391, 1987.

Kauer JMG: Functional anatomy of the carpometacarpal joint of the thumb, Clin Orthop 220:7, 1987.

Kessler FB, Hemsy CA, Berkeley ME, et al: Obliteration of traumatically induced articular surface defects using a porous implant, J Hand Surg 5:328, 1980.

Kessler I: A new silicone implant for replacement of destroyed metacarpal heads, Hand 6:308, 1974.

Kessler I and Axter A: Arthroplasty of the first carpometacarpal joint with a silicone implant, Plast Reconstr Surg 47:252, 1971.

Kessler I and Vainio K: Posterior (dorsal) synovectomy for rheumatoid involvement of the hand and wrist: a follow-up study of sixty-six procedures, J Bone Joint Surg 48-A:1085, 1966.

Kircher T: Silicone lymphadenopathy: a complication of silicone elastomer finger joint prostheses, Hum Pathol 11:240, 1980.

Kleinert HE and Frykman G: The wrist and thumb in rheumatoid arthritis, Orthop Clin North Am 4:1085, 1973.

Kowalski MF and Manske PR: Arthrodesis of digital joints in children, J Hand Surg 13A:874, 1988.

Kulick RG et al: Long-term results of dorsal stabilization in the rheumatoid wrist, J Hand Surg 6:272, 1981.

Laine VAI, Sairanen E, and Vainio K: Finger deformities caused by rheumatoid arthritis, J Bone Joint Surg 39-A:527, 1957.

Lamberta FJ, Ferlic DD, and Clayton ML: Volz total wrist arthroplasty in rheumatoid arthritis: a preliminary report, J Hand Surg 5:245, 1980.

Lane LB and Eaton RG: Ligament reconstruction for the painful "prearthritic" thumb carpometacarpal joint, Clin Orthop 220:52, 1987.

Larmon WA: Surgical management of tophaceous gout, Clin Orthop 71:56, 1970.

Leslie BM: Rheumatoid extensor tendon ruptures, Hand Clin 5:191, 1989.

Linscheid RL: Surgery for rheumatoid arthritis: timing and techniques: the upper extremity, J Bone Joint Surg 50-A:605, 1968.

Linscheid RL and Dobyns JH: Rheumatoid arthritis of the wrist, Orthop Clin North Am 3:649, 1971.

Lipscomb PR: Surgery of the arthritic hand, Sterling Bunnell Memorial Lecture, Mayo Clin Proc 40:132, 1965.

Lipscomb PR: Synovectomy of the wrist for rheumatoid arthritis, JAMA 194:655, 1965.

Lipscomb PR: Synovectomy of the distal two joints of the thumb and fingers in rheumatoid arthritis, J Bone Joint Surg 49-A:1135, 1967.

Long C and Brown ME: Electromyographic kinesiology of the hand: muscles moving the long finger, J Bone Joint Surg 46-A:1683, 1964.

Lucht U, Vang PS, and Munck J: Soft tissue interposition arthroplasty for osteoarthritis of the CMC joint of the thumb, Acta Orthop Scand 51:767, 1980.

Lynn MD and Lee J: Periarticular tenosynovial chondrometaplasia: report of a case at the wrist, J Bone Joint Surg 54-A:650, 1972.

Madden JW, DeVore G, and Arem AJ: A rational postoperative management program for metacarpophalangeal joint implant arthroplasty, J Hand Surg 2:358, 1977.

Mannerfelt L: On surgery of the rheumatoid hand: consensus and controversy (editorial) J Hand Surg 14B:259, 1989.

Mannerfelt L and Andersson K: Silastic arthroplasty of the metacarpophalangeal joints in rheumatoid arthritis: long-term results, J Bone Joint Surg 57-A:484, 1975.

Mannerfelt L and Malmsten M: Arthrodesis of the wrist in rheumatoid arthritis: a technique without external fixation, Scand J Plast Reconstr Surg 5:124, 1971.

Marmor L: The role of hand surgery in rheumatoid arthritis, Surg Gynecol Obstet 116:335, 1963.

Marmor L: Surgical treatment for arthritic deformities of the hands, Clin Orthop 39:171, 1965.

McFarland GB Jr: Early experience with the silicone rubber prosthesis (Swanson) in the reconstructive surgery of the rheumatoid hand, South Med J 65:1113, 1972.

McMaster M: The natural history of the rheumatoid metacarpophalangeal joint, J Bone Joint Surg 54-B:687, 1972.

Medl WT: Tendonitis, tenosynovitis, "trigger finger," and Quervain's disease, Orthop Clin North Am 1:375, 1970.

Mehiman CT, Zachary SV, and Barre PS: Total wrist arthroplasty in the rheumatoid patient: a clinical review, Contemp Orthop 17:39, 1988.

Melone CP Jr and Taras JS: Distal ulna resection, extensor carpi ulnaris tenodesis, and dorsal synovectomy for the rheumatoid wrist, Hand Clin 7:335, 1991.

Melone CP Jr, Beavers B, and Isani A: The basal joint pain syndrome, Clin Orthop 220:58, 1987.

Menkes CJ, Tubiana R, Galmiche B, and Delbarre F: Intra-articular injection of radioisotopic beta emitters: application to the treatment of the rheumatoid hand, Orthop Clin North Am 4:1113, 1973.

Menon, J Schoene HR, and Hohl JC: Trapeziometacarpal arthritis: results of tendon interpositional arthroplasty, J Hand Surg 6:442, 1981.

Meuli HC: Arthroplasty of the wrist, Clin Orthop 149:118, 1980.

Meuli H Ch: Meuli total wrist arthroplasty, Clin Orthop 187:107, 1984.

Mikkelsen OA: Arthrodesis of the wrist joint in rheumatoid arthritis, Hand 12:149, 1980.

Milford LW: Some thoughts on the use of finger implant arthroplasty, Orthop Rev 4:11, 1975.

Millender LH and Nalebuff EA: Arthrodesis of the rheumatoid wrist: functional evaluation of a modified technique Orthop Rev 1:13, 1972.

Millender LH and Nalebuff EA: Metacarpophalangeal joint arthroplasty utilizing the silicone rubber prosthesis, Orthop Clin North Am 4:349, 1973.

Millender LH and Nalebuff EA: Evaluation and treatment of early rheumatoid hand involvement, Orthop Clin North Am 6:697, 1975.

Millender LH and Nalebuff EA: Preventive surgery: tenosynovectomy and synovectomy, Orthop Clin North Am 6:765, 1975.

Millender LH and Nalebuff EA: Reconstructive surgery in the rheumatoid hand, Orthop Clin North Am 6:709, 1975.

Millender LH, Nalebuff EA, Amadio P, and Philips C: Interpositional arthroplasty for rheumatoid carpometacarpal joint disease, J Hand Surg 3:533, 1978.

Millender LH et al: Posterior interosseous-nerve syndrome secondary to rheumatoid synovitis, J Bone Joint Surg 55-A:753, 1973.

Millender LH et al: Dorsal tenosynovectomy and tendon transfer in the rheumatoid hand, J Bone Joint Surg 56-A:601, 1974.

Millender LH et al: Infection after silicone prosthetic arthroplasty in the hand, J Bone Joint Surg 57-A:825, 1975.

Minami A, Ogino T, and Tohyama H: Multiple ruptures of flexor tendons due to hypertrophic change at the distal radio-ulnar joint: a case report, J Bone Joint Surg 71-A:300, 1989.

Moore JR, Weiland AJ, and Valdata L: Tendon ruptures in the rheumatoid hand: analysis of treatment and functional results in 60 patients, J Hand Surg 12A:9, 1987.

Nalbandian RM: Letter to editor, J Bone Joint Surg 65-A:280, 1983.

Nalebuff EA: Present status of rheumatoid hand surgery, Am J Surg 122:304, 1971.

Nalebuff EA: The rheumatoid swan-neck deformity, Hand Clin 5:203, 1989.

Nalebuff EA and Garrod KJ: Present approach to the severely involved rheumatoid wrist, Orthop Clin North Am 15:368, 1984.

Nalebuff EA and Millender LH: Surgical treatment of the swan neck deformity in rheumatoid arthritis, Orthop Clin North Am 6:733, 1975.

Nalebuff EA and Millender LH: Surgical treatment of the boutonnière deformity in rheumatoid arthritis, Orthop Clin North Am 6:753, 1975.

Nalebuff EA and Patel MR: Flexor digitorum sublimis transfer for multiple extensor tendon ruptures in rheumatoid arthritis, Plast Reconstr Surg 52:530, 1973.

Nalebuff EA, Feldon PG, and Millender LH: Rheumatoid arthritis. In Green DP, editor: Operative hand surgery, ed 1, New York, 1982, Churchill Livingstone.

Newman RJ: Excision of the distal ulnar in patients with rheumatoid arthritis, J Bone Joint Surg 69-B:203, 1987.

O'Donovan TM and Ruby LK: The distal radioulnar joint in rheumatoid arthritis, Hand Clin 5:249, 1989.

Oster LH, Blair WF, and Steyers CM: Crossed intrinsic transfer, J Hand Surg 14A:963, 1989.

Pahle JA and Raunio P: The influence of wrist position on finger deviation in the rheumatoid hand: a clinical and radiological study, J Bone Joint Surg 51-B:664, 1969.

Paplanus SH and Payne CM: Axillary lymphadenopathy 17 years after digital silicone implants: study with x-ray microanalysis, J Hand Surg 13A:411, 1988.

Peimer CA: Long-term complications of trapeziometacarpal silicone arthroplasty, Clin Orthop 220:86, 1987.

Pelligrini VD Jr and Burton RI: Osteoarthritis of the proximal interphalangeal joint of the hand: arthroplasty or fusion? J Hand Surg 15A:194, 1990.

Polio JL and Stern PJ: Digital nerve calcification in CREST syndrome, J Hand Surg 14A:201, 1989.

Poppen NK and Niebauer JJ: "Tie-in" trapezium prosthesis: long-term results, J Hand Surg 3:445, 1978.

Posner MA and Ambrose L: Excision of the distal ulna in rheumatoid arthritis, Hand Clin 7:383, 1991.

Resnick D: Arthrography in the evaluation of arthritic disorders of the wrist, Radiology 113:331, 1974.

Riordan DC: Finger deformities and tendon repairs in rheumatoid arthritis, Orthop Rev 2:11, July 1973.

Rogers WD and Watson HK: Degenerative arthritis at the triscaphe joint, J Hand Surg 15A:232, 1990.

Savill DL: Assessment of the rheumatoid hand for reparative and reconstructive surgery, J Bone Joint Surg 46-B:786, 1964.

Schumacher HR, Zweiman B, and Bora FW Jr: Corrective surgery for the deforming hand arthropathy of systemic lupus erythematosus, Clin Orthop 117:292, 1976.

Simmons BP and Nutting JT: Juvenile rheumatoid arthritis, Hand Clin 5:157, 1989.

Smith RJ and Kaplan EB: Rheumatoid deformities at the metacarpophalangeal joints of the fingers: a correlative study of anatomy and pathology, J Bone Joint Surg 49-A:31, 1967.

Snow JW, Boyes JG, and Greider JL Jr: Implant arthroplasty of the distal interphalangeal joint of the finger for osteoarthritis, Plast Reconstr Surg 60:558, 1977.

Souter WA: Planning treatment of the rheumatoid hand, Hand 11:3, 1979.

Spar I: Flexor tendon ruptures in the rheumatoid hand: bilateral flexor pollicis longus rupture, Clin Orthop 122:186, 1977.

Stark HH et al: Fusion of the first metacarpotrapezial joint for degenerative arthritis, J Bone Joint Surg 59-A:22, 1977.

Steinberg VL and Parry CB: Electromyographic changes in rheumatoid arthritis Br Med J 1:630, 1961.

Steindler A: Arthritic deformities of the wrist and fingers, J Bone Joint Surg 33-A:849, 1951.

Stirrat CR: Treatment of tenosynovitis in rheumatoid arthritis, Hand Clin 5:169, 1989.

Straub LR: The rheumatoid hand, Clin Orthop 15:127, 1959.

Straub LR: Surgery of the arthritic hand, West J Surg 68:5, 1960.

Straub LR and Wilson EH Jr: Spontaneous rupture of extensor tendons in the hand associated with rheumatoid arthritis, J Bone Joint Surg 38-A:1208, 1956.

Straub LR, Campbell RD JR, Inglis AE, and Griffin G: The ulnar drift deformity in rheumatoid arthritis, J Bone Joint Surg 48-A:1650, 1966.

Swanson AB: Silicone rubber implants for replacement of arthritic or destroyed joints in the hand, Surg Clin North Am 48:1113, 1968.

Swanson AB: Arthroplasty in traumatic arthritis of the joints of the hand, Orthop Clin North Am 1:285, 1970.

Swanson AB: Silicone rubber implants for the replacement of the carpal scaphoid and lunate bones, Orthop Clin North Am 1:299, 1970.

Swanson AB: Disabling arthritis at the base of the thumb: treatment by resection of the trapezium and flexible (silicone) implant arthroplasty, J Bone Joint Surg 54-A:456, 1972.

Swanson AB:Flexible implant arthroplasty for arthritic finger joints: rationale, technique, and results of treatment, J Bone Joint Surg 54-A:435, 1972.

Swanson AB: Treatment of the stiff hand and flexible implant arthroplasty in the fingers, AAOS Instr Course Lect 21:73, 1972.

Swanson AB: Disabilities of the thumb joints and their surgical treatment, including flexible implant arthroplasty, AAOS Instr Course Lect 22:88, 1973.

Swanson AB: Flexible implant arthroplasty for arthritic disabilities of the radiocarpal joint: a silicone rubber intramedullary stemmed flexible hinge implant for the wrist joint, Orthop Clin North Am 4:383, 1973.

Swanson AB: Implant arthroplasty for disabilities of the distal radioulnar joint: use of a silicone rubber capping implant following resection of the ulnar head, Orthop Clin North Am 4:373, 1973.

Swanson AB: Implant resection arthroplasty of the proximal interphalangeal joint, Orthop Clin North Am 4:1007, 1973.

Swanson AB and deGroot-Swanson G: Pathogenesis and pathomechanics of rheumatoid deformities in the hand and wrist, Orthop Clin North Am 4:1039, 1973.

Swanson AB and deGroot-Swanson G: Reconstruction of the thumb basal joints: development and current status of implant techniques, Clin Orthop 220:68, 1987.

Swanson AB, deGroot-Swanson G, and Frisch EE: Flexible (silicone) implant arthroplasty in the small joints of the extremities: concepts, physical and biological considerations, experimental and clinical results. In Rubin LR, editor: Biomaterials in reconstructive surgery, St Louis, 1983, Mosby–Year Book, Inc.

Swanson AB, deGroot-Swanson G, and Maupin BK: Flexible implant arthroplasty of the radiocarpal joint: surgical technique and long-term study, Clin Orthop 187:94, 1984.

Swanson AB, deGroot-Swanson G, Maupin BK, et al: Failed carpal bone arthroplasty: causes and treatment, J Hand Surg 14Λ:417, 1989.

Swanson AB, deGroot-Swanson G, and Watermeier JJ: Trapezium implant arthroplasty: long-term evaluation of 150 cases, J Hand Surg 6:125, 1981.

Swanson AB, Meester WD, deGroot-Swanson G, et al: Durability of silicone implants: an in vivo study, Orthop Clin North Am 4:1097, 1973.

Taleinsnik J: Rheumatoid synovitis of the volar compartment of the wrist joint: its radiological signs and its contribution to wrist and hand deformity, J Hand Surg 4:526, 1979.

Taleisnik J: Rheumatoid arthritis of the wrist, Hand Clin 5:257, 1989.

Terranova W and Morgan RF: Late rupture of the flexor tendons as a complication of replacement arthroplasty, J Hand Surg 12A:15, 1987.

Terrono A and Millender LH: Surgical treatment of the boutonniere rheumatoid thumb deformity, Hand Clin 5:239, 1989.

Thompson TC: A modified operation for opponens paralysis, J Bone Joint Surg 42:632, 1942.

Trumble TE, Wu RK, and Ruwe PA: Paget's disease in the hand: correlation of magnetic resonance imaging with histology, J Hand Surg 15A:504, 1990.

Tubiana R: The hand, vol 1, Philadelphia, 1981, WB Saunders Co.

Urbaniak JR, McCollum DE, and Goldner JL: Metacarpophalangeal and interphalangeal joint reconstruction: use of silicone rubber-Dacron prostheses for replacement of irreparable joints of the hand, South Med J 63:1281, 1970.

Urbaniak JR: Prosthetic arthroplasty of the hand, Clin Orthop 104:9, 1974.

Vainio K: Vainio arthroplasty of the metacarpophalangeal joints in rheumatoid arthritis, J Hand Surg 14-A:367, 1989.

Vainio K, Reiman I, and Pulkki T: Results of arthroplasty of the metacarpophalangeal joints in rheumatoid arthritis, Reconstr Surg Traumatol 9:1, 1967.

Vaughan-Jackson OJ: Rupture of extensor tendons by attrition at the inferior radio-ulnar joint: report of two cases, J Bone Joint Surg 30-B:528, 1948.

Vaughan-Jackson OJ: Rheumatoid hand deformities considered in the light of tendon imbalance IJ Bone Joint Surg 44-B:764, 1962.

Volz RG: The development of a total wrist arthroplasty, Clin Orthop 116:209, 1976.

Volz RG: Total hip arthroplasty: a new approach to wrist disability, Clin Orthop 128:180, 1977.

Volz RG: Total wrist arthroplasty, a review of 100 patients (abstract), Orthop Trans 3:268, 1979.

Volz RG: Total wrist arthroplasty: a clinical review, Clin Orthop 187:112, 1984.

Wagner CJ: Method of treatment of Bennett's fracture dislocation, Am J Surg 80:230, 1950.

Walton RL, Brown RE, and Giansiracusa DF: Psoriatic arthritis mutilans: digital distraction lengthening: pathophysiologic and current therapeutic review, J Hand Surg 13A:510, 1988.

Weeks PM: Volar approach for metacarpophalangeal joint capsulotomy, Plast Reconstr Surg 46:473, 1970.

Weilby A and SØndorf J: Results following removal of silicone trapezium metacarpal implants, J Hand Surg 3:154, 1978.

Wilde AH: Synovectomy of the proximal interphalangeal joint of the finger in rheumatoid arthritis, J Bone Joint Surg 56-A:71, 1974.

Wilkinson MC and Lowry JH: Synovectomy for rheumatoid arthritis, J Bone Joint Surg 47-B:482, 1965.

Wilson JN: Arthroplasty of the trapezio-metacarpal joint, Plast Reconstr Surg 49:143, 1972.

Wilson RL and Carlblom ER: The rheumatoid metacarpophalangeal joint, Hand Clin 5:223, 1989.

Wise KS: The anatomy of the metacarpo-phalangeal joints, with observations of the aetiology of ulnar drift J Bone Joint Surg 57-B:485, 1975.

Wolock BS, Moore JR, and Weiland AJ: Arthritis of the basal joint of the thumb: a critical analysis of treatment options, J Arthroplasty 4:65, 1989.

Wood VE, Ichtertz DR, and Yahiku H: Soft tissue metacarpophalageal reconstruction for treatment of rheumatoid hand deformity, J Hand Surg 14A:163, 1989.

Zancolli EA, Ziadenberg C, and Zancolli E Jr: Biomechanics of the trapeziometacarpal joint, Clin Orthop 220:14, 1987.

CHAPTER 73

Volkmann's Contracture and Compartment Syndromes

MARK T. JOBE

HISTORY AND ETIOLOGY

In 1881 Volkmann stated in his classic paper that the paralytic contractures that could develop in only a few hours after injury were caused by arterial insufficiency or ischemia of the muscles. Neural injuries were initially thought to be the cause, but these were then accepted as occurring at a later stage. He suggested that tight bandages were the cause of the vascular insufficiency. This concept of extrinsic pressure as the primary cause of paralytic contracture persisted for some time in the English literature.

In 1909 Thomas studied 107 paralytic contractures. He found that some followed severe contusion of the forearm alone. In these, fractures were absent, and a splint or bandage was not applied to the limb. The idea thus was established that extrinsic pressure was not necessarily the sole cause of the ischemia. In 1914 Murphy reported that hemorrhage and effusion into the muscles could cause internal pressures to rise within the unyielding deep fascial compartments of the forearm with subsequent obstruction of the venous return. In 1928 Sir Robert Jones concluded that Volkmann's contracture could be caused by pressure from within, from without, or from both.

Compartment syndrome, already alluded to above, is the usual cause of Volkmann's contracture. It may be defined as a condition in which the circulation within a closed compartment is compromised by an increase in pressure within the compartment resulting in tissue death. This necrosis may involve not only the muscles and nerves but also eventually the skin because of excessive swelling.

Compartment syndrome may also occur as a secondary physiologic response to primary ischemia of muscle. The initial ischemia may have been incomplete, but secondary changes, including the development of massive edema within the compartment, may make it complete. The causes of compartment syndrome include crush injuries such as wringer injuries; prolonged external compression (Fig. 73-1); internal bleeding, especially after injury to a person with hemophilia; fractures; excessive exercise; burns; and intraarterial injections of drugs or sclerosing agents.

Volkmann's contracture thus is the result of an injury to the deep tissues of the limb, producing ischemia primarily of the muscles and secondarily of the nerves. Initially it is accompanied by an acute episode of severe pain that is aggravated by stretching of the muscles. Compartment syndrome thus is caused by an elevation in pressure of the tissue fluids within the closed fascial compartments of the limb, especially the volar compartment of the forearm in the upper extremity and the anterior compartment of the leg in the lower. The pressure interferes with circulation of the blood to the muscles and nerves in the compartment, and if it is untreated, the pressure may cause Volkmann's contracture or even gangrene.

The cycle of increasing muscle ischemia is depicted by Eaton and Green in Fig. 73-2. In the upper extremity, the

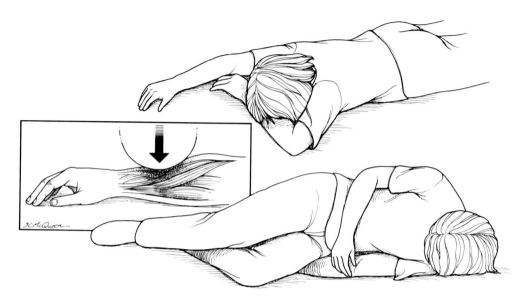

Fig. 73-1 These postures prolonged by oversedation may result in necrosis of forearm muscles, nerves, and skin.

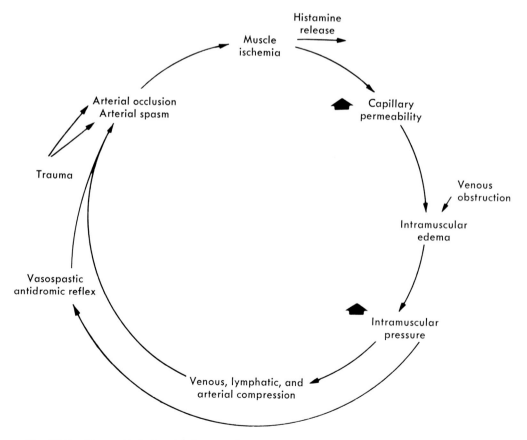

Fig. 73-2 Traumatic ischemia-edema cycle in Volkmann's contracture. (From Eaton RG and Green WT: Orthop Clin North Am 3:175, 1972.)

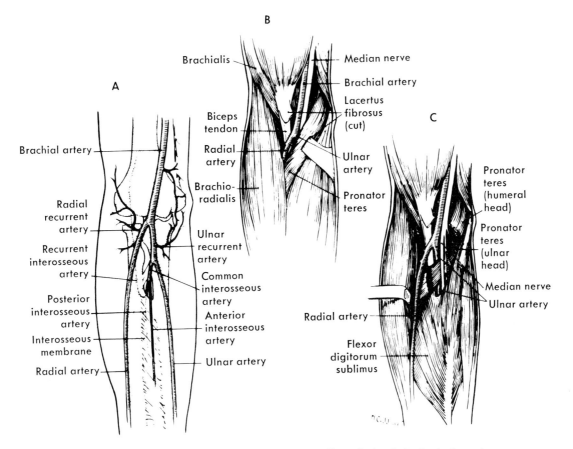

Fig. 73-3 Anatomy of Volkmann's ischemia. **A,** "Collateral circulation" of elbow does not communicate with vessels within flexor compartment. These elbow collaterals join radial and ulnar arteries proximal to pronator teres, proximal guardian of flexor compartment. **B,** Brachial artery and median nerve enter forearm through tight opening formed by biceps tendon insertion laterally and pronator teres muscle medially and are tightly covered by lacertus fibrosus. Proximal angulation, hematoma, or muscle swelling within this cruciate tendon-muscle portal is capable of major compression of neurovascular bundle. **C,** Radial artery, arising from brachial artery, passes distally superficial to pronator teres and all flexor muscles. It is not crossed by any structure along this route. Ulnar artery, however, passes beneath pronator teres and lies in deepest portions of compartment. Median nerve usually passes between humeral and ulnar heads of fleshy pronator teres, and, emerging, it becomes compressed against firm arcuate band of flexor sublimis origin (see text). (From Eaton RG and Green WT: Orthop Clin North Am 3:175, 1972.)

anterior compartment of the forearm is most commonly involved (Fig. 73-3) but the posterior compartment can be involved alone or in addition to the anterior. The intrinsic muscle compartments of the hand may also be involved (see Fig. 73-5).

An arterial injury usually results in an absent pulse, decreased skin temperature, and blanching of the skin. The treatment here is the repair of the artery.

DIAGNOSIS

Vascular deficiency in *Volkmann's ischemia* may involve only a portion of an extremity, and in the upper extremity it is usually the anterior forearm. In these in-

stances the pulse of the radial artery at the wrist may still be palpable; this may be misleading. The ischemia may be the result of a forearm fracture in an adult or child but more typically of a supracondylar fracture of the humerus in a child. Forearm fractures accounted for 22% of the contractures reported in 1967 by Eichler and Lipscomb and for 15% reported by Mubarak and Carroll in 1979. The diagnosis of ischemia in the forearm or elsewhere depends largely on the correct evaluation of the symptom of unrelenting pain. This, however, should be supported by the entire clinical picture, including swelling and any neurologic changes found by examination repeated at regular intervals if necessary. Measurements of the tissue pressure as discussed below may be useful.

A crush injury or fracture of the forearm or elbow, especially in the supracondylar area of the humerus, should cause suspicion that a forearm *compartment syndrome* may develop. The early diagnosis of impending ischemia is essential, since sometimes complete paralysis of the involved musculature may develop in only 6 to 8 hours. Pain is the most consistent symptom, although obviously it may not be discovered in a comatose patient. The forearm is tense with swelling, and sensibility of the fingertips may be diminished. Passive extension of the fingers increases the pain. The radial pulse may or may not be palpable. The dorsal compartment of the forearm may also be involved and consequently palpation with the fingers over both compartments is important. In addition, the intrinsic muscles of the hand may be involved.

The diagnosis of acute Volkmann's ischemia or acute compartment syndrome is confirmed by demonstrating an increase in compartmental pressures. In a comatose or uncooperative patient or when the diagnosis is uncertain, the tissue pressure may be measured with a wick catheter. The correlation of the clinical findings with the pressure measurements is dependable. Whitesides et al. and Whitesides, Harada, and Morimoto, in 1975 and 1977, described a method of measuring tissue pressure, which has since been improved. Other methods have evolved but the accepted pressure readings are basically the same.

MANAGEMENT
Impending Volkmann's Contracture and Compartment Syndrome

Impending tissue ischemia may be considered when the tissue pressure reaches between 30 and 10 mm Hg below the diastolic blood pressure. A higher pressure is a strong indication that fasciotomy should be recommended. In a hypotensive patient, of course, the acceptable pressure is lower. As a general rule, when in doubt, the compartment should be released. If it proves later to have been unnecessary only a scar is the result. However, if a fasciotomy should have been done but was not, loss of muscle tissue and worse may result.

FASCIOTOMY AND ARTERIAL EXPLORATION

■ *TECHNIQUE.* Make an anterior curvilinear incision medial to the biceps tendon. The incision may cross the crease directly or at an angle. Incise the deep fascia and possibly the lacertus fibrosus. Evacuate any hematoma. Expose the brachial artery and determine whether there is a free blood flow. If the flow is not satisfactory, the adventitia may be removed to expose an underlying clot or spasm or intimal tear. The adventitia may have to be resected, and the artery reanastomosed. If, however, the artery appears to be normal, continue by opening the fascia of the forearm by extending the incision and then inserting a slightly opened scissors to be cer-

tain that the fascia is completely free over the forearm muscles. Should the muscles appear gray, it is of prognostic significance. However, with release within the first several hours and establishment of blood flow, this should not be a permanent condition. Observe the median nerve to be certain that it is not severed by a fracture. This may be repaired if operative conditions permit. In a supracondylar fracture, reduce the fracture and pin it in place with Kirschner wires and control the bleeding. The skin need not be closed at this time, but anticipate secondary closure later. The elbow should not be left flexed beyond 90 degrees. In the postoperative period the elbow and hand should be elevated. In some instances a dorsal incision may be required in addition to the volar incision. Usually the volar incision releases the fascia sufficiently. Dorsal compartment pressure measurement may be helpful in making the decision.

Established Volkmann's Contracture of Forearm

Volkmann's ischemic contracture is the result of several different degrees of tissue injury; however, the earliest changes usually involve the flexor digitorum profundus muscles in the middle third of the forearm. Tsuge has classified established Volkmann's contracture into three types for purposes of treatment: mild, moderate, and severe.

A *mild contracture*, also termed *localized Volkmann's contracture*, results from partial ischemia of the profundus mass with flexion contractures usually involving only two or three fingers. Sensory changes are usually mild or absent. Intrinsic muscle contractures and joint contractures are absent. During the early stages of a mild contracture, dynamic splinting to prevent wrist contracture, physical training, and active use of the muscles may be helpful. After 3 months, the involved muscle-tendon units may be released and lengthened. However, when multiple tendon units are involved, the muscle sliding operation is better than lengthening of multiple tendons, wrist resection, or other possible procedures. An involved pronator teres may require excision.

A *moderate contracture* usually involves not only the long finger flexors but also the flexor pollicis longus and possibly the wrist flexors. Median and ulnar nerve sensory changes as well as intrinsic minus deformities are present. In this instance the muscle sliding operation, a careful neurolysis of the median and ulnar nerves without injuring their branches, and the excision of any fibrotic muscle mass encountered may be done. When no useful amplitude of movement of the finger flexors has been retained, volar transfers of such dorsal wrist extensors as the brachioradialis and extensor carpi radialis longus and a complete release of the wrist and finger flexors may be required.

A *severe contracture* involves both the flexors and extensors of the forearm. Fractures of the forearm bones and scars about the skin also may be present. Sensory feedback is usually impaired because the nerves are strangulated by the contracted and scarred muscles surrounding them. The preferred treatment in these instances is early excision of all necrotic muscles, combined with complete median and ulnar neurolysis to restore sensibility and possibly intrinsic function. Tsuge believes that this should be carried out no sooner than 3 months and no later than 1 year after the ischemic event. Tendon transfers to restore function should be performed as a secondary procedure. These may include transfer of the brachioradialis to the flexor pollicis longus and the extensor carpi radialis longus to the flexor digitorum profundus tendons. If motors to restore finger flexion are not available, a free innervated muscle transfer may be considered (see Chapter 49).

MUSCLE SLIDING OPERATION OF FLEXORS FOR ESTABLISHED VOLKMANN'S CONTRACTURE. This procedure was first described by Page in 1923 and was endorsed by Scaglietti in 1957. It has been used for Volkmann's and other contractures caused by conditions such as brain damage and burns.

■ *TECHNIQUE.* Apply a pneumatic tourniquet high on the upper arm. Make an incision beginning proximal to the elbow on the medial side and extending distally along the ulnar side of the forearm and ending at the flexor crease of the wrist where it may be carried laterally over the palmaris longus tendon (see Fig. 73-4); we prefer a straight incision. Spare all subcutaneous veins if possible and any intact cutaneous nerves such as the medial cutaneous nerve of the forearm. Beginning at the cubital fossa, incise the fascia over the musculature. Locate the ulnar nerve behind the medial epicondyle and the median nerve and brachial artery and vein as the deep dissection is carried across the elbow. Free the ulnar nerve at this level and dissect distally across the forearm, carrying the proximal origin of the flexor carpi ulnaris. Protect the median nerve as dissection is carried further distally. Release the proximal origin of the pronator teres, and using a scalpel or sharp elevator, subperiosteally release the origin of the profundus finger flexors. Then release the distal origin of the pronator teres and the origins of the palmaris longus and flexor carpi radialis. Next free the origin of the flexor digitorum sublimis. This should expose the elbow joint capsule. Release now the most distal origin of the flexor carpi ulnaris, again protecting the ulnar nerve. The interosseous membrane should now be visible. Repeated passive flexion of the fingers will help determine what further parts of the muscle origins should be detached. Mature fibrous masses within the muscles may require complete excision. Avoid injuring the intact

interosseous artery, vein, and nerve. Most of the blood supply enters the muscle mass at the junction of its upper and middle fourths. Individual branches of the vessels need not be dissected, only the origins of the muscles themselves. After releasing the muscle origins, including the flexor carpi ulnaris down to the wrist level, displacing the muscle mass distally 3 cm should be possible. Now transpose the ulnar nerve to the anterior side of the medial epicondyle. Although rare, it may be necessary also to lengthen one or two tendons at the wrist, usually those of the middle or ring finger profundus. Before closure, release the tourniquet and compress the muscle masses with sponges for 3 to 5 minutes. Then control any active bleeding by cautery, taking care not to damage the nerves. Reinflate the tourniquet and close the skin. After final release of the tourniquet, be sure that the color of the fingers returns to normal. Then wrap the arm with a bulky pad, and with the elbow at 90 degrees, the fingers in full extension, and the forearm in mild supination, apply a cast.

AFTERTREATMENT. The cast is worn for 4 weeks, and a night splint is used for several additional months. Active finger motion is begun when the cast is removed.

EXCISION OF NECROTIC MUSCLES COMBINED WITH NEUROLYSIS OF MEDIAN AND ULNAR NERVES FOR SEVERE CONTRACTURE

■ *TECHNIQUE.* Make an extensive volar forearm incision (Fig. 73-4) and excise all avascular masses of the flexor profundus and sublimis muscles, leaving any muscle that might survive or appears viable. Perform a neurolysis of the median and ulnar nerves. Then correct the finger and wrist flexion deformities by releasing the musculotendinous units at their origins. At this time at least the functional position of the hand will have been restored. At a second-stage procedure, any viable extensor muscles may be transferred to the finger flexors. Remember, however, that at least one wrist extensor must be retained. Otherwise, any wrist flexor or extensor may be transferred to power the profundus and flexor pollicis longus tendons. Sometimes a free muscle transplant from the lower extremity or from the pectoralis major may be used. This, of course, is a salvage procedure that may result in only modest improvement. If the contracture is diffuse but incomplete throughout all digital and wrist flexors, the muscle sliding technique may be considered.

Acute Ischemic Contracture of Intrinsic Musculature of Hand

Acute ischemia of the intrinsic muscles of the hand, like the larger muscles in the forearm, may result in con-

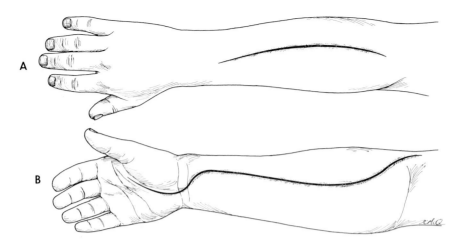

Fig. 73-4   Incisions used in forearm in severe Volkmann's contracture. **A,** Extensive opening of fascia of dorsum of forearm in dorsal compartment syndromes. **B,** Incision used for anterior forearm compartment syndromes in which skin and underlying fascia are released completely throughout. (After Gelberman RH et al: Clin Orthop 134:225, 1978.)

tracture or necrosis of the muscle bellies. It may occur after compression injuries of the hand without fracture. The hand is swollen and tense, and the fingers are held almost rigidly in a partially flexed position with the wrist in neutral. Any passive movement of the fingers causing metacarpophalangeal joint extension usually causes considerable pain. The thenar muscles rarely are involved. The hand should be decompressed immediately.

RELEASE OF ACUTE ISCHEMIC CONTRACTURE OF INTRINSIC MUSCULATURE OF HAND

■ *TECHNIQUE.* Make three dorsal parallel incisions through the skin beginning at the level of the metacarpophalangeal joints and extending to just distal to the wrist. Make the first incision radial to the second metacarpal to allow access to the first web. Make each incision down to the musculofascial area. Through each incise the fascia and release the compression of the distended muscles by allowing them to extrude into the wound if necessary. Each muscle should be identified individually to make certain that a complete release is carried out. Then passively flex the metacarpophalangeal joints and extend the proximal interphalangeal joints to stretch the muscles, being sure that all are adequately released. Do not attempt to close the wounds at this time. They may be permitted to granulate and heal, or after the swelling has decreased, they may be closed secondarily. This procedure may be done in conjunction with other more proximal releases.

Established Intrinsic Muscle Contractures of Hand

The proper surgical release of established intrinsic muscle contractures depends on the severity of the con-

tractures. When the contractures are mild (Fig. 73-5)—the metacarpophalangeal joints can be passively extended completely but while they are held extended the proximal interphalangeal joints cannot be flexed (positive intrinsic tightness test)—then the distal intrinsic release of Littler may be indicated.

In contractures that are more severe, the interosseus muscles are viable but contracted, and the intrinsic tightness test is positive. Active spreading of the fingers may be possible. In these instances the contracted muscles may be released from the metacarpal shafts by a muscle sliding operation (Fig. 73-6).

In the most severe contractures the intrinsic muscles may be not only contracted but also necrotic and fi-

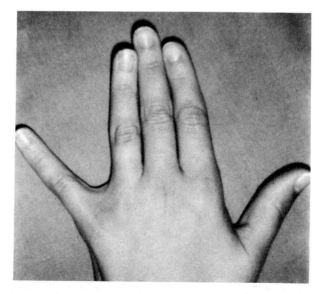

Fig. 73-5   Abduction contracture of fifth finger in patient who developed fibrosis in abductor digiti quinti, probably secondary to ischemic myositis from compressive bandage.

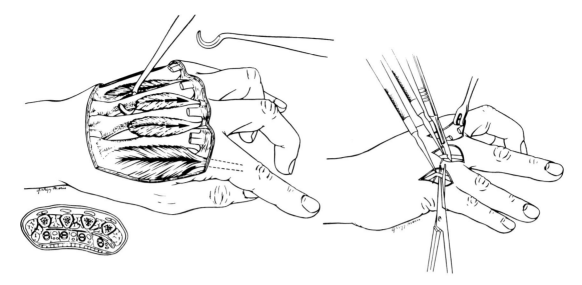

Fig. 73-6   Method of stripping and advancing interosseus muscles to slacken them, thus allowing proximal finger joints to extend and distal two to flex. Interosseus muscles of two clefts have been stripped. *Inset,* shows a cross section through middle of hand. Stripping of interossei is done only when muscles still retain considerable function. Nerve supply should be spared. (From Bunnell S: J Bone Joint Surg 35-A:88, 1953.)

brosed so that any useful muscle excursion is absent. In these instances the tendon of each muscle must be divided to release the contractures. Other procedures such as capsulotomies and tendon transfers may also be necessary.

RELEASE OF ESTABLISHED INTRINSIC MUSCLE CONTRACTURES OF HAND

■ *TECHNIQUE (LITTLER).* The same procedure is carried out on any finger as needed. Make a single midline incision on the dorsum of the proximal phalanx extending from the metacarpophalangeal joint to the proximal interphalangeal joint; thus good exposure of both sides of the extensor aponeurosis is possible. Incise the insertion of the oblique fibers of the extensor aponeurosis into the extensor tendon; make the incision parallel with the tendon (Fig. 73-7, *A*). Preserve the transverse fibers to avoid hyperextension of the metacarpophalangeal joint with its resultant clawhand deformity and limitation of extension of the interphalangeal joints. Now test the adequacy of the operation before excising any of the hood; if the dissection has not been carried far enough proximally, the interphalangeal joints cannot be fully flexed while the metacarpophalangeal joint is extended; on the other hand, if the dissection has been carried too far proximally, the metacarpophalangeal joint can be hyperextended while the interphalangeal joints are fully flexed, and a part of the aponeurosis should be sutured back to the long extensor tendon. After dissection has been extended more proximally or part of the hood has been sutured, if either is indicated, excise that part

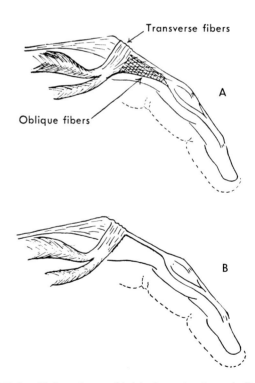

Fig. 73-7   Littler release of intrinsic contracture. **A,** Extensor aponeurosis at level of metacarpophalangeal joint consists of long extensor tendon, transverse fibers (which flex metacarpophalangeal joint), and oblique fibers (which extend interphalangeal joint). *Crosshatched* part is resected from each side of hood. **B,** Appearance of aponeurosis after release. (From Harris C Jr and Riordan DC: J Bone Joint Surg 36-A:10, 1954.)

of the hood that remains as a flap. After the correct amount of hood has been resected, the interphalangeal joints can be fully flexed, and the metacarpophalangeal joint cannot be hyperextended (Fig. 73-7, *B*). Close the incision with a running suture of fine stainless steel wire. Apply a volar plaster splint from the elbow to the middle of the proximal phalanges, immobilizing the metacarpophalangeal joints in extension and permitting full motion of the interphalangeal joints.

AFTERTREATMENT. Active motion of the interphalangeal joints is begun the day after surgery, and the splint and sutures are removed at 10 to 14 days.

RELEASE OF SEVERE INTRINSIC CONTRACTURES WITH MUSCLE FIBROSIS

■ *TECHNIQUE (SMITH).* Make a dorsal transverse incision just proximal to the metacarpophalangeal joints. Resect the lateral tendons of all the interossei and the abductor digiti quinti at the level of the metacarpophalangeal joints. If these joints remain flexed, retract the sagittal bands distally and divide each accessory collateral ligament at its insertion into the volar plate. Then free the volar plate from its attachments to the base of the proximal phalanx. With a blunt probe, separate any adhesions between the volar plate and the metacarpal head. If maintaining extension of the proximal phalanx is difficult after soft tissue release, insert a Kirschner wire obliquely through the metacarpophalangeal joint with the joint in maximum extension. When the phalanx is extended be certain that its base articulates properly with the metacarpal head before inserting the wire. If passive flexion of the proximal interphalangeal joints is incomplete with the metacarpophalangeal joints extended, resect the lateral bands at the distal half of the proximal phalanges through separate dorsal incisions.

AFTERTREATMENT. Passive and active flexion exercises of the proximal interphalangeal joints are begun within 1 day of surgery. The Kirschner wires are removed at about 3 weeks.

Adducted Thumb

Only complete loss of the thumb causes more disability in the hand than a fixed severe adduction of the thumb (web contracture). The thumb is the only digit with the ability to bring its terminal sensory pad over the entire surface of any chosen finger or over the distal palmar eminence. The saddlelike first carpometacarpal joint provides the circumductive movement of the thumb necessary for pinch or grasp (Fig. 73-8). The intrinsic muscles of the thumb and the extrinsic flexors and extensors are all important in the balanced control required in performing these functions effectively: the short abductor muscle positions and stabilizes the thumb metacarpal for

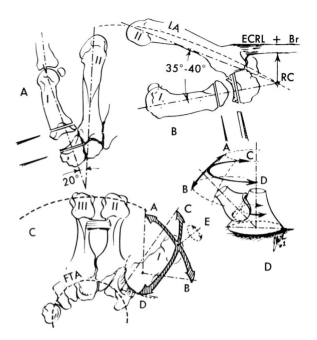

Fig. 73-8   Sketches to show optimum position in which to stabilize first metacarpal (thumb) and to show normal movements of first carpometacarpal joint. **A,** Optimum position of first metacarpal as seen from *dorsal* surface. **B,** Optimum position of first metacarpal as seen from *lateral* surface. **C,** Positions that first carpometacarpal joint allows first metacarpal to assume: *A,* palmar flexion; *B,* palmar abduction; *C,* extension abduction; *D,* flexion adduction; *E,* rotation. **D,** Geometric representation of mechanics of first carpometacarpal joint. (Redrawn by JW Littler from Littler JW: Clin Orthop 13:182, 1959.)

pinch; the adductor muscle supplies power for pinch by acting on the proximal phalanx; the long extrinsic flexor positions the distal phalanx in varying degrees of flexion and consequently controls the type of pinch, whether it be fingernail-to-fingernail opposition or pulp-to-pulp opposition with another digit. The thumb web must be supple if these important movements of the thumb are to be possible. Any contracture of the thumb web causes limited opposition of varying degrees. In severe contracture the thumb is in a position of adduction and external rotation.

The thumb web consists of skin, subcutaneous tissue, muscle, fascia, and joint capsule. Contracture of any one of these tissues may cause a secondary contracture of the others; rarely is there contracture of only one. Scarring of the skin, burns, infection, crush injuries, congenital webbing, paralysis, Dupuytren's contracture, and faulty immobilization for some injuries are causes.

The proper treatment of a contracted web is determined by which structures of the web are involved; little is accomplished by releasing the skin alone when deeper structures such as muscle, fascia, or joint capsule are also contracted. When the skin alone is contracted from a hypertrophic scar after a surgical incision or a laceration along the border of the web, it sometimes may be released by a Z-plasty (p. 2976) or a local flap (p. 2992). Dupuytren's contracture, with a fascial band causing adduction of the thumb, may be treated by Z-plasty and division or excision of the band (Fig. 73-9).

Crushing injuries, infections, or deep burns result in extensive fibrosis within the thumb web that cannot be treated by release of the skin alone; rather, the scarred components of the contracted skin, muscle, fascia, and capsule must be excised with care to avoid damaging the radial artery near the carpometacarpal joint. This excision produces a deep fissure that must be filled with skin and subcutaneous fat to provide an elastic functioning

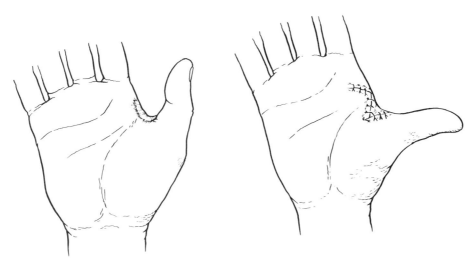

Fig. 73-9 Contracted thumb web caused by superficial scar or by Dupuytren's contracture may be released by excising abnormal tissue and performing a Z-plasty. Z-plasty may be much larger and multiple.

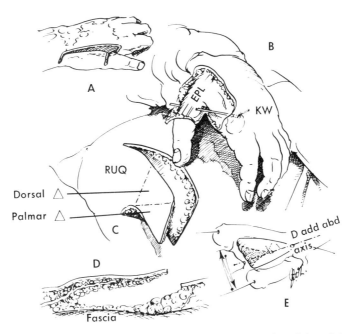

Fig. 73-10 Technique of releasing contracted thumb web and of applying abdominal flap to first intermetacarpal space. **A,** Incision to mobilize first metacarpal. **B,** Scarred skin has been excised, and first metacarpal has been abducted and fixed in this position with Kirschner wire. **C** and **D,** Flap that contains thoracoepigastric vein has been raised from right upper quadrant of abdomen (see text). **E,** Abdominal flap has been detached (at 3 weeks) and is sutured in place. (Redrawn by JW Littler from Littler JW: Clin Orthop 13:182, 1959.)

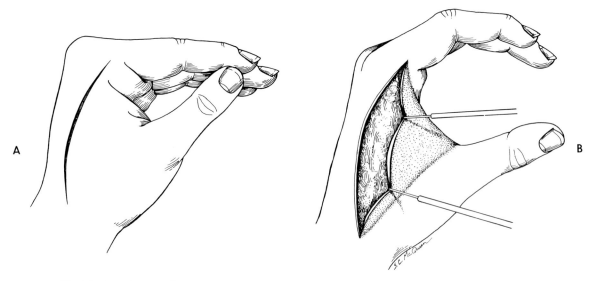

Fig. 73-11   One method of releasing dorsal skin of adducted thumb (see text) (Brand). **A,** Skin incision. **B,** Skin grafting covers defect after release has been accomplished by undermining dissection.

web: usually a direct pedicle skin graft from the abdomen. The abdominal flap is fashioned as a double triangle, one on the dorsal and one on the volar surface of the web, to eliminate any line of scar paralleling the border of the web. The first and second metacarpals are fixed in the desired position with Kirschner wires (Fig. 73-10). When motion in the carpometacarpal joint can be restored, any necessary tendon transfers for opposition may be carried out later, but if motion cannot be restored, the carpometacarpal joint must be arthrodesed to maintain permanently the new position of the thumb (p. 3190). Excellent articles on this subject by Howard and by Littler are recommended.

Paralysis of the muscles of opposition may result in secondary contracture of the skin and joint capsule and hence in contracture of the thumb web, requiring release by a Z-plasty or by a local flap and a skin graft as described by Brand (Fig. 73-11). Contracted fascia and bands of muscle must be released and capsulotomy of the carpometacarpal joint must be carried out at the same time.

Occasionally a useless index finger may provide a filleted pedicle with which a satisfactory thumb web may be constructed in one stage. This procedure not only widens the web in that the index metacarpal is excised but also provides skin that may be repositioned over a nearby defect or scar (see discussion of filleted graft, p. 3000).

REFERENCES
Volkmann's contracture (late ischemic myositis)

Braun RM, Newman J, and Thacher B: Injury to the brachial plexus as a result of diagnostic arteriography, J Hand Surg 3:90, 1978.

Brower TD: Volkmann's ischemic paralysis, Surg Clin North Am 40:491, 1960.

Brumback RJ: Compartment syndrome complicating avulsion of the origin of the triceps muscle, J Bone Joint Surg 69-A: 1445,1987.

Bunnell S: Ischaemic contracture, local, in the hand, J Bone Joint Surg 35-A:88, 1953.

Bunnell S, Doherty EW, and Curtis RM: Ischaemic contracture, local, in the hand, Plast Reconstr Surg 3:424, 1948.

Eaton RG and Green WT: Epimysiotomy and fasciotomy in the treatment of Volkmann's ischemic contracture, Orthop Clin North Am 3:175, 1972.

Eichler GR and Lipscomb PR: The changing treatment of Volkmann's ischemic contractures from 1955 to 1965 at the Mayo Clinic, Clin Orthop 50:215, 1967.

Fazi B, Raves JJ, Young JC, and Diamond DL: Fasciotomy of the upper extremity in the patient with trauma, Surg Gynecol Obstet 165:447, 1987.

Gainor BJ: Closed avulsion of the flexor digitorum superficialis origin causing compartment syndrome: a case report, J Bone Joint Surg 66-A:467, 1984.

Gardner RC: Impending Volkmann's contracture following minor trauma to the palm of the hand: a theory of pathogenesis, Clin Orthop 72:261, 1970.

Gelberman RH et al: Decompression of forearm compartment syndrome, Clin Orthop 134:225, 1978.

Green TL and Louis DS: Compartment syndrome of the arm: a complication of the pneumatic tourniquet: a case report, J Bone Joint Surg 65-A:270,1983.

Gross ES and Louis DS: Doppler hemodynamic assessment of obscure symptomatology in the upper extremity, J Hand Surg 3:467, 1978.

Halpern AA et al: Compartment syndrome of the interosseous muscles: early recognition and treatment, Clin Orthop 140:23, 1979.

Harris C Jr and Riordan DC: Intrinsic contracture in the hand and its surgical treatment, J Bone Joint Surg 36-A:10, 1954.

Holden DEA: The pathology and prevention of Volkmann's ischemic contracture, J Bone Joint Surg 61-B:296, 1979.

Ikuta Y, Kubo T, and Tsuge K: Free muscle transplantation by microsurgical technique to treat severe Volkmann's contracture, Plast Reconstr Surg 58:404, 1976.

Jones Sir R: Address on Volkmann's contracture with specific reference to treatment, Br Med J 2:639, 1928.

Joshi BB and Chaudhari SS: Dorsal relaxation incision in burst fingers, Hand 5:135, 1973.

Kulowski J: Tendon lengthening for Volkmann's ischemic clawhand, South Med J 53:1241, 1960.

Lancourt JE, Gilbert MS, and Posner MA: Management of bleeding and associated complication of hemophilia in the hand and forearm, J Bone Joint Surg 59-A:451, 1977.

Lipscomb PR: The etiology and prevention of Volkmann's ischemic contracture, Surg Gynecol Obstet 103:353, 1956.

Littler JW: The hand and upper extremity. In Converse JM, editor: Reconstructive plastic surgery, Philadelphia, 1977, WB Saunders Co.

Lord JW Jr: Post-traumatic vascular disorders and upper extremity sympathectomy, Orthop Clin North Am 12:393, 1970.

Matsen FA, Winquist RA, and Krugmire RB: Diagnosis and management of compartmental syndromes, J Bone Joint Surg 62-A:286, 1980.

Mubarak SJ and Carroll NC: Volkmann's contracture in children: aetiology and prevention, J Bone Joint Surg 61-B:285, 1979.

Murphy JB: Myositis, JAMA 63:1240, 1914.

Newmeyer WL and Kilgore ES Jr: Volkmann's ischemic contracture due to soft tissue injury alone, J Hand Surg 1:221, 1976.

Nisbet NW: Volkmann's ischaemic contracture benefited by muscle slide operation: report of a case, J Bone Joint Surg 34-B:245, 1952.

Page CM: An operation for the relief of flexion-contracture in the forearm, J Bone Joint Surg 5:233, 1923.

Parkes A: The treatment of established Volkmann's contracture by tendon transplantation, J Bone Joint Surg 33-B:359, 1951.

Reid RL and Travis RT: Acute necrosis of the second interosseous compartment of the hand, J Bone Joint Surg 55-A:1095, 1973.

Robson MC et al: Forearm compression syndrome, Orthop Rev 5:57 May 1976.

Rorabeck CH: Tourniquet-induced nerve ischemia: an experimental investigation, J Trauma 20:280, 1980.

Scaglietti O: Sindromi cliniche immediate e tardive da lesioni vascolari nelle fratture degli arti, Riforma Med 71:749, 1957.

Seddon HJ: Volkmann's contracture: treatment by incision of the infarct, J Bone Joint Surg 38-B:152, 1956.

Smith RJ: Intrinsic contracture. In Green DP: Operative hand surgery, vol 1, New York, 1982, Churchill Livingstone.

Spinner M et al: Impending ischemic contracture of the hand: early diagnosis and management, Plast Reconstr Surg 50:341, 1972.

Thomas JJ: Nerve involvement in the ischaemic paralysis and contracture of Volkmann, Ann Surg 49:330, 1909.

Tsuge K: Treatment of established Volkmann's contracture, J Bone Joint Surg 57-A:925, 1975.

Volkmann R: Die ischaemischen Muskellahmungen und Kontrakturen, Zentralbl Chir 8:801, 1881.

Weiner B: Ischemic contracture local in the hand: a complication of cardiac catheterization, Clin Orthop 90:137, 1973.

Whitesides TE Jr, Haney TC, Morimoto K, and Harada H: Tissue pressure measurements as a determinant for the need of fasciotomy, Clin Orthop 113:43, 1975.

Whitesides TE Jr, Harada H, and Morimoto K: Compartment syndromes and the role of fasciotomy, its parameters and techniques, AAOS Instr Course Lect 26:179, 1977.

Wolfort FG, Cochran TC, and Filtzer H: Immediate interossei decompression following crush to the hand, Arch Surg 106:826, 1973.

Zancolli E: Tendon transfers after ischemic contracture of the forearm: classification in relation to intrinsic muscle disorders, Am J Surg 109:356, 1965.

Adducted thumb

Araico J, Valdes JL, and Ortiz JM: An internal wire splint for adduction contracture of the thumb, Plast Reconstr Surg 48:399, 1971.

Bonola A and Fiocchi R: Cross-arm double flap in the repair of severe adduction contracture of the thumb, Hand 7:287, 1975.

Brand PW and Milford LW: Web deepening with sliding flap for adducted thumb in the hand. In Crenshaw AH, editor: Campbell's operative orthopaedics, ed 4, St Louis, 1963, Mosby–Year Book, Inc.

Brown PW: Adduction-flexion contracture of the thumb: correction with dorsal rotation flap and release of contracture, Clin Orthop 88:161, 1972.

Flatt AE and Wood VE: Multiple dorsal rotation flaps from the hand for thumb web contractures, Plast Reconstr Surg 45:258, 1970.

Flynn JE: Adduction contracture of the thumb, N Engl J Med 254:677, 1956.

Howard LD Jr: Contracture of the thumb web, J Bone Joint Surg 32-A:267, 1950.

Littler JW: The prevention and the correction of adduction contracture of the thumb, Clin Orthop 13:182, 1959.

CHAPTER 74

Congenital Anomalies of Hand

MARK T. JOBE
PHILLIP E. WRIGHT II

PRINCIPLES OF MANAGEMENT

The difficulties in treating congenital anomalies of the hand have long been recognized. Flatt cautioned that "congenital malformations are some of the most difficult problems confronting the hand surgeon." Milford observed that "a single surgical procedure cannot be standardized to suit even similar anomalies." Space precludes discussion of every treatment of every anomaly presented in this chapter. Included here are those procedures that have been shown to be safe and effective in most situations.

Treatment for the child with a congenital hand deformity may be sought at birth or later in the child's development. Involvement may be unilateral or bilateral; the anomaly may be an isolated condition, or it may be a single manifestation of a malformation syndrome or skeletal dysplasia. Early evaluation by a hand surgeon usually is desirable, not because of urgency to begin treatment but to help the parents with their concerns. Parents usually have considerable anxiety concerning the appearance of the hand, the future function of the hand, and the possibility of subsequent siblings being similarly affected; they may also have personal guilt feelings. To adequately inform the parents and to dispel as much anxiety as possible, it is helpful for the surgeon to be familiar with the modes of inheritance, as well as the preferred treatment and prognosis, of each condition. Although specific considerations and indications for surgical and nonsurgical treatment are discussed for each individual condition, the amazing ability of children to compensate functionally for deformity should be remembered.

INCIDENCE AND CLASSIFICATION

Congenital malformations of the hand encompass a myriad of deformities, all of which carry different functional and cosmetic implications for the patient and parents. Unfortunately, they occur with relative frequency. In 1982 the Congenital Malformations Committee of the

Table 74-1 Distribution of primary diagnoses: in descending order of incidence

Type of anomaly		No. of cases	Percent
Syndactyly		443	17.5
Polydactyly — all		361	14.3
Polydactyly, radial	162		6.4
Polydactyly, ulnar	130		5.2
Polydactyly, central	69		2.7
Amputation — all		179	7.1
Amputation, hand/digits	77		3.0
Amputation, arm/forearm	75		3.0
Amputation, wrist	27		1.1
Camptodactyly		173	6.9
Clinodactyly		142	5.6
Brachydactyly		131	5.2
Radial clubhand		119	4.7
Central defects		99	3.9
Thumb, hypoplastic		90	3.6
Acrosyndactyly		83	3.3
Trigger digit		59	2.3
Poland syndrome		56	2.2
Apert syndrome		52	2.1
Constriction bands		51	2.0
Musculotendinous defects		49	1.9
Madelung deformity		43	1.7
Thumb, absent		34	1.4
Ulnar finger/metacarpal absent		31	1.2
Ulnar hypoplasia		31	1.2
Synostosis, radioulnar		29	1.2
Ulnar clubhand		25	1.0
Thumb, triphalangeal		21	0.8
Hypoplasia, whole hand		21	0.8
Macrodactyly		21	0.8
Phocomelia		19	0.8
Thumb, adducted		18	0.7
Radial hypoplasia		17	0.7
Symphalangism		13	0.5
Other		115	4.6
		2525	100.0

From Flatt A: The care of congenital hand anomalies, St Louis, 1977, Mosby–Year Book, Inc.

Table 74-2 Diagnoses in Yokohama patients

Type of anomaly	No. of cases	Percent
Syndactyly	23	10.1
Polydactyly	65	28.6
Brachydactyly	19	8.4
Brachysyndactyly	10	4.4
Symphalangism	1	0.5
Annular grooves	3	1.3
Ectrodactyly		
Cleft hand	12	5.3
Ectrosyndactyly	17	7.5
Amputation	16	7.0
Microdactyly	5	2.2
Floating thumb	5	2.2
Hypoplasia of the thumb	3	1.3
Five finger	2	0.9
Monodactyly	1	0.5
Floating small finger	1	0.5
Defect of fifth metacarpus	1	0.5
Macrodactyly	3	1.3
Clinodactyly	3	1.3
Clubhand	14	6.1
Phocomelia	2	0.9
Others	21	9.3
	227	

Modified from Yamaguchi S et al: Incidence of various congenital anomalies of the hand from 1961 to 1972. In Proceedings of the sixteenth annual meeting of the Japanese Society for Surgery of the Hand. Fukuoka, 1973.

International Federation of Societies for Surgery of the Hand reported an incidence of approximately 11 anomalies per 10,000 population. These data were accumulated in seven centers located in the United Kingdom, Japan, and the United States. A similar incidence was reported earlier by Conway and Bowe (1:626 live births). The most commonly encountered anomalies of the hand are syndactyly, polydactyly, congenital amputations, camptodactyly, clinodactyly, and radial clubhand. The most common anomaly reported in the Iowa study (Flatt) was

syndactyly, as opposed to polydactyly in the Asian series (Tables 74-1 and 74-2).

The classification system devised by Swanson, Barsky, and Entin, which currently is accepted by the American Society for Surgery of the Hand and the International Federation of Societies for Surgery of the Hand, separates congenital anomalies of the hand into seven categories (see box). This classification is based on specific embryologic failures and has eliminated confusing Greek and Latin terms and eponyms. It is based in part on the system outlined by Frantz and O'Rahilly in which four patterns of deficiencies were identified on the basis of certain skeletal deficiencies: terminal transverse, terminal longitudinal, intercalary transverse, and intercalary longitudinal. After extensive clinical application and testing, Flatt found that this system permitted full categorization of complex deformities. It does not delineate etiologic factors, treatment, or prognosis.

Isolated deformities that commonly are nongenetic include unilateral transverse failure of formation, deficiencies as a result of constriction bands, longitudinal radial and ulnar dysplasias, macrodactyly, and preaxial polydactyly. Isolated deformities that usually are autosomal dominant include lobster claw deformity, symphalangism, brachydactyly, triphalangeal thumb, camptodactyly, and postaxial polydactyly. Syndactyly may occur sporadically or as a dominant trait. The malformation syn-

---

CLASSIFICATION OF CONGENITAL ANOMALIES OF THE HAND

    I. Failure of formation of parts (arrest of development)

   II. Failure of differentiation (separation) of parts

  III. Duplication

  IV. Overgrowth (gigantism)

   V. Undergrowth (hypoplasia)

  VI. Congenital constriction band syndrome

 VII. Generalized skeletal abnormalities

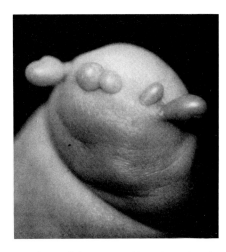

Fig. 74-1 Failure of formation (digital nubbins). Wrist motion allows use as assisting hand.

dromes and skeletal dysplasias have different patterns of inheritance.

FAILURE OF FORMATION (ARREST OF DEVELOPMENT)
Transverse Deficiencies

Transverse deficiencies include those deformities in which there is complete absence of parts distal to some point on the upper extremity, producing amputation-like stumps that allow further classification by naming the level at which the remaining stump terminates. Wynne-Davies and Lamb reported the incidence of transverse deficiencies to be 6.8 per 10,000. Most transverse deficiencies (98%) are unilateral, and the most common level is the upper third of the forearm. There is no particular sex predilection. Except for thalidomide, no particular cause has been established, and in the usual unilateral transverse deficiency there is no genetic basis, although the rare bilateral or multiple transverse deficiencies may be inherited as an autosomal recessive trait. Transverse deficiencies usually do not occur in association with malformation syndromes, but anomalies reported to occur in association with transverse deficiencies include hydrocephalus, spina bifida, myelomeningocele, clubfoot, radial head dislocation, and radioulnar synostosis.

The newborn with a transverse deficiency usually has a slightly bulbous, well-padded stump. In the more distal deficiencies rudimentary, vestigal digital "nubbins" are common (Fig. 74-1). Hypoplasia of the more proximal muscles helps differentiate these deficiencies from those associated with congenital bands. In the more common upper forearm amputation the forearm usually is no more than 7 cm long at birth and can be expected to measure no more than 10 cm by skeletal maturity. In midcarpal amputations, the second most frequent level of deficiency, the rudimentary digital remnants usually are nonfunctional. Although the affected forearm may be relatively shorter than the normal side, pronation and supination usually are possible. These children generally are of normal intelligence.

PROSTHETIC MANAGEMENT. For those patients who do not require surgery, treatment usually consists of early prosthetic fitting of the deficient limb, preferably by the time the child is crawling and certainly by the time of independent ambulation. The child's development of manual and bimanual skills progresses in an orderly and predictable pattern. Until the age of 9 months, prehension is achieved primarily by bilateral palmar grasp. Single-hand grasp develops next, and by the age of 12 to 18 months, thumb-to-finger pinch is possible. The ability to grasp an object is believed to precede the ability to release. By the age of 24 months, the child should have developed coordinated shoulder positioning, grasp, and release. The fitting of the upper limb prosthesis should complement and enhance these developmental milestones. The choice of prosthetic design is based on the level of amputation, the age and mental capacity of the child, and occasionally certain socioeconomic conditions that may determine availability and practicality of more complicated prostheses.

For the rare child with complete arm amputation, especially if the amputation is bilateral, conventional body-powered prostheses that include an elbow are unlikely to be of functional benefit. For most children with congenital above-elbow amputations, a rigid elbow is used initially. When the passive mitten initially used as a terminal device is exchanged for an actively opened split hook, usually at age 18 months, the rigid elbow is replaced by a friction elbow. At about 3 years of age, dual-terminal devices and elbow controls may be tried. For bilateral above-elbow amputations, only the preferred or dominant side is fitted with a dual-control, articulated prosthesis.

For the child with an amputation at the upper third of the forearm, a passive plastic mitten prosthesis (Fig. 74-2) is introduced between the ages of 3 and 6 months, followed by the addition of an actively opened, Plastisol-

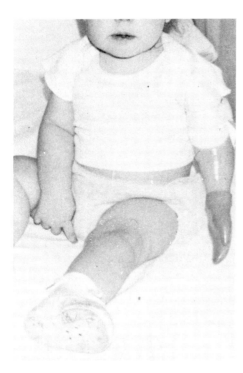

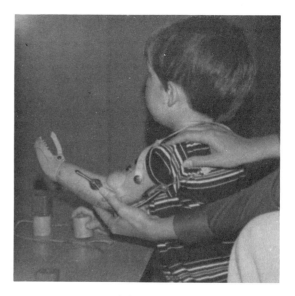

Fig. 74-3 CAPP terminal device, actively opened by patient.

Fig. 74-2 Passive plastic mitten prosthesis. (From Pellicore RJ and Tooms RE: The juvenile amputee: prosthetic management. Section I. Upper limb prosthetic management. In AAOS: Atlas of limb prosthetics: surgical and prosthetic principles, St Louis, 1981, Mosby–Year Book, Inc.)

covered, split hook at 12 to 18 months of age. A Child Amputee Prosthetic Program (CAPP) terminal device (Fig. 74-3) may be substituted if preferred. Training with a functional device is begun at 18 months of age. The CAPP device can be used until the child is about 6 years old. The prosthesis also is of some benefit in providing stability during sitting and may assist the child in pulling to a standing position. Although standard prosthetic fitting usually is satisfactory, a myoelectric prosthesis (Fig. 74-4) has been shown to be useful and appropriate for the preschool-aged child and may be considered between the ages of 2 and 4 years.

Prosthetic treatment for the child with a midcarpal amputation is somewhat more controversial. Although the carpal bones cannot be seen roentgenographically until about the age of 6 to 8 months, their presence improves the prognosis because minimal shortening of the forearm can be expected. Delay in carpal bone maturation rarely is encountered. The long, below-elbow stump is so useful for stabilizing objects and assisting in bimanual functions for which sensibility is required that the benefits of a prosthesis are debatable. Options include use of an open-ended volar plate secured to the forearm, which permits simple grip between stump and plate; an open-ended volar plate with a terminal hook; and an artificial hand driven by the radiocarpal motion. Terminal sensibility is sacrificed with the last option, but a good

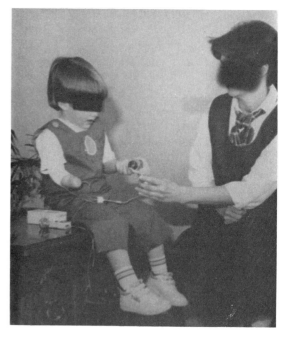

Fig. 74-4 Myoelectric prosthesis. Practice sessions are essential for child to learn to use this prosthesis effectively.

cosmetic effect is achieved. Regardless of the prosthesis chosen, therapist-supervised training sessions are essential. These sessions should be scheduled at regular intervals, particularly when a new prosthesis is introduced, and coordinated follow-up should be maintained among patient, family, therapist, orthotist, and physician. Most children do well with prostheses, although it is common for adolescents, particularly boys, to reject the prosthesis for a time before resuming its use.

SURGICAL TREATMENT. There are few indications for surgical intervention in children with transverse deficiencies of the upper extremity. Epps, Burkhalter, and McCollough in 1980 reported only 85 operations performed on 1077 children with upper extremity congenital amputations.

Amputation of nonfunctional digital remnants often is performed for psychologic and cosmetic benefits. Complete amputation of all digits often gives the hand the bizarre appearance of a little paw with small nubbins attached. As stated by Littler and emphasized by Flatt, it often is wise to alter the "stigma of congenitalism" and make the deformity appear acquired. Simple elliptic excision is appropriate.

Krukenberg reconstruction and Nathan and Trung modification. Krukenberg in 1917 described a procedure consisting of separation of the radius and ulna to allow a sensate, "chopstick"-like forearm. The Krukenberg reconstruction (Fig. 74-5) is best for the child with bilateral below-elbow amputation who is visually impaired and for the child with unilateral amputation in an underdeveloped country with limited prosthetic resources. Swanson and Swanson reported that persons with bilateral amputations found this adaptation much more useful than mechanical prostheses and that they transferred dominance to this limb when a prosthesis was used on the other limb. Chan et al. also emphasized that younger children adapt more quickly and that parents readily accept the procedure as they see their children advance from a one-handed activity pattern to a two-handed pattern. This reconstruction does not preclude the use of a prosthesis for cosmesis when desired. Surgical prerequisites include a stump length of at least 8 cm from the insertion of the biceps, relatively normal forearm musculature, and a patient and family who are willing to undergo a somewhat disfiguring operation to improve function. Nathan and Trung described a modification of this procedure that requires extensive excision of muscle and allows closure of skin flaps without the use of skin grafts.

■ *TECHNIQUE (KRUKENBERG; SWANSON AND SWANSON).* Make a longitudinal incision on the flexor surface of the forearm slightly toward the radial side (Fig. 74-6, *A*); make a similar one on the dorsal surface slightly toward the ulnar side, but on this surface elevate a V-shaped flap to form a web at the junction of the rays (Fig. 74-6, *B*). Now separate the forearm muscles into two groups (Fig. 74-6, *C* and *D*): on the radial side carry the radial wrist flexors and extensors, the radial half of the flexor digitorum sublimis, the radial half of the extensor digitorum communis, the brachioradialis, the palmaris longus, and the pronator teres; on the ulnar side carry the ulnar wrist flexors and extensors, the ulnar half of the flexor digitorum sublimis, and the ulnar half of the extensor digitorum communis. If they make the

stump too bulky or the wound hard to close, resect as necessary the pronator quadratus, the flexor digitorum profundus, the flexor pollicis longus, the abductor pollicis longus, and the extensor pollicis brevis; take care here not to disturb the pronator teres. Next incise the interosseous membrane throughout its length along its ulnar attachment, taking care not to damage the interosseous vessel and nerve. The radial and ulnar rays now can be separated 6 to 12 cm at their tips depending on the size of the forearm; motion at their proximal ends occurs at the radiohumeral and proximal radioulnar joints. The opposing ends of the rays should touch; if not, perform an osteotomy of the radius or ulna as necessary. Now the adductors of the radial ray are the pronator teres, the supinator, the flexor carpi radialis, the radial half of the flexor digitorum sublimis, and the palmaris longus; the abductors of the radial ray are the brachioradialis, the extensor carpi radialis longus, the extensor carpi radialis brevis, the radial half of the extensor digitorum communis, and the biceps. The adductors of the ulnar ray are the flexor carpi ulnaris, the ulnar half of the flexor digitorum sublimis, the brachialis, and the anconeus; the abductors of the ulnar ray are the extensor carpi ulnaris, the ulnar half of the extensor digitorum communis, and the triceps.

Remove the tourniquet, obtain hemostasis, and observe the circulation in the flaps. Now excise any excess fat, rotate the skin around each ray, and close the skin over each so that the suture line is not on the opposing surface of either (Fig. 74-6, *E* and *F*). Excise any scarred skin at the ends of the rays and, if necessary to permit closure, shorten the bones; in children the skin usually is sufficient for closure and the bones must not be shortened because growth at the distal epiphyses will still be incomplete. Preserve any remaining rudimentary digit. Next suture the flap in place at the junction of the rays and apply any needed split-thickness graft. Insert small rubber drains and, with the tips of the rays separated 6 cm or more, apply a compression dressing.

AFTERTREATMENT. The limb is constantly elevated for 3 to 4 days. The sutures are removed at about 2 weeks. At 2 to 3 weeks rehabilitation to develop abduction and adduction of the rays is begun.

■ *TECHNIQUE (NATHAN AND TRUNG)* (Fig. 74-7). Under tourniquet control, make an incision beginning on the dorsoulnar aspect of the forearm at the junction of the proximal and middle thirds. Continue this incision distally in an **S**-shaped fashion to create proximal ulnar and distal radial-based flaps. Continue this incision palmarward and proximally to create opposing distal ulnar and proximal radial-based flaps, again in an **S**-shaped fashion. Sharply incise the underlying fascia in line with the skin in-

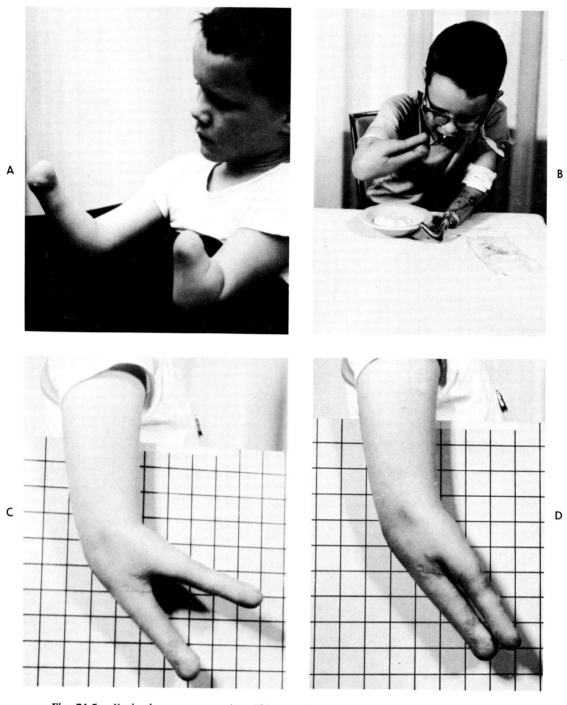

Fig. 74-5 Krukenberg reconstruction. This procedure is usually best for visually impaired children with bilateral below-elbow amputations, **A,** especially in regions with limited prosthetic resources. **B,** After reconstruction, child uses reconstructed limb as dominant hand. **C** and **D,** Tips of rays can be separated about 7.5 cm, and pinch and grasp are excellent. (From Swanson AB: J Bone Joint Surg 46-A:1540, 1964.)

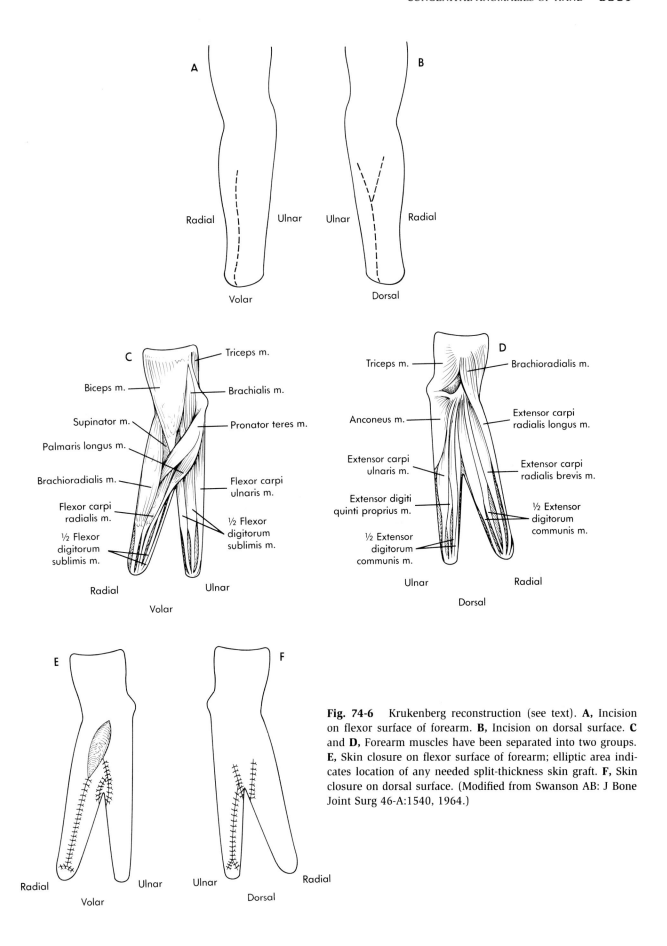

Fig. 74-6 Krukenberg reconstruction (see text). **A,** Incision on flexor surface of forearm. **B,** Incision on dorsal surface. **C** and **D,** Forearm muscles have been separated into two groups. **E,** Skin closure on flexor surface of forearm; elliptic area indicates location of any needed split-thickness skin graft. **F,** Skin closure on dorsal surface. (Modified from Swanson AB: J Bone Joint Surg 46-A:1540, 1964.)

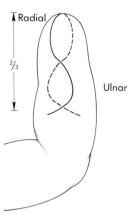

Fig. 74-7 Modified S-shaped incisions for Krukenberg reconstruction (see text). *Solid line,* Volar incision; *dotted line,* dorsal incision. (From Nathan PA and Trung NB: J Hand Surg 2:127, 1977.)

cision, taking care to preserve the cutaneous nerves. Excise the palmaris longus, the flexor carpi radialis, and the entire flexor digitorum superficialis muscles. Be careful to preserve the blood supply to the flexor digitorum profundus. Divide the flexor digitorum profundus into radial and ulnar halves by blunt dissection. Excise the pronator quadratus, carefully preserving the anterior interosseous artery and nerve. Dorsally, identify and preserve the brachioradialis. The extensor carpi radialis longus and brevis, abductor pollicis longus, and extensor pollicis brevis may be excised to allow for primary skin closure. Next make an opening between the radial and ulnar halves of the extensor digitorum communis. Gently divide the interosseous membrane by pulling apart the stumps of the radius and ulna, thus splitting the fibers. Close the wound over rubber drains, beginning distally and closing the radial stump first. A flap or graft should not be necessary for closure. Release the tourniquet after closure and check that the skin blanches and fills. Apply a compressive dressing, separating the tips of the rays 6 cm or more.

AFTERTREATMENT. The limb is elevated continuously for 48 hours. The drains are removed in routine fashion, and the sutures are removed at 2 weeks. Two to three weeks after surgery, rehabilitation is begun to develop abduction and adduction of the rays.

Metacarpal lengthening. Metacarpal lengthening usually is reserved for transverse deficiencies at the level of the metacarpophalangeal joints in the child with at least one remaining digit. Osteotomy of a digital ray with gradual distraction and subsequent bone grafting was first described by Matev in 1967 for a deficient thumb, and there have been few reports advocating this procedure for congenital absence of fingers. The procedure requires judgment and experience and should be performed by surgeons knowledgeable in the special needs and expectations of these patients and in the techniques and realistic results of the procedure. According to Kessler, Baruch, and Hecht, as well as Cowen and Loftus, metacarpal lengthening is best performed between the ages of 5 and 11 years. An average of 4 to 5 cm of length may be gained, but improved function and cosmesis may not be achieved. Complications include pin tract infection, neurovascular compromise, and distal ulcerations. Ilizarov of Russia has reported gains in length and improved function with his distraction/fixation apparatus, but reports in the English literature are presently insufficient for definitive conclusions.

■ *TECHNIQUE (KESSLER ET AL.).* Under tourniquet control, make longitudinal dorsal incisions over or between the metacarpals to be lengthened. Perform an osteotomy of the appropriate metacarpals and insert two wires transversely through the skin and metacarpals, both proximal and distal to the osteotomy (Fig. 74-8). Close the incisions in a routine manner and apply the distraction apparatus.

AFTERTREATMENT. The hand is elevated continuously for 48 hours. Distraction is done at a rate of 1 mm per day and should be painless. Distraction is terminated at any sign of vascular or neurologic impairment. Bone grafting is performed after maximum safe lengthening has been accomplished.

Longitudinal Deficiencies

Longitudinal deficiencies include all failure-of-formation anomalies that are not considered transverse deficiencies. In this category are phocomelia, radial ray dysplasia, ulnar ray dysplasia, and central dysplasia. To further identify these malformations, all absent or deficient bones are named. Any bone not named is assumed to be present. In the Iowa study these deformities constituted 9.3% of reported malformations, compared with the 7.1% incidence of transverse deficiencies.

PHOCOMELIA. Phocomelia is derived from the Greek words for "seal limb" or "flipper." It represents the most profound expression of longitudinal reduction of a limb because an intercalated segment is absent. The term is used to describe a condition in which the hand is suspended from the body near the shoulder; the hand usually is deformed and contains only three or four digits. No definite inheritance pattern has been established; the anomaly was extremely rare until the appearance of thalidomide-related deformities in the 1950s. In 1977 Flatt reported an incidence of phocomelia of 0.8% in 2525 congenital hand malformations. In 1962 Taussig reported an incidence of 60% in infants born to mothers taking thalidomide between days 38 and 54 after conception.

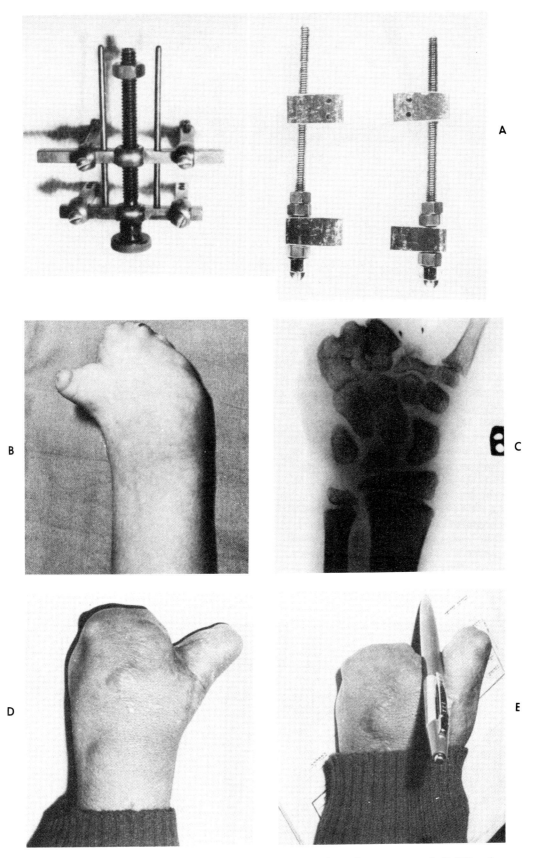

Fig. 74-8 Metacarpal lengthening with distraction. **A,** Distraction apparatus. *Left,* Older design; *right,* currently used design, consisting of two separate and independently acting parts. **B,** Aplasia of all digits and hypoplastic thumb. **C,** Thumb metacarpal is fully developed, but all other digits have only remnants of bases. **D** and **E,** Appearance and function after reconstruction. (From Kessler I, Baruch A, and Hecht O: J Hand Surg 2:394, 1977.)

Frantz and O'Rahilly described three anatomic types of phocomelia: (1) complete phocomelia with absence of all limb bones proximal to the hand, (2) absence or extreme hypoplasia of proximal limb bones with forearm and hand attached to the trunk, and (3) hand attached directly to the humerus (Fig. 74-9). Associated deformities include radial ray deficiencies in thalidomide-related phocomelia, cleft lip, and cleft palate (Robert's syndrome). Scoliosis and cardiac, skin, chromosomal, and calcification aberrations also have been reported.

Although children with phocomelia show slight differences in the overall length and appearance of the limb and different degrees of humeral, forearm, and hand deficiencies, the clavicle and scapula always are present.

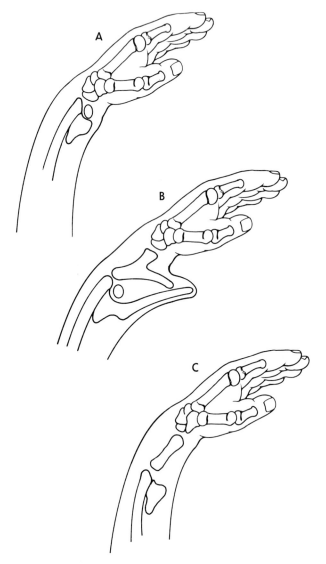

Fig. 74-9   Three types of phocomelia described by Frantz and O'Rahilly. **A,** Hand attached to shoulder with no intermediate humeral or forearm segment. **B,** Hand attached to shoulder with abnormal humeral, radial, and ulnar segment intervening. **C,** Hand attached to shoulder with intervening humeral segment without forearm segment. (Redrawn from Frantz CH and O'Rahilly R: J Bone Joint Surg 43-A:1202, 1961.)

The scapula often is deficient laterally, and active abduction of the extremity is difficult; it is usually achieved by a sudden, jerking type of motion. The abducted position usually can be maintained only by the patient gripping his ear. There is no true elbow joint. The hand usually has only three or four digits, and the thumb usually is absent. Active and passive motion at the metacarpophalangeal and proximal interphalangeal joints varies considerably. Marked difficulty in moving the hand to the midline progresses as the patient grows and the chest widens. By maturity the patient usually is unable to reach the mouth, face, and genitalia and is unable to clasp the hands together, creating considerable functional and psychologic impairment.

Treatment. Treatment of these patients generally is conservative. Various ingenious devices have been developed to assist in hygiene, feeding, and dressing, and these play a major role in the child's achieving independence. Conventional prostheses designed to increase length usually are rejected. Surgery plays a minor role in treatment of phocomelia and generally is indicated only for shoulder instability, limb shortening, or inadequate thumb opposition. The clavicular turn-down operation described by Sulamaa and Ryoppy to gain length and shoulder stability has had disappointing results and has not been shown to improve the overall function of the limb. Rotational osteotomy of one of the digits with web space deepening may improve thumb opposition, but the specific technique for phocomelia has not been well described or tested.

RADIAL CLUBHAND–RADIAL DEFICIENCIES. Radial ray deficiencies include all malformations with longitudinal failure of formation of parts along the preaxial or radial border of the upper extremity: deficient or absent thenar muscles; a shortened, unstable, or absent thumb; and a shortened or absent radius, commonly referred to as *radial clubhand.* These conditions may occur as isolated deficiencies, but more commonly they occur to some degree in association with each other. Radial clubhand occurs in an estimated 1:100,000 live births. It constituted 4.7% of congenital anomalies in the Iowa series and 6.1% in the Yokohama series. Bilateral deformities occur in approximately 50% of patients; when the deformity is unilateral, the right side is more commonly affected. Both sexes are equally affected. Complete radial absence is more common than partial absence.

In most cases of radial clubhand the cause is unknown, and the deformities are believed to occur sporadically. Of 35 patients with radial clubhand, Lamb (1977) found no blood relatives to at least the third degree with similar deficiencies; 12 of 35 had mothers who were known to have taken thalidomide. In a later study Wynne-Davies and Lamb found a higher proportion of a first-degree relative with minor congenital anomalies than would be expected from a random survey, which suggests a genetic contribution. They also found that twice as many of their patients were born during the summer quarter than during the winter quarter, and they presumed some environmental factor. Radial deficiencies in association with Fanconi's anemia and thrombocytopenia are inherited as an autosomal recessive trait; in association with Holt-Oram syndrome they are inherited in an autosomal dominant pattern.

The currently accepted and most useful classification

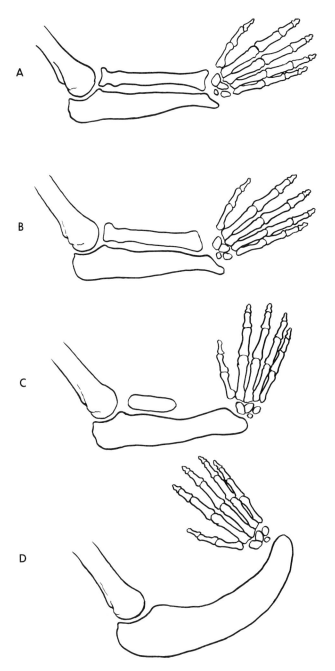

Fig. 74-10 Heikel's classification of radial dysplasia. **A,** Type I — short distal radius. **B,** Type II — hypoplastic radius. **C,** Type III — partial absence of radius. **D,** Type IV — total absence of radius. (Redrawn from Heikel HV: Acta Orthop Scand Suppl 39:1, 1959.)

of congenital radial dysplasias is a modification of that proposed by Heikel, in which four types are described (Fig. 74-10). In type I (short distal radius) the distal radial epiphysis is present but is delayed in appearance, the proximal radial epiphysis is normal, the radius is only slightly shortened, and the ulna is not bowed. In type II (hypoplastic radius) both distal and proximal radial epiphyses are present but are delayed in appearance, which results in moderate shortening of the radius and thickening and bowing of the ulna. Type III deformity (partial absence of the radius) may be proximal, middle, or distal, with absence of the distal third being most common; the carpus usually is radially deviated and unsupported, and the ulna is thickened and bowed. The type IV pattern (total absence of the radius) is the most common, with radial deviation of the carpus, palmar and proximal subluxation, frequent pseudoarticulation with the radial border of the distal ulna, and a shortened and bowed ulna. Variable degrees of thumb deficiencies are frequent with all patterns.

Associated cardiac, hemopoietic, gastrointestinal, and renal abnormalities occur in approximately 25% of patients with radial clubhand and may pose significant morbidity and mortality risks. The most frequently associated syndromes are Holt-Oram syndrome, Fanconi's anemia, thrombocytopenia–absent radius (TAR) syndrome, and the VATER syndrome, which consists of vertebral segmentation deficiencies, anal atresia, tracheoesophageal fistula, esophageal atresia, renal abnormalities, and radial ray deficiencies. In the Holt-Oram syndrome the cardiac abnormality (most commonly an atrial septal defect) requires surgical correction before any upper limb reconstruction. Children with Fanconi's anemia, a pancytopenia of early childhood, have a very poor prognosis, and death usually occurs 2 to 3 years after onset of the disease. In the TAR syndrome the thrombocytopenia usually resolves by the age of 4 to 5 years and, although it may delay reconstruction, is not a contraindication to surgical treatment. Approximately half these patients also have cardiac defects. Successful treatment of the associated abnormalities usually is possible, and upper extremity reconstruction may be appropriate in selected patients. Radial deficiency also is associated with trisomy 13 and trisomy 18; these children have multiple congenital defects and mental deficiency that may make reconstruction inappropriate despite significant deformity.

The anatomic pathology of congenital absence of the radius has been extensively reviewed by Kato, by Heikel, and by Flatt. The scapula, clavicle, and humerus often are reduced in size, and the ulna is characteristically short, thick, and curved, with an occasional synostosis with any radial remnant. Total absence of the radius is most frequent, but in partial deficiencies the proximal end of the radius is present most often. The scaphoid and trapezium are absent in more than half of these patients; the lunate, trapezoid, and pisiform are deficient in 10%;

and the thumb, including the metacarpal and its phalanges, is absent in more than 80%, although a rudimentary thumb is not uncommon. The capitate, hamate, triquetrum, and the ulnar four metacarpals and phalanges are the only bones of the upper extremity that are present and free from deficiencies in nearly all patients. The muscular anatomy always is deficient, although the deficiencies are highly variable. Muscles that frequently are normal are the triceps, extensor carpi ulnaris, extensor digiti quinti proprius, lumbricals, interossei (except for the first dorsal interossei), and hypothenar muscles. The long head of the biceps is almost always absent, and the short head is hypoplastic. The brachialis often is deficient or absent as well. The brachioradialis is absent in nearly 50% of patients. The extensors carpi radialis longus and brevis frequently are both absent or may be fused with the extensor digitorum communis. The pronator teres often is absent or rudimentary, inserting into the intermuscular septum. The palmaris longus often is defective. The flexor digitorum superficialis usually is present and is abnormal more frequently than is the flexor digitorum profundus. The pronator quadratus, extensor pollicis longus, abductor pollicis longus, and flexor pollicis longus muscles usually are absent. The peripheral nerves generally have an anomalous pattern, with the median nerve being the most clinically significant. The nerve is thicker than normal and runs along the preaxial border of the forearm just beneath the fascia. In 25% of patients it bifurcates distally, with a dorsal branch running a course similar to that of the dorsal cutaneous branch of the superficial radial nerve, which frequently is absent. This nerve is at considerable risk during radial dissections because it is quite superficial and, as stated by Flatt, "represents a strong and unyielding bowstring of the radially bowed forearm and hand." The radial nerve frequently terminates at the level of the lateral epicondyle just after innervating the triceps. The ulnar nerve characteristically is normal according to most authors, and the musculocutaneous nerve usually is absent. The vascular anatomy usually is represented by a normal brachial artery, a normal ulnar artery, a well-developed common interosseous artery, and an absent radial artery.

The obvious deformity of a short forearm and radially deviated hand is almost invariably present at birth. A prominent knob at the wrist usually is caused by the distal end of the ulna. The forearm is between 50% and 75% of the length of the contralateral forearm, a ratio that usually remains the same throughout periods of growth. The thumb characteristically is absent or severely deficient; the contralateral thumb is deficient in both unilateral and bilateral cases. Duplication of the thumb has been reported by Kummel. The hand often is relatively small. The metacarpophalangeal joints usually have limited flexion and some hyperextensibility. Flexion contractures often occur in the proximal interphalangeal joints. Stiffness of the elbow in extension, probably the

result of weak elbow flexors, frequently is associated with a radial clubhand. Most authors emphasize the elbow extension contracture as an extremely important consideration in evaluating these patients for reconstruction. Because of the radial deviation of the hand, the child usually can reach the mouth without elbow flexion. If untreated, the deformity does not appear to worsen over time, but prehension is limited and the hand is used primarily to trap objects between it and the forearm. Lamb found that unilateral involvement did not significantly affect the activities of daily living, but bilateral involvement reduced activities by one third. Associated cardiac or hematologic problems may worsen the overall prognosis.

Nonsurgical management. Immediately after birth the radial clubhand often can be corrected passively, and early casting and splinting generally are recommended (Fig. 74-11). A light, molded plastic, short arm splint is applied along the radial side of the forearm and is removed only for bathing until the infant begins to use the hands; then it is worn only during sleep. Riordan recommends applying a long arm corrective cast as soon after birth as possible. The cast is applied in three stages by means of a technique similar to that used for clubfoot casting. The hand and wrist are corrected first, then the elbow is corrected as much as possible. Although correction usually is achieved in the infant, Milford concluded that casting and splinting in a child younger than 3 months of age often is impractical. Lamb reported that elbow extension contracture can be improved by splinting with the hand and wrist in neutral position; 20 of his 27 patients improved to 90 degrees. He also cautioned that elbow flexion never improves after centralization procedures. As the child matures and ulnar growth continues, splinting is inadequate to maintain correction. There is no satisfactory conservative therapy for the significant thumb deformities associated with radial clubhand.

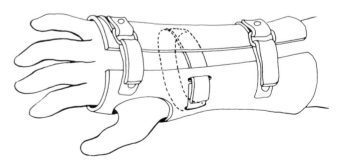

Fig. 74-11 Plastic splint for congenital absence of radius. Note, especially, middle strap that is placed over wrist at apex of angulation. Splint is useful for hands that can be properly aligned passively and for maintaining proper position after surgery.

Surgical treatment. Although surgery may be postponed for 2 to 3 years with adequate splinting, there is general agreement favoring surgical correction at 3 to 6 months of age in children with inadequate radial support of the carpus. Pollicization, when indicated, follows at 9 to 12 months of age if possible. Specific contraindications to surgical treatment include severe associated anomalies not compatible with long life, inadequate elbow flexion, mild deformity with adequate radial support (type I and some type II deformities), and older patients who have accepted the deformities and have adjusted accordingly. Reconstruction of these limbs requires familiarity with the concepts and surgical details of three types of procedures: centralization of the carpus on the forearm, thumb reconstruction, and occasionally transfer of the triceps to restore elbow flexion.

Centralization of hand. Centralization of the hand over the distal ulna was first reported in 1893 by Sayre, who suggested sharpening the distal end of the ulna to fit into a surgically created carpal notch. Lidge modified this method by leaving the ulnar epiphysis intact, providing the forerunner of modern centralization techniques. Other procedures have been performed in an attempt to stabilize the hand on the forearm. Hoffa in 1890 performed a distal transverse osteotomy of the ulna to simply realign the ulna. Bardenheuer in 1894 suggested splitting the distal ulna longitudinally to allow the carpus to become wedged between the two halves. Albee in 1919 attempted to create a radius with a free tibial graft. Starr (1945) and Riordan (1955) used a nonvascularized fibular graft to support the carpus, but fibular growth did not continue and the deformity recurred. Delorme (1969) suggested intramedullary fixation of the carpus on the ulna.

Incisions and surgical approaches also have varied. Manske and McCarroll prefer transverse ulnar incisions, as described by Riordan, removing an ellipse of skin. Watson, BeeBe, and Cruz prefer ulnar and radial Z-plasty incisions to allow removal of the distal radial anlage, which they believe is essential. The creation of a carpal notch to stabilize the carpus on the ulna also is controversial. Lamb believes this is essential and recommends that the depth of the notch equal the transverse diameter of the distal ulna, which usually requires removal of all the lunate and most of the capitate. Watson et al. do not excise any of the carpus because of the possibility of affecting growth of the forearm. In 12 patients with centralization procedures, about 30 degrees of radial deviation had recurred at an average follow-up of 10 years, a result comparable to procedures that create a carpal notch. Buck-Gramcko (1985) and Bayne and Klug also do not remove any of the carpus. When a carpal notch is not created, the distal ulna is reported to broaden and take on the roentgenographic appearance of a normal distal radius. Bora et al. recommend adjunctive tendon transfers in which the flexor digitorum superfi-

cialis from the central digits is transferred around the postaxial side of the forearm into the dorsal aspect of the metacarpal shafts, the hypothenar muscles are transferred proximally along the ulnar shaft, and the extensor carpi ulnaris is transferred distally along the shaft of the metacarpal of the little finger; however, according to their report this failed to prevent the 25 to 35 degrees of recurrent radial deviation. Bayne and Klug recommend transfer of the flexor carpi ulnaris into the distally advanced extensor carpi ulnaris to help prevent radiovolar deformity. Most authors agree that it is beneficial to use a Kirschner wire to secure alignment of the long or index metacarpal with the ulna for at least 6 weeks. Ulnar osteotomy is required if the ulna is so bowed that the Kirschner wire cannot be passed along its medullary canal. This usually is when bowing is greater than 30 degrees. When the radius is absent bilaterally, one hand should be surgically fixed in about 45 degrees of pronation and the other in about 45 degrees of supination. Prokopovitch, as well as Kessler, reported small series of radial deficiencies treated by applying external fixators to gradually stretch the soft tissues and facilitate centralization; however, we have no experience with this technique.

Centralization has been shown to improve function, particularly in bilateral involvement. Bora et al. reported total active digital motion of 54% of normal after surgery, compared with 27% in untreated patients. Forearm length was functionally doubled, and the metacarpal-ulnar angle averaged 35 degrees after surgery, compared with 100 degrees in untreated patients. Tsuyuguchi et al., however, reported that only 6 of their 12 patients were satisfied with the results despite obvious functional gains. Bayne and Klug reported that 52 of 53 patients believed that cosmesis and function had been improved by centralization. Good results had the following factors in common: (1) all had adequate preoperative soft tissue stretching; (2) surgical goals were obtained; (3) there were no problems with postoperative bracing; (4) most had less severe soft tissue contractures; and (5) most were younger than 3 years of age at the time of centralization.

Complications of centralization include growth arrest of the distal ulna, ankylosis of the wrist, recurrent instability of the wrist, damage to neural structures (particularly the anomalous median nerve), vascular insufficiency of the hand, wound infection, necrosis of wound margins, fracture of the ulna, and pin migration and breakage. Major neurovascular complications are rare.

■ **TECHNIQUE (MANSKE, McCARROLL, AND SWANSON).** Begin the incision just radial to the midline on the dorsum of the wrist at the level of the distal ulna and proceed ulnarward in a transverse direction to a point radial to the pisiform at the volar wrist crease. Pass the incision through the bulbous soft tissue mass on the ulnar side of the wrist, incising considerable fat and subcutaneous tissue (Fig. 74-12, *A*. Identify and preserve the dorsal sensory

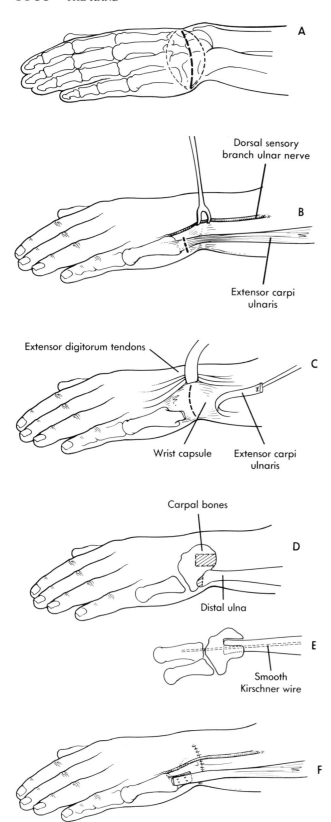

Fig. 74-12 Centralization arthroplasty technique, transverse ulnar approach (see text). **A,** Incision. **B,** Exposure of muscle, tendon, and nerve. **C,** Capsular incision. **D,** Exposure of carpoulnar junction and excision of segment of carpal bones. **E,** Insertion of Kirschner wire. **F,** Reattachment of extensor carpi ulnaris tendon. (Redrawn from Manske PR, McCarroll HR Jr, and Swanson K: J Hand Surg 6:423, 1981.)

branch of the ulnar nerve, which is deep in the subcutaneous tissue and lies near the extensor retinaculum. Expose the extensor retinaculum and the base of the hypothenar muscles. It is not necessary to identify the ulnar artery or nerve on the volar aspect of the wrist (Fig. 74-12, *B*). Identify and dissect free the extensor carpi ulnaris tendon at its insertion on the base of the fifth metacarpal, and detach and retract it proximally. Next identify and retract radially the extensor digitorum communis tendons. This exposes the dorsal and ulnar aspects of the wrist capsule. Incise the capsule transversely, thus exposing the distal ulna (Fig. 74-12, *C*).

The carpal bones are a cartilaginous mass deep in the wound on the radial side of the ulna. The carpoulnar junction is most easily identified by dissecting from proximal to distal along the radial side of the distal ulna. Take care not to mistake one of the intercarpal articulations for the carpoulnar junction. Now define the cartilaginous mass of carpal bones and excise a square segment of its midportion (measuring approximately 1 × 1 cm) to accommodate the distal ulna. Dissect free the distal ulnar epiphysis from the adjacent soft tissue and square it off by shaving perpendicular to the shaft (Fig. 74-12, *D*). Take care not to injure the epiphysis or the attached soft tissue.

Place the distal ulna in the carpal defect and stabilize it with a smooth Kirschner wire (Fig. 74-12, *E*). In practice, this usually is accomplished by passing the Kirschner wire proximally down the shaft of the distal ulna to emerge at the olecranon (or at the midshaft if the ulna is bowed.) Then pass the wire distally across the carpal notch into the third metacarpal. Cut off the proximal end of the wire beneath the skin.

Stabilize the ulnar side of the wrist by imbricating the capsule or by suturing the distal capsule to the periosteum of the shaft of the distal ulna. (If there is insufficient distal capsule, suture the cartilaginous carpal bones to the periosteum.) Obtain additional stabilization by advancing the extensor carpi ulnaris tendon distally and reattaching it to the base of the fourth or fifth metacarpal (Fig. 74-12, *F*). Also advance the origin of the hypothenar musculature proximally and suture it to the ulnar shaft to provide additional stability to the wrist. Excise the bulbous excess of the skin and soft tissue and suture the skin. This results in a pleasing cosmetic closure and helps stabilize the hand in the ulnar position (Fig. 74-13).

AFTERTREATMENT. The wrist is immobilized in a plaster cast for 6 weeks and then is placed in a removable orthoplast splint. The Kirschner wire is removed at 6 to 12 weeks. Children are encouraged to wear the splint until they reach skeletal maturity.

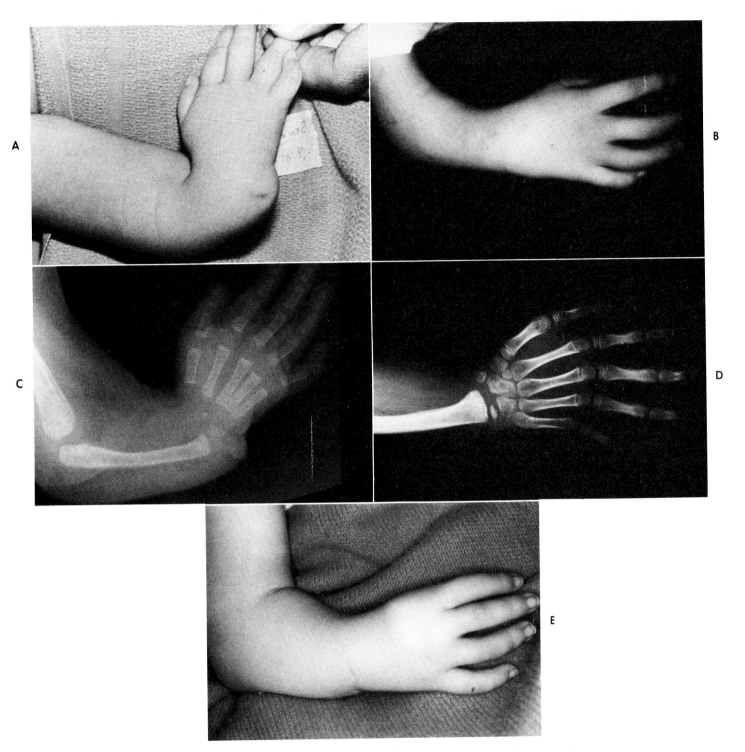

Fig. 74-13   **A,** Preoperative photograph of radial clubhand deformity. **B,** Five years after centralization arthroplasty of radial clubhand. **C,** Preoperative roentgenogram of radial clubhand deformity. **D,** Five years after centralization arthroplasty of radial clubhand. **E,** Pleasing scar is produced by transverse incision as recommended by Riordan. Ulna was placed centrally in carpus and held with medullary wire. (**A** to **D** from Manske PR, McCarroll HR Jr, and Swanson K: J Hand Surg 6:423, 1981.)

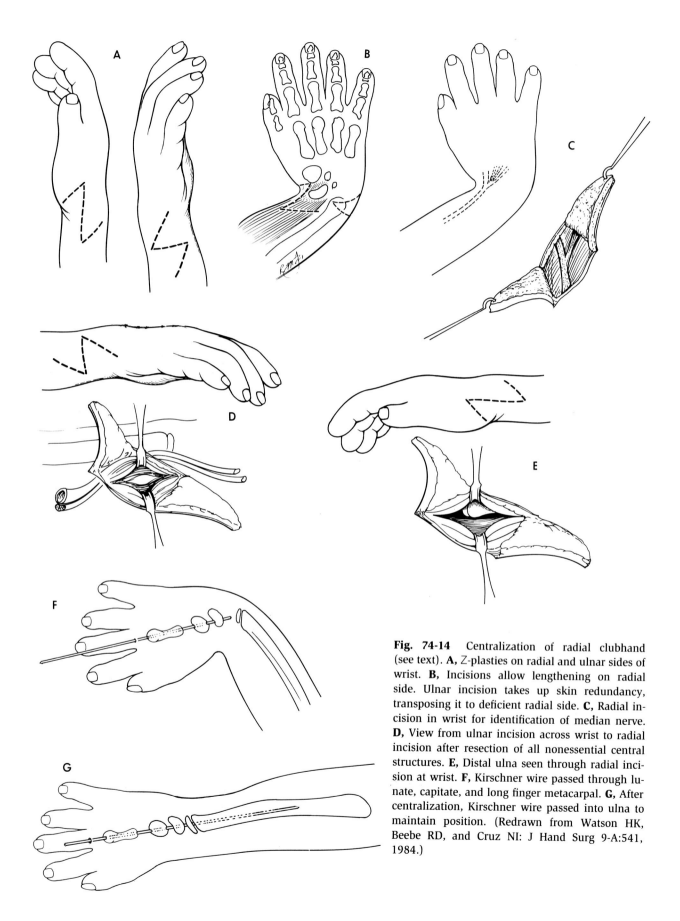

Fig. 74-14 Centralization of radial clubhand (see text). **A,** Z-plasties on radial and ulnar sides of wrist. **B,** Incisions allow lengthening on radial side. Ulnar incision takes up skin redundancy, transposing it to deficient radial side. **C,** Radial incision in wrist for identification of median nerve. **D,** View from ulnar incision across wrist to radial incision after resection of all nonessential central structures. **E,** Distal ulna seen through radial incision at wrist. **F,** Kirschner wire passed through lunate, capitate, and long finger metacarpal. **G,** After centralization, Kirschner wire passed into ulna to maintain position. (Redrawn from Watson HK, Beebe RD, and Cruz NI: J Hand Surg 9-A:541, 1984.)

■ *TECHNIQUE (WATSON, BEEBE, AND CRUZ).* Under pneumatic tourniquet control, make two skin incisions (Fig. 74-14, *A*). On the radial aspect perform a standard 60-degree Z-plasty with a longitudinal central limb to obtain lengthening along the longitudinal axis of the forearm. On the ulnar aspect perform a similar Z-plasty but with a transverse central limb to take up skin redundancy in this area, transposing the excess tissue to the deficient radial wrist area (Fig. 74-14, *B*). Once the skin incisions are completed, carry the dissection along the radial side, identifying the median nerve (Fig. 74-14, *C*). The median nerve is more radially located than usual and may be the most superficial structure encountered after the radial skin incision is made. Identification and preservation of the "radial-median" nerve are vital to the resulting functional capacity of the hand. Continue the dissection ulnarward, resecting the fibrotic distal radial anlage, which may act as a restricting band, to maintain the hand in radial deviation (Fig. 74-14, *D*). Next identify and protect the ulnar nerve and artery through the ulnar incision to allow complete dissection around the distal ulna without damage to critical structures (Fig. 74-14, *E*). Perform a complete capsular release of the ulnocarpal joint, taking care to avoid injury to the ulnar epiphysis. At this point the hand should be fully movable, attached to the forearm only by the skin, the dorsal and palmar tendons, and the preserved neurovascular structures.

Take care to remove all the fibrotic material in the "center" of the wrist and forearm area. The ulna and ulnar incision should be clearly visible through the radial incision, and the reverse also should be true. It should not be necessary to remove any carpal bones or to remodel the distal ulna to maintain the hand in a centralized position. Pass a 0.045-inch Kirschner wire through the lunate, capitate, and long finger metacarpal, exiting through the metacarpophalangeal joint (Fig. 74-14, *F*). Centralize the hand in the desired position and pass the Kirschner wire in a retrograde fashion into the ulna to maintain the position of the hand (Fig. 74-14, *G*). Deflate the tourniquet and obtain hemostasis before skin closure, or deflate the tourniquet immediately after the application of the dressing and splint. Apply a bulky hand dressing with a dorsal plaster splint extending above the elbow. Before discontinuing anesthesia, ensure that circulation in the hand is satisfactory.

AFTERTREATMENT. The hand is elevated for 24 to 48 hours. The dressing is changed and sutures are removed 2 weeks after surgery. A long arm cast is applied and worn for an additional 4 weeks. The Kirschner wire is removed at 6 weeks, and a short arm cast is applied to be worn for an additional 3 weeks. Night splinting is continued until epiphyseal closure to avoid recurrence of radial deviation.

Centralization of hand and tendon transfers

■ *TECHNIQUE (BORA ET AL; Fig. 74-15).* Bora et al. suggest that treatment be started immediately after birth with corrective casts to stretch the radial side of the wrist. At the age of 6 to 12 months the hand is centralized surgically over the distal end of the ulna, and tendon transfers are carried out 6 to 12 months later.

Stage I. Make a radial S-shaped incision and excise the radiocarpal ligament. Isolate and excise the lunate and capitate. Then make a longitudinal incision over the distal ulnar epiphysis, free it from the surrounding tissue, and preserve the tendons of the extensor carpi ulnaris and extensor digitorum quinti minimus. Transpose the distal end of the ulna through the plane between the flexor and extensor tendons and into a slot formed by the removal of the lunate and capitate. With the distal end of the ulna at the base of the long finger metacarpal, transfix it with a smooth Kirschner wire. Check the position of the ulna and carpus by roentgenograms in the operating room to ensure that the ulna is aligned with the long axis of the long finger metacarpal. Now suture the dorsal radiocarpal ligament over the neck of the ulna, close the skin, and apply a long arm cast with the elbow at 90 degrees. When the deformity is unilateral, the wrist and hand should be placed in neutral, and when it is bilateral, they should be placed in 45 degrees of pronation on one side and 45 degrees of supination on the other. The cast is removed at 6 weeks, and a splint is applied for night wear.

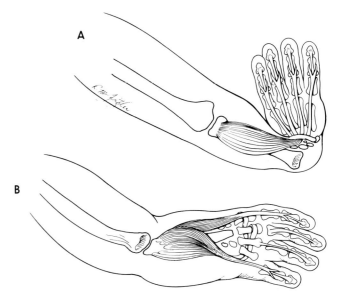

Fig. 74-15 Centralization of hand and tendon transfer (see text). **A,** Volar aspect of radial clubhand deformity showing right-angle relationship of hand and forearm and acute angulation of extrinsic flexor tendons. **B,** Volar aspect after centralization and transfer of sublimis tendons of ring and long fingers. (Redrawn from Bora FW Jr: J Bone Joint Surg 52-A:966, 1970.)

Stage II (Fig. 74-15, *B*). Three tendon transfers are performed 6 to 12 months after the centralization procedure. Before attempting to transfer the flexor digitorum sublimis tendons, test for function, because in some instances the sublimis tendon is nonfunctioning in one or more of the three ulnar digits. Passively maintain the metacarpophalangeal joints and the wrist joint in hyperextension and the interphalangeal joints in extension, and release one finger at a time. An intact sublimis tendon will flex the proximal interphalangeal joint of the released finger.

Make a midlateral incision on the ulnar side of the long finger at the level of the proximal interphalangeal joint. Divide the sublimis tendon at the level of the middle phalanx and divide also the chiasm of the decussating fibers. Perform a similar procedure on the ring finger. Next make a short transverse incision on the volar aspect of the forearm and pull the two tendons into it. At the site of previous dorsal incision reenter the wrist and transfer the sublimis tendons subcutaneously around the ulnar side of the ulna to the dorsum of the hand. Loop the tendon from the long finger around the shaft of the index finger metacarpal and the tendon from the ring finger around the shaft of the long finger metacarpal (Fig. 74-15). Transpose the tendons extraperiosteally and suture them back to themselves with the wrist in 15 degrees of dorsiflexion and maximum ulnar deviation. Now transfer the extensor carpi ulnaris tendon distally along the shaft of the little finger metacarpal and transfer the origin of the hypothenar muscles proximally along the ulnar shaft. Thus an effort is made to maintain balance and prevent recurrence of the deformity.

AFTERTREATMENT. A cast is applied after the procedure and is worn for 1 month; after this a night splint is worn for at least 3 months. Careful follow-up should be made to observe for possible recurrence of deformity. A night splint may be used for several years.

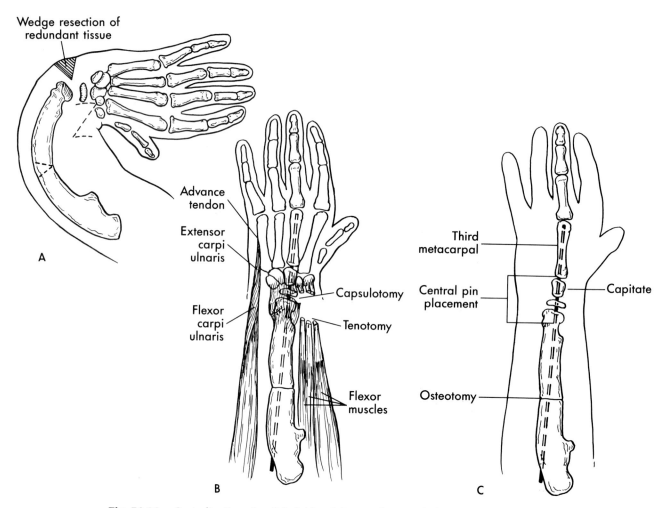

Fig. 74-16   Centralization of radial clubhand (see text). **A**, Radial release and resection of redundant soft tissue. **B**, Radial capsular release and tendon transfer. **C**, Centralization and pin fixation with ulnar osteotomy. (Redrawn from Bayne LG and Klug MS: J Hand Surg 12-A:169, 1987.)

■ *TECHNIQUE (BAYNE AND KLUG).* Make a transverse wedge incision over the end of the ulna to excise the redundant skin and fibrofatty tissue (Fig. 74-16, *A*). A Z-plasty incision also may be necessary on the radial surface of the distal forearm and wrist to give extra length to the tight skin on the radial side and make the wrist flexors and tight capsular attachments more accessible. If the radial contracture has been corrected before surgery, a Z-plasty incision may not be necessary.

Through the ulnar incision identify the dorsal sensory branch of the ulnar nerve, the extensor carpi ulnaris, and the flexor carpi ulnaris. Expose the distal ulna, taking care not to damage the epiphyseal blood supply. Develop a distally based ulnocarpal flap. Locate the interval between the carpus and the radial aspect of the ulna. Using sharp dissection, free the capsular attachments to the carpal structures, flex the elbow, and reduce the carpus over the end of the ulna. If this cannot be done easily, use the radial incision. Elevate the skin flaps, and identify and protect the anomalous superficial branch of the median nerve. The flexor carpi radialis and frequently the brachioradialis are attached to the radial carpal bones, producing a strong tethering force; release these if necessary.

If reduction is still difficult, lightly shave the cartilage of the distal ulna to flatten the surface, taking care not to expose the epiphyseal bone. Because carpal bone excision or excessive shaving often leads to intercarpal fusion and a stiff wrist, Bayne and Klug prefer ulnar osteotomy to carpal bone excision if reduction cannot be obtained. Select a Kirschner wire slightly smaller than the one that will be used for final fixation and use it to make a pilot channel from distal to proximal through the center of the ulna. Then introduce the larger Kirschner wire into the carpal bones and the third metacarpal, crossing the metacarpophalangeal joint. Place the proximal end of the wire in the pilot hole in the central portion of the end of the ulna and drive it retrograde proximally through the ulna (Fig. 74-16, *C*). Withdraw the pin so that it does not block motion of the third metacarpophalangeal joint. Obtain roentgenograms to ensure that the carpus is perfectly centralized on the distal ulna; failure to achieve perfect reduction is a common cause of subsequent loss of centralization.

After fixation of the hand, advance the ulnocarpal flap proximally and suture it in place. Advance the extensor carpi ulnaris as far distally as possible on the fifth metacarpal. Suture the flexor carpi ulnaris into the extensor carpi ulnaris as far distally and dorsally as possible (Fig. 74-16, *B*). The force of the transfer should be directed dorsally and ulnarward to counteract the palmar and radial deviating structures and balance the hand dynamically on the end

of the ulna (Fig. 74-16, *B*). Close the incisions. Place the hand in a neutral position, release the tourniquet and evaluate circulation, and apply a bulky dressing and long arm plaster splint.

If the ulna is severely bowed, a closing wedge osteotomy may be necessary; bowing of more than 30 degrees should be corrected. Make the osteotomy at the apex of angulation of the ulna.

AFTERTREATMENT. The dressing is changed in 2 weeks, and sutures are removed. A long arm plaster cast is applied. Mobilization of the fingers is encouraged. The cast and Kirschner wire are removed at 6 to 8 weeks. A short arm orthoplast splint is applied with the fingers and elbow free. The splint is worn full time until the child is 6 years old, after which time it is used at night until skeletal maturity is reached.

Pollicization for reconstruction of thumb with radial clubhand. Although the thumb frequently is absent or severely deficient in radial dysplasia, children usually are able to adapt to the thumbless hand with ulnar-side-of-index to radial-side-of-middle finger prehension and finger-to-palm prehension after centralization. Despite this adaptability, overall function and self-care activities are impaired and can be improved with successful pollicization. Because normal, as well as compensatory, prehensile patterns are firmly established within the first year of life, it is desirable that surgical reconstruction be performed early. Pollicization is recommended for both unilateral and bilateral cases. If a "floating" thumb deformity is present, with inadequate musculotendinous and bony elements, the remnant should be amputated before pollicization to allow reconstruction of a stable thumb. The parents must be clearly informed that the floating thumb is of no functional use and will be discarded after the operation.

Gossett in 1949 was the first to report replacement of the thumb with the index finger, and the index finger continues to be the preferred donor digit if it is not too deficient. Despite reports of successful single-stage toe-to-hand transfers, in the congenitally deficient thumb the index is preferred because the appearance is more acceptable and there is less donor site morbidity (Fig. 74-

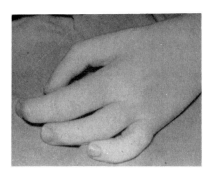

Fig. 74-17 Appearance of hand after pollicization.

17). Buck-Gramcko (1971) reported that results were better when pollicization was performed in the first year of life; his youngest patient was 11 weeks old. Side-to-side grip between index and middle fingers, particularly for smaller objects, persisted in children whose reconstruction was performed later in life. This author emphasized the importance of removing the entire index metacarpal except for the head, which acts as the new trapezium. The index finger must be rotated 160 degrees and placed in 40 degrees of palmar abduction for optimal function and appearance. Hyperextension instability at the index metacarpophalangeal joint is prevented by positioning the metacarpal head in 70 to 80 degrees of hyperextension before fixation. The reattached intrinsic muscles are important in the function of the thumb and in the formation of a new thenar eminence for cosmesis. Milford stressed the importance of suturing the intrinsic tendons into the lateral bands to enhance extension.

■ *TECHNIQUE (BUCK-GRAMCKO).* Make an **S**-shaped incision down the radial side of the hand just onto the palmar surface. Begin the incision near the base of the index finger on the palmar aspect and end it just proximal to the wrist. Make a slightly curved transverse incision across the base of the index finger on the palmar surface, connecting at right angles to the distal end of the first incision (Fig. 74-18, *A*). Make a third incision on the dorsum of the proximal phalanx of the index finger from the proximal interphalangeal joint, extending proximally to end at the incision around the base of the index finger (Fig. 74-18, *B*). Through the palmar incision, free the neurovascular bundle between the index and middle fingers by ligating the artery to the radial side of the middle finger. Then separate the common digital nerve carefully into its component parts for the two adjacent fingers so that no tension will be present after the index finger is rotated. Sometimes an anomalous neural ring is found around the artery; split this ring carefully so that angulation of the artery after transposition of the finger will not occur. When the radial digital artery to the index finger is absent, it is possible to perform the pollicization on a vascular pedicle of only one artery. On the dorsal side preserve at least one of the great veins.

Now, on the dorsum of the hand, sever the tendon of the extensor digitorum communis at the metacarpophalangeal level. Detach the interosseus muscles of the index finger from the proximal phalanx and the lateral bands of the dorsal aponeurosis. Partially strip subperiosteally the origins of the interosseus muscles from the second metacarpal, being careful to preserve the neurovascular structures.

Now perform an osteotomy and resect the second metacarpal as follows. If the phalanges of the index finger are of normal length, resect the whole metacarpal with the exception of the base of the metacar-

pal, which must be retained to obtain the proper length of the new thumb. When the entire metacarpal is resected except for the head, rotate the head as shown in Fig. 74-18, *E,* and attach it by sutures to the joint capsule of the carpus and to the carpal bones, which in young children can be pierced with a sharp needle. Rotate the digit 160 degrees to allow apposition (Fig. 74-18, *F*). Bony union is not essential, and fibrous fixation of the head is sufficient for good function. When the base of the metacarpal is retained, fix the metacarpal head to its base with one or two Kirschner wires, again in the previously described position. In attaching the metacarpal head, bring the proximal phalanx into complete hyperextension in relation to the metacarpal head for maximum stability of the joint. Unless this is done, hyperextension is likely at the new "carpometacarpal" joint (Fig. 74-18, *G*). Suture the proximal end of the detached extensor digitorum communis tendon to the base of the former proximal phalanx (now acting as the first metacarpal) to create the new "abductor pollicis longus." Section the extensor indicis proprius tendon, shorten it appropriately, and then suture it by end-to-end anastomosis.

Suture the tendinous insertions of the two interosseus muscles to the lateral bands of the dorsal aponeurosis by weaving the lateral bands through the distal part of the interosseus muscle and turning them back distally to form a loop that is sutured to itself. In this way, the first palmar interosseus will become an "adductor pollicis" and the first dorsal interosseus will become an "abductor brevis" (Fig. 74-18, *H*).

Close the wound by fashioning a dorsal skin flap to close the defect over the proximal phalanx and fashion the rest of the flaps as necessary for skin closure as in Fig. 74-18, *C* and *D*.

AFTERTREATMENT. The hand is immobilized for 3 weeks, and then careful active motion is begun.

Opponensplasty. Abductor digiti minimi opponensplasty, as described by Huber, may be appropriate for the rare patient with only isolated thenar asplasia in association with the radial clubhand or for patients with weakness in apposition after pollicization. Manske and McCarroll reported improvement in appearance, dexterity, strength, and usefulness of the thumb in 20 of 21 patients with an average age at operation of 4 years, 9 months.

■ *TECHNIQUE (MANSKE AND McCARROLL).* Make an incision beginning over the ulnar border of the proximal phalanx of the little finger and palm, curving radialward proximal to the metacarpophalangeal joint, and crossing the wrist crease on the radial side of the pisiform (Fig. 74-19, *A*). Detach the tendinous insertions into the extensor hood and the proximal phalanx of the little finger, retaining as

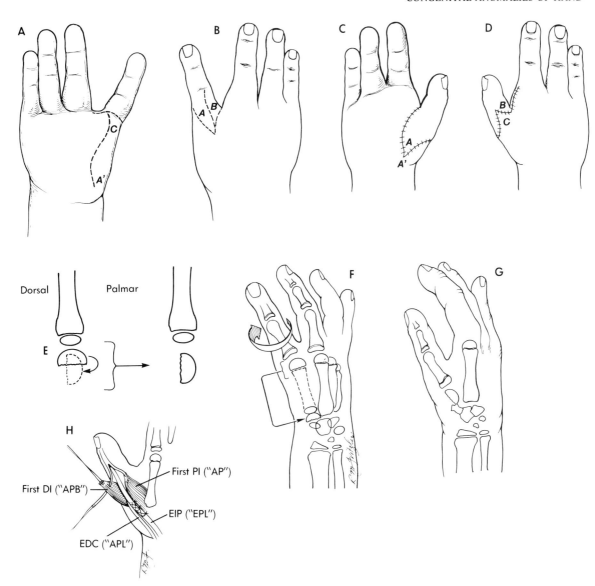

Fig. 74-18   Pollicization of index finger. **A** and **B,** Palmar and dorsal skin incisions. **C** and **D,** Appearance after wound closure. **E,** Rotation of metacarpal head into flexion to prevent postoperative hyperextension. **F,** Index finger rotated about 160 degrees along long axis to place finger pulp into position of opposition. **G,** Final position of skeleton in about 40 degrees of palmar abduction with metacarpal head secured to metacarpal base or carpus. **H,** Reattachment of tendons to provide control of new thumb. First palmar interosseus *(PI)* functions as adductor pollicis *(AP)*; first dorsal interosseus *(DI),* as abductor pollicis brevis *(APB)*; extensor digitorum communis *(EDC),* as abductor pollicis longus *(APL)*; and extensor indicis proprius *(EIP),* as extensor pollicis longus *(EPL)*. (Redrawn from Buck-Gramcko D: J Bone Joint Surg 53-A:1605, 1971.)

much tendon length as possible (Fig. 74-19, *B*). Starting distally, dissect the abductor digiti minimi muscle out of its fascial sheath to its origin at the pisiform, taking care to avoid dissection on the proximal and radial sides of the muscle where the neurovascular structures enter. Make a second incision over the dorsoradial aspect of the metacarpophalangeal joint of the thumb and pass the muscle through a large subcutaneous tunnel between

the thumb incision and the proximal ulnar incision (Fig. 74-19, *C*). Be certain that the muscle glides freely in the tunnel and is not restricted by soft tissue.

The method of insertion of the transferred tendon at the metacarpophalangeal joint (Fig. 74-20, *A*) depends on the patient's deformity. In patients with thenar aplasia with other radial anomalies, suture one of the transferred slips to the soft tissue at the

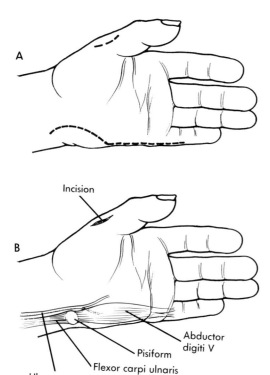

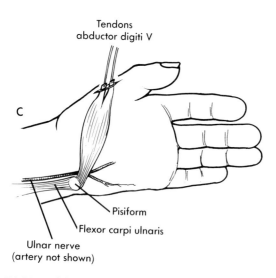

Fig. 74-19 Abductor digiti minimi opponensplasty (see text). **A,** Incisions. **B,** Detachment of tendinous insertions. **C,** Abductor digiti minimi passed through subcutaneous tunnel. (Redrawn from Manske PR and McCarroll HR Jr: J Hand Surg 3:552, 1978.)

radial aspect of the base of the proximal phalanx and the other to the extensor pollicis longus muscle at the level of the metacarpophalangeal joint as recommended by Riordan, Powers, and Hurd (Fig. 74-20, *B*). In patients with isolated thenar aplasia, stabilize the metacarpophalangeal joint by imbricating the ulnar capsule in a pants-over-vest fashion (Fig. 74-20, *C*). Then suture one of the tendinous inser-

tions to the radial capsule and the other to the imbricated ulnar capsule and to the extensor pollicis longus tendon. If the opponensplasty is performed after pollicization, suture one slip to the radial lateral band and the other to the central slip at the proximal interphalangeal joint of the pollicized finger (Fig. 74-20, *D*). Close the incisions in routine fashion and apply a bulky dressing and splint, holding the thumb in opposition.

AFTERTREATMENT. Three weeks after surgery the bulky dressing is removed and the thumb is taped into opposition for an additional 3 weeks; the child is encouraged to use the hand. Six weeks after surgery all dressings are discontinued. Formal retraining of the transfer usually is not necessary.

Triceps transfer to restore elbow flexion. An elbow stiff in extension is a contraindication to centralization; rarely, however, a child may have passive elbow flexion but minimal or no active flexion because of complete absence of elbow flexors. Menelaus reported that triceps transfer restored elbow flexion in two patients when performed 2 to 3 months after centralization; both improved from a preoperative passive range of motion of 0 to 45 degrees to a postoperative active range of motion of 0 to 90 degrees.

■ *TECHNIQUE (MENELAUS).* Make a lateral incision to expose the lower end of the triceps muscle and the anterior, lateral, and posterior aspects of the proximal end of the ulna. Identify the triceps insertion and dissect a tongue of periosteum from the proximal end of the ulna in continuity with the triceps tendon. Dissect the triceps proximally to the midarm level. Identify and mobilize the ulnar nerve; then perform a posterior capsulotomy of the elbow. Roll the periosteal tongue and the triceps tendon and pass this through a tunnel created in the coronoid process of the ulna. Secure the transfer with a nonabsorbable suture. Close the wound and apply a splint or cast with the elbow in 120 degrees of flexion.

AFTERTREATMENT. The transfer is protected in a long arm cast for 4 to 6 weeks. The sutures are removed at 2 weeks. After cast removal, gentle active exercises are begun, supporting the limb in a 90-degree, long arm, posterior splint that is worn between exercise periods and during sleep.

CLEFT HAND–CENTRAL DEFICIENCIES. Central deficiencies of the hand include those malformations in which there is a longitudinal failure of formation of the second, third, or fourth ray. Also included in this category are those deformities in which there is severe suppression of the radial four rays, leaving a one-digit (fifth-ray) hand. Further suppression that results in the digitless hand is considered a transverse deficiency. Common names for this deformity include ectrodactyly, crab claw,

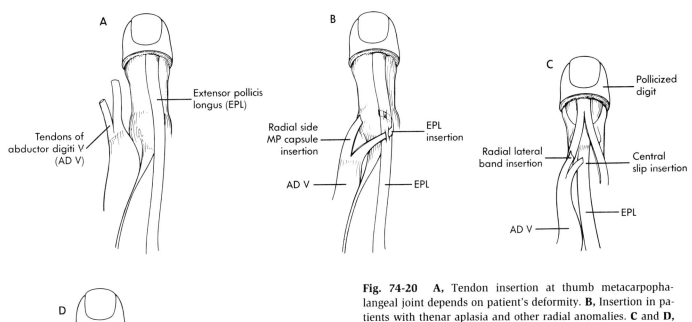

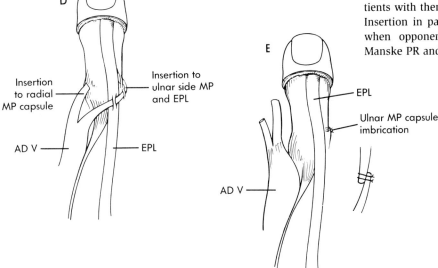

Fig. 74-20 **A,** Tendon insertion at thumb metacarpophalangeal joint depends on patient's deformity. **B,** Insertion in patients with thenar aplasia and other radial anomalies. **C** and **D,** Insertion in patients with isolated thenar aplasia. **E,** Insertion when opponensplasty follows pollicization. (Redrawn from Manske PR and McCarroll HR Jr: J Hand Surg 3:552, 1978.)

lobster claw, and cleft hand. It is exceedingly rare, with an incidence of approximately 1:90,000 live births. This group of malformations constituted 3.9% of the Iowa series. The first description of central deficiencies was published in 1770 by Hartsinck, who reported on certain blacks called *Touvingas,* or "two-fingered Negroes," in Dutch Guiana who had similar bilateral hand and foot deformities.

Central deficiencies are commonly classified into two main patterns of deformity: typical and atypical. The typical pattern is a central V-shaped cleft with variable degrees of deficiency of the middle ray (Fig. 74-21). Syndactyly between the ulnar and radial two digits is common. The deformity typically is bilateral with similar bilateral foot deformities. The atypical pattern, initially described by Lange, is a severe U-shaped deficiency that involves the index, middle, and ring ray, leaving only a thumb and little finger attached to the hand (Fig. 74-22). This deformity usually is unilateral without associated

foot deformities. Flatt suggested that the typical and atypical forms are distinctly different, not only in appearance but also in cause, and that the term *cleft hand* should refer only to typical patterns and the term *lobster claw* should refer to the fully developed atypical pattern. Flatt's classification of these malformations includes four groups: group 0, all bones present; group 1, one ray involved; group 2, two rays involved; and group 3, three rays involved. These groups are further divided into three subgroups based on the degree of finger involvement (Fig. 74-23). This classification is more complicated but helps eliminate some confusion.

The cause of central deficiencies is unknown, and most cases occur sporadically. An autosomal dominant mode of inheritance frequently is seen in the typical pattern, but penetrance often is incomplete. Maisels suggested a centripetal suppression theory according to which milder deformities have only a simple cleft without significant tissue loss, but as the severity of suppres-

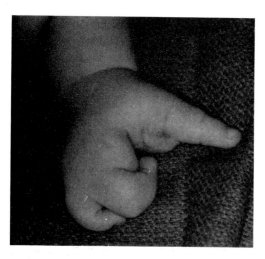

Fig. 74-21 Typical pattern of central deficiency with central V-shaped cleft.

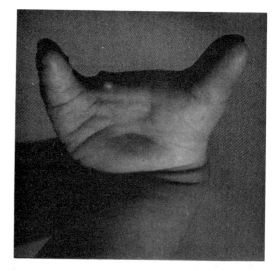

Fig. 74-22 Atypical pattern of central deficiency with U-shaped deficiency involving index, middle, and ring fingers.

EXAMPLES OF CLASSIFICATION GROUPS

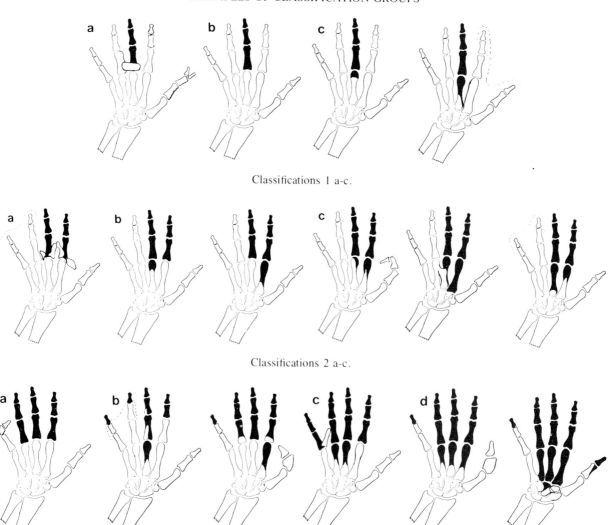

Classifications 1 a-c.

Classifications 2 a-c.

Classifications 3 a-d.

Fig. 74-23 Flatt's classification of central deficiencies. Group 0 — all bones present; group 1 — one ray involved; group 2 — two rays involved; and group 3 — three rays involved. (From Nutt JN and Flatt AE: J Hand Surg 6:48, 1981.)

sion increases, absence of the central ray is seen first, followed by loss of the radial rays and eventually loss of all rays (Fig. 74-24). Müller emphasized the etiologic differences between cleft hand and symbrachydactyly, noting that cleft hand seems to result from primary insufficiency of the central ectodermal ridge, whereas symbrachydactyly may result from primary failure of formation of the underlying bone. This would explain the absence of terminal digital remnants in pure central longitudinal deficiencies. The association of cleft hand and central polydactyly also has been established, emphasizing the complexity of these deformities.

Anomalies that occur most often in association with central hand deficiencies include cleft foot, cleft lip, and cleft palate; congenital heart disease, imperforate anus, anonychia, cataracts, and deafness also have been reported. Barsky reported that five of nine patients had cleft foot and three of nine had cleft lip and palate. In Flatt's series major musculoskeletal anomalies in addition to hand deformities included hypoplasia or pseudarthrosis of the clavicle, absent pectoralis major muscle, short humerus, synostosis of the elbow, short forearm, absent ulna, radioulnar synostosis, bilateral absence of

the tibia, bilateral dislocation of the hip, short femur, hypoplastic patella, clubfoot, calcaneovalgus foot, cavovarus foot, deviated nasal septum, and congenital ptosis. Five patients had associated genitourinary system anomalies.

The typical cleft hand pattern of a central V-shaped defect in the palm is present at birth. The middle finger usually is entirely missing, and frequently the two remaining digits on each side of the cleft have varying degrees of webbing, often causing a thumb adduction contracture. Similar foot deformities are frequent. Occasionally the index finger may be missing as well, but rarely are the ring and middle fingers absent. In the atypical pattern only two fingers are present, one along the radial border and one along the ulnar border. A shallow U-shaped defect intervenes along the distal palm. The most lateral (radial) ray often lies in the same plane as the most medial (ulnar) ray. The deformity usually is unilateral, without associated foot deformity. In the most severe forms all digits except for the small finger may be absent.

Roentgenographic findings are highly variable. Transversely oriented bones and occasionally a delta phalanx

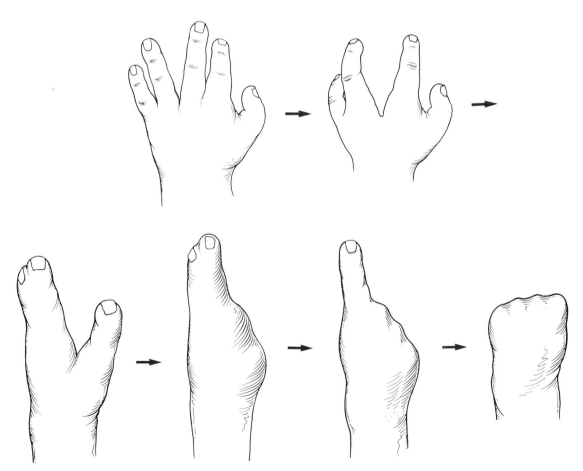

Fig. 74-24 Maisels' suppression theory. Milder deformities have only simple cleft without significant tissue loss, but as severity of suppression increases, absence first of central ray is followed by loss of radial rays and eventually loss of all rays. (Redrawn from Maisels DO: Br J Plast Surg 23:269, 1970.)

may be seen. There may appear to be two metacarpals supporting one digit or a split metacarpal supporting two digits. Carpal coalition is present in older children.

Children with these deformities develop amazing dexterity but frequently hide their hand in a pocket to avoid drawing attention to its clawlike appearance. This is particularly true in grade school and in new surroundings but seems to diminish as the patient matures. Even patients with the atypical pattern may develop adequate pinch and grasp.

Treatment. There is no appropriate nonsurgical treatment for these deformities, and the use of prostheses, as recommended in the early writing of Fort, has been essentially abandoned except on rare occasions when they are requested for cosmesis. The surgical management must be individualized according to the deformity and available anatomy. General principles of hand surgery are applicable, in that good pinch and grasp are the primary goals, followed by acceptable cosmesis if possible. Surgical reconstruction includes closure of the cleft, release of syndactyly, correction of thumb adduction contracture, removal of transverse or other deforming bony elements, and correction of delta phalanx. In the atypical pattern, deepening of the palm for grasp, osteotomies of the ulnar or radial metacarpals to allow better opposition, tendon transfers in the hypoplastic hand to restore digital motion, and possibly single-stage toe-to-hand transfer for the one-digit hand occasionally are needed.

In planning the sequence and timing of surgery, the recommendations of Flatt should be carefully reviewed. Syndactyly should be released in the normal time sequence: the border digits by 6 months of age and the central digits by 18 months of age. After a recovery period of 6 months, closure of the cleft alone or closure of the cleft with correction of thumb adduction contracture may be performed. Often it is difficult to determine the extent of thumb mobility required by the patient. A minor adduction contracture usually does not require correction. To close the cleft, bony elements that block closure should be removed sparingly because central metacarpal loss may weaken the palm and lead to cleft recurrence. If cleft closure is performed simultaneously with first–web space deepening, the index metacarpal may be transferred to the long metacarpal position by means of the Snow and Littler, or Miura and Komada technique. The technique described by Miura and Komada is less demanding technically and produces comparable results with less risk of complications. Ueba also described a technique helpful for palmar cleft with absence of the long finger, especially when the cleft hand is combined with a narrow thumb web. All functioning digits with any proximal phalanx should be spared, because these usually significantly improve grasp. A delta phalanx should be corrected at about 3 years of age, especially if it is causing radial deviation of the thumb or ulnar deviation of the little finger.

In the atypical pattern the thumb or little finger, or both, usually are hypoplastic to some extent, making pinch impossible; deepening of the palm and possibly metacarpal osteotomies performed between the ages of 2 and 3 years should improve grasp. In hands of nearly normal size, tendon transfers usually are unnecessary; however, in severely hypoplastic hands (less than 50% of normal), tendon transfers may be needed to supplement the available motors. These transfers should be delayed until the age of 3 years.

If only one digit exists, a single-stage toe-to-hand transfer may be performed around the age of 18 months. The strongest indications for this procedure in a child are complete adactyly, complete absence of a thumb, or a nonfunctional thumb with two or fewer fingers on the same hand. Although Gilbert has reported success with this technique, there are a number of problems associated with the procedure: incorporation of the transferred digit into a functional pattern may be difficult for a child who has never had a thumb; tendon transfers may be required because of deficient donor tendons; anomalous vascular patterns may be present; identification of a recipient branch of the median nerve may be difficult; and a branch of the superficial radial nerve or an adjacent digital nerve may be required to reinnervate the transferred toe.

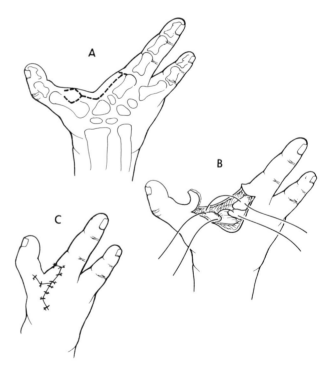

Fig. 74-25 Barsky technique of cleft closure (see text). **A,** Skin incision. **B,** Approximation of metacarpals with heavy sutures passed through holes drilled in bone. **C,** Flap used to create new web and skin on dorsal and palmar surfaces. (Redrawn from Barsky AJ: J Bone Joint Surg 46-A:1707, 1964.)

Cleft closure

■ ***TECHNIQUE (BARSKY).*** Under tourniquet control, sharply elevate a distally based diamond-shaped flap from one side of the opposing sides of the involved fingers (Fig. 74-25, *A*). Place the flap slightly dorsally to allow for a gentle slope of the commissure. Make the flap approximately 1 cm at the base and 1.5 times longer than wide. Defat the flap down to the subdermal vascular plexus. Make an incision from the free end of the flap along the opposing surfaces of the cleft. Expose the metacarpals extraperiosteally. Excise excess soft tissue and bony elements that will prevent apposing of the metacarpals. Drill two holes in each metacarpal just proximal to the heads and place a heavy suture through the holes (Fig. 74-25, *B*). Approximate the metacarpals and tie the suture to secure the correction. Close the dorsal and palmar skin incisions from proximal to distal. Excise excess skin to create interdigitating flaps along the dorsal and palmar surfaces. Place the finger flap into the commissure and, before suturing the flap, excise excess skin from the dorsum of the hand rather than from the flap (Fig. 74-25, *C*). Apply a well-molded, long arm cast to the level of the metacarpal heads over a minimum amount of bandages.

AFTERTREATMENT. The cast is worn for 3 to 4 weeks. If the thumb tends to separate excessively, apply another cast for an additional 2 to 3 weeks; then allow regular use of the hand. Special therapy usually is not required.

Combined cleft closure and release of thumb adduction contracture

■ ***TECHNIQUE (SNOW AND LITTLER).*** First, make incisions that outline the sides of the cleft on the dorsal surfaces of the index and ring fingers, joining the incisions where the V-shaped apex extends proximal to the level of the metacarpal head. Then make a small, straight incision on the ulnar side of the index finger to accommodate a small flap that will be used to make a commissure (Fig. 74-26, *A*). Raise this flap on the radial side of the ring finger. As the incisions pass the metacarpal heads, curve them back proximally onto the palm, almost parallel with each other and lying to the cleft side of the midline of the two fingers (Fig. 74-26, *B*). Do not extend the incisions any further into the palm than a point opposite the V-shaped apex of the dorsal incision. This is the palmar flap that will create the new thumb web.

To release the thumb adduction contracture, make another incision beginning on the dorsum of the thumb web at the same level as the V-shaped cleft incision. Extend the incision distally, parallel with the index split incision until it reaches the distal edge of the thumb-index web. This creates a strip of dorsal skin that is left connected to the index finger and the dorsum of the hand and that will cover the dorsal veins and extensor tendons of the index finger.

Develop the split flap from the dorsum, carefully tying the dorsal veins in the incision; do not dissect them off the flap. The flap will be compromised unless venous drainage is good. Also carefully protect and preserve the branches of the median nerve.

Next develop the thumb-index incision and release the fibrous bands between the two metacarpals. Detach the origins of the first dorsal interosseus from these bones. The adductor muscle and the radial belly of the flexor pollicis brevis muscle may have to be elevated from their origins; the radial artery must be protected during this step. Occasionally the dissection will have to be carried down to the capsule of the carpometacarpal joint, and sometimes the capsule must be incised to permit full thumb abduction.

Now perform an osteotomy of the index ray at its base and transfer it to the third metacarpal (Fig. 74-26, *C*). If the third metacarpal is small, shape the index ray into a peg and impale it into the base of the third metacarpal. If enough bone is present, fix the index metacarpal to the base of the third metacarpal with Kirschner wire (Fig. 74-26, *D*). Carefully align the metacarpals so that the transposed ray maintains the transverse and longitudinal arches of the hand and allows the fingers to flex into the palm normally without overlap (Fig. 74-26, *D*).

Suture the skin between the ring and index fingers. Inset the small, longitudinal incision on the ulnar side of the index finger to make a commissure. Use a small drain in the wound as needed. Place the large palmar-based cleft flap between the index finger and the newly abducted thumb (Fig. 74-26, *E*). If this flap does not completely cover the area of defect, use a split-skin graft for complete coverage. Never place these flaps under tension; if necessary, use a skin graft over the index finger. Apply a well-padded long arm cast, maintaining the arches of the hand and leaving the fingers and thumb enough freedom to move.

AFTERTREATMENT. The cast is worn for 6 weeks. Sutures are removed at about 2 weeks and the Kirschner wire at about 6 weeks, or after bone healing has occurred. After cast and pin removal normal activities are permitted on a graduated basis over a period of 6 to 8 weeks.

■ ***TECHNIQUE (MIURA AND KOMADA;*** Fig. 74-27). Make a linear incision beginning on the radial side of the base of the ring finger and continuing to the ulnar side of the base of the index finger and crossing the cleft space. Make a curved incision around the base of the index finger at the level desired for the new thumb web space. Then detach the index

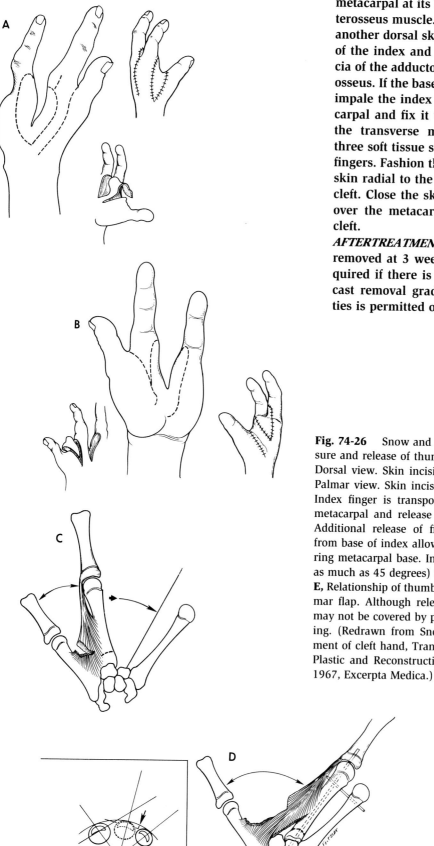

metacarpal at its base, along with the first dorsal interosseus muscle. If exposure is not adequate, make another dorsal skin incision to expose just the bases of the index and long metacarpals. Release the fascia of the adductor pollicis and the first dorsal interosseus. If the base of the third metacarpal is present, impale the index ray on the base of the third metacarpal and fix it with Kirschner wires. Reconstruct the transverse metacarpal ligament with two or three soft tissue sutures between the index and ring fingers. Fashion the flap for the thumb web from the skin radial to the curved incision along the original cleft. Close the skin. Apply a long arm cast molded over the metacarpals to prevent separation of the cleft.

AFTERTREATMENT. The cast and skin sutures are removed at 3 weeks. Additional casting may be required if there is any laxity in the cleft. After final cast removal gradual resumption of normal activities is permitted over a period of 6 to 8 weeks.

Fig. 74-26 Snow and Littler technique of combined cleft closure and release of thumb adduction contracture (see text). **A,** Dorsal view. Skin incisions; flap elevation; wound closure. **B,** Palmar view. Skin incisions; flap elevation; wound closure. **C,** Index finger is transposed after osteotomy of base of index metacarpal and release of first dorsal interosseus muscle. **D,** Additional release of first dorsal interosseus subperiosteally from base of index allows transposition of index metacarpal to ring metacarpal base. Inset shows rotation necessary (possibly as much as 45 degrees) for transposed digit to prevent overlap. **E,** Relationship of thumb adduction contracture release and palmar flap. Although release allows thumb mobility, area at *C* may not be covered by palmar flap and may require skin grafting. (Redrawn from Snow JW and Littler JW: Surgical treatment of cleft hand, Transactions of the International Society of Plastic and Reconstructive Surgeons, Fourth Congress, Rome, 1967, Excerpta Medica.)

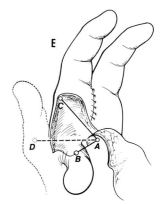

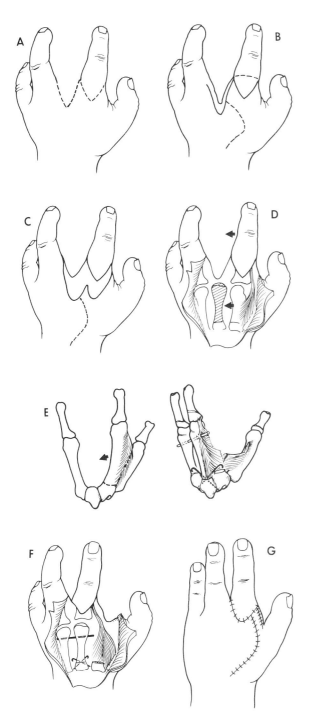

Fig. 74-27 Reconstruction of cleft hand with adducted thumb. **A,** Initial skin incision on dorsum of hand. **B,** Additional incisions *(broken line)* to expose metacarpal dorsally and finger on palmar surface. **C,** Index finger skin flaps. **D,** Scheme for transposing index metacarpal to middle metacarpal position. **E,** Bone transposition: fasciae of first dorsal interosseus and adductor pollicis are released, and muscle may require release. **F,** Transposition of index and release of thumb completed. **G,** Appearance after wound closure. (Redrawn from Miura T and Komada T: Plast Reconstr Surg 64:65, 1979.)

■ *TECHNIQUE (UEBA).* Make a V-shaped skin incision, in the form of a triangular skin flap, on the radial side of the ring finger (Fig. 74-28, *A*). This flap is used to form the commissure. Make a second skin incision beginning from the palmar end of the previous skin incision and extending to the ulnar side of the palm (Fig. 74-28, *B*). Make a third skin incision around the base of the index finger; then place an incision at the bottom of the cleft to connect the previous incisions (Fig. 74-28, *C*). Elevate the interdigital palmar and dorsal skin flaps and sever the fibrous bands between the thumb and index finger to widen the thumb web as much as possible (Fig. 74-28, *D*). Elevate the periosteum around the second metacarpal and transfer the metacarpal ulnarward, taking care not to injure the ulnar nerve. Shift the second metacarpal slightly ulnarward and supinate it so that the index finger flexes without overlapping the ring finger. Fix the second metacarpal to the fourth metacarpal with one or two Kirschner wires and a nonabsorbable suture or long-lasting absorbable suture around the metacarpal necks.

Then connect the common extensor tendons to the index and ring fingers with a free tendon graft taken from the palmaris longus muscle. Pass this tendon graft through the extensor tendons at the level of the metacarpophalangeal joints, reflect its ends, and suture them to the extensor aponeurosis (Fig. 74-28, *E*). After rotating the flaps (Fig. 74-28, *F*), make suture lines transversely to conceal the original cleft and deepen the thumb web (Fig. 74-28, *G*). Close the skin with absorbable sutures. Apply a long arm cast, molded to avoid recurrence of the cleft.

AFTERTREATMENT. The cast and any remaining sutures are removed at 3 weeks when a second cast is applied. The cast and Kirschner wires are removed at about 6 weeks or when bone healing is complete. Resumption of normal activities is allowed during the next 4 to 6 weeks.

Deepening of web and metacarpal osteotomy

■ *TECHNIQUE.* It usually is safer to undertake correction in two stages. First, deepen the web by Z-plasty and remove any redundant bone segments or rudimentary digits. Later, shorten a metacarpal if needed or rotate one or both to provide appositional pinch between the digits. Apply a long arm cast.

AFTERTREATMENT. The sutures are removed at 2 weeks and the cast at 4 to 6 weeks. Normal activities are resumed during the next 4 to 6 weeks.

Tendon transfer for type II deformities

■ *TECHNIQUE (FLATT).* This procedure requires a good, stable, passive range of motion in the border digits. Identify the donor tendons, either wrist flex-

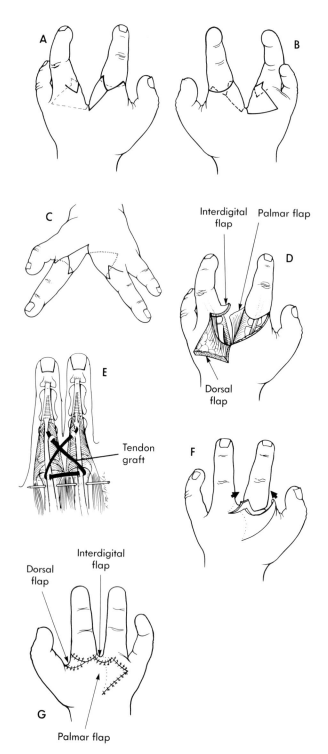

Fig. 74-28 Ueba technique for cleft hand. **A,** Dorsal view of incisions. *Solid line,* Dorsal incisions; *broken line,* palmar incisions. **B,** Palmar view of incisions. *Solid line,* Palmar incisions; *broken line,* dorsal incisions. **C,** Incisions from web space. *Solid line,* Dorsal incisions; *broken line,* palmar incisions. **D,** Flaps developed and elevated. **E,** Reconstruction of extensor tendon with graft; Kirschner wire stabilizes index to ring metacarpal. **F,** Flaps rotated. **G,** Appearance of palm after wound closure. (Redrawn from Ueba Y: J Hand Surg 6:557, 1981.)

ors or extensors, through appropriate incisions. Harvest the palmaris longus tendon to be used as a graft for the transfers. Secure the graft to the donor tendons with a Pulvertaft weave and secure the distal ends into the terminal phalanges of the border digits with pull-out wire.

AFTERTREATMENT. The wrist is splinted in mild flexion for 3 weeks; then the pull-out wire and skin sutures are removed. Normal activities are gradually resumed during the next 4 to 6 weeks.

ULNAR CLUBHAND–ULNAR DEFICIENCIES. Ulnar deficiencies are those malformations in which there is longitudinal failure of formation along the postaxial border of the upper extremity. The most common form is a partial deficiency of the ulna and the ulnar two digits, commonly referred to as *ulnar clubhand.* Other terms for this deformity include ulnar dysmelia, paraxial ulnar hemimelia, and congenital absence of the ulna. Ulnar deficiencies are among the rarest of congenital hand anomalies, with a relative incidence one tenth to one third that of radial deficiencies.

The cause of this rare anomaly is unknown, and its occurrence is sporadic. The only report that suggests a familial pattern is that of Roberts in 1886 in which he reported the deformity in three successive generations.

Swanson, Tada, and Yonenobu recognize four types of ulnar deficiency (Fig. 74-29): type 1, hypoplasia or partial defect of the ulna; type 2, total defect of the ulna; type 3, total or partial defect of the ulna with humeroradial synostosis; and type 4, total or partial defect of the ulna associated with congenital amputation at the wrist. Partial absence of the ulna is more common than total absence, the reverse of radial deficiencies. In Swanson et al.'s series 53.4% of patients had humeroradial synostosis and 5.7% had congenital amputations at the wrist.

Anomalies associated with ulnar deficiencies, unlike radial deficiencies, are almost solely limited to the musculoskeletal system and include clubfoot, fibular deficiencies, spina bifida, femoral agenesis, mandibular defects, and absence of the patella. Carpal bone deformities are common because of severe deformity and coalition. Digital malformation occurs in 89% of patients, and radial head dislocation is frequent.

Varying degrees of deficiency along the ulnar side of the hand are present at birth. The forearm usually is shortened and frequently bowed. The small and ring fingers usually are absent. Syndactyly of the remaining digits is common. The middle and index fingers, as well as the thumb, are absent in about two thirds of patients. Forearm bowing with radial convexity is caused by the tethering effect of the ulnar anlage. Ulnar deviation of the hand usually correlates with the degree of radial bowing and increased ulnar slope to the distal radius, as does supination deformity of the forearm. The elbow usually is restricted in motion and may be fused. The deformity is more commonly unilateral.

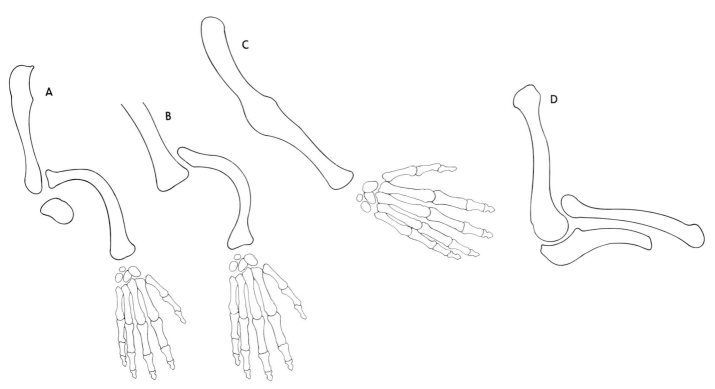

Fig. 74-29 Swanson's classification of ulnar deficiency. **A,** Type 1 — hypoplasia or partial defect of ulna. **B,** Type 2 — total defect of ulna. **C,** Type 3 — total or partial defect of ulna with humeroradial synostosis. **D,** Type 4 — total or partial defect of ulna with congenital amputation at wrist. (Redrawn from Swanson BA, Tada K, and Yonenobu K: J Hand Surg 9-A:658, 1984.)

Roentgenograms usually show a typical pattern (Fig. 74-30) of an absent distal ulna and a bowed radius with an increased ulnar slope along its distal articular surface. The pisiform and hamate usually are absent, and frequently there are coalitions of the other carpal bones. It often is difficult to determine the presence or absence of the proximal ulna because mineralization may not occur until the child is 1 year of age.

Nonsurgical management. Initial management of ulnar clubhand in the infant consists of corrective casting and splinting. A long arm cast is applied in the method of Riordan, applying the hand section first, then joining the hand to the forearm in the corrected position, and finally joining the forearm to the arm in 90 degrees of elbow flexion. Frequent cast changes are necessary and should be continued until correction is achieved. Removable splints may be used to maintain correction. This should be continued until the child is 6 months of age, at which time exploration and excision of the ulnar anlage should be considered if significant radial bowing is present.

Surgical treatment. Indications for surgical intervention are syndactyly, radial bowing and presence of an ulnar anlage, dislocation of the radial head with limited el-

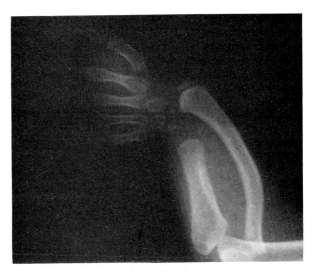

Fig. 74-30 Roentgenographic appearance of type I ulnar clubhand.

bow extension and forearm pronation and supination, and internal rotation deformity of the humerus. Surgical separation of the syndactyly should be performed in accordance with standard syndactyly protocol: separation of the thumb and index finger by 6 months of age and of the central syndactyly by 18 months of age. Malrotation, as well as syndactyly, of the thumb may require first metacarpal derotational osteotomy to correct the supination deformity. This procedure usually requires a local rotational flap to create the web and should be performed 6 months after syndactyly release.

Most authors agree that an ulnar anlage should be excised to prevent further radial bowing and shortening. Straub first called attention to the fibrocartilage anlage that spans the gap between proximal ulna and distal radius and ulnar carpus. This anlage does not appear to grow and acts as a tether to deform the radius and carpus with subsequent bowing of the radial shaft and dislocation of the radial head. Ogden, Watson, and Bohne recommend routine resection of the distal end of the fibrocartilaginous mass before the age of 2 to 3 years. Riordan recommends resection before 6 months of age. Broudy and Smith recommend removal of the distal ulnar anlage when there is progressive or severe ulnar deviation of the hand at the radiocarpal joint, increased radial bowing, or gradual dislocation of the radial head. If bowing is severe, wedge osteotomy of the radius may be necessary at the time of anlage excision.

If radial head dislocation blocks extension of the elbow, creation of a one-bone forearm should be considered. If the block in extension is acceptable and functional pronation and supination are preserved, then surgical treatment probably will not improve function. If there is marked shortening and bowing of the radius with considerable forearm instability and restriction of elbow motion, then creation of a one-bone forearm probably will improve function. For this procedure to be successful, some proximal ulna must be present. The proximal radius usually is excised several months before the creation of the one-bone forearm because simultaneous performance of the two procedures might be too extensive.

Internal rotation deformity of the humerus may be present with humeroradial synostosis and requires correction if it impairs function.

Rotational osteotomy of first metacarpal

■ *TECHNIQUE (BROUDY AND SMITH).* Under tourniquet control, make a transverse, racquet-shaped skin incision on the volar aspect and extend it to a V-shaped tongue at the middorsum of the first metacarpal. The apex of the V lies at the level of the first metacarpal base (Fig. 74-31, *A*) to allow adequate exposure for osteotomy. Make a proximal longitudinal incision on the radiovolar side of the first metacarpal, 120 degrees from the apex of the V (Fig. 74-31, *B*). Perform an osteotomy of the base of the first

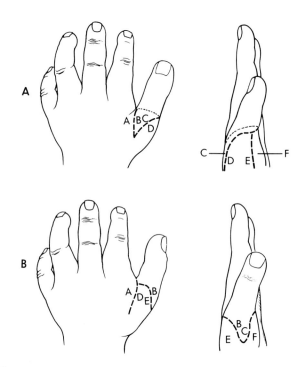

Fig. 74-31 Rotational osteotomy of first metacarpal. **A,** Incision. **B,** After osteotomy, dorsal V-flap is rotated volarly. (Redrawn from Broudy AS and Smith RJ: J Hand Surg 4:304, 1979.)

metacarpal and position the metacarpal in the desired amount of pronation. Fix the metacarpal in position with Kirschner wires, suture the V flap into the opened linear incision, and close the V defect in a side-to-side manner. Apply a long arm cast.
AFTERTREATMENT. The cast is removed 6 weeks after surgery, and progressive activity is begun. Kirschner wires are removed 6 weeks after surgery or when bone healing is complete. A removable, short arm, thumb spica splint is worn during sleep for another 6 weeks.

Excision of ulnar anlage

■ *TECHNIQUE (FLATT).* Under tourniquet control, make a lazy-S incision along the postaxial border, carrying it across the wrist crease to the midcarpal level. Because of the absence of the extrinsic flexor muscles, the ulnar neurovascular bundle and the anlage lie close together in the subcutaneous tissues. Free and protect the neurovascular bundle before dissecting the anlage off its carpal attachment. Remove at least one third of the forearm length. Incise the soft tissues on the ulnar side of the wrist joint sufficiently to allow full correction of the hand on the distal radial articular surface. The hand should flop over into neutral or even slight radial deviation; if it must be pushed into neutral, release more of the soft tissue. Close the wound with nonab-

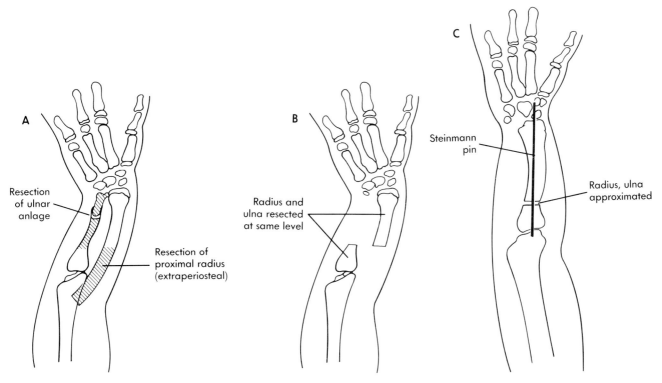

Fig. 74-32 Creation of one-bone forearm. **A,** Resection of distal ulnar anlage and proximal radius *(shaded areas).* **B,** Alignment of distal radius and proximal ulna. **C,** Kirschner wire extending into carpals used to stabilize radial and ulnar segments.

sorbable sutures and apply a well-molded, long arm cast.

AFTERTREATMENT. The sutures are removed at 3 weeks, and the cast is changed. The cast is removed 6 weeks after surgery, and normal activities are resumed gradually during the next 4 to 6 weeks.

Creation of one-bone forearm

■ *TECHNIQUE (STRAUB).* Make a curved longitudinal dorsoradial incision beginning just proximal to the elbow and ending at the middle or distal third of the forearm. Expose and excise the fibrocartilaginous band that extends distally from the ulnar fragment; in excising this band, free its proximal end by performing an osteotomy on the distal end of the fragment. Next expose the radial nerve at the elbow and trace it distally to its interosseous branch; this branch and its enclosing supinator muscle may be grossly displaced by the dislocation of the proximal radius. Develop the cleavage between the dorsal and volar muscles of the forearm while carefully protecting the important neurovascular structures in the antecubital area. Then at the level of the distal end of the ulnar fragment, divide the radial shaft and excise its proximal part, including the radial head (Fig. 74-32, *A*). Place the proximal end of the distal radial fragment against the distal end of the ulnar fragment (Fig. 74-32, *B*) and fix them together with

a Kirschner wire passed distally through the olecranon (Fig. 74-32, *C*). Close the skin with absorbable or nonabsorbable sutures. Apply a long arm cast with the elbow flexed about 90 degrees.

AFTERTREATMENT. The cast is changed 2 weeks after surgery, and any remaining sutures are removed. A long arm cast is worn for a total of 8 weeks after surgery. The cast and Kirschner wire or Steinmann pin fixation are removed at 8 weeks or when bone healing is complete. Normal activities are resumed after another 6 to 8 weeks.

FAILURE OF DIFFERENTIATION
Syndactyly

Syndactyly, or "webbed fingers," is due to the failure of the fingers to separate during embryologic development. It is the most common congenital anomaly of the hand, occurring in 1:2000 births. The specific cause is unknown, but it is believed to result from an abnormal slowing of growth and development of the finger buds during the seventh and eighth weeks of gestation. Although most are sporadic occurrences, Flatt found a family history of syndactyly in 40% of his patients, which suggests heredity as one factor. Several pedigrees have shown an autosomal dominant trait for long–ring finger syndactyly, but penetrance has been incomplete.

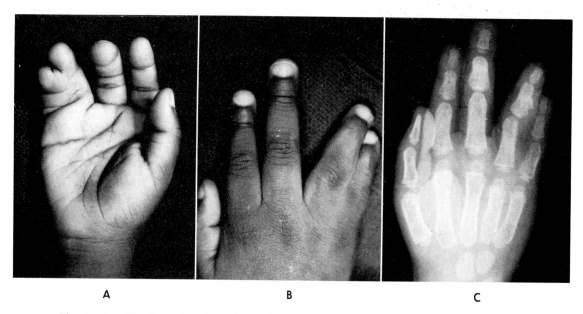

Fig. 74-33 Simple syndactyly in 5-year-old child. Fingers are bridged only by skin and other soft tissues. **A,** Palmar view. **B,** Dorsal view. **C,** Roentgenogram. Note angular deformity of ring finger.

Syndactylies are classified as complete or incomplete and as simple or complex. Complete syndactyly is present when the fingers are joined from the web to the fingertip; incomplete syndactyly indicates that the fingers are joined from the web to a point proximal to the fingertips. Simple syndactyly exists when only skin or other soft tissue bridges the fingers (Fig. 74-33); complex syndactyly occurs when there are common bony elements shared by involved fingers (Fig. 74-34). Acrosyndactyly refers to lateral fusion of adjacent digits at their distal ends with proximal fenestrations between the joined digits. Brachysyndactyly denotes associated shortening of the syndactyl digits. Anomalies that may be found in association with syndactyly include webbing of the toes, polydactyly, constriction rings, brachydactyly, cleft feet, hemangioma, absence of muscles, spinal deformities, funnel chest, and heart disorders. Apert's syndrome and Poland's syndrome characteristically include multiple syndactylies.

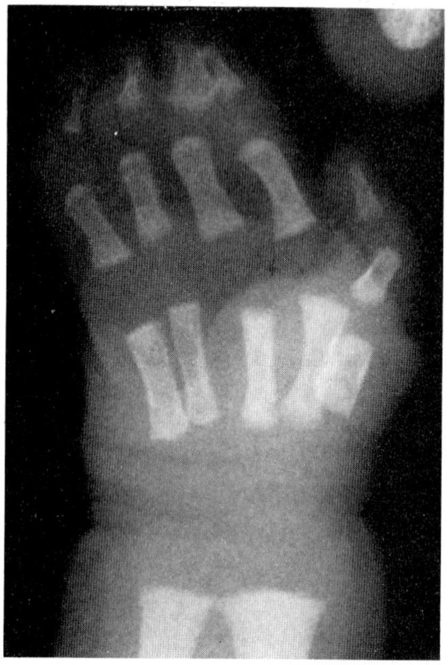

Syndactyly occurs between the long and ring fingers

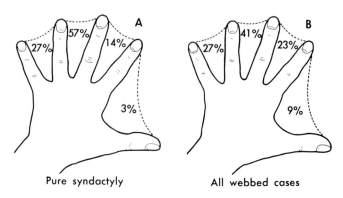

Fig. 74-35 Site of syndactyly. **A,** Percentage incidence when only true syndactyly of simple or complex type is considered. **B,** Total count incidence in which associated conditions (all webbed digits) are included. (From Flatt AE: Practical factors in the treatment of syndactylism. In Littler JW et al: Symposium of reconstructive hand surgery, vol 9, St Louis, 1974, Mosby–Year Book, Inc.)

Fig. 74-34 Complex syndactyly. Common bony elements are shared by involved fingers.

in more than 50% of patients (Fig. 74-35); the fourth web, second web, and first web are affected in diminishing frequencies. The syndactyly is bilateral in about half the patients, and boys are more frequently affected than are girls. The intervening skin usually is normal although deficient in surface area compared with the normal hand, a fact that is important in the consideration of surgical correction. The two nails may be completely separate, or the digits may share a common nail without intervening eponychium. If the fingers are of relatively similar length, flexion and extension usually are normal. Abnormally tight fascial bands usually are present within the web, minimizing any lateral movement between the involved digits. Frequently there are anomalous sharings of musculotendinous units, nerves, and vessels between joined digits. The phalanges usually are normal in the simple pattern; in the complex pattern, however, various interosseous connections range from duplication patterns, to branching patterns, to shared patterns. Differentiation of the joints also may be incomplete. Rarely is there any angular deformity of the digits at birth unless a delta phalanx is present. If a central syndactyly involves the middle and ring or middle and index fingers, angular deformities develop slowly. If, however, the syndactyly involves the ring and little fingers or index finger and thumb, then a gradual flexion contracture, lateral deviation, and rotation deformity usually develop in the longer of the two digits within the first year of life. In Poland's syndactyly or syndrome the sternocostal portion of the ipsilateral pectoralis major muscle is absent. The hand deformity includes unilateral shortening of the index, long, and ring fingers; multiple simple incomplete syndactylies; and hypoplasia of the hand (Fig. 74-36).

TREATMENT. Surgical intervention is not urgent. While awaiting the appropriate age for reconstruction, parents should be encouraged to massage the web in an attempt to stretch the intervening skin to facilitate later surgery. Surgical reconstruction is best done before the child is of school age. Kettlekamp and Flatt found results to be better in children older than 18 months at the time of correction, especially in the final appearance of the commissure. There is a tendency for the web to migrate distally and the commissure to contract if surgery is performed at an earlier age. If the syndactyly involves the second or third web space and there are no other deformities of the involved fingers, surgery should be delayed until the child is at least 18 months of age. When digits of different sizes are completely involved, whether the syndactyly is simple or complex, early separation, between the ages of 6 and 12 months, is best because of the likelihood of angular, rotational, and flexion deformities. These deformities are difficult to correct, and preventing them takes precedence over the possibility of distal web migration and commissure contracture. When multiple digits are involved, the border digits should be

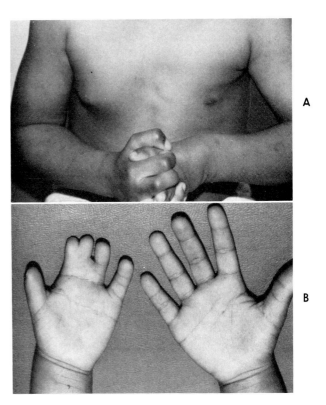

Fig. 74-36   Poland's syndrome in 9-year-old child. **A,** Hypoplasia of pectoralis major muscle. **B,** Brachysyndactyly. (Courtesy Dr. George L Burruss, Memphis.)

released early, followed by subsequent releases after a 6-month waiting period. Simultaneous releases of the radial and ulnar sides of a finger are contraindicated and may jeopardize the viability of the finger.

The surgical procedure includes three technical steps: separation of the digits, commissure reconstruction, and resurfacing of the intervening borders of the digits. Early attempts at separation incorporated such techniques as passage of setons, use of ligatures, and straight linear incisions. Pieri in 1949 condemned the use of straight incisions and favored a zigzag incision to prevent linear contracture along the long axis of the finger; all currently accepted methods incorporate this principle. Shared digital nerves are carefully split longitudinally to preserve innervation to both digits. Common digital arteries may extend into the web and require ligation of one of more branches. Care should be taken to avoid devascularizing the digit. When the nail is shared, an additional longitudinal strip of nail and underlying matrix usually must be removed to match the normal nail width. Osseous structures usually are divided longitudinally with a scalpel if the procedure is performed at an early age.

Special attention must be given to the reconstruction of the web commissure. The normal commissure has a sloping configuration from proximal dorsal to distal palmar. Dorsally it begins at about the level of the transverse metacarpal ligament and extends distally and palmarward to about the level of the proximal digital flexion crease, usually at about the midpoint of the bony proximal phalanx. Distally the commissure forms a rectangle between the small, ring, index, and middle fingers. In some hands the commissure between the middle and ring fingers forms a V or ∪ shape. The distal web span must be greater than the proximal web span to allow abduction of the fingers about the axis of the metacarpophalangeal joint. In recreating a commissure with normal appearance and function, a properly designed local flap generally is preferable to a skin graft to minimize commissure contracture. Numerous local flaps have been designed, but the most commonly used are the dorsal "pantaloon" flap described by Bauer, Tondra, and Trusler, the matching volar and dorsal proximally based V-shaped flaps conceived by Zeller and popularized by Cronin and by Skoog, and the "butterfly" flap devised by Shaw et al. Woolf and Broadbent described the butterfly flap as useful for partial simple syndactyly that ends proximal to the proximal interphalangeal joint (Fig. 74-37).

Regardless of flap design, in resurfacing the intervening borders of the digits, there never is enough skin for primary closure of each digit. This phenomenon can be clearly demonstrated to the parents by comparing the sum of the circumferences of two individual fingers with that of the circumference of two fingers held together; the latter is always less. The zigzag incision is designed to create interdigitating volar and dorsal flaps for one finger; the other finger requires either full- or split-thickness skin grafting (full-thickness grafting usually is preferred). Grafts should be avoided at the base of the ring finger where wearing of a ring may be bothersome. The parents should be informed that recurrence and angular deformity are possible despite a well-designed and well-executed reconstruction and that future revision may be necessary. Toledo and Ger found reoperation necessary

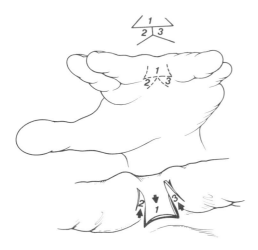

Fig. 74-37 Butterfly flap technique for release of syndactyly. Flaps are designed in web space to form dorsal rectangle; then flaps are rotated to deepen web. (Redrawn from Woolf RM and Broadbent TR: Plast Reconstr Surg 49:48, 1972.)

in 59% of patients with major associated anomalies and in 30% of patients with syndactyly as the primary abnormality.

The most common complication of syndactyly reconstruction is scar deformity of the digit or web. Distal migration of the web may occur, particularly if surgery is performed before the child is 18 months old. The most catastrophic complication is circulatory insufficiency to the finger, resulting in loss of the digit. This rarely has been reported and should not occur if the syndactyly on each side of the finger is released in stages.

Syndactyly release with dorsal flap

■ **TECHNIQUE (BAUER ET AL).** Outline all incisions carefully with a skin-marking pen (Fig. 74-38, *A* and *B*). First, cut a single rectangular skin flap from the dorsal surface of the two webbed fingers for the new web between these fingers. Base it proximally at the level of an adjacent normal web; make it wide enough to form a normal web and long enough to reach the palmar edge of the new web. Now separate the fingers with longitudinal dorsal and palmar incisions on the ring finger along the ulnar side of the abnormal web (toward the radial side of the ring finger); locate and curve these incisions so that they outline the flaps that will cover the ulnar side of the middle finger. Take care not to injure the digital nerve of the ring finger. Raise these flaps and remove from them any excess subcutaneous fat to give the middle finger a more normal shape. Suture them together on the ulnar side of the middle finger; then suture the web flap in place (Fig. 74-38, *C*). Cover the defect on the ring finger with a full-thickness free graft taken from the groin. If the fingernails are confluent, they should be separated, and the matrix at their margins should be removed so that the grafts can be brought around to the edge of each nail. When a finger is webbed on both sides, it is safer to separate only one side at a time.

Place Xeroform gauze over the grafts and then carefully insert a wet contour dressing between the fingers; begin at the web space and pack distally so that the fingers are held in wide abduction and extension. Then apply a dry dressing and a plaster splint to immobilize the fingers and wrist.
AFTERTREATMENT. The hand is elevated for a week or more before redressing.

Syndactyly release with matching volar and dorsal proximally based V-shaped flaps

■ **TECHNIQUE (SKOOG).** With a skin pencil outline the incisions to be made on the fingers. Design dorsal and volar flaps so that when mobilized they will cover most of the denuded side of one finger without tension (Fig. 74-39, *A* and *B*). Make the free borders of the flaps irregular by designing small triangular points at the level of the interphalangeal joints. In planning the flaps so that they fit each other, first outline the incision on one side and then establish the key points for the incision on the opposite side by pushing straight needles vertically through the web. Then elevate the tourniquet and raise the flaps consisting mainly of the skin that forms the abnormal web. In raising the flaps preserve all subcutane-

ous tissue and be careful not to sever digital nerves and arteries. Then release the tourniquet and control all bleeding. Using the triangular flaps, reconstruct the web space (Fig 74-39, *C*). On one finger close the flaps as planned and cover the small remaining defect at the dorsomedial aspect of the base of this finger (Fig. 74-39, *D*) by a full-thickness skin graft obtained from the inguinal region. Then make a pattern of the denuded area on the adjacent finger and on the new web and obtain a matching full-thickness graft again from the inguinal region. Carefully suture the graft in place (Fig. 74-39, *E*) and close the donor area. Then apply a pressure dressing: place Xeroform gauze over the grafts and suture lines, spread the fingers widely and place between them wet cotton pressed to fit the contours of the

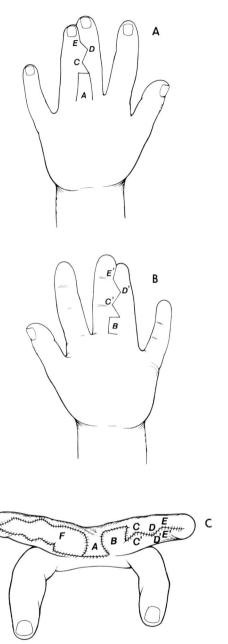

Fig. 74-38 Syndactyly release. **A,** Dorsal skin incisions. Rectangular dorsal flap *(A)* is designed for web; alternating flaps *(C, D,* and *E)* are arranged to interdigitate with volar flaps. **B,** Palmar skin incisions. Rectangular flap *(B)* is arranged to cover radial side of ring finger; remaining flaps *(C', D', E')* are arranged to interdigitate with dorsal flaps. **C,** Separation is completed; flaps have been sutured into place, covering radial side of ring finger and web. Skin graft is required for ulnar side of middle finger. (Redrawn from Bauer TB, Tondra JM, and Trusler HM: Plast Reconstr Surg 17:385, 1956.)

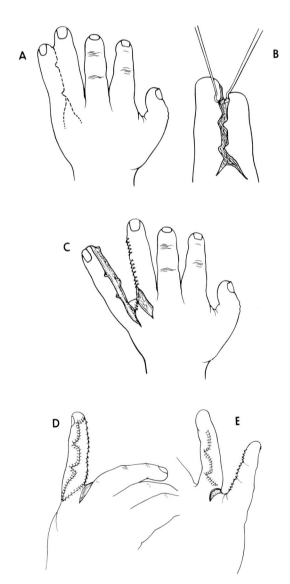

Fig. 74-39 Skoog technique for syndactyly. **A** and **B,** Dorsal and volar skin incisions. **C,** Web space reconstruction; closure of ring finger. **D** and **E,** Dorsal and volar views: skin graft in place on little finger and graft in web space.

fingers and web, and then wrap on dry gauze and Webril. Next apply a plaster splint; extend it proximal to the elbow if necessary to ensure sufficient immobilization.

When more than two fingers are involved in the syndactyly, it is safer to separate only one side of a single finger at a time.

AFTERTREATMENT. The hand is elevated for at least 3 days after surgery. At 10 to 14 days the dressing is changed, with the patient under general anesthesia if necessary. Sutures may be removed at this time. Another bandage is maintained for an additional 10 to 14 days, and gradual resumption of normal activities is allowed.

Apert's Syndrome

In 1906 Apert described a patient with a group of deformities that included atypical facies and multiple complex syndactylies of the hand, which he called *acrocephalosyndactyly.* Despite its rarity (1:200,00 births), much has been written about the management of the complex hand deformities in this syndrome. The condition is believed to result from a single gene mutation in one of the parents and can be passed in dominant and recessive forms; sporadic occurrences also are possible. Apert's syndrome was classified into two main categories by Blank: true or typical, characterized by multiple complex syndactylies, and atypical, with only partial syndactylies.

At birth these patients have a high, broad forehead and a flattened occiput. The eyes are widely set, with the outer canthus lower than the inner canthus. The lower jaw is prominent, and the maxilla is shortened (Fig. 74-40, *A*). Mental retardation is common but not universal. There may be associated visceral abnormalities. These patients usually can be expected to live well into adulthood. The hand deformities are typically symmetric. The hand is spoon shaped, with a tapering terminal end and complex syndactyly of the index, middle, and ring fingers (Fig. 74-40, *B*). The little finger usually shows complete simple syndactyly with the ring finger. Often a nail is shared between the index, long, and ring fingers. Syndactyly also may occur between the thumb and index finger. The fingers have limited motion because of incomplete joint development, and they usually are shortened. Five digits usually are present, distinguishing Apert's syndrome from Carpenter's syndrome (acrocephalopolysyndactyly), in which polydactyly also is present. The arm and forearm frequently are shortened with limited elbow motion. The untreated hand functions in a spoonlike fashion with either a two-handed or a thumb-to-side-of-index finger prehensile pattern.

TREATMENT. Reconstructive surgery usually improves hand function in these patients by creating a three-fingered hand with an opposable thumb. The surgical management should follow the protocol outlined by

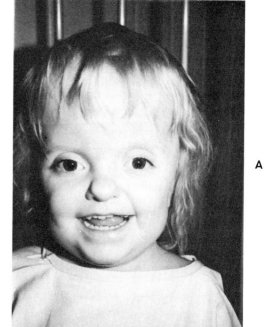
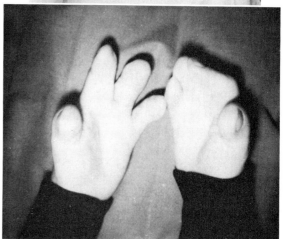

Fig. 74-40 Apert's syndrome. **A,** Characteristic facial features of high forehead and wide-set eyes. **B,** Complex syndactyly involving all fingers of both hands; left hand has had syndactyly release.

Flatt. In the child younger than 2 years, bilateral simultaneous reconstructive procedures may be carried out because the child is not dependent on self-care. In the older child only one hand at a time should be reconstructed. The border digits should be released before the child is 1 year old. If the thumb is not included in the syndactyly, a simple four-part Z-plasty is used to deepen the first web. Six to 9 months later, release of the central syndactylies and deletion of the middle finger at the metacarpophalangeal joint are performed. This deletion provides the necessary skin coverage and good sensibility to the remaining digits. Flatt found more deformity in patients with a ray amputation of the middle finger and ulnar transposition of the index finger, and this procedure is not recommended.

■ *TECHNIQUE (FLATT)*. Stage I, release of the border digits, is performed before the age of 1 year. After application and inflation of a tourniquet, incise the border syndactylies as described by Bauer et al. to release the small, ring, and index fingers and the thumb. If the thumb is not included in the syndactyly, deepen the web with a four-part Z-plasty (p. 3403). Close the skin flaps with interrupted sutures and cover the remaining defects with a full-thickness skin graft.

Stage II is performed 6 to 9 months later to allow for revascularization and softening of the tissues. Make the incisions on the long finger to create flaps as described by Bauer et al. (p. 3388), using all the skin overlying the middle digit. After the flaps are elevated, amputate the middle digit at the metacarpophalangeal joint. Use the overlying skin to reconstruct the remaining commissure between the index and ring fingers and to cover the fingers. Close the flaps in routine fashion and use a full-thickness skin graft if necessary to cover the remaining defects. Apply sterile dressings of moistened cotton batting between the webs and apply a plaster splint to maintain positioning. The splint is worn for 4 weeks, and then active motion of the hand is encouraged.

DUPLICATION (POLYDACTYLY)

Duplication of digits, or polydactyly, is a common and conspicuous hand anomaly. It was recorded in biblical literature as long ago as 3000 years, and approximately 9000 to 10,000 new cases are recorded each year. Polydactyly is classified into three main categories: preaxial — duplication of the thumb (bifid thumb); central — duplication of the index, middle, or ring fingers; and postaxial — duplication of the small finger. Also included in the general category of duplication is ulnar dimelia, or mirror hand, an exceedingly rare anomaly.

Preaxial Polydactyly (Bifid Thumb)

The bifid thumb represents a complete or partial duplication of the thumb (Fig. 74-41). It is the most common duplication pattern in white and Oriental populations, occurring in 1:3000 births. It usually is unilateral; only 9 of 70 patients in Wassel's series had bilateral involvement. The cause of the bifid thumb is unknown. Most occur sporadically, which suggests environmental factors rather than genetic predisposition. Preaxial polydactyly has been produced in the offspring of rats by the administration of cytosine arabinoside during pregnancy. When the thumb duplication is associated with a triphalangeal thumb, an autosomal dominant pattern and sporadic occurrence have been identified. Bifid thumb typically occurs as an isolated deformity unassociated with other malformation syndromes, but visceral anomalies have been rarely reported, particularly hand-heart or Holt-Oram syndrome.

Wassel described a group of 70 patients with bifid thumbs and suggested a now widely used classification (Fig. 74-42): type I, partial duplication of the distal phalanx and a common epiphysis; type II, complete duplication, including the epiphysis of the distal phalanx; type III, duplication of the distal phalanx and bifurcation of the proximal phalanx; type IV, complete duplication of the distal and proximal phalanges; type V, complete duplication of the distal and proximal phalanges with bifurcation of the metacarpal; type VI, complete duplication of the distal and proximal phalanges and the metacarpal; and type VII, variable degrees of duplication associated with a triphalangeal thumb. In Wassel's series type IV was the most common pattern (47%), followed by type VII (20%) and type II (15%). Wood found that type IV and type VII deformities could be further subdivided depending on the extent of duplication and triphalangism.

The deformity usually is unilateral, and clinical appearance varies from mild widening of the thumb tip to complete duplication of the entire thumb. Typically there is some degree of hypoplasia of both duplicates, and more commonly the radial duplicate is the more hypoplastic. There may be convergence or divergence of the duplications. Occasionally the thumb has decreased pronation, placing it in the same plane as the other digits. Anatomic dissections have revealed fibrous interconnections between the two thumbs. The nail may be one large, conjoined nail with a central longitudinal groove, or it may be completely duplicated. The ulnar-innervated intrinsic muscles to the thumb (adductor pollicis and deep head of the flexor pollicis brevis) typically insert on the ulnarmost thumb duplicate, and the median-innervated intrinsic muscles to the thumb (abductor pollicis, superficial head of the flexor pollicis brevis, and opponens pollicis) typically insert on the radialmost thumb duplicate. Extrinsic flexor and extensor tendons may be duplicated and usually are eccentrically placed along each thumb. The phalanges may be angulated, and there may be an associated delta phalanx. The joints usually are stiff, with a widened joint surface. The collateral ligaments of the duplicated joints often are shared, with insufficiency in the space along the adjacent sides. Wide variations may occur in the neurovascular anatomy. Both radial and ulnar neurovascular bundles to the digits may be completely duplicated or may be shared with small separate branches that supply the individual digits.

TREATMENT. Surgical correction of the bifid thumb almost always is indicated, not only for the obvious cosmetic improvement but also for better function. Occasionally, if the thumb appears only slightly broader than expected, with underlying roentgenographic evidence of duplication, then surgery might not improve the condi-

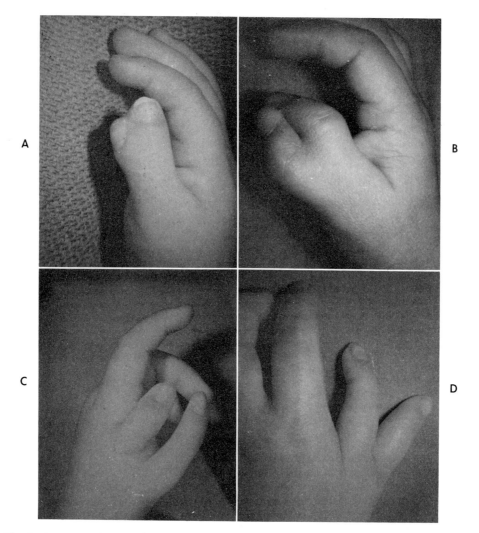

Fig. 74-41   Varied manifestations of bifid thumb ranging from partial (**A**) to complete (**D**) duplication of thumb. Wassel's type IV (**B**) is the most common.

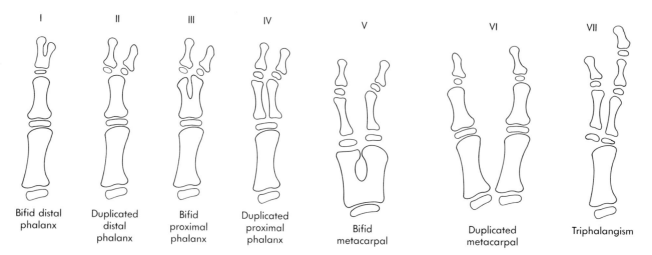

I	II	III	IV	V	VI	VII
Bifid distal phalanx	Duplicated distal phalanx	Bifid proximal phalanx	Duplicated proximal phalanx	Bifid metacarpal	Duplicated metacarpal	Triphalangism

Fig. 74-42   Wassel's classification of thumb polydactyly. (Redrawn from Wassel HD: Clin Orthop 64:175, 1969.)

tion. Surgical reconstruction generally is performed when the child is about 18 months of age but no later than 5 years of age if possible. Later revisions may be required, and fusions needed for late angular deformities and instability may be performed at around 8 to 10 years of age. Simple excision of the more hypoplastic digit rarely results in a satisfactory thumb because of progressive angulation and instability. For types I and possibly II bifid thumbs in which there is only partial duplication of the nail, a combination procedure (Bilhaut-Cloquet) is recommended. More proximal duplication requires excision of the most hypoplastic thumb, narrowing of the widened proximal articular surface, ligament reconstruction, intrinsic transfer, and centralization of the extrinsic flexor and extensor tendons if necessary. In general, the ulnarmost thumb should be preserved. Preoperative splinting, as recommended by Isasawa et al., may be beneficial; however, we have not attempted this.

Late angular deformity and instability are the most frequent complications, and these may require further ligament reconstruction, corrective closing wedge osteotomy, or perhaps arthrodesis. Miura has successfully treated this Z-collapse at the thumb interphalangeal joint with a rotation skin flap on the concave side of the deformity, combined with excision of the radial half of the extensor tendon and transfer of the flexor tendon into the ulnar side of the distal phalanx. Other reported complications include infection and deformity, scar contracture, joint stiffness, inadequate tendon excursion, residual prominence at the previous site of duplication, and a narrowed first web space. Loss of sensibility or viability of the digit rarely is encountered if surgical details are carefully observed.

Types I and II bifid thumbs

■ *TECHNIQUE* (*BILHAUT-CLOQUET;* Fig. 74-43). Under tourniquet control, make a central wedge-shaped incision from dorsal to palmar over the involved thumb tip, extending proximally to the level of bifurcation. The dorsal component of the incision will pass through the nail and nail bed. Incise the cen-

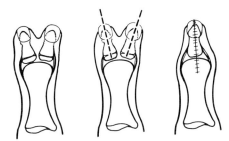

Fig. 74-43 Bilhaut-Cloquet technique for symmetric thumb duplication in which duplicate digits are joined at midline after excision of excess central soft and osseous tissue (see text). (Redrawn from Marks TW and Bayne LG: J Hand Surg 3:107, 1978.)

tral component of the underlying tendon and bone of the duplicated structures in line with the skin incision. Carefully approximate the articular surface and epiphysis of the remaining parts of the distal phalanx and secure them with a transverse Kirschner wire. This may be difficult because of tightening of the collateral ligaments. Carefully suture the nail bed with 6-0 absorbable suture and close the skin with interrupted sutures. Apply a short or long arm thumb spica cast, depending on the patient's age. Younger children require the long arm cast.

AFTERTREATMENT. The cast is removed 4 to 6 weeks after surgery, and the Kirschner wire may be removed 6 weeks after surgery. Progressively increased use is allowed after removal of the cast and wire.

Types III through VI bifid thumbs

■ *TECHNIQUE (LAMB; MARKS AND BAYNE).* Under tourniquet control, make a racquet-shaped incision over the most hypoplastic thumb (usually the radialmost digit). If the ulnar thumb is the more affected, it should be removed instead. Through the incision expose the abductor pollicis brevis tendon as it inserts into the proximal phalanx of the radialmost thumb and carefully preserve this tendon. If the ulnar thumb is to be excised, then identify the adductor pollicis and carefully preserve it. Detach the collateral ligament distally from the phalanx that is to be excised. Strip the collateral ligament proximally off the metacarpal or phalanx with a strip of periosteum to allow adequate exposure of the joint. Excise the supernumerary digit with the part of the metacarpal or phalanx with which it articulates (Fig. 74-44, *A*). Centralize the remaining digit over the remaining articular surface (Fig. 74-44, *B*) and suture the collateral ligament and intrinsic tendon securely to the phalanx (Fig. 74-44, *C*). Secure this alignment with a longitudinal Kirschner wire placed across the joint (Fig. 74-44, *D*). Check the alignment of the extensor and flexor tendons to ensure that they track centrally along the digit. Partial resection or transfer of the tendons may be required to achieve a central line of pull. Close the skin with simple interrupted sutures. A Z-plasty also may be required if there is inadequate skin along the ulnar border for a tension-free closure.

AFTERTREATMENT. The thumb is immobilized for about 4 weeks, at which time the wire may be removed and the hand mobilized. A protective splint may be required for another 3 to 4 weeks.

Triphalangeal Thumb

As the name implies, the triphalangeal thumb has three phalanges instead of the normal two. This uncom-

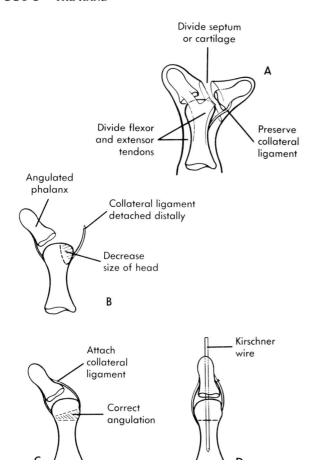

Fig. 74-44 Technique for asymmetric duplication (see text). **A,** Removal of less functional component. **B,** Transfer of collateral ligament. **C,** Osteotomy of proximal phalanx. **D,** Kirschner wire fixation. (Redrawn from Marks TW and Bayne LG: J Hand Surg 3:107, 1978.)

mon anomaly, which can be inherited as an autosomal dominant trait, has been associated with maternal use of thalidomide. Two major types of triphalangeal thumbs are most common: one has a small, wedge-shaped extra ossicle (delta phalanx, p. 3418) that causes an angular deformity without significantly increasing thumb length; the other has an extra phalanx that is normal or nearly normal and creates the appearance of a five-fingered hand (Fig. 74-45). Buck-Gramcko described a transitional type in which a trapezoidal extra phalanx causes both increased length and angular deformity (Fig. 74-46). The triphalangeal thumb also has been classified as opposable or nonopposable. The most common hand anomaly associated with triphalangeal thumb is a bifid

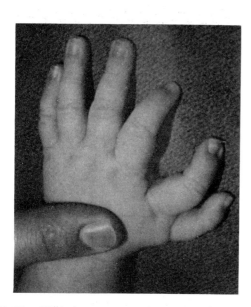

Fig. 74-45 Clinical appearance of triphalangeal thumb associated with duplication (Wassel's type VII).

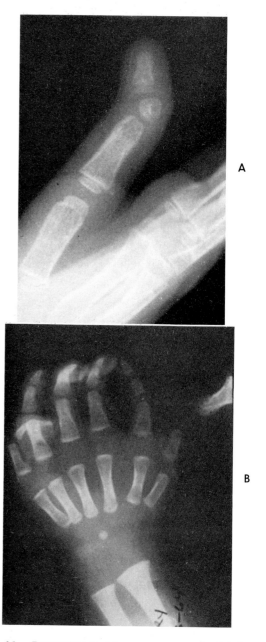

Fig. 74-46 Roentgenographic appearance of triphalangeal thumb. **A,** Type I. **B,** Type II with associated duplication.

thumb; other associated conditions include cleft foot, tibial defects, congenital heart disease, Fanconi's anemia, anomalies of the gastrointestinal tract, and chromosomal anomalies.

In type I deformities (delta phalanx) the thumb is deviated ulnarward in the area of the interphalangeal joint. Roentgenograms show either a delta phalanx or a trapezoidal extra phalanx. In type II deformities (five-fingered hand) the thumb is longer than normal and lies in the same plane as the other fingers. Extra skin creases overlie the additional interphalangeal joint. Patients with type II deformities are unable to oppose the thumb to the other digits and tend to use side-to-side prehension. Hypoplasia of the thenar muscles often is associated with type II deformities and further hinders opposition. Polydactyly usually is present, and 60% of patients have significant web space contractures. Roentgenograms show a complete extra, rectangular phalanx; the duplicated phalanx typically is the middle phalanx.

TREATMENT. Although nonsurgical treatment does not correct the condition, surgical intervention is not required for all children with triphalangeal thumbs, especially those with type I deformities. The goals of surgical treatment are correction of angular deformity, restoration of normal length, correction of web contracture, and improvement of opposition. Removal of the abnormal phalanx along with reconstruction of the collateral ligament allows remodeling of the joint surfaces and usually provides adequate stability, especially if performed during the first year of life; however, Wood reported late instability and angular deformity in 10 of 29 patients after ligamentous reconstruction. Reduction osteotomy, as described by Peimer, will correct the angulation deformity with less chance of ligamentous instability. This osteotomy is best performed when the child is between 24 and 30 months of age and the epiphysis is clearly visible on the roentgenogram. Late instability can be treated with arthrodesis. Contracture of the first web space may be released with a four-part Z-plasty as described by Woolf and Broadbent (p. 3403). Severe contracture may require a dorsal rotation flap as described by Strauch and Spinner. Thenar hypoplasia may require opponensplasty with the use of the abductor digiti minimi (p. 3372) or ring sublimis (p. 3404). For type II deformity (five-fingered hand), pollicization of the radialmost digit, as described by Buck-Gramcko (p. 3372), is recommended.

Surgical correction also may be required for associated anomalies such as polydactyly. Wood outlined treatment guidelines for duplication associated with triphalangism of the thumb. If the duplication is Wassell's type IV (p. 3391), the radialmost digit should be excised when the child is about 6 months old. In Wassell's type VII duplication (complete duplication), the triphalangeal thumb should be removed. The remaining thumb may require web reconstruction and metacarpal osteotomy to complete the pollicization.

Reduction osteotomy

■ *TECHNIQUE (PEIMER).* Mark the preoperative roentgenograms, or make a sketch of the phalangeal and epiphyseal deformities, to plan the location of the osteotomies and the amount to be resected. Use a skin-marking pen to mark the curved dorsal incision, including the nail and matrix that must be removed (Fig. 74-47, *A*). Make a curved incision through the nail, matrix, and skin down to the level of the paratenon. Elevate skin flaps and expose the middle and distal phalanges by dividing and reflecting the extensor pollicis longus tendon just proximal to its insertion on the distal phalanx. Use a scalpel or fine bone-cutting forceps to narrow the distal phalanx to the desired width, taking care to avoid fragmenting the phalanx. Expose the distal phalangeal epiphysis with the first longitudinal cut (Fig. 74-47, *B*). With a scalpel perform a transverse osteotomy, completely excising the epiphysis (Fig. 74-47, *C*). Perform a second transverse osteotomy in the middle of the middle phalanx distal to the normal horizontal portion of the epiphysis. Confirm that the second osteotomy is parallel with the proximal interphalangeal joint by inserting a thin hypodermic needle into the joint to determine the joint

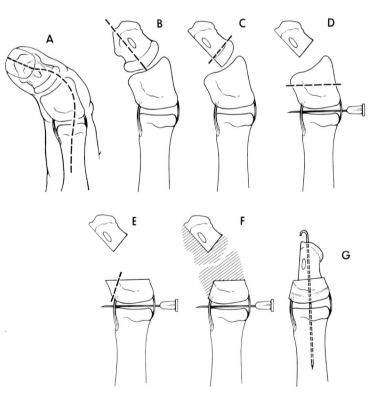

Fig. 74-47 Reduction osteotomy (see text). **A,** Dorsal incision. **B,** Narrowing of distal phalanx. **C,** Excision of distal epiphysis. **D,** Needle placed across interphalangeal joint to orient transverse osteotomy. **E,** Completion of osteotomy. **F,** Combined osteotomies form closing wedge to shorten and realign thumb. **G,** Bone ends are fixed with smooth wires. (Redrawn from Peimer CA: J Hand Surg 10-A:376, 1985.)

line (Fig. 74-47, *D*). With the second transverse osteotomy, expose the abnormal longitudinal portion of the **C**-shaped middle phalangeal epiphysis and completely excise the distal portion of the middle phalanx and the abnormal epiphysis without cutting the collateral ligament (Fig. 74-47, *E*). After removing the bone fragments, place the remaining bone in a closing-wedge position to realign and shorten the thumb (Fig. 74-47, *F* and *G*). If necessary, use bone-cutting forceps or a small rasp to contour the bony surfaces. Align the bone ends and fix them with one or two smooth 0.028-inch or 0.035-inch Kirschner wires. Transfix the retained interphalangeal joint if additional stability is needed. Check the adequacy of resection and realignment, and confirm the Kirschner wire placement and phalangeal position with roentgenograms. Shorten and repair the extensor pollicis longus tendon with fine sutures. Release the tourniquet, excise redundant skin, and close the wound. Cut and bend the Kirschner wires, leaving them protruding through the skin. Apply a long plaster, opponens gauntlet splint that extends above the elbow.

AFTERTREATMENT. If necessary, the splint can be removed for wound inspection during the first 2 to 3 weeks after surgery, but the hand is kept well splinted for 6 to 8 weeks. The Kirschner wires are removed after 6 to 8 weeks or when bone healing is evident on roentgenograms. Splinting usually is not required after pin removal. Physical therapy may be helpful in regaining motion in older patients.

Postaxial Polydactyly

Duplication of the small finger is the most common pattern of duplication in the black population. It occurs in approximately 1:300 black births, with a relative frequency of 8:1 compared with duplication of other digits. The true incidence is impossible to determine because many of these children have the extra digit removed in the nursery, although this probably is done less frequently than in the past. Stelling, as well as Turek, classified postaxial polydactyly into three types based on the degree of duplication: type 1, duplication of soft parts only; type 2, partial duplication of the digit, including the osseous structures (Fig. 74-48); and type 3, complete duplication of the ray, including the metacarpal. Type 3 duplication is rare.

Duplication of the small finger is believed to be genetically determined. Types 2 and 3 duplications are believed to be inherited as dominant traits with marked penetrance. The type 1 pattern is multifactorial, involving two genes with incomplete penetrance. Persons with type 2 or 3 deformities may produce offspring with any of the three types, whereas those with type 1 deformities produce only children with type 1 patterns. Autosomal recessive inheritance also has been identified in association with multiple abnormalities.

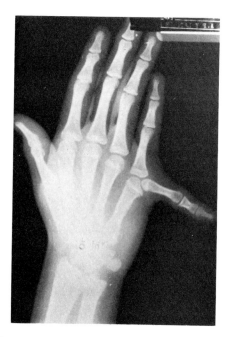

Fig. 74-48   Type 2 postaxial polydactyly: partial duplication of digit, including osseous structures.

The typical black child with a supernumerary digit likely inherited it as an autosomal dominant trait and has no other abnormalities; postaxial polydactyly in the white child frequently is associated with more serious abnormalities. The most common local associated anomaly is syndactyly, but there may be multiple deformities, as well as chromosomal abnormalities.

Infants with postaxial polydactyly may have a well-formed extra digit along the ulnar border of the small finger (type 2) or may have only a rudimentary soft tissue tag (type 1). Both digits usually are hypoplastic to some degree. Angular deformity may be present at birth or may occur later during growth.

TREATMENT. The use of ligatures around the base of type 1 postaxial duplication is not recommended because of reports of fatal hemorrhage. In type 2 duplications the extra digit should be excised through an elliptic incision, usually when the child is about 1 year old. A frequent complication is an unsightly bump caused by a retained segment of duplicated metacarpal head.

■ *TECHNIQUE.* Under tourniquet control, make an elliptic incision around the base of the extra digit. Leave excess skin at the time of initial incision and excise this as appropriate at the time of closure. Identify, ligate, and divide the neurovascular bundle to the extra digit. For type 1 duplication, complete the excision at this point and close the skin with simple closure. For type 2 duplication, identify and preserve the abductor digiti quinti minimi tendon. Expose the area of bone bifurcation subperiosteally. Identify and preserve the ulnar collateral ligament if the bifurcation is in the area of the joint. Amputate the extra digit and trim any excess bone in the area of the bifurcation. Reconstruct the collateral ligament and abductor insertion if violated. Close the skin with simple interrupted sutures. Apply a soft bandage.

AFTERTREATMENT. A very young child may require a cast for a short time (10 days), but generally no immobilization is necessary. Sutures are removed at 2 weeks, and unlimited activity is allowed.

Central Polydactyly

Central polydactyly refers to duplication of the index, middle, or ring finger. It rarely occurs as a solitary deformity and usually is associated with complex syndactyly. The most typical pattern is type 2 central polydactyly concealed within a syndactyly between the middle and ring fingers. Polydactyly of the index finger and polysyndactyly of the middle and ring fingers probably are inherited as autosomal dominant traits. Associated anomalies include polydactyly and syndactyly of the toes.

TREATMENT. In isolated central polydactyly excision of the most hypoplastic digit is performed in keeping with surgical principles of polydactyly reconstruction. In the central polysyndactyly pattern surgical options include syndactyly reconstruction with excision of the extra digit or creation of a three-fingered hand, which Flatt believes gives better results. The complexity of these deformities requires astute surgical judgment and an individualized approach. Surgical reconstruction should be performed by the time the child is 6 months old to prevent further angular deformity. As many normal-appearing fingers as possible should be reconstructed. Amputation of a functionless digit may be performed later.

Ulnar Dimelia

Ulnar dimelia, commonly called *mirror hand,* occurs as radial and ulnar clusters of fingers in the same hand that are near mirror images of each other (Fig. 74-49). It is considered a duplication phenomenon of the ulnar half of the forearm, wrist, and hand, but because there is complete substitution of the radial components as well, this anomaly is not so easily classified as pure duplication. It is an exceedingly rare anomaly, with few reports in the literature. The largest reported series is that of Harrison, Pearson, and Roaf, in which they describe the deformity in three patients. The cause is unknown, but its occurrence usually is sporadic. It is believed to result from an aberration in the control process of the apical ectodermal ridge of the limb bud. When associated with fibular dimelia, it may be explained as a single gene mutation transmitted as an autosomal dominant trait. Ulnar dimelia usually is associated with some degree of hypoplasia of the arm and scapula. The only distant associated anomaly is fibular dimelia with absence of the tibia.

The deformity usually is unilateral and grotesque, with multiple fingers dangling from a somewhat normal palm. The hand usually has six to eight well-formed fingers that may all lie in nearly the same plane or with slight opposition between the two halves. The postaxial digits appear slightly more normal than the preaxial digits. There is no thumb. Syndactyly may be present. The digits may be somewhat flexed because of deficient extensors, the hand usually is radially deviated at the wrist, and extension of the wrist may not be possible. The wrist and elbow appear thick, elbow motion is decreased, and the arm is shortened. The ulna and ulnar carpal bones are completely duplicated, the scaphoid and trapezium are replaced, and the distal ulnar epiphysis is broadened. At the elbow each of the duplicated ulnae articulates with the distal humerus separately, and they tend to face each other. There is no capitellum on the distal humerus.

TREATMENT. Parents should be encouraged to maintain passive range of motion in the fingers, wrist, elbow, and shoulder by gentle stretching exercises until the child reaches an appropriate age for reconstruction, usually by the age of 2 years. During this period the child should be carefully observed during play to determine which radial digit may function best as the thumb. Surgical intervention should be performed early to prevent the inevitable psychologic trauma to the parents, which also may be sensed by the child. No single surgeon has accumulated enough experience to clearly delineate the best method of treating the many complex problems involved with this deformity. Problems that require correction include limited movement of the elbow, limited pronation and supination, limited movement of the wrist, excessive number of fingers, inadequate finger extension, absence of the thumb, and inadequate first web space.

To improve elbow flexion, Harrison et al. excised the upper 1-inch portion of the lateral ulna in a 1-year-old patient and achieved 40 degrees of elbow flexion; by the time the child was 12 years old, however, the elbow again had stiffened into extension. Most authors recommend this treatment method for limited elbow flexion but emphasize postoperative muscle strengthening. Pronation and supination also may be improved, but rotation osteotomy may be required to place the forearm in a more functional position. Limitation of wrist extension by palmar and radial contractures may require Z-plasty and lengthening of the contracted tendons and capsule. The flexor carpi radialis muscle may be transferred to the dorsum to aid extension, and Gorriz recommends transferring the flexor digitorum superficialis of the pollicized finger to the dorsum of the index metacarpal. Wrist arthrodesis may be necessary for recurrent wrist instability; this procedure can be performed when the child is about 12 years of age. Pollicization may be performed in one stage according to the principles of Buck-Gramcko (p. 3372), using the most functional of the radial digits. The excess radial digits are deleted, including the metacarpal and carpal bones. The excess skin is used as a filleted flap to recreate a first web space. Entin

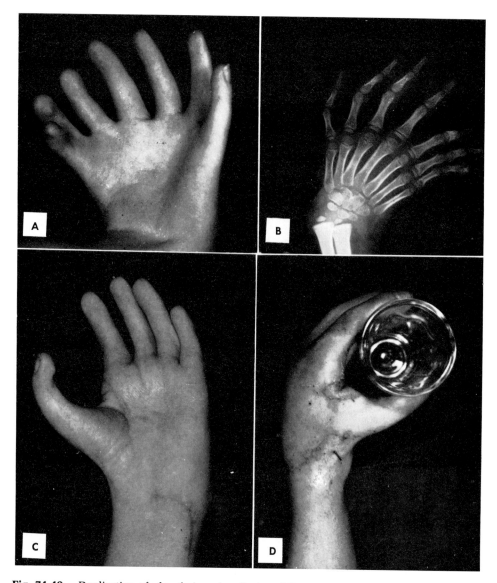

Fig. 74-49 Duplication of ulna (mirror hand). **A** and **B,** Appearance before surgery. Middle digit corresponds to normal index finger; on each side of this digit is set of ulnar digits. **C** and **D,** Same hand 6 months after reconstruction by procedures illustrated in Fig. 74-50. (From Entin MA: Surg Clin North Am 40:497, 1960.)

recommeded deleting the first and third rays, with pollicization of the second digital ray (Fig. 74-50). Tendon transfers, with the use of donor tendons from the amputated digits or the flexor carpi ulnaris if duplicated, may be necessary to improve finger extension.

Excision of proximal ulna

■ *TECHNIQUE.* Under tourniquet control if possible, place a longitudinal incision over the proximal aspect of the preaxial ulnar bone. Expose the proximal ulna extraperiosteally, preserving a sufficient periosteal and ligamentous strip to reconstruct a collateral ligament. Excise a sufficient amount of the ulna, along with its remaining periosteum, to allow

adequate extension and flexion, usually approximately 1 inch of bone. Check the stability of the elbow, close the incision in layers, and apply a long arm cast with the elbow in 90 degrees of flexion.

AFTERTREATMENT. The cast is worn for 3 to 6 weeks depending on the stability of the elbow. The neurovascular status must be carefully monitored. After the cast is removed, active assisted flexion and extension exercises are begun. A night splint is recommended to hold the elbow in 90 degrees of flexion until the child can actively flex the elbow against resistance. Emphasis should be placed on strengthening the elbow flexors and extensors to maintain the motion achieved at surgery.

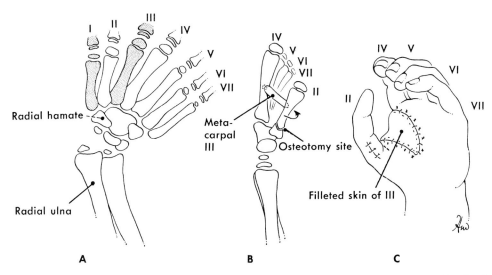

Fig. 74-50   Reconstructive procedures for duplication of ulna (mirror hand). **A,** Sketch of roentgenogram shown in Fig. 74-49. In reconstruction digits I and III were discarded; digit II was retained for pollicization. **B,** Sketch of pollicization of digit II. This digit was properly positioned by osteotomy through base of its metacarpal and by intermetacarpal graft cut from metacarpal of discarded digit III. **C,** Filleted skin of digit III was used as flap to cover space created by pollicization. (From Entin MA: Surg Clin North Am 40:497, 1960.)

Reconstruction of hand and wrist

■ *TECHNIQUE.* Before inflation of the tourniquet, carefully plan the incision to allow pollicization of the most functional digit, as well as fillet-type amputations of the excessive digits and exposure of the neurovascular bundles to the digit chosen for pollicization. After the incisions and skin flaps have been designed, exsanguinate the limb and inflate the tourniquet. Make the incisions and carefully dissect the common neurovascular bundles to the middle digit in each web space. Ligate the bifurcation to each adjacent digit. Carefully dissect the common digital nerves to the thenar level before division. Carefully preserve the digital nerves and dorsal veins to the pollicized digit. Next dissect out the tendons to the pollicized digit; if there are bifurcations of these tendons, divide the abnormal insertions to the neighboring tendons. Amputate the extra digits, including the metacarpal and articulating carpal bones. Preserve the extensor tendons to the excised digits, if present, to use later to reinforce finger extension or thumb abduction. Shorten the metacarpal of the pollicized digit by performing an osteotomy just proximal to the metacarpal neck and scarring the remaining shaft. Rotate the head of the metacarpal into 120 degrees of flexion and 90 degrees of pronation, and secure it in this position with two sutures or a Kirschner wire, which allows appropriate shortening and opposition of the pollicized digit. Then suture the intrinsic muscles to the lateral bands of the extensor mechanism of the pollicized digit to augment adduction and abduction. Now use the fillet flaps from the deleted digits to reconstruct a first web space. Remove any excess skin to allow appropriate closure of the shortened, pollicized digit. If increased extension of the wrist is needed, divide the flexor digitorum sublimis muscle at the level of the A-1 pulley into the pollicized digit and transfer it to the dorsal base of the second metacarpal. Deflate the tourniquet, check the viability of the remaining digits and flaps, and apply a bulky dressing with a long arm posterior splint supporting the elbow at 90 degrees, the wrist at neutral or in slight extension, and the thumb in the abducted position. *AFTERTREATMENT.* The splint is worn for 3 weeks but may be changed for suture removal and wound inspection. After splint removal an exercise program is begun and a removable night splint is used to hold the thumb in the opposed position for an additional 3 months.

OVERGROWTH (MACRODACTYLY)

Macrodactyly is a rare congenital anomaly in which there is enlargement of the finger. Flatt found macrodactyly in only 19 of 1476 patients with congenital hand anomalies, an incidence of 0.9%. The index finger is involved most frequently. Macrodactyly does not appear to be an inherited condition. Although its cause is uncertain, three possible factors are strongly suspected: abnormal nerve supply, abnormal blood supply, and abnormal humoral mechanism. Some have postulated that macrodactyly is an aborted type of neurofibromatosis; however, other manifestations of this disease usually are not seen in these patients. Barsky described two types of true macrodactyly: static enlargement of the digit without progression as the child grows and progressive enlargement out of proportion to normal growth. The latter form may not enlarge during infancy but begins to enlarge rapidly during early childhood; this form frequently is associated with angular deformity. Macrodactyly most commonly exists without other conditions, but syndactyly is associated with macrodactyly in about 10% of patients. Macrodactyly involving both the hands and feet has been reported by Keret, Ger, and Marks. Some patients with neurofibromatosis will develop macrodactyly.

In static macrodactyly the deformity is present in infancy. There usually is diffuse enlargement of the digit; however, the distal and palmar tissues usually appear more enlarged than the dorsal and proximal tissues. The finger grows but in proportion to normal digital growth. Progressive macrodactyly occurs in early childhood as a rapidly enlarging digit, frequently with an angular deformity that makes the finger banana shaped (Fig. 74-51). The skin may be thickened and the nails hypertrophied. The phalanges always are involved, and the metacarpals may be enlarged as well. With maturity the enlarged digit begins to lose motion. Later in life symptoms of carpal tunnel syndrome may develop, with complaints of paresthesias and hypesthesias. Trophic ulcers also may develop over the involved digit. Involvement usually is unilateral, and multiple digits are affected two to three times as often as single digits. If the thumb is involved, a characteristic abduction and hyperextension deformity results. It generally is believed that all the tissues of the involved finger are enlarged; however, some have noted sparing of the tendons and vessels. The nerves that innervate the involved territory are characteristically enlarged. In a rare type of macrodactyly, which Kelikian called *hyperostotic variety,* there may be osteocartilaginous deposits around the joints. Schuind suggested the possibility of a traumatic etiology for this condition.

Treatment

There are no satisfactory nonsurgical methods of controlling macrodactyly. Attempts to compress the digit with elastic wrapping have been unsuccessful. Indications for surgery include enlargement, angulation, carpal tunnel syndrome, and causalgia. For the progressively enlarging digit, a debulking procedure usually is needed. With this procedure as much excess tissue as possible is excised from one half the digit; 3 months later the other half is debulked. This procedure may be required several times during the growth period. Tsuge proposed that the disproportionate growth is a result of excessive neural input and recommended that the digital nerves be stripped of one half their fascicles at the time of debulking. He also recommended complete excision of the enlarged digital nerves during debulking as the most effective way of controlling progressive macrodactyly, believing that this causes only minimal neural impairment in children. Kelikian recommended segmental resection of the tortuous digital nerves with end-to-end repair.

Epiphyseal arrest after the digit has reached estimated adult length also is frequently recommended. Clifford recommends holes drilled through the epiphyses, Jones recommends resection of the epiphyses, and Wood uses a high-speed drill for epiphysiodesis of all phalanges. Various methods of digital shortening also have been described, including simple amputation of the distal phalanx and filleting of the distal phalanx, with transfer of

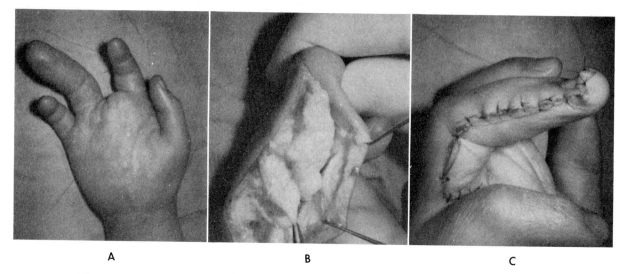

A B C

Fig. 74-51 **A,** Recurrent macrodactyly in 6-year-old child 2 years after debulking procedure of ring finger and amputation of middle finger. **B,** Intraoperative photograph shows enlargement of digital nerve. **C,** Wound closure after debulking.

the nail and matrix onto the end of the middle phalanx, with or without some of the underlying distal phalanx. In the angulated finger, closing wedge osteotomies through either the proximal or middle phalanx are necessary for correction. Millesi described a complicated technique for shortening the enlarged thumb, in which parts of the distal and proximal phalanges are removed and the distal interphalangeal joint is preserved. Amputation is used to provide relief only as a last resort in the adult with a severe and bothersome deformity.

The most common complication is recurrence, which is expected after debulking. Flap necrosis is a major surgical complication, and some have recommended excision of the overlying skin and replacement with a full-thickness skin graft to avoid this problem. Careful attention to flap design may help prevent skin necrosis. Operating on only one side of the finger at a time minimizes the risk of circulatory disturbance.

DEBULKING

■ *TECHNIQUE (TSUGE).* Under tourniquet control, make a midlateral incision the length of the involved digit. Identify and dissect out the digital nerve. Excise all excessive adipose tissue. If the digital nerve is grossly enlarged, half the fascicles may be stripped and excised as recommended by Tsuge. If the digital nerve is excessively tortuous, then a

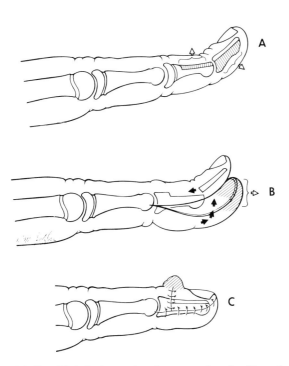

Fig. 74-52 Digital shortening for macrodactyly (Tsuge). **A,** Matching sections *(shaded areas)* of volar half of distal phalanx and dorsal half of middle phalanx are removed. **B,** Distal phalanx is reduced on middle phalanx, with preservation of dorsal skin bridge but removal of excess soft tissue. **C,** Soft tissue closure is completed, accepting some excess dorsal soft tissue. (Redrawn from Tsuge K: J Hand Surg 10-A:968, 1985.)

section may be resected and an end-to-end repair performed as described by Kelikian. Resect matching sections of the volar half of the distal phalanx and the dorsal half of the middle phalanx (Fig. 74-52, *A*) and reduce the fragments (Fig. 74-52, *B*). Remove excessive skin, close the incision (Fig. 74-52, *C*), and apply a bulky hand dressing. No particular postoperative protection is required. Debulking of the opposite side of the digit can be performed 3 months after the first procedure.

EPIPHYSIODESIS

■ *TECHNIQUE.* Under tourniquet control, make a midlateral incision the length of the entire finger. Identify the epiphyses of the proximal, middle, and distal phalanges and perform epiphysiodesis of these with a high-speed burr or curet and cautery. Close the incision and apply a finger splint, which is worn for 3 weeks.

DIGITAL SHORTENING

■ *TECHNIQUE.* Under tourniquet control, make an L-shaped incision beginning at the midlateral aspect of the proximal interphalangeal joint and extending distally to a level just proximal to the germinal matrix (Fig. 74-53, *A*). Carry the incision transversely across the dorsum of the finger. Remove the distal half of the middle phalanx and the proximal part of the distal phalanx. Using a rongeur, sharpen the distal end of the remaining middle phalanx to a point to fit into the medullary canal of the distal phalanx (Fig. 74-53, *B*). Place the distal phalanx onto the middle phalanx and fix it with a Kirschner wire to recess the finger (Fig. 74-53, *C*). Excess volar soft tissue can be removed at a later stage. Close the incision and apply a finger splint to be worn for 3 weeks.

THUMB SHORTENING

■ *TECHNIQUE (MILLESI).* Under tourniquet control, excise the distal half of the nail and nail matrix, as well as the underlying distal phalangeal tuft (Fig. 74-54, *A*). Through a dorsal longitudinal incision overlying the proximal and distal phalanx, remove the middle third of the proximal phalanx and the middle third of the overlying nail and matrix. Next remove the middle third of the middle phalanx by performing parallel oblique osteotomies (Fig. 74-54, *B*). Reduce the two remaining longitudinal components of the distal phalanx and pin them with a transverse Kirschner wire. Reduce the distal and proximal fragments of the proximal phalanx in a shortened fashion and pin them with an oblique Kirschner wire (Fig. 74-54, *C*). Close the wound by carefully approximating the skin edges, as well as the nail matrix, leaving the Kirschner wires protruding through the skin. Apply a thumb splint.

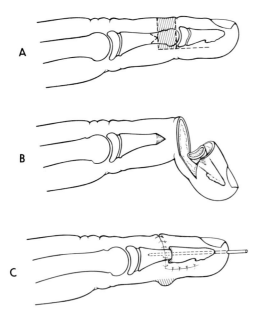

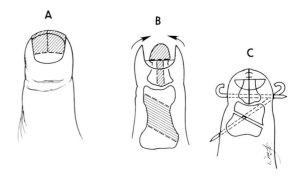

Fig. 74-54 Thumb reduction for macrodactyly (Millesi). **A,** Removal of distal half of nail and distal phalanx, preserving eponychial tissue. **B,** Reduction osteotomies performed through dorsal incision. **C,** Remaining bone reduced and pinned. (Redrawn from Millesi H: Macrodactyly: a case study. In Littler JW et al: Symposium on reconstructive hand surgery, St Louis, 1974, Mosby–Year Book, Inc.)

Fig. 74-53 Digital shortening for macrodactyly (Barsky). **A,** L-shaped midlateral and dorsal incisions allow removal of excess dorsal tissue, distal half of middle phalanx, and proximal portion of distal phalanx *(shaded area)*. **B,** Bone ends are prepared for pencil-cone reduction. **C,** Distal phalanx is reduced on middle phalanx and secured with Kirschner wire. (Redrawn from Barsky AJ: J Bone Joint Surg 49-A:1255, 1967.)

AFTERTREATMENT. The splint is worn for 3 weeks. The Kirschner wires are removed when the osteotomy incisions are healed, usually by 4 to 6 weeks.

UNDERGROWTH

Congenital hand anomalies classified as *undergrowth* deformities are those in which development is incomplete, making the entire upper extremity or any of its parts smaller or deficient. Hypoplasia of digital parts often occurs with other deformities of the hand, such as radial clubhand, syndactyly, and even macrodactyly. Its use as a separate category is best limited to those deformities that present a formed but deficient part without other anomalies.

Hypoplastic Thumb

The designation *hypoplastic thumb* generally applies to any thumb with some degree of deficiency in any of its anatomic parts — osseous, musculotendinous, or ectodermal. The thumb may be functional but simply shorter than normal or, in the most severe manifestation, totally absent. The hypoplastic thumb constituted 3.6% of anomalies in Flatt's series and 1.3% in the Yokohama series; hypoplasia of the whole hand represented 0.8% in Flatt's series and absence of the thumb, 1.4%. Because of the wide variety of deformities produced by hypoplasia

of the thumb, etiologic factors also are varied. Many of these deformities are sporadic occurrences, but some are transmitted genetically or are associated with specific syndromes. The six types of hypoplastic thumb are based on the appearance of the deformity and the deficient structures. They include short thumb, adducted thumb, abducted thumb, floating thumb, absent thumb, and clasped thumb.

SHORT THUMB. The normal thumb extends to about the level of the proximal interphalangeal joint of the index finger; a thumb is considered "short" if its length is less than this. Hypoplasia of any or all osseous components produces a thumb that is significantly shorter than normal. The short thumb frequently is associated with other anomalies and syndromes. When the metacarpal is short and slender, it may be a manifestation of a syndrome such as Fanconi's, Holt-Oram, or Juberg-Hayward syndrome; it also may be associated with other malformations of the spine and cardiovascular and gastrointestinal systems. When the metacarpal is short and broad, it may be associated with Cornelia de Lange's syndrome, hand-foot-uterus syndrome, diastrophic dwarfism, or myositis ossificans progressiva. Shortening of the proximal phalanx of the thumb may be associated with brachydactyly. The distal phalanx may be broad and short in association with Rubinstein-Taybi, Apert's, Carpenter's, or hand-foot-uterus syndrome. The thumb may be radially deviated ("hitchhiker's thumb") or very short and stubby ("potter's thumb" or "murderer's thumb"). A slender distal phalanx may be associated with Fanconi's or Holt-Oram syndrome.

Treatment. If the hypoplastic thumb is only short, surgical correction rarely is indicated. If prehension is significantly limited, deepening of the web space may be sufficient to create a relative lengthening of the thumb in relation to objects that are grasped. This may be achieved with a two- or four-limb Z-plasty.

ADDUCTED THUMB. The adducted thumb usually is caused by absence or partial absence of the thenar muscles, which results in deficient opposition. Strauch and Spinner noted that these thumbs often lack a functional flexor pollicis longus muscle. The radial collateral ligament of the thumb metacarpophalangeal joint also may be deficient. The thumb usually is shortened and tapered, with a flattened thenar eminence and a deficient first web space. The deformity usually is transmitted as an autosomal dominant trait and usually is unilateral.

Treatment. The goals of surgical reconstruction of the adducted thumb are correction of the adduction contracture and restoration of opposition. The adduction contracture may be corrected by a two- or four-limb Z-plasty or a sliding dorsal flap raised from the radial side of the index finger. The two-limb Z-plasty rarely attains adequate correction. The two most popular techniques for restoration of opposition are the ring flexor superficialis tendon opponensplasty and the abductor digiti quinti opponensplasty, as described by Huber and popularized by Littler and Cooley. The Huber procedure allows creation of a more nearly normal-appearing thenar eminence. Littler also described the use of an abdominal flap (Fig. 74-55) for reconstruction of the adducted thumb.

Simple Z-plasty of thumb web

■ *TECHNIQUE.* Before inflating the tourniquet, diagram the appropriate skin incision, designing the flap with its longitudinal axis along the distal ridge of the first web space and extending from the proximal thumb crease to approximately 1 cm proximal to the proximal digital crease of the index finger at a point that corresponds to the radial confluence of the proximal and middle palmar creases. Draw an oblique proximal palmar limb, as well as a distal dorsal limb, at an approximately 60-degree angle, with the lengths of both limbs corresponding to the longitudinal incision (Fig. 74-56, *A*). In designing these flaps, keep in mind the basic principle of all Z-plasty procedures: all flap sides must be of equal lengths. Now inflate the tourniquet and make the appropriate incisions as outlined. Elevate the flaps sharply, carefully undermining to avoid vascular compromise. If additional depth is needed, sharply dissect the distal edge of the web space musculature to obtain a partial recession. Reverse the flaps and carefully suture them with interrupted 6-0 nylon sutures or absorbable skin sutures (Fig. 74-56, *B*). Mattress sutures may be used to help prevent tip necrosis. Deflate the tourniquet, check for adequate blood supply to the flaps, and apply a sterile dressing with the thumb splinted in the abducted, opposed position.

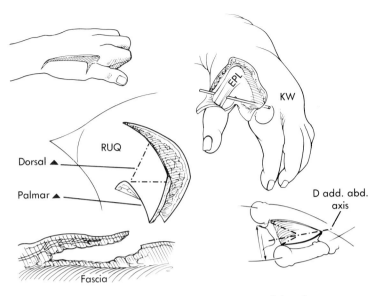

Fig. 74-55   Correction of adduction contracture of thumb using abdominal flap based on thoracoepigastric vessels. (Redrawn from Littler JW: Clin Orthop 13:182, 1959.)

AFTERTREATMENT. The splint and sutures are removed 2 weeks after surgery, and free use of the hand is allowed if healing has progressed adequately.

Four-limb Z-plasty

■ *TECHNIQUE (MODIFIED FROM BROADBENT AND WOOLF).* Before inflating the tourniquet, outline the flaps. Make the longitudinal axis of the Z-plasty along the distal edge of the thumb web ridge, extending from the ulnar margin of the proximal thumb crease to an area approximately 1 cm proximal to the proximal digital crease of the index finger. Draw proximal palmar and distal dorsal limbs at 90-degree angles to the longitudinal axis; the lengths of these limbs should equal that of the longitudinal incision (Fig. 74-57, *A*). Bisect each angle with an additional oblique limb, again with the

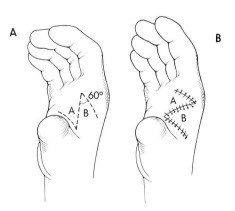

Fig. 74-56   Simple Z-plasty of thumb web. **A,** Incisions. **B,** Closure after reversal of flaps.

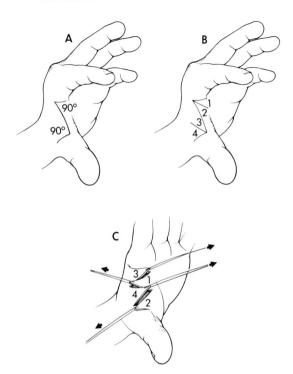

Fig. 74-57 Four-flap Z-plasty for lengthening first web in adducted thumb. **A,** Ninety-degree dorsal and volar flaps are marked in first web. **B,** These are then bisected to create four flaps. **C,** Flaps are elevated, transposed, and interdigitated to complete lengthening. (Redrawn from Woolf RM and Broadbent TR: Plast Reconstr Surg 49:48, 1972.)

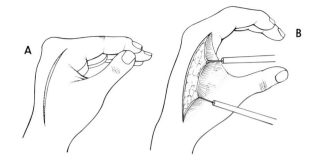

Fig. 74-58 Dorsal sliding flap for correction of adduction deformity of first web. **A,** Incision. **B,** Radial flap is undermined, and dorsal defect is covered with split-thickness skin graft.

length corresponding to the length of the other flap margins (Fig. 74-57, *B*). Then inflate the tourniquet and make the appropriate incisions. Sharply elevate the flaps, elevating the skin, as well as a small amount of subcutaneous tissue. For further deepening perform a small recession of the thumb web musculature in its midsubstance. Do not perform a complete myotomy. Interdigitate the appropriate flaps and suture them with 6-0 monofilament nylon. It is helpful to label the flaps before incision; if the flaps are labeled *1, 2, 3,* and *4,* beginning from the radialmost flap and ending at the ulnarmost flap, the sequence after interdigitation should be *3, 1, 4, 2,* (Fig. 74-57, *C*). Then deflate the tourniquet, inspect the flaps for viability, and apply a bulky dressing with the thumb splinted in the abducted position.

AFTERTREATMENT. The sutures and splint are removed 2 weeks after surgery. If desired, a small web-spacer splint may be used for an additional 2 weeks.

Web deepening with sliding flap

■ *TECHNIQUE (BRAND; Fig. 74-58).* Before inflating the tourniquet, design the flaps by drawing a line dorsally from the apex of the first and second metacar-

pals and extending it distally to the radial side of the proximal phalanx of the index finger. Then curve the line back across the web space into the palm proximally to the apex of the first and second metacarpals. Exsanguinate the arm, inflate the tourniquet, and make the skin incisions as outlined. Sharply elevate the skin flaps with a small amount of subcutaneous tissue. Release any thickened dorsal and volar fascia carefully to avoid injury to the neurovascular structures. If severe contracture is present, incise the capsule of the carpometacarpal joint of the thumb. Pull the thumb away from the palm and hold it with a Kirschner wire. Allow the flap to slide with the thumb and use it to cover the thumb and palmar web. Cover the dorsal defect with a split-thickness skin graft. Suture the flaps in place with interrupted 6-0 nylon sutures, and secure and bolster the skin graft. Deflate the tourniquet, inspect the flaps for viability, and apply a sterile dressing with the thumb splinted in the abducted position.

AFTERTREATMENT. Sutures are removed at 2 weeks, and the Kirschner wire is removed at 4 weeks, after which unrestricted motion of the thumb is allowed.

Ring sublimis opponensplasty

■ *TECHNIQUE (RIORDAN).* Expose the sublimis tendon of the ring finger through an ulnar midlateral incision over the proximal interphalangeal joint and divide the tendon at the level of the joint or just proximal to it. Divide the chiasm, thus separating the two slips of tendon at the level of the joint so that they will pass around the profundus and can be easily withdrawn at the wrist. Now expose the flexor carpi ulnaris tendon through an L-shaped incision that extends proximally along the flexor carpi ulnaris tendon and distally turns radialward, parallel with the flexor creases of the wrist. To make a pulley, cut halfway through the flexor carpi ulnaris tendon at a point approximately 6.3 cm proximal to the pisiform (Fig. 74-59). Then strip the radial half of

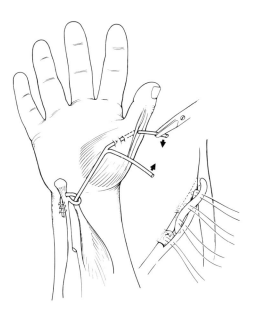

Fig. 74-59 Opponensplasty of ring sublimis for adduction contracture of thumb (see text).

the tendon distally almost to the pisiform and create a loop large enough for the sublimis tendon to pass through easily; carry the end of the radial segment of the flexor carpi ulnaris through a split in the remaining half of the tendon, loop it back, and suture it to the remaining half. Now make a wide **C**-shaped incision on the thumb as follows. Begin on the dorsum of the thumb just proximal to the interphalangeal joint and proceed proximally and volarward around to the radial aspect of the thumb. At a point just proximal to the metacarpophalangeal joint, curve the incision dorsalward in line with the major skin creases of the thenar eminence. Preserve on the dorsoradial aspect of the thumb the fine sensory nerve from the superficial branch of the radial nerve. Expose and define the extensor pollicis longus tendon over the proximal phalanx, the extensor aponeurosis over the metacarpophalangeal joint, and the tendon of the abductor pollicis brevis. Now at the wrist identify the sublimis tendon to the ring finger and withdraw it into the forearm incision. Pass the tendon through the loop fashioned from the flexor carpi ulnaris. Then, with a small hemostat or a tendon carrier, pass the tendon subcutaneously across the thenar eminence in line with the fibers of the abductor pollicis brevis.

Now make a small tunnel for insertion of the transfer by burrowing between two small parallel incisions in the abductor pollicis brevis tendon. Split the end of the sublimis tendon for approximately 2.5 cm, or more if necessary, and pass one half of it through the tunnel. Now separate the extensor aponeurosis from the periosteum of the proximal phalanx of the thumb, make a small incision in

it 6 mm distal to the first tunnel, and pass the same strip of sublimis through it. Bring the slip out from beneath the aponeurosis through a small longitudinal slit in the long extensor tendon about 3 mm proximal to the interphalangeal joint.

Now determine the proper tension for the transfer. Grasp the two slips of sublimis with small hemostats and cross them. With the thumb in full opposition and the wrist in a straight line, place the two overlapping slips of sublimis under some tension. Releasing the thumb and passively flexing the wrist should completely relax the transfer so that the thumb can be brought into full extension and abduction; extending the wrist 45 degrees should place enough tension on the transfer to bring the thumb into complete opposition and the tip of the thumb into complete extension. If the tension is insufficient, increase it and repeat the test. When the correct tension has been determined, suture the slips of sublimis together with the cut ends buried (Fig. 74-59, *inset*). Now anchor the transfer and the tendon of the abductor pollicis brevis to the joint capsule with a single nylon or wire suture so that the transfer passes over the exact middle of the metacarpal head; this prevents later displacement of the tendon toward the palmar aspect of the joint during opposition. Close the wound with nonabsorbable sutures and immobilize the hand in a pressure dressing and a dorsal plaster splint as follows. Place the wrist in 30 degrees of flexion, the fingers in the functional position, and the thumb in full opposition with the distal phalanx extended; place a few layers of gauze between the individual fingers to prevent maceration of the skin.

AFTERTREATMENT. At 3 weeks the dressing and splint are removed and active motion is begun, but the thumb is supported with an opponens splint for an additional 6 weeks. Many patients can oppose the thumb as soon as the splint is removed. When the sublimis of the ring finger has been used for the transfer, as in the Riordan technique, training in its use may be facilitated by asking the patient to place the tip of the thumb against the ring finger; this maneuver produces flexion of the ring finger and an automatic attempt to oppose the thumb with the transferred sublimis. In patients with weak quadriceps muscles who habitually rise from a sitting position by pushing up with the flattened hands or in patients who use crutches, the transfer must be protected for 3 months or longer, or it will be overstretched and cease to function.

Abductor digiti quinti opponensplasty

■ *TECHNIQUE (HUBER; LITTLER AND COOLEY).* Make a curved palmar incision along the radial border of the abductor digiti quinti muscle belly, extending from the proximal side of the pisiform proximally to the ulnar border of the little finger distally. Free both tendinous insertions of the muscle, one from the extensor expansion and the other from the base of the proximal phalanx. Lift the muscle from its fascial compartment and carefully expose its neurovascular bundle. Isolate the bundle, taking care not to damage the veins. Next free the origin of the muscle from the pisiform but retain the origin on the flexor carpi ulnaris tendon; now the muscle can be mobilized enough for its insertion to reach the thumb. Make a curved incision on the radial border of the thenar eminence and create across the palm a subcutaneous pocket to receive the transfer. Now fold the abductor digiti quinti muscle over about 170 degrees (like a page of a book) and pass it subcutaneously to the thumb. Suture its tendons of insertion to the insertion of the abductor pollicis brevis. Throughout the procedure avoid compression of and undue tension on the muscle and its neurovascular pedicle. Apply a carefully formed light compression dressing and then a volar plaster splint to hold the thumb in abduction and the wrist in slight flexion.

ABDUCTED THUMB. The abducted thumb deformity was described in 1919 by Tupper, who reported four patients with mildly hypoplastic thumbs and associated abduction deformities. He called this *pollex abductus* and believed it resulted from an abnormal insertion of the flexor pollicis longus muscle into an otherwise normal extensor pollicis longus muscle, causing marked abduction of the proximal phalanx of the thumb. This was verified at the time of reconstruction, when he also noted deficiencies in the thenar musculature, adduction contracture of the first metacarpal with web space deficiency, marked laxity of the ulnar collateral ligament, radial and superficial displacement of the flexor pollicis longus, and inability to flex the interphalangeal joint of the thumb. This is an extremely rare deformity, and since the first report only five more cases have been reported.

Treatment. There have been almost as many surgical procedures described for the abducted thumb as there have been cases reported: release of the bifurcated tendon insertion and reattachment to the metacarpal neck; release of the tendon distally, withdrawal at the wrist, and reattachment to the distal phalanx; and release of the anomalous slip to the extensor pollicis longus muscle, with an ulnarward shift of the extensor pollicis longus at the metacarpophalangeal joint. All procedures have been combined with release of the radial collateral ligament and reefing of the ulnar collateral ligament of the metacarpophalangeal joint, and some have required a secondary opponensplasty. Blair and Omer described a technique in which the flexor pollicis longus is released from its abnormal tendinous insertion and centralized by being moved ulnarward. To complete the transfer, the

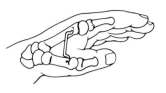

Fig. 74-60 Staged reconstruction for abducted thumb in which adduction contracture is released and maintained with interposed Kirschner wire; this may be followed in 6 weeks by reconstruction of ulnar collateral ligament and ring sublimis opponensplasty. (Redrawn from Dobyns JH, Wood VE, and Bayne LG: Congenital hand deformities. In Green DP, editor: Operative hand surgery, ed 2, New York, 1988, Churchill Livingstone, Inc.)

abductor pollicis brevis musculotendinous junction is divided, the flexor pollicis longus tendon is transferred under the intrinsic muscle, and the intrinsic muscle is reattached. They did not find it necessary to reconstruct the ulnar collateral ligament. For severe web space contracture Bayne recommends a staged procedure in which the web space is first released and maintained with a Kirschner wire (Fig. 74-60), followed in 6 weeks by a Riordan opponensplasty that uses the ring sublimis and by reconstruction of the ulnar collateral ligament that uses one slip of the sublimis.

Rerouting of flexor pollicis longus

■ **TECHNIQUE (BLAIR AND OMER).** Under tourniquet control, make a zigzag palmar incision along the thumb to allow exploration of the flexor pollicis longus, the ulnar collateral ligament, and the extensor pollicis longus. Develop the flaps, and identify and protect the digital nerves. Identify the abnormal tendinous slip of the flexor pollicis longus that passes over the radial border of the thumb and into the extensor pollicis longus, usually between the metacarpophalangeal joint and the interphalangeal joint. Release this abnormal insertion sharply. Release the insertion of the abductor pollicis brevis (Fig. 74-61, *A*). Transfer the flexor pollicis longus tendon ulnarward under the abductor pollicis brevis tendon (Fig. 74-61, *B*). If the abduction deformity of the thumb metacarpophalangeal joint cannot be corrected, release the radial collateral ligament. Suture the abductor pollicis brevis tendon into its normal insertion (Fig. 74-61, *C*). This technique centralizes the flexor pollicis longus and constructs a sling at the metacarpophalangeal joint. If there is continued laxity of the ulnar collateral ligament of the thumb metacarpophalangeal joint, use the abnormal tendon slip to reinforce the ligament. Suture the skin with simple interrupted sutures and apply a modified thumb spica cast that extends beyond the interphalangeal joint dorsally and stops proximal to the metacarpophalangeal joint on the volar side. This

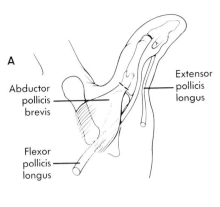

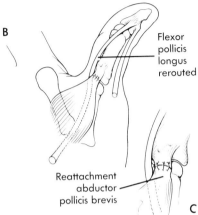

Fig. 74-61 Rerouting of flexor pollicis longus for abducted thumb (see text). Flexor pollicis is centralized after tenotomy and reattachment of abductor pollicis brevis. (Redrawn from Blair W and Omer G: J Hand Surg 6:241, 1981.)

prevents hyperextension and abduction of the thumb but allows metacarpophalangeal flexion and flexor tendon excursion.

AFTERTREATMENT. The cast is removed at 6 weeks, and unlimited motion of the hand is allowed.

FLOATING THUMB (POUCE FLOTTANT). Floating thumb refers to a small, slender thumb that appears to dangle from the radial border of the hand. Typically there are two phalanges, a fingernail, no metacarpophalangeal joint, and no first metacarpal (Fig. 74-62). The trapezium and scaphoid also often are absent. The thumb takes origin somewhat more distally than usual, and there is neither extrinsic nor intrinsic muscle function.

Treatment. Amputation is the treatment of choice, followed by index finger pollicization. Despite gallant attempts to restore stability and function to these severely deficient and useless thumbs, the results have not been as rewarding as with pollicization. In bilateral cases pollicization of one side should be performed early; the parents then may decide what to do concerning the other side.

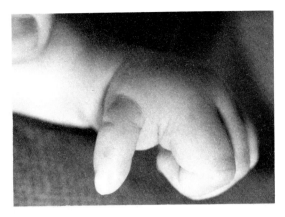

Fig. 74-62 Floating thumb (pouce flottant) deformity.

ABSENT THUMB. This is the most severe manifestation of the hypoplastic thumb and may be associated with radial ray deficiencies, ring D chromosome abnormalities, Holt-Oram syndrome, trisomy 18 syndrome, Rothmund-Thomson syndrome, and thalidomide use. Radial clubhand also is associated with an absent thumb except in the thrombocytopenia–absent radius (TAR) syndrome. Absence of the thumb creates an extreme functional impairment, particularly if the anomaly is bilateral. The development of a strong lateral pinch between the index and long fingers compensates for the absence of the thumb, and a fairly strong grip may be developed. Rotational deformity of the fingers allows limited opposition.

Treatment. Function and appearance can be improved with satisfactory pollicization of the index finger. The timing of pollicization is based on the child's natural development of prehensile activities. Because this develops early, beginning at the age of 3 months, the best time for pollicization is between the ages of 6 and 12 months to allow some growth of the hand before surgery. The choice of procedure usually is between recession and pollicization of the index finger. Recession is preferable in the older child with a strong lateral pinch between the index and long fingers because this pattern may persist despite pollicization. This operation recesses the index finger to make it more resemble a thumb and provides a wider gap between the index and long fingers.

Recession of index finger

■ *TECHNIQUE (FLATT).* Under tourniquet control, make a dorsal longitudinal 1 cm incision in the first web space. Divide the deep transverse metacarpal ligament, palmar and dorsal fascia, and intertendinous connections between the index and middle finger metacarpals. Take care to avoid injury to the neurovascular structures. Make a second short, curved dorsoradial incision at the base of the index metacarpal. Expose the base of the index metacarpal

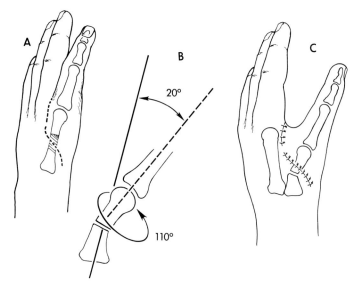

Fig. 74-63 Recession of index finger. **A,** Two incisions are required: intermetacarpal ligament is cut through distal incision, and osteotomy of index metacarpal is performed through proximal incision. **B,** Distal portion of index is rotated 110 degrees and abducted 20 degrees palmarward. **C,** Skin closure. (Redrawn from Flatt AE: The care of congenital hand anomalies, St Louis, 1977, Mosby–Year Book, Inc.)

and perform an osteotomy (Fig. 74-63, *A*). The metacarpal now may be easily grasped and maneuvered. Reposition the metacarpal into 20 degrees of radial abduction, 35 degrees of palmar abduction, and 100 to 110 degrees of axial rotation (Fig. 74-63, *B*). Recess the metacarpal by removing 1.5 to 2 cm of the metacarpal shaft. When the desired position and recession are achieved, pass a Kirschner wire into adjacent metacarpals to fix the index metacarpal in this position. Close the incision routinely (Fig. 74-63, *C*) and apply a well-padded, long arm cast that holds the repositioned index finger in abduction.

AFTERTREATMENT. The cast is changed 2 weeks after the operation, and the skin sutures are removed. A long arm cast that supports the pollicized index finger is applied and worn for 4 more weeks. The Kirschner wire is removed when bone healing is complete, usually 4 to 6 weeks after the operation, and progressively increasing activities are allowed. The thumb is splinted in a resting position for another 4 to 6 weeks.

CONGENITAL CLASPED THUMB. Congenital clasped thumb is an unusual condition in which the thumb is positioned in adduction and extreme flexion at the metacarpophalangeal joint. Underlying hypoplasia or absence of the extensor pollicis brevis muscle is usual, and the extensor pollicis brevis or extensor pollicis longus may be absent. Some degree of total thumb hypoplasia may be present. This may be an isolated deformity, or it may be associated with clubfoot deformities and several well-de-

fined syndromes. There is no single cause, but the deformity results from an imbalance between the flexors and extensors of the thumb. Weckesser, Reed, and Heiple called this deformity a syndrome and classified it into four distinct types on the basis of etiologic factors: group 1, deficient extension only; group 2, flexion contracture combined with deficient extension; group 3, hypoplasia of the thumb, including tendon and muscle deficiencies; and group 4, those deformities that do not easily fit any of the other three categories. Group 1 syndrome appears to be transmitted as a sex-linked recessive gene because it is more common in boys and frequently is bilateral.

At birth the thumb usually is flexed into the palm, with the deformity typically located at the metacarpophalangeal joint (Fig. 74-64, *B*), unlike trigger thumb deformity. During the first few weeks of life, it is typical for an infant to clutch the thumb, but normally the thumb is released intermittently. If no active extension at the metacarpophalangeal joint is demonstrated after prolonged observation and particularly by the age of 3 months, the diagnosis of congenital clasped thumb is established.

Nonsurgical management. Most clasped thumb deformities are deficiencies of extension only (group 1) and usually respond to early splinting in extension and abduction. Weckesser et al. recommend the use of a plaster splint, which is changed every 6 weeks and continued for 3 to 6 months. The long-term results of this protocol appear satisfactory if the initial response to splinting is good. If at the end of 3 to 6 months of splinting there is no evidence of active extension of the metacarpophalangeal joint, further splinting will probably not be beneficial. This lack of response to splinting usually indicates that the extrinsic extensors are extremely deficient (the usual case) or totally absent and that a tendon transfer is required to restore function.

Surgical treatment. Useful donor tendons for an inadequate extensor pollicis longus muscle are the palmaris longus, brachioradialis, extensor carpi radialis longus, extensor indicis proprius, and flexor superficialis muscles. The extensor pollicis longus is an ideal motor muscle, but it may be absent as well. Flatt prefers to use the brachioradialis with a tendon graft. The extensor pollicis brevis muscle may be replaced with the extensor indicis proprius muscle. Significant web space contracture also may require reconstruction.

For group 3 deformities with significant hypoplasia of the thenar muscles and abductor pollicis longus and instability of the metacarpophalangeal joint (Fig. 74-64), Neviaser recommends a single-stage operation involving chondrodesis of the metacarpophalangeal joint, replacement of the extensor pollicis longus with the extensor indicis proprius, replacement of the abductor pollicis longus with the palmaris longus, and a Huber opponensplasty (p. 3405). Web space reconstruction usually is necessary in these patients. With this protocol Neviaser

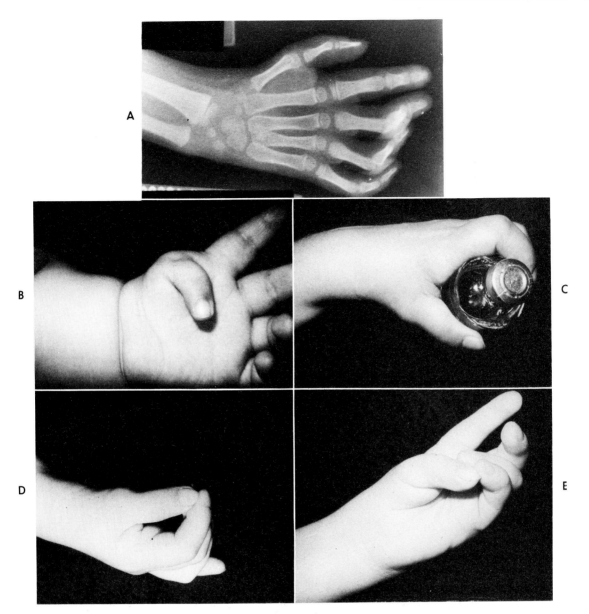

Fig. 74-64 **A,** Typical deformity demonstrating skeletal hypoplasia. **B,** Hypoplastic thumb with metacarpophalangeal instability, adduction contracture of web space, and absence of extrinsic extensors, long abductor, and thenar muscles. **C,** After operation, child's grasp improved. **D,** Stability also was present. **E,** Child's thumb could be opposed to tip of little finger after operation. (From Neviaser RJ: J Hand Surg 4:301, 1979).

obtained useful grasp and pinch in eight patients with no complications, despite the magnitude of the surgery. These procedures should be performed after the first year of life and before the child reaches school age.

Group 2 clasped thumb deformity

■ *TECHNIQUE.* Stage I is release of web space contracture, which is performed as described on p. 3403. Stage II is restoration of thumb extension (Fig. 74-65) with the use of the extensor indicis proprius.

Under tourniquet control, make a short transverse incision at the base of the index metacarpal and locate the extensor indicis proprius tendon. Divide the tendon at its confluence with the extensor hood. Next make a short transverse incision over the dorsum of the wrist in line with the extensor indicis proprius tendon and withdraw the tendon into this wound. Make a bayonet-shaped incision over the dorsoulnar aspect of the thumb centered over the metacarpophalangeal joint. Identify the extensor pollicis longus tendon, if present, and retract it to one side. Create a tunnel through the base of the proximal phalanx from the ulnar aspect to the radial aspect distal to the epiphysis. Reroute the tendon of the extensor indicis proprius subcutaneously from the wrist to the base of the thumb, passing it

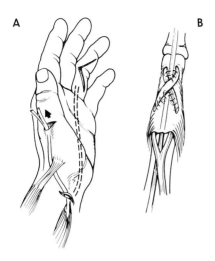

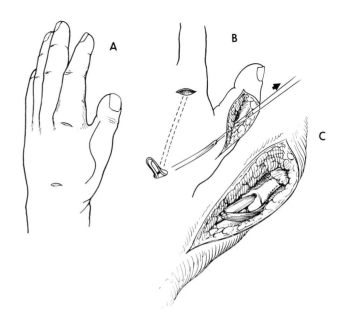

Fig. 74-65 Littler's technique for correction of congenital clasped thumb. **A,** Path of transferred tendon. **B,** Suture of transferred tendon. (Redrawn from Crawford HH, Horton CE, and Adamson JE: J Bone Joint Surg 48-A:82, 1966.)

Fig. 74-66 Transfer of extensor indicis proprius for absent extensor pollicis brevis. **A,** Incisions. **B,** Extensor indicis proprius is passed through bony tunnel in proximal phalanx of thumb and, **C,** sutured to itself. (Redrawn from Roselius (Copyright, 1988) from Dobyns JH, Wood VE, and Bayne LG: Congenital hand deformities. In Green DP, editor: Operative hand surgery, ed 2, New York, 1988, Churchill Livingstone, Inc.)

through the osseous tunnel and suturing it back onto itself. If the extensor pollicis longus is absent or severely deficient, choose either the flexor digitorum sublimis to the ring finger or the brachioradialis, with a palmaris longus tendon graft for the donor muscle. If the flexor digitorum sublimis is selected, make a transverse incision at the base of the ring finger on the palmar aspect and release the sublimis tendon just proximal to Camper's chiasm. Make a short longitudinal incision over the palmar aspect of the wrist proximal to the flexion crease and identify the ring sublimis tendon (Fig. 74-65, *A*). Deliver the sublimis tendon into this wound, reroute it subcutaneously around the radial border of the wrist deep to the abductor pollicis longus tendon, and suture it into the remnants of the extensor pollicis longus at the distal phalanx (Fig. 74-65, *B*). If there is no distal tendon in which to suture the donor, create a periosteal flap to anchor the distal insertion of the tendon. Fix the thumb in extension with a Kirschner wire, close the incision in routine fashion, and apply a splint with the thumb in extension and abduction.

AFTERTREATMENT. Six weeks after surgery the Kirschner wire is removed. The hand is held in a plaster splint for an additional 2 months. Some type of thumb support, such as a removable splint, should be continued for about 4 months before unrestricted activity is allowed.

Group 3 clasped thumb deformity

■ *TECHNIQUE (NEVIASER MODIFIED).* Under tourniquet control, make a dorsal incision over the thumb metacarpophalangeal and interphalangeal joints (Fig. 74-66, *A*). If the metacarpophalangeal joints

are unstable to both radial and ulnar stresses, perform a dorsal capsulotomy and identify the articular surfaces of the metacarpal and proximal phalanx. Shave the articular cartilage with a scalpel to expose the epiphyseal bone and pin the joint with a Kirschner wire. Next make a short transverse dorsal incision at the base of the index finger to expose the extensor indicis proprius tendon. Make a transverse dorsal incision over the wrist in line with the tendon, divide the tendon distally, and deliver it into the wound (Fig. 74-66, *B*). Reroute the tendon subcutaneously and suture it into the soft tissue around the base of the distal phalanx or beneath a periosteal flap. Now make a short transverse palmar incision at the wrist over the palmaris longus tendon. Divide this tendon at its insertion into the palmar fascia and route it subcutaneously, passing it through an osseous tunnel created at the base of the thumb proximal phalanx just distal to the epiphysis; suture the tendon back onto itself (Fig. 74-66, *C*). Next perform an opponensplasty as described on p. 3404, perform a **Z**-plasty reconstruction of the web space contracture (p. 3403), and derotate the thumb metacarpal, if necessary, by sharply incising the capsule of the trapeziometacarpal joint and pronating the thumb 90 degrees. Fix this with a Kirschner wire. Close the incisions in routine fashion and apply a splint with the thumb in the corrected position.

AFTERTREATMENT. The Kirschner wires are removed 6 weeks after surgery, and progressive motion is allowed. The thumb is protected in a night splint for another 3 to 4 weeks.

Hypoplastic Hands and Digits

Hypoplastic hands or digits are those in which development of the part is defective or incomplete. Like syndactyly, elements of hypoplasia are seen in almost all hand deformities, and this term is best limited to those fingers and hands in which there is relatively symmetric deficiency of the part without associated deformity. Hypoplasia of the entire hand accounted for 0.8% of the deformities in the Iowa series, and brachydactyly ("short fingers") accounted for 5.2%. The single most commonly hypoplastic bony segment is the middle phalanx (brachyphalangia or brachymesophalangia). Brachymetacarpia ("short metacarpal") also is included with the hypoplastic deformities if it is present early, but this is extremely rare; it usually is not noted until after the adolescent growth spurt.

Brachydactyly has played an important role in the genetic literature as the first example of mendelian inheritance demonstrated in human beings. Shortening of the fingers usually is considered a dominant trait, but further genetic variations also have been described. If a person with brachydactyly marries a normal individual, their offspring have a 50% chance of having brachydactyly. Sporadic cases do occur, but no specific etiologic factor has been identified.

Brachyphalangia usually occurs alone, but it may occur in association with similar toe deformities. Shortening of the middle phalanges is common in malformation syndromes such as Treacher Collins, Bloom's, Cornelia de Lange's, Holt-Oram, Silver's, and Poland's syndromes. In Poland's syndrome the shortening usually is unilateral. Brachydactyly E, as defined by Bell, consists of brachymetacarpia of the long, ring, and little fingers in association with pseudohypoparathyroidism. Other conditions associated with brachymetacarpia include Turner's, Biemond, and Silver's syndromes.

There is no useful classification for the hypoplastic hand or digits. Geneticists have devised several detailed groupings of this disorder in an attempt to better record patterns of inheritance, but for the most part these serve no useful purpose in determining management of the deformities.

Hypoplasia of the digits may range from simple shortening (most common) to a small hand with nothing more than nubbins for fingers. In some patients this may represent an intermediate entity between congenital amputation and hypoplastic digits. There usually is some degree of hypoplasia of all tissues, not just the osseous structures. Except for the nubbinlike fingers, function usually is near normal. Brachymetacarpia usually is noted during the teenage growth spurt as a depression of

one or more metacarpal heads with the fist clenched. The ulnar two fingers are most commonly affected.

NONSURGICAL MANAGEMENT. Single-digit shortening, particularly of the little finger, requires no surgical correction. Although a single short digit surrounded by digits of normal length may be cosmetically unsatisfactory, functional limitation usually is minimal; also, digital lengthening will not improve function and may result in stiffness.

SURGICAL TREATMENT. Lengthening procedures have been recommended for brachymetacarpia to improve appearance of the metacarpal row and increase grip strength. Wood found that more than 1 cm of shortening may disrupt the metacarpal arch and cause decreased grip strength. Tajima described a single-stage lengthening using a V-shaped metacarpal osteotomy with an interpositional bone graft. Buck-Gramcko (1971) detaches the interossei and intermetacarpal ligaments at the time of osteotomy (Fig. 74-67). Despite success with lengthening procedures, these should be discouraged for the adult patient whose only concern is the appearance of the hand.

For the hypoplastic hand with no functioning digits or with preservation of only one digit, consideration may be given to more complex and less predictable procedures, but this is a controversial area of reconstructive hand surgery. It generally is accepted that, with the exception of the soft tissue nubbin, any digit regardless of size will be of some use to the patient. The musculotendinous structures in these fingers usually are extremely deficient, with little if any excursion. Added length created by distraction techniques or web deepening may produce a sense of improved function. A one-stage, nonvascularized, toe-phalanx transplantation as an interpositional or terminal graft may be beneficial for the extremely hypoplastic digit. Even if the periosteum and epiphysis are

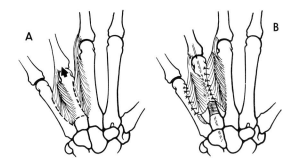

Fig. 74-67 Buck-Gramcko technique for lengthening brachymetacarpia in hypoplastic hand. **A,** Detachment of interossei and intermetacarpal ligaments, and metacarpal osteotomy. **B,** Interposition bone graft fixed with Kirschner wire. (Redrawn from Roselius (Copyright, 1988) from Dobyns JH, Wood VE, and Bayne LG: Congenital hand deformities. In Green DP, editor: Operative hand surgery, ed 2, New York, 1988, Churchill Livingstone, Inc.)

preserved, growth of the transferred phalanx is limited. The 1970 report of Matev of an average 3.3 cm lengthening of the thumb metacarpal in three adult patients with traumatic amputations sparked interest in the use of similar techniques for lengthening the severely hypoplastic digit. The usual technique includes division of the metacarpal bone and periosteum, application of external fixation, and gradual distraction of approximately 1 mm per day until the desired length is achieved or neurovascular or cutaneous limits are reached. Cowen and Loftus reported lengthening of the entire palm through the carpometacarpal joints with the use of distal metacarpal and proximal carpal pins. Although the usual length achieved is from 25 to 50 mm, Cowen and Loftus reported gaining as much as 7 cm. Ilizarov, Shtin, and Ledyaev also have reported lengthening of hand and forearm bones with their distraction apparatus. Lengthening within a digit should be avoided; the shortest bone to which the device can be applied is about 3 cm.

Metacarpal lengthening

■ **TECHNIQUE (TAJIMA) (Fig 74-68).** Under tourniquet control, make a dorsal longitudinal incision over the shortened metacarpal. Retract the extensor tendon to one side and expose the metacarpal shaft subperiosteally. Perform two **V**-shaped osteotomies at the junction of the proximal and middle thirds of the bone. Expose the deep transverse metacarpal ligament distally and incise it. Sharply detach the interosseus muscle on both sides of the metacarpal. Now manually distract the metacarpal to ensure that the osteotomy incisions are adequate. Harvest the iliac crest bone graft and fashion it to fill the gap in the lengthened bone. Insert the graft and secure it with a longitudinal Kirschner wire. Reattach the interosseus muscle to the periosteum through separate drill holes into either the bone graft or the metacar-

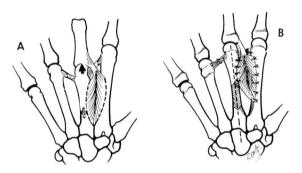

Fig. 74-68 Tajima technique for metacarpal lengthening in hypoplastic hand. **A,** Chevron osteotomy is made in shortened metacarpal; interosseus muscle and transverse metacarpal ligaments are released. **B,** Bone graft is interposed and secured with axial Kirschner wire; transverse metacarpal ligaments are repaired if possible. (Redrawn from Roselius (Copyright, 1988) from Dobyns JH, Wood VE, and Bayne LG: Congenital hand deformities. In Green DP, editor: Operative hand surgery, ed 2, New York, 1988, Churchill Livingstone, Inc.)

pal, depending on where the interosseus muscle falls into place after lengthening. Suture the skin in routine fashion and apply a cast or splint.

AFTERTREATMENT. The osteotomy is protected with a cast or splint until union occurs, but motion of the finger is begun 3 weeks after surgery. The Kirschner wire may be removed at 6 weeks.

Toe-phalanx transplantation

■ *TECHNIQUE.* Under tourniquet control, make a dorsal longitudinal incision over the second toe, which usually is excessively long and is the donor of choice; similar grafts may be harvested from the third or fourth toes if desired. Carry the incision through the skin, subcutaneous tissue, and extensor mechanism. Harvest the proximal phalanx, including the periosteum, as described by Goldberg and Watson, in an attempt to retain epiphyseal growth. Close the donor site with simple sutures. The cartilage over each end of the donor phalanx may or may not be retained, depending on whether some pseudojoint function is desirable. Make a dorsal longitudinal incision over the hypoplastic digit, which may be represented only by an empty skin tube. Place the toe phalanx within the hypoplastic digit in axial alignment with the adjacent bone and secure it with a longitudinal Kirschner wire. This may be used as an interpositional graft or terminal graft. Close the skin with interrupted sutures and apply a supportive dressing. After the digit viability is certain, apply a cast of appropriate length.

AFTERTREATMENT. The cast is maintained for approximately 6 weeks. Kirschner wires are removed and activities are gradually increased.

Lengthening with distraction

■ *TECHNIQUE (COWEN AND LOFTUS)*

Stage I. Under tourniquet control, make a **Z**-type incision on the dorsum of the hand and perform an osteotomy of the involved metacarpal or metacarpals. Manually distract the bone to ensure complete release of the soft tissues. Insert a transverse 0.062-inch Kirschner wire through the metacarpal distal to the osteotomy site. Insert this wire into the rectangular blocks of the distraction device. Using the device as a drill guide, place two additional Kirschner wires transversely through the metacarpal if possible. Use the same technique to insert the proximal wires. Release the tourniquet and observe circulation. Make a few turns of the distraction device. Close the incision in routine fashion. If complete closure is not possible after distraction, the open portion of the incision may be allowed to granulate or may be covered with a split-thickness graft.

AFTERTREATMENT. The patient is kept in the hospital for a few days after the procedure for careful observation. The patient or parents are instructed to increase the distraction by one third of a turn three times daily or one half turn twice daily. This amounts to approximately 1 mm of lengthening per day. This process is continued until the desired length is achieved and may require as much as 3 months. Close observation by the surgeon and the family during this process is mandatory to recognize any neurovascular compromise. When desired lengthening is obtained or neurovascular or cutaneous limits have been reached, the second stage of the procedure is performed.

■ *TECHNIQUE (COWEN AND LOFTUS)*

Stage II. Make a dorsal incision over the metacarpal or metacarpals that are to be grafted. Harvest donor bone graft from the iliac crest, ulna, fibula, or toe phalanx and insert this into the bony defect created by distraction. Stabilize the graft with a longitudinal Kirschner wire or leave the external fixator in place. Close the incision, deflate the tourniquet, and apply a short arm cast with a protective plaster bow in older children or a long arm cast in infants. *AFTERTREATMENT.* After 1 to 2 weeks the cast is replaced by a sling or wrap that covers the entire hand and distraction device. The apparatus and Kirschner wires are removed when sufficient time has passed to allow bone healing, usually after 8 or more weeks. The hand is protected with a cast or splint as needed, depending on the roentgenographic and clinical progress.

CONGENITAL RING SYNDROME

Congenital ring, or congenital constriction band, syndrome occurs when deep cutaneous creases encircle a limb as if a string were tightly tied around the part (Fig. 74-69). Its frequent association with congenital amputations and acrosyndactyly led to this malformation's designation as a syndrome. Other terms used to describe this condition include Streeter bands or dysplasia, annular grooves or defects, and intrauterine amputation. Patterson reported an incidence of 1:15,000 births. Constriction bands represented 2% of anomalies in Flatt's series. The more distal rings are more common, as is involvement of the central digits.

There is no evidence that congenital ring syndrome is an inherited condition. Kino believes the cause to be an external effect of amniotic adhesions formed in utero after hemorrhages in the distal rays. Patterson and also Streeter theorize failure of development of subcutaneous tissue in the same manner that normal skin creases are formed. There is general agreement that these malformations occur somewhat later than 5 to 7 weeks' gestation, when the majority of hand anomalies occur. The youngest fetus described by Potter was at 10 weeks of gestation.

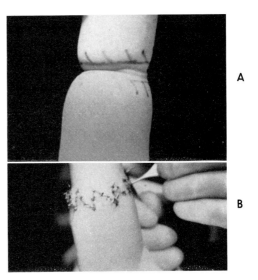

Fig. 74-69 A, Congenital ring syndrome in 3-month-old child. B, Z-plasty's release of constrictures.

Patterson includes four types of deformity in constriction ring syndrome: (1) a simple ring usually occurring transversely, but occasionally obliquely, around the limb or digit; (2) a deeper ring often associated with abnormality of the part distally, usually lymphedema; (3) fenestrated syndactyly (acrosyndactyly) or lateral fusion of adjacent digits at their distal ends with proximal fenestrations between the intervening skin and soft tissue; and (4) intrauterine amputation in which the soft tissues are more affected than the bone, which may protrude as in a guillotine amputation—there are no rudimentary parts distally and the proximal limb parts are normally developed. These four types may be present in any combination in a single child, but they do not occur constantly with any other type of anomaly of the limbs. Syndactyly, hypoplasia, brachydactyly, symphalangism, symbrachydactyly, and camptodactyly have been reported in up to 80% of patients with congenital ring syndrome, and clubfoot, cleft lip, cleft palate, and cranial defects have been reported in 40% to 50% of patients with this syndrome. Generally, there are no associated visceral malformations, but one of Flatt's patients had a patent ductus arteriosus.

These malformations usually are asymmetric. The grooves, or rings, vary in circumferential extent and depth and at times appear as normal but misplaced skin creases. Lymphedema distal to the crease is frequent. With shallow rings the skin often is normal but subcutaneous tissue usually is deficient. With deeper rings the superficial blood vessels that run across the ring are absent, although deep vessels are intact. Digits distal to the rings may be shortened or completely amputated. Terminal simple syndactyly with small fenestrations through the proximal web is frequent; Miura reported acrosyndactyly in 26 of 55 patients with congenital constriction band syndrome. The rings are not static in their effect. If the ring is deep and unrelenting, there may be progressive necrosis beneath the ring, with increased scarring, constriction, and vascular impairment. In 58% of Flatt's patients distal lymphedema, cyanosis, and worsening at the site of constriction occurred before surgical intervention. Rarely does the ring progress to cause frank necrosis of the distal part.

Treatment

For very shallow, incomplete creases with no distal lymphedema, surgical intervention usually is unnecessary except to improve appearance. The creases should be observed for gradual improvement in appearance, which may occur as "baby fat" is lost. If creases are deep enough to cause lymphedema or impairment of circulation, they should be excised down to normal tissue and the defect should be closed with multiple Z-plasty procedures. If the ring completely encircles the part, the safer approach is staged excision of one half of the groove with Z-plasty closure, followed by a second operation 2 to 3 months later. Lymphedema and cyanosis usually improve gradually after release. Simple excision of the groove with simple everting closure generally is inadequate because circumferential scar contracture may occur.

Acrosyndactyly is a frequent component of this syndrome. Because all fingertips frequently are bound together, permanent deformity will result unless early syndactyly reconstruction is performed. Release of the border digits should be done within the first 6 months of life, followed by release of the central digits when the child is about 18 months of age. Finger stiffness at the proximal interphalangeal joints is common after syndactyly release. Short digits may require lengthening by osteotomy and distraction. The shortened thumb may require deepening of the web space or lengthening by the method of Solland, in which an extremely shortened index finger is added to the top of the thumb. Amputations in this syndrome usually have adequate or abundant soft tissue coverage and rarely require surgical reconstruction.

MULTIPLE Z-PLASTY RELEASE OF CONGENITAL RING

■ *TECHNIQUE.* If the congenital ring is deep and completely encircles the limb or finger, plan to correct only half of the ring in the initial procedure. Before inflating the tourniquet, mark out the multiple Z-plasty sites along the constricting ring (Fig. 74-70, *A*). Exsanguinate the limb and inflate the tourniquet. Excise half the constricting ring and then sharply incise the Z-plasty sites to elevate the flaps. Suture the flaps in an appropriate interdigitating fashion to allow for lengthening of the constricting ring (Fig. 74-70, *B*). Deflate the tourniquet and ap-

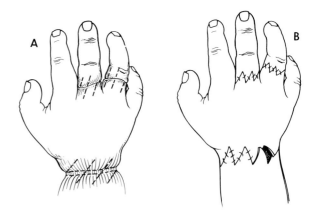

Fig. 74-70 Multiple Z-plasties for severe congenital ring syndrome. **A,** Band is completely excised after it is ascertained that no deep fascial constriction remains. Only volar half of ring should be corrected at initial procedure. **B,** Z-plasty closure. (Redrawn from Roselius (Copyright, 1988) from Dobyns JH, Wood VE, and Bayne LG: Congenital hand deformities. In Green DP, editor: Operative hand surgery, ed 2, New York, 1988, Churchill Livingstone, Inc.)

ply a bulky dressing with a short arm or long arm splint.
AFTERTREATMENT. The splinting is maintained for 2 to 3 weeks. Sutures are removed after 10 to 14 days. The other half of the constricting ring can be similarly reconstructed after 2 to 3 months.

MISCELLANEOUS ANOMALIES
Congenital Trigger Digits

Congenital trigger digit occurs when the normal gliding movement of the flexor tendon is impeded within the digital flexor sheath. Unlike the situation in adults with stenosing tenovaginitis, the congenitally involved finger usually shows a persistent flexion deformity rather than actual "triggering" (Fig. 74-71, *A*). This is a relatively rare condition and was found in only 2.3% of Flatt's patients. It occurs far more commonly in the thumb and is bilateral in about 25% of patients. The condition occurs sporadically and is not believed to be an inherited trait. Trigger digits typically occur without other anomalies, but an association with trisomy 13 has been reported.

Approximately 25% of trigger digits are noted at birth; frequently the condition is not noted until the age of 1 or 2 years, at which time the child has a relatively fixed flexion posture of the interphalangeal joint of the thumb. Even with some force, it may not be possible to fully extend the interphalangeal joint of the thumb. Dellon and Hansen reported an occasional extension posture of the thumb and involvement of multiple digits. The abnormal clicking or snapping usually is not the presenting complaint commonly seen in adults. This condition must be differentiated from the clasped thumb deformity, in which there is primarily metacarpophalangeal flexion.

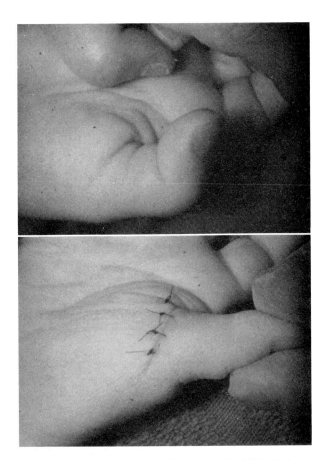

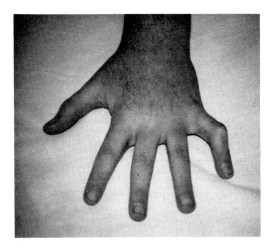

Fig. 74-72   Camptodactyly (flexion deformity of proximal interphalangeal joint) involving only little finger.

Fig. 74-71   A, Trigger thumb in 2-year-old child. **B,** Appearance after release.

The pathologic anatomy responsible for trigger digits includes narrowing and thickening of the sheath, with occasional formation of a ganglion cyst. An intratendinous nodule may be present proximal to the first annular pulley. Chronic inflammation also is frequent. Fixed contractures are unlikely if the condition resolves or is corrected before the child is 3 years old. Spontaneous resolution occurs in about 30% of children whose condition appears within the first year of life and in about 12% of those in whom the condition appears between the ages of 6 months and 2 years.

TREATMENT. Because spontaneous resolution can be expected in about 30% of children whose condition becomes apparent within the first year of life, observation and gentle manipulation are appropriate. Splinting may be attempted but has not been shown to be of benefit. If the condition does not resolve spontaneously, surgical intervention should not be delayed beyond the age of 3 years. Surgical release of the first annular pulley should be performed at about the age of 2 years if spontaneous resolution has not occurred. In the rare instance in which multiple trigger digits fixed in extension prevent the child from making a fist, surgical intervention should be earlier (around the age of 1 year). Accidental nerve

injury may be avoided by first making a shallow incision and identifying the digital nerves. Lacerated digital nerves and tendons should be repaired. Recurrence is unlikely if release is adequate.

Release of congenital trigger thumb

■ *TECHNIQUE.* Under tourniquet control, make a transverse incision at the volar crease of the metacarpophalangeal joint of the thumb. Carefully protect the two digital nerves. The flexor sheath usually is quite prominent just beneath the subcutaneous fat. Identify the proximal edge of the first annular pulley and completely incise it longitudinally under direct vision. Shaving the nodule and excising a segment of the A-1 pulley usually are unnecessary. Close the wound (Fig. 74-71, *B*) and apply a soft dressing. No particular immobilization is required. This procedure may be performed in a similar fashion in other involved digits.

Camptodactyly

Camptodactyly is a flexion deformity of the proximal interphalangeal joint that usually involves only the little finger (Fig. 74-72). This type of bent finger deformity should be distinguished from clinodactyly, in which the finger is bent either radialward or ulnarward. Camptodactyly occurs in fewer than 1% of the population and was found in 6.9% of the anomalies in Flatt's series. There is a strong hereditary predisposition in many patients, in whom the deformity is transmitted as an autosomal dominant trait. Sporadic cases also occur. All structures that could possibly cause flexion deformity at the proximal interphalangeal joint have been considered as possible etiologic factors. Kilgore and Graham found a stout band of tissue in association with Landsmeer's ligament. McFarlane, Curry, and Evans found an abnormal insertion of the lumbrical tendon into the flexor superficialis tendon, the capsule of the metacarpophalangeal joint, or the extensor expansion of the adjacent finger in all 21 of their patients. This appears to support the view of Millesi that camptodactyly is due to a relative imbalance between the flexors and extensors. Smith and Kaplan suggested relative shortening in the flexor superficialis muscle/tendon unit because the deformity usually could be corrected with simultaneous flexion of the wrist (Fig. 74-73). Other theories include contractures of the collateral ligaments or volar plate, insufficient palmar skin, and congenital fibrous substrata in the subcutaneous tissues.

There appear to be two types of camptodactyly, based on the age at which the deformity occurs. The first type occurs in infancy and affects both sexes equally. This is the more common type and occurs in about 80% of patients. The second type occurs during adolescence and affects mostly girls. Camptodactyly commonly is associated with many syndromes, including trisomy 13, oculodentodigital, orofaciodigital, Aarskog, and cerebrohepatorenal syndromes. Koman, Toby, and Poehling recently reported a subgroup of camptodactyly in which severe flexion deformities of the proximal interphalangeal joints are present at birth. Often several digits of the same hand are affected, and there is no predilection for the small finger. Pathologic findings in this subtype primarily involve the extension mechanism (attenuation of the central slip, palmar subluxation of the lateral bands, and hypoplasia of the radial extensor structure). Koman et al. noted postoperative impingement only in those patients whose extensor mechanism was realigned and augmented by release or transfer of the flexor digitorum superficialis.

Most patients are seen with a flexion deformity of the proximal interphalangeal joint during the first year of life. About two thirds have bilateral deformities, which are not necessarily symmetric in severity. The metacarpophalangeal joint usually is held in hyperextension to compensate for the flexed posture. Rotational deformity may cause mild overlapping of fingers. In young children the deformity disappears when the wrist is flexed, but in older children the flexion deformity usually is fixed. If left untreated, 80% will worsen, especially during the pe-

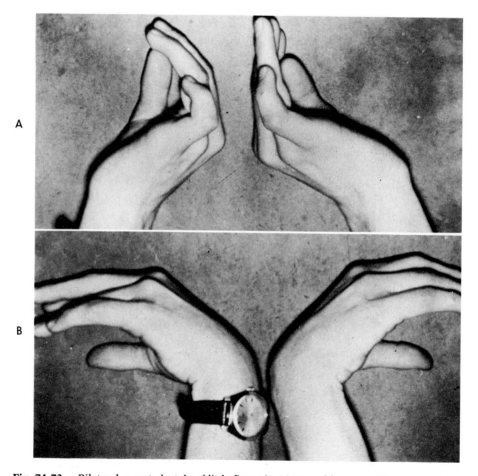

Fig. 74-73 Bilateral camptodactyly of little finger in 18-year-old man. **A,** Flexion contractures of proximal interphalangeal joints were increased when wrists were extended. **B,** Contractures almost disappeared when wrists were flexed. (From Smith RJ and Kaplan EB: J Bone Joint Surg 50-A:1187, 1968.)

riod of growth acceleration. The deformity usually does not progress after the age of 18 to 20 years. Rarely, pain and swelling are present.

TREATMENT. Neither nonsurgical nor surgical treatment of camptodactyly has been particularly predictable or satisfying. Engber and Flatt reported that 20% of patients improved with nonsurgical treatment and only 35% improved with surgical treatment. Miura reported full-time dynamic splinting in 24 patients until full extension was achieved, followed by splinting for 8 hours a day. Good results were obtained as long as splinting was continued, but some flexion deformity recurred when splinting was discontinued. It is reasonable to advise patients with mild deformities to live with their deformities. For young children in whom the deformity disappears with wrist flexion and for whom the parents desire surgical correction, release of the sublimis tendon may correct the deformity and prevent worsening during growth. This usually should be performed by the age of 4 years. In older children and young adults in whom the deformity can be corrected with splinting but who continue to have weak extension at the proximal interphalangeal joint, release of the flexor digitorum sublimis muscle and transfer into the extensor apparatus, as advocated by Millesi and by Lankford, is advised. A volar release, including local skin flap and volar plate release, has been used before tendon transfer to allow passive correction of the flexion deformity.

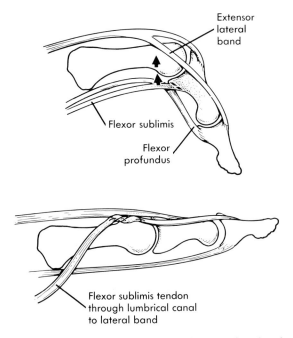

Fig. 74-74 Technique for correction of camptodactyly. Flexor sublimis tendon is transferred to extensor apparatus. (Redrawn from Roselius (Copyright, 1988) from Dobyns JH, Wood VE, and Bayne LG: Congenital hand deformities. In Green DP, editor: Operative hand surgery, ed 2, New York, 1988, Churchill Livingstone, Inc.)

Transfer of flexor superficialis tendon to extensor apparatus

■ ***TECHNIQUE (McFARLANE ET AL.; Fig. 74-74).*** Under tourniquet control, make a straight midline incision over the finger so that a Z-plasty closure can be achieved as necessary. Divide the flexor digitorum sublimis tendon just proximal to the vinculum longum and transfer it through the lumbrical canal to the dorsal surface of the finger. Suture the sublimis tendon to the extensor apparatus with nonabsorbable sutures. Tension the transferred tendon so that normal stance of the digit is achieved in all wrist positions. If correction of the deformity is not complete, consideration can be given to a proximal release of the volar plate; however, it is best to accept a flexion deformity of approximately 20 degrees. Insert a Kirschner wire through the proximal interphalangeal joint to maintain extension. Close the skin with single or multiple Z-plasty procedures. Apply a short arm cast with the metacarpophalangeal joints in 90 degrees of flexion and the digits fully extended.

AFTERTREATMENT. The cast and Kirschner wire are removed 4 weeks after surgery. A dorsal splint with a metacarpal stop to prevent overstretching of the transferred tendon is worn for another 4 weeks.

Kirner's Deformity

This anomaly, originally described by Kirner in 1927, consists of palmar and radial curving of the distal phalanx of the little finger. It is an unsightly deformity that occurs only infrequently; David and Burwood determined an incidence of 1:410 live births in their survey of 3000 patients. The deformity occurs more frequently in girls and may rarely affect several fingers. Sporadic, as well as familial, occurrences have been reported, and there is no known specific etiologic factor. A similar deformity may result from frostbite, epiphyseal fracture, and infection. Kirner's deformity has been associated with Cornelia de Lange's, Silver's, and Turner's syndromes.

The deformity typically is seen when the child is around the age of 8 to 10 years and appears as a beaked little fingertip with increased convexity of the fingernail (Fig. 74-75). The fingertip curves radially and toward the palm. The deformity usually is bilateral and symmetric. Although it may be progressive, usually it is not painful. Roentgenograms reveal a broadened epiphysis with irregularities of the metaphysis. The typical curvature can be seen within the distal phalanx (Fig. 74-76, *A*).

TREATMENT. For mild deformities either splinting or no treatment may be appropriate. More severe deformities in skeletally mature patients require one or more osteotomies of the terminal phalanx, as described by Carstam and Eiken. No effective treatment has been described for correction of the nail deformity.

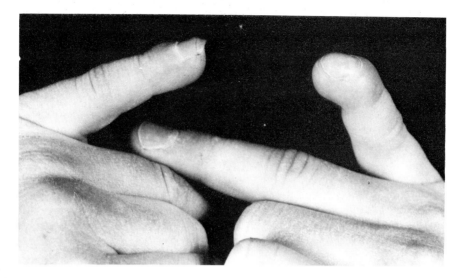

Fig. 74-75   Kirner's deformity (see text). (From Carstam N and Eiken O: J Bone Joint Surg 52-A:1663, 1970.)

Opening wedge osteotomy of terminal phalanx

■ *TECHNIQUE (CARSTAM AND EIKEN; Fig. 74-76, B).* Under tourniquet control, make a radial midlateral incision over the distal phalanx of the involved finger. Expose the distal phalanx subperiosteally and perform two osteotomies through the volar three fourths of the diaphysis. Using a periosteal hinge left intact on the dorsum of the phalanx, correct the deformity. This periosteal hinge also helps control rotation of the fragments. Complete correction of the deformity may be blocked by a curved nail deformity. Place a longitudinal Kirschner wire through the phalanx and the distal interphalangeal joint to hold the correction. If the phalanx is extremely small, insert a Kirschner wire extraperiosteally along the volar aspect of the phalanx to act as an internal splint. Close the incisions in routine fashion and apply a long arm or short arm splint.

AFTERTREATMENT. The splint and Kirschner wire are removed 4 to 6 weeks after surgery. Usually no specific postoperative therapy is necessary. Activities are permitted depending on the clinical and roentgenographic signs of healing.

Delta Phalanx

The delta phalanx is an abnormal, trapezoidal-shaped phalanx that appears triangular on roentgenograms (Fig. 74-77) and derives its name from the Greek letter *delta*. The abnormal epiphysis is C- or J-shaped and tends to

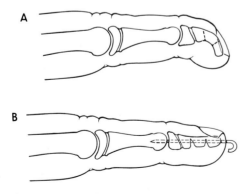

Fig. 74-76   Correction of Kirner's deformity. **A,** Deformity. **B,** Multiple opening wedge osteotomy cuts in distal phalanx fixed with Kirschner wire. (Redrawn from Carstam N and Eiken O: J Bone Joint Surg 52-A:1663, 1970.)

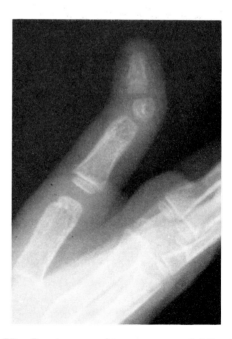

Fig. 74-77   Roentgenographic appearance of delta phalanx.

bracket one side of the phalanx. The incidence of this deformity in the general population has not been established. The specific cause is not known, but in as many as 44% of patients there is a strong family history and autosomal dominant transmission. Delta phalanx rarely is an isolated anomaly and usually occurs in association with such entities as polydactyly, syndactyly, symphalangism, cleft foot, triphalangeal thumb, central hand deficiency, ulnar clubhand, Apert's syndrome, Poland's syndrome, diastrophic dwarfism, and Holt-Oram syndrome.

The delta phalanx causes an angular deformity of the digit in the frontal plane (clinodactyly). When the deformity is in the border digits, the finger tends to deviate toward the hand. The angulation frequently is mild, but when it is severe, it may cause an unacceptable appearance. According to Flatt this anomaly most commonly occurs in the proximal phalanx of the thumb in association with triphalangeal thumb and in the middle phalanx of the small finger. The next most frequent location is the proximal phalanx of the ring finger. Progressive angulation is inevitable.

TREATMENT. Moderate angulation of the finger produced by the delta phalanx is awkward and unsightly. Nonsurgical treatment will not alter progression, and surgical intervention should be aimed at narrowing the digit, straightening the phalanx, and destroying the abnormal portion of the epiphysis. If it is associated with central polydactyly, the delta phalanx should be excised along with the extra digit with a syndactyly-type reconstruction. If it is associated with a triphalangeal thumb, the delta phalanx should be excised and the joint ligaments reconstructed. The deformity may recur after osteotomy. Reverse wedge osteotomy, as described by Carstam and Theander, is preferable to simple opening wedge osteotomy. Carstam and Theander reported elimination or marked reduction of clinodactyly in all of their patients. Vickers described a procedure in which he resected the isthmus of the continuous epiphysis and inserted an interpositional fat graft. He reported spontaneous angular correction and growth of the phalanx in 11 patients. Smith described a technique in which he performed an opening wedge osteotomy of the delta phalanx and inserted a bone graft obtained from the distal phalanx (Fig. 74-78).

Reverse wedge osteotomy

■ *TECHNIQUE (CARSTAM AND THEANDER; Fig. 74-79).* Under tourniquet control, make a curved dorsal incision over the involved phalanx, extending from the distal portion of the proximal phalanx, over the entire length of the middle phalanx, and onto the proximal portion of the distal phalanx. Carefully mobilize the edges of the extensor tendon so that both borders of the delta phalanx in the middle phalanx can be seen. Identify and protect the insertion

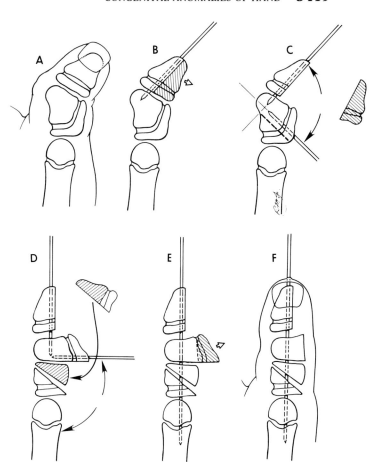

Fig. 74-78 Modified opening wedge technique for correction of delta phalanx as described by Smith. (Redrawn from Dobyns JH, Wood VE, and Bayne LG: Congenital hand deformities. In Green DP, editor: Operative hand surgery, ed 2, New York, 1988, Churchill Livingstone, Inc.)

of the central extensor slip. Remove a wedge-shaped piece of bone from the central portion of the delta phalanx, either by using a scalpel if it is mostly cartilaginous or by carefully picking away at it with sharp bone cutters, as described by Flatt. Reverse this wedge-shaped piece of bone and insert it into the defect after correcting the angular deformity. Place a longitudinal Kirschner wire through the distal phalanx and into the proximal phalanx to hold the corrected position; leave the wire protruding through the distal end of the finger. Close the incision in routine fashion and apply a long or short arm splint.

AFTERTREATMENT. The splint and Kirschner wire are removed 4 to 6 weeks after surgery. Gradually increased activity is permitted depending on clinical and roentgenographic healing.

Madelung's Deformity

Madelung's deformity is an abnormality of the palmar ulnar part of the distal radial epiphysis in which progres-

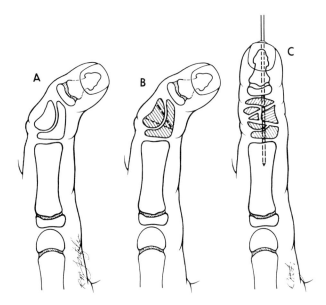

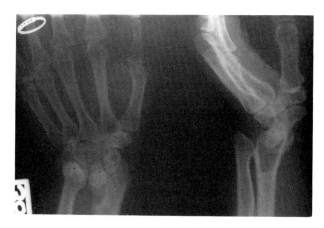

Fig. 74-80 Roentgenographic appearance of Madelung's deformity. Note abnormalities of radius, ulna, and carpal bones.

Fig. 74-79 Reverse wedge osteotomy for correction of delta phalanx. **A,** Delta phalanx involving middle phalanx. **B,** Wedge-shaped piece of bone is removed from central portion. **C,** Wedge is reversed and reinserted after correction of angular deformity; Kirschner wire is used for fixation. (Redrawn from Carstam N and Theander G: Scand J Plast Reconstr Surg 9:199, 1975.)

sive ulnar and volar tilt develops at the distal radial articular surface, with dorsal subluxation of the distal ulna. The deformity probably was first described by Malgaigne in 1855 and later by Madelung in 1878. It is believed to be a congenital disorder, although it seldom is obvious until late childhood or adolescence. It is a rare anomaly, accounting for only 1.7% of hand anomalies in Flatt's series. The cause of Madelung's deformity is uncertain; however, it has been shown to be transmitted in an autosomal dominant pattern. Other Madelung-like deformities have occurred after trauma, as reported by Vender and Watson in a gymnast, and after infection or neoplasm. There is no definitive method of distinguishing these from idiopathic Madelung's deformity. Vender and Watson classified Madelung's and Madelung-like deformities into four groups: posttraumatic, dysplastic (dyschondrosteosis or diaphyseal aclasis), genetic (for example, Turner's syndrome), and idiopathic. They believe that acquired deformities usually can be distinguished by a lack of appropriate physical findings, unilaterality, less severe carpal deformities, and the appropriate history of repetitive injury or stress.

A deformity of the wrist similar to Madelung's deformity frequently is associated with dyschondrosteosis, the most common form of mesomelic dwarfism. This disorder consists of mild shortness of stature, shortness of the middle segment of the upper and lower extremities, and Madelung's deformity. Other associated conditions include mucopolysaccharidosis, Turner's syndrome,

achondroplasia, multiple exostoses, multiple epiphyseal dysplasia, and dyschondroplasia (Ollier's disease).

Madelung's deformity typically consists of volar subluxation of the hand, with prominence of the distal ulna and volar and ulnar angulation of the distal radius. It is more commonly bilateral and affects girls more frequently than boys. A family history of the deformity often is present. The deformity usually manifests in late childhood or early adolescence, with decreased motion and minimal pain. As growth occurs, the deformity worsens in appearance. Roentgenographic abnormalities are seen in the radius, ulna, and carpal bones (Fig. 74-80). The radius is curved, with its convexity dorsal and radial, and there is a similar angulation of the distal radial articular surface. The forearm is relatively short. The distal radial epiphysis is triangular in shape because of the failure of growth in the ulnar and volar aspects of the epiphysis; early closure of these aspects of the epiphysis also is frequent. Osteophyte formation may be visible at the volar ulnar border of the radius. The ulna is subluxated dorsally, the ulnar head is enlarged, and the overall length of the ulna is decreased. The carpus appears to have subluxated ulnarward and palmarward into the distal radioulnar joint, which usually is spread apart. The carpus appears wedge shaped, with its apex proximal within the lunate.

TREATMENT. Because children with Madelung's deformity usually have minimal pain and excellent function, a conservative approach is warranted initially. Surgery should be considered for severe deformity or persistent pain, usually from ulnocarpal impingement of the carpus. Distal radial osteotomy with ulnar shortening (Milch recession) is a preferred treatment in skeletally immature patients. The radial osteotomy may be a closing or opening wedge as needed for alignment. Osteotomy combined with a judicious Darrach excision of the distal ulnar head may be used in skeletally mature pa-

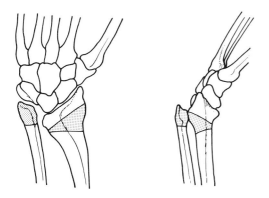

Fig. 74-81   Reconstruction of Madelung's deformity. Dorsal- and radial-based closing wedge osteotomy of radius is performed in conjunction with Darrach excision. Correct alignment is obtained, and plate and screws are used for fixation. (Redrawn from Ranawat CS, DeFiore J, and Straub LR: J Bone Joint Surg 57-A:772, 1975.)

tients. White and Weiland reported good results in one patient with radial osteotomy combined with a Laurenstein procedure. The deformity may recur after either procedure, and range of motion of the forearm usually does not improve after surgery.

Closing wedge osteotomy combined with Darrach excision of distal ulnar head

■ **TECHNIQUE** (*RANAWAT, DEFIORE, AND STRAUB; Fig. 74-81*). Make a dorsal longitudinal incision over the distal forearm, detach the extensor retinaculum from the radius over the extensor digitorum communis tendons, and reflect the retinaculum and the tendon of the extensor digiti minimi ulnarward. If the patient is skeletally mature, expose the distal radioulnar joint and excise about 1 cm of the distal ulna. If the patient is skeletally immature, expose the ulnar shaft and perform an appropriate cuff recession as described by Milch. Next perform an osteotomy parallel with the distal articular surface of the radius. Resect an appropriate wedge of bone based radially and dorsally from the distal end of the proximal fragment of the radius and appose the raw surfaces. Stabilize the osteotomy with Kirschner wires so that the distal articular surface of the radius is facing volarward 0 to 15 degrees to the long axis of the radius and ulnarward 60 to 70 degrees. Close the incision in routine fashion and apply a long arm cast.

AFTERTREATMENT. The cast and pins are removed 4 weeks after surgery, and active exercises of the wrist are begun. The osteotomy incision is protected with a cast or splint until there are sufficient roentgenographic and clinical signs of bone healing. Normal activities are progressively resumed. After the final cast is removed, protective splinting may be necessary for 8 to 10 weeks after surgery.

REFERENCES
General

Beals RK and Crawford A: Congenital absence of the pectoral muscles, Clin Orthop 119:166, 1976.

Birch-Jensen A: Congenital deformities of the upper extremities, Odense, Denmark, 1949, Ejnar Muntsgaads Forleg.

Cheng JCY, Chow SK, and Leung PC: Classification of 578 cases of congenital upper limb anomalies with the IFSSH system — a 10 years' experience, J Hand Surg 12-A:1055, 1987.

Conway H and Bowe J: Congenital deformities of the hands, Plast Reconstr Surg 18:286, 1956.

Dobyns JH, Wood VE, and Bayne LG: Congenital hand deformities. In Green DP, editor: Operative hand surgery, ed 2, New York, 1988, Churchill Livingstone, Inc.

Flatt AE: The care of congenital hand anomalies, St Louis, 1977, Mosby–Year Book, Inc.

Frantz CH and O'Rahilly R: Congenital skeletal limb deficiencies, J Bone Joint Surg 43-A:1202, 1961

Huber E: Hilfsoperation bei Medianuslahmung, Dtsch Z Chir 162:271, 1921.

Imamura T and Miura T: The carpal bones in congenital hand anomalies: a radiographic study in patients older than ten years, J Hand Surg 13-A:650, 1988.

Lamb DW: The practice of hand surgery, ed 2, Oxford, 1989, Blackwell Scientific Publications.

Lamb DW and Scott H: Management of congenital and acquired amputation in children, Orthop Clin North Am 12:997, 1981.

Littler JW: Introduction to surgery of the hand, Plast Reconstr Surg 4:1543, 1964.

MacDonnell JA: Age of fitting upper extremity prostheses in children, J Bone Joint Surg 40-A:655, 1958.

Marcer E: Intervento per correggere la clinodattilia metacarpofalangia, Clin Orthop 1:111, 1949.

Matev IB: Thumb reconstruction in children through metacarpal lengthening, Plast Reconstr Surg 64:665, 1979.

Milford L: The hand: congenital anomalies. In Crenshaw AH, editor: Campbell's operative orthopaedics, ed 7, St Louis, 1987, Mosby–Year Book, Inc.

Ogino T: A clinical and experimental study of teratogenic mechanism of cleft hand, polydactyly and syndactyly, Nippon Seikeigeka Gakkai Zasshi 53:535, 1979.

O'Rahilly R: Morphologic patterns in limb deficiencies and duplications, Am J Anat 89:135, 1956.

Silverman ME, Copeland AJ Jr, and Hurst JW: The Holt-Oram syndrome: the long and short of it, Am J Cardiol 25:11, 1970.

Stelling F: The upper extremity. In Ferguson AB, editor: Orthopedic surgery in infancy and childhood, Baltimore, 1963, Williams & Wilkins.

Stetten DW: Idiopathic progressive curvature of the radius, or so-called Madelung's deformity of the wrist (carpus varus and carpus valgus), Surg Gynecol Obstet 8:4, 1909.

Swanson AB: A classification for congenital limb malformations, J Hand Surg 1:8, 1976.

Swanson AB, Barsky AJ, and Entin M: Classification of limb malformations on the basis of embryological failures, Surg Clin North Am 48:1169, 1968.

Temtamy SA and McKusick VA: Absence deformities as isolated malformations, Birth Defects 14:36, 1978.

Temtamy SA and McKusick VA: Absence deformities as part of syndromes, Birth Defects 14:73, 1978.

Turek SI: Orthopaedic principles and their application, Philadelphia, 1967, JB Lippincott Co.

Watson-Jones R: Fractures and joint injuries, ed 3, vol 2, Baltimore, 1943, Williams & Wilkins.

Wynne-Davies R, Kuczynski K, Lamb DW, and Smith RJ: Congenital abnormalities of the hand. In Lamb DW, Hooper G, and Kuczynski K, editors: The practice of hand surgery, ed 2, Oxford, 1989, Blackwell Scientific Publications.

Wynne-Davies R and Lamb DW: Congenital upper limb anomalies: an etiologic grouping of clinical, genetic, and epidemiologic data from 382 patients with "absence" defects, constriction bands, polydactylies, and syndactylies, J Hand Surg 10-A (6, pt 2):958, 1985.

Yamaguchi S et al: Restoration of function to congenitally deformed hands. Proceedings of the sixteenth annual meeting of the Japanese Society for Surgery of the Hand, Fukuoka, 1973.

Transverse deficiencies

Chan KM, Ma GFY, Cheng JCY, and Leung PC: The Krukenberg procedure: a method of unilateral anomalies of upper limb in Chinese children, J Hand Surg 9-A:548, 1984.

Cowen NJ and Loftus JM: Distraction augmentation manoplasty: technique for lengthening digits for the entire hand, Orthop Rev 7:45, 1978.

Epps C, Burkhalter W, and McCollough NC III: Modern amputation surgery and prosthetic techniques. In The American Academy of Orthopaedic Surgeons: Instructional course lectures, Presented in Atlanta, 1980.

Ilizarov GA: Clinical application of the tension-stress effect of limb-lengthening, Clin Orthop 250:8, 1990.

Kessler I, Baruch A, and Hecht O: Experience with distraction lengthening of digital rays in congenital anomalies, J Hand Surg 2:394, 1977.

Krukenberg H: Uber Platiches Unwertung von Amputationstumpen, Stuttgart, 1917, Ferdinand Enk.

Matev I: A new method of thumb reconstruction. Paper presented at the Anglo-Scandinavian Symposium of Hand Surgery, Lausanne, Switzerland, May 26-27, 1967.

Nathan PA and Trung NB: The Krukenberg operation: a modified technique avoiding skin grafts, J Hand Surg 2:127, 1977.

Swanson AB and Swanson G deG: The Krukenberg procedure in the juvenile amputee, Clin Orthop 148:55, 1980.

Phocomelia

Lamb DW, MacNaughtan AK, and Fragiadakis EG: Phocomelia of the upper limb, Hand 3:200, 1971.

Sulamaa M and Ryoppy S: Early treatment of congenital bone defects of the extremities: aftermath of thalidomide disaster, Lancet 1:130, 1964.

Taussig HB: A study of the German outbreak of phocomelia: the thalidomide syndrome, JAMA 180:1106, 1962.

Radial deficiencies

Albee FH: Formation of radius congenitally absent: condition seven years after implantation of bone graft, Ann Surg 87:105, 1928.

Bayne LG and Klug MS: Long-term review of the surgical treatment of radial deficiencies, J Hand Surg 12-A:169, 1987.

Bora FW, Osterman AL, Kaneda RR, and Esterhai J: Radial clubhand deformity: long-term follow-up, J Bone Joint Surg 63-A:741, 1981.

Buck-Gramcko D: Pollicization of the index finger: method and results in aplasia and hypoplasia of the thumb, J Bone Joint Surg 53-A:1605, 1971.

Buck-Gramcko D: Radialization as a new treatment for radial club hand, J Hand Surg 10-A (pt 2):964, 1985.

DeLorme TL: Treatment of congenital absence of radius by transepiphyseal fixation, J Bone Joint Surg 51-A:117, 1969.

Goldberg MJ and Meyn M: The radial clubhand, Orthop Clin North Am 7:341, 1976.

Gosset J: La pollicisation de l'index, J Chir 65:403, 1949.

Harrison SH: Pollicization in cases of radial club hand, Br J Plast Surg 23:192, 1970.

Heikel HVA: Aplasia and hypoplasia of the radius, Acta Orthop Scand Suppl 39:1, 1959.

Kato K: Congenital absence of the radius, with review of the literature and report of three cases, J Bone Joint Surg 6:589, 1924.

Kessler I: Centralization of the radial club hand by gradual distraction, J Hand Surg 14-B:37, 1989.

Kummel W: Die Missbildungen der Extremitäten durch Defekt, Verwachsung und Ueberzahl, Heft 3, Kassel, Germany, 1895, Bibliotheca Medica.

Lamb DW: The treatment of radial club hand: absent radius, aplasia of the radius, hypoplasia of the radius, radial paraxial hemimelia, Hand 4:22, 1972.

Lamb DW: Radial club hand, a continuing study of sixty-eight patients with one hundred and seventeen club hands, J Bone Joint Surg 59-A:1, 1977.

Lamb DW, Wynne-Davies R, and Soto L: An estimate of the population frequency of congenital malformations of the upper limb, J Hand Surg 7:557, 1982.

Lidge RT: Congenital radial deficient club hand, J Bone Joint Surg 51-A:1041, 1969.

Manske PR and McCarroll HR Jr: Abductor digiti minimi opponensplasty in congenital radial aplasia, J Hand Surg 3:522, 1978.

Manske PR, McCarroll HR Jr, and Swanson K: Centralization of the radial club hand: ulnar surgical approach, J Hand Surg 6:423, 1981.

Menelaus MB: Radial club hand with absence of the biceps muscle treated by centralization of the ulna and triceps transfer: report of two cases, J Bone Joint Surg 58-B:488, 1976.

Prokopovich VS: Aligning of length of the forearm bones in the congenital club-hand in children, Orthop Travmatol Protez 1:51, 1980.

Riordan DC: Congenital absence of the radius, J Bone Joint Surg 37-A:1129, 1955.

Riordan DC: Congenital absence of the radius, a 15-year follow-up, J Bone Joint Surg 45-A:1783, 1963.

Riordan DC, Powers RC, and Hurd RA: The Huber procedure for congenital absence of thenar muscle. Paper presented at the annual meeting of the American Society for Surgery of the Hand, San Francisco, Feb 27, 1975.

Sayre RH: A contribution to the study of club-hand, Trans Am Orthop Assoc 6:208, 1893.

Skerik SK and Flatt AE: The anatomy of congenital radial dysplasia: its surgical and functional implications, Clin Orthop 66:125, 1969.

Starr DE: Congenital absence of the radius: a method of surgical correction, J Bone Joint Surg 27:572, 1945.

Tsuyuguchi Y, Yukioka M, Kawabata Y, et al: Radial ray deficiency, J Pediatr Orthop 7:699, 1987.

Watson HK, Beebe RD, and Cruz NI: Centralization procedure for radial clubhand, J Hand Surg 9-A:541, 1984.

Wynne-Davies R and Lamb DW: Congenital upper limb anomalies, J Hand Surg 10-A (6, pt 2):958, 1985.

Central deficiencies

Barsky AJ: Cleft hand: classification, incidence, and treatment, J Bone Joint Surg 46-A:1707, 1964.

Flatt AE and Wood VE: Multiple dorsal rotation flaps from the hand for thumb web contractures, Plast Reconstr Surg 45:258, 1970.

Fort AJA: Des difformities congenitales et acquises des doigts, et des Boyens d'y remedier, Paris, 1869, Adrien Delahaye.

Gilbert A: Toe transfers for congenital hand defects, J Hand Surg 7-A:118, 1982.

Hartsinck JJ: Beschryving van Guiana, of de wilde Kust in Zuid-America, vol 2, Amsterdam, 1770, Gerrit Tielenburg.

Lange M: Grundsatzliches uber die Beurteilung der Enstehung und Bewertung atypischer Handund Fussmissbildungen, Verh Dtsch Orthop Ges 31, Kongress Konigsberg/Pr Z Orthop (suppl) 31:80, 1936.

Maisels DO: Lobster-claw deformities of the hands and feet, Br J Plast Surg 23:269, 1970.

Manske PR: Cleft hand and central polydactyly in identical twins: a case report, J Hand Surg 8:906, 1983.

Milford L: The split (cleft) hand. Paper presented at Symposium on Congenital Hand Deformities, American Society for Surgery of the Hand, Atlanta, 1978.

Miura T: Cleft hand involving only the ring and small fingers, J Hand Surg 13A:530, 1988.

Miura T and Komada T: Simple method for reconstruction of the cleft hand with an adducted thumb, Plast Reconstr Surg 64:65, 1979.

Müller W: Die angeborenen Fehlbildugen der menschlichen Hand, Leipzig, Germany, 1937, Thieme.

Nutt JN III and Flatt AE: Congenital central hand deficit, J Hand Surg 6:48, 1981.

Snow JW and Littler JW: Surgical treatment of cleft hand. Transactions of the International Society for Plastic Reconstructive Surgery, Fourth Congress, Rome, 1967, Excerpta Medical Foundation.

Tada K, Yonenobu K, and Swanson AB: Congenital central ray deficiency in the hand: a survey of 59 cases and subclassification, J Hand Surg 6:434, 1981.

Ueba Y: Plastic surgery for cleft hand, J Hand Surg 6:557, 1981.

Watari S and Tsuge K: A classification of cleft hands, based on clinical findings, Plast Reconstr Surg 64:381, 1979.

Ulnar deficiencies

Broudy AS and Smith RJ: Deformities of the hand and wrist with ulnar deficiency, J Hand Surg 4:304, 1979.

Ogden JA, Watson HK, and Bohne W: Ulnar dysmelia, J Bone Joint Surg 58-A:467, 1976.

Roberts AS: A case of deformity of the forearm and hands with an unusual history of hereditary congenital deficiency, Ann Surg 3:135, 1886.

Straub LR: Congenital absence of ulna, Am J Surg 109:300, 1965.

Swanson AB, Tada K, and Yonenobu K: Ulna ray deficiency: its various manifestations, J Hand Surg 9-A:658, 1984.

Syndactyly

Bauer TB, Tondra JM, and Trusler HM: Technical modification in repair of syndactylism, Plast Reconstr Surg 17:385, 1956.

Cronin TD: Syndactylism: results of zig-zag incision to prevent postoperative contracture, Plast Reconstr Surg 18:460, 1956.

Keret D and Ger E: Evaluation of a uniform operative technique to treat syndactyly, J Hand Surg 12-A (2, pt 2):727, 1987.

Kettlekamp DB and Flatt AE: An evaluation of syndactyly repair, Surg Gynecol Obstet 133:471, 1961.

Miura T: Syndactyly and split hand, Hand 8:125, 1976.

Percival NJ and Sykes PJ: Syndactyly: a review of the factors which influence surgical treatment, J Hand Surg 14-B:196, 1989.

Pieri G: Processo operatorio per la cura sindattilia grave, Chir Ital 3-4:258, 1949.

Shaw DT, Li CS, Richey DG, and Nahigian JH: Interdigital butterfly flap in the hand (the double-opposing Z-plasty), J Bone Joint Surg 55-A:1677, 1973.

Skoog T: Syndactyly: a clinical report on repair, Acta Chir Scand 130:537, 1965.

Sugiura Y: Poland's syndrome: clinicoroentgenographic study on 45 cases, Cong Anom 16:17, 1976.

Toledo LC and Ger E: Evaluation of the operative treatment of syndactyly, J Hand Surg 4:556, 1979.

Wilson MR, Louis DS, and Stevenson TR: Poland's syndrome: variable expression and associated anomalies, J Hand Surg 13-A:880, 1988.

Woolf RM and Broadbent TR: The four-flap Z-plasty, Plast Reconstr Surg 49:48, 1972.

Zeller S: Abhandlung uber die ersten Erscheinungen venerischer Lokal-Krankheits-Formen, und deren Behandlung, sammt einer kurzen Anzeige zweier neuen Operazions-Methoden, nahmlich: die angebornen verwachsenen Finger, und die Kastrazion betreffend, Wien, 1810, JG Binz.

Zoltie N, Verlende P, and Logan A: Full thickness grafts taken from the plantar instep for syndactyly release, J Hand Surg 14-B:201, 1989.

Apert's syndrome

Apert E: De l'acrocephalosyndactylie, Bull Mem Soc Med Hop Paris 23:1310, 1906.

Blank CE: Apert's syndrome: a type of acrocephalosyndactyly: observations on a British series of thirty-nine cases, Ann Hum Genet 24:151, 1960.

Hoover GH, Flatt AE, and Weiss MW: The hand in Apert's syndrome, J Bone Joint Surg 52-A:877, 1970.

Preaxial polydactyly

Andrew JG and Sykes PJ: Duplicate thumbs: a survey of results in twenty patients, J Hand Surg 13-B:50, 1988.

Bilhaut M: Guerison d'un pouce bifide per un nouveau procede operatoire, Cong Fren Chir 4:576, 1890.

Iwasawa M, Matsuo K, Hirose T, and Sakaguchi Y: Improvement in the surgical results of treatment of duplicated thumb by preoperative splinting, J Hand Surg 14-A:941, 1989.

Kawabata H, Tada K, Masada K, et al: Revision of residual deformities after operations for duplication of the thumb, J Bone Joint Surg 72-A:988, 1990.

Manske PR: Treatment of duplicated thumb using a ligamentous/periosteal flap, J Hand Surg 14-A:728, 1989.

Marks TW and Bayne LG: Polydactyly of the thumb: abnormal anatomy and treatment, J Hand Surg 3:107, 1978.

Miura T: Non-traumatic flexion deformity of the proximal interphalangeal joint — its pathogenesis and treatment, Hand 15:25, 1983.

Ogino T, Ishii S, and Minami M: Radially deviated type of thumb polydactyly, J Hand Surg 13-B:315, 1988.

Wassel HD: The results of surgery of polydactyly of the thumb: a review, Clin Orthop 64:175, 1969.

Triphalangeal thumb

Aase JM and Smith DW: Congenital anemia and triphalangeal thumbs, J Pediatr 74:417, 1969.

Abramowitz I: Triphalangeal thumb: a case report and evaluation of its importance in the morphology and function of the thumb, S Afr Med J 41:104, 1967.

Ezaki M: Radial polydactyly, Hand Clin 6:577, 1990.

Milch H: Triphalangeal thumb, J Bone Joint Surg 33-A:692, 1951.

Miura T: Triphalangeal thumb, Plast Reconstr Surg 58:587, 1976.

Peimer CA: Combined reduction osteotomy for triphalangeal thumb, J Hand Surg 10-A:376, 1985.

Phillips RS: Congenital split foot (lobster claw) and triphalangeal thumbs, J Bone Joint Surg 53-B:247, 1971.

Shiono H and Ogino T: Triphalangeal thumb and dermatoglyphics, J Hand Surg 9-B:151, 1984.

Swanson AB and Brown KS: Hereditary triphalangeal thumb, J Hered 53:259, 1962.

Wood VE: Polydactyly and the triphalangeal thumb, J Hand Surg 3:436, 1978.

Postaxial polydactyly

Barsky AJ, Kahn S, and Simon BE: Congenital anomalies of the hand, Plast Reconstr Surg 4:1704, 1964.

Frazier TM: A note on race-specific congenital malformation rates, Am J Obstet Gynecol 80:184, 1960.

Handforth JR: Polydactylism of the hand in southern Chinese, Anat Rec 106:119, 1950.

Kanavel AB: Congenital malformations of the hands, Arch Surg 25:282, 1932.

Odiorne JM: Polydactylism in related New England families, J Hered 34:45, 1943.

Ruby L and Goldberg MJ: Syndactyly and polydactyly, Orthop Clin North Am 7:361, 1976.

Simmons BP: Polydactyly, Hand Clin 1:545, 1985.

Sverdrup A: Postaxial polydactylism in six generations of a Norwegian family, J Genet 12:217, 1922.

Temtamy S and MsKusick VA: Synopsis of hand malformations with particular emphasis on genetic factors, Birth Defects 3:125, 1969.

Wassel HD: The results of surgery for polydactyly of the thumb, Clin Orthop 64:175, 1969.

Central polydactyly

Manske PR: Cleft hand and central polydactyly in identical twins: a case report, J Hand Surg 8:906, 1983.

Miura T, Nakamura R, and Imamura T: Polydactyly of the hands and feet, J Hand Surg 12-A:474, 1987.

Tada K, Kurisaki E, Yonenobu K, et al: Central polydactyly: a review of 12 cases and their surgical treatment, J Hand Surg 7:460, 1982.

Ulnar dimelia

Buck-Gramcko D: Operative Behandlung einer Spiegelbild-Deformität der hand (mirror hand — doppelte ulna mit polydaktylie): Traitement operatoire d'une difformite en miroir de l'avant-bras (deboublement du cutitus et des doigts cubitaux), Ann Chir Plast 9:180, 1964.

Entin MA: Reconstruction of congenital abnormalities of the upper extremity, J Bone Joint Surg 41-A:681, 1959.

Gorriz G: Ulnar dimelia — a limb without anteroposterior differentiation, J Hand Surg 7-A:466, 1982.

Harrison RG, Pearson MA, and Roaf R: Ulnar dimelia, J Bone Joint Surg 42-B:549, 1960.

Perini G: Dimelia ulnare e suo trattamento chirurgico, Arch Putti Chir Organi Mov 6:363, 1965.

Stalling F: The upper extremity. In Ferguson AB, editor: Orthopedic surgery in infancy and childhood, Baltimore, 1963, Williams & Wilkins.

Turek SL: Orthopaedic principles and their application, Philadelphia, 1967, JB Lippincott Co.

Macrodactyly

Barsky AJ: Macrodactyly, J Bone Joint Surg 49-A:1255, 1967.

Clifford RH: Treatment of macrodactylism: case report, Plast Reconstr Surg 23:245, 1959.

Greenberg BM, Pess GM, and May JW Jr: Macrodactyly and the epidermal nevus syndrome, J Hand Surg 12-A (2, pt 2):730, 1987.

Jones KG: Megalodactylism: case report of a child treated by epiphyseal resection, J Bone Joint Surg 45-A:1704, 1963.

Kelikian H: Congenital deformities of the hand and forearm, Philadelphia, 1974, WB Saunders Co.

Keret D, Ger E, and Marks H: Macrodactyly involving both hands and both feet, J Hand Surg 12-A:610, 1987.

Millesi H: Macrodactyly: a case study. In Littler JW, Cramer LM, and Smith JW, editors: Symposium on reconstructive hand surgery, St Louis, 1974, Mosby–Year Book, Inc.

Pho RWH, Patterson M, and Lee YS: Reconstruction and pathology in macrodactyly, J Hand Surg 13-A:78, 1988.

Schuind F, Merle M, Dap F, et al: Hyperostotic macrodactyly, J Hand Surg 13-A:544, 1988.

Tsuge K: Treatment of macrodactyl, J Hand Surg 10-A:968, 1985.

Wood VE: Macrodactyly, J Iowa Med Soc 59:922, 1969.

Hypoplastic thumb

Bayne LG: Abducted thumb (congenital hand deformities). In Green DP, editor: Operative hand surgery, New York, 1988, Churchill Livingstone, Inc.

Blair WF and Omer GE Jr: Anomalous insertion of the flexor pollicis longus, J Hand Surg 6:241, 1981.

Bonatz E, Masear VR, Meyer RD, and Cohen S: Degenerative arthritis of the carpus associated with congenital hypoplastic thumb, J Hand Surg 14-A:734, 1989.

Brand PW and Milford LW: Web deepening with sliding flap for adducted thumb in the hand. In Crenshaw AH, editor: Campbell's operative orthopaedics, ed 4, St Louis, 1963, Mosby–Year Book, Inc.

Broadbent TR and Woolf RM: Flexion-abduction deformity of the thumb: congenital clasped thumb, Plast Reconstr Surg 34:612, 1964.

Cheng JCY, Chan KM, Ma GFY, and Leung PC: Polydactyly of the thumb: a surgical plan based on 95 cases, J Hand Surg 9-A:155, 1984.

DeHaan MR, Wong LB, and Peterson DP: Congenital anomaly of the thumb: aplasia of the flexor pollicis longus, J Hand Surg 12-A:108, 1987.

Dobyns JH, Lipscomb PR, and Cooney WP: Management of thumb duplication, Clin Orthop 195:26, 1985.

Egloff DV and Verdan CL: Pollicization of the index finger for reconstruction of the congenitally hypoplastic or absent thumb, J Hand Surg 8:839, 1983.

Fitch RD, Urbaniak JR, and Ruderman RJ: Conjoined flexor and extensor pollicis longus tendons in hypoplastic thumb, J Hand Surg 9-A:417, 1984.

Gilbert A: Congenital absence of the thumb and digits, J Hand Surg 14-B:6, 1989.

Lipskeir E and Weizenbluth M: Surgical treatment of the clasped thumb, J Hand Surg 14-B:72, 1989.

Littler JW and Cooley SGE: Opposition of the thumb and its restoration by abductor digiti quinti transfer, J Bone Joint Surg 45-A:1389, 1963.

Manske PR: Redirection of the extensor pollicis longus in the treatment of spastic thumb-in-palm deformity, J Hand Surg 10-A:533, 1985.

Miura T: An appropriate treatment for postoperative Z-formed deformity of the duplicated thumb, J Hand Surg 2:380, 1977.

Neviaser RJ: Congenital hypoplasia of the thumb with absence of the extrinsic extensors, abductor pollicis longus, and thenar muscles, J Hand Surg 4:301, 1979.

Riordan DC: Tendon transfers in hand surgery, J Hand Surg 8 (5, pt 2):748, 1983.

Strauch B and Spinner M: Congenital anomaly of the thumb: absent intrinsics and flexor pollicis longus, J Bone Joint Surg 58-A:115, 1976.

Tada K, Yonenobu K, Tsuyuguchi Y, et al: Duplication of the thumb: a retrospective review of 237 cases, J Bone Joint Surg 65-A:584, 1983.

Tsuyuguchi Y, Masada K, Kawabata H, et al: Congenital clasped thumb: a review of forty-three cases, J Hand Surg 10-A:613, 1985.

Tupper JW: Pollex abductus due to congenital malposition of the flexor pollicis longus, J Bone Joint Surg 51-A:1285, 1969.

Usami F: Bilateral congenital absence of the flexor pollicis longus with craniofacial abnormalities, J Hand Surg 12-A:603, 1987.

Weckesser EC, Reed JR, and Heiple KG: Congenital clasped thumb (congenital flexion-adduction deformity of the thumb), J Bone Joint Surg 50-A:1417, 1968.

Wenner SM and Shalvoy RM: Two-stage correction of thumb adduction contracture in Freeman-Sheldon syndrome (craniocarpotarsal dysplasia), J Hand Surg 14-A:937, 1989.

Hypoplastic hands and digits

Bell J: On brachydactyly and symphalangism. In Penrose LS, editor: The treasury of human inheritance, vol 5, Cambridge, 1951, Cambridge University Press.

Buck-Gramcko D: Pollicization of the index finger: method and results in aplasia and hypoplasia of the thumb, J Bone Joint Surg 53-A:1605, 1971.

Buck-Gramcko D: The role of neurovascular toe-phalanx transplants, Hand Clin 6:643, 1990.

Carroll RE and Green DP: Reconstruction of hypoplastic digits using two phalanges, J Bone Joint Surg 57-A:727, 1975.

Cowen NJ: Surgical management of the hypoplastic hand. In Cowen NJ, editor: Practical hand surgery, Miami, 1980, Symposia Specialties, Inc.

Cowen NJ and Loftus JM: Distraction augmentation manoplasty: technique for lengthening digits for the entire hand, Orthop Rev 7:45, 1978.

Goldberg NH and Watson HK: Composite toe (phalanx with epiphysis) transplants in the reconstruction of the aphalangic hand, J Hand Surg 7:454, 1982.

Huber E: Hilfsoperation bei onedianuslahmung, Dtsch Z Chir 162:271, 1921.

Ilizarov GA, Shtin VP, and Ledyaev VI: The course of reparative regeneration of cortical bone in distraction osteosynthesis under various conditions of fragment fixation, Eksp Khr Anesteziol 14:3, 1969.

Matev IB: Thumb reconstruction after amputation at the metacarpophalangeal joint by bone lengthening, J Bone Joint Surg 52-A:957, 1970.

Tajima T: Operative treatment of congenital hand anomalies, Clin Orthop Surg 11:475, 1976.

Tupper JW: Pollex abductus due to congenital malposition of the flexor pollicis longus, J Bone Joint Surg 51-A:1285, 1969.

Congenital ring syndrome

Kino Y: Clinical and experimental studies of the congenital constriction band syndrome with emphasis on its etiology, J Bone Joint Surg 57-A:636, 1975.

Miura T: Congenital constriction band syndrome, J Hand Surg 9-A:82, 1984.

Ogino T and Saitou Y: Congenital constriction band syndrome and transverse deficiency, J Hand Surg 12-B:343, 1987.

Patterson TJS: Congenital ring-constrictions, Br J Plast Surg 14:1, 1961.

Potter EL: Pathology of the foetus and the newborn, St Louis, 1953, Mosby–Year Book, Inc.

Richardson GA and Humphrey MS: Congenital compression of the radial nerve, J Hand Surg 14-A:901, 1989.

Salama R and Weisman SL: Congenital bilateral anomalous band between flexor and extensor pollicis longus tendons, Hand 7:25, 1975.

Sølland H: Lengthening a finger with the "on the top" method, Acta Chir Scand 122:184, 1961.

Streeter GL: Focal deficiencies in fetal tissues and their relation to intra-uterine amputation. In Contributions to embryology, No 126, vol 22, Washington, DC, 1930, Carnegie Institute of Washington.

Temtamy SA and McKusick VA: Digital and other malformations associated with congenital ring constrictions, Birth Defects 14:547, 1978.

Congenital trigger digits

Dellon AL and Hansen FC: Bilateral inability to grasp due to multiple (ten) congenital trigger fingers, J Hand Surg 5:470, 1980.

Dinham JM and Meggitt DF: Trigger thumbs in children, J Bone Joint Surg 56-B:153, 1974.

Camptodactyly

Engber WM and Flatt AE: Camptodactyly: an analysis of sixty-six patients and twenty-four operations, J Hand Surg 2:216, 1977.

Hori M, Nakamura R, Inoue G, et al: Nonoperative treatment of camptodactyly, J Hand Surg 12-A:1061, 1987.

Kilgore ES Jr and Graham WP III: Camptodactyly. In The hand, Philadelphia, 1977, Lea & Febiger.

Koman LA, Toby EB, and Poehling GG: Congenital flexion deformities of the proximal interphalangeal joint in children: a subgroup of camptodactyly, J Hand Surg 15-A:582, 1990.

Lankford LL: Correspondence club letter, No 1975-1, Dallas, May 1975.

McFarlane RM, Curry GJ, and Evans HB: Anomalies of the intrinsic muscles in camptodactyly, J Hand Surg 8:531, 1983.

Millesi H: Camptodactyly. In Littler JW, Cramer LM, and Smith JW, editors: Symposium on reconstructive hand surgery, St Louis, 1974, Mosby–Year Book, Inc.

Miura T: Non-traumatic flexion deformity of the proximal interphalangeal joint: its pathogenesis and treatment, Hand 15:25, 1983.

Oldfield MC: Campdactodactyly: flexor contractures of the fingers in young girls, Br J Plast Surg 8:312, 1956.

Smith RJ and Kaplan EB: Camptodactyly and similar atraumatic flexion deformities of the proximal interphalangeal joints of the fingers, J Bone Joint Surg 50-A:1187, 1968.

Kirner's deformity

Carstam N and Eiken O: Kirner's deformity of the little finger, J Bone Joint Surg 52-A:1663, 1970.

David TJ and Burwood RL: The nature and inheritance of Kirner's deformity, J Med Genet 9:430, 1972.

Dykes RG: Kirner's deformity of the little finger, J Bone Joint Surg 60-B:58, 1978.

Kirner J: Doppelseitige Verkrummung des Kleinfingergrundgliedes als selbstandiges Krankheitsbild, Fortschr Rontgenstr 36:804, 1927.

Todd AH: Case of hereditary contracture of the little fingers, Lancet 2:1088, 1929.

Delta phalanx

Carstam N and Theander G: Surgical treatment of clinicodactyly caused by longitudinally bracketed diaphysis (delta phalanx), Scand J Plast Reconstr Surg 9:199, 1975.

Smith RJ: Osteotomy for "delta-phalanx" deformity, Clin Orthop 123:91, 1977.

Vickers D: Clinodactyly of the little finger: a simple operative technique for reversal of the growth abnormality, J Hand Surg 12-B:335, 1987.

Wood VE: Clinodactyly: an unusual presentation, J Hand Surg 14-B:449, 1989.

Madelung's deformity

Darrach W: Habitual forward dislocation of the head of the ulna, Ann Surg 57:928, 1913.

Gelberman RH and Bauman T: Madelung's deformity and dyschondrosteosis, J Hand Surg 5:338, 1980.

Madelung V: Die spontane Subluxation der Hand nach vome, Verh Dtsch Ges Chir 7:259, 1878.

Malgaigne JF: Traité des fractures et des luxations, 2:711, 1855.

Milch H: Cuff resection of the ulna for malunited Colles' fracture, J Bone Joint Surg 23:311, 1941.

Ranawat CS, DeFiore J, and Straub LR: Madelung's deformity: an end-result study of surgical treatment, J Bone Joint Surg 57-A:722, 1975.

Vender MI and Watson HK: Acquired Madelung-like deformity in a gymnast, J Hand Surg 13-A:19, 1988.

Vickers DW: Langenskiöld's operation (physiolysis) for congenital malformations of bone producing Madelung's deformity and clinicodactyly, J Bone Joint Surg 66-B:778, 1984.

White GM and Weiland AJ: Madelung's deformity: treatment by osteotomy of the radius and Lauenstein procedure, J Hand Surg 12-A:202, 1987.

Dupuytren's Contracture

MARK T. JOBE

Dupuytren's contracture is caused by a proliferative fibroplasia of the subcutaneous palmar tissue, occurring in the form of nodules and cords and resulting in secondary flexion contractures of the finger joints. Other secondary changes include thinning of the overlying subcutaneous fat, adhesion of the skin to the lesion, and later pitting or dimpling of the skin.

The activity of the lesion, and thus the rate of development of the deformity, are variable. Occasionally a finger may become markedly flexed within a few weeks or months, but the development of a severe deformity usually requires several years. In some patients, the lesion progresses steadily; in others, exacerbations and remissions occur. However, regression is rare.

Approximately 5% of patients with Dupuytren's contractures have similar lesions in the medial plantar fascia of one or both feet, known as Ledderhose's disease, and 3% of patients demonstrate plastic induration of the penis, known as Peyronie's disease."Knuckle pads" are common on the dorsum of the proximal interphalangeal joints. Patients with these associated findings are considered to have a Dupuytren's diathesis and are prone to progressive and recurrent disease.

Commonly occurring in the fifth to seventh decades of life Dupuytren's contracture occurs 10 times more frequently in men than in women. It is most common in those of Scandinavian and Celtic origin, although it has occasionally been reported in blacks and rarely in Orientals. The lesion is more frequent and severe in persons with epilepsy (42%) and those suffering from alcoholism. The involvement, although often bilateral (45%), is rarely symmetrical.

The cause of Dupuytren's contractures remains unknown. Evidence points to heredity as a factor; the lesion seems to occur earlier and more frequently in some families. James suggested an autosomal dominant pattern. The possibility that trauma and manual labor may be factors has been studied extensively. The presence in the lesion of hemosiderin suggests hemorrhage from tears, but in whites the lesion occurs as often in the minor hand as in the major one, thus making trauma an unlikely cause. Vascular insufficiency and cigarette smoking have been linked to Dupuytren's disease as possible causative factors.

The lesion usually begins in line with the ring finger at the distal palmar crease and progresses to involve the ring and little fingers, these digits being affected more frequently than all others combined. Flexion contractures of the metacarpophalangeal and proximal interphalangeal joints gradually develop, their severity depending on the extent and maturity of the fibroplasia. Discomfort is rare and usually consists of itching or occasional pain over the nodules.

PATHOGENESIS

In 1972 Gabbiani and Majno implicated the myofibroblast as the dominant cell type in Dupuytren's contracture. This is a contractile cell with increased type 3 collagen possibly originating from a transformed perivascular smooth muscle cell. Most investigators now agree that in Dupuytren's contracture the subcutaneous nodules and cords are formed by fibroplasia and by hypertrophy of already existing fibers of the palmar fascia. Millesi believes that the pathologic tissue arises only through changes in the existing fibers of the palmar fascia and not by the formation of new tissue. Luck has suggested that the subcutaneous nodules develop first and mature later to become cords. However, Gosset suggested that the nodules and cords do not represent two stages of the disease but two forms of it originating in two different tissues, the subcutaneous fat and palmar fascia. Further, Hueston concluded that the nodules develop subcutaneously and only later may involve the palmar fascia and overlying skin. Contracture of the metacarpophalangeal and proximal interphalangeal joints and displacement of a neurovascular bundle in a digit result from the pattern of contracture of the fascial cords.

The fascial structures that may become involved in the

3427

fibroproliferative process have been clearly outlined by McFarlane and include the pretendinous band, the superficial transverse ligament, the spiral band, the natatory ligament, the lateral digital sheet, and Grayson's ligament. Thomine also describes a longitudinally oriented fascia located dorsal to the neurovascular bundle, which he terms the *retrovascular cord*. This structure is often involved in the disease. Cleland's ligament is generally believed to be spared. The pretendinous cord (Fig. 75-1) is nearly always responsible for contracture of the metacarpophalangeal joint. It may attach to the base of the proximal phalanx or to the tendon sheath at this level, or it may extend to attach to the base of the middle phalanx or the skin. A spiral cord, composed of abnormal pretendinous band, spiral band, lateral digital sheet, and Grayson's ligament, may project from the midline at the level of the metacarpophalangeal joint to insert either into the area distal to the proximal interphalangeal joint or just proximal to it. It may continue around the neurovascular bundle and rejoin the pretendinous cord. In its course it may displace the neurovascular bundle toward the midline of the finger, making dissection somewhat tedious, but it must be dissected to its insertion to afford complete release of the flexed position of the proximal interphalangeal joint. Neurovascular displacement is most

commonly found on the ulnar aspect of the little and ring fingers.

The lateral cord may extend distally and contribute to a flexion contracture of the distal interphalangeal joint. Although a plane exists between it and the overlying skin it is minimal and must be developed sharply. The retrovascular cord is not believed to significantly contribute to flexion contracture of the proximal interphalangeal joint; however, it may be responsible for some residual flexion contracture or recurrence if not excised.

Skoog believes that in the palmar fascia only the longitudinal pretendinous bands are involved and that the superficial transverse palmar ligament is always spared. McFarlane believes that it may become involved in the first web space and contribute to a thumb web contracture requiring excision.

PROGNOSIS

The prognosis in Dupuytren's contracture seems to be dependent on the following factors, which in turn may determine the extent of any operation.

1. *Heredity.* A family history of the disease is an indication that the lesion is likely to progress more rapidly than usual, especially if the onset is early.
2. *Sex.* In women the lesion usually begins later and progresses more slowly, and women often accommodate better to the inconvenience of the resulting deformity. Zemel et al. have shown, however, that long-term results after operation are worse in women than in men with postoperative flare reaction being twice as likely.
3. *Alcoholism or epilepsy.* In these conditions the lesion is more severe, progresses more rapidly, and recurs more frequently.
4. *Location and extent of disease.* When the disease is bilateral and especially when it is associated with knuckle pads and with nodules in the plantar fascia, it progresses more rapidly and recurs more frequently; further, it usually progresses more rapidly in the ulnar side of the hand than in the radial side.
5. *Behavior of disease.* How the disease has behaved in the past, whether treated or not, is an indication of its probable behavior in the future.

When the proximal interphalangeal joint begins to contract, it usually progresses to a fixed deformity that becomes increasingly difficult to correct completely. Severe metacarpophalangeal joint contracture is more easily corrected surgically than is moderate proximal interphalangeal joint contracture.

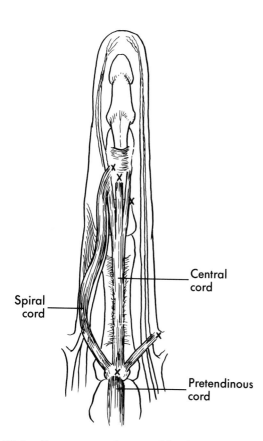

Fig. 75-1   Frequent attachments (*x*) of deforming fibrous cords are noted here. Note distorted course of digital nerve on left. (Redrawn from Chiu HF and McFarlane RM: J Hand Surg 3:1, 1978.)

TREATMENT

Although many medical remedies have been tried, the best treatment known is surgical. Roentgen therapy would be of value in the earliest fibroblastic phase, except that it destroys subcutaneous glands and may even burn the skin; thus the risk is too great. No treatment at all may be indicated in the absence of contracture or when a contracture is progressing slowly and is not disabling; then the patient should be observed every 3 months. Any operation is technically easier early in the disease when the skin is more normal, but it should be delayed until the development of proximal interphalangeal joint contracture or metatarsophalangeal joint contracture of 30 degrees or greater. Rarely is the presence of a palmar nodule alone an indication for surgery; however, if it is causing sufficient discomfort, pitting, and maceration, surgery may be indicated.

The five surgical procedures used in treating Dupuytren's contracture are (1) subcutaneous fasciotomy, (2) partial (selective) fasciectomy, (3) complete fasciectomy, (4) fasciectomy with skin grafting, and (5) amputation. In choosing the best procedure for a given patient, the degree of contracture, the patient's age, occupation, and general health, the nutritional status of the palmar skin, and the presence or absence of arthritis should all be considered. In general, the more severe the involvement and the more grave the prognosis, the more extensive any indicated fasciectomy should be. However, the fasciectomy may be carried out in stages and may be preceded by a subcutaneous fasciotomy.

The least extensive procedure, *subcutaneous fasciotomy*, is used for patients who are elderly or arthritic or whose general health is poor. The results of this procedure are more permanent when dense, mature cords are severed than when the lesion is more diffuse; when the lesion is in the involutional stage, recurrence is likely. Since this procedure will allow stretching of the palmar skin, it may also be useful as a preliminary operation to fasciectomy. Fasciotomy should be considered a temporary measure since 72% of contractures so treated recur to a degree requiring further surgery according to Rodrigo et al.

Partial (selective) fasciectomy is usually indicated when only the ulnar one or two fingers are involved. It is the operation used more frequently because postsurgically morbidity is less and complications are fewer than after complete fasciectomy. Even though the rate of recurrence after partial fasciectomy is high (50%), the need for another surgical procedure is only 15%. In this operation only the mature deforming tissue is excised. It must be emphasized, however, that this does not represent all diseased fascia since fascia may become biochemically or microscopically involved long before it becomes clinically apparent (Albin et al., 1975). Several incisions as shown in Fig. 75-3 are useful. We prefer the zigzag incision on the fingers (see Fig. 75-3, *B*) or a variant of it because it exposes the diseased tissue better. Whatever the incision used, it should be fashioned to fit the needs of the individual patient, considering the contractures of the skin and the adherence of skin to the underlying fascia. When tightness of the palmar skin limits

extension of a finger, a midline incision converted to appropriate Z-plasties is indicated (see Fig. 75-3, *A*); this incision allows quicker dissection under direct vision and exposes digital nerves that may have been pulled from their normal position by the fascia. Regardless of the incision, dissection is made easier by magnification, ideal lighting, and a stable surface. Pressing the knife against the taut unyielding fascial cords in a feathering motion is safer than the usual cutting movements.

Sometimes after fasciectomy, extension of the proximal interphalangeal joint is incomplete. This may be caused by a projection of the involved fascia that passes along the proximal phalanx to the fascial structures on the dorsum of the joint; the projection can be carefully excised. When a flexion contracture of the joint is severe, a volar capsulotomy as described by Curtis in Chapter 68 may be indicated.

The technique of Skoog is a partial or selective fasciectomy because in it only the pretendinous fibers of the palmar fascia are excised. According to Skoog, there is a definite plane between the pretendinous longitudinal fibers of the palmar fascia and the transverse palmar ligament that is limited to the midpalmar area; thus in Dupuytren's contracture the pretendinous fibers can be dissected from this ligament. He emphasizes, however, that the pretendinous fibers may seem attached to the ligament. Further, according to Skoog, the interdigital or natatory ligaments do become involved in Dupuytren's contracture and prevent the fingers from spreading normally; they are indistinguishable from the transverse palmar ligament, except for their anatomic location.

Complete fasciectomy is rarely if ever indicated since it is associated frequently with complications of hematoma, joint stiffness, and delayed healing, and it does not completely prevent recurrence of the disease.

Fasciectomy with skin grafting as advocated by Hueston may be indicated for young people in whom the prognosis is poor because of such factors as epilepsy, alcoholism, or the presence of the disease elsewhere in the body, and in whom the lesion has recurred after one excision. The skin and underlying abnormal fascia are excised, and a full-thickness or thick split skin graft is applied. Recurrence has not been reported in areas of the palm treated in this manner.

Amputation, although rarely necessary, may be indicated if flexion contracture of the proximal interphalangeal joint, especially of the little finger, is severe and cannot be corrected enough to make the finger useful. A 40-degree flexion contracture is usually tolerated fairly well. Then the skin from the involved finger may be used to cover the defect in the palmar skin; the finger is filleted (p. 3000), and the skin is folded into the palm as a pedicle with normal neurovascular bundles.

Another alternative for the severely contracted proximal interphalangeal joint is joint resection and arthrodesis. This results in a much shortened little finger but avoids the complication of an amputation neuroma.

Subcutaneous Fasciotomy

■ *TECHNIQUE (LUCK)*. Using a pointed scalpel, make 3.2 mm skin puncture wounds on the ulnar side of the palmar fascia at the following levels: (1) the apex of the palmar fascia between the thenar and hypothenar eminences, (2) at or near the level of the proximal palmar crease, and (3) at the level of the distal palmar crease. (Digital nerves are more likely to be cut at the distal palm where they become more superficial and may be intertwined with the diseased collagen.) Insert a small tenotomy knife or a fasciatome (Luck) that resembles a myringotome, its blade parallel with the palm, through each of the puncture wounds in turn and pass it across the palm beneath the skin but superficial to the fascia (Fig. 75-2). Then turn the edge of the blade toward the palmar fascia and extend the fingers to tighten the involved tissue. Carefully divide the fascial cords by pressing the fasciatome through them, using direct finger pressure over the blade or at most a gentle rocking motion; never use a sawing motion. Whenever a cord is divided, the sense of gritty firm resistance disappears, indicating that the blade has passed completely through the fascia. Now using the fasciatome blade in a plane parallel with the skin, free the latter from the underlying fascia. The corrugated skin, even though very thin at times, can be safely undermined and released as necessary with little fear of necrosis.

In the fingers subcutaneous fasciotomy is safe only for a fascial cord located in the midline. Insert the blade through a puncture wound adjacent to the cord and divide it obliquely. For a laterally placed cord use a short longitudinal incision and excise a segment under direct vision. Also enucleate larger nodules in both fingers and palm under direct vision.

AFTERTREATMENT. A pressure dressing is used for 24 hours; then a smaller dressing is applied, and active motion of the hand and fingers is encouraged.

Partial Fasciectomy

■ *TECHNIQUE.* Outline the proposed incision with a skin pencil before inflation of the tourniquet (Fig. 75-3). Take into consideration the pits and other areas of skin with diminished vascularity by making an incision over or near these areas, thus avoiding their presence at the base of a flap. These areas may sometimes be excised when the final rotation of the skin takes place in closure.

Make a zigzag or vertical incision over the deforming pathologic structure. Zigzag incisions tend to straighten out, causing tension lines at the creases; however, the flaps created by zigzag incisions may heal more securely. Design the Z-plasty flaps to be created later for the vertical incisions so that a transverse central segment is within or near each joint crease. Continue the incision proximally into the palm, avoiding crossing the palmar creases at a right angle.

Elevate the skin and underlying normal subcutaneous tissue from the pathologic fascia from proximal to distal (Fig. 75-4). Do not create the Z-plasty flaps until the wound is ready for closure.

Excise the pathologic fascia from proximal palm

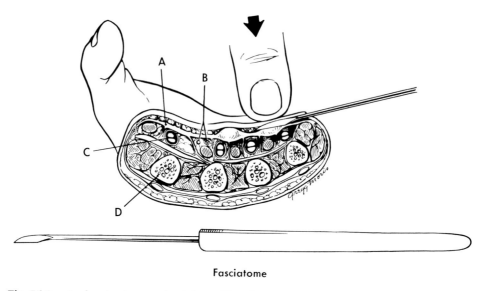

Fasciatome

Fig. 75-2 Luck subcutaneous fasciotomy. *Top,* Cross section of hand to show relations of palmar fascia and technique of subcutaneous fasciotomy. *A,* Palmar fascia; *B,* neurovascular bundle; *C,* flexor tendons; *D,* metacarpal. Fasciatome is being pressed, *arrow,* through a fascial cord. *Bottom,* Fasciatome. (From Luck JV: J Bone Joint Surg 41-A:635, 1959.)

to distal finger. Carefully cauterize small bleeding points, but avoid heating or burning digital nerves. Excision of all transverse palmar fascial fibers may not be necessary. Avoid entering tendon sheaths so that blood does not enter later and cause irritation; this is more difficult to do proximal to the pulley at the metacarpophalangeal joint. Carefully excise the fascia by placing it under tension and pressing a sharp knife against it rather than using a less precise cutting motion. A frequent change of knife

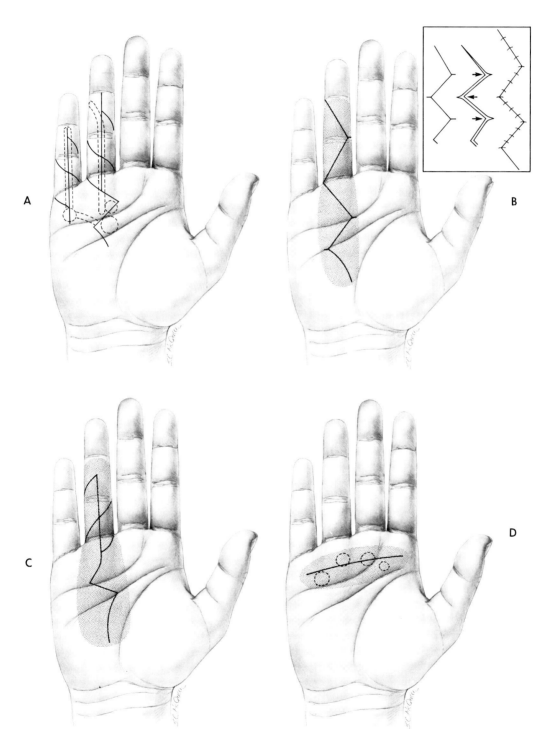

Fig. 75-3 **A,** Multiple Z-plasties may be employed to provide exposure and convert vertical incision to zigzag closures. Only one extension is made into palm. **B,** When skin contracture is not a major problem, a zigzag pattern may be used in making exposure, with extended corners as shown to make use of redundant skin. **C,** Extent of possible undermining of skin is shown in shaded area. **D,** When only palm is involved, a transverse incision only may be used.

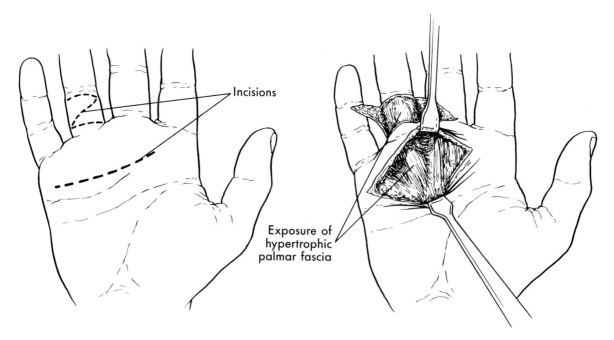

Fig. 75-4   Approaches to palmar fascia for partial fasciectomy (see text).

blades is helpful. Avoid cutting displaced digital nerves by carefully locating each nerve at the fatty pad at the level of the metacarpophalangeal joint and following it distally. Excise the natatory ligament if it is contracted. Be certain to follow all the bands of contracted fascia to their distal insertion. Insertions may be into tendon sheaths, bone, and skin; occasionally they are dorsolateral to the proximal interphalangeal joint. When excision of the pathologic fascia has been completed, all joints should permit full passive extension or nearly so.

Now fashion the skin flaps. If there is any extra skin, the pitted or thinned areas may be excised. Before closing, elevate the hand, compress the wound, release the tourniquet, hold for 10 minutes, and then check for and control bleeding. Using skin hooks and with minimal handling of the flaps, suture them in place with No. 5-0 or No. 6-0 monofilament nylon. Place few sutures in the palm to allow necessary drainage around a rubber drain. Apply one layer of nonadherent gauze and then a large wet cotton mass dressing that is compressed gently against the wound to conform to the contours of the palm and fingers. Apply a compression dressing over this, and use a volar plaster splint to support the wrist but leave finger motion unencumbered.

AFTERTREATMENT. All drains are removed within 48 hours. Early proximal interphalangeal motion is encouraged. The hand is kept elevated for a minimum of 48 hours. The shoulder is moved actively at intervals during this period to avoid cramping. Should there be undue pain in the hand or fever af-

ter 48 hours, the wound should be inspected for a hematoma. If a hematoma is found elevating the skin, the patient should be taken back to surgery immediately if necessary to evacuate the hematoma; the involved area of the wound should be left open. Otherwise, the first dressing is removed after about 1 week; the hand is redressed and splinted at the wrist for another week. During this second week with the wrist still splinted, the patient is encouraged to move all the finger joints.

At 2 weeks, the sutures are removed, and the hand is left free of all dressings. The patient is warned not to place the hand in a dependent position for rest and not to soak the hand in hot water. Active exercise in warm water is permissible, but no passive stretching is allowed. Moderate use of the hand is permitted at 3 weeks; however, several months of rehabilitation may be necessary. Silicone putty is a valuable adjunct to an exercise program.

■ *TECHNIQUE (SKOOG).* Outline the proposed incision with a skin pencil. First make a transverse incision in the distal palmar crease long enough to expose the part of the palmar fascia to be excised (Fig. 75-5). Then over the cords make distal extensions of the incision and carry them to the base of the fingers. On the fingers make Z-plasty incisions. Now, from the transverse palmar incision and in a crease in the center of the palm, make a proximal extension of the incision. Raise the proximal triangular flaps thus formed no more than necessary to expose the border of the palmar fascia on either or both sides. Now excise the involved pretendinous fascia

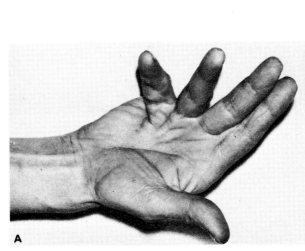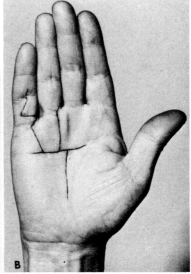

Fig. 75-5 Skoog technique of partial fasciectomy. **A,** Dupuytren's contracture that developed during period of 15 years in 55-year-old patient. **B,** Result after partial fasciectomy. **B** illustrates locations of transverse and longitudinal palmar skin incisions and of Z-plasty incision on little finger. (From Skoog T: Surg Clin North Am 47:433, 1967.)

but leave intact the transverse palmar ligament and the underlying peritendinous septa. At the base of the fingers and adjacent parts of the palm, free and protect the neurovascular bundles and excise any diseased fascia here and in the fingers. Now close the incision with interrupted stitches, placing a few mattress sutures along the transverse part of the incision to fix the skin edges to the transverse palmar ligament and obliterate a pocket in which a hematoma can form.

When the deformity is severe, modify the incision and use a full-thickness skin graft if necessary.

AFTERTREATMENT. The aftertreatment is as described for partial fasciectomy.

REFERENCES

Albin R, Brickely D, Glimcher MJ, and Smith RJ: Dupuytren's contracture: an active cellular process, J Bone Joint Surg 57-A:726, 1975.

An HS, Southworth SR, Jackson T, and Russ B: Cigarette smoking and Dupuytren's contracture of the hand, J Hand Surg 13-A:872, 1988.

Badalamente MA, Hurst LC, and Sampson SP: Prostaglandins influence myofibroblast contractility in Dupuytren's disease, J Hand Surg 13-A:867, 1988.

Berg E, Marino AA, and Becker RO: Dupuytren's contracture: some associated biophysical abnormalities, Clin Orthop 83:144, 1972.

Boswick JA Jr, Kilgore ES, Watson HK, et al: Symposium: Dupuytren's contracture, Contemp Orthop 16:71, 1988.

Boyes JH: Dupuytren's contracture: notes on the age at onset and the relationship to handedness, Am J Surg 88:147, 1954.

Boyes JH and Jones FE: Dupuytren's disease involving the volar aspect of the wrist, Plast Reconstr Surg 41:204, 1968.

Brickley-Parsons D, Glimcher M, Smith R, et al: Biochemical changes in the collagen of the palmar fascia in patients with Dupuytren's disease, J Bone Joint Surg 63-A:787, 1981.

Browne WE: Dupuytren's contracture: a report of surgical correction in 83 cases (1945-1957), Clin Orthop 13:255, 1959.

Carr TL: Local radical fasciectomy for Dupuytren's contracture, Hand 6:40, 1974.

Chiu HF and McFarlane RM: Pathogenesis of Dupuytren's contracture: a correlative clinical pathological study, J Hand Surg 3:1, 1978.

Colville J: Dupuytren's contracture: the role of fasciotomy, Hand 15:162, 1984.

Crawford HR: Surgical correction of Dupuytren's contracture, Surg Clin North Am 36:793, 1956.

Davis JE: One surgery of Dupuytren's contracture, Plast Reconstr Surg 36:277, 1965.

Deming EG: Y-V advancement pedicles in surgery for Dupuytren's contracture, Plast Reconstr Surg 29:581, 1962.

Freehafer AA and Strong JM: The treatment of Dupuytren's contracture by partial fasciectomy, J Bone Joint Surg 45-A:1207, 1963.

Fromison AI and Zahrawi F: Treatment of compression neuropathy of the ulnar nerve at the elbow by epicondylectomy and neurolysis, J Hand Surg 5:391, 1980.

Gabbiani G and Majno G: Dupuytren's contracture: fibroblast contraction? An ultrastructural study, Am J Pathol 66:131, 1972.

Gelberman RH, Amiel D, Rudolph RM, and Vance RM: Dupuytren's contracture: an electron microscopic, biochemical, and clinical correlative study, J Bone Joint Surg 62-A:425, 1980.

Gosset J: Maladie de Dupuytren et anatomie des aponevroses palmodigitales. In Maladie de Dupuytren, Paris, 1966, L'Expansion Scientifique.

Hamlin E Jr: Limited excision of Dupuytren's contracture: a follow-up study, Ann Surg 155:454, 1962.

Heyse WE: Dupuytren's contracture and its surgical treatment: clinical study of a local resection method, JAMA 174:1945, 1960.

Hill NA: Current concepts review: Dupuytren's contracture, J Bone Joint Surg 67-A:1439, 1985.

Honner R et al: Dupuytren's contracture: long-term results after fasciectomy, J Bone Joint Surg 53-B:240, 1971.

Hoopes JE et al: Enzymes of glucose metabolism in palmar fascia and Dupuytren's contracture, J Hand Surg 2:62, 1977.

Howard LD Jr: Dupuytren's contracture: a guide for management, Clin Orthop 15:118, 1959.

Hueston JT: Dupuytren's contracture, Edinburgh, 1963, E & S Livingstone, Ltd.

Hueston JT: Dupuytren's contracture: medicolegal aspects, Med J Aust (special supplement), November 16, 1987.

Iwasaki H, Muller H, and Stutte HJ: Palmar fibromatosis (Dupuytren's contracture): ultrastructural and enzyme histochemical studies of 43 cases, Virchows Arch 405:41, 1984.

James JIP: The genetic pattern of Dupuytren's disease and idiopathic epilepsy. In Hueston JT and Tubiana R, editors: Dupuytren's disease, ed 2, Edinburgh, 1985, Churchill-Livingstone.

James WD and Odom RB: The role of myofibroblast in Dupuytren's contracture, Arch Dermatol 116:807, 1980.

Kasdan ML and Chipman JR: Dupuytren's contracture: wound irrigation to prevent hematoma, Orthop Rev 16:525, 1987.

Kelly AP Jr and Clifford RH: Subcutaneous fasciotomy in the treatment of Dupuytren's contracture, Plast Reconstr Surg 24:505, 1959.

King EW, Bass DB, and Watson HK: Treatment of Dupuytren's contracture by extensive fasciectomy through multiple Y-V-plasty incisions: short-term evaluation of 170 consecutive operations, J Hand Surg 4:234, 1979.

Kischer CW and Speer DP: Microvascular changes in Dupuytren's contracture, J Hand Surg 9-A:58, 1984.

Larsen RD and Posch JL: Dupuytren's contracture: with special reference to pathology, J Bone Joint Surg 40-A:773, 1958.

Larsen RD, Takagishi N, and Posch JL: The pathogenesis of Dupuytren's contracture: experimental and further clinical observations, J Bone Joint Surg 42-A:993, 1960.

Legge JWH and McFarlane RM: Prediction of results of treatment of Dupuytren's disease, J Hand Surg 5:608, 1980.

Luck JV: Dupuytren's contracture: a new concept of the pathogenesis correlated with surgical management, J Bone Joint Surg 41-A:635, 1959.

Luck JV: Dupuytren's contracture: pathogenesis and surgical management: a new concept, AAOS Instr Course Lect 16:70, 1959.

Lueders HW, Shapiro RL, and Lee H: Cross-finger pedicle flaps for recurrent Dupuytrens, Orthop Rev 4:39, July 1975.

MacCallum P and Hueston JT: The pathology of Dupuytren's contracture, Aust NZ J Surg 31:241, 1962.

Matev LB: Asymmetric Z-plasty in the operative treatment of Dupuytren's contracture, Am Dig Foreign Orthop Lit, p 11, First quarter, 1970.

McFarlane RM: Patterns of the diseased fascia in the fingers in Dupuytren's contracture: displacement of the neurovascular bundle, Plast Reconstr Surg 54:31, 1974.

McFarlane RM and Jamieson WG: Dupuytren's contracture: the management of one hundred patients, J Bone Joint Surg 48-A:1095, 1966.

McIndoe A and Beare RLB: The surgical management of Dupuytren's contracture, Am J Surg 95:197, 1958.

Mennen U and Grabe RP: Dupuytren's contracture in a Negro: a case report, J Hand Surg 4:451, 1979.

Millesi H: The clinical and morphological course of Dupuytren's disease. In Maladie de Dupuytren, Paris, 1966, L'Expansion Scientifique.

Moberg E: Three useful ways to avoid amputation in advanced Dupuytren's contracture, Orthop Clin North Am 4:1001, 1973.

Murrell GAC, Francis MJO, and Howlett CR: Dupuytren's contracture: fine structure in relation to aetiology, J Bone Joint Surg 71-B:367, 1989.

Rayan GM: Rheumatoid arthritis and Dupuytren's contracture, Plast Reconstr Surg 81:50, 1988.

Reumert T and Zachariae L: Continued investigations into the effect of diuretics upon oedema of the hand following operation for Dupuytren's contracture (Bumetanide, Leo), Acta Orthop Scand 44:410, 1973.

Rhode CM and Jennings WD Jr: Dupuytren's contracture, Am J Surg 33:855, 1967.

Richards HJ: The surgical treatment of Dupuytren's contracture, J Bone Joint Surg 36-B:90, 1954.

Rodrigo JJ et al: Treatment of Dupuytren's contracture: long-term results after fasciotomy and fascial excision, J Bone Joint Surg 58-A:380, 1976.

Sennwald GR: Fasiectomy for treatment of Dupuytren's disease and early complications, J Hand Surg 15-A:755, 1990.

Shum DT and McFarlane RM: Histogenesis of Dupuytren's disease: an immunohistochemical study of 30 cases, J Hand Surg 13-A:61, 1988.

Skoog T: Dupuytren's contracture, Postgrad Med 21:91, 1957.

Skoog T: Dupuytren's contracture: pathogenesis and surgical treatment, Surg Clin North Am 47:433, 1967.

Snyder CC: The contracture of Dupuytren, Am Surg 23:487, 1957.

Spiegel D and Chase RA: The treatment of contractures of the hand using self-hypnosis, J Hand Surg 5:428, 1980.

Stein A et al: Dupuytren's contracture: a morphologic evaluation of the pathogenesis, Ann Surg 151:577, 1960.

Thomine JM: Le fascia digital: development et anatomie. In Tubiana R, editor: La maladies de Dupuytren, ed 2, Paris, 1972, Expansion Scientific Francais.

Tomasek JJ, Schultz RJ, and Haaksma CJ: Extracellular matrix-cytoskeletal connections at the surface of the specialized contractile fibroblast (myofibroblast) in Dupuytren disease, J Bone Joint Surg 69-A:1400, 1987.

Tubiana R: Limited and extensive operations in Dupuytren's contracture, Surg Clin North Am 44:1071, 1964.

Tubiana R, Thomine JM, and Brown S: Complications in surgery of Dupuytren's contracture, Plast Reconstr Surg 39:603, 1967.

Ushijima M, Tsuneyoshi M, and Enjoji M: Dupuytren's fibromatoses: a clinicopathologic study of 62 cases, Acta Pathol Jpn 34:991, 1984.

Wakefield AR: Dupuytren's contracture, Surg Clin North Am 40:483, 1960.

Wang MKH et al: Dupuytren's contracture, an analytic and etiologic study, Plast Reconstr Surg 25:323, 1960.

Webster GV: A useful incision in Dupuytren's contracture, Plast Reconstr Surg 19:514, 1957.

Weckesser EC: Results of wide excision of the palmar fascia for Dupuytren's contracture: special reference to factors which adversely affect prognosis, Ann Surg 160:1007, 1964.

Zachariae L: Operation for Dupuytren's contracture by the method of McCash, Acta Orthop Scand 41:433, 1970.

Zachariae L et al: The effect of a diuretic (Centyl, Leo) on the oedema of the hand following surgical treatment of Dupuytren's contracture, Acta Orthop Scand 41:411, 1970.

Zemel NP, Balcomb TV, Stark HH, et al: Dupuytren's disease in women: evaluation of long-term results after operation, J Hand Surg 12-A:1012, 1987.

CHAPTER 76

Carpal Tunnel and Ulnar Tunnel Syndromes and Stenosing Tenosynovitis

PHILLIP E. WRIGHT II*

CARPAL TUNNEL SYNDROME

Carpal tunnel syndrome, also known as tardy median nerve palsy, results from compression of the median nerve within the carpal tunnel. It occurs most often in patients between 30 and 60 years old and is five times more frequent in women than in men. Any condition that crowds or reduces the capacity of the carpal tunnel may initiate the symptoms; malaligned Colles' fracture and edema from infection or trauma are among the more obvious, and tumors or tumorous conditions such as a ganglion, lipoma, or xanthoma are among the more frequent. In Colles' fracture, immobilizing the wrist in marked flexion and ulnar deviation may cause acute compression of the median nerve within the carpal tunnel immediately after reduction. Systemic conditions such as obesity, diabetes mellitus, thyroid dysfunction, amyloidosis, and Raynaud's disease are sometimes associated with the syndrome. Occasionally a patient will have symptoms of carpal tunnel syndrome caused by an habitual sleeping posture at night in which the wrist is kept acutely flexed. Trauma caused by repetitive hand motions has been identified as a cause of carpal tunnel syndrome, especially in patients whose work requires repeated forceful finger and wrist flexion and extension. Laborers using vibrating machinery are at risk, as are office workers, especially typists and data entry clerks, who spend long hours with the wrists flexed.

This syndrome may occur during pregnancy but usually disappears after delivery.

Aberrant muscles of the forearm are another cause of median nerve compression. Acute median nerve symptoms with no obvious cause may be associated with an acute thrombosis of the median artery.

The cause is obscure in some patients, and hence the term *spontaneous* median neuropathy. The syndrome is frequently associated with nonspecific and rheumatoid tenosynovitis, as are trigger finger and de Quervain's disease. Schuind, Ventura, and Pasteels studied biopsy specimens of the flexor tendon synovium from 21 patients with "idiopathic" carpal tunnel syndrome. The findings were similar in all and were typical of a connective tissue undergoing degeneration under repeated mechanical stress.

Diagnosis

Paresthesia over the sensory distribution of the median nerve is the most frequent symptom; it occurs more often in women and frequently causes the patient to awaken several hours after getting to sleep with burning and numbness of the hand that is relieved by exercise. Tinel's sign may also be demonstrated in most patients by percussing the median nerve at the wrist. Atrophy to some degree of the median-innervated thenar muscles has been reported in about half of the patients treated by operation. Acute flexion of the wrist for 60 seconds (Phalen's test) in some but not all patients or strenous use of the hand increases the paresthesia. Application of a blood pressure cuff on the upper arm sufficient to produce venous distention may initiate the symptoms. Gellman et al. evaluated the clinical usefulness of commonly administered provocative tests, including wrist flexion, nerve percussion, and the tourniquet test, in 67 hands with electrical proof of carpal tunnel syndrome and in 50 control hands. The most sensitive test was the wrist flexion test, whereas nerve percussion was the most specific

---

*Revision of chapter by Lee W. Milford, M.D.

and the least sensitive. Because of its insensitivity and nonspecificity, the tourniquet test was not recommended. They also found that with the wrist in neutral the mean pressure within the carpal tunnel in 15 patients with carpal tunnel syndrome was 32 mm Hg. This pressure increased to 99 mm Hg with 90 degrees of wrist flexion and increased to 110 mm Hg with the wrist at 90 degrees of extension. The pressures in the control subjects with the wrist in neutral were 2.5 mm Hg, 31 mm Hg with the wrist in flexion, and 30 mm Hg with the wrist in extension.

Durkan described a "new" carpal compression test in which direct compression is applied to the medial nerve for 30 seconds with the thumbs or an atomizer bulb attached to a manometer. Patients with the carpal tunnel syndrome usually have symptoms of numbness, pain, or paresthesias in the median nerve distribution. When compared with the Tinel nerve percussion and Phalen's wrist flexion test, the carpal compression test was more specific (90%) and more sensitive (87%) than either of these tests.

Sensibility testing in peripheral nerve compression syndromes was investigated by Gelberman et al. who found that threshold tests of sensibility correlated accurately with symptoms of nerve compression and electrodiagnostic studies. They found Semmes-Weinstein monofilament pressure testing to be the most accurate in determining early nerve compression. Koris et al. combined the Semmes-Weinstein monofilament test with the wrist flexion test for a "quantitative provocational" diagnostic test. This combined test was reported to have 82% sensitivity and 86% specificity.

According to most authors, the most reliable confirmatory tests are nerve conduction studies. However, these studies occasionally are normal when clinical signs of carpal tunnel syndrome are present, and they may be abnormal in asymptomatic patients. Nerve conduction studies are reported to be as high as 90% sensitive and 60% specific for the diagnosis of carpal tunnel syndrome. Computerized tomographic scanning displays the bony structures clearly, but does not define the soft tissues accurately. Ultrasonography has been used to show the movement of the flexor tendons within the carpal tunnel, but does not clearly show soft tissue planes. Early reports of magnetic resonance imaging (MRI) in carpal tunnel syndrome are promising. A major advantage of MRI is its high soft tissue contrast, which gives detailed images of both bones and soft tissues. Healy et al. reported that of 11 wrists with carpal tunnel syndrome evaluated with MRI, operative findings correlated with MRI evidence of synovial disease, carpal tunnel stenosis, and median nerve compression in 10.

Care should be taken not to confuse this syndrome with nerve compression caused by a cervical disc herniation, thoracic outlet structures, and median nerve compression proximally in the forearm and at the elbow.

Treatment

If mild symptoms have been present and there is no thenar muscle atrophy, the injection of hydrocortisone into the carpal tunnel may afford relief. Great care should be taken not to inject directly into the nerve. Injection may also be used as a diagnostic tool in patients without bony or tumorous blocking of the canal; well over 65% percent of these cases are caused by a nonspecific synovitis, and these seem to respond more favorably to injection. Injection also helps to eliminate the possibility of other syndromes, especially cervical disc or thoracic outlet. Some patients prefer to be injected two or three times before a surgical procedure is carried out. If the response is positive and there is no muscle atrophy, conservative treatment with splinting and injection is reasonable.

In a study of 331 patients with carpal tunnel syndrome, Kaplan, Glickel, and Eaton identified five important factors in determining the success of nonoperative treatment: (1) age over 50 years, (2) duration of over 10 months, (3) constant paresthesias, (4) stenosing flexor tenosynovitis, and (5) a Phalen's test positive in less than 30 seconds. Two thirds of patients were cured by medical treatment when none of these factors was present, 59.6% with one factor, and 83.3% with two factors; 93.2% with three factors did not improve. No patient with four or five factors was cured by medical management.

On the basis of experimental and clinical observations, Gelberman et al. proposed that carpal tunnel syndrome be divided into early, intermediate, advanced, and acute stages. Patients with early carpal tunnel syndrome and mild symptoms responded to steroid injection. Those with intermediate and advanced (chronic) syndromes responded to carpal tunnel release. Extensive neurolysis was not shown to have any significant effect. Treatment of acute carpal tunnel syndrome should be individualized, depending on its etiology. For carpal tunnel syndrome caused by an acute increase in carpal tunnel pressure (such as after a Colles' fracture treated with flexed-wrist immobilization) relief may be obtained by a change in wrist position without surgical release of the tunnel.

When signs and symptoms are persistent and progressive, especially if they include thenar atrophy, division of the deep transverse carpal ligament is indicated. The results of surgery are good in most instances (in 85% according to Lipscomb), and benefits seem to last in most patients. Although thenar atrophy may disappear, it resolves slowly, if at all. Care should be taken to avoid the palmar sensory branch of the median nerve since, when severed, it frequently causes a painful neuroma that may later require excision from the scar.

As noted earlier, when symptoms of median nerve compression develop during treatment of acute Colles' fracture, the constricting bandages and cast should be loosened, and the wrist should be extended to neutral position. When tardy median nerve palsy develops after Colles' fracture and has been unrecognized for several weeks, surgery is indicated without further delay.

SURGICAL RELEASE OF CARPAL TUNNEL

■ *TECHNIQUE*. Make a curved incision ulnar to and paralleling the thenar crease. Extend this proximally to the flexor crease of the wrist where it may be continued farther proximally if necessary. Angle the incision toward the ulnar side of the wrist to avoid crossing the flexor creases at a right angle but especially to avoid cutting the palmar sensory branch of the median nerve that lies in the interval between the palmaris longus and the flexor carpi radialis tendons (Fig. 76-1). Should this nerve be severed, do not attempt to repair it, but section it at its origin. After incising and reflecting the skin and subcutaneous tissue, divide the transverse carpal ligament along its ulnar border to avoid damage to the median nerve and its recurrent branch, which frequently perforates the distal border of the ligament and may leave the median nerve on the volar side (Fig. 76-2). The strong fibers of the transverse carpal ligament extend distally farther than is generally suspected (Fig. 76-3). Inspect the flexor tenosynovium. Tenosynovectomy may occasionally be indicated, especially in patients with rheumatoid arthritis. Close only the skin and drain the wound.

AFTERTREATMENT. A compression dressing and a volar splint are applied. The hand is actively used as soon as possible after surgery, but the dependent position is avoided. A smaller dressing may be applied after 1 week, and normal use of the hand is then encouraged. The sutures are removed after 10 to 14 days. The splint should be maintained for 14 to 21 days.

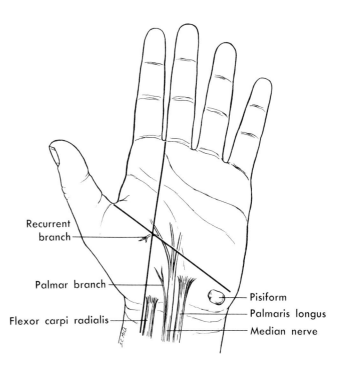

Fig. 76-2 Anatomic guidelines suggested by Kaplan to help in locating recurrent branch of median nerve.

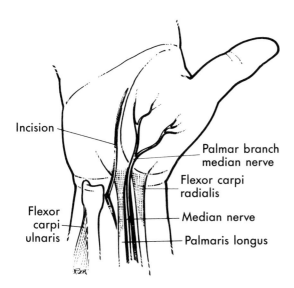

Fig. 76-1 Care should be taken in any incision about wrist to avoid cutting palmar branch of median nerve.

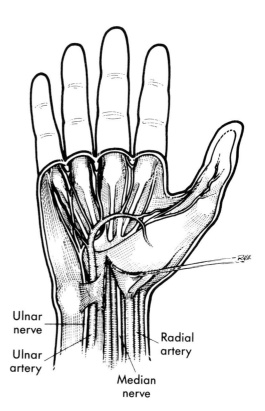

Fig. 76-3 Anatomic relations of deep transverse carpal ligament.

ENDOSCOPIC RELEASE OF CARPAL TUNNEL. Preliminary reports of endoscopic release of the transverse carpal ligament are promising, but independent evaluation of this technique is presently insufficient to determine its place in the management of carpal tunnel syndrome. Reports by Okutsu et al. Chow, and Agee suggest that the endoscopic technique results in more rapid recovery, decreased scarring and pain, and no loss of grip or pinch strength. Problems related to endoscopic carpal tunnel release include: (1) learning a technically demanding endoscopic procedure, (2) a limited visual field that prevents inspection of other structures, (3) vulnerability of the median nerve, flexor tendons, and superficial palmar arterial arch, (4) inability to easily control bleeding, and (5) limitations imposed by mechanical failure. Even if the efficacy of this technique is proven, it is doubtful that it should be used in every patient with carpal tunnel syndrome, and consideration should always be given to an open technique if endoscopic release cannot be accomplished safely.

Unrelieved, or Recurrent, Carpal Tunnel Syndrome

In a series of explorations of previously operated patients by Langloh and Linscheid, good results were reported in one half and fair results in one third. Symptoms may recur from hyperplasia of the tenosynovium. On reexploring the canal, in most instances the deep transverse carpal ligament has reformed so completely that the site of previous division cannot be identified. Symptoms from cervical disc disease and thoracic outlet syndrome should be carefully ruled out.

ULNAR TUNNEL SYNDROME

Ulnar tunnel syndrome results from compression of the ulnar nerve within a tight triangular fibroosseous tunnel about 1.5 cm long located at the carpus. The walls of the tunnel consist of the superficial transverse carpal ligament anteriorly, the deep transverse carpal ligament posteriorly, and the pisiform bone and pisohamate ligament medially (Fig. 76-4). Like the median nerve within the carpal tunnel, the ulnar nerve is subject to compression within this tunnel. Compared with carpal tunnel syndrome, ulnar tunnel syndrome is much less common because the space occupied by the ulnar nerve at the wrist is much more yielding. The more common location of ulnar nerve constriction is at the elbow.

The exact level of compression determines whether symptoms are motor or sensory or both. Compression just distal to the tunnel affects the deep branch of the nerve that supplies most of the intrinsics. A space-occupying lesion such as a ganglion or tumor may cause compression in this area. True or false aneurysm of the ulnar artery (Fig. 76-5), thrombosis of the ulnar artery, or frac-

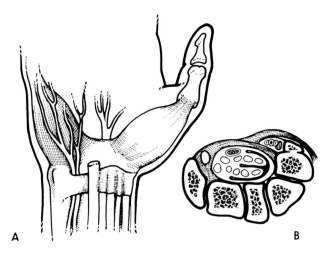

Fig. 76-4   Anatomic relations of structures within ulnar tunnel. **A**, Palmar view. Ulnar nerve lies medial to ulnar artery. **B**, Cross section of both carpal and ulnar tunnels. Ulnar tunnel at top right is bounded anteriorly by superficial transverse carpal ligament, posteriorly by deep transverse carpal ligament, and medially by pisiform bone and pisohamate ligament. Structures within this tunnel (left to right): vein, artery, vein, and nerve.

ture of the hamate with hemorrhage may be the cause of pressure on the ulnar nerve. Other reported causes are lipoma and aberrant muscles. Occasionally in rheumatoid disease, carpal tunnel and ulnar tunnel syndromes both develop in the same hand. In the differential diagnosis, herniation of a cervical disc, thoracic outlet syndrome, and peripheral neuropathy must be considered.

Treatment consists of exploration of the ulnar nerve at the wrist and removal of any ganglion or other cause of compression.

Should the ulnar artery be occluded for several millimeters, Raynaud's syndrome may be produced in the ulnar three digits because the sympathetic nerve fibers to these digits pass along the ulnar artery.

Segmental resection of the occluded section and replacement with a vein graft is the preferred procedure when it is feasible. Usually symptoms are relieved, and weakened or atrophic intrinsic muscles may recover in 3 to 12 months after surgery. For the technique of exploration, see the approach described for repair of the deep branch of the ulnar nerve (Chapter 65).

STENOSING TENOSYNOVITIS

Stenosing tenosynovitis occurs more often in the hand and wrist than anywhere else in the body. When the extensor pollicis brevis and the abductor pollicis longus tendons in the first dorsal compartment are affected, the condition is sometimes called de Quervain's disease. When the long flexor tendons are involved, trigger thumb, trigger finger, or snapping finger occurs. Less often, the extensor pollicis longus may be affected at the

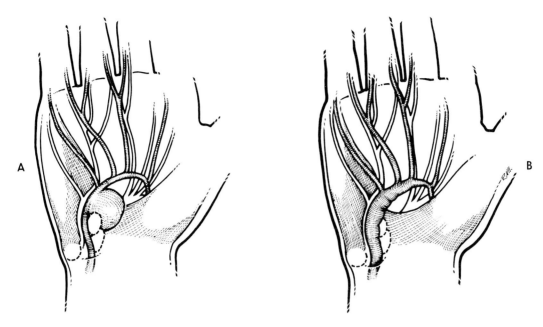

Fig. 76-5   Two types of traumatic aneurysms of ulnar artery in hand. **A**, Saccular "false" aneurysm arising from ulnar artery. **B**, "True" fusiform aneurysm of ulnar artery. (From Green DP: J Bone Joint Surg 55-A:120, 1973.)

level of Lister's tubercle. Any of the other tendons that pass beneath the dorsal wrist retinaculum may also be involved. The tenosynovitis that precedes the stenosis may result from an otherwise subclinical collagen disease, or recurrent mild trauma such as that experienced by carpenters and waitresses may be the cause. Some case histories indicate that acute trauma may initiate the pathologic condition. The stenosis occurs at a point where the direction of a tendon changes, for here a fibrous sheath acts as a pulley, and friction is maximum. Although the tenosynovium lubricates the sheath, friction may cause a reaction when the repetition of a particular movement is necessary, as in winding a fine coil of wire or stacking laundry.

In our experience many cases of tenosynovitis in various locations, even stenosing tenosynovitis, respond favorably to injections of a steroid preparation. Pain may increase temporarily during the initial 24 hours after loss of the local anesthetic effect; therefore the patient should be warned about this possibility. It may be 3 to 7 days before the steroid becomes effective, but surgery is avoided in many instances.

Before injection it should be determined that the tenosynovitis is not caused by other conditions such as gout or infection that could be worsened by steroid injections.

de Quervain's Disease

Stenosing tenosynovitis of the abductor pollicis longus and extensor pollicis brevis tendons occurs typically in adults between 30 and 50 years old. Women are affected

10 times more frequently than men. The cause is almost always related to overuse, either in the home or at work, or is associated with rheumatoid arthritis. The presenting symptoms are usually pain and tenderness at the radial styloid. Sometimes a thickening of the fibrous sheath is palpable. Finkelstein's test is usually positive: "on grasping the patient's thumb and quickly abducting the hand ulnarward, the pain over the styloid tip is excruciating."* Although Finkelstein states that this test is "probably the most pathognomonic objective sign," it is not diagnostic; the patient's history and occupation, the roentgenograms, and other physical findings must also be considered.

Conservative treatment, consisting of rest on a splint and the injection of a steroid preparation, is most successful within the first 6 weeks after onset. Harvey, Harvey, and Horsley reported 63 wrists initially treated with injections of steroids and local anesthetic into the tendon sheath. In 45 pain relief was complete (71.4%), and in 7 pain was relieved after a second injection. Only 11 (17.4%) required surgery. Christie in 1955 and Lapidus in 1972 reported similar experiences. When pain persists, surgery is the treatment of choice.

Anatomic variations are common in the first dorsal compartment. When the findings of anatomic dissections by Stein, Ramsey, and Key (11%), Keon-Cohen (33%), and Leão (24%) are combined, an incidence of 21% with separate compartments results. Reports of separate com-

*From Finkelstein H: Stenosing tendovaginitis at the radial styloid process, J Bone Joint Surg 30:509, 1930.

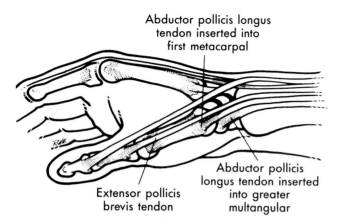

Fig. 76-6 Often abductor pollicis longus inserts on both greater multangular and base of first metacarpal through two tendons. Thus at surgery for de Quervain's disease at least one aberrant tendon is often found.

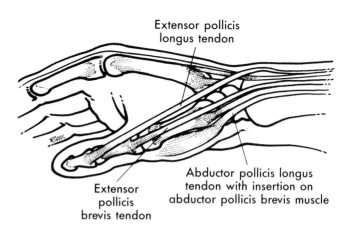

Fig. 76-7 Rarely abductor pollicis longus inserts on both fascia of abductor pollicis brevis and base of first metacarpal.

partments found at surgery vary from 20% to 58%. Over half of patients may have "aberrant" or duplicated tendons, usually the abductor pollicis longus. These tendons sometimes insert more proximally and medially than usual, into the greater multangular (Fig. 76-6), the abductor pollicis brevis muscle (Fig. 76-7), the opponens pollicis muscle, or the muscle fasica. The extensor pollicis brevis is considered a "late" tendon phylogenetically and is absent in about 5% of wrists. The presence of these variations and failure to deal with them at the time of surgery may account for any persistence of pain. In the report of Harvey, Harvey, and Horsley, 11 of 63 patients treated with injections required surgery; 10 of these were found to have the extensor pollicis brevis in a separate compartment.

■ *TECHNIQUE.* **Use a local anesthetic and a tourniquet. After sterile skin preparation and draping, use a tourniquet as needed, and infiltrate the skin in the area of the first dorsal compartment with sufficient local anesthetic agent. Make a skin incision that runs from dorsal to volar in a transverse to oblique direction, parallel with the skin creases over the area of tenderness in the first dorsal compartment (Fig. 76-8). The longitudinal incision advocated by some creates a longer area in which skin scar may adhere to the cutaneous nerves and the tendons. Carry sharp dissection just through the dermis and not into the subcutaneous fat, avoiding the branches of the superficial radial nerve. After retracting the skin edges, use blunt dissection in the subcutaneous fat. Then find and protect the sensory branches of the superficial radial nerve, usually located deep to the superficial veins. Identify the tendons proximal to the stenosing dorsal ligament and sheath and open the first dorsal compartment on its dorsoulnar side. With the thumb abducted and the wrist flexed, lift the abductor pollicis longus and the extensor**

pollicis brevis tendons from their groove. If they cannot be easily freed, look for additional "aberrant" tendons and separate compartments. Then close the skin incision only and apply a small pressure dressing.

Failure to obtain complete relief after surgery may result from (1) formation of a neuroma in a severed branch of the superficial radial nerve, (2) volar subluxation of the tendon when too much of the sheath is removed, (3) failure to find and release a separate aberrant tendon within a separate compartment, and (4) hypertrophy of scar from a longitudinal skin incision.

AFTERTREATMENT. **The small pressure dressing is removed after 48 hours, and a patch dressing is applied. Motion of the thumb and hand is immediately encouraged and is increased as tolerated.**

Trigger Finger and Thumb

Trigger thumb may be congenital, but it also occurs in adults, usually after 45 years of age. When associated with a collagen disease, several fingers may be involved — the middle and ring most often. A nodule or fusiform swelling of the flexor tendon just proximal to its theca at the distal palmar crease causes a relative stenosis of the sheath. The nodule can be palpated by the examiner's fingertip and will move with the tendon. The nodule is usually at the entry of the tendon into the proximal annulus at the level of the metacarpophalangeal joint; however, in the rheumatoid patient, a nodule distal to this point may cause triggering that will not always be relieved by sectioning the proximal annulus alone. Occasionally a partially lacerated flexor tendon at this level may heal with a nodule sufficiently large to cause triggering. Local tenderness may be present but is not a prominent complaint. Pressure accentuates the

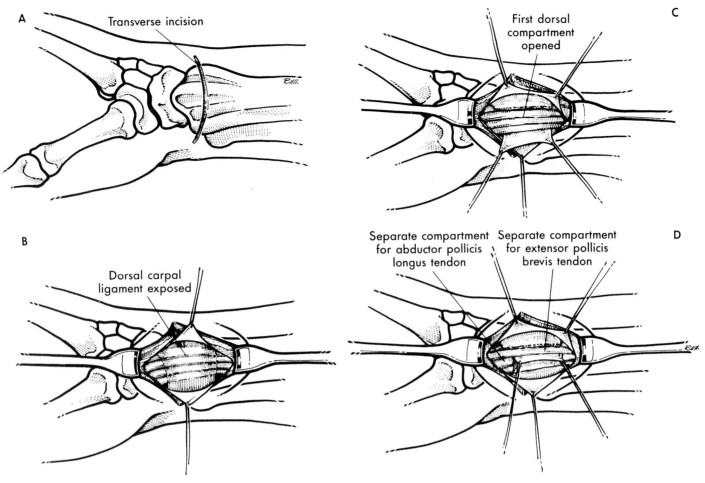

Fig. 76-8 Surgical treatment of de Quervain's disease. **A**, Skin incision. **B**, Dorsal carpal ligament has been exposed. **C**, First dorsal compartment has been opened on its ulnar side. **D**, Occasionally separate compartments are found for extensor pollicis brevis and abductor pollicis longus tendons.

snapping or triggering of the distal joints. It should be noted, particularly in the thumb, that the constriction is opposite the metacarpophalangeal joint, although the interphalangeal joint is the one that appears to lock or snap. (See also locking of joint, p. 3185.) In congenital trigger digit deformities expectant observation should be the first treatment, since many will resolve within the first 6 months and nearly all within 2 years. Rarely is trigger finger seen in a child after 2 years of age.

■ *TECHNIQUE.* Make a transverse incision about 1.9 cm long just distal to the distal palmar crease for trigger finger (Fig. 76-9, *A*) or just distal to the flexor crease of the thumb at the metacarpophalangeal joint for trigger thumb (see Fig. 61-12, *J*). Take care to avoid the digital nerves, which on the thumb are more palmar and closer to the flexor sheath than might be anticipated. Identify with a small probe the discrete proximal edge of the flexor sheath. Now place a small knife blade or one blade

of a pair of slightly opened blunt scissors just under the edge of the sheath and gently push it distally, cutting the sheath (Fig. 76-9, *B*). Thus the constriction of the tendon is released. Flex and extend the digit to be sure that the release is complete. Then close the skin and apply a small dry compression dressing.

AFTERTREATMENT. The compression dressing is removed after 48 hours, and a patch dressing is applied. Normal use of the finger or thumb is then advised.

Bowler's Thumb

Bowler's thumb is a perineural fibrosis caused by repetitious compression of the ulnar digital nerve of the thumb while grasping a bowling ball (Fig. 76-10). Bowlers with this condition are usually those who bowl 3 or 4 times a week. It is accompanied by tingling and

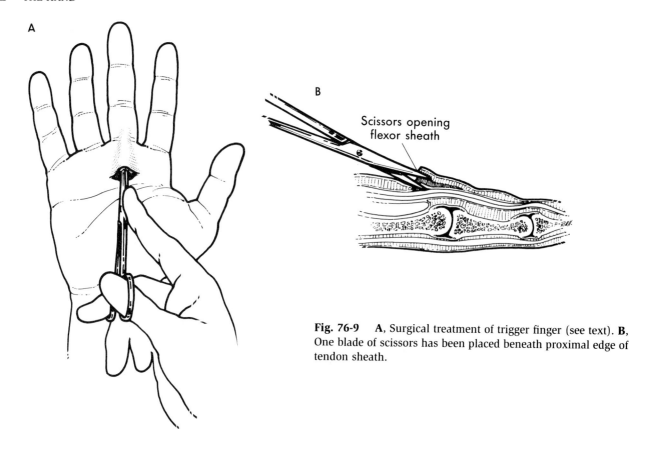

Fig. 76-9 **A,** Surgical treatment of trigger finger (see text). **B,** One blade of scissors has been placed beneath proximal edge of tendon sheath.

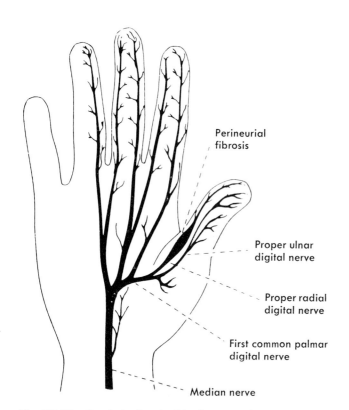

Fig. 76-10 Bowler's thumb. Distal sensory branches of median nerve in hand and location of perineural fibrosis of proper ulnar digital nerve of thumb are shown. (From Minkow FV and Bassett FH III: Clin Orthop 83:115, 1972.)

hyperesthesia about the pulp. There is usually a palpable lump that is exceedingly tender and at times accompanied by distal skin atrophy. Early awareness of the cause can lead to protection of the thumb by a shield or splint and rest from bowling to help reduce the symptoms and to prevent the condition from becoming chronic. Occasionally neurolysis and dorsal transfer of the nerve become necessary.

REFERENCES

Carpal tunnel syndrome

Adamson JE, Srouji SJ, Horton CE, and Mladick RA: The acute carpal tunnel syndrome, Plast Reconstr Surg 47:332, 1971.

Agee JM, Tortosa, RD, Palmer CA, and Berry C: Endoscopic release of the carpal tunnel: a randomized perspective multicenter study. Presented at the 45th annual meeting of the American Society of the Hand, Sept. 24-27, 1990, Toronto, Canada.

Aghasi MK, Rzetelny V, and Axer A: The flexor digitorum superficialis as a cause of bilateral carpal-tunnel syndrome and trigger wrist, J Bone Joint Surg 62-A:134, 1980.

Alegado RB and Meals RA: An unusual complication following surgical treatment of de Quervain's disease, J Hand Surg 4:185, 1979.

Ariyan S and Watson SK: The palmar approach for the visualization and release of the carpal tunnel: an analysis of 429 cases, Plast Reconstr Surg 60:539, 1977.

Barton NJ: Another cause of median nerve compression by a lumbrical muscle in the carpal tunnel, J Hand Surg 4:189, 1979.

Bauman TD, Gelberman RH, Mubarak SJ, and Garfin SR: The acute carpal tunnel syndrome, Clin Orthop 156:151, 1981.

Bell GE Jr and Goldner JL: Compression neuropathy of the median nerve, South Med J 49:966, 1956.

Berman AT and Straub RR: Importance of preoperative and postoperative electrodiagnostic studies in the treatment of the carpal tunnel syndrome, Orthop Rev 3:57, June 1974.

Brian WR, Wright AD, and Wilkinson M: Spontaneous compression of both median nerves in the carpal tunnel: six cases treated surgically, Lancet 1:277, 1947.

Brown FE and Tanzer RC: Entrapment neuropathies of the upper extremity. In Flynn JE, ed: Hand Surgery, ed 3, Baltimore, 1982, Williams & Wilkins.

Brown LP and Coulson DB: Triggering at the carpal tunnel with incipient carpal-tunnel syndrome: report of an unusual case, J Bone Joint Surg 56-A:623, 1974.

Browne EZ Jr and Snyder CC: Carpal tunnel syndrome caused by hand injuries, Plast Reconstr Surg 56:41, 1975.

Burnham PJ: Acute carpal tunnel syndrome: median artery thrombosis as cause, Arch Surg 87:645, 1963.

Butler B Jr and Bigley EC Jr: Aberrant index (first) lumbrical tendinous origin associated with carpal-tunnel syndrome: a case report, J Bone Joint Surg 53-A:160, 1971.

Caffee HH: Anomalous thenar muscle and median nerve: a case report, J Hand Surg 4:446, 1979.

Cannon BW and Love JG: Tardy median palsy: median neuritis: median thenar neuritis amenable to surgery, Surgery 20:210, 1946.

Carroll RE and Green DP: The significance of the palmar cutaneous nerve at the wrist, Clin Orthop 83:24, 1972.

Carroll RE and Hurst LC: The relationship of the thoracic outlet syndrome and carpal tunnel syndrome, Clin Orthop 164:149, 1982.

Chow JCY: Endoscopic release of the carpal ligament: a new technique for carpal tunnel syndrome, Arthroscopy 5:19, 1989.

Chow JCY: Endoscopic release of the carpal ligament for carpal tunnel syndrome: 22-month clinical results, Arthroscopy 6:288, 1990.

Chow JCY: Endoscopic release of the carpal ligament: analysis of 300 cases. Presented at the 58th Annual Meeting of the American Academy of Orthopaedic Surgeons, Anaheim, California, March 9, 1991.

Conklin JE and White WL: Stenosing tenosynovitis and its possible relation to the carpal tunnel syndrome, Surg Clin North Am 40:531, 1960.

Cseuz KA, Thomas JE, Lamber EH, et al: Long-term results of operation for carpal tunnel syndrome, Mayo Clin Proc 41:232, 1966.

Curtis RM and Eversmann WW Jr: Internal neurolysis as an adjunct to the treatment of the carpal-tunnel syndrome, J Bone Joint Surg 55-A:733, 1973.

De Abreau LB and Moreira RG: Median-nerve compression at the wrist, J Bone Joint Surg 40-A:1426, 1958.

Dellon AL: Clinical use of vibratory stimuli to evaluate peripheral nerve injury and compression neuropathy, Plast Reconstr Surg 65:466, 1980.

Dellon AL and Fine IT: A noninvasive technique for diagnosis of chronic compartment syndrome in the first dorsal interosseous muscle, J Hand Surg 15-A:1008, 1990.

DeLuca FN and Cowen NJ: Median-nerve compression complicating a tendon graft prosthesis, J Bone Joint Surg 57-A:553, 1975.

Doyle JR and Carroll RE: The carpal tunnel syndrome: a review of 100 patients treated surgically, Calif Med 108:263, 1968.

Duran JA: A new diagnostic test for carpal tunnel syndrome, J Bone Joint Surg 73-A:535, 1991.

Enger WD and Gmeiner JG: Palmar cutaneous branch of the ulnar nerve, J Hand Surg 5:26, 1980.

Eversmann WW Jr and Tirsick JA: Intraoperative changes in motor nerve conduction latency in carpal tunnel syndrome, J Hand Surg 3:77, 1978.

Freshwater MF and Arons MS: The effect of various adjuncts on the surgical treatment of carpal tunnel syndrome secondary to chronic synovitis, Plast Reconstr Surg 61:93, 1978.

Frymoyer JW and Bland J: Carpal-tunnel syndrome in patients with myxedematous arthropathy, J Bone Joint Surg 55-A:78, 1973.

Gama C and Franca CM: Nerve compression by pacinian corpuscles, J Hand Surg 5:207, 1980.

Garland H, Sumner D, and Clark JMP: Carpal-tunnel syndrome: with particular reference to surgical treatment, Br Med J 1:581, 1963.

Gelberman, RH, Aronson D, and Weisman MH: Carpal-tunnel syndrome: results of a prospective trial of steroid injection and splinting, J Bone Joint Surg 62-A:1181, 1980.

Gelberman RH, Szabo RM, Williamson RV, and Dimick MP: Sensibility testing in peripheral nerve compression syndromes: an experimental study in humans, J Bone Joint Surg 65-A:632, 1983.

Gelberman RH, Hergenroeder PT, Hargens AR, et al: The carpal tunnel syndrome: a study of carpal tunnel pressures, J Bone Joint Surg 63-A:380, 1981.

Gellman H, Gelberman RH, Tan AM, and Botte MJ: Carpal tunnel syndrome: an evaluation of the provocative diagnostic test, J Bone Joint Surg 68-A:735, 1986.

Harris CM, Tanner E, Goldstein MN, and Pettee DS: The surgical treatment of the carpal-tunnel syndrome correlated with preoperative nerve conduction studies, J Bone Joint Surg 61-A:93, 1979.

Healy C, Watson JD, Longstaff A, And Campbell MJ: Magnetic resonance imaging of the carpal tunnel,

Heathfield KWG: Acroparaesthesiae and the carpal-tunnel syndrome, Lancet 2:663, 1957.

Hecht O and Lipsker E: Median and ulnar nerve entrapment caused by ectopic calcification: report of two cases, J Hand Surg 5:30, 1980.

Herndon JH, Eaton RG, and Littler WJ: Carpal-tunnel syndrome: an unusual presentation of osteoid-osteoma of the capitate, J Bone Joint Surg 56-A:1715, 1974.

Hybbinette CH and Mannerfelt L: The carpal tunnel syndrome: a retrospective study of 400 operated patients, Acta Orthop Scand 46:610, 1975.

Inglis AE: Two unusual operative complications in the carpal-tunnel syndrome: a report of two cases, J Bone Joint Surg 62-A:1208, 1980.

Jabaley ME: Personal observations on the role of the lumbrical muscles in carpal tunnel syndrome, J Hand Surg 3:82, 1978.

Jackson IT and Campbell JC: An unusual cause of carpal tunnel syndrome: a case of thrombosis of the median artery, J Bone Joint Surg 52-B:330, 1970.

Johnson RK and Shrewsbury MM: Anatomical course of the thenar branch of the median nerve — usually in a separate tunnel through the transverse carpal ligament, J Bone Joint Surg 52-A:269, 1970.

Kaplan SJ, Glickel SZ, and Eaton RG: Predictive factors in the nonsurgical treatment of carpal tunnel syndrome, J Hand Surg 15-B:106, 1990.

Katz JN and Stirrat CR: A self-administered hand diagram for the diagnosis of carpal tunnel syndrome, J Hand Surg 15-A:360, 1990.

Kessler FB: Complications of the management of carpal tunnel syndrome, Hand Clin 2:401, 1986.

Koris M, Gelberman RH, Duncan K, et al: Carpal tunnel syndrome: evaluation of a quantitative provocational diagnostic test, Clin Orthop 251:157, 1990.

Kummel BM and Zazanis GA: Shoulder pain as the presenting complaint in carpal tunnel syndrome, Clin Orthop 92:227, 1973.

Langloh ND and Linscheid RL: Recurrent and unrelieved carpal-tunnel syndrome, Clin Orthop 83:41, 1972.

Lanz U: Anatomical variations of the median nerve in the carpal tunnel, J Hand Surg 2:44, 1977.

Lichtman DM, Florio RL, and Mack GR: Carpal tunnel release under local anesthesia: evaluation of the outpatient procedure, J Hand Surg 4:544, 1979.

Linscheid RL: Carpal tunnel syndrome secondary to ulnar bursa distention from the intercarpal joint: report of a case, J Hand Surg 4:191, 1979.

Linscheid RL, Peterson LFA, and Juergens JL: Carpal-tunnel syndrome associated with vasospasm, J Bone Joint Surg 49-A:1141, 1967.

Lipscomb PR: Tenosynovitis of the hand and the wrist: carpal tunnel syndrome, de Quervain's disease, trigger digit, Clin Orthop 13:164, 1959.

Littler JW and Li CS: Primary restoration of thumb opposition with median nerve decompression, Plast Reconstr Surg 39:74, 1967.

Lundborg G, Gelberman RH, Minteer-Convery M, et al: Median nerve compression in the carpal tunnel: functional response to experimentally induced controlled pressure, J Hand Surg 7:252, 1982.

Lynch AC and Lipscomb PR: The carpal tunnel syndrome and Colles' fractures, JAMA 185:363, 1963.

MacDonald RI, Lichtman DM, Hanlon JJ, and Wilson JN: Complications of surgical release for carpal tunnel syndrome, J Hand Surg 3:70, 1978.

MacDougal B, Weeks PM, and Wray RC Jr: Median nerve compression and trigger finger in the mucopolysaccharidoses and related diseases, Plast Reconstr Surg 59:260, 1977.

Mangini U: Some remarks on the etiology of the carpal tunnel compression of the median nerve, Bull Hosp Joint Dis 22:56, 1961.

May JW and Rosen H: Division of the sensory ramus communicans between the ulnar and median nerves: a complication following carpal tunnel release, J Bone Joint Surg 63-A:836, 1981.

McCormack RM: Carpal tunnel syndrome, Surg Clin North Am 40:517, 1960.

Nagai H: Tunnel-endoscopy, Arthroscopy 5:1, 1980.

Nissenbaum M and Kleinert HE: Treatment considerations in carpal tunnel syndrome with coexistent Dupuytren's disease, J Hand Surg 5:544, 1980.

Ogden JA: An unusual branch of the median nerve, J Bone Joint Surg 54-A:1779, 1972.

Okutsu I, Ninomiya S, Takatori Y, and Ugawa Y: Endoscopic management of carpal tunnel syndrome, Arthroscopy 5:11, 1989.

Omer GE and Spinner M: Management of peripheral nerve problems, Philadelphia, 1980, WB Saunders Co.

Orcutt SA, Kramer WG III, Howard MW, et al: Carpal tunnel syndrome secondary to wrist and finger flexor spasticity, J Hand Surg 15-A:940, 1990.

Pecket P, Gloobe H, and Nathan H: Variations in the arteries of the median nerve: with special considerations on the ischemic factor in the carpal tunnel syndrome (CTS), Clin Orthop 97:144, 1973.

Phalen GS: The carpal tunnel syndrome, AAOS Instr Course Lect 14:142, 1957.

Phalen GS: The carpal-tunnel syndrome: seventeen years' experience in diagnosis and treatment of six hundred fifty-four hands, J Bone Joint Surg 48-A:211, 1966.

Phalen GS: Reflections on 21 years' experience with the carpal-tunnel syndrome, JAMA 212:1365, 1970.

Phalen GS: The carpal-tunnel syndrome: clinical evaluation of 598 hands, Clin Orthop 83:29, 1972.

Phalen GS: The birth of a syndrome, or carpal tunnel revisited, J Hand Surg 6:109, 1981.

Phalen GS and Kendrick JI: Compression neuropathy of the median nerve in the carpal tunnel, JAMA 164:524, 1957.

Phalen GS, Gardner WJ, and LaLonde AA: Neuropathy of the median nerve due to compression beneath the transverse carpal ligament, J Bone Joint Surg 32-A:109, 1950.

Posch JL and Marcotte DR: Carpal tunnel syndrome: an analysis of 1,201 cases, Orthop Rev 5:25, May 1976.

Ragi EF: Carpal tunnel syndrome: a statistical review, Electromyogr Clin Neurophysiol 21:373, 1981.

Rowland SA: A palmar incision for release of the carpal tunnel, Clin Orthop 103:89, 1974.

Rubinstein MA: Carpal tunnel syndrome in lymphatic leukemia, JAMA 213:1037, 1970.

Schuind F, Ventura M, and Pasteels JL: Idiopathic carpal tunnel syndrome: histologic study of flexor tendon synovium, J Hand Surg 15-A:497, 1990.

Schultz RJ, Endler PM, and Huddleston HD: Anomalous median nerve and an anomalous muscle belly of the first lumbrical associated with carpal-tunnel syndrome: case report, J Bone Joint Surg 55-A:1744, 1973.

Shivde AJ, Dreizin I, and Fisher MA: The carpal tunnel syndrome: a clinical electrodiagnostic analysis, Electromyogr Clin Neurophysiol 21:143, 1981.

Skie M, Zeiss J, Ebraheim NA, and Jackson WT: Carpal tunnel changes and median nerve compression during wrist flexion and extension seen by magnetic resonance imaging, J Hand Surg 15-A:934, 1990.

Smith RJ: Anomalous muscle belly of the flexor digitorum superficialis causing carpal-tunnel syndrome: report of a case, J Bone Joint Surg 53-A:1215, 1971.

Stein AH Jr: The relation of median nerve compression to Sudeck's syndrome, Surg Gynecol Obstet 115:713, 1962.

Taleisnik J: The palmar cutaneous branch of the median nerve and the approach to the carpal tunnel: an anatomical study, J Bone Joint Surg 55-A:1212, 1973.

Tanzer RC: The carpal tunnel syndrome, Clin Orthop 15:171, 1959.

Tanzer RC: The carpal-tunnel syndrome: a clinical and anatomical study, J Bone Joint Surg 41-A:626, 1959.

Tompkins DG: Median neuropathy in the carpal tunnel caused by tumor-like conditions: report of two cases, J Bone Joint Surg 49-A:737, 1967.

Walton S and Cutler CR: Carpal tunnel syndrome: case report of unusual etiology, Clin Orthop 74:138, 1971.

Wood MR: Hydrocortisone injections for carpal tunnel syndrome, Hand 12:62, 1980.

Wood VE: Nerve compression following opponensplasty as a result of wrist anomalies: report of a case, J Hand Surg 5:279, 1980.

Yamaguchi DM, Lipscomb PR, and Soule EH: Carpal tunnel syndrome, Minn Med 48:22, 1965.

Ulnar tunnel syndrome

Baird DB and Friedenberg ZB: Delayed ulnar-nerve palsy following a fracture of the hamate, J Bone Joint Surg 50-A:570, 1968.

Cameron BM: Occlusion of the ulnar artery with impending gangrene of the fingers relieved by section of the volar carpal ligament, J Bone Joint Surg 36-A:406, 1954.

Dupont C, et al: Ulnar tunnel syndrome at the wrist: a report of four cases of ulnar-nerve compression at the wrist, J Bone Joint Surg 47-A:757, 1965.

Fahrer M and Millroy PJ: Ulnar compression neuropathy due to an anomalous abductor digiti minimi: clinical and anatomic study, J Hand Surg 6:266, 1981.

Fissette J, Onkelinx A, and Fandi N: Carpal and Guyon tunnel syndrome in burns at the wrist, J Hand Surg 6:13, 1981.

Gore DR: Carpometacarpal dislocation producing compression of the deep branch of the ulnar nerve, J Bone Joint Surg 53-A:1387, 1971.

Green DP: True and false traumatic aneurysms in the hand: report of two cases and review of the literature, J Bone Joint Surg 55-A:120, 1973.

Hayes CW Jr: Ulnar tunnel syndrome from giant cell tumor of tendon sheath: a case report, J Hand Surg 3:187, 1978.

Howard FM: Ulnar-nerve palsy in wrist fractures, J Bone Joint Surg 43-A:1197, 1961.

Jeffrey AK: Compression of the deep palmar branch of the ulnar nerve by an anomalous muscle: case report and review, J Bone Joint Surg 53-B:718, 1971.

Kleinert HE and Hayes JE: The ulnar tunnel syndrome, Plast Reconstr Surg 47:21, 1971.

Magassy CL, Newmeyer WL, Creech BJ, and Kilgore ES Jr: Ulnar tunnel syndrome, Orthop Rev 2:21, 1973.

McCarthy RE and Nalebuff EA: Anomalous volar branch of the dorsal cutaneous ulnar nerve: a case report, J Hand Surg 5:19, 1980.

McFarland GB Jr and Hoffer MM: Paralysis of the intrinsic muscles of the hand secondary to lipoma in Guyon's tunnel, J Bone Joint Surg 53-A:375, 1971.

Richmond DA: Carpal ganglion with ulnar nerve compression, J Bone Joint Surg 45-B:513, 1963.

Stein AH Jr and Morgan HC: Compression of the ulnar nerve at the level of the wrist, Am Pract 13:195, 1962.

Taylor AR: Ulnar nerve compression at the wrist in rheumatoid arthritis: report of a case, J Bone Joint Surg 56-A:142, 1974.

Wissinger HA: Resection of the hook of the hamate: its place in the treatment of median and ulnar nerve entrapment in the hand, Plast Reconstr Surg 56:501, 1975.

de Quervain's disease

Bruckschwaiger O: An atypical form of de Quervain's disease, Can Med J 71:277, 1954.

Burman M: Stenosing tendovaginitis of the dorsal and volar compartments of the wrist, Arch Surg 65:752, 1952.

Christie BGB: Local hydrocortisone in deQuervain's disease, Br Med J 1:1501, 1955.

Fenton R: Stenosing tendovaginitis at the radial styloid involving an accessory tendon sheath, Bull Hosp Joint Dis 11:90, 1950.

Finkelstein H: Stenosing tendovaginitis at the radial styloid process, J Bone Joint Surg 12:509, 1930.

Harvey FJ, Harvey PM, and Horsley MW: De Quervain's disease: surgical or nonsurgical treatment, J Hand Surg 15-A:83, 1990.

Keon-Cohen B: de Quervain's disease, J Bone Joint Surg 33-B:96, 1951.

Lacey T II, Goldstein LA, and Tobin CE: Anatomical and clinical study of the variations in the insertions of the abductor pollicis longus tendon associated with stenosing tendovaginitis, J Bone Joint Surg 33-A:347, 1951.

Lapidus PW: Symposium on ambulant surgery, stenosing tenovaginitis, Surg Clin North Am 33:1317, 1953.

Lapidus PW: Stenosing tenovaginitis of the wrist and fingers, Clin Orthop 83:87, 1972.

Lapidus PW and Guidotti FP: Stenosing tenovaginitis of the wrist and fingers, Clin Orthop 83:87, 1972.

Leao L: de Quervain's disease: a clinical and anatomical study, J Bone Joint Surg 40-A:1063, 1958.

Loomis LK: Variations of stenosing tenosynovitis at the radial styloid process, J Bone Joint Surg 33-A:340, 1951.

McMahon M, Craig SM, and Posner MA: Tendon subluxation after de Quervain's release: treatment by brachioradialis tendon flap, J Hand Surg 16-A:30, 1991.

Muckart RD: Stenosing tendovaginitis of abductor pollicis longus and extensor pollicis brevis at the radial styloid (de Quervain's disease), Clin Orthop 33:201, 1964.

Murphy ID: An unusual form of de Quervain's syndrome: report of two cases, J Bone Joint Surg 31-A:858, 1949.

Pick RY: de Quervain's disease, a clinical triad, Clin Orthop 143:165, 1979.

Strandell G: Variations of the anatomy in stenosing tenosynovitis at the radial styloid process, Acta Chir Scand 113:234, 1957.

Witczak JW, Masear VR, and Meyer RD: Triggering of the thumb with de Quervain's stenosing tendovaginitis, J Hand Surg 15-A:265, 1990.

Wood MB and Linscheid RL: Abductor pollicis longus bursitis, Clin Orthop 93:293, 1973.

Woods THE: de Quervain's disease: a plea for early operation: a report on 40 cases, Br J Surg 51:358, 1964.

Trigger thumb and trigger finger

Fahey JJ and Bollinger JA: Trigger-finger in adults and children, J Bone Joint Surg 36-A:1200, 1954.

Kolind-Sorensen V: Treatment of trigger fingers, Acta Orthop Scand 41:428, 1970.

Loomis LK: Flexion deformity of the infant thumb, South Med J 50:1259, 1957.

Lorthioir J Jr: Surgical treatment of trigger-finger by a subcutaneous method, J Bone Joint Surg 40-A:793, 1958.

Lutter LD: A new cause of locking fingers, Clin Orthop 83:131, 1972.

Rayan GM: Distal stenosing tenosynovitis, J Hand Surg 15-A:973, 1990.

Rayan GM: Stenosing tenosynovitis in bowlers, Am J Sports Med 18:214, 1990.

Rockey HC: Trigger-finger due to a tenosynovial osteochondroma, J Bone Joint Surg 45-A:387, 1963.

Sprecher EE: Trigger thumb in infants, J Bone Joint Surg 31-A:672, 1949.

Stein AH, Ramsey RH, and Key JA: Stenosing tendovaginitis at the radial styloid process (de Quervain's disease), Arch Surg 63:216, 1951.

Weilby A: Trigger finger: incidence in children and adults and the possibility of a predisposition in certain age groups, Acta Orthop Scand 41:419, 1970.

Young L and Holtmann B: Trigger finger and thumb secondary to amyloidosis, Plast Reconstr Surg 65:68, 1980.

Miscellaneous tenosynovitis

Dickson DD and Luckey C: Tenosynovitis of the extensor carpi ulnaris tendon sheath, J Bone Joint Surg 30-A:903, 1948.

Drury BJ: Traumatic tendovaginitis of the fifth dorsal compartment of the wrist, Arch Surg 80:554, 1960.

Fitton JM, Shea FW, and Goldie W: Lesions of the flexor carpi radialis tendon and sheath causing pain at the wrist, J Bone Joint Surg 40-B:359, 1968.

Ritter MA and Inglis AE: The extensor indicis proprius syndrome, J Bone Joint Surg 51-A:1645, 1969.

Steuber JB and Klineman WB: Flexor carpi radialis tunnel syndrome, J Hand Surg 6:293, 1981.

Weeks PM: A cause of wrist pain: non-specific tenosynovitis involving the flexor carpi radialis, Plast Reconstr Surg 62:263, 1978.

CHAPTER 77

Tumors and Tumorous Conditions of Hand

MARK T. JOBE

Tumors of the hand are common and varied, but each has its own peculiar incidence, malignant potential, and symptoms. Any tumor that may arise in an extremity may also occur in the hand. Because the hand is a sensitive organ, has little potential free space, and is packed with moving parts, any tumor usually is detected early because of pain, impairment of function, or obvious swelling despite often being a benign process. Malignant tumors arising from tissues of the hand other than skin are so rare that even single cases warrant publication. The hand also may be the site of distant metastasis, most commonly adenocarcinoma of the breast, lung, or kidney; the distal phalanx is the most common site.

CLASSIFICATION

Tumors involving the hand are classified in a manner similar to tumors involving the rest of the body. Benign tumors are classified as latent, active, or aggressive, according to their local biologic activity (Table 77-1). Benign latent tumors are those in which tumor growth has occurred during childhood or adolescence and has subsequently entered an inactive or healing phase. Solitary and unicameral bone cysts are examples of benign latent

tumors. A benign active tumor continues to enlarge and, although it is well encapsulated, may have an irregular or lumpy border. Most benign tumors of the hand fall into this category. A benign aggressive tumor, although non-metastasizing and innocent appearing on histologic sections, is locally destructive and is surrounded by a thin and tenuous capsule that may not contain all the tumor cells. A giant cell tumor of bone often behaves in this aggressive manner. A wide margin is often necessary for complete eradication of benign aggressive tumors.

Malignant tumors are classified as low grade (I), high grade (II), or associated with metastasis (III) (Table 77-2). Most malignant tumors of the hand are low-grade tumors. Malignant tumors are further classified, according to the degree of local extension, as either intracompartmental (A) or extracompartmental (B). In the hand, each ray forms a distinct compartment. The individual phalanges are not considered separate compartments, but rather they, along with their corresponding intrinsic muscles, form the ray compartment. The flexor tendon and sheath of each finger are part of the ray compartment as far proximally as the midpalmar space. The extensor tendon is part of the ray compartment as far as the metacarpophalangeal joint. Each metacarpal is a separate compartment. If a tumor involves the palmar space or the loose areolar tissue on the dorsum of the hand, it

*Revision of chapter by Lee W. Milford, M.D.

Table 77-1 Classification of benign tumors

Stage 1	Latent
Stage 2	Active
Stage 3	Aggressive

(Modified from Enneking WE: Musculoskeletal tumor surgery, New York, 1983, Churchill Livingstone.)

is considered extracompartmental because proximal spread is unobstructed. Tumors arising in the digits remain confined to that compartment for long periods of time and only then extend into the palm.

DIAGNOSIS

Usually a thorough history, physical examination, and routine plain roentgenograms are all that are necessary for the experienced surgeon to adequately determine the diagnosis and appropriate treatment of benign-appearing tumors in the hand. If a more aggressive process is present — causing considerable pain, inflammation, a large tumor, or bony destruction — further diagnostic and staging studies are warranted before biopsy or any definitive surgical procedure. We have found that local imaging studies such as tomograms, bone scans, angiograms, computed tomography (CT) scans, and magnetic resonance images (MRIs) are more helpful in surgical planning than in obtaining a specific diagnosis. Careful preoperative evaluation for pulmonary metastases with a chest roentgenogram and CT scan also is indicated if a malignant tumor is suspected.

TREATMENT

The treatment of tumors of the hand is surgical, with the possible exception of warts. Rarely is biopsy needed, because complete local excision is usually indicated, and the entire tumor is then available for microscopic study. Incisional biopsy is advised if a malignant tumor is suspected or if the morbidity of surgical excision outweighs the morbidity caused by the tumor itself, as may be true in some benign neural tumors. Incisions should be made directly over the mass to be harvested for biopsy and should be oriented so as not to jeopardize function of the hand or interfere with complete removal of the tumor. The way in which a tumor is removed depends on its location, its aggressiveness, its potential for metastasizing, and at times its sensitivity to adjuvant chemotherapy and radiation therapy. The various surgical margins are summarized in Table 77-3.

Benign tumors of soft tissue are treated by excisional biopsy (marginal excision). Benign tumors of bone are often treated by curettage (intracapsular) and occasionally bone grafting. Malignant tumors require a wide excision in which a tumor-free cuff of tissue (approximately

Table 77-2 Classification of malignant tumors

Stage IA	Low grade, intracompartmental
Stage IB	Low grade, extracompartmental
Stage IIA	High grade, intracompartmental
Stage IIB	High grade, extracompartmental
Stage III	Either grade with regional or distant metastasis

(Modified from Enneking WF, Spanier SS, and Goodman MA: Clin Orthop 153:106, 1980.)

2 cm) is removed with the tumor. Malignant tumors involving the distal phalanx may be treated with a transdiaphyseal amputation through the middle phalanx. Malignant tumors of the middle phalanx may be treated with a transdiaphyseal amputation through the proximal phalanx. If the malignant tumor involves the proximal phalanx, a ray amputation is usually required. Malignant tumors of the metacarpals, especially if large and extracompartmental, often require a one- to three-ray amputation to achieve adequate surgical margins. Stage IIB lesions involving the hand may require amputation through the distal third of the forearm at a level just proximal to the musculotendinous junctions. Reconstruction following wide or radical excisions for malignant tumors of the hand should be delayed until tumor-free margins have been documented. The same principles of surgical technique described in Chapter 61 are followed in treating tumors.

The following list of tumors and tumorous conditions, although not exhaustive, serves as a guide in considering those most commonly found in the hand, excluding skin blemishes, warts, and malignant skin tumors. Most of those listed in the following are discussed.

Benign tumors
Lipoma
Giant cell tumor of tendon sheath (xanthoma)
Fibroma
Recurring digital fibrous tumor of childhood
Juvenile aponeurotic fibroma
Fibromatosis (desmoid)
Pseudosarcomatous fasciitis
Glomus tumor
Hemangioma

Table 77-3 Classification of surgical margins

Type	Plane of dissection
Intracapsular	Piecemeal, debulking, or curettage
Marginal	Shell out (en bloc) through pseudocapsule or reactive zone
Wide	Intracompartmental (en bloc) with cuff of normal tissue
Radical	Extracompartmental (en bloc) with entire compartment

(Modified from Enneking WE: Musculoskeletal tumor surgery, New York, 1983, Churchill Livingstone.)

Lymphangioma
Traumatic neuroma
Multiple neurofibromas
Neurilemoma (schwannoma)
Lipofibroma
Osteoid osteoma
Enchondroma
Benign osteoblastoma
Aneurysmal bone cyst
Giant cell tumors of bone
Osteochondroma
Malignant tumors
Osteogenic sarcoma
Chondrosarcoma
Epithelioid sarcoma
Fibrosarcoma
Malignant fibrous histiocytoma
Metastatic tumors
Rhabdomyosarcoma
Ewing's sarcoma
Tumorous conditions
Ganglion
Epidermoid cyst (inclusion cyst)
Sebaceous cyst
Mucous cyst
Congenital arteriovenous fistula
Pyogenic granuloma
Foreign body granuloma
Gout
Déjerine-Sottas disease
Calcinosis
Localized calcium deposits
Turret exotosis
Carpometacarpal boss
Paget's disease
Epidermolysis bullosa

BENIGN TUMORS

LIPOMA. Lipoma, although common elsewhere in the body, is rare in the hand (Figs. 77-1 and 77-2). It may be superficial, arising from the subcutaneous tissues and having the characteristic signs of a soft, fluctuant, bulging mass or it may occur deep in the palm, arising within Guyon's canal, the carpal tunnel, and the deep palmar space. Usually a painless mass is present that impairs grasp. Lateral deviation of the fingers also may be present. Local compression of the median or ulnar nerve may cause muscular weakness or diminished sensibility. As noted by Oster, Blair, and Steyers, lipomas arising from the deep palmar space tend to present in the periphery of the hand because of the unyielding nature of the overlying palmar aponeurosis. Unhurried, careful dissection is necessary for removal because the tumor often sequesters digital nerves and is much larger than is clinically apparent. Recurrence after marginal excision is unlikely.

Intraneural lipofibroma is a rare benign tumor that usually involves the median nerve. Patients present within the first three decades of life with a mass located in the palmar aspect of the hand or wrist with median nerve deficit. Microscopically, fibroadipose tissue is seen infiltrating the epineurium, separating and compressing the fascicles. A conservative approach should be taken in treating these tumors. Incisional biopsy may be necessary for diagnosis. If extrinsic neural compression exists, surgical decompression should be performed by fasciotomy or carpal tunnel release. Intraneural excision of the tumor usually sacrifices the involved nerve.

GIANT CELL TUMOR OF TENDON SHEATH (XANTHOMA). Giant cell tumor of tendon sheath is the second most common subcutaneous tumor of the hand (Figs. 77-3 and 77-4). The reported age distribution is

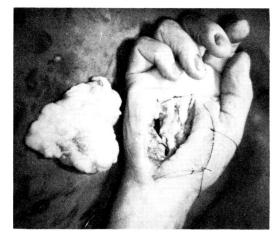

Fig. 77-1 Lipoma of palm extended through deep palmar space and between interosseus muscles to dorsum of hand.

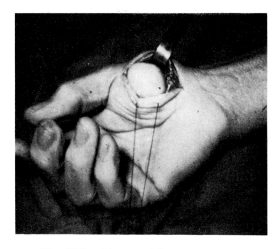

Fig. 77-2 Lipoma of thenar eminence.

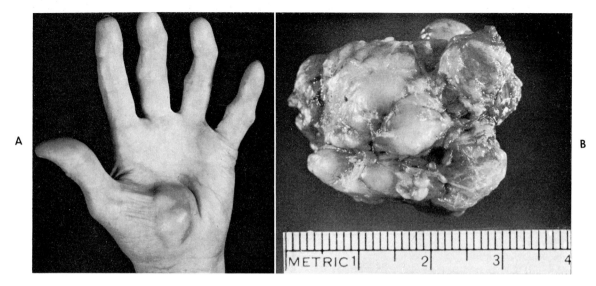

Fig. 77-3   A, Giant cell tumor of tendon sheath in palm. **B,** Gross specimen of tumor showing pseudoencapsulation. (From Phalen GS, McCormack LJ, and Gazale WJ: Clin Orthop 15:140, 1959.)

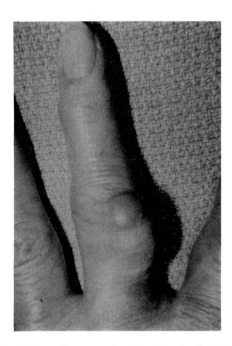

Fig. 77-4   Giant cell tumor of tendon sheath of middle finger.

from 8 to 80 years. It occurs in the hand more frequently than in any other part of the body and more often on the palmar side of the fingers than on the dorsal. Multiple xanthomas may be associated with hypercholesterolemia. Its growth is usually slow, and it may remain the same size for many years. Pain and tenderness are rare. If it occurs at a joint, often the proximal interphalangeal joint, its size may interfere with joint motion. It rarely erodes bone. Grossly, the tumors appear as a yellow or tan, lobulated mass. Histologic sections reveal spindle

cells, fibrous tissue, cholesterol-laden histiocytes, multinucleated giant cells, and hemosiderin. This lesion is always benign, but about 10% may recur even after meticulous excision of friable fragments. Excision is often difficult because the tumor may wind in and around the flexor tendons and their sheaths, the digital nerves, and even the extensor tendons and may involve as much as three fourths of the circumference of one digit.

Benign Tumors of Fibrous Origin

Fibrous tissue frequently proliferates in the hand as a response to local injury and is considered simple scar tissue; however, it may proliferate without apparent cause, and the diagnosis must be made based on the appearance of the tumor, the age of the patient, the clinical behavior of the tumor, and its histologic appearance. All tumors of fibrous origin may involve the hand and, although most are benign, they are frequently active or aggressive lesions with a tendency to recur following local excision. The differential diagnosis in benign fibrous tumors includes a simple fibroma, recurring digital fibrous tumor of childhood, juvenile aponeurotic fibroma, Dupuytren's contractures or nodules, fibromatosis or desmoid, and pseudosarcomatous fasciitis. Fibromatosis or extraabdominal desmoid, as well as pseudosarcomatous fasciitis, are especially aggressive tumors; however, they usually involve the more proximal portions of extremities.

RECURRING DIGITAL FIBROUS TUMOR OF CHILD-HOOD. In 1965 Reye described a benign fibrous tumor that develops in the fingers and toes of infants and young children (Fig. 77-5). The distinguishing feature of this tumor is the presence of intracytoplasmic inclusion bodies within proliferating fibroblasts. These inclusion bodies are not visible with routine hematoxylin and eosin staining. A viral etiologic factor has been suggested, although this is uncertain. These tumors tend to be multicentric, occurring on several digits. The dermis appears to be the site of involvement, with sparing of the overlying epidermis. No malignant potential is present, and spontaneous regression has been reported. A marginal excision is recommended when function seems compromised or appearance is bothersome, especially if tendons, joints, or nails are involved. Local recurrence following marginal excision is common, occurring in 60% of patients.

JUVENILE APONEUROTIC FIBROMA. First described by Keasbey in 1953, juvenile aponeurotic fibroma is a benign fibrous tumor typically appearing in the hands or wrists of children and young adults. It also has been called calcifying fibroma because of its cartilagenous nature, a feature that distinguishes it from other benign tumors of fibrous origin. Clinically, it is a painless, solitary, and mobile mass less than 4 cm in diameter, usually involving the palm (Fig. 77-6). It has no gender predilection and no tendency to involve the ulnar side of the hand as do Dupuytren's nodules. Juvenile aponeurotic fibromas tend to develop close to tendons and are able to infiltrate surrounding muscle and fat. On roentgenograms, calcifications may be seen within the soft tissue mass. Because juvenile aponeurotic fibroma has a distinct tendency for local recurrence after marginal excision, a wide excision, preferably without sacrifice of function, is recommended. Metastatic fibrosarcoma after locally recurrent juvenile aponeurotic fibroma has been reported and long term follow-up of these patients is necessary.

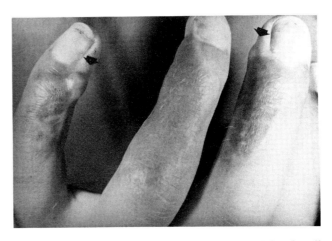

Fig. 77-5 Recurring digital fibrous tumor of childhood. Full-thickness skin grafts were applied to left long, ring, and little fingers after removal of tumor. Arrows show recurrent tumors of long and little fingers. (From Poppen NK and Niebauer JJ: J Hand Surg 2:253, 1977.)

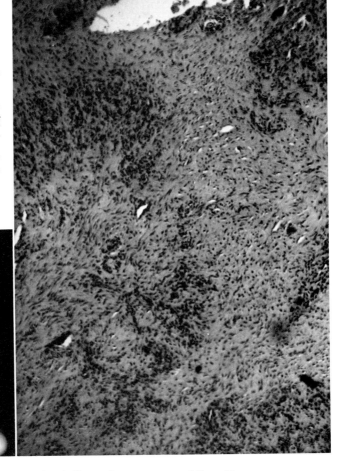

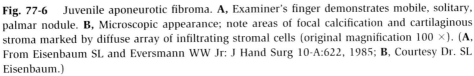

Fig. 77-6 Juvenile aponeurotic fibroma. **A,** Examiner's finger demonstrates mobile, solitary, palmar nodule. **B,** Microscopic appearance; note areas of focal calcification and cartilaginous stroma marked by diffuse array of infiltrating stromal cells (original magnification 100 ×). (**A,** From Eisenbaum SL and Eversmann WW Jr: J Hand Surg 10-A:622, 1985; **B,** Courtesy Dr. SL Eisenbaum.)

FIBROMA. Fibromas are rare in the hand and may be either deep, arising from a joint capsule, or superficial. They tend to occur early in life, growing for a limited time and then subsiding. There are no calcifications, as are seen in juvenile aponeurotic fibroma. Clinically, these tumors are distinguishable from Dupuytren's nodules because they occur earlier in life, tend not to multiply, have no predilection for the ulnar side of the hand, and are not associated with contractures. These tumors are well encapsulated and are easily dissected free from surrounding tissue by blunt dissection. They are firm, white, and composed of dense mature fibroblasts and fibrous tissue. Marginal extracapsular excision is usually curative.

• • •

GLOMUS TUMOR. Pain, cold sensitivity, and tenderness are the symptoms of a glomus tumor, a small but interesting tumor. Direct pressure on the tumor by a small firm object such as a pinhead causes excruciating pain, whereas pressure slightly to one side of it is painless. It is usually less than 1 cm in diameter and often only a few millimeters. It may be deep red or purple. It occurs more often in the hand than in any other part of the body. Glomus tumors are located beneath the fingernail in 25% to 65% of patients (Figs. 77-7 and 77-8). The tumor results from hypertrophy of a glomus, which is a normal structure of the skin — a coiled arteriovenous shunt whose function is to help regulate body temperature. It should be meticulously and completely excised but only after it has been accurately localized with the help of the conscious patient before the anesthetic is administered. The prognosis is good for relief of pain.

HEMANGIOMA. The following remarks are limited to the cavernous hemangioma (Figs. 77-9 and 77-10) and do not include the capillary superficial infantile heman-

gioma that tends to involute by the age of 7 years. A cavernous hemangioma may be slightly to moderately tender and may enlarge a digit with distended venous sinuses. It produces a bluish color when it occurs close to the surface, and it forms a soft, collapsible mass. Calcifications often may be visible on roentgenograms. Custom-fitted compression garments may be a useful conservative treatment. Radiation therapy is discouraged. Surgery is the treatment of choice for cavernous hemangiomas if symptoms justify it. The tumor may be so extensive that a two-stage procedure is required for its removal — the first to ligate the vessels and the second to excise the lesion. With careful tourniquet control, blood partially fills the sinuses and outlines the extent of the tumor at the time of surgical excision. Complete excision is usually curative if the tumor is fairly well localized; however, in diffuse lesions, recurrence is common.

LYMPHANGIOMA. Lymphangioma is a benign soft tissue tumor consisting of abnormal proliferation of lymph vessels and lymphoid tissue (Fig. 77-11). Although it is rare in the hand, its tendency to occur during childhood, its associated pain, and its tendency to recur after excision makes it especially troublesome for the patient, patient's parents, and surgeon. It has no malignant potential and overly aggressive surgery should be avoided be-

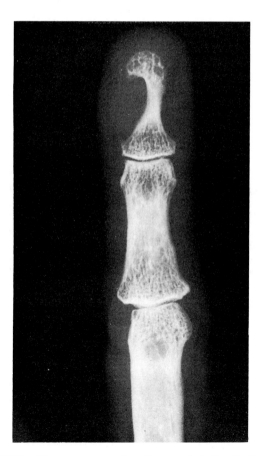

Fig. 77-8 Glomus tumor that has eroded distal phalanx. (From Posch JL: J Bone Joint Surg 38-A:517, 1956.)

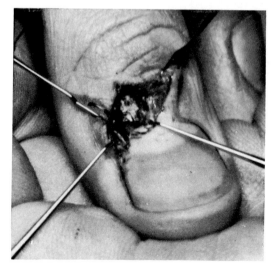

Fig. 77-7 Glomus tumor in subungual area of right thumb. (From Posch JL: J Bone Joint Surg 38-A:517, 1956.)

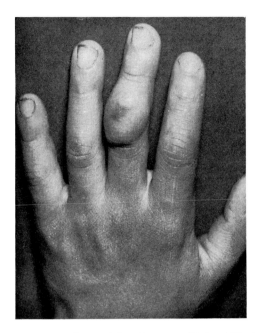

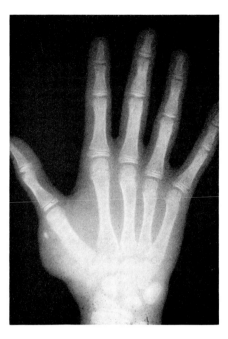

Fig. 77-9 Hemangioma of dorsal aspect of left middle finger. (From Posch JL: J Bone Joint Surg 38-A:517, 1956.)

Fig. 77-10 Cavernous hemangioma of thumb metacarpal; note calcification in soft tissue mass.

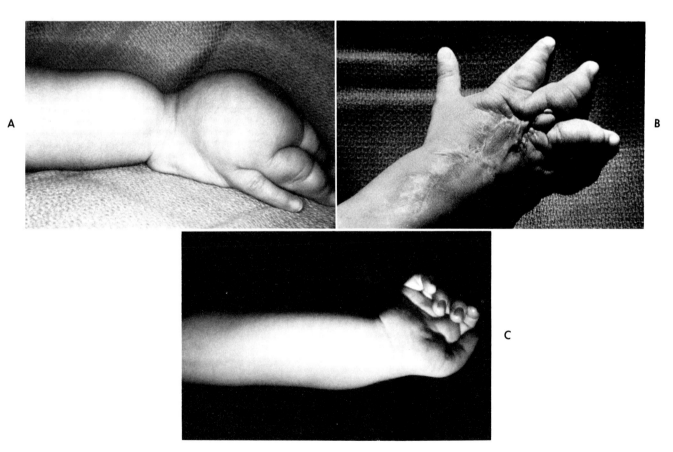

A

B

C

Fig. 77-11 **A,** Extensive lymphangioma in distal forearm, hand, and fingers of 2-year-old girl. **B,** Hypertrophic scarring of surgical incisions and margins of full-thickness skin graft. **C,** Contour of forearm of 18-year-old girl indicates residual tumor. Wrist is contracted in extension and ulnar deviation. (From Blair WF, Buckwalter JA, Michelson MR, and Omer GE: J Hand Surg 8:399, 1983.)

cause hypertrophic scarring may follow. Blair et al. emphasize the importance of both the parents and surgeon having realistic expectations and goals. They recommend excisional biopsy for diagnostic confirmation and debulking of the tumor.

TRAUMATIC NEUROMA. Traumatic neuroma is the result of an attempt by a peripheral nerve to regenerate after its fibers have been interrupted. The tumor is a bundle of all the nerve elements in one tangled mass at the distal end of the proximal nerve segment. Because this attempted growth occurs to some degree in all individuals, it is not considered a true neoplasm. It may be extremely tender, particularly when it involves a digital nerve and when it adheres to an amputation scar that is unprotected by a good pad of skin and fat. The tumor is usually invisible from the exterior and is demonstrated by pressing on the suspected area with a firm object such as a pinhead or pencil point. When a painful neuroma occurs at an amputation site, enough of the nerve should be resected (usually about 6 mm in the case of a digital nerve) that its end can be well protected by a pad of subcutaneous fat and skin (see also discussions of nerve suture in Chapter 65, and finger amputation on p. 3204). The neuroma will regenerate, of course, but will not be painful if sufficiently protected.

MULTIPLE NEUROFIBROMAS. Generalized cutaneous neurofibromas (Fig. 77-12), unlike traumatic neuromas, are not tender and are seen in clusters along the course of the nerve. They seem to be less common in the hand than in other parts of the body. The rate of malignant degeneration has been reported to be as high as 15%, but this rate was not reported specifically for the hand. Excision is curative but is indicated only if the tumors are constantly irritated or cosmetically unacceptable.

NEURILEMOMA (SCHWANNOMA). Neurilemomas arise from nerve sheaths (Fig. 77-13) and are rarely found in the hand. They are not extremely tender. They are more mobile at right angles to the course of the nerve than in line with the nerve. These tumors are frequently misdiagnosed as ganglions. They are rarely multifocal. With a careful microsurgical technique, the tumor usually can be dissected from the surrounding fascicle. Occasionally, the whole nerve may have to be sacrificed if the mass cannot be dissected free from the nerve trunk. Excision is curative.

OSTEOID OSTEOMA. Osteoid osteoma, rare in the hand, is characterized by pain that gradually increases from mild to severe, is usually worse at night, and is dramatically relieved by aspirin. Some osteoid osteomas of the phalanges are painless, presumably because of the lack of nerve fibers trapped within the tumor. Generalized swelling of the involved part and tenderness to pressure are frequent findings. The carpus, especially the scaphoid, may be the site of involvement. The roentgenographic appearance depends on the area of bone involved. A small oval or round sclerotic nidus (Figs. 77-14 and 77-15) is surrounded first by an area of less-dense bone, like a halo, and then by an area of sclerotic bone. If the lesion is in cortical bone or near the cortex, extreme sclerosis occurs and may obliterate the nidus, but at times it may be demonstrated by planograms. A bone scan may be helpful in making the diagnosis. Treatment consists of creating a cortical window for complete re-

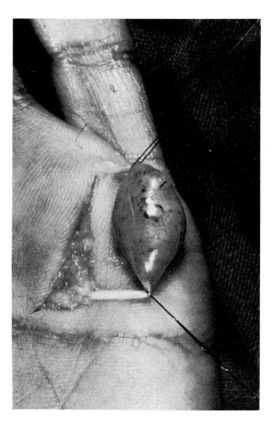

Fig. 77-13 Neurilemoma. (From Clifford RH and Kelly AP Jr: Clin Orthop 13:204, 1959.)

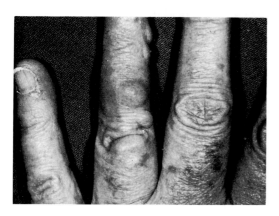

Fig. 77-12 Neurofibromas of finger. (From Gaisford JC: Surg Clin North Am 40:549, 1960.)

moval of the nidus. Recurrent symptoms may be expected if excision is incomplete.

ENCHONDROMA. Enchondroma is the most common primary bone tumor of the hand skeleton, as well as the most destructive lesion of bone found in the hand (Fig. 77-16). Occasionally some enlargement of the finger is seen if the loculated medullary tumor has expanded the

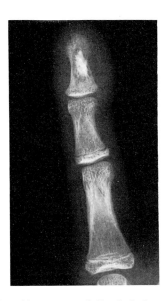

Fig. 77-14 Osteoid osteoma of distal phalanx. Note sclerotic nidus. (From Dunitz NL, Lipscomb PR, and Ivins JC: Am J Surg 94:65, 1957.)

bony cortex. Pathologic fracture is a frequent complication because only minimal trauma is needed to fracture the thin shell of bone. The fracture is usually allowed to heal, with thickening of the cortex by periosteal new bone, before excision of the tumor. At surgery a small window is made in the lateral aspect of the phalanx, and the soft cartilaginous material is curetted thoroughly; tiny flecks of calcium are often seen. The cavity is packed with bone chips, and the cortical window is replaced. Amputation may be necessary when all useful finger function has been destroyed. These tumors are found in multiplicity in Ollier's disease (Fig. 77-17). The diagnosis can usually be made from the roentgenogram, but other destructive lesions, such as inclusion cysts, giant cell tumors, and aneurysmal bone cysts, should be considered.

BENIGN OSTEOBLASTOMA. This tumor is rare. The small bones of the hand and feet are its second most common location; it is rarely considered in the differential diagnosis of bone tumors of the hand. It is similar in both clinical presentation and histologic appearance to osteoid osteoma. In general, osteoblastomas tend to be larger than osteoid osteomas, cause less pain, and are more expansile roentgenographically. Fig. 77-18, *A*, shows the ground-glass appearance of a benign osteoblastoma with gross deformity of the metacarpal from pressure from within, yet the cortical shell is intact. Histologically, areas of mature bone, osteoid, and plump osteoblasts are seen. Treatment is by curettage and bone grafting. Locally aggressive or recurrent lesions may re-

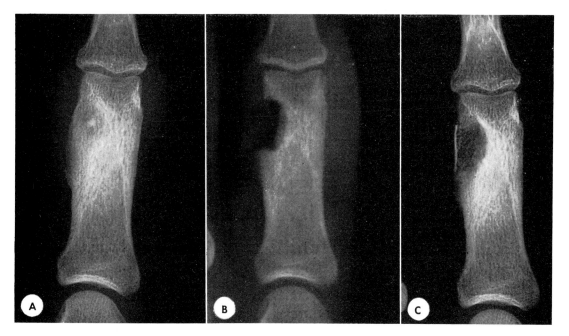

Fig. 77-15 Osteoid osteoma of proximal phalanx. **A,** Before surgery. Note sclerotic nidus surrounded by area of radiolucency. **B,** After block resection from involved part of bone. Defect was filled with graft of homogeneous iliac bone. **C,** Two months after surgery. Cortical part of graft is visible. (From Dunitz NL, Lipscomb PR, and Ivins JC: Am J Surg 94:65, 1957.)

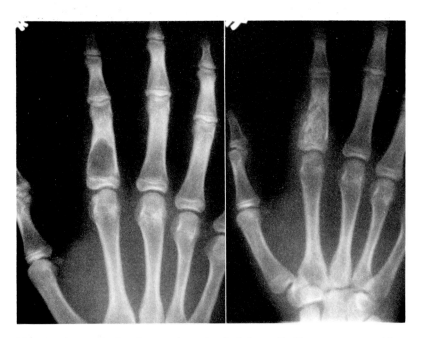

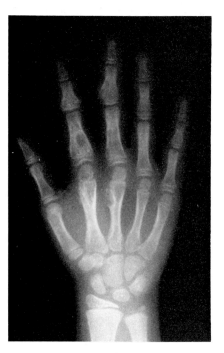

Fig. 77-16   **A,** Enchondroma of proximal phalanx. **B,** After curettage and bone grafting.

Fig. 77-17   Muiltiple enchondromatosis in metacarpals and phalanges of 6-year-old girl.

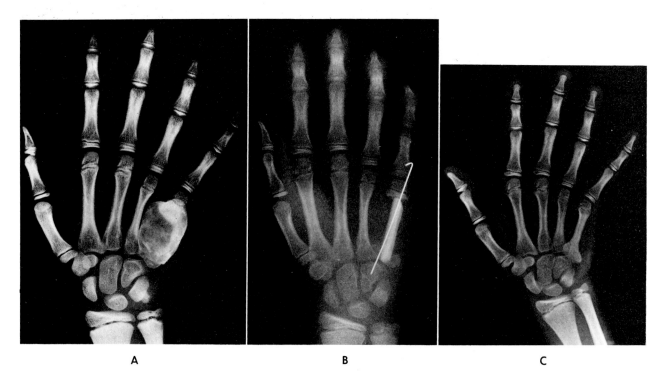

A   B   C

Fig. 77-18   **A,** Expanding intraosseous tumor of fifth metacarpal with "ground glass" appearance. Cortical shell is intact and has caused deformity of fourth metacarpal from pressure. **B,** Partial thickness fibular graft has been interposed. Epiphyseal plate and subchondral cortex of proximal metacarpal have been preserved. **C,** Graft has remodeled 15 months after operation. Evidence of tumor is absent, and growth plate and carpometacarpal joint have been maintained. (From Mosher JF and Peckham AC: J Hand Surg 3:358, 1978.)

quire excision and interpositional bone grafting as shown in Fig. 77-18, *B*.

ANEURYSMAL BONE CYST. Only about four aneurysmal bone cysts of the hand have been reported; but it has been recognized as a separate entity in any part of the body only during the last 4 decades. When it occurs as a central lesion in a phalanx, it causes enlargement, limitation of motion, and pain (Figs. 77-19 and 77-20). On roentgenograms it is almost indistinguishable from giant cell tumor or enchondroma. The treatment is curettage and filling the cavity with bone chips.

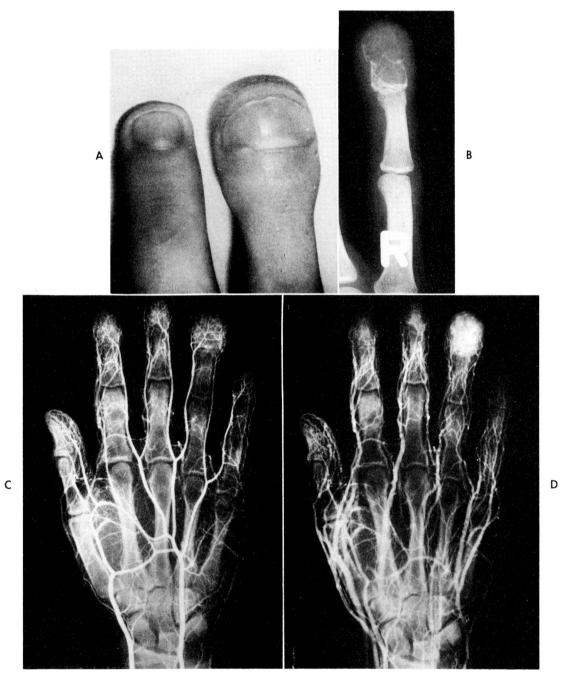

Fig. 77-19   White male, aged 17 years, first seen with swollen ring finger 1 year after tip of finger was crushed by falling railroad tie. Immediate swelling occurred with drainage from split skin at tip. Finger soon became asymptomatic as initial edema decreased; but insidious enlargement of distal phalanx, dull aching, and clubbing of nail were noted. Bulbous enlargement progressed over next 12 months. **A,** Initial examination demonstrated large bulbous distal phalanx. **B,** Roentgenogram of destroyed expanded distal phalanx. **C,** Arteriogram shows arterial filling of lesion and, **D,** venous phase with large venous channels. (From Fuhs SE and Herndon JH: J Hand Surg 4:152, 1979.)

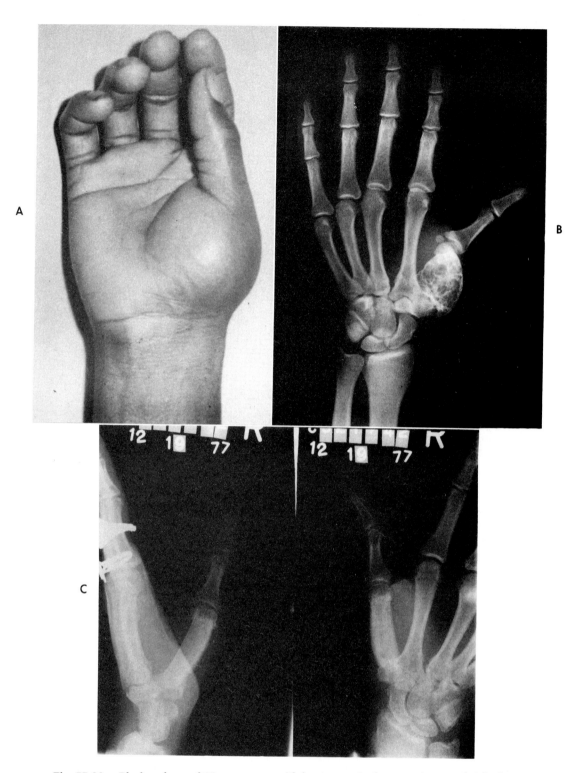

Fig. 77-20 Black male, aged 20 years, seen with bony mass in thenar eminence of right dominant hand. Two years earlier he had sustained injury to ulnar collateral ligament during high school wrestling. No medical treatment was carried out, and thumb became asymptomatic. While working on construction 5 to 6 months later, he noted dull aching about base of thumb and began having difficulty holding tools and basketball. **A,** Initial examination. Note large distorted thenar mass. **B,** Roentgenogram demonstrated cystic expanding lesion of metacarpal. Note disruption of proximal articular surface and preserved distal portion of metacarpal. **C,** Roentgenogram at 1 year after operation. Bone graft has fused to greater multangular and distal metacarpal. No tumor remains. (From Fuhs SE and Herndon JH: J Hand Surg 4:152, 1979.)

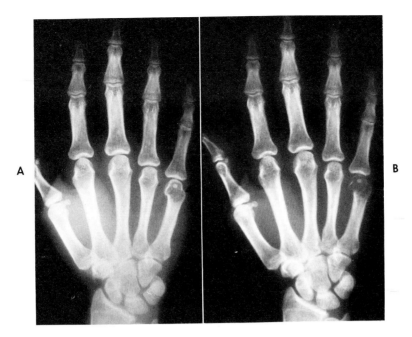

Fig. 77-21   **A,** Giant cell tumor head of fifth metacarpal. **B,** Pathologic fracture caused by tumor.

GIANT CELL TUMORS OF BONE. Giant cell tumors of bone are uncommon in the hand. In a literature review, Averell, Smith, and Campbell found 39 reported tumors. In addition, they reported a series of 28 tumors, 5 of which were eccentrically located. All lesions within the phalanges and metacarpals originated in the epiphyses; however, some later extended into the diaphysis. They noted extensive destruction of cortex and cancellous bone with marked expansion of the cortex. Most lesions had a thin covering of periosteum remaining. This tumor should not be confused with an enchondroma, and a biopsy is indicated to confirm the diagnosis.

In the 28 patients observed by Averill et al., 5 had multicentric giant cell tumors. Tumors were found in places such as the proximal humerus, the distal radius, and the distal femur, suggesting that a full bone survey is indicated to discover remote sites of tumor when a giant cell tumor is suspected.

Generally curettage and bone grafting are not sufficient treatment for this tumor. Because giant cell tumors of the hand are just as aggressive as those found elsewhere, if the cortex is not eroded, resection of the bone and reconstructive surgery are indicated (Fig. 77-21); if cortical invasion and destruction recur, ablation of the part is then indicated (Fig. 77-22). Radiation therapy for giant cell tumors of bone has been ineffective and has resulted in radiation sarcoma in as many as 20% of patients. Cryosurgery has been advocated by Marcove et al. and by Meals et al. and may be especially useful as an adjunctive treatment when simple curettage and bone grafting are performed.

OSTEOCHONDROMA. Osteochondromas are rare in the hand but are seen occasionally on a phalanx (Fig. 77-23). They are most common in the metaphyseal area and may continue to grow until skeletal maturity, at which time excisional biopsy may be indicated because of pain, deformity, or mechanical symptoms.

MALIGNANT TUMORS

In the hand, malignant tumors are rare beneath the skin. Of primary bone malignancies of the hand, chondrosarcoma is the most common. Fibrosarcoma and rhabdomyosarcoma rank first and second in frequency in soft tissues, followed by synovioma. Epithelioid sarcoma in some series is reported just as frequently as fibrosarcoma and rhabdomyosarcoma. Surgical principles discussed in the first section of this chapter should serve as a general guide for the treatment of malignant tumors. Proper surgical treatment requires the removal of some normal hand tissue and occasionally a complete below-elbow amputation. Surgical success is not dependent on how little tissue is sacrificed but whether residual tumor is left behind. Although some authors have stated that malignant bone tumors of the hand almost never metastasize, this can occur, especially after local recurrence.

The most common malignant tumors in the hand are discussed. Not every type of sarcoma is included because most of these have only been reported in the hand on rare occasions.

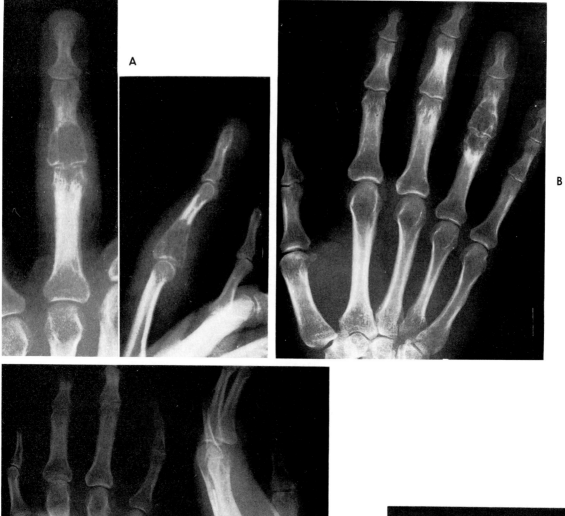

Fig. 77-22 Giant cell tumor of middle phalanx. **A,** Before excision. **B,** Status 5 years after excision. Tumor has recurred, and proximal phalanx has also become involved. **C,** After fourth ray was amputated and fifth ray was transposed laterally. (From Stein AH Jr: Surg Gynecol Obstet 109:189, 1959.)

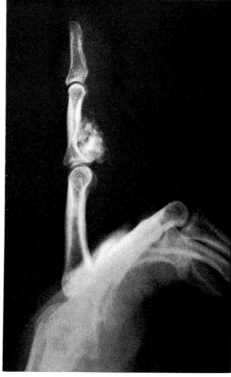

Fig. 77-23 Osteochondroma of middle phalanx.

OSTEOGENIC SARCOMA. Osteogenic sarcoma in the hand is so rare that only about 14 proven cases have been reported (Fig. 77-24). Some of these were caused by irradiation from overexposure to roentgen rays or by ingestion of radium salts. Trauma seems to play no part in the cause. Careful wide excision of the tumor offers a good prognosis; this is in contrast to the same tumor in other parts of the body. Adjuvant chemotherapy may be indicated.

CHONDROSARCOMA. Chondrosarcoma of the hand occasionally may occur in the carpus. Granberry and Bryan reported a chondrosarcoma in the greater multangular that mimicked osteoarthritis roentgenographically (Fig. 77-25). Some have been reported in preexisting enchondromas (Fig. 77-26), but this is rare.

Chondrosarcomas of the bones of the hands and feet are rare and may be difficult to differentiate from enchondromas (Fig. 77-27). Pain is a presenting symptom, whereas it occurs rarely in other chondromas. A fracture may accompany a chondroma or enchondroma as the bone is weakened. Roentgenograms then reveal the weakened or fractured bone and the tumor. A chondrosarcoma should be suspected if a lesion recurs after routine curettage of an enchondroma. Once chondrosarcoma is diagnosed, Dahlin and Salvador report that anything short of total or en bloc resection, such as ray resection, is usually unsuccessful (Fig. 77-28). However, if radical surgery is the primary procedure, recurrence of the tumor is unlikely and the prognosis is good.

EPITHELIOID SARCOMA. Epithelioid sarcoma is commonly misdiagnosed at first because of its initially benign course and appearance. It usually presents as a subcutaneous, firm mass in young adults. It has a predilection to grow along fascial or tendinous structures, forming multiple nodules, and may appear to be a simple inflammatory process. At times, the overlying skin ulcerates with necrosis of the underlying lesion. The histologic appearance of this tumor also may be confusing, but there is a basic granulomatous pattern with central necrosis and surrounding inflammatory cells. Under high magnification, tumor cells take on the appearance of epithelial cells. Metastasis to regional lymph nodes is common, and metastasis to the lungs usually follows multiple recurrences. An inadequate excision invariably is followed by recurrence. Enzinger and Weiss found an 85% incidence of local recurrence in 62 tumors, with most occurring within 6 months after excision. A primary wide excision or an amputation of a digit or entire ray is indicated. Even after a wide excision, the tumor may be present within the margins of the specimen, requiring even further excision. A below-elbow amputation may be necessary after any recurrence in the hand proximal to the metacarpophalangeal joints. Prat et al. recommend regional node dissection in combination with

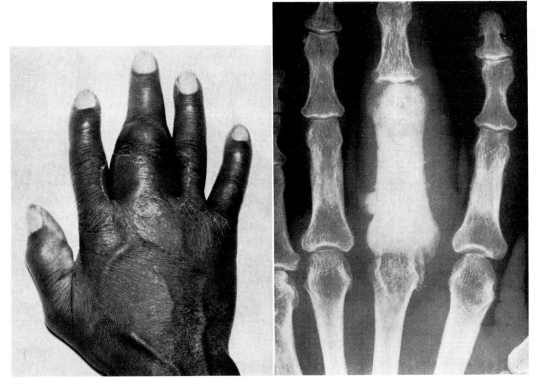

Fig. 77-24   Osteogenic sarcoma of proximal phalanx. (From Drompp BW: J Bone Joint Surg 43-A:199, 1961.)

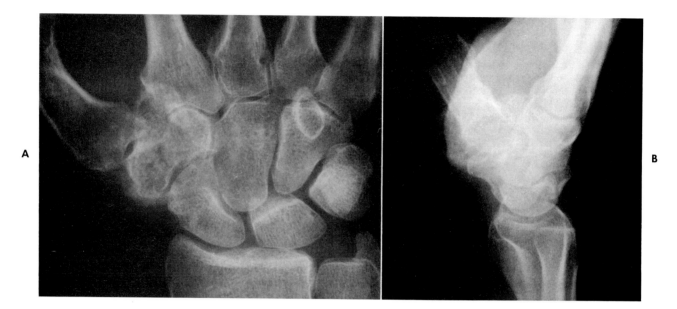

Fig. 77-25   Roentgenograms of carpus demonstrating enlargement of greater multangular with encroachment on thenar musculature. Early cystic reaction is seen in adjacent bones. Tumor at this time was thought most likely to be enchondroma. **A,** Anteroposterior view. **B,** Lateral view. (From Granberry WM and Bryan W: J Hand Surg 3:219, 1978.)

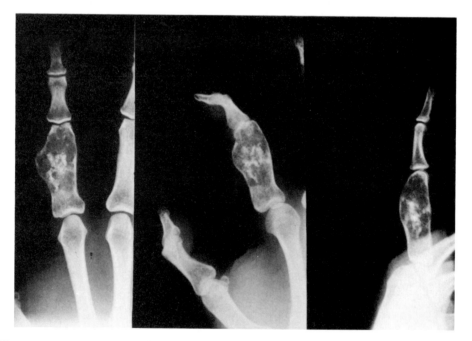

Fig. 77-26   Posteroanterior, lateral, and oblique views of right index finger, showing greatly expanded proximal phalanx in which fluffy radiopacity is clearly visible. (From Wu KK, Frost HM, and Guise EE: J Hand Surg 8:317, 1983.)

the primary excision. The role of adjuvant chemotherapy is unclear at present.

FIBROSARCOMA. Fibrosarcoma is of mesothelial origin. The enlargement of a mass on the hand or pressure on peripheral nerves may cause the patient to seek help

(Fig. 77-29). If it recurs after one wide excision, amputation is indicated.

METASTATIC TUMORS. Metastatic tumors occurring in the hand have been reported as arising most frequently from bronchogenic carcinoma, but they have

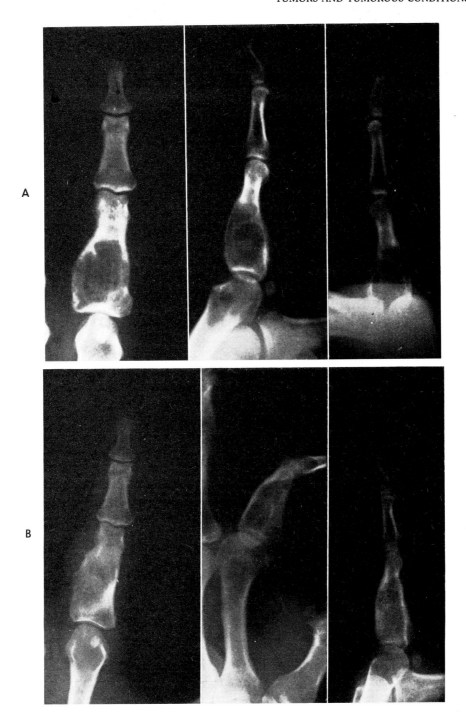

Fig. 77-27   Chondrosarcoma of proximal phalanx. **A,** Original lesion was treated by curettage and by packing cavity with bone chips. Microscopically, tumor was enchondroma. **B,** About 3 years later enlargement of bone and several areas of rarefaction are present, but nothing present was suggestive of malignancy. Microscopically, recurrent tumor was chondrosarcoma. (From Sbarbaro JL Jr and Straub LR: Am J Surg 100:751, 1960.)

also been reported as arising from carcinoma of the kidney, prostate gland, breast, uterus, and colon. They are rare, representing about 0.1% of all metastatic lesions, and occur in the phalanges and metacarpals with equal frequency but are more common at the terminal phalanx. They may be confused with infection because there usually is tenderness, swelling, and redness. Roentgeno-

grams show an osteolytic lesion that usually is destroying the adjacent cortex (Fig. 77-30). Other than infection, the differential diagnosis includes gout, giant cell tumor of bone, enchondroma, epidermoid cyst, and aneurysmal bone cyst. A tissue diagnosis is imperative. The patient's general condition will determine the treatment. If a phalangeal lesion is painful, an amputation through

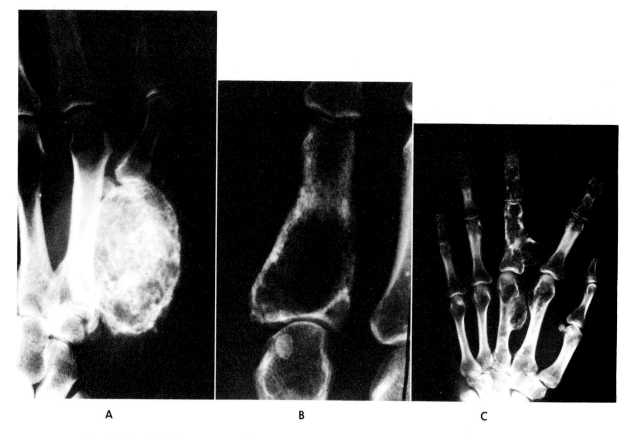

A   B   C

Fig. 77-28 Chondrosarcoma of hand. **A,** Chondrosarcoma of first metacarpal that penetrates into soft tissues proximally. **B,** Aggressive chondrosarcoma of proximal phalanx of finger. **C,** Multiple chondrosarcomas of hand. (From Dahlin DC and Salvador AH: Cancer 34:755, 1974.)

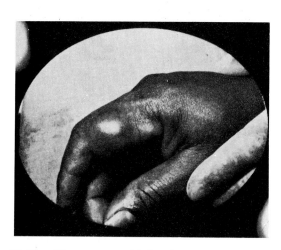

Fig. 77-29 Fibrosarcoma of index finger. (From Posch JL: J Bone Joint Surg 38-A:517, 1956.)

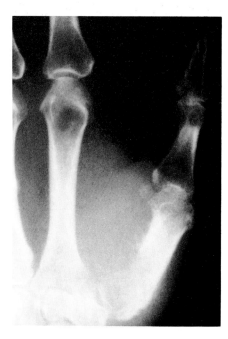

Fig. 77-30 Metastatic carcinoma of thumb metacarpal.

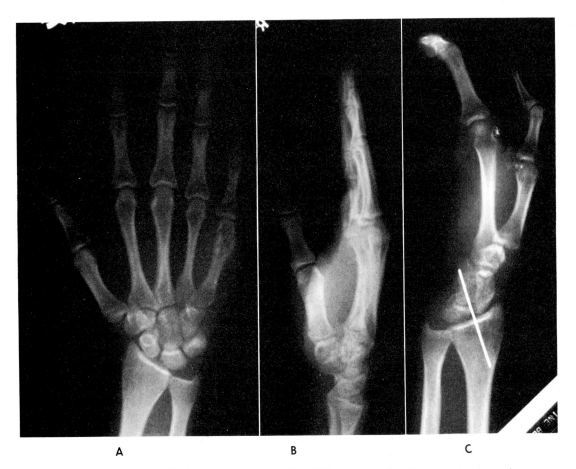

Fig. 77-31   **A** and **B,** Rhabdomyosarcoma in distal fifth metacarpal of 17-year-old girl. **C,** After amputation of ulnar side of hand with Kirschner wire fixation in distal radius. Patient died 2 years later from tumor at base of brain.

the joint proximal to the level of involvement should relieve pain and provide rapid healing. The presence of a metastatic lesion in the hand carries an ominous prognosis for patient survival with a median survival of 5 to 6 months.

RHABDOMYOSARCOMA. Another rare tumor of the hand is rhabdomyosarcoma. The few reported have all been fatal, in contrast to other malignant bone tumors in the hand. Any one of the three types may occur; it seems to be more frequent at the thenar eminence (Fig. 77-31).

EWING'S SARCOMA. Ewing's sarcoma, like other malignant tumors, rarely involves the hand, and currently only about 20 have been reported in the literature. It occurs more frequently in males and usually manifests during the second decade of life. Clinically, the tumor often is mistaken for a local infection because the patient may complain of pain, swelling, fever, and general malaise. Leukocytosis and elevation in the erythrocyte sedimentation rate are common. Roentgenograms of the hand demonstrate a permeative pattern of bone destruction with periosteal reaction. Ewing's sarcoma is a highly

aggressive tumor. In the past, 5-year survival rates were reported to be 10% to 15%; however, with newer therapeutic regimens of chemotherapy, radiation, and surgical excision, survival rates have improved to 50% to 75%. In general, Ewing's sarcoma of the hand carries a better prognosis than does more centrally located sarcoma.

TUMOROUS CONDITIONS

GANGLION. The ganglion is the most common tumor of the hand and characteristically arises either from the synovium of a joint or tendon sheath or from a tendon itself, where it may cause a snapping finger or trigger finger (p. 3440). Although the cause of ganglia is unclear, a history of acute or recurrent chronic injury, possibly occupational, is frequent.

The most frequent site of origin is the dorsum of the carpus just radial to the tendons of the common finger extensors. The second most frequent site is the volar aspect of the carpus between the tendons of the flexor carpi radialis and the abductor pollicis longus. The radial

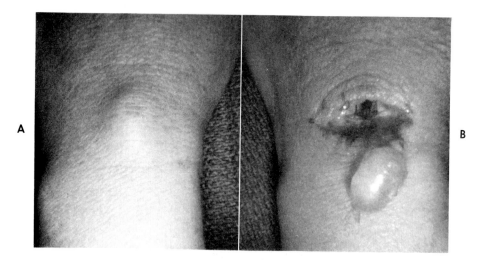

Fig. 77-32   **A,** Ganglion on dorsum of wrist. **B,** Excision of ganglion.

artery should be protected when a ganglion is excised here.

Ganglia on the dorsum of the wrist are usually firm, smooth, fluctuant, and round (Fig. 77-32, *A*). Those extending proximally along the extensor tendons are likely to be less firm and are multilocular and irregular but still contain slightly yellow gelatinous stringy fluid common to all ganglia. The most common site in a flexor tendon is at the level of the flexor skin crease of the metacarpophalangeal joint. Here the mass is round and hard and is often tender to firm pressure. A ganglion is frequently associated with aching or a feeling of weakness. Mild discomfort may sometimes be noted even before the tumor mass is detectable. Ganglia occasionally may disappear spontaneously but sometimes recur when treated by rupture or aspiration. Ganglia on the dorsum of the wrist may be ruptured by digital pressure or by striking the flexed wrist with a book. This is particularly appropriate for young people when a surgical scar is objectionable.

Nelson and co-workers have reported a significant comparative study of treatment. They reported a cure rate of 94% with operations using general anesthesia or axillary block, of 84% with local anesthesia and tourniquet, and of 65% with rupture by pressure or rupture with a needle after injection of cortisone.

Ganglia of the flexor tendon sheaths of the digits are frequently cured by multiple punctures with an 18-gauge needle with the patient under local anesthesia. Ganglia on the radial aspect of the volar side of the wrist are not ruptured easily by pressure; also needle rupture is not feasible because frequently the radial artery is intimately associated with the ganglion.

Surgical excision of a ganglion should include the removal of a generous margin about its base (Fig. 77-32, *B*), often a part of a joint capsule. No attempt is made to close the capsule. A few clusters of small ganglia may be

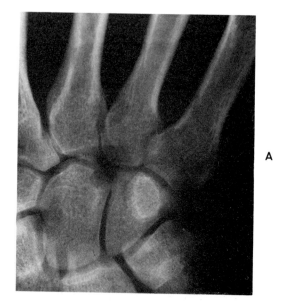

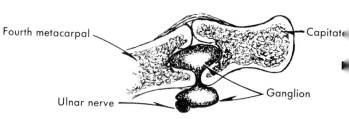

Fig. 77-33   **A,** Anteroposterior roentgenographic study demonstrates erosion at base of fourth metacarpal and distal capitate. Surgery revealed intraarticular ganglion bridging carpometacarpal joint with extensions into substance of capitate and fourth metacarpal. **B,** Ganglion viewed in sagittal section. (From Bowers WH and Hurst LC: J Hand Surg 4:375, 1979.)

seen that later may mature if not removed. The technique of careful complete excision now makes recurrence rare.

Ganglia seldom occur in the palm (Fig. 77-33). Here their presence is made known not by an external enlargement but by secondary changes caused by pressure on motor nerves. Several have been reported that caused atrophy of the muscles innervated by the deep branch of the ulnar nerve. One ganglion that we have seen (Fig. 77-34) arose in the palm deep to the flexor tendons and just ulnarward from the origin of the abductor muscle in line with the deep branch of the ulnar nerve. The atrophy of the first dorsal interosseus muscle was readily seen. Two months after excision of the ganglion, regeneration of the involved muscles began, and complete return of function was evident at 6 months.

EPIDERMOID CYST (INCLUSION CYST). It is now generally accepted that epidermoid cysts may develop from implantation of epithelial cells by trauma. The history is usually that of a penetrating wound about the palm or fingertip several months before a hard, rubbery, nontender subcutaneous mass develops (Fig. 77-35). The distal phalanx is the most common osseous site (Fig. 77-36). The cyst occurs at the base of a fingernail and looks like an enchondroma on roentgenograms; the cortex is expanded, and a central lytic lesion is the only bony reaction. Surgical removal of the cyst is curative. When the bone is involved, to curet and fill the defect with bone chips is worthwhile.

SEBACEOUS CYST. Sebaceous cysts are very rare in the hand because the palmar skin contains no sebaceous glands. They may be confused with epidermoid cysts implanted in the subcutaneous tissues, with mobile overlying skin.

MUCOUS CYST. Mucous cysts occur typically in the skin on the dorsum and to one side of the distal finger joint in an adult female (Fig. 77-37). It is thought to result from myxomatous degeneration of the corneum. The overlying skin is often so thin and translucent that clear mucoid fluid may be seen within. Mucous cysts are frequently associated with Heberden's nodes in osteoarthritis. Anteroposterior, lateral, and oblique roentgenographic views almost always will demonstrate a bony osteophyte near the cyst. This osteophyte should be sought and excised along with the cyst and its stalk, which frequently leads to the joint (Fig. 77-38). We occasionally place a small split-skin graft over the defect and stent it into place if the overlying skin requires excision. The graft is easily removed free-hand from the same arm just below the axillary hairline. Some prefer to rotate a small local skin flap over the defect (Fig. 77-39).

CONGENITAL ARTERIOVENOUS FISTULA. Congenital arteriovenous fistulas are produced by lack of differenti-

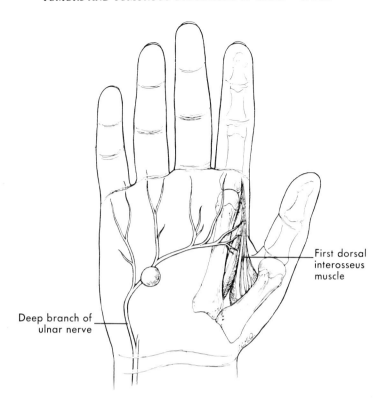

Fig. 77-34 Ganglion in palm producing pressure on deep branch of ulnar nerve causing atrophy of first dorsal interosseus muscle.

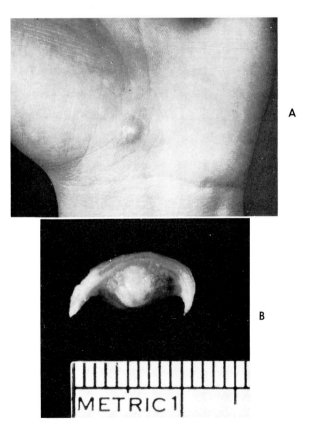

Fig. 77-35 Epidermoid cyst. **A,** Cyst beneath scar on palm. **B,** Gross specimen. (Courtesy Dr. George GS Phalen.)

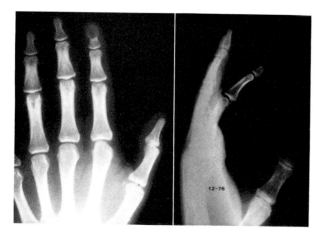

Fig. 77-36   Epidermoid inclusion cyst of bone.

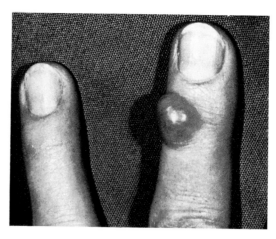

Fig. 77-37   Mucous cyst of finger. (From Gaisford JC: Surg Clin North Am 40:549, 1960.)

ation of the common embryonic anlage into a true artery and vein. Shunts exist between the arterial and venous circulation (Fig. 77-40). Several may extend over one small area, such as a finger, over a large area, or may even involve an entire extremity. Varicose veins of the upper extremity should suggest a congenital arteriovenous fistula, especially when healing is slow or absent after minor trauma. The temperature of the surrounding skin is usually elevated, and the limb may be hypertrophied.

This lesion is not characterized by pain, as is the glomus tumor; however, secondary chronic ulceration may be painful. It is most accurately diagnosed by an arteriogram that reveals dilation of the arteries just proximal to the fistula, abnormal filling of the arteries distal to it, and presence of the contrast medium within the fistula.

All communications between the arterial and venous parts of the fistula should be ligated. This is very difficult because they are so small and numerous. Early surgery is indicated to prevent destruction by infection and gangrene. It may be necessary to perform surgery in stages and at times to replace the skin that has undergone necrosis. Reading the literature on this condition is required before attacking it for the first time.

PYOGENIC GRANULOMA.   Pyogenic granuloma is a heaping up of granulation tissue, at times in the shape of a mushroom, overhanging normal skin; it tends to bleed

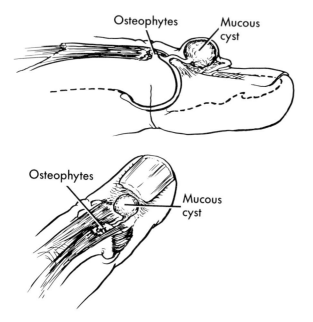

Fig. 77-38   Relationship between mucous cyst and a marginal osteophyte of distal interphalangeal joint. Note that cyst communicates with joint. This thin communication may become pinched off, but at some stage in development it is in direct communication with joint space. Marginal osteophyte produces attrition of extensor tendon expansion with motion. (From Eaton RG et al: J Bone Joint Surg 55-A:570, 1973.)

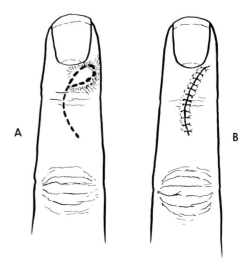

Fig. 77-39   Excision of mucous cyst from distal phalanx. **A,** Skin incision. **B,** Closure. (Modified from Atasoy E et al: J Bone Joint Surg 54-A:1455, 1972.)

easily. A history of trauma and infection usually precedes it. If the lesion is completely excised, including the vascular base, and the wound is closed, recurrence is unlikely.

FOREIGN BODY GRANULOMA. A firm fibrous capsule and deep granulomatous reaction around a foreign material accidentally introduced make the diagnosis of a foreign body granuloma easy when the history is accurate,

but it is difficult to diagnose clinically without this history. Removal of the foreign body is curative.

GOUT. Some patients with advanced gout have such large deposits of urate crystals within the ligaments, tendons, tendon sheaths, and metaphysis, causing erosion of the diaphysis, that the resultant bone destruction may resemble a lytic tumor on roentgenograms (Fig. 77-41, *A*). Usually, soft tissue swelling and other findings

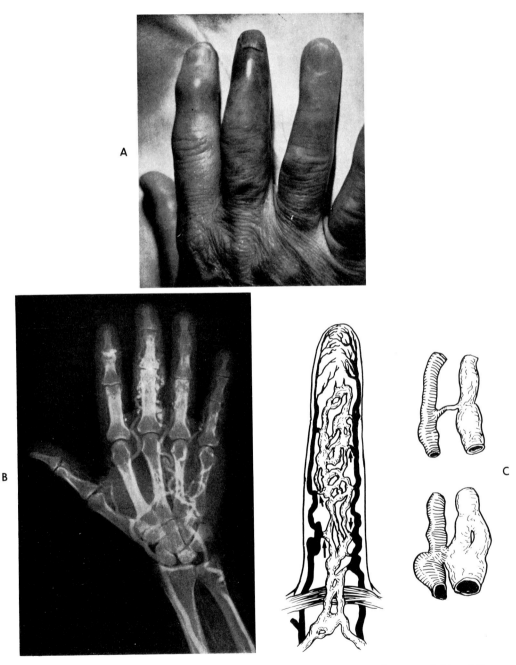

Fig. 77-40 Congenital arteriovenous fistulas of middle finger. **A,** Discoloration of skin of distal phalanx, atrophy of nail, and dilation of veins at base of finger. **B,** Arteriogram made before surgery. Puddling of contrast medium in region of the proximal interphalangeal joint locates some arteriovenous fistulas. **C,** Types and locations of fistulas found at surgery. (From Curtis RM: J Bone Joint Surg 35-A:917, 1953.)

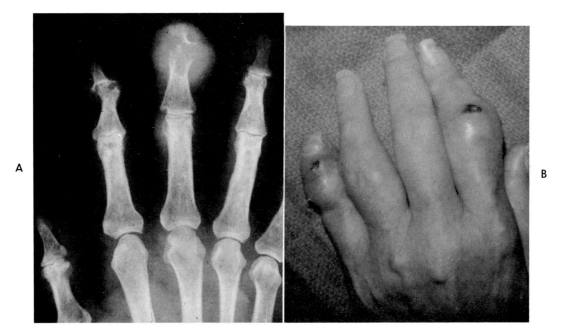

Fig. 77-41   **A,** Destructive lesions around distal interphalangeal joints in gout. **B,** Clinical appearance of hand of patient with gout.

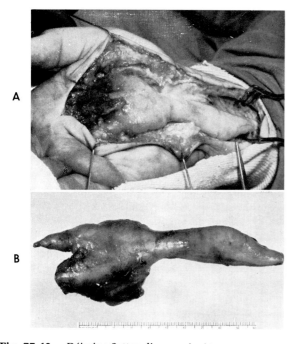

Fig. 77-42   Déjerine-Sottas disease. **A,** At surgery, severe enlargement of median nerve. In this patient, symptoms were severe enough to justify resection of nerve. **B,** Resected part of nerve. (Courtesy Dr. GS Phalen.)

quickly establish the diagnosis (Fig. 77-41, *B*). Clinically, the lesion may easily be confused with an infection because increased heat, swelling, and tenderness are present.

DEJERINE-SOTTAS DISEASE. Déjerine-Sottas disease, a rare lesion, is a localized swelling of a peripheral nerve caused by hypertrophic interstitial neuropathy. It is usually present as a tender mass at the wrist and is sometimes quite painful. Surgical exploration reveals enlargement of the median nerve (Fig. 77-42). It cannot be excised without resecting the nerve, and of course, this should not be done. Dividing the transverse carpal ligament may help to relieve pain and occasionally has resulted in a decrease in the size of the nerve distally. The swelling sometimes subsides spontaneously after surgery.

The lesion is sometimes associated with macrodactyly (Chapter 74). The same clinical picture has been caused by infiltration of the nerve by various fatty tumors.

CALCINOSIS. The exact cause of calcium deposits is obscure, but many think that they result from connective tissue degeneration and that amorphous calcium deposition is secondary. About one third of the patients give a history of trauma. Calcium deposits occur in the hand much less frequently than about the shoulder and hip, but in the hand, pain, tenderness, and erythema are more alarming. They can easily be confused with an infection because of the inflammatory reaction. Roentgenograms taken soon after the onset of symptoms may show only a light cloud, suggesting a deposit, but later the pic-

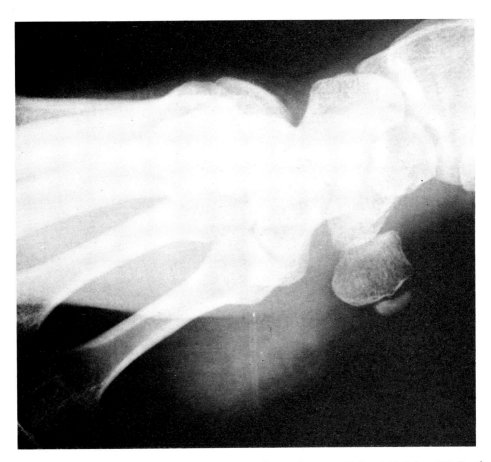

Fig. 77-43   Calcium deposit in pisiform bursa. (From Cameron BM and McGehee FO: South Med J 51:496, 1958.)

ture is usually diagnostic. Calcium deposits about the hand are more common near the insertion of the flexor carpi ulnaris tendon; the wrist area accounts for about two thirds of the cases reported (Fig. 77-43). However, deposits do occur in the collateral ligaments of the fingers and thumb (Fig. 77-44), the thumb extensor tendons, and the tendons of the intrinsic muscles. Rarely, multiple deposits are seen (Fig. 77-45).

Treatment usually consists of heat, rest, and the injection of a local anesthetic with or without a steroid preparation. Aspiration of the deposit if possible may give more immediate relief. However, the tension may be relieved by spontaneous rupture or by gradual absorption. Only large deposits require surgical treatment.

Calcinosis circumscripta. Calcinosis circumscripta is associated with collagen diseases such as lupus erythematosus, rheumatoid arthritis, dermatomyositis, and especially scleroderma, with an incidence of 50% in this disease. The pathologic mechanism of deposit of these calcific lobules in the skin and subcutaneous tissues is unknown. Calcinosis circumscripta is rare but frequently is preceded by Raynaud's phenomenon for many years. Deposits occur more densely over pressure areas such as fingertips and may at times erode through the skin. Par-

tial excision may be indicated when the deposits cause pain or interfere with function, but wound breakdown and skin necrosis are frequent when dissection is extensive (Fig. 77-46).

TURRET EXOSTOSIS. Turret exostosis is a smooth, dome-shaped extracortical mass of bone lying beneath the extensor apparatus on the middle or proximal phalanx of a finger. It is caused by traumatic subperiosteal hemorrhage that eventually ossifies. Clinically, a firm mass develops on the dorsum of the phalanx and limits excursion of the extensor apparatus (Fig. 77-47), thus limiting flexion of the interphalangeal joints distal to the lesion. Roentgenograms that reveal negative results during the first few weeks after injury later reveal subperiosteal new bone located on the dorsum of the phalanx. Conservative treatment has not been beneficial. Any indicated surgery should be delayed until the subperiosteal bone becomes mature, usually 4 to 6 months after injury; at that time recurrence is less likely.

To excise the exostosis, a midlateral incision (Chapter 61) is made, the extensor apparatus is elevated, and the periosteum is incised laterally and carefully elevated from the underlying bone; care is taken not to tear the periosteum dorsally, thus preserving a smooth surface over

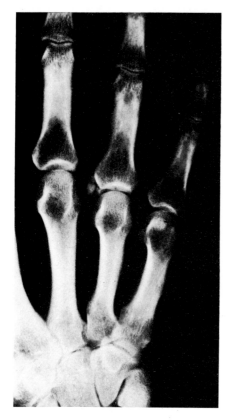

Fig. 77-44 Calcium deposit in collateral ligament of metacarpophalangeal joint of ring finger.

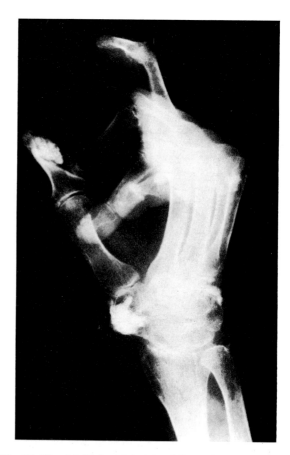

Fig. 77-45 Multiple calcinosis of digits, hand, and wrist.

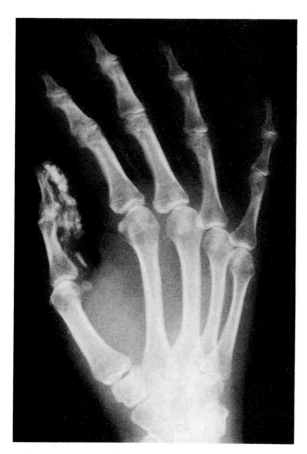

Fig. 77-46 Calcinosis circumscripta of thumb. (Courtesy Dr. EC Weckesser.)

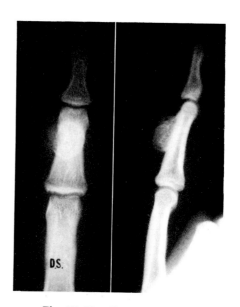

Fig. 77-47 Turret exostosis.

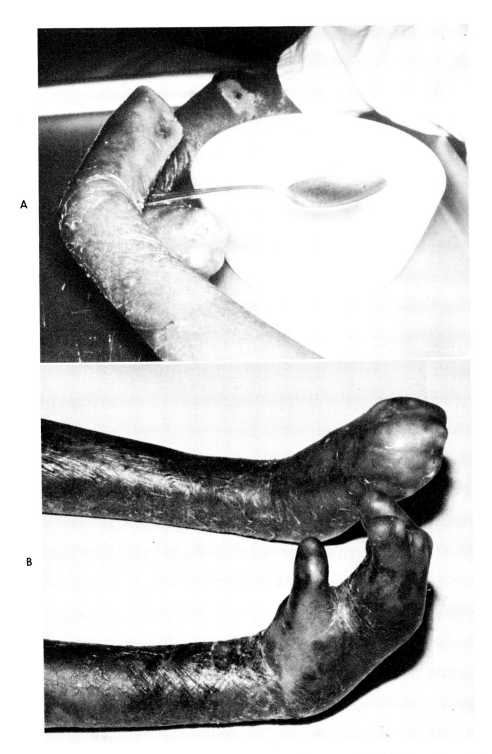

Fig. 77-48 **A,** Epidermolysis bullosa. Note total envelopment of all digits by epidermis. Patient fed himself by fixing a spoon between his deformed wrists. Enveloping epidermis had been removed from these hands approximately 1 year before photographs. **B,** Postoperative views of hands. Right hand was released with a pedicle flap to palm and split grafts to digits 3 months before photograph. (From Horner RL et al: J Bone Joint Surg 53-A:1347, 1971.)

which the extensor apparatus can glide. Next all of the new bone is resected, the periosteum and the wound are closed, and a wet cotton-compression dressing is applied.

CARPOMETACARPAL BOSS. A carpometacarpal boss is a bony, nonfluctuant, fixed lump on the dorsum of the hand at the level of the base of the second and third metacarpals and is visible on a tangential roentgenogram. It is frequently confused with a ganglion but lies distal to the common site of a ganglion. It can be confused with a fracture or tenosynovitis because an extensor tendon occasionally may subluxate over the dome of the lesion. It may cause pain on local pressure or on forced dorsiflexion of the wrist. Some lesions are asymptomatic, whereas many lesions associated with trauma are painful; either may constitute a cosmetic problem.

There has been great hesitancy in the past to resect these lesions because of the reportedly high rate of recurrence. Recent authors do not support this but warn that, even though the lesion is usually proximal to the base of the second and third metacarpals, it may involve the insertion of the extensor carpi radialis brevis muscle.

EPIDERMOLYSIS BULLOSA. Epidermolysis bullosa of the severe type, a hereditary disorder, occurs in 1 out of every 300,000 births. At birth or soon after, bullae are present over the extremities because the process affects the entire dermis and, at times, the mucous membranes. Its ultimate course is chronic infection of the bullae and

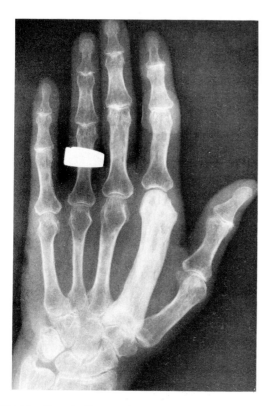

Fig. 77-49   Paget's disease of second metacarpal. (From Haverbush TJ et al: J Bone Joint Surg 54-A:173, 1972.)

the continuing formation of a cocoonlike epidermis over all the fingers of each hand. Surgical release of these digits is very discouraging because recurrence of the webbing and flexion contractures of the fingers is rapid. Free-skin grafts and distant flaps have been used to limited advantage, but no effective treatment of the disease process is known. These patients are poor surgical risks because of chronic infection. Some authors have reported a death rate of 25% during childhood or adolescence, apparently because of debilitation. Surgical procedures, if any are indicated, are repetitious degloving procedures that give limited hand function over a limited period of time. The less severe types of the disease may not need surgical treatment. Splinting after degloving may be of some value (Fig. 77-48).

PAGET'S DISEASE. Paget's disease may occur in the long bones of the hand, although this is very rare, especially as compared with the 3% incidence of Paget's disease of bone in the general population. Roentgenograms reveal the same sclerotic fusiform enlargement of the long bones as elsewhere in the body. It should not be confused with fibrous dysplasia (Fig. 77-49).

REFERENCES
General

Bogumill GP, Sullivan DJ, and Baker GI: Tumors of the hand, Clin Orthop 108:214, 1975.

Butler ED, Hamill JP, Seipel RS, and DeLorimer AA: Tumors of the hand: a ten-year survey and report of 437 cases, Am J Surg 100:293, 1960.

Caulfield PA: Common premalignant and malignant lesions of the hand, Surg Clin North Am 30:1675, 1950.

Clifford RH and Kelly AP Jr: Diagnosis and treatment of tumors of the hand, Clin Orthop 13:204, 1959.

Enneking WE: Musculoskeletal tumor surgery, New York, 1983, Churchill Livingstone.

Gaisford JC: Tumors of the hand, Surg Clin North Am 40:549, 1960.

Haber MH, Alter AH, and Wheelock MC: Tumors of the hand, Surg Gynecol Obstet 121:1073, 1965.

Howard JM: Tumors of the hand, Surg Clin North Am 31:1307, 1951.

Howard LD Jr: Tumors of the hand. In Bunnell S, editor: Surgery of the hand, ed 3, Philadelphia, 1956, JB Lippincott Co.

Mangini U: Tumors of the skeleton of the hand, Bull Hosp Joint Dis 28:61, 1967.

Mason ML: Tumors of the hand, Surg Gynecol Obstet 64:129, 1937.

Mason ML: Tumors of the hand, Minn Med 37:600, 1954.

Posch JL: Tumors of the hand, J Bone Joint Surg 38-A:517, 1956.

Shellito JG and Dockerty MB: Cartilaginous tumors of the hand, Surg Gynecol Obstet 86:465, 1948.

Smith RJ: Tumors of the hand: who is best qualified to treat tumors of the hand? J Hand Surg 2:251, 1977 (editoral).

Stein AH, Jr: Benign neoplastic and nonneoplastic destructive lesions in the long bones of the hand, Surg Gynecol Obstet 109:189, 1959.

Strickland JW and Steichen JB: Nerve tumors of the hand and forearm, J Hand Surg 2:285, 1977.

Benign tumors

Acharya G, Merritt WH, and Theogaraj SD: Hemangioendotheliomas of the hand: case reports, J Hand Surg 5:181, 1980.

Allen PW and Enzinger FM: Juvenile aponeurotic fibroma, Cancer 26:857, 1970.

Amadio PC, Reiman HM, and Dobyns JH: Lipofibromatous hamartoma of nerve, J Hand Surg 13-A:67, 1988.

Averill RM, Smith RJ, and Campbell CJ: Giant-cell tumors of the bones of the hands, J Hand Surg 5:39, 1980.

Barre PS, Shaffer JW, Carter JR, and Lacey SH: Multiplicity of neurilemomas in the upper extremity, J Hand Surg 12-A:307, 1987.

Baruch A, Haas A, Lifschitz-Mercer B, and Zeligowsky A: Simple bone cyst of the metacarpal, J Hand Surg 12-A:1103, 1987.

Bauer RD, Lewis MM, and Posner MA: Treatment of enchondromas of the hand with allograft bone, J Hand Surg 13-A:908, 1988.

Becker H and Chait L: Fibromatosis of the upper limb, J Hand Surg 4:264, 1979.

Ben-Menachem Y and Epstein MJ: Post-traumatic capillary hemangioma of the hand: a case report, J Bone Joint Surg 56-A:1741, 1974.

Blair WF: Granular cell schwannoma of the hand, J Hand Surg 5:51, 1980.

Blair WF, Buckwalter JA, Mickelson MR, and Omer GE: Lymphangioma of the forearm and hand, J Hand Surg 8-A:399, 1983.

Bolem JJ, Vuzevski VD, and Huffstadt AJC: Recurring digital fibroma of infancy, J Bone Joint Surg 56-B:746, 1974.

Booher RJ: Tumors arising from blood vessels in the hands and the feet, Clin Orthop 19:71, 1961.

Booher RJ and McPeak CJ: Juvenile aponeurotic fibromas, Surgery 46:924, 1959.

Booher RJ: Lipoblastic tumors of the hands and feet: review of the literature and report of thirty-three cases, J Bone Joint Surg 47-A:727, 1965.

Bosch DT and Bernhard WG: Lipoma of the palm, Am J Clin Pathol 20:262, 1950.

Burkhalter WE, Schroeder FC, and Eversmann WW Jr: Aneurysmal bone cysts occurring in the metacarpals: a report of three cases, J Hand Surg 3:579, 1978.

Burry AF, Kerr JFR, and Pope JH: Recurring digital fibrous tumor of childhood: an electron microscopic and virological study, Pathology 2:287, 1970.

Carroll RE: Osteoid osteoma in the hand, J Bone Joint Surg 35-A:888, 1953.

Carroll RE and Berman AT: Glomus tumors of the hand: review of the literature and report on twenty-eight cases, J Bone Joint Surg 54-A:691, 1972.

Davidson SF, Das SK, and Smith EE: Cellular schwannoma of the hand, J Hand Surg 14-A:907, 1989.

Dellon AL, Weiss SW, and Mitch WE: Bilateral extraosseous chondromas of the hand in a patient with chronic renal failure, J Hand Surg 3:139, 1978.

DiFazio F and Mogan J: Intravenous pyogenic granuloma of the hand, J Hand Surg 14-A:310, 1989.

Doyle JR: Tendon xanthoma: a physical manifestation of hyperlipidemia, J Hand Surg 13-A:238, 1988.

Duinslaeger L, Vierendeels T, and Wylock P: Vascular leiomyoma in the hand, J Hand Surg 12-A:624, 1987.

Dunitz NL, Lipscomb PR, and Ivins JC: Osteoid osteoma of the hand and wrist, Am J Surg 94:65, 1957.

Eisenbaum SL and Eversmann WW Jr: Juvenile aponeurotic fibroma of the hand, J Hand Surg 10-A:622, 1985.

Entin MA and Wilkinson RD: Scleroderma hand: a reappraisal, Orthop Clin North Am 4:1031, 1973.

Ewald FC: Bone cyst in a phalanx of a two-and-a-half-year-old child: case report and discussion, J Bone Joint Surg 54-A:399 1972.

Feinberg MS: Fibroma of a tendon causing limited finger motion: a case report, J Hand Surg 4:386, 1979.

Fisher ER, Gruhn J, and Skerrett P: Epidermal cyst in bone, Cancer 11:643, 1958.

FitzPatrick DJ and Bullough PG: Giant cell tumor of the lunate bone: a case report, J Hand Surg 2:269, 1977.

Fletcher AG Jr and Horn RC Jr: Giant cell tumors of tendon sheath origin: a consideration of bone involvement and report of two cases with extensive bone destruction, Ann Surg 133:374, 1951.

Fuhs SE and Herndon JH: Aneurysmal bone cyst involving the hand: a review and report of two cases, J Hand Surg 4:152, 1979.

Geiser JH and Eversmann WW Jr: Closed system venography in the evaluation of upper extremity hemangiomas, J Hand Surg 3:173, 1978.

Ghiam GF and Bora FW Jr: Osteoid osteoma of the carpal bones, J Hand Surg 3:280, 1978.

Giannikas AC: Treatment of metacarpal enchondromata: report of three cases, J Bone Joint Surg 48-B:333, 1966.

Grant GH: Methods of treatment of neuromata of the hand, J Bone Joint Surg 33-A:841, 1951.

Grundberg AB: Osteoid osteoma of the thumb: report of a case, J Hand Surg 2:266, 1977.

Heiple KG and Elmer RM: Chondromatous hamartomas arising from the volar digital plates: a case report, J Bone Joint Surg 54-A:393, 1972.

Herrick RT, Godsil RD Jr, and Widener JH: Lipofibromatous hamartoma of the radial nerve: a case report, J Hand Surg 5:211, 1980.

Houpt P, Storm van Leeuwen JB, and van den Bergen HA: Intraneural lipofibroma of the median nerve, J Hand Surg 14-A:706, 1989.

Jablon M, Horowitz A, and Bernstein DA: Magnetic resonance imaging of a glomus tumor of the fingertip, J Hand Surg 15-A:507, 1990.

Jacob RA and Buchino JJ: Lipofibroma of the superficial branch of the radial nerve, J Hand Surg 14-A:704, 1989.

Jamra FNA and Rebeiz JJ: Lipofibroma of the median nerve, J Hand Surg 4:160, 1979.

Janecki CJ, Rouston G, and Depapp EW: Extraarticular synovial chondrometaplasia: locking of the proximal interphalangeal joint of the finger, J Hand Surg 5:473, 1980.

Jewusiak EM, Spence KF, and Sell KW: Solitary benign enchondroma of the long bones of the hand: results of curettage and packing with freeze-dried cancellous-bone allograft, J Bone Joint Surg 53-A:1587, 1971.

Johnson RJ and Bonfiglio M: Lipofibromatous hamartoma of the median nerve, J Bone Joint Surg 51-A:984, 1969.

Jones WA and Ghorbal MS: Benign tendon sheath chondroma, J Hand Surg 11-B:276, 1986.

Keasbey LE: Juvenile aponeurotic fibroma (calcifying fibroma): a distinctive tumor arising in the palms and soles of young children, Cancer 6:338, 1953.

Keasbey LA and Fanselau HA: The aponeurotic fibroma, Clin Orthop 19:115, 1961.

Kline SC, Moore JR, and deMente SH: Glomus tumor originating within a digital nerve, J Hand Surg 15-A:98, 1990.

Lafferty KA, Nelson EL, Demuth RJ, et al: Juvenile aponeurotic fibroma with disseminated fibrosarcoma, J Hand Surg 11-A:737, 1986.

Laing PW: A tendon tumour presenting as a trigger finger, J Hand Surg 11-B:275, 1986.

Langa V, Posner MA, and Steiner GE: Lipofibroma of the median nerve: a report of two cases, J Bone Joint Surg 12-B:221, 1987.

Lewis MM, Marshall JL, and Mirra JM: Synovial chondromatosis of the thumb: a case report and review of the literature, J Bone Joint Surg 56-A:180, 1974.

Louis DS and Dick HM: Ossifying lipofibroma of the median nerve, J Bone Joint Surg 55-A:1082, 1973.

Louis DS, Hankin FM, and Braunstein EM: Giant cell tumour of the triquetrum, J Hand Surg 11-B:279, 1986.

Louis DS, Hankin FM, Greene TL, and Dick HM: Lipofibromas of the median nerve: long-term follow-up of four cases, J Hand Surg 10-A:403, 1985.

Love JG: Glomus tumors: diagnosis and treatment, Mayo Clin Proc 19:113, 1944.

Lucas GL: An intratendinous cyst in the extensor digitorum brevis manus tendon, J Hand Surg 4:176, 1979.

Mackenzie DH: Intraosseous glomus tumors: report of two cases, J Bone Joint Surg 44-B:648, 1962.

Maher DP: Granular cell tumor in the hand, J Hand Surg 12-A:800, 1987.

Marcove RC, Lyden JP, Huvos AG, and Bullough PG: Giant cell tumors treated by cryosurgery, J Bone Joint Surg 55-A:1633, 1973.

Marshall JH, Sonsire JM, Neilsen PE, et al: Digital angiography and osteoblastoma of the triquetrum, J Hand Surg 12-A:256, 1987.

Mason ML and Wheelock MC: Aneurysmal bone cyst of the hand, Q Bull Northwestern Univ Med School 32:268, 1958.

Match RM and Leffert RD: Massive neurofibromatosis of the upper extremity with paralysis, J Hand Surg 12-A:718, 1987.

Maxwell GP, Curtis RM, and Wilgis EFS: Multiple digital glomus tumors, J Hand Surg 3:363, 1978.

Meals RA, Mirra JM, and Bernstein AJ: Giant cell tumor of metacarpal treated by cryosurgery, J Hand Surg 14-A:130, 1989.

Medlar RC and Sprague HH: Osteochondroma of the carpal scaphoid, J Hand Surg 4:150, 1979.

Meyerding HW and Jackson AE: Benign giant cell tumors: a report of seven cases in which the bones of the hands and feet were involved, Surg Clin North Am 30:1201, 1950.

Mikhail IK: Median nerve lipoma in the hand, J Bone Joint Surg 46-B:726, 1964.

Miller SH, Smith RL, and Shochat SJ: Compression treatment of hemangiomas, Plast Reconstr Surg 58:573, 1976.

Morley GH: Intraneural lipoma of the median nerve in the carpal tunnel: report of a case, J Bone Joint Surg 46-B:734, 1964.

Mosher JF and Peckham AC: Osteoblastoma of the metacarpal: a case report, J Hand Surg 3:358, 1978.

Mullis WF, Rosato FE, and Rosato EF, et al: The glomus tumor, Surg Gynecol Obstet 135:705, 1972.

Murphy AF and Wilson JN: Tenosynovial osteochondroma in the hand, J Bone Joint Surg 40-A: 1236, 1958.

Murray JA and Schlafly B: Giant-cell tumors in the distal end of the radius: treatment by resection and fibular autograft interpositional arthrodesis, J Bone Joint Surg 68-A:687, 1986.

Neviaser RJ and Newman W: Dermal angiomyoma of the upper extremity, J Hand Surg 2:271, 1977.

Neviaser RJ and Wilson JN: Benign chondroblastoma in the finger, J Bone Joint Surg 54-A:389, 1972.

Olazabal A and Sormann GW: A giant cell tumor of the thumb: a case report, J Hand Surg 11-A:56, 1986.

Oster LH, Blair WF, and Steyers CM: Large lipomas in the deep palmar space, J Hand Surg 14-A:700, 1989.

Patel MR and Desai SS: Pseudomalignant osseous tumor of soft tissue: a case report and review of the literature, J Hand Surg 11-A:66, 1986.

Patel MR, Desai SS, Gordon SL, et al: Management of skeletal giant cell tumors of the phalanges of the hand, J Hand Surg 12-A:70, 1987.

Patel ME, Silver JW, Lipton DE, and Pearlman HS.: Lipofibroma of the median nerve in the palm and digits of the hand, J Bone Joint Surg 61-A:393, 1979.

Peled I, Iosipovich Z, Russo M, and Wexler MR: Hemangioma of the median nerve, J Hand Surg 5:363 1980.

Phalen GS: Neurilemomas of the forearm and hand, Clin Orthop 114:219, 1976.

Phalen GS, McCormack LJ, and Gazale WJ: Giant-cell tumor of tendon sheath (benign synovioma) in the hand: evaluation of 56 cases, Clin Orthop 15:140, 1959.

Poppen NK and Niebauer JJ: Recurring digital fibrous tumor of childhood, J Hand Surg 2:253, 1977.

Pulvertaft RG: Unusual tumors of the median nerve: report of two cases, J Bone Joint Surg 46-B:731, 1964.

Rask MR, Barnes AG, and Kopf EH: Glomus tumor treated by prostaglandin inhibition: report of a case, Clin Orthop 143:171, 1979.

Rettig AC and Strickland JW: Glomus tumor of the digits, J Hand Surg 2:261, 1977.

Reye RDK: Recurring digital fibrous tumors of childhood, Arch Pathol 80:228, 1965.

Riveros M and Pack GT: The glomus tumor: report of 20 cases, Ann Surg 133:394, 1951.

Rosenfeld K, Bora WF Jr, and Lane JM: Osteoid osteoma of the hamate: a case report and review of the literature, J Bone Joint Surg 55-A:1085, 1973.

Rowland SA: Lipofibroma of the median nerve in the palm, J Bone Joint Surg 49-A:1309, 1967.

Rowland SA: Case report: ten year follow-up of lipofibroma of the median nerve in the palm, J Hand Surg 2:316, 1977.

Rusko RA and Larsen Rd: Intraneural lipoma of the median nerve: case report and literature review, J Hand Surg 6:388, 1981.

Saito H, Tajima T, Watanabe H, and Yamamoto H: An epidermoid cyst of the tendon, J Hand Surg 4:448, 1979.

Schajowicz F, Aiello CL, and Slullitel I: Cystic and pseudocystic lesions of the terminal phalanx with special reference to epidermoid cysts, Clin Orthop 68:84, 1970.

Schmitz RL and Keeley JL: Lipomas of the hand, Surgery 42:696, 1957.

Sevitt S and Horn JS: A painless and calcified osteoid osteoma of the little finger, J Pathol Bacteriol 67:571, 1954.

Shereff MJ, Posner MA, and Gordon MH: Upper extremity hypertrophy secondary to neurofibromatosis: a case report, J Hand Surg 5:355, 1980.

Siegel D, Gebhardt M, and Jupiter MB: Spontaneous rupture of the extensor pollicis longus tendon, J Hand Surg 12-A:1106, 1987.

Sieracki JC and Kelly AP Jr: Traumatic epidermoid cysts involving digital bones: epidermoid cysts of the distal phalanx, Arch Surg 78:597, 1959.

Silverman TA and Enzinger FM: Fibrolipomatous hamartoma of nerve, Am J Surg Pathol 9:7, 1985.

Smith JA and Millender LH: Treatment of recurrent giant-cell tumor of the digit by phalangeal excision and toe phalanx transplant: a case report, J Hand Surg 4:164, 1979.

Smith RJ and Mankin HJ: Allograft replacement of distal radius for giant cell tumor, J Hand Surg 2:299, 1977.

Sondergaard G and Mikkelsen S: Fibrolipomatous hamartoma of the median nerve, J Hand Surg 12-B:224, 1987.

Specht EE and Staheli LT: Juvenile aponeurotic fibroma, J Hand Surg 2:256, 1977.

Stern RE and Gauger DW: Pigmented villonodular tenosynovitis: a case report, J Bone Joint Surg 59-A:560, 1977.

Stevenson TW: Xanthoma and giant cell tumor of the hand, Plast Reconstr Surg 5:75, 1950.

Strauss A: Lipoma of the tendon sheaths: with report of a case and review of the literature, Surg Gynecol Obstet 35:161, 1922.

Strong ML Jr: Chondromas of the tendon sheath of the hand: report of a case and review of the literature, J Bone Joint Surg 57-A:1164, 1975.

Szepesi J: Synovial chondromatosis of the metacarpophalangeal joint, Acta Orthop Scand 46:926, 1975.

Takigawa K: Carpal chondroma: report of a case, J Bone Joint Surg 53-A:1601, 1971.

Takigawa K: Chondroma of the bones of the hand: a review of 110 cases, J Bone Joint Surg 53-A:1591, 1971.

Tang J, Ishii S, Usui M, and Naito T: Multifocal neurilemomas in different nerves of the same upper extremity, J Hand Surg 15-A:788, 1990.

Terrill RQ, Groves J, and Cohen MB: Two cases of chondroid syringoma of the hand, J Hand Surg 12-A:1094, 1987.

Tupper JW and Booth DM: Treatment of painful neuromas of sensory nerves in the hand: a comparison of traditional and newer methods, J Hand Surg 1:144, 1976.

Wallace PF and Fitzmorris CS Jr: Juvenile aponeurotic fibroma: a case report, J Hand Surg 2:258, 1977.

Watson-Jones R: Encapsulated lipoma of the median nerve at the wrist, J Bone Joint Surg 46-B:736, 1964.

Wenner SM and Johnson K: Giant cell reparative granuloma of the hand, J Hand Surg 12-A:1097, 1987.

Whiston TB: Neurofibroma eroding the carpus: report of a case, J Bone Joint Surg 35-B:260, 1953.

Yeoman PM: Fatty infiltration of the median nerve, J Bone Joint Surg 46-B:737, 1964.

Zadek I and Cohne HG: Epidermoid cyst of the terminal phalanx of a finger with a review of literature, Am J Surg 85:771, 1953.

Zook EG: Extensive giant cell tumor of the finger: a case history, J Hand Surg 2:267, 1977.

Malignant tumors

Amadio PC and Lombardi RM: Metastatic tumors of the hand, J Hand Surg 12-A:311, 1987.

Basora J and Fery A: Metastatic malignancy of the hand, Clin Orthop 108:182, 1975.

Bell JL and Mason ML: Metastatic tumors of the hand: report of two cases, Q Bull Northwestern Univ Med School 27:114, 1953.

Block RS and Burton RI: Multiple chondrosarcomas in a hand: a case report, J Hand Surg 2:310, 1977.

Bryan RS, Soule EH, Dobyns JH, et al: Metastatic lesions of the hand and forearm, Clin Orthop 101:167, 1974.

Bryan RS, Soule EH, Dobyns JH, et al: Primary epitheloid sarcoma of the hand and forearm: a review of thirteen cases, J Bone Joint Surg 56-A:458, 1974.

Button M: Epitheloid sarcoma: a case report, J Hand Surg 4:368, 1979.

Carroll RE: Epidermoid (epithelial) cyst of the hand skeleton, Am J Surg 85:327, 1953.

Carroll RE: Osteogenic sarcoma in the hand, J Bone Joint Surg 39-A:325, 1957.

Carroll RE: Squamous cell carcinoma of the nail bed, J Hand Surg 1:92, 1976.

Clifford RH and Kelly AP Jr: Primary malignant tumors of the hand, Plast Reconstr Surg 15:227, 1955.

Culver JE Jr, Sweet DE, and McCue FC: Chondrosarcoma of the hand arising from a pre-existent benign solitary enchondroma: case report and pathological description, Clin Orthop 113:128, 1975.

Dahlin D and Salvador AH: Chondrosarcoma of the bones and feet, Cancer 34:758, 1974.

Drompp BW: Bilateral osteosarcoma in the phalanges of the hand: a solitary case report, J Bone Joint Surg 43-A:199, 1961.

Dryer RF, Buckwalter JA, Flatt AE, and Bonfiglio M: Ewing's sarcoma of the hand, J Hand Surg 4:372, 1979.

Enneking WF, Spanier SS, and Goodman MA: The surgical staging of musculoskeletal sarcoma, Clin Orthop 153:106, 1980.

Enneking WF, Spanier SS, and Goodman MA: The surgical staging of musculosceletal sarcoma, J Bone Joint Surg 62-A:1027, 1980.

Enzinger FM and Weiss SW: Soft tissue tumors, ed 2, St Louis, 1988, Mosby-Year Book, Inc.

Euler E, Wilhelm K, Permanetter W, and Kreusser TH: Ewing's sarcoma of the hand: localization and treatment, J Hand Surg 15-A:659, 1990.

Frassica FJ, Amadio PC, Wold LE, et al: Primary malignant bone tumors of the hand, J Hand Surg 14-A:1022, 1989.

Gelberman RH, Stewart WR, and Harrelson JM: Hand metastasis from melanoma: a case study, Clin Orthop 136:264, 1978.

Gottschalk RG and Smith RT: Chondrosarcoma of the hand: report of a case with radioactive sulphur studies and review of literature, J Bone Joint Surg 45-A:141, 1963.

Granberry WM and Bryan W: Chondrosarcoma of the trapezium: a case report, J Hand Surg 3:277, 1978.

Greene MH: Metastasis of pulmonary carcinoma to the phalanges of the hand, J Bone Joint Surg 39-A:972, 1957.

Hankin FM, Hankin RC, and Louis DS: Malignant fibrous histiocytoma involving a digit, J Hand Surg 12-A:83, 1987.

Heymans M, Jardon-Heghers C, and Vanwijck R: Hand metastases from urothelial tumor, J Hand Surg 15-A:509, 1990.

Hindley CJ and Metcalfe JW: A colonic metastatic tumor in the hand, J Hand Surg 12-A:803, 1987.

Hubbard LF and Burton RI: Malignant fibrous histiocytoma of the forearm: report of a case and review of the literature, J Hand Surg 2:292, 1977.

Jokl P, Albright JA, and Goodman AH: Juxtacortical chondrosarcoma of the hand, J Bone Joint Surg 53-A:1370, 1971.

Kerin R: Metastatic tumors of the hand, J Bone Joint Surg 40-A:263, 1958.

Kerin R: The hand in metastatic disease, J Hand Surg 12-A:77, 1987.

Lansche WE and Spjut HJ: Chondrosarcoma of the small bones of the hand, J Bone Joint Surg 40-A:1139, 1958.

Marcove RC and Charosky CB: Phalangeal sarcomas simulating infections of the digits: review of the literature and report of four cases, Clin Orthop 83:224, 1972.

Marmor L and Horner RL: Metastasis to a phalanx simulating infection in a finger, Am J Surg 97:236, 1959.

McDowell CL and Henceroth WD: Malignant fibrous histiocytoma of the hand: a case report, J Hand Surg 2:297, 1977.

McGraw JM and Stern PJ: Flexion contracture of the thumb: a malignant etiology, J Hand Surg 14-A:736, 1989.

Mutz SB and Curl W: Alveolar cell rhabdomyosarcoma of the hand: case report with four year survival and no evidence of recurrence, J Hand Surg 2:283, 1977.

Nelson DL, Abdul-Karim FW, Carter JR, and Makley JT: Chondrosarcoma of small bones of the hand arising from enchondroma, J Hand Surg 15-A:655, 1990.

Nissenbaum M, Kutz JE, and Lister GD: Clear-cell carcinoma of the lung metastatic to the hamate: a case report, Clin Orthop 134:293, 1978.

Palmieri TJ: Chondrosarcoma of the hand, J Hand Surg 9-A:332, 1984.

Patel MR, Pearlman HS, Engler J, and Wollowick BS: Chondrosarcoma of the proximal phalanx of the finger: review of the literature and report of a case, J Bone Joint Surg 59-A:401, 1977.

Patel MR, Srinivasan KC, and Pearlman HS: Malignant hemangioendothelioma in the hand: a case report, J Hand Surg 3:585, 1978.

Peimer CA, Smith RJ, Sirota RL, and Cohen BE: Epithelioid sarcoma of the hand and wrist: patterns of extension, J Hand Surg 2:275, 1977.

Potenza AD and Winslow DJ: Rhabdomyosarcoma of the hand, J Bone Joint Surg 43-A:700, 1961.

Prat J, Woodruff JM, and Marcove RC: Epithelioid sarcoma: an analysis of 22 cases indicating the prognostic significance of vascular invasion and regional lymph node metastasis, Cancer 41:1472, 1978.

Ream JR, Corson JM, Holdsworth DE, and Millender LH: Chondrosarcoma of the extraskeletal soft tissue of the finger, Clin Orthop 97:148, 1973.

Roberts PH and Price CHG: Chondrosarcoma of bones of the hands and feet: a study of 30 cases, Cancer 34:755, 1974.

Sbarbaro JL Jr and Straub LR: Chondrosarcoma in a phalanx: report of a case, Am J Surg 100:751, 1960.

Schiavon M, Mazzoleni F, Chiarelli A, and Matano P: Squamous cell carcinoma of the hand: fifty-five case reports, J Hand Surg 13-A:413, 1988.

Shapiro L and Baraf CS: Subungual epidermoid carcinoma and keratoacanthoma, Cancer 25:141, 1970.

Trias A, Basora J, Sanchez G, and Madarnas P: Chondrosarcoma of the hand, Clin Orthop 134:297, 1978.

Wilson KM, Jubert AV, and Joseph JI: Sweat gland carcinoma of the hand (malignant acrospiroma), J Hand Surg 14-A:531, 1989.

Wu KK and Guise ER: Metastatic tumors of the hand: a report of six cases, J Hand Surg 3:271, 1978.

Wu KK and Kelly AP: Periosteal (juxtacortical) chondrosarcoma: report of a case occurring in the hand, J Hand Surg 2:314, 1977.

Wu KK, Collon DJ, and Guise EE: Extraosseous chondrosarcoma, J Bone Joint Surg 62-A:189, 1980.

Wu KK, Frost HM, and Guise EE: A chondrosarcoma of the hand arising from an asymptomatic benign solitary enchondroma of 40 years' duration, J Hand Surg 8:317, 1983.

Tumorous conditions

Aitken AP and Magill HK: Calcareous tendinitis of the flexor carpi ulnaris, N Engl J Med 244:434, 1951.

Altner PC and Singh SK: An unusual case of ectopic ossification in a finger, J Hand Surg 6:142, 1981.

Andren L and Eiken O: Arthrographic studies of wrist ganglions, J Bone Joint Surg 53-A:299, 1971.

Angelides AC and Wallace PF: The dorsal ganglion of the wrist: its pathogenesis, gross and microscopic anatomy, and surgical treatment, J Hand Surg 1:228, 1976.

Arner O, Lindholm A, and Romanus R: Mucous cysts of the fingers: report of 26 cases, Acta Chir Scand 111:314, 1956.

Artz TD and Posch JL: The carpometacarpal boss, J Bone Joint Surg 55-A:747, 1973.

Barnes WE, Larsen RD, and Posch JL: Review of ganglia of the hand and wrist with analysis of surgical treatment, Plast Reconstr Surg 34:570, 1964.

Bowers WH and Hurst LC: An intraarticular-intraosseous carpal ganglion, J Hand Surg 4:375, 1979.

Calin A: Reiter's syndrome. In Kelley WN, Harris ED Jr, Ruddy S, and Sledge CB, editors: Textbook of rheumatology, vol 2, Philadelphia, 1981, WB Saunders.

Cameron BM and McGehee FO: Calcification of the pisiform bursae: report of two cases, South Med J 51:496, 1958.

Carroll RE, Sinton W, and Garcia A: Acute calcium deposits in the hand, JAMA 157:422, 1955.

Constantian MB, Zuelzer WA, and Theogaraj SD: The dorsal ganglion with anomalous muscles, J Hand Surg 4:84, 1979.

Cooper W: Calcareous tendinitis in the metacarpophalangeal region, J Bone Joint Surg 24:114, 1942.

Curtis RM: Congenital arteriovenous fistulae of the hand, J Bone Joint Surg 35-A:917, 1953.

De Orsay RH, Mccray PM Jr, and Ferguson LK: Pathology and treatment of ganglion, Am J Surg 36:313, 1937.

Eaton RG, Dobranski AI, and Littler JW: Marginal osteophyte excision in treatment of mucous cysts, J Bone Joint Surg 55-A:570, 1973.

Gondos B: Calcification about the wrist associated with acute pain (periarthritis calcarea), Radiology 60:244, 1953.

Haverbush TJ, Wilde AH, and Phalen GS: The hand in Paget's disease of bone: report of two cases, J Bone Joint Surg 54-A:173, 1972.

Holt EP and Odell RT: Peritendinitis calcarea, South Med J 45:400, 1952.

Horner RL, Wiedel JD, and Bralliar F: Involvement of the hand in epidermolysis bullosa, J Bone Joint Surg 53-A:1347, 1971.

Johnson MK and Lawrence JF: Metaplastic bone formation (myositis ossificans) in the soft tissues of the hand: case report, J Bone Joint Surg 57-A:999, 1975.

Kleinert HE, Kutz JE, Fishman JH, and McCraw LH: Etiology and treatment of the so-called mucous cyst of the finger, J Bone Joint Surg 54-A:1455, 1972.

Lamp JC, Graham JH, Urbach F, et al: Keratoacanthoma of the subungual region: a clinicopathological and therapeutic study, J Bone Joint Surg 46-A:1721, 1964.

Landon GC, Johnson KA, and Dahlin DC: Subungual exostoses, J Bone Joint Surg 61-A:256, 1979.

Lee BS and Kaplan R: Turret exostosis of the phalanges, Clin Orthop 100:186, 1974.

Lewin DW: Congenital arteriovenous fistulae, Lancet 2:621, 1930.

MacCullom MS: Dorsal wrist ganglions in children, J Hand Surg 2:325, 1977.

Maguire JK, Milford LW, and Pitcock JA: Focal myositis in the hand, J Hand Surg 13-A:140, 1988.

Matthews P: Ganglia of the flexor tendon sheaths in the hand, J Bone Joint Surg 55-B:612, 1973.

Mendelson BC, Linscheid RL, Dobyns JH, and Muller SA: Surgical treatment of calcinosis cutis in the upper extremity, J Hand Surg 2:318, 1977.

Morgan JB, Newberg AH, and Davis PH: Intraosseous ganglion of the lunate, J Hand Surg 6:61, 1981.

Nelson CL, Sawmiller S, and Phalen GS.: Ganglions of the wrist and hand, J Bone Joint Surg 54-A:1459, 1972.

Newmeyer WL, Kilgore ES Jr, and Graham WP III: Mucous cysts: the dorsal distal interphalangeal joint ganglion, Plast Reconstr Surg 53:313, 1974.

Phalen GS: Calcification adjacent to the pisiform bone, J Bone Joint Surg 34-A:579, 1952.

Pollen AG: Calcareous deposits about the metacarpo-phalangeal joints, J Bone Joint Surg 43-B:250, 1961.

Schlenker JD, Clark DD, and Weckesser EC: Calcinosis circumscripta of the hand in scleroderma, J Bone Joint Surg 55-A:1051, 1973.

Seddon HJ: Carpal ganglion as a cause of paralysis of the deep branch of the ulnar nerve, J Bone Joint Surg 34-B:386, 1952.

Seidenstein H: Acute pain in the wrist and hand associated with calcific deposits: report of fifteen cases, J Bone Joint Surg 32-A:413, 1950.

Spar I and Maenza R: Pseudocyst in a finger of a patient with scleroderma, J Bone Joint Surg 59-A:559, 1977.

Straub LR, Smith JW, Carpenter GK Jr, and Dietz GH.: The surgery of gout in the upper extremity, J Bone Joint Surg 43-A:731, 1961.

Tophoj K and Henriques U: Ganglion of the wrist: a structure developed from the joint: a histological study with serial sections, Acta Orthop Scand 42:244, 1971.

Wissinger HA, McClain EJ, and Boyers JH: Turret exostosis: ossifying hematoma of the phalanges, J Bone Joint Surg 48-A:105, 1966.

Yelton CL and Dickey LE Jr: Calcification about the hand and wrist, South Med J 51:489, 1958.

CHAPTER 78

Infections of Hand

PHILLIP E. WRIGHT II*

FACTORS INFLUENCING HAND INFECTIONS

The clinical course of most hand infections is affected by anatomic, local, and systemic factors, in addition to bacterial virulence and size of the inoculum.

Anatomic factors that to some extent determine the ease of penetration, localization, and spread of infections include: (1) the thin layer of skin and subcutaneous tissue over the tendons, bones, and joints; (2) the closed space of the distal digital pulp; (3) the proximity of the flexor tendon sheath to bone and joint; (4) the proximal extent of the flexor sheath into the palm, connecting with the radial and ulnar bursae; and (5) the location of the thenar and midpalmar spaces in the hand and Parona's space proximal to the wrist near the flexor tendon sheaths.

Local factors predisposing to infection include: (1) the extent and nature of soft tissue damage, (2) the amount and virulence of bacterial contamination, and (3) the type and amount of foreign material that is present and persistent in the wound.

Systemic factors generally include: (1) nutritional status of the patients, (2) systemic diseases such as diabetes, (3) the chronic use of medications such as cortisone that might predispose to infection, and (4) the use and nature of immunosuppressive medications.

Treatment of hand infections depends on the specific identification of the organism, the specific anatomic area involved, location of the infection in the hand and fingers, and the type of inflammation, areas of tenderness, and erythema determined by palpation and observation. Identification of organisms with culture and antibiotic sensitivity studies allows proper medical treatment.

The infections discussed here do not include all possible infections in the hand, but each has a characteristic pattern of potential spread determined by the anatomy, type of infection, and host resistance.

GENERAL APPROACH TO HAND INFECTIONS

With a careful history and physical examination, the location of the infection, extent of spread, presence of swelling, lymphangitis, lymphadenitis, and joint involvement may be determined. An attempt should be made to determine the presence of an abscess that requires drainage. Fluctuance may be difficult to identify in the hand. Roentgenograms, complete blood count, and erythrocyte sedimentation rate usually are obtained. If any fluid or tissue is obtained, it is sent to the laboratory for Gram stain, culture, and antibiotic sensitivity determinations. Specific requests usually are made of the laboratory to culture for aerobic and anaerobic bacteria, as well as for mycobacteria and fungi.

Initial antibiotic therapy traditionally has been empiric, depending on the Gram stain and the most likely organism. Increasingly it appears that consideration should be given to the possibility of mixed flora as the cause of hand infections. The organism most commonly isolated from hand infections in *Staphylococcus aureus*. Typically 80% or more of wounds cultured from swabs produce multiple organisms, whereas tissue specimens

---

*Revision of chapter by Lee W. Milford, M.D.

may produce a single causative organism in about 75%. Streptococci, enterobacteria, pseudomonas, enterococci, and bacterioides are other organisms commonly causing hand infections. Less common causes include the various mycobacteria, *Gonococcus, Pasturella multocida* (in cat or dog bites), *Eikenella corrodens* (in human bites), *Aeromonas hydrophila* from standing in fresh water, *Haemophilus influenzae* (in children from 2 months to 3 years of ages), a variety of anaerobic organisms (including the clostridia), and other rare bacteria, such as anthrax, erysipeloid, and brucella.

Antibiotics traditionally recommended for hand infections include a penicillinase-resistant penicillin or cephalosporin. Addition of antibiotics effective against gram-negative organisims has been recommended for high-risk situations such as infections in intravenous drug users and contaminated outdoor or farm injuries.

Following a protocol of early, aggressive surgical incision and drainage and a combination of intravenous penicillin G and cefazolin with gentamicin, when indicated, Spiegel and Szabo reported a shorter hospital stay, faster healing, and fewer complications in 69 patients compared to 107 patients treated before institution of the protocol. Because of the constantly changing inventory of antibiotics and the variations in patient populations and wound flora, antibiotic selection should be based on a variety of indications, including the assistance of an infectious disease specialist when needed.

Glass, Kilgore, and Linscheid and Dobyns, as well as others, have identified the failure to recognize the polymicrobial nature of hand infections and inadequate surgical debridement as frequent causes of poor results. The importance of adequate surgical treatment cannot be overemphasized because antibiotics alone may be insufficient to control the infection.

Incision and Drainage

■ *TECHNIQUE.* Use a general anesthetic or distant regional block, since a local anesthetic may not function in the septic environment, may spread the infection, and adds to an already swollen part. Use a tourniquet, but, before inflating it, elevate the hand for 3 to 6 minutes to avoid limb exsanguinuation with an elastic wrap because of the potential for proximal spread of the infection. After properly preparing and draping, make the incision for drainage as described for specific infections. After making the skin incision, always spread the deeper structures with blunt dissection to avoid injury to important nerves, vessels, and tendons.

Although an incision for drainage relieves pain and reduces the spread of infection, it also creates an open infected wound subject to further contamination. Copious irrigation with a pulsatile irrigator is an effective way to decrease contamination. Although wound closure after abscess drainage has been advocated, it probably is safer to return to the

surgical suite in 3 to 5 days and close the wound secondarily, condition of the wound permitting. However, if joints or flexor tendons have been exposed by skin necrosis, cover them at once to preserve their vital functions. In most instances leave the wound open. Infections involving the tendon sheaths and joints usually result in some loss of function, but those more superficial usually do not, unless surgical scars have adhered to adjacent structures such as nerves or tendons or have resulted in hypertrophy from tension.

AFTERTREATMENT. Immediately after surgery the hand is wrapped with bulky layers of gauze to hold it in the position of function and to pad the wound. A metal or plaster splint is applied to support the wrist. The hand is continuously elevated after surgery. Active motion of digits is begun as soon as possible. The dressing usually is first changed between 24 and 48 hours after drainage and then is changed daily or every other day. Moist dressings may help remove infected drainage. Mask and gloves should be worn during dressings to avoid further contamination. After several days further debridement of necrotic material may be necessary if the infection is extensive. As soon as drainage has ceased and healthy granulation tissue appears, the wound is secondarily closed; a free skin graft may be necessary, but usually only when a skin slough has occurred.

ABSCESSES
Paronychia

A "runaround" infection usually is caused by the introduction of *Staphylococcus aureus* into the eponychium

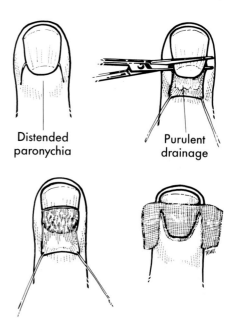

Distended paronychia

Purulent drainage

Fig. 78-1 Incision and drainage of paronychia (see text).

by a hangnail or poor nail hygiene. When an abscess forms in the eponychial or paronychial fold, it is known as a paronychia. It usually begins at one corner of the horny nail and travels either under the eponychium or under the nail toward the opposite side. When an abscess is on one side only, incise it, angling the knife away from the nail to avoid cutting the nail bed, which would cause a ridge later. If the abscess lies under one corner of the nail root, remove this corner. If it has already migrated to the opposite side and under the nail, make a second incision there, fold back the skin proximally, and excise the proximal one third of the nail. Then loosely pack the wound open for 48 hours for drainage (Fig. 78-1). A chronic infection should be treated in the same manner; fungus and yeast infections should be considered if the course has been prolonged.

Felon

The distal finger pulp is divided into tiny compartments by strong fibrous septa that traverse it from skin to bone. A fibrous curtain is also present at the distal flexor finger crease. Because of these septa, any swelling causes immediate pain that is intensified because of increased pressure within the pulp. The pulp abscess (felon) may extend into the periosteum, around the nail bed, or proximally through the fibrous curtain or through the skin to the exterior over the pulp. Those beginning deep are likely to penetrate the periosteum and cause osteomyelitis; the more superficial ones cause skin necrosis.

The treatment consists of antibiotics and incision for drainage. The diagnosis of an abscess in this area is sometimes difficult, but one is usually present if severe pain has lasted for 12 hours or more. When the abscess points volarward, causing necrosis of the overlying skin, drain it by excising the necrotic skin. When the abscess is in the distal pulp area pointing volarward toward the whorl of the fingerprint, it is best drained by a vertical incision begun distal to the skin crease and placed precisely in the midline to avoid the lateral branches of the digital nerve and to allow healing with minimal scar (Fig. 78-2).

If the abscess is deep and is partitioned by the septa, make a longitudinal incision, cutting through the partitions (Fig. 78-3). This incision must be accurate: make it dorsal to the tactile surface of the finger and not more than 3 mm from the distal free edge of the nail; otherwise the ends of the digital nerve will be painfully damaged. An incision like a ⌐ is sufficient; a fishmouth incision around the whole fingertip is slow to heal and may result in painful scarring, especially if it is placed too far palmar.

Web Space Infection (Collar Button Abscess)

Web space infection usually localizes in one of the three fat-filled spaces just proximal to the superficial transverse ligament at the level of the metacarpophalangeal joints. Typically the infection begins beneath palmar calluses in laborers. It may begin near the palmar surface, but, because the skin and fascia here are less yielding, it may localize to drain dorsally. Here the tissue becomes obviously swollen, but the significant amount of the abscess remains nearer the palm. This may be the more dangerous part because, unless drained, it may spread through the lumbrical canal into the middle palmar space. Two longitudinal incisions usually are necessary for drainage: one on the dorsal surface between the metacarpal heads and the other on the palm, beginning distal to the distal palmar crease and curving proximally. The web should not be incised.

Deep Fascial Space Infections

The palmar fascial space lies between the fascia covering the metacarpals and their contiguous muscles and the fascia dorsal to the flexor tendons. Its ulnar border is the fascia of the hypothenar muscles, and its radial border is the fascia of the adductor and other thenar mus-

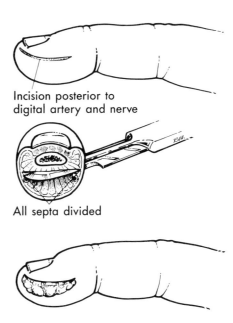

Incision posterior to digital artery and nerve

All septa divided

Fig. 78-3   Incision and drainage of felon (see text).

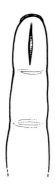

Fig. 78-2   Midline vertical incision for draining an abscess pointing volarward in distal pulp of finger (see text).

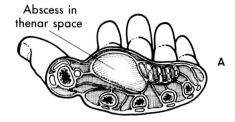

Abscess in
thenar space

A

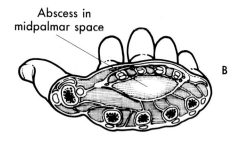

Abscess in
midpalmar space

B

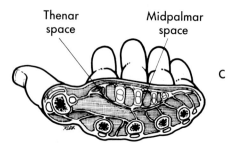

Thenar
space

Midpalmar
space

C

Fig. 78-4 Boundaries of deep palmar space. This space is divided into thenar space and middle palmar space (see text). **A,** Abscess in thenar space. **B,** Abscess in middle palmar space. **C,** Relations of spaces when not distended by pus.

cles. This space is divided into a middle palmar space and a thenar space by a fascial membrane that passes obliquely from the third metacarpal shaft to the fascia dorsal to the flexor tendons of the index finger (Fig. 78-4). Parona's space is bordered by the pronator quadratus dorsally, the flexor pollicis longus laterally, the flexor carpi ulnaris medially, and the flexor tendons on the palmar aspect; it rarely is the site of abscess formation. Fortunately, infections in these spaces are now rare, since less extensive infections nearby are usually controlled by antibiotics before they spread. Abscesses in these spaces usually result from the spread of infection from other parts of the hand, typically from purulent flexor tenosynovial infections.

A middle palmar abscess causes a severe systemic reaction, local pain and tenderness, inability to actively move the long and ring fingers because of pain, and generalized swelling of the hand and fingers so that they resemble an inflated rubber glove. A thenar abscess causes similar symptoms, but the thumb web is more swollen, the index finger is held flexed, and active motion of both the index finger and thumb is impaired because of pain.

Drain the middle palmar space through a curved incision beginning at the level of the distal palmar crease, in line with the middle finger and extending ulnarward to just inside the hypothenar eminence. Enter the space on either side of the long flexor tendon of the ring finger with a blunt instrument such as a hemostat to avoid injury to neurovascular structures. Leave a drain in place if needed.

Drain the thenar space through a curved incision in the thumb web parallel to the border of the first dorsal interosseus muscle or along the proximal side of the thenar crease. Avoid the recurrent branch of the median nerve at the proximal end of this crease. Avoid sharp, deep dissection, using blunt dissection to delineate the extent of the abscess.

Tenosynovitis

An infection within the theca of a flexor tendon results from the spread of adjacent pulp infections or from puncture wounds of the flexor creases. Kanavel considered tenderness over the involved sheath, rigid positioning of the finger in flexion, pain on attempts to hyperextend the fingers, and swelling of the involved part to be the four "cardinal" signs of suppurative tenosynovitis. Of these, tenderness over the flexor sheath is considered the most significant. When early tenosynovitis is suspected, immediate treatment with antibiotics and splinting may abort spread of the infection if the patient's symptoms have been present for less than 48 hours. The prognosis for function is poor when an infection here produces pus that must be drained. If drainage is required, either an open or closed irrigation technique may be used. If the open technique is used, healing and rehabilitation are prolonged and full motion may not be regained.

CLOSED IRRIGATION. Neviaser has popularized a closed irrigation technique that is similar to that advocated by Carter, Burman, and Mersheimer.

■ *TECHNIQUE (NEVIASER, MODIFIED).* **With the patient under suitable anesthesia and after appropriately preparing and draping the hand and arm, inflate a pneumatic tourniquet; but, to decrease the risk of spread of infection, do not wrap the limb. Expose the proximal end of the flexor sheath in the region of the A1 pulley by either a straight transverse incision parallel to the distal palmar crease or by a zigzag incision in this area (Fig. 78-5). Expect to see serosanguinous or purulent fluid in the sheath. Open the sheath proximal to the A1 pulley and swab the fluid to send for cultures. Make a second incision in the midaxial line on either side of the finger in the distal portion of the middle segment of the digit. As an alternative, carefully make a transverse incision over the distal flexion crease. Open the flexor sheath distal to the A4 pulley. Using smooth forceps or hemostats, pass a 16- or an 18-gauge**

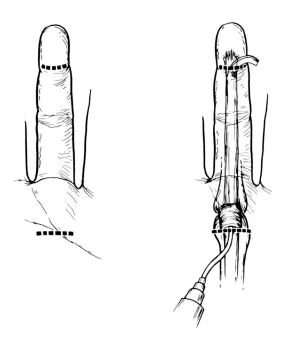

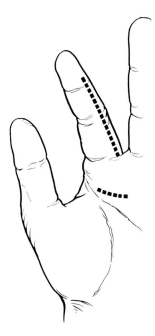

Fig. 78-5   Closed irrigation for tenosynovitis. (Neviaser, modified).

Fig. 78-6   Open drainage for advanced infection and necrosis of tendon and sheath.

polyethylene catheter beneath the A1 pulley from distal to proximal in the flexor sheath for 1.5 to 2 cm. Distally place a small piece of rubber drain beneath the A4 pulley and bring it out through the skin incision. Irrigate the sheath from proximal to distal with saline. Close the wounds around the catheter and the rubber drain, leaving the distal wound sufficiently loose to allow fluid to drain. Suture the catheter to the palmar skin. Test the system for patency by irrigating freely with saline. Wrap the hand in a bulky dressing supported with a splint, leaving the tip of the rubber drain exposed to observe outflow. Bring the inflow catheter out through the dressing, tape it to the dressing, and attach it to a 30 ml syringe.

When the radial or ulnar bursa is involved, place a second catheter in the palmar wound and pass it proximally in the sheath, securing it to the palmar skin with a suture to prevent dislodgement. Open the respective bursa proximally through a longitudinal incision on the radial or ulnar side of the distal forearm just proximal to the wrist, place a piece of rubber drain in the bursa, and bring it out through the skin. Irrigate in both proximal and distal directions for these combined digital and bursal infections.

AFTERTREATMENT. The wounds are irrigated with 30 ml of saline every 2 hours, and the distal end of the fingers are checked for patency and flow. After 48 hours the dressing is removed to examine the fingers. If signs of persistent infection are present, irrigation is continued for another 24 hours. The dressings are removed at that time and the fingers

are examined. If no residual signs of infection remain, the catheter and drain are removed, a lighter dressing is applied, and active motion exercises are begun. If pain or drainage persists, irrigation for several days may be necessary.

OPEN DRAINAGE. Open drainage rarely is used, but may be necessary in fingers with advanced infection and necrosis of the tendon and sheath that requires debridement.

■ *TECHNIQUE.* With the patient under suitable anesthesia, inflate the tourniquet but do not wrap the limb. Use two incisions. Make the first incision midaxial on either side of the finger, extending from the distal flexion crease nearly to the web (Fig. 78-6). Make the second incision on the palm, parallel to and near the palmar crease over the A1 pulley. Identify the flexor sheath in the distal wound, open the sheath, and obtain swabs or fluid to send for culture determination. Irrigate from the proximal wound distally with saline. Leave the wound open, wrap the hand in a bulky dressing, and place it in a splint.

AFTERTREATMENT. Active finger motion is encouraged as soon as possible after about 36 to 48 hours. The bandages are removed, the wounds are inspected, and whirlpool treatments are begun daily or twice daily. Active motion exercises are encouraged during and between treatments. Although delayed closure may be considered, usually resolution of drainage is so prolonged that secondary healing is allowed to take place to minimize the recurrence of infection.

Infections of Radial and Ulnar Bursae

The radial and ulnar bursae are the tenosynovial sheaths of the flexor tendons at the wrist (Fig. 78-7). The proximal prolongation of the thumb flexor sheath is the radial bursa. The flexor sheaths communicate from the proximal palmar crease to the level of the pronator quadratus and then extend distally as the tendon sheath of the little finger to form the ulnar bursa. Often the two bursae communicate with each other and allow inflammation to spread from one to the other in a "horseshoe abscess."

To drain the radial bursa, first make a lateral incision along the proximal phalanx of the thumb and open the bursa at its distal end. Introduce a probe here, advance it proximally to the wrist, and make a second incision over its end. Insert small 16- or 18-gauge polyethylene drainage tubes proximally and rubber drains distally for irrigation. Make a palmar incision and pass drainage tubes proximally as described for tenosynovitis. Open the ulnar bursa on the ulnar side of the little finger and again proximal to the wrist with the help of a probe. If both bursae are involved, one proximal ulnar incision may be sufficient to drain both, since the two bursae communicate proximally in most patients.

Finger Joint Infections (Septic Arthritis)

Finger joint infections usually result from spread of infection in adjacent structures, direct penetration of the

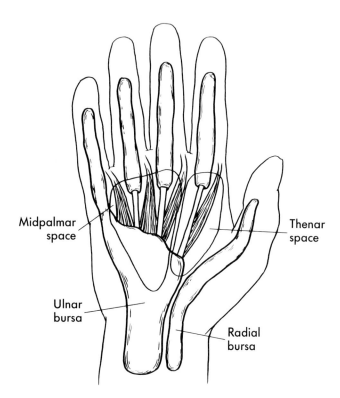

Fig. 78-7 Flexor tendon sheaths and proximal extensions into the radial and ulnar bursae. (Redrawn from Neviaser RJ and Gunther SF: AAOS Instr Course Lect 29:108, 1980.)

joint, and less commonly hematogenous spread. When hematogenous spread occurs, the primary source should be identified. In addition to the history and physical and roentgenographic evaluations, diagnosis is accomplished by joint aspiration and synovial fluid analysis, Gram stain, and cultures. Fluid obtained from a septic joint usually is turbid, opaque, or grossly purulent. The joint fluid white blood cell count usually is over 50,000/mm³. The polymorphonuclear count usually is over 75%, and the synovial fluid glucose is 40 mg or lower.

Septic arthritis may cause articular cartilage destruction and osteomyelitis in the underlying phalanx. This may be delayed or avoided if incision and drainage are performed and appropriate antibiotics are used once pus is identified in the joint. If the joint and adjacent bone are destroyed and require removal, antibiotic impregnated polymethylmethacrylate may be a useful adjunct in reconstruction with arthrodesis or bone grafting, as advocated by Asche and by Freeland and Senter. Amputation may be required to salvage the hand. Usually little is lost by such an amputation because the chronically infected finger retains little useful function. In children antibiotics, drainage, and splinting are continued longer than in adults in an attempt to salvage the hand.

OPEN DRAINAGE OF SEPTIC FINGER JOINTS

■ *TECHNIQUE.* **With the patient under appropriate anesthesia, apply and inflate a tourniquet but do not wrap the arm. To drain the metacarpophalangeal joint, make an incision on either side of the metacarpal head, retract the extensor expansion distally, and open the joint capsule dorsal to the collateral ligament sufficiently to allow free drainage and irrigation of the joint. Leave the capsule and skin incisions open.**

To drain the thumb and finger interphalangeal joints and the thumb metacarpophalangeal joints, use a midaxial incision on either side of the joint. Avoid injury to the neurovascular bundles. In the fingers, section the transverse retinacular ligament, retract the extensor lateral band dorsally, and retract the neurovascular bundle toward the palm. Identify the collateral ligament and make a longitudinal incision parallel to the ligament and palmar to it, separating the accessory collateral ligament from it. Remove a portion of the accessory collateral ligament, drain the joint, and send specimens for aerobic and anerobic cultures. Irrigate the wound with saline and leave it open. Apply a bulky dressing and a splint.

AFTERTREATMENT. **The hand is elevated for about 24 hours. Then the bandage is changed and motion exercises are begun. The dressing is changed daily or twice daily and exercise periods in a whirlpool bath are begun. When the wound is satisfactorily clean, it may be closed secondarily; otherwise, it should be allowed to heal by secondary intention.**

Osteomyelitis

Osteomyelitis of the metacarpals and phalanges is usually caused by infection of neighboring soft tissues or by an open fracture. Hematogenous osteomyelitis is rare in the hand. The principles of diagnosis and treatment, including drainage, intravenous antibiotics, and early mobilization, that apply to large bones apply here (see Chapter 4). If diagnostic measures, including roentgenograms and radionuclide studies, suggest bone infection with no sequestrum formation, the process is considered acute or subacute and may resolve without surgical drainage if appropriate, antibiotics are instituted for organisms obtained by needle aspiration. If no organisms can be obtained, open drainage of pus and debridement of necrotic material provides adequate material for culture and ensures decompression of abscesses. When the process has lingered and sequestra have formed, it is considered a chronic infection. Although salvage of digits is possible with diaphysectomy, sequestrectomy, external fixation, the use of antibiotic-impregnated polymethylmethacrylate, and subsequent bone grafting, frequently it is difficult to preserve a functioning digit and hand because of the severe stiffness that develops in the involved digit, as well as in the remaining digits. Especially in adults, unless the infection can be controlled to preserve satisfactory function in the involved digit and hand, amputation should be considered. The amputation should be at the joint proximal to the involved bone; merely nibbling off part of the bone involved rarely will prevent spread of the infection.

Infection of the distal finger pulp may erode the distal phalanx, as roentgenograms will show, especially when

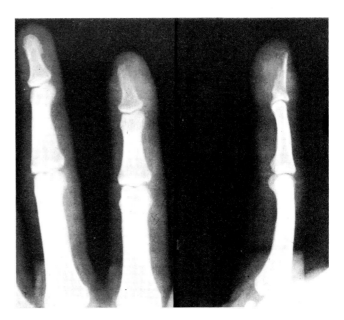

Fig. 78-8   Osteitis of distal phalanx caused by finger pulp infection.

the abscess is deep and is located proximally (Fig. 78-8). This area of osteitis will regenerate to some extent after the abscess is drained, especially in children, and should not be confused with sequestrating osteomyelitis (Fig. 78-9).

Human Bite Injuries

Human bite injuries occur in two ways. The first is inadvertent and relatively innocent, involving nail biting

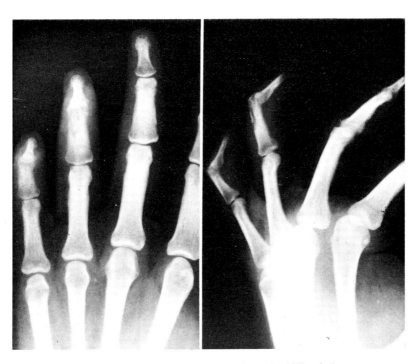

Fig. 78-9   Sequestrating osteomyelitis of middle phalanx.

and similar activities. The second, though at times accidental, usually involves intentionally violent attacks and includes the more common full-thickness bites, bite amputations, and injuries related to striking a tooth with the clenched fist. Clenched-fist injuries account for some of the most severe infections related to human tooth wounds. Most often the third and fourth digits are injured at the metacarpophalangeal joint. Although fractures of the metacarpal neck may be seen, chondral and osteochondral fractures may occur in 6% to 59% of patients. The chance of inoculating the hand with virulent organisms is great because 42 different bacterial species have been identified in the normal human mouth flora. The most common infecting organism is *Staphylococcus aureus,* and the second most common is *Streptococcus.* Other organisms found are *Eikenella, Micrococcus, Clostridia, Spriochetes,* and *Neisseria. Malinowski et al.* reported an average 2½-day delay in seeking medical attention, and the patients frequently were noncompliant. Reported complications from the injury include osteomyelitis, fracture, pain, permanent joint stiffness, arthritis, digital amputation, systemic sepsis, and death. The incidence of complications varies from 25% to 50%.

The mechanism for introducing anaerobic bacteria into the joint is understood best by realizing that the injury occurs when the hand is in a fist. When the finger is extended, the injured joint is closed as the tendon that was lacerated by the tooth glides proximally (Fig. 78-10). This provides an anaerobic environment for growth of the bacteria introduced. Some surgeons advise that all human bite patients be admitted to the hospital.

Generally all patients with small lacerations over the metacarpophalangeal joint should be assumed to have tooth injuries, regardless of the history given. Roentgenograms should be obtained to rule out fractures and foreign bodies, and the wound should be explored to rule out intraarticular injury. Several authors have observed that patients presenting less than 24 hours after injury usually to not have signs of sepsis, so that joint exploration, swabbing for cultures (aerobic and anerobic with attention to *Eikenella corrodens*), treatment with antibiotics, and close observation usually are sufficient. Patients presenting 24 hours or more after injury may have definite signs and symptoms of sepsis and may require open joint drainage and irrigation, close observation usually in the hospital, and intravenous antibiotics. At this time antibiotics usually recommended include either penicillin G, ampicillin, carbenicillin, or tetracycline for *E. corrodens* and a cephalosporin for *Staphylococcus.* Antibiotics may be changed at 36 to 48 hours, depending on culture and sensitivity reports. Tetanus prophylaxis is ensured and the wound is left open.

If the healing is progressing satisfactorily, motion exercises may be started at 24 hours after drainage. Daily washing of the wound with soap and water usually provides sufficient cleansing. In some patients with other problems such as diabetes and in those taking corticosteroids, final resolution and healing may be prolonged, leading to some of the previously mentioned complications. A 7- to 10-day course of antibiotics usually is followed, depending on the course of the infection.

Dog bites to the hand may present as puncture wounds or as superficial or deep lacerations. Canine oral flora include *S. aureus, Streptococcus viridans, Bacteroides ssp.,* and *Pasturella multocida.* Most are usually sensitive to penicillin. Tetanus prophylaxis should be accompanied by the use of antibiotics in healing dog bites. Deep wounds should be debrided, cleansed, irrigated, and left open for secondary closure. More superficial lacerations may be loosely closed after the wound has been

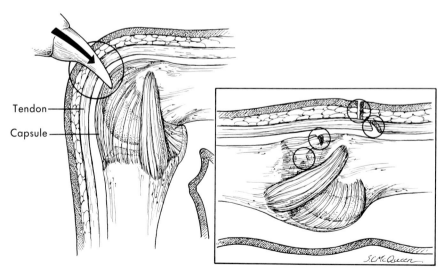

Fig. 78-10 Entry of tooth is made through skin, tendon, and joint capsule while metacarpophalangeal joint is flexed. When joint is extended, these tissues shift to occupy a different site. This causes an inoculated closed intraarticular wound.

thoroughly cleansed, the margins debrided, and the wound irrigated thoroughly with copious amounts of normal saline.

Cat bites more often present as puncture wounds. *P. multocida* is commonly isolated from cat bites and usually is sensitive to penicillin. If the bites are minor or superficial, treatment includes cleansing and observation. If the cat bites are deep, they may be connected with a scalpel blade to allow thorough wound debridement and irrigation. A severe wound is left open, whereas more superficial wounds may be loosely closed.

Snyder has summarized treatment for other land and marine animal bites, as well as snake and insect bites.

MISCELLANEOUS AND UNUSUAL INFECTIONS
Herpetic Infections

Herpes simplex was first reported by Adamson in 1909. It often resembles a pyogenic infection and frequently involves the paronychial region, but it may involve the palm, usually distal to the metacarpophalangeal joint. It occurs most often on the thumb and index finger. Herpes simplex virus I and II are the most common in the hand. The lesions begin as swelling with pain and the development of vesicles (Fig. 78-11). The vesicles progress to ulcers over about 2 weeks. In the next 7 to 10 days the vesicles begin to dry and heal; however, viral shedding may make the lesions infective for another 12 days or so. Recurrence is possible. Laboratory techniques to confirm the diagnosis include viral

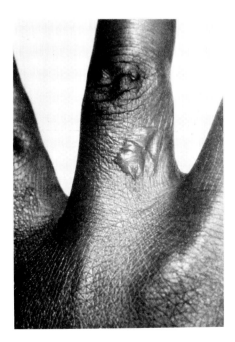

Fig. 78-11 Vesicular eruption of dorsal aspect of the proximal phalanx, left long finger. (From Sehayik RI and Bassett FH III: Clin Orthop 166:138, 1982.)

cultures, Tzanck and other smears and stains, and serological tests for primary infections. Diagnosis can be confirmed by herpes antibody titers. It is often found in persons involved in the care of the oral or respiratory system such as dental hygienists and medical personnel. It may be accompanied by axillary and epitrochlear adenopathy with lymphangitis of the forearm. Surgical drainage is not indicated for herpetic infections. The lesions should be kept clean to avoid bacterial infection. Treatment presently is medical and includes the use of the drug acyclovir in some patients.

Infections in Drug Addicts

The lack of asepsis in cleaning the skin and preparation of injectable substances probably accounts for most infections associated with intravenous drug abuse. Although infection may present as septicemia, usually the sepsis is localized because of subcutaneous extravasation. Reyes categorized such hand infections into four types, depending on the depth and location of infection. Type I infection is in the skin and subcutaneous tissues, usually on the dorsum of the fingers. Type II infection includes the extensor tendon and possibly the periosteum and bone. Type III involves the flexor tendon sheath of the finger and has the worst prognosis. Type IV includes the seqeulae of arterial injection, such as digital necrosis and pain. Dorsal swelling may be caused by chronic lymphedema and fibrosis instead of infection.

Treatment includes hospitalization, aggressive incision, drainage and debridement, culturing for aerobic and anaerobic organisms, copious lavage, leaving the wound open, splinting, multiple daily dressing changes, appropriate intravenous antibiotics, and progressive rehabilitation of the hand.

Infections in Patients with Acquired Immunodeficiency Syndrome (AIDS)

Although little has yet been written about the incidence and natural history of hand infections in patients with AIDS, with the epidemic nature of this syndrome hand surgeons are almost certain to see more and more of these patients with hand infections. Glickel in 1988 reported eight patients with hand infections and AIDS or AIDS-related complex. Three patients had herpes, two had osteomyelitis, one had septic arthritis, and two had bacterial abscesses. He stressed the atypical presentation and course of the infections. Herpetic infections were more virulent than usual and did not resolve spontaneously; intravenous antiviral therapy was necessary. Dorsal bacterial abscesses did not respond to early drainage and progressed to osteomyelitis in one patient. Because five of the eight infections occurred either before or at the time of diagnosis of AIDS, he suggests that an "atypical" hand infection in a patient who is at risk for AIDS should arouse suspicion that a human immunovirus infection is present.

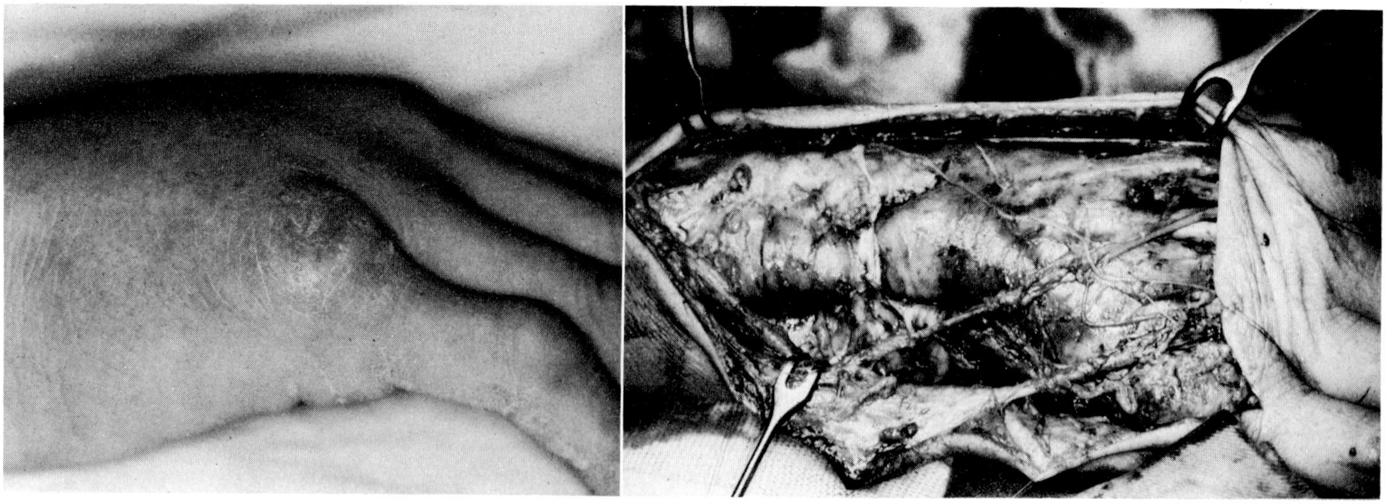

A

B

Fig. 78-12 **A,** Fisherman experienced swelling over dorsum of right hand and near metacar-pophalangeal joint of small finger after crab bite. **B,** View at surgery showing extensive synovi-tis of extensor tendons from wrist to fingers. (From Chow SP, Stroebel AB, Lau JHK, and Collins RJ: J Hand Surg 8:568, 1983.)

Mycobacterial Infections

TUBERCULOSIS. The most common presentation of *Mycobacterium tuberculosis* in the hand is tenosynovitis. Presenting frequently as an extensive palmar "ganglion," it may cause median nerve compression in the carpal tunnel. Although uncommon in the hand, tuberculosis infection should be considered when unexplained tenos-ynovitis is encountered, and tissue cultures and speci-mens should be examined for *M. tuberculosis.* A combi-nation of antituberculous medication and tenosynovec-tomy generally is recommended. Tuberculosis also may involve the bones of the fingers and wrist.

NONTUBERCULOUS MYCOBACTERIA. The nontuber-culosis mycobacteria that most commonly infect the hand are *Mycobacterium marinum* and *Mycobacterium kansasii.* Hand infections by *Mycobacterium fortuitum, Mycobacterium chelonei,* and other mycobacterial species rarely have been reported. *M. marinum* and *M. kansasii* may cause infections in the skin, tenosynovium, and deeper structures.

Any poorly healing ulcer on the hand should have a culture for *M. marinum* at 30° to 32° C on Lowenstein-Jensen medium. Skin testing is not as reliable for this or-ganism as it is for tuberculosis. In the early stages the in-fection is frequently confused with gout or rheumatoid arthritis, and nearly all of the reported cases have had a cortisone injection. Typically the organism is found around swimming pools or fish tanks, from whence it derives its name, "swimming pool granuloma," and may infect an open wound or abrasion. It can attack bone, joint, synovium, or skin (Fig. 78-12).

M. kansasii may behave in a similar manner and

should be considered when a chronic synovitis is not ob-viously a complication of rheumatoid arthritis, especially if only a single digit or joint is involved. A typical case is one in which a synovectomy of the wrist has been done for compression of the median nerve only to be followed by recurrence of swelling and compression of the nerve several weeks later. A slowly healing sinus may also be present. Thus, when a persistent or recurring synovitis of the wrist or finger is encountered, a mycobacterial infec-tion should be suspected. When a part is aspirated for routine bacterial cultures, fungus cultures and those for tuberculosis should also be ordered. The results of the cultures may not be known for several weeks, since these organisms grow slowly.

Treatment is by synovectomy or other excisional sur-gery for diagnostic and therapeutic reasons. If the diag-nosis has not already been established, material is sent for bacteriologic and histologic identification of the or-ganisms. When the diagnosis is established, appropriate antimicrobial therapy is started. The help of an infectious disease consultant for this therapy usually is requested.

Fungal Infections

Three types of manifestations of fungal infections in the extremities have been described: (1) cutaneous infec-tions caused by dermatophytes, (2) subcutaneous infec-tions, and (3) deep or systemic infections. Usual causes of deep or systemic infections include sporotrichosis, ma-duromycosis, histoplasmosis, coccidioidomycosis, and blastomycosis. In addition to appropriate medical treat-ment, surgical therapy is indicated for flexor or extensor tenosynovitis, fungal arthritis, and osteomyelitis.

REFERENCES

Anouchi YS and Froimson I: Hand infections with *Mycobacterium chelonei*: a case report and review of the literature, J Hand Surg 13-B:331, 1988.

Asche G: Treatment of hand infections with gentamycin-PMMA-minichains, Tech Orthop 1:55, 1986.

Badger SJ, Butler T, and Kim CK: Experimental *Eikenella corrodens* endocarditis in rabbits, Infect Immun 23:751, 1979.

Becton JL and Niebauer JJ: Nocardia infection of the hand, J Bone Joint Surg 52-A:1443, 1970.

Belsole R and Fenske N: Cutaneous larva migrans in the upper extremity, J Hand Surg 5:178, 1980.

Behr JT, Daluga DJ, Light TR, and Lewis NS: Herpetic infections in the fingers of infants: report of five cases, J Bone Joint Surg 69-A:137, 1987.

Bielejeski TR: Granular-cell tumor (myoblastoma) of the hand: report of a case, J Bone Joint Surg 55-A:841, 1973.

Bilos ZJ, Eskestrand T, and Shivaram MS: Deep fasciitis of the biceps region, J Hand Surg 4:378, 1979.

Bilos ZJ, Kucharchuk A, and Metzger W: *Eikenella corrodens* in human bites, Clin Orthop 134:320, 1978.

Bingham DLC: Acute infections of the hand, Surg Clin North Am 40:1285, 1960.

Bolton H, Fowler PJ, and Jepson RP: Natural history and treatment of pulp space infection and osteomyelitis of the terminal phalanx, J Bone Joint Surg 31-B:499, 1949.

Burgess RC: Chronic tenosynovitis caused by *Actinobacillus actinomycetemcomitans*, J Hand Surg 12-A:294, 1987.

Burkhalter WE: Deep space infections, Hand Clin 5:553, 1989.

Canales FL, Newmeyer WL III, and Kilgore ES Jr: The treatment of felons and paronychias, Hand Clin 5:515, 1989.

Carter SJ and Mersheimer WL: Infections of the hand, Orthop Clin North Am 1:455, 1970.

Carter SJ, Burman SO, and Mersheimer WL: Treatment of digital tenosynovitis by irrigation with peroxide and oxytetracycline: review of nine cases, Ann Surg 163:645, 1966.

Chow SP, Stroebel AB, Lau JHK, and Collins RJ: *Mycobacterium marinum* infection of deep structures of hand, J Hand Surg 8:568, 1983.

Chow SP, Ip FK, Lau JHK, et al: *Mycobacterium marinum* infection of the hand and wrist: results of conservative treatment in twenty-four cases, J Bone Joint Surg 69-A:1161, 1987.

Chuinard RG and D'Ambrosia RD: Human bite infections of the hand, J Bone Joint Surg 59-A:416, 1977.

Coleman DA: Human bite wounds, Hand Clin 5:561, 1989.

Cortez LM and Pankey GA: *Mycobacterium marinum* infections of the hand: report of three cases and review of the literature, J Bone Joint Surg 55-A:363, 1973.

Covey DC, Nossaman BD, and Albright JA: Ischemic injury of the hand from intra-arterial propylhexedrine injection, J Hand Surg 13-A:58, 1988.

Deenstra W: Synovial hand infection from *Mycobacterium terrae*, J Hand Surg 13-B:335, 1988.

Defibre BK Jr: Bowen's disease of the nail bed: a case presentation and review of the literature, J Hand Surg 3:182, 1978.

Dehaven KE, Wilde AH, and O'Duffy JD: Sporotrichosis arthritis and tenosynovitis: report of a case cured by synovectomy and amphotericin B, J Bone Joint Surg 54-A:874, 1972.

Dellinger EP, Wertz MJ, Miller SD, and Coyle MB: Hand infections: bacteriology and treatment: a prospective study, Arch Surg 123:745, 1988.

DeMello FJ and Leonard MS: *Eikenella corrodens*: a new pathogen, Oral Surg 47:401, 1979.

DiFazio F and Mogan J: Intravenous pyogenic granuloma of the hand, J Hand Surg 14A:310, 1989.

Dreyfuss UY and Singer M: Human bites of the hand: a study of one hundred six patients, J Hand Surg 10-A:884, 1985.

Ellis W: Multiple bone lesions caused by Avian-Battey mycobacteria: report of a case, J Bone Joint Surg 56-B:323, 1974.

Enna CD: Skeletal deformities of the denervated hand in Hansen's disease, J Hand Surg 4:227, 1979.

Entin MA: Infections of the hand, Surg Clin North Am 44:981, 1964.

Feldman F, Auerbach R, and Johnston A: Tuberculous dactylitis in the adult, Am J Roentgenol Radium Ther Nucl Med 112:460, 1971.

Fitzgerald RH Jr, Cooney WP, Washington JA, et al: Bacterial colonization of mutilating hand injuries and its treatment, J Hand Surg 2:85, 1977.

Flynn JE: Modern considerations of major hand infections, N Engl J Med 252:605, 1955.

Fowler JR: Viral infections, Hand Clin 5:613, 1989.

Freeland AE and Senter BS: Septic arthritis and osteomyelitis, Hand Clin 5:533, 1989.

Gang RK; Herpes of a digit, J Hand Surg 14-B:441, 1989.

Glass KD: Factors related to the resolution of treated hand infections, J Hand Surg 7:388, 1982.

Glickel SZ: Hand infections in patients with acquired immunodeficiency syndrome, J Hand Surg 13-A:770, 1988.

Goldner JL: Thumb and finger infections, Am J Surg 28:12, 1962.

Goldstein EJC, Kirby BD, and Finegold SM: Isolation of *Eikenella corrodens* from pulmonary infections, Am Rev Resp Dis 119:55, 1979.

Goldstein EC, Miller T, Citron DM, and Finegold S: Infections following clenched-fist injury: a new perspective, J Hand Surg 3:455, 1978.

Grayson MJ and Saldana MJ: Toxic shock syndrome complicating surgery of the hand, J Hand Surg 12-A:1082, 1987.

Gropper PT, Pisesky WA, Bowen V, and Clement PB: Flexor tenosynovitis caused by *Coccidiodes immitis*, J Hand Surg 8:344, 1983.

Gunther S: *Mycobacterium kansasii* infection in the deep structure. In Flynn JE: Hand surgery, ed 3, Baltimore, 1982, Williams & Wilkins.

Gunther SS and Levy CS: Mycobacterial infections, Hand Clin 5:591, 1989.

Gunther SF, Elliot RC, Brand RL, et al: Experience with atypical mycobacterial infection in the deep structures of the hand, J Hand Surg 2:90, 1977.

Haedicke GJ, Grossman JAI, and Fisher AE: Herpetic whitlow of the digits, J Hand Surg 14-B:443, 1989.

Hennessy MJ and Mosher TF: Mucormycosis infection of an upper extremity, J Hand Surg 6:249, 1981.

Hitchcock TF and Amadio PC: Fungal infections, Hand Clin 5:599, 1989.

Holms W and Ali MA: Acute osteomyelitis of index finger caused by dog bite, J Hand Surg 12-B:137, 1987.

Hooker RP, Eberts TJ, and Strickland JA: Primary inoculation tuberculosis, J Hand Surg 4:270, 1979.

Hurst LC, Amadio PC, Badalamente MA, et al: *Mycobacterium marinum* infections of the hand, J Hand Surg 12-A:428, 1987.

Iverson RE and Vistnes LM: Coccidioidomycosis tenosynovitis in the hand, J Bone Joint Surg 55-A:413, 1973.

Janes PC and Mann RJ: Extracutaneous sporotrichosis, J Hand Surg 12-A:441, 1987.

Jones MW, Wahid IA, and Matthews JP: Septic arthritis of the hand due to *Mycobacterium marinum*, J Hand Surg 13-B:333, 1988.

Kanavel AB: Infections of the hand: a guide to the surgical treatment of acute and chronic suppurative processes in the fingers, hand, and forearm, ed 6, Philadelphia, 1933, Lea & Febiger.

Kaplan JE, Zoschke D, and Kisch AL: Withdrawal of immunosuppressive agents in the treatment of disseminated coccidioidomycosis, Am J Med 68:624, 1980.

Kilgore ES: Hand infections, Part 2, J Hand Surg 5:723, 1983.

Linscheid RL and Dobyns JH: Common and uncommon infections of the hand, Orthop Clin North Am 6:1063, 1975.

Liseki EJ, Curl WW, and Markey KL: Hand and forearm infections caused by *Aeromonas hydrophilia*, J Hand Surg 5:605, 1980.

Long WT, Filler BC, Cox E II, and Stark HH: Toxic shock syndrome after a human bite to the hand, J Hand Surg 13-A:957, 1988.

Loudon JB, Miniero JD, and Scott JC: Infections of the hand, J Bone Joint Surg 30-B:409, 1948.

Louis DS and Silva J Jr: Herpetic whitlow: herpetic infections of the digits, J Hand Surg 4:90, 1979.

Malinowski RW, Strate RG, Perry JF Jr, and Fischer RP: The management of human bite injuries of the hand, J Trauma 19:655, 1979.

Maloon S, de Beer J de V, Opitz M, and Singer M: Acute flexor tendon sheath infections, J Hand Surg 15-A:474, 1990.

Mandel MA: Immune competence and diabetes mellitus: pyogenic human hand infections, J Hand Surg 3:458, 1978.

Mann RJ, Hoffeld TA, and Farmer CB: Human bites of the hand: twenty years of experience, J Hand Surg 2:97, 1977.

Marr JS, Beck AM, and Lugo JA Jr: An epidemiologic study of the human bite, Public Health Rep 94:514, 1979.

Mathews RE, Gould JS, and Kashlan MB: Diffuse pigmented villonodular tenosynovitis of the ulnar bursa, J Hand Surg 6:64, 1981.

McCabe SJ, Murray JF, Ruhnke HL, and Rachlis A: Mycoplasma infection of the hand acquired from a cat, J Hand Surg 12-A:1085, 1987.

McConnell CM and Neale HW: Two-year review of hand infections at a municipal hospital, Am Surg 45:643, 1979.

McDonald I: Eikenella corrodens infection of the hand, Hand 11:224, 1979.

McKay D et al: Infections and sloughs in the hands of drug addicts, J Bone Joint Surg 55-A:741, 1973.

Minkin BI, Mills CL, Bullock DW, and Burke FD: Mycobacterium kansasii osteomyelitis of the scaphoid, J Hand Surg 12-A:1092, 1987.

Nee PA and Lunn PG: Isolated anterior interosseous nerve palsy following herpes zoster infection: case report and review of the literature, J Hand Surg 14-B:447, 1989.

Neviaser RJ: Closed tendon sheath irrigation for pyogenic flexor tenosynovitis, J Hand Surg 3:462, 1978.

Neviaser RJ: Tenosynovitis, Hand Clin 5:525, 1989.

Neviaser RJ and Gunther SF: Tenosynovial infections of the hand—diagnosis and management. I. Acute pyogenic tenosynovitis of the hand, AAOS Instr Course Lect 29:108, 1980.

Newman ED, Harrington TM, Torretti D, and Bush DC: Suppurative extensor tenosynovitis caused by Staphylococcus aureus, J Hand Surg 14-A:849, 1989.

Patzakis MJ, Wilkins J, and Bassett RL: Surgical findings in clenched-fist injuries, Clin Orthop 220:237, 1987.

Peeples E, Boswick JA Jr, and Scott FA: Wounds of the hand contaminated by human or animal saliva, J Trauma 20:393, 1980.

Perlman R, Jubelirer RA, and Schwarz J: Histoplasmosis of the common palmer tendon sheath, J Bone Joint Surg 54-A:676, 1972.

Phair IC and Quinton DN: Clenched fist human bite injuries, J Hand Surg 14-B:86, 1989.

Prince H, Ispahani P, and Baker M: A Mycobacterium malmoense infection of the hand presenting as a carpal tunnel syndrome, J Hand Surg 13-B:328, 1988.

Rayan GM, Flournoy DJ, and Cahill SL: Aerobic mouth flora of the rhesus monkey, J Hand Surg 12-A:299, 1987.

Rayan GM, Putnam JL, Cahill SL, and Flournoy DJ: Eikenella corrodens in human mouth flora, J Hand Surg 13-A:953, 1988.

Reyes FA: Infections secondary to intravenous drug abuse, Hand Clin 5:629, 1989.

Rhode CM: Treatment of hand infections, Am Surg 27:85, 1961.

Robins RHC: Infections of the hand: a review based on 1,000 consecutive cases, J Bone Joint Surg 34-B:567, 1952.

Sanger JR, Stampfl DA, and Franson TR: Recurrent granulomatous synovitis due to Mycobacterium kansasii in a renal transplant recepient, J Hand Surg 12-A:436, 1987.

Schecter WP, Markison RE, Jeffrey RB, et al: Use of sonography in the early dectection of suppurative flexor tenosyonvitis, J Hand Surg 14-A:307, 1989.

Schmidt DR and Heckman JD: Eikenella corrodens in human bite infections of the hand, J Trauma 23:478, 1983.

Scott JC and Jones BV: Results of treatment of infections of the hand, J Bone Joint Surg 34-B:581, 1952.

Sehayik RI and Bassett FH III: Herpes simplex infection involving the hand, Clin Orthop 166:138, 1982.

Shankar S: Diabetes mellitus presenting as "acute osteomyelitis" of the index finger, J Hand Surg 12-B:133, 1987.

Simmons EH, Van Peteghem K, and Trammell TR: Onchocerciasis of the flexor compartment of the forearm: a case report, J Hand Surg 5:502, 1980.

Singer RM and Gorosh JE: Purpura fulminans, J Hand Surg 15-A:172, 1990.

Sinkovics JG, Plager C, and Mills K: Eikenella corrodens as pathogen, Ann Intern Med 90:991, 1979.

Smith J and Ruby LK: Nocardia asteroides thenar space infection: a case report, J Hand Surg 2:109, 1977.

Snyder CC: Animal bite wounds, Hand Clin 5:571, 1989.

Southwick GJ and Lister GD: Actinomycosis of the hand: a case report, J Hand Surg 4:360, 1979.

Spiegel JD and Szabo RM: A protocol for the treatment of severe infections of the hand, J Hand Surg 13-A:254, 1988.

Stark RH: Group B β-hemolytic streptococcal arthritis and osteomyelitis of the wrist, J Hand Surg 12-A:296, 1987.

Stark RH: Mycobacterium avium complex tenosynovitis of the index finger, Orthop Rev 19:345, 1990.

Suso S, Peidro L, and Ramon R: Tuberculosis synovitis with "rice bodies" presenting as carpal tunnel syndrome, J Hand Surg 13-A:574, 1988.

Swanson E, Freiberg A, and Salter DR: Radial artery infections and aneurysms after catherization, J Hand Surg 15-A:166, 1990.

Williams CS and Riordan DC: Mycobacterium marinum (atypical acid-fast bacillus) infections of the hand: a report of six cases, J Bone Joint Surg 55-A:1042, 1973.

Young VL, Fernando B, Tabas M, et al: A case study of pyoderma gangrenosum, J Hand Surg 13-A:259, 1988.

PART XVIII

THE SPINE

CHAPTER 79

Spinal Anatomy and Surgical Approaches

MARVIN R. LEVENTHAL

ANATOMY OF VERTEBRAL COLUMN

The vertebral column is composed of alternating bony vertebrae and fibrocartilaginous discs that are connected by strong ligaments and supported by musculature that extends from the skull to the pelvis and provides axial support to the body. There are 33 vertebrae (7 cervical, 12 thoracic, 5 lumbar, 5 sacral, and 4 coccygeal) (Fig. 79-1). The sacral and coccygeal vertebrae form the sacrum and coccyx. A typical vertebra is composed of an anterior body and a posterior arch made up of two pedicles and two laminae that are united posteriorly to form the spinous process. To either side of the arch of the vertebral body is a transverse process and superior and inferior articular processes. The articular processes articulate with adjacent vertebrae to form synovial joints. The relative orientation of the articular processes accounts for the degree of flexion, extension, or rotation possible in each segment of the vertebral column. The spinous and transverse processes serve as levers for the numerous muscles attached to them. The vertebral bodies increase in size from cephalic to caudal, and this is believed to be the result of the increasing weights and stresses borne by successive segments. The intervertebral discs connecting the vertebral bodies absorb many of the stresses applied to the vertebral column. A disc consists of an outer concentric layer of fibrous tissue known as the *anulus fibrosis* and a central gelatinous portion, the *nucleus pulposus*. At birth the vertebral column is convex dorsally, which forms the predominant sagittal contour; however, when the erect position is acquired compensatory cervical and lumbar lordotic curves develop opposite the primary thoracic and sacral kyphotic curves. The length of the vertebral column averages 72 cm in adult males and 7 to 10 cm less in adult females. The vertebral canal extends throughout the length of the column and provides protection for the spinal cord, conus medullaris, and cauda equina. Nerves and vessels pass through the intervertebral foramina formed by the superior and inferior borders of the pedicles of adjacent vertebrae.

ANATOMY OF THORACIC AND LUMBAR PEDICLES

Pedicle dimensions and angles change progressively from the upper thoracic spine distally. A thorough knowledge of these relationships is important when considering the use of the pedicle as a screw purchase site. Pedicle dimensions have been studied by Zindrick et al., Saillant, and others, and data obtained from these studies have added to the knowledge of pedicle morphologic characteristics and provided information about the depth to which screws may be safely inserted at levels throughout the thoracolumbar spine. In 2905 pedicle measurements made from T1 to L5, pedicles were widest at L5 and narrowest at T5 in the horizontal plane (Fig. 79-2). The widest pedicles in the sagittal plane were at T11, and the narrowest were at T1. Because of the oval shape of the pedicle, the sagittal plane width was generally larger than the horizontal plane width. The largest pedicle angle in the horizontal plane was at L5. In the sagittal plane, the pedicles angle caudad at L5 and cephalad

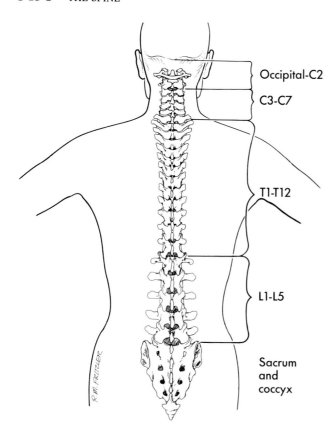

Fig. 79-1 Vertebral column: upper cervical vertebrae (occiput to C2), lower cervical vertebrae (C3-7), thoracic vertebrae (T1-12), lumbar vertebrae (L1-5), sacrum, and coccyx.

Occipital-C2

C3-C7

T1-T12

L1-L5

Sacrum and coccyx

at L3 through T1. The depth to the anterior cortex was significantly longer along the pedicle axis than along a line parallel to the midline of the vertebral body at all levels, with the exception of T12 and L1. The locations for screw insertion have been identified and described by Roy-Camille, Saillant, and Mazel and by Louis. The respective facet joint space and the middle of the transverse process are the most important reference points. An opening is made in the pedicle with a drill or handheld curet, after which a self-tapping screw is passed through the pedicle into the vertebral body. The pedicles of the thoracic and lumbar vertebrae are tube-like bony structures that connect the anterior and posterior columns of the spine. Medial to the medial wall of the pedicle lies the dural sac. Inferior to the medial wall of the pedicle is the nerve root in the neural foramen. The lumbar roots usually are situated in the upper third of the foramen; therefore, it is more dangerous to penetrate the pedicle medially or inferiorly as opposed to laterally or superiorly.

There are three techniques for localization of the pedicle that we use routinely: (1) the intersection technique, (2) the pars interarticularis technique, and (3) the mamillary process technique. It is important in preoperative planning to assess individual spinal anatomy with the use of high-quality anteroposterior and lateral roentgenograms of the lumbar and thoracic spine, as well as

with axial computed tomography (CT) scanning at the level of the pedicle. The intersection technique is perhaps the most commonly used method of localizing the pedicle. It involves dropping a line from the lateral aspect of the facet joint, which intersects a line that bisects the transverse process at a spot overlying the pedicle (Figs. 79-3 and 79-4). The pars interarticularis is that area of bone where the pedicle connects to the lamina. Because the laminae and the pars interarticularis can be easily identified at surgery, they provide landmarks by which a pedicular drill starting point can be made. The mamillary process technique is based on a small prominence of bone at the base of the transverse process. This mamillary process can be used as a starting point for transpedicular drilling. Usually the mamillary process is more lateral than the intersection technique starting point, which is also more lateral than the pars interarticularis starting point. With this in mind, a different angle must be used when drilling from these sites. With the help of preoperative CT scanning at the level of the pedicle and intraoperative roentgenograms, the angle of the pedicle to the sagittal and horizontal planes may be determined.

CIRCULATION OF SPINAL CORD

The arterial supply to the spinal cord has been determined from gross anatomic dissection, latex arterial injections, and intercostal arteriography. Dommisse has contributed most significantly to our knowledge of the blood supply, stating that the principles that govern the blood supply of the cord are constant, whereas the patterns vary with the individual. He emphasizes the following factors:

1. *Dependence on three vessels:* these are the anterior median longitudinal arterial trunk and a pair of posterolateral trunks near the posterior nerve rootlets.
2. *Relative demands of gray matter and white matter:* the longitudinal arterial trunks are largest in the cervical and lumbar regions near the ganglionic enlargements and are much smaller in the thoracic region. This is because the metabolic demands of the gray matter are greater than those of the white matter, which contains fewer capillary networks.
3. *Medullary feeder (radicular) arteries of the cord:* these reinforce the longitudinal arterial channels. There are from 2 to 17 anteriorly and from 6 to 25 posteriorly. The vertebral arteries supply 80% of the radicular arteries in the neck; those in the thoracic and lumbar areas arise from the aorta. The lateral sacral arteries, as well as the fifth lumbar, the iliolumbar, and the middle sacral arteries, are important in the sacral region.
4. *Supplementary source of blood supply to the spinal cord:* the vertebral and posteroinferior cerebellar arteries are important sources of arterial supply. Sacral medullary feeders arise from the lateral sacral

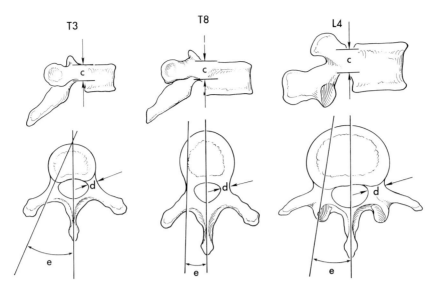

Fig. 79-2   Pedicle dimensions of T3 (**A**), T8 (**B**), and L4 (**C**) vertebrae. Vertical diameter (c) increases from 0.7 to 1.5 cm, horizontal diameter (d) increases from 0.7 to 1.6 cm with minimum of 0.5 cm in T5. Direction is almost sagittal from T4 to L4. Angle (e) seldom extends beyond 10 degrees. More proximally direction is more oblique: T1 = 36 degrees, T2 = 34 degrees, T3 = 23 degrees. L5 is oblique (30 degrees) but is large and easy to drill. (Redrawn from Roy-Camille R, Saillant G, and Mazel Ch: Orthop Clin North Am 17:147, 1986.)

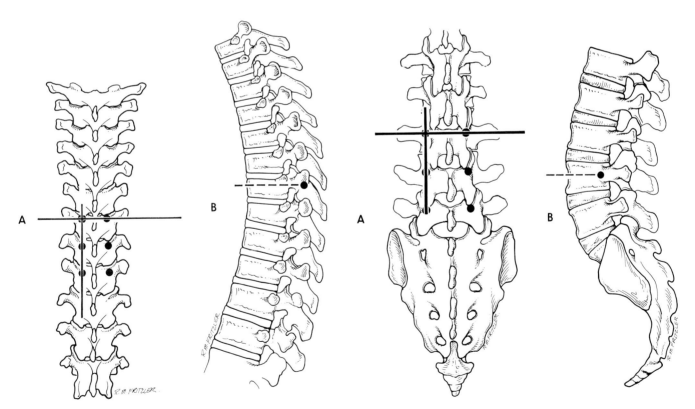

Fig. 79-3   Pedicle entrance point in thoracic spine at intersection of lines drawn through middle of inferior articular facet and middle of insertion of transverse processes (1 mm below facet joint). **A**, Anteroposterior view. **B**, Lateral view. (Redrawn from Roy-Camille R, Saillant G, and Mazel Ch: Orthop Clin North Am 17:147, 1986.)

Fig. 79-4   Pedicle entrance point in lumbar spine at intersection of two lines (see Fig. 79-3). On typical bony crest it is 1 mm below articular joint. **A**, Anteroposterior view. **B**, Lateral view. (Redrawn from Roy-Camille R, Saillant G, and Mazel Ch: Orthop Clin North Am 17:147, 1986.)

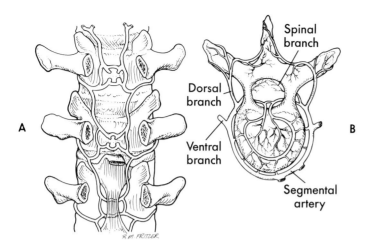

Fig. 79-5 Vertebral blood supply. **A**, Posterior view; laminae removed to show anastomosing spinal branches of segmental arteries. **B**, Cross-sectional view; anastomosing arterial supply of vertebral body, spinal canal, and posterior elements. (Redrawn from Bullough PG and Oheneba B-A: Atlas of spinal diseases, Philadelphia, 1988, JB Lippincott Co.)

arteries and accompany the distal roots of the cauda equina. The flow in these vessels seems reversible and the volume adjustable in response to the metabolic demands.

5. *Segmental arteries of the spine:* at every vertebral level a pair of segmental arteries supplies the extraspinal and intraspinal structures. The thoracic and lumbar segmental arteries arise from the aorta; the cervical segmental arteries arise from the vertebral arteries as well as the costocervical and thyrocervical trunks. In 60% of people an additional source arises from the ascending pharyngeal branch of the external carotid artery. The lateral sacral arteries and to a lesser extent the fifth lumbar, iliolumbar, and middle sacral arteries supply segmental vessels in the sacral region.

6. *"Distribution point" of the segmental arteries:* the segmental arteries divide into numerous branches at the intervertebral foramen, which has been termed the *distribution point* (Fig. 79-5). A second anastomotic network lies within the spinal canal in the loose connective tissue of the extradural space. This occurs at all levels, with the greatest concentration in the cervical and lumbar regions. Undoubtedly the presence of the rich anastomotic channels offers alternative pathways for arterial flow, preserving spinal cord circulation after the ligation of segmental arteries.

7. *Artery of Adamkiewicz:* the artery of Adamkiewicz is the largest of the feeders of the lumbar cord; it is located on the left side, usually at the level of T9-11 (in 80% of people). It is clear that the anterior longitudinal arterial channel of the cord rather than any single medullary feeder is crucial. Equally clear is that the preservation of this large feeder does not

ensure continued satisfactory circulation for the spinal cord. In principle it would seem of practical value to protect and preserve each contributing artery as far as is surgically possible.

8. *Variability of patterns of supply of the spinal cord:* the variability of blood supply is a striking feature, yet there is absolute conformity with a principle of a rich supply for the cervical and lumbar cord enlargements. The supply for the thoracic cord from approximately T4-9 is much poorer.

9. *Direction of flow in the blood vessels of the spinal cord:* the three longitudinal arterial channels of the spinal cord can be compared with the circle of Willis at the base of the brain, but it is more extensive and more complicated, although it functions with identical principles. These channels permit reversal of flow and alterations in the volume of blood flow in response to metabolic demands. This internal arterial circle of the cord is surrounded by at least two outer arterial circles, the first of which is situated in the extradural space and the second in the extravertebral tissue planes. It is by virtue of the latter that the spinal cord enjoys reserve sources of supply through a degree of anastomosis lacking in the inner circle. The "outlet points," however, are limited to the perforating sulcal arteries and the pial arteries of the cord.

In summary, the blood supply to the spinal cord is rich, but the spinal canal is narrowest and the blood supply is poorest from T4-9. This should be considered the critical vascular zone of the spinal cord, a zone in which interference with the circulation is most likely to result in paraplegia.

The dominance of the anterior spinal artery system has been challenged by the fact that much anterior spinal surgery has been performed in recent years with no increase in the incidence of paralysis. This would seem to indicate that a rich anastomotic supply does exist and that it protects the spinal cord. The evidence suggests that the posterior spinal arteries may be as important as the anterior system but are as yet poorly understood. Venous drainage of the spinal cord is more difficult to clearly define than is the arterial supply (Fig. 79-6). It is well-known that the venous system is highly variable. Dommisse points out that there are two sets of veins: those of the spinal cord and those that fall within the plexiform network of Batson. The veins of the spinal cord are a small component of the entire system and drain into the plexus of Batson. Batson's plexus is a large and complex venous channel extending from the base of the skull to the coccyx. It communicates directly with the superior and inferior vena caval system and the azygos system. The longitudinal venous trunks of the spinal cord are the anterior and posterior venous channels, which are the counterparts of the arterial trunks. The three components of Batson's plexus are the extradural vertebral venous plexus; the extravertebral venous

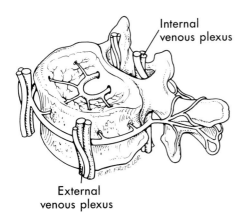

Internal
venous plexus

External
venous plexus

Fig. 79-6   Venous drainage of vertebral bodies and formation of internal and external vertebral venous plexuses. (Redrawn from Bullough PG and Oheneba B-A: Atlas of spinal diseases, Philadelphia, 1988, JB Lippincott Co.)

plexus, which includes the segmental veins of the neck, the intercostal veins, the azygos communications in the thorax and pelvis, the lumbar veins, and the communications with the inferior vena caval system; and the veins of the bony structures of the spinal column. The venous system plays no specific role in the metabolism of the spinal cord; it communicates directly with the venous system draining the head, chest, and abdomen. This interconnection allows metastatic spread of neoplastic or infectious disease from the pelvis to the vertebral column.

During anterior spinal surgery, we empirically follow these principles: (1) ligate segmental spinal arteries only as necessary to gain exposure; (2) ligate segmental spinal arteries near the aorta rather than near the vertebral foramina; (3) ligate segmental spinal arteries on one side only when possible, leaving the circulation intact on the opposite side; and (4) limit dissection in the vertebral foramina to a single level when possible so that collateral circulation is disturbed as little as possible.

SURGICAL APPROACHES
Anterior Approaches

With the posterior approach for correction of spinal deformities well established, in recent years more attention has been placed on the anterior approach to the spinal column. Many pioneers in the field of anterior spinal surgery recognized that anterior spinal cord decompression was necessary in spinal tuberculosis and that laminectomy not only failed to relieve anterior pressure but also removed important posterior stability and produced worsening of kyphosis. Advances in major surgical procedures, including anesthesia and intensive care, have made it possible to perform spinal surgery with acceptable safety.

Common use of the anterior approach for spinal surgery did not evolve until the 1950s. Leaders in the anterior approach to the cervical and lumbar areas have been Cloward; Southwick and Robinson; Bailey and Badgley; Bohlman; and others. The transthoracic approach to the thoracic spine has developed more slowly. Nachlas and Borden, and Smith, von Lackum, and Wylie were among the first to report their experiences; however, the major proponents of this technique were Hodgson et al. of Hong Kong. Their reports of success with this method received worldwide acceptance.

In general, anterior approaches to the spine are indicated for decompression of the neural elements (spinal cord, conus medullaris, cauda equina, or nerve roots) when anterior neural compression has been documented by myelography, postmyelogram CT scanning, or magnetic resonance imaging (MRI). A number of pathologic entities can cause significant compression of the neural elements, including traumatic, neoplastic, inflammatory, degenerative, and congenital lesions.

Anterior approaches to the spine generally are performed by an experienced spine surgeon and, as a rule, this type of surgery is not appropriate for those who only occasionally perform spinal techniques. In many centers, a team approach is preferred to use the skill of the orthopaedic surgeon, neurosurgeon, thoracic surgeon, or head and neck surgeon. The orthopaedic surgeon still must have a working knowledge of the underlying viscera, fluid balance, physiology, and other elements of intensive care. Complications of anterior spine surgery are rare; however, there is a high risk of significant morbidity and these approaches should be used with care and only in appropriate circumstances. Potential dangers include iatrogenic injury to vascular, visceral, or neurologic structures.

The exact incidence of serious complications from anterior spinal surgery is not known. A thorough understanding of anatomic tissue planes and meticulous surgical technique are necessary to prevent serious complications. The choice of approach depends on the preference and experience of the surgeon, the patient's age and medical condition, the segment of the spine involved, the underlying pathologic process, and the presence or absence of signs of neural compression. Commonly accepted indications for anterior approaches are listed in Table 79-1.

ANTERIOR APPROACH FROM OCCIPUT TO C3. The anterior approach to the upper cervical spine (occiput to C3) may be either transoral or retropharyngeal, depending on the pathologic process present and the experience of the surgeon.

Anterior Transoral Approach

■ *TECHNIQUE (SPETZLER) (FIG. 79-7).* Position the patient supine using a Mayfield head-holding device or with skeletal traction through Gardner-Wells tongs. Monitoring of the spinal cord through somatosensory evoked potentials is recommended. The surgeon may sit directly over the patient's head. Pass a

Table 79-1 Relative indications for anterior spinal approaches

A. Traumatic
  1. Fractures with documented neurocompression secondary to bone or disc fragments anterior to dura
  2. Incomplete spinal cord injury (for cord recovery) with anterior extradural compression
  3. Complete spinal cord injury (for root recovery) with anterior extradural compression
  4. Late pain or paralysis after remote injuries with anterior extradural compression
  5. Herniated intervertebral disc
B. Infectious
  1. Open biopsy for diagnosis
  2. Debridement and anterior strut grafting
C. Degenerative
  1. Cervical spondylitic radiculopathy
  2. Cervical spondylitic myelopathy
  3. Thoracic disc herniation
  4. Cervical, thoracic, and lumbar interbody fusions
D. Neoplastic
  1. Extradural metastatic disease
  2. Primary vertebral body tumor
E. Deformity
  1. Kyphosis — congenital or acquired
  2. Scoliosis — congenital, acquired, or idiopathic

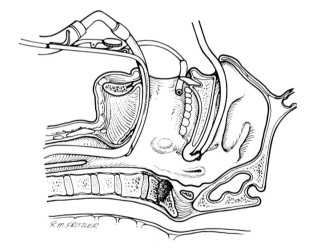

Fig. 79-7 Anterior transoral approach (see text). (Redrawn from Spetzler RF: Transoral approach to the upper cervical spine. In Evarts CM, editor: Surgery of the musculoskeletal system, New York, 1983, Churchill Livingstone.)

red rubber catheter down each nostril and suture it to the uvula. Apply traction to the catheters to pull the uvula and soft palate out of the operative field, taking care not to necrose the septal cartilage by excessive pressure. Insert a McGarver retractor into the open mouth and use it to retract and hold the endotracheal tube out of the way. The operating microscope is useful to improve the limited exposure. Prepare the oropharynx with pHisoHex and Betadine. Palpate the anterior ring of C1 beneath the posterior pharynx, and make an incision in the wall of the posterior pharynx from the superior aspect of C1 to the top of C3. Obtain hemostasis with bipolar electrocautery, taking care not to overcauterize, thereby producing thermal necrosis of tissue and increased risk of infection.

With a periosteal elevator subperiosteally dissect the edges of the pharyngeal incision from the anterior ring of C1 and the anterior aspect of C2. Use traction stitches to maintain the flaps out of the way. Next, under direct vision, with either the operating microscope or with magnification loupes and headlights, perform a meticulous debridement of C1 and C2 with a high-speed air drill, rongeur, or curet. When approaching the posterior longitudinal ligament, a diamond burr is safer to use in removing the last remnant of bone. Once adequate debridement of infected bone and necrotic tissue has been accomplished, decompress the upper cervical spinal cord. If the cervical spine is to be fused anteriorly, harvest a corticocancellous graft from the patient's iliac crest, fashion it to fit, and insert it. Irrigate the operative site with antibiotic solution and close the posterior pharynx in layers.

AFTERTREATMENT. An endotracheal tube is left in place overnight to maintain an adequate airway. A halo vest can then be applied or skeletal traction may be maintained before mobilization.

Anterior retropharyngeal approach. This approach to the upper cervical spine, as described by McAfee et al., is excellent for anterior debridement of the upper cervical spine and allows placement of bone grafts for stabilization if necessary. Unlike the transoral approach, it is entirely extramucosal and is reported to have fewer complications of wound infection and neurologic deficit.

■ *TECHNIQUE (McAFEE ET AL.).* Position the patient supine, preferably on a turning frame with skeletal traction through tongs or a halo ring. Somatosensory evoked potential monitoring of cord function is suggested during the procedure. Perform fiberoptic nasoltracheal intubation to prevent excessive motion of the neck and to keep the oral pharynx free of tubes that could depress the mandible and interfere with subsequent exposure.

Make a right-sided transverse skin incision in the submandibular region with a vertical extension as

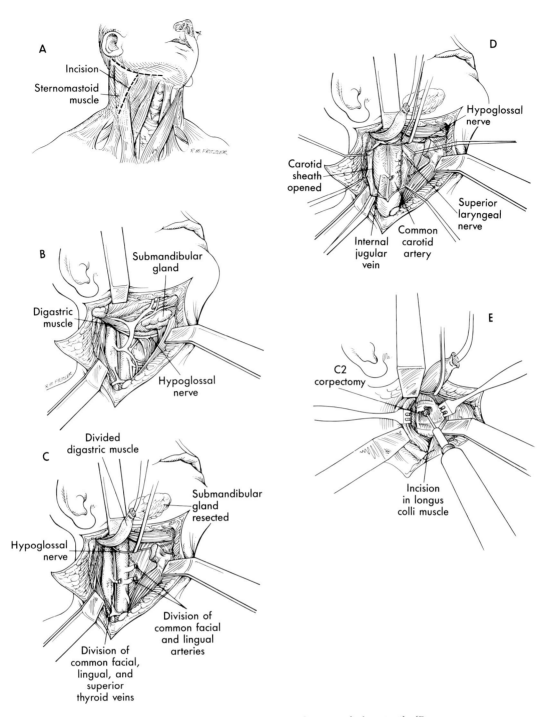

A
Incision
Sternomastoid muscle

B
Submandibular gland
Digastric muscle
Hypoglossal nerve

C
Divided digastric muscle
Submandibular gland resected
Hypoglossal nerve
Division of common facial, lingual, and superior thyroid veins
Division of common facial and lingual arteries

D
Hypoglossal nerve
Carotid sheath opened
Superior laryngeal nerve
Internal jugular vein
Common carotid artery

E
C2 corpectomy
Incision in longus colli muscle

Fig. 79-8   Anterior retropharyngeal approach (see text). (Redrawn from McAffee PC, Bohlman HH, Riley LH Jr, et al: J Bone Joint Surg 69-A:1371, 1987.)

long as required to provide adequate exposure (Fig. 79-8, *A*). If the approach does not have to be extended below the level of the fifth cervical vertebra, there is no increased risk of damage to the recurrent laryngeal nerve.

Carry the dissection through the platysma muscle with the enveloping superficial fascia of the neck and mobilize flaps from this area. Identify the marginal mandibular branch of the seventh nerve with the help of a nerve stimulator and ligate the retromandibular veins superiorly. Keep the dissection deep to the retromandibular vein to prevent injury to the superficial branches of the facial nerve. Ligate the retromandibular vein as it joins the internal jugular vein. Next, mobilize the anterior border of the sternocleidomastoid muscle by longitudinally dividing the superficial layer of the deep cervical fascia. Feel for the pulsations of the carotid artery and take care to protect the contents of the carotid sheath. Resect the submandibular gland (Fig. 78-8, *B*) and ligate the duct to prevent formation of a salivary fistula. Identify the digastric and stylohyoid muscles and tag and divide the tendon of the former. It is important to emphasize that the facial nerve can be injured by superior retraction on the stylohyoid muscle; however, by dividing the digastric and stylohyoid muscles, the hyoid bone and hypopharynx can be mobilized medially, preventing exposure of the esophagus, hypopharynx, and nasopharynx. Next, identify the hypoglossal nerve and retract it superiorly. Continue dissection to the retropharyngeal space between the carotid sheath laterally and the larynx and pharynx medially. Increase exposure by ligating branches of the carotid artery and internal jugular vein, which prevent retraction of the carotid sheath laterally (Fig. 79-8, *C* and *D*). Identify and mobilize the superior laryngeal nerve. Following adequate retraction of the carotid sheath laterally, divide the alar and prevertebral fascial layers longitudinally to expose the longus colli muscles. Take care to maintain the head in a neutral position and accurately identify the midline. Remove the longus colli muscles subperiosteally from the anterior aspect of the arch of C1 and the body of C2, taking care to avoid injury to the vertebral arteries. Next, meticulously debride the involved osseous structures (Fig. 79-8, *E*) and, if needed, perform bone grafting with either autogenous iliac or fibular bone.

Close the wound over suction drains and repair the digastric tendon. Close the platysma and skin flaps in layers.

AFTERTREATMENT. The patient is maintained in skeletal traction with the head of the bed elevated to reduce swelling. Intubation is continued until pharyngeal edema has resolved, usually by 48 hours. The patient may then be extubated and mobilized in a halo vest or if indicated a posterior stabilization procedure may be performed before mobilization.

Extended maxillotomy and subtotal maxillectomy. Cocke et al. have described an extended maxillotomy and subtotal maxillectomy as an alternative to the transoral approach for exposure and removal of tumor or bone anteriorly at the base of the skull and cervical spine to C5. This approach has been used in a limited number of procedures and the indications are not firmly established. It is technically demanding and requires a thorough knowledge of head and neck anatomy. It should be performed by a team of surgeons, including an otolaryngologist, a neurosurgeon, and an orthopaedist.

Before surgery the size, position, and extent of the tumor or bone to be removed should be determined, using the appropriate imaging techniques. Three to five days before the surgery nasal, oral, and pharyngeal secretions are cultured to determine the proper antibiotics needed. Cephalosporin and aminoglycoside antibiotics are given before and after surgery if the floral cultures are normal, and are adjusted if the flora is abnormal or resistant to these drugs.

Subtotal maxillectomy

■ *TECHNIQUE (COCKE ET AL.).* Position the patient on the operating table with the head elevated 25 degrees. Intubate the patient orally and move the tube to the contralateral side of the mouth. Perform a percutaneous endoscopic gastrostomy (PEG) if the wound is to be left open or if problems are anticipated. Perform a tracheostomy if the exposure may be limited or if there are severe pulmonary problems. This step is usually unnecessary.

Insert a Foley catheter and suture the eyelids closed with 6-0 nylon. Infiltrate the soft tissues of the upper lip, cheek, gingiva, palate, pterygoid fossa, nasopharynx, nasal septum, nasal floor, and lateral nasal wall with 1% lidocaine with 1:100,000 epinephrine. Pack each nasal cavity with cottonoid strips saturated with 4% cocaine and 1% phenylephrine. Prepare the skin with Betadine, dried with alcohol. Drape the operative site with cloth drapes held in place with sutures or surgical clips and covered with a transparent surgical drape.

Expose the superior maxilla through a modified Weber-Ferguson skin incision (Fig. 79-9, *A*). Make a vertical incision through the upper lip in the philtrum from the nasolabial groove to the vermilion border. Extend the lower end to the midline and then vertically in the midline through the buccal mucosa to the gingivobuccal gutter. Divide the upper lip and ligate the labial arteries. Extend the external skin incision transversely from the upper end of the lip incision in the nasolabial groove to beyond the nasal ala and then superiorly along the nasofacial groove to the lower eyelid. Extract the central incisor tooth (Fig. 79-9, *B*). Make a vertical midline incision through the mucoperiosteum of the anterior maxilla from the gingivobuccal gutter to the central incisor defect, and then transversely through the buccal gingiva adjacent to the teeth to the retromolar region. Elevate the skin, subcutaneous tissues, periosteum, and mucoperiosteum of the maxilla to expose the anterior and lateral walls of the maxilla, nasal bone, piriform aperture of the nose, inferior orbital nerve, malar bone, and masseter muscle. Divide the anterior margin of the masseter muscle at its malar attachment and remove a wedge of malar bone. Use this wedge to accommodate the Gigli saw as it divides the maxilla (Fig. 79-9, *C*). Make an incision in the lingual, hard palate mucoperiosteum adjacent to the teeth from the central incisor defect to join the retromolar incision. Extend the retromolar incision medial to the mandible lateral to the tonsil and to the retropharyngeal space to the level of the hyoid bone or lower pharynx, if necessary. Elevate the mucoperiosteum of the hard palate from the central incisor defect and alveolar ridge to and beyond the midline of the hard palate. Detach the soft palate with its nasal lining from the

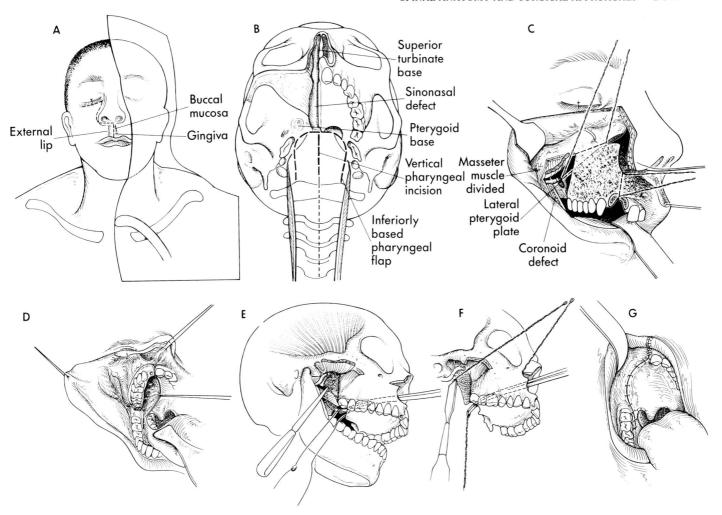

Fig. 79-9 Extended maxillotomy and subtotal maxillectomy (see text). (Redrawn from Cocke EW Jr, Robertson JH, Robertson JR, and Crook JP Jr: Arch Otolaryngol Head Neck Surg 116:92, 1990.)

posterior margin of the hard palate. Divide and electrocoagulate the greater palatine vessels and nerves. Pack the palatine foramen with bone wax. Retract the mucoperiosteum of the hard palate, the soft palate, anterior tonsillar pillar, tonsil, and pharynx medially from the prevertebral fascia. It is usually unnecessary to detach and retract the soft palate from the posterior or lateral pharyngeal walls. Expose the nasal cavity by detaching the nasal soft tissues from the lateral margin and base of the nasal piriform aperture (Fig. 79-9, *B*). Remove a bony wedge of the ascending process of the maxilla to accommodate the upper Gigli saw (Fig. 79-9, *C*). Remove the coronoid process of the mandible above the level of entrance of the inferior alveolar vessels and nerves, after dividing its temporalis muscle attachment, to expose the lateral pterygoid plate and the internal maxillary artery. Divide the pterygoid muscles with the Shaw knife or the cutting current of the Bovie cautery until the sharp, posterior bone edge of the lateral pterygoid plate is seen or palpated. Mobilize,

clip, ligate, and divide the internal maxillary artery near the pterygoid plate. Position the upper Gigli saw (Fig. 79-9, *C*) using a sharp-pointed, medium-sized, curved, right-angled ligature carrier threaded with a No. 2 black silk suture. Direct the suture behind the lateral pterygoid plate into the nasopharynx and behind the posterior margin of the hard palate into the oropharynx. Pass a Kelly forceps through the nose to behind the hard palate to retrieve the medial end of the silk suture in the ligature carrier. Attach a Gigli saw to the lateral end of the suture. Thread the saw into position to divide the upper maxilla. Engage the medial arm of the saw into the ascending process wedge and its lateral arm into the malar wedge. Take care to position the saw as high as possible behind the pterygoid plate. Use a broad periosteal elevator beneath the saw on the pterygoid plate to maintain the elevated position (Fig. 79-9, *D*). Position the lower Gigli saw by passing a Kelly forceps (Fig. 79-9, *E*) through the nose into the nasopharynx behind the posterior naring of the hard palate. Engage the saw between the blades of the clamp and thread it through the nose into position for division of the hard palate. Divide the bony walls of the maxilla (Fig. 79-9, *E*). First divide the hard palate and then the upper maxilla. Take care to avoid entangling the saws and protect the soft tissues from injury. Remove the maxilla after division of its muscle attachments. Ligate the distal end of the internal maxillary artery. Place traction sutures in the soft tissues of the lip on either side of the initial lip incision and in the mucoperiosteum of the hard and soft palates. The posterior pharynx is now fully exposed.

Infiltrate the mucous membrane covering the posterior wall of the nasopharynx, oropharynx, and the tonsillar area to the level of the hyoid bone with 1% lidocaine and epinephrine 1:100,000. Make a vertical midline incision through the soft tissues of the posterior wall of the nasopharynx extending from the sphenoid sinus to the foramen magnum. Another option is to make a transverse incision from the sphenoid to the lateral nasopharyngeal wall posterior to the eustacian tube along the lateral pharyngeal wall inferiorly posterior to the posterior tonsillar pillar behind the soft palate. Duplicate this incision on the opposite side producing an inferiorly based pharyngeal flap (Fig. 79-9, *F*). Make a more extensive exposure by extending the lateral pharyngeal wall incision through the anterior tonsillar pillar to join the retromolar incision. Extend this incision into the retropharyngeal space and retract the anterior tonsillar pillar, tonsil, and soft palate toward the midline with a traction suture. It is unnecessary to completely separate the soft palate from the pharyngeal wall. Extend the pharyngeal wall incision inferiorly to the level of the hyoid bone or beyond. Elevate, divide, and separate the superior constrictor muscle, prevertebral fascia, longus capitus muscle, and anterior longitudinal ligaments from the bony skull base and upper cervical spine ventrally. Expose the amount of bone to be operated on up to the foramen magnum to C5. Use an operating microscope and/or loupe magnification for improved vision. Remove the offending bone with a high-speed burr, taking care to avoid penetration of the dura.

Close the nasopharyngeal mucous membrane and the subcutaneous tissue in one layer with interrupted sutures. Use a split-thickness skin or dermal graft from the thigh to resurface the buccal mucosa and any defects in the nasal surface of the hard palate. Use a quilting stitch to hold the graft in place without packing. Replace the zygoma and stabilize it with wire if it was mobilized. Return the maxilla to its original position and hold it in place with wire or compression plates. Place a nylon sack impregnated with antibiotic into the nasal cavity. Close the

oral cavity incision with vertical interrupted mattress 3-0 polyglycolic acid sutures (Fig. 79-9, *G*). Close the facial wound with 5-0 chromic and 6-0 nylon sutures.

Extended maxillotomy

■ *TECHNIQUE.* Expose the base of the skull and upper cervical spine as by the maxillectomy technique, but omit the extraction of the central incisor and the gingivolingual incision. Use a degloving procedure for elevation of the facial skin over the maxilla and nose to avoid facial scars. Divide the fibromuscular attachment of the soft palate to the pterygoid plate and hard palate exposing the nasopharynx. Place the upper Gigli saw with the aid of a ligature carrier for division of the maxilla beneath the infraorbital nerve. Elevate the mucoperiosteum of the adjacent floor of the nose from the piriform aperture to the soft palate. Extend this elevation medially to the nasal septum and laterally to the inferior turbinate. Divide the bone of the nasal floor with a Stryker saw without lacerating the underlying hard palate periosteum. Hinge the maxilla on the hard palate and nasal mucoperiosteum as well as the soft palate and rotate it medially.

AFTERTREATMENT. Continuous spinal fluid drainage is maintained and the head is elevated 45 degrees if the dura was repaired or replaced. These are omitted if there was no dural tear or defect. An ice cap is used on the cheek and temple to reduce edema. Antibiotic therapy is continued until the risk of infection is minimized. Half-strength hydrogen peroxide is used for mouth irrigations to help keep the oral cavity clean. The endotracheal tube is removed when the risk of occlusion by swelling is minimized. The nasopharyngeal cavity is cleaned with saline twice daily for 2 months after pack removal. Facial sutures are removed at 4 to 6 days and oral sutures at 2 weeks.

ANTERIOR APPROACH TO C3-7. Exposure of the middle and lower cervical region of the spine is most commonly carried out through an anterior approach medial to the carotid sheath. A thorough knowledge of anatomic fascial planes, as described by Southwick and Robinson in 1957, allows a safe, direct approach to this area.

■ *TECHNIQUE (SOUTHWICK AND ROBINSON).* As with other approaches to the cervical spine, skeletal traction is suggested and spinal cord monitoring should be employed. Exposure may be carried out through either a transverse or longitudinal incision, depending on the surgeon's preference (Fig. 79-10, *A*). A left-sided skin incision is preferred because of more constant anatomy of the recurrent laryngeal nerve and less risk of inadvertent injury to the nerve. In general, an incision 3 to 4 fingerbreadths above the clavicle will be needed to expose C3-5 and an inci-

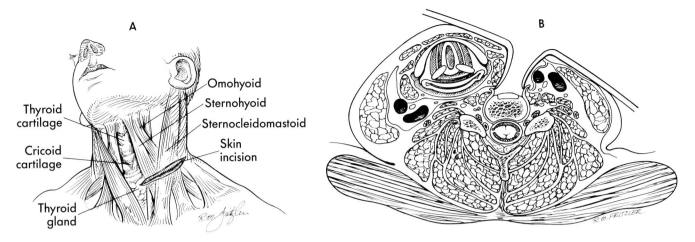

Fig. 79-10 Anterior approach to C3-7 (see text). **A**, Incision. **B**, Thyroid gland, trachea, and esophagus have been retracted medially, and carotid sheath and its contents retracted laterally in opposite direction.

sion 2 to 3 fingerbreadths above the clavicle will allow exposure of C5-7.

Center a transverse incision over the medial border of the sternocleidomastoid muscle. Infiltration of the skin and subcutaneous tissue with a 1:500,000 epinephrine solution will assist with hemostasis. Incise the platysma muscle in line with the skin incision or open it vertically for more exposure. Identify the anterior border of the sternocleidomastoid muscle and longitudinally incise the superficial layer of the deep cervical fascia and localize the carotid pulse by palpation. Carefully divide the middle layer of deep cervical fascia that encloses the omohyoid medial to the carotid sheath. As the sternomastoid and carotid sheath are retracted laterally, the anterior aspect of the cervical spine can be palpated. Identify the esophagus lying posterior to the trachea and retract the trachea, esophagus, and thyroid medially (Fig. 79-10, *B*). Bluntly divide the deep layers of the deep cervical fascia consisting of the pretracheal and prevertebral fascia overlying the longus colli muscles. Subperiosteally reflect the longus colli from the anterior aspect of the spine out laterally to the level of the uncovertebral joints. The resulting exposure is sufficient for wide debridement and bone grafting.

Close the wound over a drain to prevent hematoma formation and possible airway obstruction. Approximate the platysma and skin edges in routine fashion.

ANTERIOR APPROACH TO CERVICOTHORACIC JUNCTION, C7 TO T1. The cervicothoracic junction is without ready anterior access. The rapid transition from cervical lordosis to thoracic kyphosis results in an abrupt change in the depth of the wound. Also this is a confluent area of vital structures that are not readily retracted. The three approaches to this area include (1) low anterior cervical, (2) high transthoracic, and (3) transsternal.

The low anterior cervical approach provides access to T1 at the inferior extent and the lower cervical spine at the superior extent of the dissection. Exposure is limited at the upper thoracic region, but generally is adequate for placement of a strut graft if needed. Individual anatomic structure should be considered carefully in preoperative planning.

Low anterior cervical approach

■ *TECHNIQUE.* Enter on the left side by a transverse incision placed 1 fingerbreadth above the clavicle. Extend it well across the midline, taking particular care when dissecting about the carotid sheath in the area of entry of the thoracic duct. The latter approaches the jugular vein from its lateral side, but variations are not uncommon. Further steps in exposure follow those of the conventional anterior cervical approach.

High transthoracic approach

■ *TECHNIQUE.* A kyphotic deformity of the thoracic spine tends to force the cervical spine into the chest, in which instance a high transthoracic approach is a logical choice. Make a periscapular incision (Fig. 79-11) and remove the second or third rib; removing the latter is necessary to provide sufficient working space in a child or if a kyphotic deformity is present. This exposes the interval between C6 and T4. Excision of the first or second rib is adequate in adults or in the absence of an exaggerated kyphosis.

• • •

For equal exposure of the thoracic and cervical spine from C4 to T4, the sternal splitting approach described by Hodgson et al. and Fang, Ong, and Hodgson is recommended; it is commonly used in cardiac surgery.

Transsternal approach

■ *TECHNIQUE.* Make a Y-shaped or straight incision with the vertical segment passing along the midster-

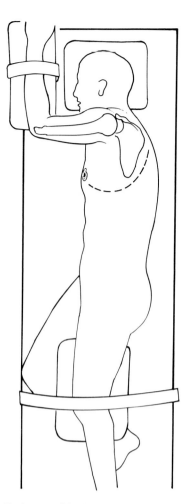

Fig. 79-11 Patient positioning and periscapular incision for high transthoracic approach.

nal area from the suprasternal notch to just below the xiphoid process (Fig. 79-12, *A*). Next, extend the proximal end diagonally to the right and left along the base of the neck for a short distance. To avoid entering the abdominal cavity, take care to keep the dissection beneath the periosteum while exposing the distal end of the sternum. At the proximal end of the sternal notch take care to avoid the inferior thyroid vein. By blunt dissection reflect the parietal pleura from the posterior surfaces of the sternum and costal cartilages, and develop a space. Pass one finger or an instrument above and below the suprasternal space, insert a Gigli saw, and split the sternum. Now spread the split sternum and gain access to the center of the chest (Fig. 79-12, *B*). In children the upper portion of the exposure will be posterior to the thymus and bounded by the innominate and carotid arteries and their venous counterparts. Next, develop the left side of this area bluntly. In patients with kyphotic deformity the innominate vein may now be divided as it crosses the field; it may be very tense and subject to rupture. This division is recommended by Fang et al.. The disadvantage of ligation is that it leaves a slight postoperative enlargement of the left upper extremity that is not apparent unless carefully assessed. This approach

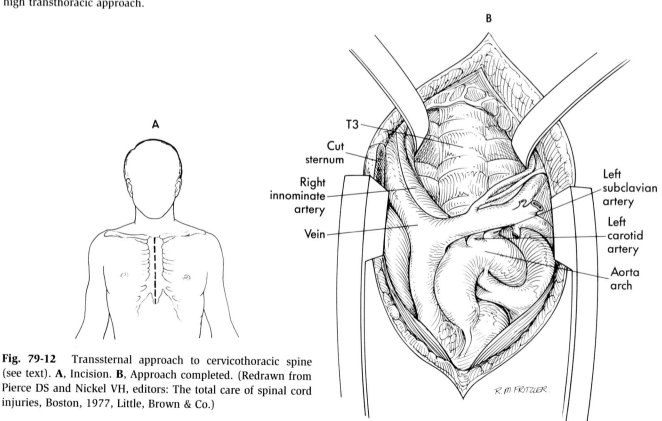

Fig. 79-12 Transsternal approach to cervicothoracic spine (see text). **A**, Incision. **B**, Approach completed. (Redrawn from Pierce DS and Nickel VH, editors: The total care of spinal cord injuries, Boston, 1977, Little, Brown & Co.)

provides limited access, and its success depends on accuracy in preoperative interpretation of the deformity and a high degree of surgical precision.

ANTERIOR APPROACH TO THORACIC SPINE. The transthoracic approach to the thoracic spine provides direct access to the vertebral bodies from T2-12. Clearly, the midthoracic vertebral bodies are best exposed by this approach, while views of the upper and lower extremes of the spine are more limited. In general, a left-sided thoracotomy incision is preferred, although some surgeons favor a right-sided thoracotomy for approaching the upper thoracic spine to avoid the subclavian and carotid arteries in the left superior mediastinum. In a left-sided thoracotomy approach the heart may be retracted anteriorly, whereas in the right-sided approach the liver may present a significant obstacle to exposure. The level of the incision should be positioned to meet the level of exposure required. Ordinarily an intercostal space is selected at or just above the involved segment. When only one vertebral segment is involved, the rib at that level can be removed; however, if multiple levels are involved the rib at the upper level of the proposed dissection should be removed. Because of the normal thoracic kyphosis, dissection is easier from proximal to distal. Exposure is improved by resection of a rib, and the rib provides a satisfactory bone graft, but resection is not necessary if a limited exposure is adequate for biopsy, decompression, or fusion. The transthoracic approach adds a significant operative risk and certainly is more hazardous than the more commonly used posterior or posterolateral approaches. The increased risk of thoracotomy must be weighed against the more limited exposure provided by alternative posterior approaches.

■ *TECHNIQUE.* Place the patient in the lateral decubitus position with the right side down; an inflatable beanbag is helpful in maintaining the patient's position and the table may be flexed to increase exposure (Fig. 79-13, *A*). Make an incision over the rib corresponding to the involved vertebra and expose it subperiosteally. Use electrocautery to maintain hemostasis during the exposure. Disarticulate the rib from the transverse process and the hemifacets of the vertebral body. Take care to identify and preserve the intercostal nerve lying along the inferior aspect of the rib as it localizes the neural foramen leading into the spinal canal. Incise the parietal pleura and reflect it off of the spine, usually one vertebra above and one below the involved segment to allow adequate exposure for debridement and grafting (Fig. 79-13, *B*). Identify the segmental vessels crossing the midportion of each vertebral body and ligate and divide these (Fig. 79-13, *C*). Carefully reflect the periosteum overlying the spine with elevators to expose the involved vertebrae. Use a small elevator to clearly delineate the pedicle of the vertebrae and a Kerrison rongeur to remove the pedicle,

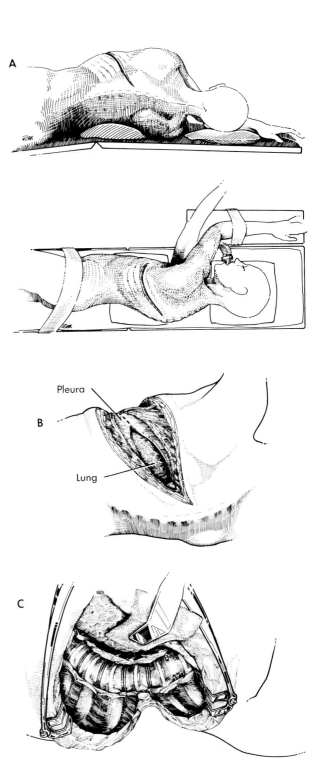

Fig. 79-13 Transthoracic approach (see text). **A**, Positioning of patient and incision. **B**, Rib removal and division of pleura, exposing lung. **C**, Exposure of spine and division of segmental vessels over one vertebral body.

thus exposing the dural sac. Identify the disc spaces above and below the vertebrae and incise the anulus. Remove disc material using rongeurs and curets. An entire cross section of the vertebral body is thus developed, and the anterior margin of the neural canal is identified with the posterior longitudinal ligament lying in the slight concavity on the back of the vertebral body. Expose sufficient segmental vessels and disc spaces to accomplish the intended procedure — usually corpectomy and strut grafting.

ANTERIOR APPROACH TO THORACOLUMBAR JUNCTION. Occasionally, it may be necessary to expose simultaneously the lower thoracic and upper lumbar vertebral bodies. Technically this is a more difficult exposure because of the presence of the diaphragm and the increased risk involved in simultaneous exposure of the thoracic cavity and the retroperitoneal space. In most instances, thoracic lesions should be exposed through the chest, while lesions predominantly involving the upper lumbar spine may be exposed through an anterior retroperitoneal incision. The diaphragm is a dome-shaped organ that is muscular in the periphery and tendinous in the center. Posteriorly, it originates from the upper lumbar vertebrae through crura, the arcuate ligaments, and the twelfth ribs. Anteriorly and laterally, it attaches to the cartilaginous ends of the lower six ribs and xiphoid. The diaphragm is innervated by the phrenic nerve, which descends through the thoracic cavity on the pericardium. The phrenic nerve joins the diaphragm adjacent to the fibrous pericardium, dividing into three major branches that extend peripherally in anterolateral and posterior directions. Division of these major branches may interfere with diaphragmatic function. It is best to make an incision around the periphery of the diaphragm to minimize interference with function when performing a thoracoabdominal approach to the spine. We recommend a left-sided approach at the thoracolumbar junction, since the vena cava on the right is less tolerant of dissection and may result in troublesome hemorrhage and, in addition, the liver may be hard to retract.

■ *TECHNIQUE.* Place the patient in the right lateral decubitus position and place supports beneath the buttock and shoulder. Make the incision curvilinear with ability to extend either the cephalad or caudal end (Fig. 79-14, *A*). To best gain access to the interval of T12 to L1, resect the tenth rib, which allows exposure between T10 and L2. The only difficulty is in identifying the diaphragm as a separate structure; it tends to closely approximate the wall of the thoracic cage, allowing the edge of the lung to penetrate into the space beneath the knife as the pleura is divided (Fig. 79-14, *B*). Now take care in entering the abdominal cavity. Since the transversalis fascia and the peritoneum do not diverge, dissect with caution and identify the two cavities on either side of

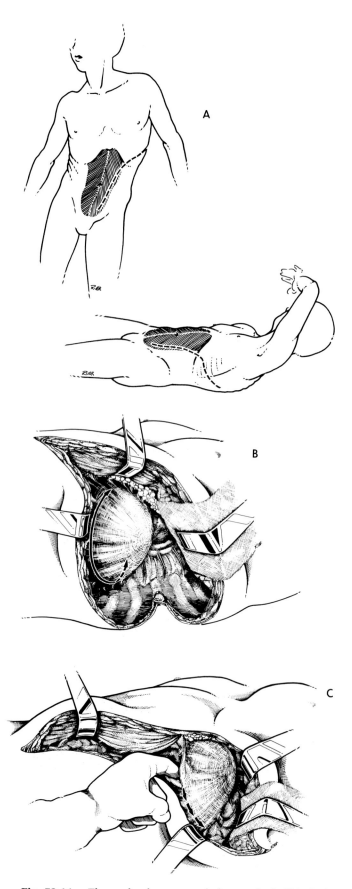

Fig. 79-14 Thoracolumbar approach (see text). **A,** Skin incision. **B,** Transthoracic detachment of diaphragm. **C,** Retroperitoneal detachment of diaphragm.

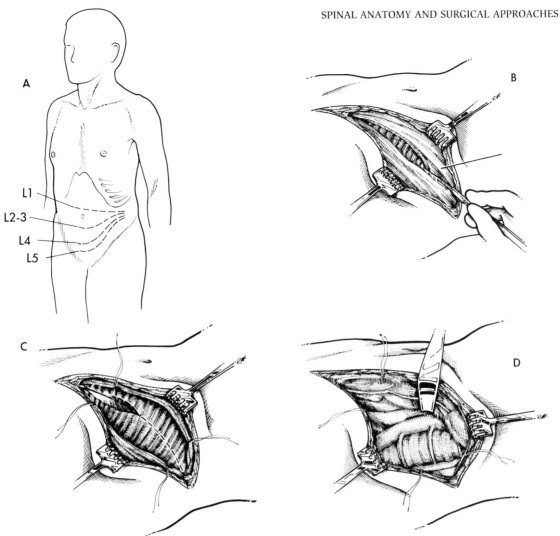

Fig. 79-15 Anterior retroperitoneal approach (see text). **A,** Skin incisions for lumbar vertebrae. **B,** Incision of fibers of external oblique muscle. **C,** Incision into fibers of internal oblique muscle. **D,** Exposure of spine before ligation of segmental vessels.

the diaphragm. To achieve confluence of the two cavities, reflect the diaphragm from the lower ribs and the crus from the side of the spine (Fig. 79-14, *C*). Alternatively, incise the diaphragm 2.5 cm away from its insertion and tag it with sutures for later accurate closure. Incise the prevertebral fascia. Take care to identify the segmental arteries and veins over the midportion of each vertebral body. Isolate these, ligate them in the midline, and expose the bone as previously described.

ANTERIOR RETROPERITONEAL APPROACH, L1-5. The anterior retroperitoneal approach to the lumbar vertebral bodies is a modification of the anterolateral approach commonly used by general surgeons for sympathectomy. It is an excellent approach that should be considered for extensive resection, debridement, or grafting at multiple levels in the lumbar spine. Depending on which portion of the lumbar spine is to be approached, the incision may be varied in placement between the twelfth rib and the superior aspect of the iliac crest. The

major dissection in this approach is behind the kidney in the potential space between the renal fascia and the quadratus lumborum and psoas muscles.

■ *TECHNIQUE.* Position the patient in the lateral decubitus position, generally with the right side down. The approach is made most often from the left side to avoid the liver and the inferior vena cava, which is more difficult to repair than the aorta should vascular injury occur during the approach to the spine. Flex the table to increase exposure between the twelfth rib and the iliac crest. Flex the hips slightly to release tension on the psoas muscle. Make an oblique incision over the twelfth rib from the lateral border of the quadratus lumborum to the lateral border of the rectus abdominus muscle to allow exposure of the first and second lumbar vertebrae (Fig. 79-15, *A*). Alternatively, place the incision several fingerbreadths below and parallel to the costal margin when exposure of the lower lumbar vertebrae (L3-5) is necessary. Use electrocautery to divide the subcutaneous tissue, fascia, and muscle of the external oblique, internal oblique, transversus abdominus, and transversalis fascia in line with the skin incision (Fig. 79-15, *B* and *C*). Carefully protect the peritoneum and reflect it anteriorly by blunt dissection. If the peritoneum is entered during the approach, it must be repaired. Identify the psoas muscle in the retroperitoneal space and allow the ureter to fall anteriorly with the retroperitoneal fat. The sympathetic chain is found between the vertebral bodies and the psoas muscle laterally, while the genitofemoral nerve is lying on the anterior aspect of the psoas muscle. Place a Finochietto rib retractor between the costal margin and the iliac crest to aid exposure. Palpate the vertebral bodies from T12 to L5 and identify and protect with a Deaver retractor the great vessels lying anterior to the spine. It is important to note that the lumbar segmental vessels are lying in the midportion of the vertebral bodies and that the relatively avascular discs are prominent on each adjacent side of the vessels (Fig. 79-15, *D*). Once the appropriate involved vertebra is identified, elevate the psoas muscle bluntly off the lumbar vertebrae and retract it laterally to the level of the transverse process with a Richardson retractor. Sometimes removal of the transverse process with a rongeur is helpful in allowing adequate retraction of the psoas muscle. Ligate and divide the lumbar segmental vessel overlying the involved vertebrae. Clearly delineate the pedicle of the involved vertebrae with a small elevator and locate the neuroforamen with the exiting nerve root. Bipolar coagulation of vessels around the neuroforamen is recommended. Then remove the pedicle with an angled Kerrison rongeur and expose the dura.

After completion of the spinal procedure, obtain meticulous hemostasis and close the wound in layers over a drain in the retroperitoneal space.

ANTERIOR APPROACH TO LUMBOSACRAL JUNCTION

Transperitoneal exposure of lumbar spine, L5 to S1. Transperitoneal exposure of the lumbar spine is an alternative to the retroperitoneal approach. The advantage of the transperitoneal route is a somewhat more extensive exposure, especially at the L5 to S1 level. A disadvantage is that the great vessels and hypogastric nerve plexus must be mobilized before the spine is exposed. The superior hypogastric plexus contains the sympathetic function for the urogenital systems, and especially in males may result in complications such as retrograde ejaculation. Damage to the superior hypogastric plexus should not produce impotence or failure of erection, however. Injury to the hypogastric plexus can be avoided by careful opening of the posterior peritoneum and blunt dissection of the prevertebral tissue from left to right and by opening the posterior peritoneum higher over the bifurcation of the aorta and then extending the opening down

over the sacral promontory. In addition, electrocautery should be kept to a minimum when dissecting within the aortic bifurcation, and until the anulus of the L5 to S1 disc is clearly exposed no transverse scalpel cuts on the front of the disc should be made.

■ *TECHNIQUE.* Position the patient supine on the operating table and make either a vertical midline incision or a transverse incision (Fig. 79-16, *A*). The transverse incision is cosmetically superior and gives excellent exposure; it requires transection of the rectus abdominus sheath. Identify and open the sheath and transect the rectus abdominus muscle. The posterior rectus sheath, abdominal fascia, and peritoneum are conjoined in this area. Open the posterior rectus sheath and abdominal fascia to the peritoneum. Carefully open the peritoneum to avoid damage to bowel content. Carefully pack off the abdominal contents and identify the posterior peritoneum over the sacral promontory. Palpate the aorta and the common iliac vessels through the posterior peritoneum. Make a longitudinal incision in the posterior peritoneum in the midline about the aortic bifurcation. Extend the incision distally and to the right along the right common iliac artery to its bifurcation at the external and internal iliac arteries. Identify the right ureter, crossing the right iliac artery, and curve the incision medially to avoid this structure. Avoid the use of electrocautery anterior to the L5-S1 disc space to prevent damage to the superior hypogastric plexus. The left common iliac vein often lies as a flat structure across the L5-S1 disc within the aortic bifurcation. After identification of the left common iliac artery and vein, use blunt dissection to the right of the artery and hypogastric plexus and mobilize the soft tissue from left to right. Carefully dissect the middle sacral artery and vein from left to right (Fig. 79-16, *B*). Longitudinal blunt dissection allows better mobilization of these vascular structures. If bleeding is encountered, use direct finger and sponge pressure rather than electrocautery. If electrocautery is used in this area we recommend the bipolar rather than the unipolar machine because there is less likelihood of injuring the hypogastric plexus with a thermal burn. Following adequate exposure of the L5-S1 disc, obtain a roentgenogram after inserting a 22-gauge spinal needle into the disc space. Because the L5-S1 disc and the sacrum often are angled horizontally, the body of L5 may be mistaken for the sacrum. Further development of the exposure proceeds as in other anterior approaches to the lumbar vertebrae.

Posterior Approaches

The posterior approach through a midline longitudinal incision provides access to the posterior elements of the spine at all levels, including cervical, thoracic, and lumbosacral. It is the most direct access to the spinous pro-

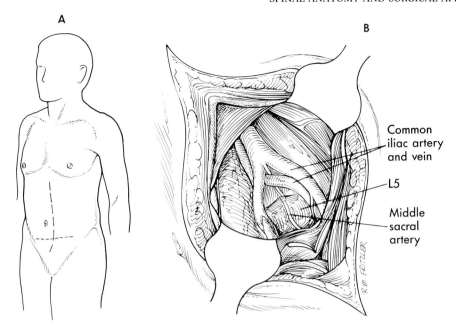

Fig. 79-16 Transperitoneal approach to lumbar and lumbosacral spine (see text). **A,** Median longitudinal or transverse Pfannenstiel's incision. **B,** Dissection of middle sacral artery and vein.

cesses, laminae, and facets and, in addition, the spinal canal may be explored and decompressed over a large area after laminectomy. Under most circumstances, the choice of approach to the spine should be dictated by the site of the primary pathologic condition. Posterior approaches to the spine rarely are indicated when the anterior spinal column is the site of an infectious process or a metastatic disease. The posterior elements usually are not involved in the pathologic process and provide stabilization for the uninvolved structures of the spinal column. Removal of the uninvolved posterior elements, as in laminectomy, may result in subluxation, dislocation, or severe angulation of the spine, causing increased compression of the neural elements and worsening of any neurologic deficit. Posterior approaches to the spine commonly are used for degenerative or traumatic spinal disorders and allow excellent exposure to carry out a wide variety of fusion techniques, with or without internal stabilization.

POSTERIOR APPROACH TO CERVICAL SPINE, OCCIPUT TO C2

■ *TECHNIQUE.* Position the patient prone on a turning frame with skeletal traction through tongs, taking care to avoid excessive pressure on the eyes. Alternatively, a three-point head rest may be used to provide rigid immobilization of the cervical spine during surgery. After routine skin preparation, attach the drapes to the neck with stay sutures or staples. Make a midline longitudinal skin incision from the occiput to C2 (Fig. 79-17). Infiltration of the skin and subcutaneous tissue with a dilute 1:500,000 epinephrine solution is helpful to provide hemostasis. Using electrocautery and elevators, expose the pos-

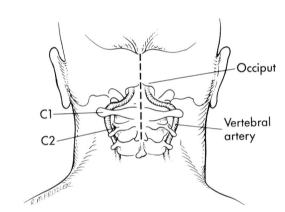

Fig. 79-17 Posterior approach to upper cervical spine (see text).

terior elements subperiosteally and insert self-retaining retractors. It is important to deepen the incision in the midline through the thin white median raphe and avoid cutting muscle tissue. The median raphe of the cervical spine is a wandering avascular ligament and does not follow a straight midline incision. In children, expose no spinal levels unnecessarily to avoid spontaneous fusion at adjacent levels, including the occiput. When exposing the upper cervical spine, take care not to carry the dissection further than 1.5 cm laterally on either side to avoid the vertebral arteries. When necessary, expose the occiput with elevators, insert the self-retaining re-

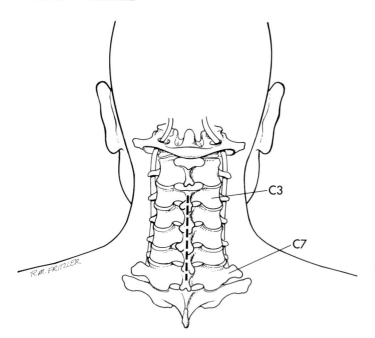

Fig. 79-18 Posterior approach to lower cervical spine (see text).

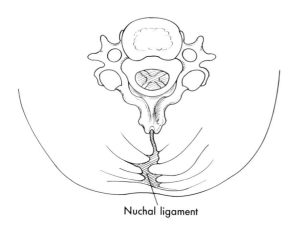

Nuchal ligament

Fig. 79-19 Posterior approach to lower cervical spine. Nuchal ligament is irregular. To maintain dry field, surgeon must stay within ligament.

tractors to expose the base of the skull and the dorsal spine of C2. The area in between will contain the ring of C1; this is often deep compared with the spinous process of C2. While maintaining lateral retraction of the soft tissues, identify the posterior tubercle of C1 longitudinally in the midline and begin subperiosteal dissection to the bone. Often the ring of C1 is thin and direct pressure can fracture it or cause the instrument to slip off the ring and penetrate the atlanto-occipital membrane. The dura may be vulnerable on both the superior and inferior edges of the ring of C1. The second cervical ganglion is an important landmark on the ring of C1 laterally.

It lies approximately 1.5 cm laterally on the lamina of C1 in the groove for the vertebral artery. There is little, if any, indication for dissection lateral to this groove. The vertebral artery may be damaged by penetration of the atlanto-occipital membrane off the superior border of the ring of C1 more lateral than the usually safe 1.5 cm from the midline. Below C2 the lateral margins of the facet joints are the safe lateral extent of dissection. After exposure of the posterior occiput, the ring of C1, and the posterior elements of C2, the intended surgical procedure may be performed. After this, the wound is closed in layers over a drain.

POSTERIOR APPROACH TO CERVICAL SPINE, C3-7

■ *TECHNIQUE.* Position the patient prone on a turning frame with skeletal traction through tongs or with the head positioned in the three-point head fixation device that is attached to the table. The large spinous processes of C2 and C7 are prominent and can be identified by palpation. It is important to note on preoperative roentgenograms any posterior element deficiencies, such as an occult spina bifida, before exposure of the posterior elements. Make a midline skin incision over the appropriate vertebrae (Fig. 79-18) and inject the skin and subcutaneous tissues with a 1:500,000 epinephrine solution to aid in hemostasis. Deepen the dissection in the midline, using the electrocautery knife and staying within the thin white median raphe to avoid cutting the vascular muscle tissue (Fig. 79-19). It is helpful to maintain tension on the soft tissue by inserting self-retaining retractors. Using electrocautery and elevators, detach the ligamentous attachments to the spinous processes and expose the posterior elements subperiosteally to the lateral edge of the facet joints, which is the extent of dissection on either side of the midline. After identifying the lateral edge of the facet joint, pack each level with a taped sponge to keep blood loss to a minimum. It is helpful to expose the spinous processes from distally to proximally because the muscles may then be stripped from the spinous processes in the acute angle between their insertions and the bone. If exposure in the opposite direction is attempted, the knife blade or periosteal elevator will tend to follow the direction of the fibers into the muscle and divide the vessels, thus increasing hemorrhage.

POSTERIOR APPROACH TO THORACIC SPINE, T1-12.
Posterior approach to the thoracic spine can be made through a standard midline longitudinal exposure with reflection of the erector spinae muscle laterally to the tips of the transverse processes. Alternatively, the thoracic vertebrae may be approached through a costotransversectomy when direct access to the transverse processes and pedicles of the thoracic spine and limited ac-

cess to the vertebral bodies are indicated. Costotransversectomy should be considered for simple biopsy or local debridement. It should be noted, however, that this approach does not provide the working operative area or length of exposure to the thoracic vertebral bodies that is afforded by a transthoracic approach or the midlongitudinal posterior approach.

■ *TECHNIQUE.* Position the patient prone on a padded spinal operating frame. Make a long midline incision over the area to be exposed (Fig. 79-20). Infiltration of the skin, subcutaneous tissue, and erector spinae to the level of the laminae with a 1:500,000 epinephrine solution is helpful in providing hemostasis. Deepen the dissection in the midline using either a scalpel or the electrocautery knife through the superficial and lumbodorsal fasciae to the tips of the spinous processes. Expose subperiosteally the posterior elements by reflecting the erector spinae muscle laterally to the tips of the transverse processes from distally to proximally, using periosteal elevators. Repeat the procedure until the desired number of vertebrae are exposed and where both sides of the spine require exposure use the same technique on each side. Pack each segment with a taped sponge immediately after exposure to lessen bleeding. After satisfactory exposure of the posterior elements, obtain a roentgenogram to confirm proper localization of the intended level. After completion of the spinal procedure, close the wound in layers over a suction drain.

COSTOTRANSVERSECTOMY

■ *TECHNIQUE.* Place the patient prone on a padded spinal operating frame. Make a straight longitudinal incision about 2.5 inches (6.3 cm) lateral to the spinous processes centered over the level of the desired vertebral dissection (Fig. 79-21, *A*). (Alternatively, make a curved incision with its apex lateral to the midline.) Palpate the slight depression between the dorsal paraspinal muscle mass and the prominent posterior angle of the rib and center the incision over this groove lateral to the spinous processes. Deepen the dissection through the subcutaneous tissues and the trapezius and latissimus dorsi muscles and the lumbodorsal fasciae, which are divided longitudinally. Dissect the paraspinal muscles sharply from their insertions on the ribs and transverse processes, and retract them medially. Expose the transverse process and posterior aspects of the associated rib subperiosteally and remove a section of rib 5 to 7.5 cm long at the level of involvement. The rib generally is transected with rib cutters about 3.5 inches lateral to the vertebrae at its prominent posterior angle. The costotransverse ligament and joint capsule are quite strong and increase the inherent stability of the thoracic spine. Take care to remain subperiosteally and extrapleural during this

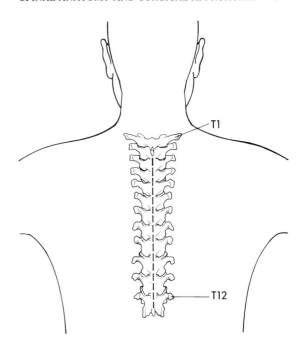

Fig. 79-20   Posterior approach to thoracic spine (see text).

part of the exposure and to protect the intercostal neurovascular bundle. Anterior to the transverse process is the vertebral pedicle, and above and below the pedicle lie the neuroforamina. The nerve roots emerge from the superior portion of the foramina, giving off a dorsal and ventral ramus. The ventral ramus becomes the intercostal nerve and is joined by the intercostal vessels. Once the pedicles, neuroforamina, and neurovascular structures have been identified, proceed with dissection directly anteriorly on the pedicle to the vertebral body along a path that is relatively free of major vessels or nerve (Fig. 79-21, *B*). Carefully dissect the parietal pleura with elevators anteriorly to expose the anterolateral aspect of the vertebral body, raising the sympathetic trunk and parietal pleura. Exposure may be increased by removal of the transverse process, pedicle, and facet joints as necessary. After completion of the spinal procedure, fill the wound with saline and inflate the lungs to check for air leaks. Close the wound in layers over a drain to prevent hematoma collection. Obtain a chest roentgenogram to document the absence of air in the pleural space, which may occur if the pleura is inadvertently entered during the exposure.

POSTERIOR APPROACH TO LUMBAR SPINE, L1-5. The posterior approach to the lumbar spine provides access directly to the spinous processes, laminae, and facet joints at all levels. In addition, the transverse processes and pedicles may be reached through this approach. Recently, Wiltse and Spencer refined the paraspinal approach to the lumbar spine, which involves a longitudi-

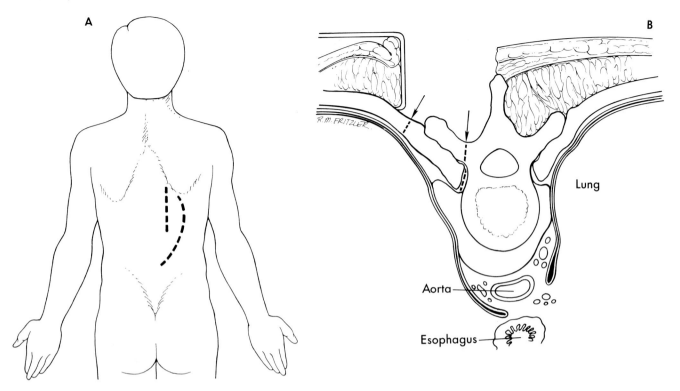

Fig. 79-21 Costotransversectomy. **A**, Straight longitudinal incision about 2.5 inches (6.3 cm) lateral to spinous processes, centered over level of vertebral dissection. **B**, Resection of costotransverse articulation.

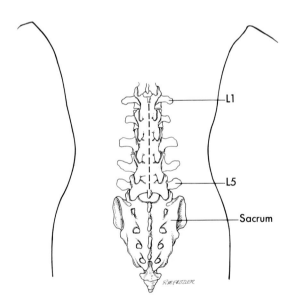

Fig. 79-22 Posterior approach to lumbar spine (see text).

nal separation of the sacrospinalis muscle group to expose the posterolateral aspect of the lumbar spine. This approach is especially useful in removing far lateral disc herniation, decompressing a "far-out" syndrome, and inserting pedicle screws.

■ *TECHNIQUE.* Position the patient prone or in the kneeling position on a padded spinal frame. By allowing the abdomen to hang free, intravenous pressure is decreased and blood loss is decreased as a result of collapse of the epidural venous plexus. Make a midline skin incision centered over the involved lumbar segment (Fig. 79-22.) Infiltration of the skin and subcutaneous tissue with a 1:500,000 epinephrine solution aids hemostasis. Carry the dissection down in the midline through the skin, subcutaneous tissue, and lumbodorsal fascia to the tips of the spinous processes. Use self-retaining retractors to maintain tension on soft tissues during exposure. Subperiosteally expose the posterior elements from distally to proximally using electrocautery and periosteal elevators to detach the muscles from the posterior elements. Pack each segement with a taped sponge immediately after exposure to lessen bleeding. If the procedure requires exposure of both sides of the spine, use the same technique on each side. We recommend accurate localization of the involved segment with a permanent roentgenogram in the operating room. After completion of the spinal procedure, close the wound in layers over a drain.

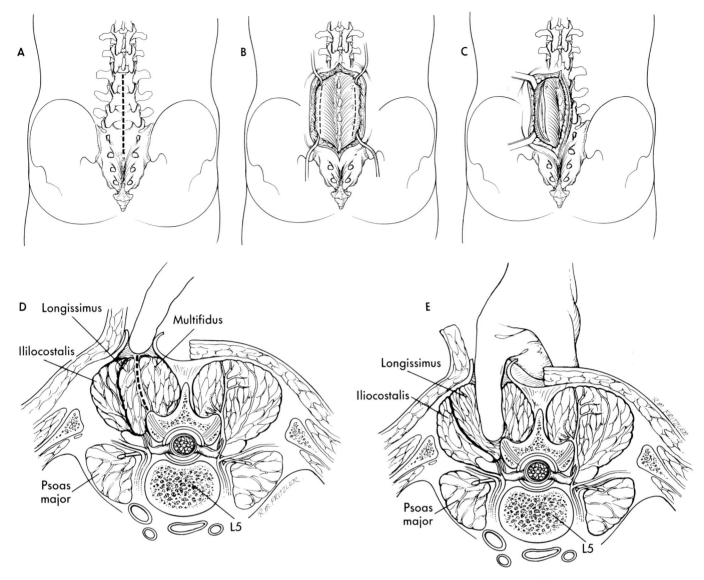

Fig. 79-23   Paraspinal approach to lumbar spine (see text). **A**, Midline skin incision. **B** and **C**, Fascial incisions. **D** and **E**, Blunt finger dissection between muscle groups to palpate facet joints. (Redrawn from Wiltse LL and Spencer CW: Spine 13:696, 1988.)

Paraspinal approach to lumbar spine

■ *TECHNIQUE (WILTSE AND SPENCER).* Position the patient prone or in the kneeling position on a spinal frame. By allowing the abdomen to hang free, intravenous pressure is decreased and blood loss is decreased as a result of collapse of the epidural venous plexus. Make a midline skin incision centered over the involved lower lumbar segment (Fig. 79-23, *A*). Infiltration with 1:500,000 epinephrine- solution is helpful in providing hemostasis. Carry dissection down to the lumbodorsal fascia and retract the skin and subcutaneous tissue laterally on either side. Then make a fascial incision approximately 2 cm lateral to the midline (Fig. 79-23, *B* and *C*). Once the fascial layers have been divided, a natural cleavage plane is entered lying between the multifidus and longissimus muscles. Using blunt finger dissection between the muscle groups (Fig. 79-23, *D* and *E*), palpate the facet joints at L4-5. Place self-retaining Gelpi retractors between the two muscle groups. Using either electrocautery or an elevator, separate the transverse fibers of the multifidus from their heavy fascial attachments. Expose the lumbar transverse processes, facet joints, and lamina subperiosteally and denude them of soft tissue. Take care not to carry the dissection anterior to the transverse processes, since the exiting spinal nerves lie just in front of the transverse processes and can be injured. Use bipolar cautery to control bleeding from the lumbar arteries and veins coursing above the base of the transverse processes. Perform unilateral or bilateral decompression and fusion of the lumbosacral spine. Close the wound over a suction drain and suture the skin flaps down to the fascia to remove dead space.

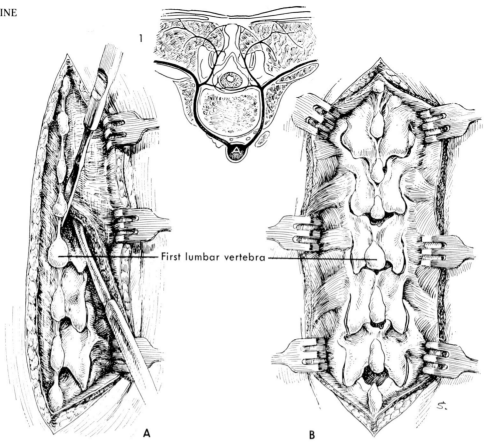

First lumbar vertebra

A   B

Fig. 79-24   Approach to posterior aspect of spine. **A,** Muscle insertions are freed subperiosteally from lateral side of spinous processes and interspinous ligaments; dissection proceeds proximally, the periosteal elevator being held against bases of spinous processes. **B,** Spinous processes, laminae, and articular facets exposed. **1,** Courses of arteries supplying posterior spinal muscles, showing proximity of internal muscular branches to spinous processes. (Modified from Wagoner G: J Bone Joint Surg 19:469, 1937.)

POSTERIOR APPROACH TO LUMBOSACRAL SPINE, L1 TO SACRUM

■ *TECHNIQUE (WAGONER).* Make a longitudinal incision over the spinous processes of the appropriate vertebrae and incise the superficial fascia, the lumbodorsal fascia, and the supraspinous ligament longitudinally, precisely over the tips of the processes. With a scalpel divide longitudinally the ligament between the two spinous processes in the most distal part of the wound. Insert a small, blunt periosteal elevator through this opening so that its end rests on the junction of the spinous process with the lamina of the more proximal vertebra. Move the handle of the elevator proximally and laterally to place under tension the muscles attached to this spinous process. Then with a scalpel moving from distally to proximally strip the muscles subperiosteally from the lateral surface of the process. Then place the end of the elevator in the wound so that its end rests on the junction of the spinous process with the lamina of the next most proximal vertebra and repeat the procedure as described. Repeat the procedure until the desired number of vertebrae have been exposed (Fig. 79-24). For operations requiring exposure of both sides of the spine, use the same technique on each side.

This approach exposes the spinous processes and medial part of the laminae. Increase the exposure, if desired, by further subperiosteal reflection along the laminae; expose the posterior surface of the laminae and the articular facets. Pack each segment with a tape sponge immediately after exposure to lessen bleeding. Divide the supraspinous ligament precisely over the tip of the spinous processes and denude subperiosteally the sides of the processes because this route leads through a relatively avascular field; otherwise the arterial supply to the muscles will be encountered (Fig. 79-24). Blood loss may be further decreased by using an electrocautery and a suction apparatus. Replace blood as it is lost. Expose the spinous processes from distally to proximally as just described because the muscles may then be stripped from the spinous processes in the acute angle between their insertions and the bone. If exposure in the opposite direction is attempted, the knife blade or periosteal elevator will tend to follow the direction of the fibers into the muscle and divide the vessels, thus increasing hemorrhage.

REFERENCES

Anatomy and biomechanics

Aspden RM: The spine as an arch: a new mathematical model, Spine 14:266, 1989.

Bick EM and Copel JW: Longitudinal growth of the human vertebra: a contribution to human osteogeny, J Bone Joint Surg 32-A:803, 1950.

Bullough PG and Oheneba B-A: Atlas of spinal diseases, Philadelphia, 1988, JB Lippincott Co.

Di Chiro G: Angiography of obstructive vascular disease of the spinal cord, Radiology 100:607, 1971.

Dickson RA and Deacon P: Annotation: spinal growth, J Bone Joint Surg 69-B:690, 1987.

Dommisse GF: The blood supply of the spinal cord: a critical vascular zone in spinal surgery, J Bone Joint Surg 56-B:225, 1974.

Esses SI and Bednar DA: The spinal pedicle screw: techniques and systems, Orthop Rev 18:676, 1989.

Kardjieve V, Symeonov A, and Chankov I: Etiology, pathogenesis, and prevention of spinal cord lesions in selective angiography of the bronchial and intercostal arteries, Radiology 112:81, 1974.

Karlström G, Olerud S, and Sjöstrom L: Transpedicular fixation of thoracolumbar fractures, Contemp Orthop 20:285, 1990.

Keim HA and Hilal SK: Spinal angiography in scoliosis patients, J Bone Joint Surg 53-A:904, 1971.

Louis R: Single staged posterior lumbosacral fusion by internal fixation with screw plates. Presented at the Annual Meeting of the International Society for the Study of the Lumbar Spine, Sidney, Australia, 1985.

Macnab I and Dall D: The blood supply of the lumbar spine and its application to the technique of intertransverse lumbar fusion, J Bone Joint Surg 53-B:628, 1971.

Mazzara JT and Fielding JW: Effect of C1-C2 rotation on canal size, Clin Orthop 237:115, 1988.

Pasternak BM, Boyd DP, and Ellis FH Jr: Spinal cord injury after procedures on the aorta, Surg Gynecol Obstet 135:29, 1972.

Roy-Camille R, Saillant G, and Mazel Ch: Plating of thoracic, thoracolumbar, and lumbar injuries with pedicle screw plates, Orthop Clin North Am 17:147, 1986.

Saillant G: Anatomic study of vertebral pedicles: surgical application, Rev Chir Orthop 62:151, 1976.

Zindrick MR, Wiltse LL, Doornik A, et al: Analysis of the morphometric characteristics of the thoracic and lumbar pedicles, Spine 12:160, 1987.

Zindrick MR, Wiltse LL, Widell EH, et al: A biomechanical study of intrapeduncular screw fixation in the lumbosacral spine, Clin Orthop 203:99, 1986.

Surgical approaches

Bailey RW and Badgley CE: Stabilization of the cervical spine by anterior fusion, J Bone Joint Surg 42-A:565, 1960.

Bohlman HH, Ducker TB, and Lucas JT: Spine and spinal cord injuries. In Rothman RH and Simeone FA, editors: The spine, ed 2, Philadelphia, 1982, WB Saunders Co.

Bohlman HH and Eismont FJ: Surgical techniques of anterior decompression and fusion for spinal cord injuries, Clin Orthop 154:57, 1981.

Bonney G and Williams JPR: Trans-oral approach to the upper cervical spine: a report of 16 cases, J Bone Joint Surg 67-B:691, 1985.

Burrington JD et al: Anterior approach to the thoracolumbar spine: technical considerations, Arch Surg 111:456, 1976.

Cauchoix J and Binet JP: Anterior surgical approaches to the spine, Ann R Coll Surg 21:237, 1957.

Charles R and Govender S: Anterior approach to the upper thoracic vertebrae, J Bone Joint Surg 71-B:81, 1989.

Cloward RB: The anterior approach for ruptured cervical discs, J Neurosurg 15:602, 1958.

Cocke EW Jr, Robertson JH, Robertson JR, and Crook JP Jr: The extended maxillotomy and subtotal maxillectomy for excision of skull base tumors, Arch Otolaryngol Head Neck Surg 116:92, 1990.

Codivilla A: Sulla scoliosi congenita, Arch di Ortop 18:65, 1901.

Colletta AJ and Mayer PJ: Chylothorax: an unusual complication of anterior thoracic interbody spinal fusion, Spine 7:46, 1982.

Compere EL: Excision of hemivertebrae for correction of congenital scoliosis: report of two cases, J Bone Joint Surg 14:555, 1932.

Fang HSY and Ong GB: Direct anterior approach to the upper cervical spine, J Bone Joint Surg 44-A:1588, 1962.

Fang HSY, Ong GB, and Hodgson AR: Anterior spinal fusion: the operative approaches, Clin Orthop 35:16, 1964.

Fielding JW and Stillwell WT: Anterior cervical approach to the upper thoracic spine: a case report, Spine 1:158, 1976.

Fraser RD: A wide muscle-splitting approach to the lumbosacral spine, J Bone Joint Surg 64-B:44, 1982.

Freeman BL: The pediatric spine. In Canale ST and Beaty JH, editors: Operative pediatric orthopaedics, St Louis, 1991, Mosby–Year Book, Inc.

Hall JE: The anterior approach to spinal deformities, Orthop Clin North Am 3:81, 1972.

Hall JE, Denis F, and Murray J: Exposure of the upper cervical spine for spinal decompression by a mandible and tongue-splitting approach: case report, J Bone Joint Surg 59-A:121, 1977.

Harmon PC: Results from the treatment of sciatica due to lumbar disc protrusion, Am J Surg 80:829, 1950.

Henry AK: Extensile exposure, ed 2, Edinburgh, 1957, Churchill Livingstone.

Hodgson AR, Stock FE, Fang HYS, and Ong GB: Anterior spinal fusion: the operative approach and pathological findings in 412 patients with Pott's disease of the spine, Br J Surg 48:172, 1960.

Johnson RM and McGuire EJ: Urogenital complications of anterior approaches to the lumbar spine, Clin Orthop 154:114, 1981.

Johnson RM and Southwick WO: Surgical approaches to the cervical spine. In Rothman RH and Simeone FA, editors: The spine, ed 2, Philadelphia, 1982, WB Saunders Co.

Leventhal MR: Surgical approaches in the treatment of spinal infections. In Wood GW, editor: SPINE: State of the art reviews 3:385, 1989.

McAfee PC, Bohlman HH, Riley LH Jr, et al: The anterior retropharyngeal approach to the upper part of the cervical spine, J Bone Joint Surg 69-A:1371, 1987.

Michele AA and Krueger FJ: Surgical approach to the vertebral body, J Bone Joint Surg 31-A:873, 1949.

Micheli LJ and Hood RW: Anterior exposure of the cervicothoracic spine using a combined cervical and thoracic approach, J Bone Joint Surg 65-A:992, 1983.

Mirbaha MM: Anterior approach to the thoraco-lumbar junction of the spine by a retroperitoneal-extrapleural technic, Clin Orthop 91:41, 1973.

Nachlas IW and Borden JN: The cure of experimental scoliosis by directed growth control, J Bone Joint Surg 33-A:24, 1951.

Perry J: Surgical approaches to the spine. In Pierce DS and Nickel VH, editors: The total care of spinal cord injuries, Boston, 1977, Little, Brown & Co.

Pierce DS and Nickel WH, editors: The total care of spinal cord injuries, Boston, 1977, Little, Brown & Co.

Riley LH Jr: Surgical approaches to the anterior structures of the cervical spine, Clin Orthop 91:16, 1973.

Riseborough EJ: The anterior approach to the spine for the correction of deformities of the axial skeleton, Clin Orthop 93:207, 1973.

Robinson RA and Riley LH Jr: Techniques of exposure and fusion of the cervical spine, Clin Orthop 109:78, 1975.

Rothman RH and Simeone FA, editors: The spine, ed 2, Philadelphia, 1982, WB Saunders Co.

Royle ND: The operative removal of an accessory vertebra, Med J Australia 1:467, 1928.

Smith AD, von Lackum WH, and Wylie R: An operation for stapling vertebral bodies in congenital scoliosis, J Bone Joint Surg 36-A:342, 1954.

Southwick WO and Robinson RA: Surgical approaches to the vertebral bodies in the cervical and lumbar regions, J Bone Joint Surg 39-A:631, 1957.

Spetzler RF: Transoral approach to the upper cervical spine. In Evarts CM, editor: Surgery of the musculoskeletal system, vol 4, New York, 1983, Churchill Livingstone.

Sundaresan N, Shah J, and Feghali JG: A transsternal approach to the upper thoracic vertebrae, Am J Surg 148:473, 1984.

Turner PL and Webb JK: Surgical approach to the upper cervical spine, J Bone Joint Surg 69-B:542, 1987.

von Lackum HL and Smith AF: Removal of vertebral bodies in the treatment of scoliosis, Surg Gynecol Obstet 57:250, 1933.

Wagoner G: A technique for lessening hemorrhage in operations on the spine, J Bone Joint Surg 19:469, 1937.

Warner WC: Cervical spine anomalies. In Canale ST and Beaty JH, editors: Operative pediatric orthopaedics, St Louis, 1991, Mosby–Year Book, Inc.

Watkins RG: Surgical approaches to the spine, New York, 1983, Springer-Verlag.

Whitesides TE Jr and Kelly RP: Lateral approach to the upper cervical spine for anterior fusion, South Med J 59:879, 1966.

Wiltberger BR: Resection of vertebral bodies and bone grafting for chronic osteomyelitis of the spine, J Bone Joint Surg 34-A:215, 1952.

Wiltberger BR: The dowel intervertebral-body fusion as used in lumbar disc surgery, J Bone Joint Surg 39-A:284, 1957.

Wiltse LL: The paraspinal sacrospinalis-splitting approach to the lumbar spine, Clin Orthop 91:48, 1973.

Wiltse LL and Spencer CW: New uses and refinements of the paraspinal approach of the lumbar spine, Spine 13:696, 1988.

Wood GW: Anatomic, biologic, and pathophysiologic aspects of spinal infections. In Wood GW, editor: SPINE: State of the art reviews 3:385, 1989.

CHAPTER 80

Fractures, Dislocations, and Fracture-Dislocations of Spine

MARVIN R. LEVENTHAL

Fractures and dislocations of the spine are serious injuries that most commonly occur in young people. Nearly 43% of patients with spinal cord injuries sustain multiple injuries. Kraus et al. in 1975 estimated that each year 50 people in 1 million sustain a spinal cord injury. Of those who die within 1 year of their accidents, 90% die en route to the hospital. With the development of regional trauma centers and increased training of paramedics and emergency medical technicians, the chances of survival after serious spinal cord injury have increased. The National Institute of Disability and Rehabilitation Research estimates that 14,000 Americans suffer spinal cord injury each year, that about 8000 to 10,000 are left paralyzed, and that in the United States alone there are approximately 300,000 wheelchair-bound paraplegics and quadriplegics. No accurate accounting of the monetary cost of these devastating injuries has been made, but estimates are as high as 4 billion dollars per year in health care costs and lost productivity.

EVALUATION OF SPINAL INJURY
History

A detailed history of the mechanism of injury is important but frequently is unobtainable at the initial exami-

nation. The most common causes of severe spinal trauma are motor vehicle accidents, falls, diving accidents, and gunshot wounds. Bohlman, in a review of over 300 cervical spinal injuries, found that delays in diagnosis were common and that one of three severe cervical spinal injuries were not initially recognized. The most common causes for misdiagnoses were head trauma, acute alcoholic intoxication, and multiple injuries. Patients with decreased levels of consciousness or comatose patients often do not complain of neck pain. Severe facial or scalp lacerations bleed profusely and divert attention from the cervical spinal injury. A Brown-Séquard type of hemiparesis may be mistaken for a stroke. Spinal injury should be suspected in any patient with a head injury or severe facial or scalp lacerations.

Physical Examination

A general physical examination is performed with the patient supine. The head should be examined for lacerations and contusions and palpated for facial fractures. The ear canals should be inspected to rule out leakage of spinal fluid or blood behind the tympanic membrane, suggestive of a skull fracture. The spinous processes should be palpated from the upper cervical to the lumbosacral region. A painful spinous process may indicate a spinal injury. Palpable defects in the interspinous ligaments may indicate disruption of the supporting ligamentous complex. Careful and gentle rotation of the head may elicit pain; however, excessive flexion and extension of the neck should be avoided. The elbows may be flexed if a spinal cord injury causes loss of function below the biceps, or they may be extended if the paralysis is higher. Penile erection and incontinence of the bowel or bladder suggest a significant spinal injury. Quadriplegia is indicated by flaccid paralysis of the extremities. Initial blood pressure may be decreased without a compensatory increase in pulse because of spinal cord shock. The chest, abdomen, and extremities should be examined for occult injuries. The spine should be protected during this initial assessment; however, once spinal cord injury is identified and the appropriate precautions taken, the patient should be moved from the spine board as soon as possible to decrease the risk of decubitus ulcers.

Neurologic Evaluation

Bohlman, Stauffer, and Meyer all emphasize the importance of accurate and detailed neurologic evaluation of patients with spinal cord injuries. The level of consciousness should be determined quickly, including pupillary size and reaction. Epidural or subdural hematoma, a depressed skull fracture, or other intracranial pathologic conditions may cause progressive deterioration in neurologic function. The Glasgow Coma Scale (Table 80-1) is useful in determining the level of consciousness. A detailed, initial neurologic examination, including sensory, motor, and reflex function, is important in determining prognosis and treatment. The presence of an incomplete or complete spinal cord injury must be determined and documented by meticulous neurologic examination. Sensory examination is performed with pinpricks beginning at the head and neck and progressing distally to examine specific dermatome distributions (Fig. 80-1). Important dermatome landmarks are the nipple line (T4), xiphoid process (T7), umbilicus (T10), inguinal region (T12, L1), and the perineum and perianal region (S2, S3, and S4). The skin should be marked where sensation is present before proceeding to motor examination. Evidence of sacral sensory sparing can establish the diagnosis of an incomplete spinal cord injury. The only area of sensation distal to an obvious cervical lesion in a quadriplegic patient may be in the perianal region (Fig. 80-2). Motor examination should be systematic, beginning with the upper extremities. During motor examination it is important to differentiate between complete and incomplete spinal cord injuries and pure nerve root lesions. A protruded cervical disc or a unilateral dislocated facet may produce an isolated nerve root paralysis. Some lumbar spine injuries may present as isolated root injuries with weakness of the foot or leg, depending on the specific root involved. Table 80-2 shows the cor-

Table 80-1   Glasgow Coma Scale

Eyes open	Spontaneous	4
	To sound	3
	To pain	2
	Never	1
Best verbal response	Oriented	5
	Confused conversation	4
	Inappropriate words	3
	Incomprehensible words	2
	None	1
Best motor response	Obeys commands	6
	Localizes pain	5
	Flexion withdrawal	4
	Abnormal	3
	Extension	2
	None	1

From Teasdale G and Jennett B: Acta Neurochirurg 34:45, 1976. With permission.

relation between neurologic function and the level of intactness. After examination of the extremities and trunk, the presence or absence of sacral motor sparing should be determined by voluntary rectal sphincter or toe flexor contractions. If voluntary contraction of the sacrally innervated muscles is present, then prognosis for recovery of motor function is good. Finally reflexes should be documented. Usually paralyzed patients are areflexic and flexion withdrawal of the legs to pinprick does not indicate voluntary motion.

Spinal shock rarely lasts longer than 24 hours but may last for days or weeks. A positive bulbocavernosus reflex (Fig. 80-3) or return of anal wink reflex (Fig. 80-4) indicates the end of spinal shock. If no motor or sensory function below the injured level can be documented when spinal shock ends, a complete spinal cord injury is present and the prognosis is poor for recovery of distal motor or sensory function.

Roentgenographic Examination

The initial roentgenograms should include a lateral view of the cervical spine and anteroposterior views of the chest and pelvis. The most frequently missed cervical spine fractures on roentgenograms involve the odontoid process or the cervicothoracic junction. Roentgenographic views of the injured neck should include standard anteroposterior, lateral, and right and left oblique projections with the patient immobilized and unmoved during examination. Weir, in a study of 360 normal adults, established the criteria for roentgenographic evaluation of the cervical spine. This included the prevertebral soft tissue shadow, which should not exceed 5 mm in width at the level of the anteroinferior border of the third cervical vertebra. A width of more than 5 mm is

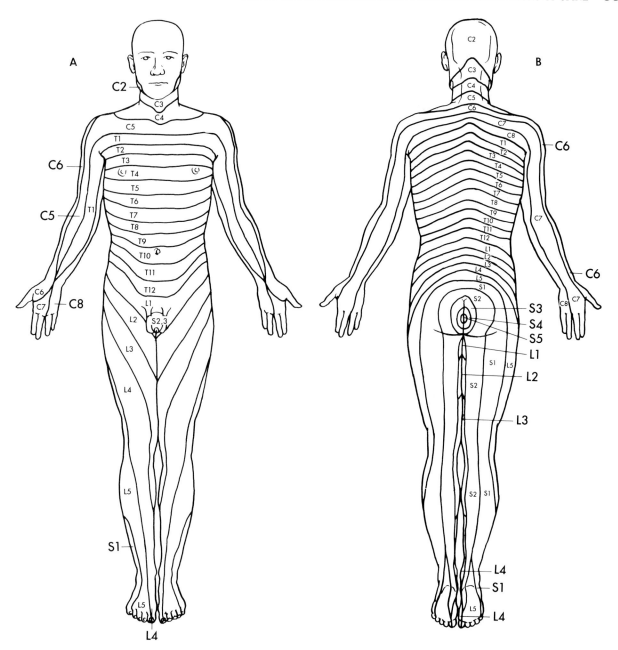

Fig. 80-1   Dermatome distributions (see text).

Fig. 80-2   Examination of perianal skin for sensation in cervical cord injury. Discrimination between sharpness and dullness may be only indication of incomplete injury. (Redrawn from Stauffer ES: Clin Orthop 112:9, 1975.)

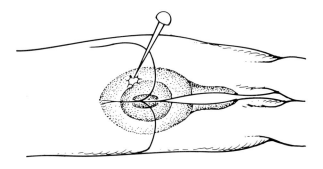

Table 80-2 Neurologic function: level of intactness

Motor-sensory response	Intact level
Motor	
Diaphragm	C3-5
Shrug shoulders	C4
Deltoids (and flex elbows)	C5
Extend wrist	C6
Extend elbow/flex wrist	C7
Abduct fingers	C8
Active chest expansion	T1-12
Hip flexion	L2
Knee extension	L3-4
Ankle dorsiflexion	L5-S1
Ankle plantar flexion	S1-2
Sensory	
Anterior thigh	L2
Anterior knee	L3
Anterolateral ankle	L4
Dorsum of great and second toe	L5
Lateral side of foot	S1
Posterior calf	S2
Perianal sensation (perineum)	S2-5

From Meyer PR Jr, editor: Surgery of spine trauma, New York, 1989, Churchill Livingstone.

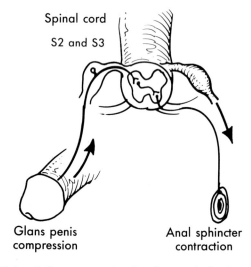

Fig. 80-3 Bulbocavernosus reflex (see text). (Redrawn from Stauffer ES: Clin Orthop 112:9, 1975.)

strongly suggestive of injury with soft tissue swelling. Loss of the cervical lordotic curve is not in itself indirect evidence of cervical spine injury with resultant muscle spasm but may be simply a normal variant. Lateral flexion and extension views can be made to determine the stability of the cervical spine, but these are not routinely recommended in the initial examination. If flexion and extension views are made, they should be obtained under the supervision of a physician, and the patient should be carefully observed for pain response or any change in neurologic status. If the cervicothoracic junction cannot be seen adequately on lateral views, a swimmer's view or computed tomography (CT) scans should

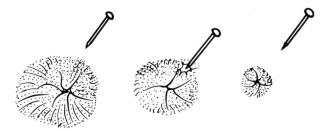

Fig. 80-4 Anal wink. Contracture of external sphincter caused by pinprick (see text). (Redrawn from Stauffer ES: Clin Orthop 112:9, 1975.)

be obtained. The cervical spine is the most easily examined because the thoracic and lumbar areas are less accessible with the patient supine. Fractures of the thoracic spine and at the cervicothoracic or thoracolumbar junction are easily overlooked, but with sophisticated imaging techniques, including tomography, water-soluble contrast myelography, postmyelogram CT with sagittal reconstructions, and magnetic resonance imaging (MRI), injuries to osseous, ligamentous, and neurologic structures can be evaluated accurately. Tomography can be used to clarify questionable findings on plain roentgenograms, to reveal an otherwise occult injury, and to further evaluate a known fracture or fracture-dislocation. Usually excellent bony detail of the fracture pattern can be obtained with routine tomography. CT is helpful in evaluating the degree of compromise of the spinal canal. The addition of water-soluble contrast material to the subarachnoid space improves the contrast between bone fragments and neural elements. We prefer routine CT to standard tomography for the initial evaluation of spinal injuries. MRI has the advantages of being noninvasive, having no risk of ionizing radiation, and not requiring frequent repositioning as for routine myelography. MRI allows examination of the intervertebral discs, supporting ligamentous structures, and neural elements. Its role in spinal trauma is still evolving, but it appears to provide superior images of lesions of the craniocervical and cervicothoracic regions. Several studies have suggested that MRI can help determine the prognosis for neurologic recovery.

Multiple Spinal Fractures

If a spinal fracture is identified at any level, the entire spine should be examined with anteroposterior and lateral views to document the presence or absence of spinal fractures at other levels. Multiple-level spinal fractures, which may be contiguous or separated, are estimated to occur in 3% to 5% of patients with spinal fractures (Fig. 80-5). Multiple noncontiguous spinal fractures rarely occur without injury to the spinal cord. In 710 patients admitted to a regional spinal cord injury unit, Calenoff, Geimer, and Rosen found an incidence of 4.5%. They described three patterns of injury (Fig. 80-6). In pattern A

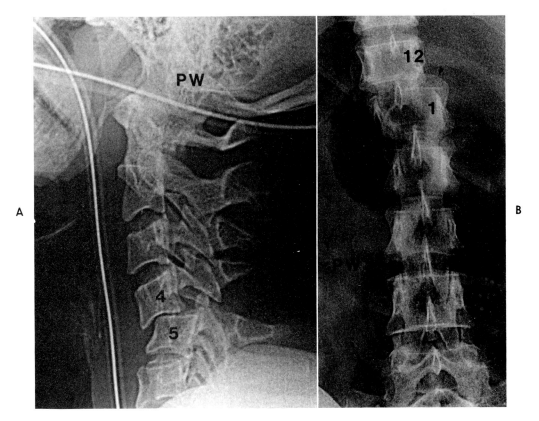

Fig. 80-5 **A,** Fracture-dislocation of cervical spine at C4-5 and complete spinal cord injury in 38-year-old woman. **B,** Anteroposterior view of thoracolumbar spine shows noncontiguous translation injury at T12-L1 level. This combination of injuries is consistent with pattern A described by Calenoff (see text).

the primary lesion occurs between C5 and C7, with secondary injuries at T12 or the lumbar spine. In pattern B the primary injury occurs at T2 and T4, with secondary injuries in the cervical spine. In pattern C the primary injury occurs between T12 and L2, with secondary injuries from L4 to L5. They noted that patients with multiple-level, noncontiguous fractures had a disproportionate number of primary vertebral injuries in the middle and upper thoracic spine. If a fracture is identified at this level, a secondary vertebral injury should be suspected. The secondary lesions tended to cluster at L4 and L5 and at C1 and C2: approximately 43% of the secondary fractures occurred at the extremes of the spine. Recognition of these secondary injuries is important to avoid increasing neurologic deficit, chronic pain, or progressive deformity.

SPINAL CORD SYNDROMES

Spinal cord syndromes resulting from incomplete traumatic lesions have been described by Schneider and Kahn and by Bosch, Stauffer, and Nickel. The following generalizations can be made from their investigations: (1) the greater the sparing of motor and sensory functions distal to the injury, the greater the expected recovery; (2) the more rapid the recovery, the greater the

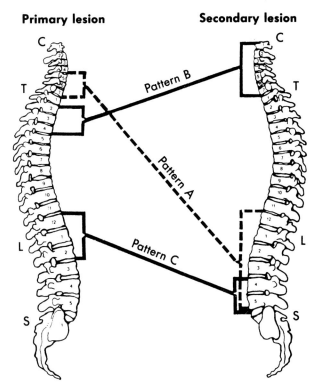

Fig. 80-6 Three patterns of multiple-level injury described by Calenoff et al. (see text). (From Calenoff L, Chessare JW, Rogers LF, et al: AJR 130:665, 1978.)

amount of recovery; and (3) when new recovery ceases and a plateau is reached, no further recovery can be expected. The importance of determining whether a patient has a complete or incomplete cord injury cannot be over-emphasized in the overall prognosis (Tables 80-3 to 80-5). By definition, an incomplete spinal cord injury is one in which some motor or sensory function is spared distal to the cord injury. A complete spinal cord injury is manifested by total motor and sensory loss distal to the injury. When the bulbocavernosus relfex is positive and no sacral sensation or motor function has returned, the paralysis will be permanent and complete in most patients. An incomplete spinal cord syndrome may be a Brown-Séquard syndrome, central cord syndrome, anterior cord syndrome, posterior cord syndrome, or rarely monoparesis of the upper extremity. Ninety percent of incomplete lesions produce either a central cord syndrome, a Brown-Séquard syndrome, or an anterior cervical cord syndrome (Fig. 80-7).

The *central cord syndrome* is the most common. It consists of destruction of the central area of the spinal cord, including both gray and white matter (Fig. 80-7, *B*). The centrally located arm tracts in the cortical spinal area are the most severely affected, and the leg tracts are affected to a lesser extent. Generally patients have a quadriparesis involving the upper extremities to a greater degree than the lower. Sensory sparing is variable, but usually sacral pinprick sensation is preserved. Frequently these patients show immediate partial recovery after being placed in skeletal traction through skull tongs. Prognosis is variable, but more than 50% of patients have return of bowel and bladder control, become ambulatory, and have improved hand function. This syndrome usually results from a hyperextension injury in an older person with pre-existing osteoarthritis of the spine. The spinal cord is pinched between the vertebral body anteriorly and the buckling ligamentum flavum posteriorly (Fig. 80-7, *A*). It also may occur in younger patients with flexion injuries.

The *Brown-Séquard syndrome* is an injury to either half of the spinal cord (Fig. 80-7, *C*) and is usually the result of a unilateral laminar or pedicle fracture, penetrating injury, or a rotational injury resulting in a subluxation. It is characterized by motor weakness on the side of the lesion and the contralateral loss of pain and temperature sensation. Prognosis for recovery is good with significant neurologic improvement often occurring.

Anterior cord syndrome usually is caused by a hyperflexion injury with bone or disc fragments compressing the anterior spinal artery and cord. It is characterized by complete motor loss and loss of pain and temperature discrimination below the level of injury. The posterior columns are spared to varying degrees (Fig. 80-7. *D*), resulting in preservation of deep touch, position sense, and vibratory sensation. Prognosis for significant recovery in this injury is poor.

Posterior cord syndrome involves the dorsal columns of the spinal cord and produces loss of proprioception vibrating sense while preserving other sensory and motor functions. This syndrome is rare and usually is caused by an extension injury.

A *mixed syndrome* usually is an unclassifiable combination of several syndromes. It describes the small percentage of incomplete spinal cord injuries that do not fit one of the previously described syndromes.

Conus medullaris syndrome, or injury of the sacral cord (conus) and lumbar nerve roots within the spinal canal, usually results in areflexic bladder, bowel, and lower extremities. Most of these injuries occur bewtween T11 and L2 and result in flaccid paralysis in the perineum and loss of all bladder and perianal muscle control. The irreversible nature of this injury to the sacral segments is evidenced by the absence of the bulbocaver-

Table 80-3 Function attained following central cord lesion*

	Admission (%)	Present at discharge (%)	Follow-up (%)
Ambulation	33.3	77	59
Hand function	26	42	56
Bladder function	17	—	53
Bowel function	9.5	—	53

From Bosch A, Stauffer ES, and Nickel VL: JAMA 216:473, 1971.
*Chronic sequelae of central cord damage: (1) increased spasticity and pyramidal tract involvement, (2) incidence of 23.8%, and (3) prognosis poor with progressive neurologic loss.

Table 80-4 Function attained following hemisection cord lesion

	Admission (%)	Present at discharge (%)	Follow-up (%)
Ambulation	60	100	80
Hand function	60	80	100
Bowel function	80	80	100
Bladder function	100	100	100

From Bosch A, Stauffer ES, and Nickel VL: JAMA 216:473, 1971.

Table 80-5 Function attained following anterior cord lesion

	Admission (%)	Present at discharge (%)	Follow-up (%)
Ambulation	0	0	0
Hand function	16	16	16
Bladder function	0	0	0
Bowel function	0	0	0

From Bosch A, Stauffer ES, and Nickel VL: JAMA 216:473, 1971.

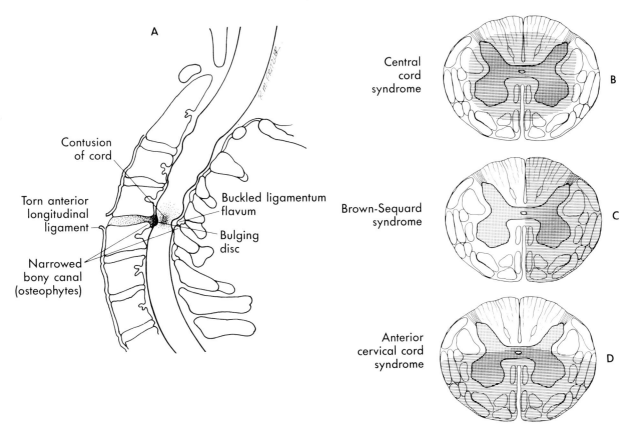

Fig. 80-7 Spinal cord lesions. **A** and **B,** Central cord syndrome; spinal cord is pinched between vertebral body and buckling ligamentum flavum. **C,** Brown-Séquard syndrome. **D,** Anterior cervical cord syndrome.

nosus reflex and the perianal wink. Motor function in the lower extremities between L1 and L4 may be present if nerve root sparing occurs.

Cauda equina syndrome, or injury between the conus and the lumbosacral nerve roots within the spinal canal, also results in areflexic bladder, bowel, and lower limbs. With a complete cauda equina injury, all peripheral nerves to the bowel, bladder, perianal area, and lower extremities are lost, and the bulbocavernosus reflex, anal wink, and all reflex activity in the lower extremities are absent, indicating absence of any function in the cauda equina. It is important to remember that the cauda equina functions as the peripheral nervous system, and there is a possibility of return of function of the nerve rootlets if they have not been completely transected or destroyed. Most often the cauda equina syndrome presents as a neurologically incomplete lesion.

EMERGENCY ROOM MANAGEMENT

The initial examination of a trauma patient with suspected spinal injury is performed by general surgery, anesthesia, respiratory, neurosurgery, and orthopaedic specialists. Although cardiovascular, respiratory, and neuro-

logic functions generally are evaluated by the appropriate specialists, the orthopaedist should remember three changes in vital signs that suggest a cervical or upper thoracic fracture with spinal cord injury above the level of T6: hypotension, hypothermia, and brachycardia.

A National Acute Spinal Cord Injury study reported the results of a double-blind, randomized, controlled clinical trial of very high-dose methylprednisolone in the treatment of acute spinal cord injury. Compared with a control group, patients who had methylprednisolone infusion within 8 hours of injury showed significantly more improvement in motor function and pinprick and touch sensation at 6 weeks and at 6 months after injury. At this time, all patients seen at our level 1 trauma center who have a confirmed acute spinal cord injury and have no contraindications for administation of a corticosteroid are treated with a protocol of methylprednisolone administration consisting of a bolus dose of 30 mg per kilogram of body weight administered over 15 mintues, followed by a 45-minute pause, and then a 23-hour continuous infusion of 5.4 mg per kilogram per hour. Bracken et al. reported 55% overall improvement in motor function, with more significant improvement if methylprednisolone therapy was begun within 8 hours of injury. Because of the massive dose of steroid administered over a 24-hour period, there is the potential for increased incidences of wound infection and gastrointestinal hemorrhage.

CERVICAL SPINE INJURIES

The cervical spinal column is extremely vulnerable to injury. The seven cervical vertebrae, whose specific facet joint articulations allow movement in the planes of flexion, extension, lateral bending, and rotation, have attached at the cephalic aspect the skull and its contents. Injury occurs when forces applied to the head and neck result in loads that exceed the ability of the supporting structures to dissipate energy. Many cervical spine injuries are caused by hyperextension in older patients with spondylolitic disease or in younger patients with congenitally narrowed spinal canals.

Jefferson found that injuries to the cervical spine involve two particular areas: C1 to C2 and C5 to C7. Meyer identified C2 and C5 as the two most common areas of cervical spine injury. Injuries of the cervical spine produce neurologic damage in approximately 40% of patients. Approximately 10% of traumatic cord injuries have no obvious roentgenographic evidence of vertebral injury.

Classification

Numerous classifications of cervical spine injuries have been formulated, but the mechanistic classification proposed by Allen et al. appears to be the most complete. In a review of 165 lower cervical spine injuries, they identified the following six common patterns of injury, each of which is subdivided into stages based on the degree of injury to osseous and ligamentous structures.

Compressive flexion (five stages)

- CF stage 1: blunting of the anterosuperior vertebral margin to a rounded contour, and no evidence of failure of the posterior ligamentous complex.
- CF stage 2: obliquity of the anterior vertebral body with loss of some anterior height of the centrum, in addition to the changes seen in stage 1. The anteroinferior vertebral body has a "beak" appearance, concavity of the inferior end plate may be increased, and the vertebral body may have a vertical fracture.
- CF stage 3: fracture line passing obliquely from the anterior surface of the vertebra through the centrum and extending through the inferior subchondral plate, and a fracture of the beak, in addition to the characteristics of a stage 2 injury.
- CF stage 4: deformation of the centrum and fracture of the beak with mild (less than 3 mm) displacement of the inferoposterior vertebral margin into the spinal canal.
- CF stage 5: bony injuries as in stage 3 but with more than 3 mm of displacement of the posterior portion of

the vertebral body posteriorly into the spinal canal. The vertebral arch remains intact, the articular facets are separated, and the interspinous process space is increased at the level of injury, suggesting a posterior ligamentous disruption in a tension mode.

Vertical compression (three stages)

- VC stage 1: fracture of the superior or inferior end plate with a "cupping" deformity. Failure of the end plate is central rather than anterior, and posterior ligamentous failure is not evident.
- VC stage 2: fracture of both vertebral end plates with cupping deformities. Fracture lines through the centrum may be present, but displacement is minimal.
- VC stage 3: progression of the vertebral body damage described in stage 2. The centrum is fragmented, and the displacement is peripheral in multiple directions. Most commonly the centrum fails with significant impaction and fragmentation. The posterior aspect of the vertebral body is fractured and may be displaced into the spinal canal. The vertebral arch may be intact with no evidence of ligamentous failure, or it may be comminuted with significant failure of the posterior ligamentous complex; the ligamentous disruption is between the fractured vertebra and the one below it.

Distractive flexion (four stages)

- DF stage 1: failure of the posterior ligamentous complex, as evidence by facet subluxation in flexion, with abnormal divergence of the spinous process.
- DF stage 2: unilateral facet dislocation (the degree of posterior ligamentous failure ranges from partial failure sufficient only to permit the abnormal displacement to complete failure of both the anterior and posterior ligamentous complexes, which is uncommon). Subluxation of the facet on the side opposite the dislocation suggests severe ligamentous injury. In addition, a small fleck of bone may be displaced from the posterior surface of the articular process, which is displaced anteriorly. Widening of the uncovertebral joint on the side of the dislocation and displacement of the tip of the spinous process toward the side of the dislocation may be seen. Beatson serially divided the posterior interspinous ligaments, facet capsule, posterior longitudinal ligament, anulus fibrosus, and anterior longitudinal ligament and found that unilateral facet dislocation can occur with rupture of only the posterior interspinous ligament and the facet capsule.
- DF stage 3: bilateral facet dislocations, with approximately 50% anterior subluxation of the vertebral body. Blunting of the anterosuperior margin of the inferior vertebra to a rounded corner may or may not be present. Beatson demonstrated that rupture of the interspinous ligament, the capsules of both facet joints, the posterior longitudinal ligament, and the anulus fibrosus of the intervertebral disc were necessary to create this lesion.
- DF stage 4: full vertebral body width displacement an-

teriorly or a grossly unstable motion segment, giving the appearance of a "floating" vertebra.

Compression extension (five stages)

- CE stage 1: unilateral vertebral arch fracture, with or without anterorotatory vertebral displacement. Posterior element failure may consist of a linear fracture through the articular process, impaction of the articular process, and ipsilateral pedicle and lamina fractures, resulting in the "transverse facet" appearance on anteroposterior roentgenograms, or a combination of ipsilateral pedicle and articular process fractures.
- CE stage 2: bilaminar fractures without evidence of other tissue failure. Typically the laminar fractures occur at multiple contiguous levels.
- CE stage 3: bilateral vertebral arch fractures with fracture of the articular processes, pedicles, lamina, or some bilateral combination, without vertebral body displacement.
- CE stage 4: bilateral vertebral arch fractures with partial vertebral body width displacement anteriorly.
- CE stage 5: bilateral vertebral arch fracture with full vertebral body width displacement anteriorly. The posterior portion of the vertebral arch of the fractured vertebra does not displace, and the anterior portion of the arch remains with the centrum. Ligament failure occurs at two levels: posteriorly between the fractured vertebra and the one above it and anteriorly between the fractured vertebra and the one below it. Characteristically, the anterosuperior portion of the vertebra below is sheared off by the anteriorly displaced centrum.

Distractive extension (two stages)

- DE stage 1: either failure of the anterior ligamentous complex or a transverse fracture of the centrum. The injury usually is ligamentous, and there may be a fracture of the adjacent anterior vertebral margin. The roentgenographic clue to this injury is abnormal widening of the disc space.
- DE stage 2: evidence of failure of the posterior ligamentous complex, with displacement of the upper vertebral body posteriorly into the spinal canal, in addition to the changes seen in stage 1 injuries. Because displacement of this type tends to reduce spontaneously when the head is placed in a neutral position, roentgenographic evidence of the displacement may be minimal, rarely greater than 3 mm on initial films with the patient supine.

Lateral flexion (two stages)

- LF stage 1: asymmetric compression fracture of the centrum and ipsilateral vertebral arch fracture, without displacement of the arch on the anteroposterior view. Compression of the articular process or comminution of the corner of the vertebral arch may be present.
- LF stage 2: lateral asymmetric compression of the centrum and either ipsilateral displaced vertebral arch fracture or ligamentous failure on the contralateral

side with separation of the articular processes. Both ipsilateral and compressive and contralateral disruptive vertebral arch injuries may be present.

Instability

White and Panjabi defined clinical instability as the loss of the ability of the spine under physiologic loads to maintain relationships between vertebrae in such a way that the spinal cord or nerve roots are not damaged or irritated and deformity or pain does not develop. Clinical instability may be caused by trauma, neoplastic or infectious disorders, or iatrogenic causes. Instability may be acute or chronic. Acute instability is caused by bone or ligament disruption that places the neural elements in danger of injury with any subsequent loading or deformity. Chronic instability is the result of progressive deformity that may cause neurologic deterioration, prevent recovery of injured neural tissue, or cause increasing pain or decreasing function.

In a series of cadaver studies, White and Panjabi systematically cut the various supporting structures and noted the resulting instabilities of the spine. The supporting structures of the lower cervical spine can be divided into two groups: anterior and posterior (Fig. 80-8). A motion segment is made up of two adjacent vertebrae and the intervening soft tissues. If a motion segment has all the anterior elements and one posterior element intact, or all the posterior elements and one anterior element intact, it will remain stable under physiologic loads. White and Panjabi suggest that a motion segment

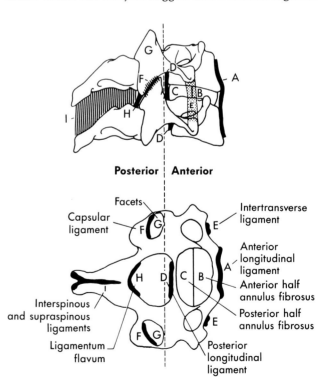

Fig. 80-8 Important anterior and posterior supporting structures of the spine. (Redrawn from White AA, Southwick WO, and Panjabi MM: Spine 1:15, 1976.)

Table 80-6 Checklist for diagnosis of clinical instability in lower cervical spine*

Element	Point value
Anterior elements destroyed or unable to function	2
Posterior elements destroyed or unable to function	2
Relative sagittal plane translation >3.5 mm	2
Relative sagittal plane rotation >11 degrees	2
Positive stretch test	2
Medullary (cord) damage	2
Root damage	1
Abnormal disc narrowing	1
Dangerous loading anticipated	1

From White AA, Southwick WO, and Panjabi MM: Spine 1:15, 1976.
*Total of 5 or more = unstable.

should be considered unstable if all the anterior or posterior elements are not functional. They developed a checklist for the diagnosis of clinical instability of the lower cervical spine (Table 80-6), in which a score of 5 or more indicates instability.

Roentgenographically, cervical spine instability is indicated by the horizontal translation of one vertebra relative to an adjacent vertebra in excess of 3.5 mm on the lateral flexion-extension view (Fig. 80-9). Instability also

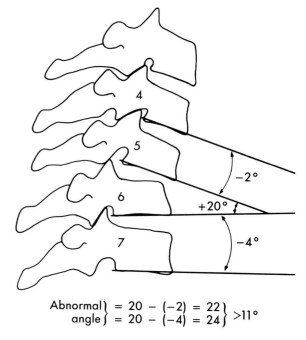

$$\begin{matrix} \text{Abnormal} \\ \text{angle} \end{matrix} \Bigg\} = \begin{matrix} 20 - (-2) = 22 \\ 20 - (-4) = 24 \end{matrix} \Bigg\} > 11°$$

Fig. 80-10 Significant sagittal plane rotation (more than 11 degrees) suggests instability. (Redrawn from White AA, Johnson RM, and Panjabi MM: Clin Orthop 120:85, 1975.)

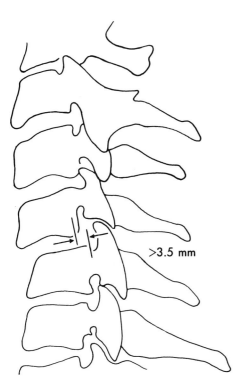

Fig. 80-9 Sagittal plane translation of more than 3.5 mm suggests clinical instability. (Redrawn from White AA, Johnson RM, and Panjabi MM: Clin Orthop 120:85, 1975.)

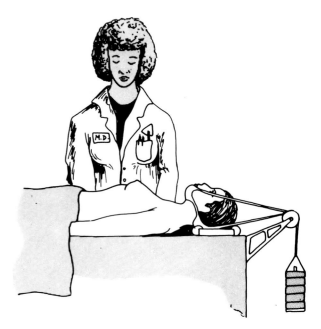

Fig. 80-11 Stretch test to determine cervical spine instability. This test must be closely monitored by physician and is contraindicated when spine is obviously unstable. (Redrawn from White AA III and Panjabi MM: Clinical biomechanics of the spine, Philadelphia, 1978, JB Lippincott Co.)

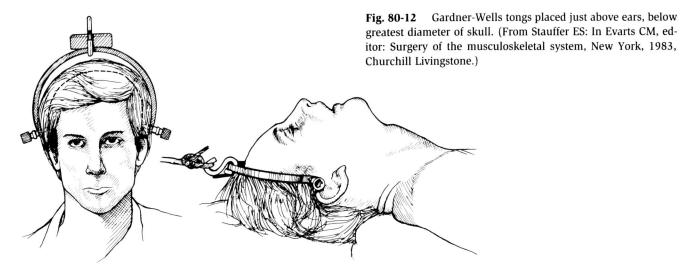

Fig. 80-12 Gardner-Wells tongs placed just above ears, below greatest diameter of skull. (From Stauffer ES: In Evarts CM, editor: Surgery of the musculoskeletal system, New York, 1983, Churchill Livingstone.)

is indicated by more than 11 degrees of angulation of one vertebra relative to another (Fig. 80-10).

STRETCH TEST. The stretch test (Fig. 80-11) may be useful for determining clinical instability in the lower cervical spine, but it is contraindicated in an obviously unstable injury. This test measures the displacement patterns of the spine under carefully controlled conditions and identifies anterior or posterior disrupted ligaments. The stretch test should always be done under supervision of the attending physician.

■ *TECHNIQUE.* Apply traction through secured skeletal traction or a head halter. If the latter is used, place a small piece of gauze sponge between the molars for patient comfort. Place a roller under the patient's head. Place the roentgenographic film as close as possible to the patient's neck, position the roentgen tube 72 inches from the film, and make a lateral exposure. Add weight up to 10 pounds and increase traction in 5-pound increments, repeating the lateral views after each addition until either one third of the body weight or 65 pounds is reached. After each addition of weight, check for any change in neurologic status. The test is considered positive and should be discontinued if any neurologic changes occur or if any abnormal separation of the anterior or posterior vertebral elements occurs. Allow at least 5 minutes between incremental weight applications for developing the film, evaluating neurologic status, and checking for creep of the viscoelastic structures involved. White, Southwick, and Panjabi suggest that a stretch test is abnormal if differences in interspace separation are more than 1.7 mm or if the angle between the prestretched condition and that after application of maximum weight is more than 7.5 degrees.

Treatment

The goals of treatment of cervical spine injuries are (1) to realign the spine, (2) to prevent loss of function of undamaged neurologic tissue, (3) to improve neurologic recovery, (4) to obtain and maintain spinal stability, and (5) to obtain early functional recovery. After initial medical stabilization and documentation of neurologic function, spinal alignment can be obtained by skeletal traction through spring-loaded Gardner-Wells tongs or a halo ring. Continuous monitoring during reduction is essential to prevent iatrogenic injury from overdistraction of an unstable motion segment. Ten pounds of traction weight is applied, then weight is added in 5-pound increments, with lateral roentgenograms after each addition, until the spine is realigned (Fig. 80-12). Although there is no agreement on the safe upper limit of traction, most surgeons do not apply more than 40 to 50 pounds of traction. A general guideline is 10 pounds for the head and 5 pounds for each additional level of injury (Table 80-7). If spinal realignment cannot be obtained by traction, open reduction and stabilization, usually through a posterior approach, are indicated. If spinal realignment is

Table 80-7 Traction recommended for levels of injury

Level	Minimum weight in pounds (kg)	Maximum weight in pounds (kg)
First cervical vertebra	5 (2.3)	10 (4.5)
Second cervical vertebra	6 (2.7)	10-12 (4.5-5.4)
Third cervical vertebra	8 (3.6)	10-15 (4.5-6.8)
Fourth cervical vertebra	10 (4.5)	15-20 (6.8-9.0)
Fifth cervical vertebra	12 (5.4)	20-25 (9.0-11.3)
Sixth cervical vertebra	15 (6.8)	20-30 (9.0-13.5)
Seventh cervical vertebra	18 (8.1)	25-35 (11.3-15.8)

obtained with traction and is documented roentgenographically, weight is reduced by 50% to maintain alignment and the course of treatment is determined. Usually tomograms, CT scanning, and MRI provide additional information about ligamentous, intervertebral disc, and osseous injuries. The pathologic anatomy must be carefully defined before treatment is determined. Arena, Eismont, and Green reported that 8.8% of patients had extrusion of a cervical disc in addition to cervical facet subluxations or dislocations. They recommend preoperative evaluation with myelography, CT scanning, or MRI. If a disc is herniated, anterior discectomy and interbody fusion should be performed before posterior cervical wiring and fusion to avoid neurologic deterioration.

NONOPERATIVE TREATMENT. Many cervical spine injuries can be treated without surgery. Immobilization in a rigid cervical orthosis for 8 to 12 weeks may be sufficient. For a stable cervical spine injury with no compression of the neural elements, a rigid cervical brace or halo for 8 to 12 weeks usually produces a stable, painless spine without residual deformity. Stable compression fractures of the vertebral bodies and undisplaced fractures of the laminae, lateral masses, or spinous processes also can be treated with immobilization in a cervical orthosis. Unilateral facet dislocations that are reduced in traction may be immobilized in a halo vest for 8 to 12 weeks. Patients with spinal fractures that are treated nonoperatively must be observed closely. Serial roentgenograms should be obtained weekly for the first 3 weeks, and then at 6 weeks, 3 months, 6 months, and 1 year. Herkowitz and Rothman demonstrated subacute instability of the cervical spine after initial roentgenographic evaluation that showed no bony or soft tissue abnormalities. The elastic and plastic deformation of the ligamentous structures and discs of the cervical spine is believed responsible for this subacute instability. Because subacute instability may occur despite adequate initial physical and roentgenographic examinations, a second complete evaluation should be performed within 3 weeks of injury.

Halo vest immobilization. The halo orthosis was first used by Perry and Nickel in 1959 for the stabilization after cervical spine fusion in patients with poliomyelitis. The use of the halo vest has expanded considerably since then, and it is used in the treatment of many cervical spine injuries.

Complications of halo immobilization have been reported to occur in as many as 30% of patients (Table 80-8). Recurrence of the spinal deformity secondary to loss of reduction also has been reported. Garfin et al. suggest that many of the complications of halo use can be avoided or minimized by the following measures:

1. Before insertion of the anterolateral pins, the patient should be requested to close his eyes tightly; if not, traction on the skin and muscles of the eyelids may prevent full closure of the eyes.

Table 80-8 Complications with halo immobilization

Complication	Patients (%)
Pin loosening	36
Pin infection	20
Pin site pain	18
Pressure sores under vest or cast	11
Disfiguring scars	9
Nerve injury	2
Dysphagia	2
Bleeding at pin site	1
Dural puncture	1

From Garfin SR, editor: Complications of spine surgery, Baltimore, 1989, Williams & Wilkins.

2. The pins should be routinely retightened after 24 to 48 hours. A loose pin should only be retightened once. Retightening efforts should be discontinued if no resistance is met during this procedure.
3. If a pin is to be replaced, a new pin should be inserted satisfactorily before the loose pin is removed to maintain the position of the halo ring and the alignment of the spine.
4. The recommended torque for insertion of the four halo pins is 8 inch-pounds instead of 4 or 6 inch-pounds. Increasing the insertional torque to 10 pounds increases the penetration of the pin but does not significantly improve the structural properties of the pin-bone interface. Ballock, Botte, and Garfin noted marked reductions in pin loosening and pin infection rates when the pins were inserted at 8 inch-pounds compared with 6 inch-pounds.
5. The risk of dislodgement of the halo ring is minimized by proper placement of the ring above the orbit but below the greatest circumference of the calvarium.
6. Local pin care should be meticulous to prevent pin site infection. The pin site should be cleaned daily with povidone-iodine or hydrogen peroxide. If pin site infection occurs, the wound should be cultured, antibiotic sensitivities should be obtained, and appropriate antibiotic therapy should be initiated.
7. The most commonly injured nerves are the supraorbital and supratrochlear. These injuries may be avoided by not placing pins over the medial third of the orbit.
8. Inserting the anterolateral pins behind the hairline in hopes of obtaining a more cosmetically acceptable scar should be avoided if possible. This location places the pin within the temporal fossa where the skull is the thinnest. Pins located in the temporal fossa also pierce the temporalis muscle and often lead to painful mastication.
9. Application of a well-molded plaster body jacket attached to the halo, which may be extended down over the iliac crest for additional support, may be

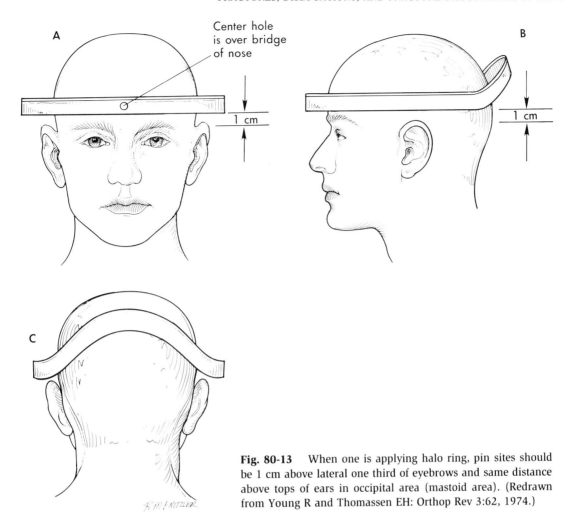

Fig. 80-13   When one is applying halo ring, pin sites should be 1 cm above lateral one third of eyebrows and same distance above tops of ears in occipital area (mastoid area). (Redrawn from Young R and Thomassen EH: Orthop Rev 3:62, 1974.)

substituted for the premolded polyethylene vest if increased stability is desired.

■ *TECHNIQUE FOR APPLICATION OF THE HALO.* Place the patient supine with his head supported just over the end of the stretcher by an assistant or by an application device that is attached to the stretcher and that will also hold the halo ring. Prepare the skin and scalp by washing the hair with a surgical preparation such as povidone-iodine. Have an assistant hold a halo of appropriate size about the patient's head or place the halo in the application device. Hold the halo below the area of greatest diameter of the skull, about at the level of the eyebrows and approximately 1 cm above the tips of the ears (Fig. 80-13). Inject a local anesthetic into the four areas selected for pin insertion, and place the two anterior pins in bare skin and not within the hairline. The bone is extremely thin just anterior to the ears, and anchorage here is not good. Also, the supraorbital nerve should be avoided. Posteriorly the central channels are usually the best sites. Introduce the pins and tighten two diagonally opposed pins simultaneously. Be certain that the patient closes his eyes during the insertion of the two anterolateral pins. Continue to tighten the pins until all four engage the skin and bone. Continue tightening diagonal pairs of pins with a torque screwdriver. Alternate tightening of the pins to prevent migration of the halo to an asymmetric position. Tighten all pins to 8 inch-pounds. Secure the pins to the halo with appropriate lock nuts or set screws. Attach the halo ring to the halo vest through the anterior and posterior uprights or attach the halo ring to a well-molded plaster body jacket. Anteroposterior and lateral radiographs should be obtained to document the alignment of the spine.

SURGICAL TREATMENT. Unstable injuries of the cervical spine, with or without neurologic deficit, require operative treatment. In most patients, early open reduction and internal fixation are indicated to obtain stability. Cervical spine fractures may be stabilized through an anterior or posterior approach; usually a posterior approach is used with triple-wire stabilization and fusion with iliac bone grafting. This allows rapid mobilization of the patient in a cervical orthosis, and healing usually

A   B   C

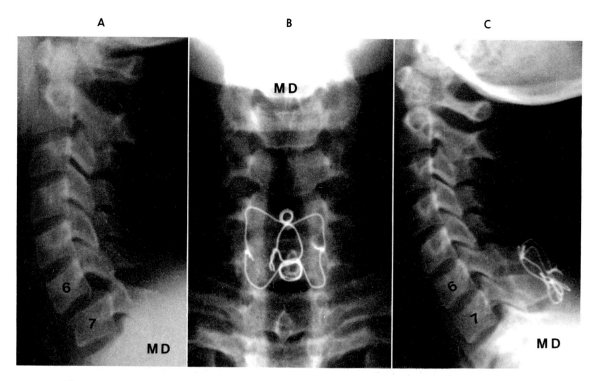

Fig. 80-14   A, Distraction flexion lesion at C6-7 in 18-year-old patient. Note widening of inter-spinous process space, moderate anterior subluxation at C6-7, and perched facets bilaterally. **B** and **C,** After posterior stabilization with triple-wire technique and autogenous iliac bone graft, spinal alignment is restored. Patient was mobilized early in rigid cervical orthosis and had full functional recovery.

occurs within 8 to 12 weeks. If the spinal cord or nerve roots are compressed by retropulsed bone fragments or disc material, anterior decompression may be indicated to improve neurologic recovery. Stauffer and Kelly, however, reported instability and recurrent deformity after anterior decompression and strut grafting in posteriorly unstable fractures. Posterior stability should be obtained first, followed by anterior decompression and fusion if indicated. The exception to this is the rare patient with a subluxation or dislocation that cannot be reduced by traction and that produces minimal or no neurologic symptoms. MRI, CT scanning, or myelography should be performed to determine if a disc is herniated. If so, anterior discectomy and interbody fusion are indicated, followed by a posterior procedure. Anderson, Bohlman, and Freehafer reported improved neurologic recovery in patients with both incomplete and complete cord injuries after anterior decompression and fusion.

When decompression or stabilization is indicated, several basic principles should be followed:

1. The injury must be clearly defined before surgery by plain roentgenograms, high-resolution CT scanning with sagittal and coronal reconstruction, or MRI.
2. Laminectomy has a limited role in the treatment of cervical fractures or dislocations and may contribute to clinical instability and neurologic deficit. It

may be occasionally indicated if posterior bone fragments from the neural arch are compressing the neural elements.
3. Compression of the cervical cord or roots by retropulsed bone fragments or disc material usually is anterior, and anterior decompression and fusion are indicated.
4. For posterior ligamentous or bony instability, posterior fusion with triple-wire fixation and iliac bone grafting is indicated.

The choice of surgical approaches depends on the pattern of injury. Posterior approaches usually are indicated for ligamentous instability (Fig. 80-14). Anterior decompression and fusion are most often indicated for burst fractures of the cervical spine with documented compression of the neural elements by retropulsed bone or disc fragments and an incomplete neurologic deficit (Fig. 80-15). Combined anterior decompression and posterior fusion are indicated for posterior instability and anterior compression of the neural elements (Fig. 80-16).

INJURIES TO UPPER CERVICAL SPINE (OCCIPUT TO C2)

Dislocations of atlanto-occipital joint. Dislocations of the atlanto-occipital joint are uncommon (Fig. 80-17). The injury may be either anterior or posterior and usually is fatal, although there are reports in the literature of

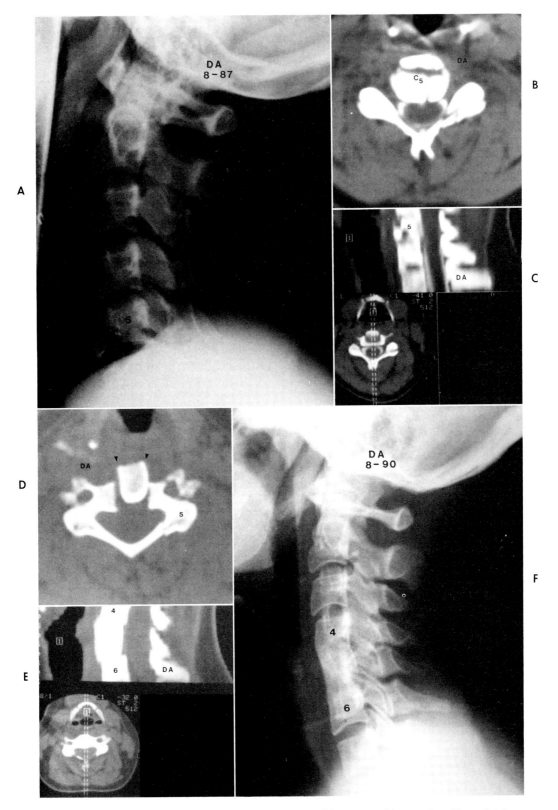

Fig. 80-15   **A,** Compressive flexion injury in 20-year-old woman with complete C5 quadriplegia. **B,** CT scan shows encroachment on subarachnoid space and flattening of cervical cord,
with fractures of left lateral mass. **C,** CT scan with sagittal reconstruction shows fracture of C5
vertebral body with mild displacement of posterior vertebral margin into spinal canal; no widening of interspinous process space, suggestive of posterior ligamentous instability, is apparent.
D, CT scan after anterior decompression and iliac crest strut grafting. **E,** CT scan with sagittal
reconstruction shows adequate decompression of spinal cord and proper position of graft from
C4 to C6. **F,** Three years after surgery, lateral roentgenogram shows incorporation of graft and
solid arthrodesis from C4 to C6. Patient had single-level root recovery and is functional C6
quadriplegic.

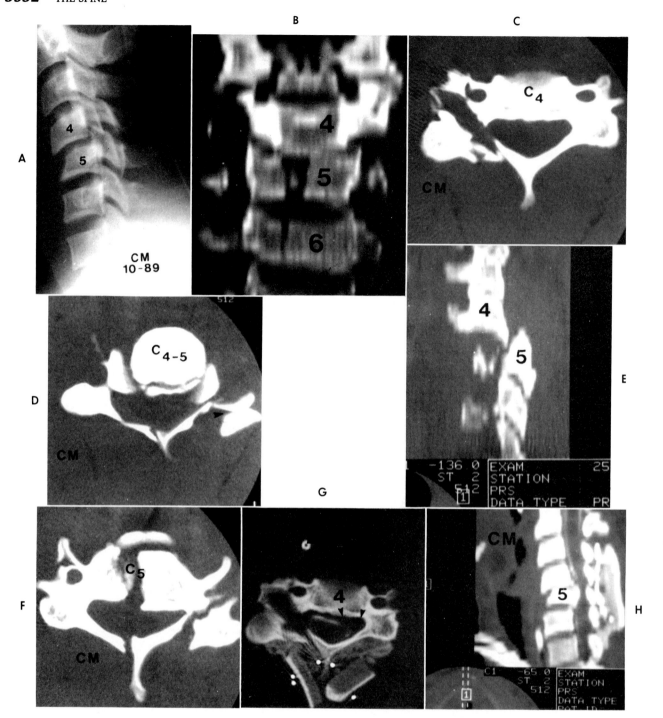

Fig. 80-16 Collegiate defensive back sustained axial loading injury to cervical spine while making tackle; he was rendered complete C5 quadriplegic. **A,** Lateral roentgenogram shows mild anterior subluxation of C4 and C5 caused by left unilateral facet dislocation. **B,** CT scan with coronal reconstruction shows significant fractures of bodies of C5 and C6 that were not noted on lateral roentgenogram. **C,** CT scan through C4 vertebral body shows fractures through ipsilateral right pedicle and lamina with free-floating lateral mass at this level. **D,** CT scan through C4 and C5 shows unilateral left-sided C4-5 facet dislocation *(arrow)*. **E,** CT scan with sagittal reconstruction shows left-sided unilateral C4-5 facet dislocation. **F,** CT scan through C5 vertebral body shows significant fractures of anterior and posterior elements and marked narrowing of spinal canal. **G,** CT scan with sagittal reconstruction shows significant narrowing of spinal canal resulting from retropulsed bone and disc material. **H,** CT scan with contrast in subarachnoid space shows disc material retropulsed into spinal canal to left of midline behind body of C4. This was believed to impair function of left C4 nerve root and cause paralysis of left hemidiaphragm. Note also large, cortical cancellous bone graft wired into place posteriorly.

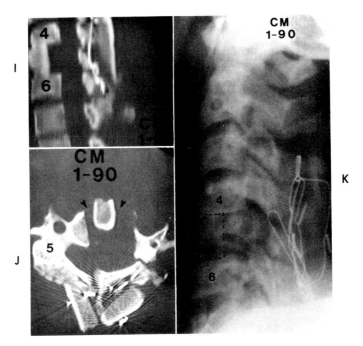

Fig. 80-16, cont'd **I**, CT scan with sagittal reconstruction shows adequate decompression at C5 and placement of iliac strut graft from C4 to C6. **J**, Axial scan confirms adequate anterior decompression and proper placement of strut grafts *(arrow)*. Spinal alignment has been restored and stability achieved. **K**, Lateral roentgenogram shows final alignment of spine after combined anterior and posterior fusions; note oblique facet wire used for additional rotational stability.

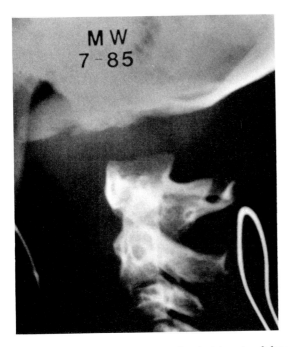

Fig. 80-17 Lateral roentgenogram of pedestrian struck by car who sustained fatal atlanto-occipital dislocation. Note marked widening of space between base of skull and atlas.

patients who survived this injury. Davis et al., in an extensive study of fatal cranial spinal injuries, demonstrated that many spinal injuries occurred between the occiput and C3. For this injury to occur, the alar and apical ligaments, the tectorial membrane, and the posterior atlanto-occipital ligaments must be disrupted. Fractures of the atlanto-occipital joint may accompany the dislocation. Many patients die immediately from complete respiratory arrest caused by brain stem compression. Treatment of these injuries requires reduction of the dislocation and stabilization of the atlanto-occipital joint. Cervical traction is contraindicated because of severe instability. Immediate application of a halo vest is recommended to stabilize the joint. The patient's respiratory and neurologic status must be carefully monitored. We recommend early surgical stabilization of the atlanto-occipital joint because ligamentous healing in a halo vest is not predictable and many of these injuries are so unstable that displacement may occur even in the halo vest. Stabilization is obtained by posterior cervical arthrodesis using large cortical cancellous bone grafts wired in place as described by Wertheim and Bohlman (Fig. 80-18).

■ *TECHNIQUE (WERTHEIM AND BOHLMAN).* After careful fiberoptic nasal tracheal intubation and with somatosensory evoked potential monitoring equipment in place, position the patient prone on a Stryker frame with a previously applied halo vest in

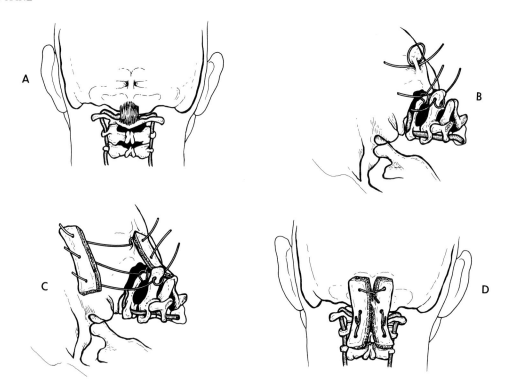

Fig. 80-18   Wertheim and Bohlman method of occipitocervical fusion. **A,** Burr is used to create ridge in external occipital protuberance and then hole is made in ridge. **B,** Wires are passed through outer table of occiput, under arch of atlas, and through spinous process of axis. **C,** Grafts are placed on wires. **D,** Wires are tightened to secure grafts in place. (Redrawn from Wertheim SB and Bohlman HH: J Bone Joint Surg 69-A:833, 1987.)

place. The posterior shell of the halo vest and the uprights may be removed for exposure of the neck. Prepare and drape the patient in the usual manner. Infiltrate the skin and subcutaneous tissues with a 1:500,000 epinephrine solution to aid hemostasis, and make a midline skin incision from the occiput to C3. Carry dissection down in the midline from the inion distally to the level of the third cervical spinous process. Subperiosteally expose the posterior elements from the occiput to C2 using periosteal elevators and electrocautery to reduce interfascial and periosteal bleeding. Take care not to extend the dissection farther than 1.5 cm laterally at the level of the C1 vertebra to avoid injury to the vertebral arteries. Using a high-speed burr, drill a transverse hole across the keel region of the occiput below the inion in the midline overlying the cerebellum (Fig. 80-18, *A*), and place a wire for fixation of the bone graft to the calvaria. If this bony prominence, the inion, does not exist, drill the hole closer to the border of the foramen magnum. Drill a second hole through the base of the spinous process of C2, and place a 20-gauge wire through the transverse hole beneath the inion and loop it on itself to fix the bone graft to the base of the skull. Place additional 20-gauge wires sublaminally beneath the ring of C1 and through the hole in the base of C2

and loop each around the inferior aspect of the spinous process (Fig. 80-18, *B*). Remove a thick, unicortical, cancellous bone graft from the posterior aspect of the ilium. The shape of the iliac wing allows the graft to curve and more nearly match the area to be spanned across the occipitocervical junction.

Lightly decorticate with a Hall high speed burr. Drill matching holes in the graft for the insertion of the wires and tighten the graft into place with the cancellous portion of the graft adjacent to the posterior elements of the occiput and C1-2 (Fig. 80-18, *C* and *D*). Tighten the wire through the base of the occiput to its adjacent free end, the free ends of the sublaminar wire beneath the ring of C1, and the wires through the base of the spinous process of C2 to lock the bone grafts in place. Thoroughly irrigate the wound with antibiotic solution, insert a closed suction drain, and close the wound in layers.

AFTERTREATMENT. Halo traction may be used after surgery or the posterior shell of the halo vest may be reapplied. Consolidation of the bone grafts generally occurs by 12 to 16 weeks.

Fractures of the atlas. Jefferson first described burst fractures of the atlas in 1920, attributing the fracture to axial loading to the top of the head. Levine and Edwards, in a review of 144 patients with 163 injuries of the C1-2 complex, found that 53% of patients with fractures of the atlas also had other cervical spinal fractures, most commonly type I traumatic spondylolisthesis of the axis and posteriorly displaced type II and type III dens fractures. They also emphasize the difficulty of accurate roentgenographic diagnosis of these injuries. The lateral cervical spine view usually shows fractures through the posterior arch of C1. However, when the fracture is extremely anterior to the junction of the lateral mass of C1, the fracture may not be visible on the lateral view. They found anteroposterior and lateral tomography to be accurate in detecting fractures in both the anterior and posterior portions of the ring of C1, but CT scans failed to demonstrate all fractures in 6 of 11 patients.

Three primary types of fractures of the ring of C1 have been identified: (1) posterior arch fracture, which usually occurs at the junction of the posterior arch and the lateral mass; (2) lateral mass fracture, which usually occurs on one side only with the fracture line passing either through the articular surface or just anterior and posterior to the lateral mass on one side; a fracture through the posterior arch on the opposite side sometimes occurs; and (3) burst fracture (Jefferson fracture), which is characterized by four fractures, two in the posterior arch and two in the anterior arch.

Most fractures of the atlas can be treated with immobilization in a rigid cervical orthosis or a halo vest. Isolated posterior arch fractures are stable injuries that can be treated in a cervical collar for 8 to 12 weeks. In the 53% of patients with additional cervical spinal injuries in their series, Levine and Edwards reported loss of reduction of some C2 fractures after surgery because of a failure to recognize a fracture in the posterior arch of C1. In some patients an occiput to C2 stabilization resulted in severe restriction of cervical spine motion. We agree with Levine and Edwards that external immobilization of the cervical spine until healing of the C1 ring fracture occurs should be done before proceeding with surgical stabilization of the C2 fracture.

Nondisplaced or minimally displaced fractures of the lateral mass and Jefferson fractures can be treated by collar immobilization to prevent displacement and allow fracture healing. Fractures in which the lateral mass of the atlas is displaced laterally more than 7 mm beyond the articular surfaces of the axis should be reduced with halo traction (Fig. 80-19). Halo traction should be maintained for 3 to 6 weeks before application of a halo vest if the lateral mass is severely displaced, because displacement may recur if a halo vest is applied immediately after reduction. Spence, Decker, and Cell determined that if the lateral mass overhangs the aritcular surfaces of the axis more than 7 mm a tear of the transverse ligament is likely, resulting in clinical C1-2 instability (Fig. 80-20). In axial loading of the C1-2 complex, the supporting alar ligaments, apical ligaments, and facet capsules usually remain intact, and significant instability is prevented by these remaining intact structures. Fielding et al. have shown that in severe flexion injuries with isolated transverse ligament ruptures, the alar ligament, facet capsules, and transverse ligament are rendered incompetent, resulting in gross clinical instability. However, Levine and Edwards on flexion and extension views of all their patients with lateral mass and Jefferson fractures found no significant C1-2 instability after fracture healing.

Rupture of the transverse ligament. This injury is a purely ligamentous injury and is different from other injuries involving the C1-2 complex. It most commonly results from a fall with a blow to the back of the head. The transverse ligament may be avulsed with a bony fragment from the lateral mass on either side, or it may rupture in its mid substance. Usually the anterior subluxation of the ring of C1 can be detected on flexion films and the instability can be reduced in extension (Fig. 80-21). Lateral views should be carefully checked for retropharyngeal hematoma, which suggests an acute injury, and for small flecks of bone avulsed off the lateral masses of C1, which may indicate avulsion of the ligament. The primary indication of this injury is instability at C1-2 on flexion and extension films. Anterior widening of the atlanto-dens interval of more than 5 mm on the flexion view suggests that the transverse ligament is incompetent. Flexion and extension views should be made under the supervision of the physician, and the patient must be closely monitored for alterations in neurologic or respiratory function.

Because rupture of the transverse ligament is primarily a ligamentous injury, nonoperative treatment is ineffective in obtaining stability. Surgical stabilization of the C1-2 complex is the treatment of choice. Initial treatment consists of immobilization through skull traction and then posterior stabilization of the C1-2 complex with a Gallie type of fusion. This type of fusion directs a vector force posteriorly to pull C1 into a reduced position in reference to C2. The dens prevents C1 from being pulled too far posteriorly and therefore overreduction is impossible. If a bone block technique, such as the Brooks-Jenkins fusion, is performed, the ring of C1 may redisplace anteriorly. If the posterior arch of C1 is fractured, a halo vest should be used for 8 to 12 weeks to allow healing of the posterior arch before proceeding with a standard C1-2 posterior arthrodesis. In 12 patients with ruptures of the transverse ligament, Levine and Edwards found an average loss of correction of 4 mm after bone block techniques and 1 mm after Gallie wiring.

Rotary subluxation of C1 on C2. This injury is uncommon in adults and is a different entity from rotatory subluxation in children (Fig. 80-22). The injury in adults usually is caused by motor vehicle accidents and often is not recognized at initial evaluation because the patient presents with torticollis and restricted neck motion. An open-mouth odontoid roentgenogram may reveal the

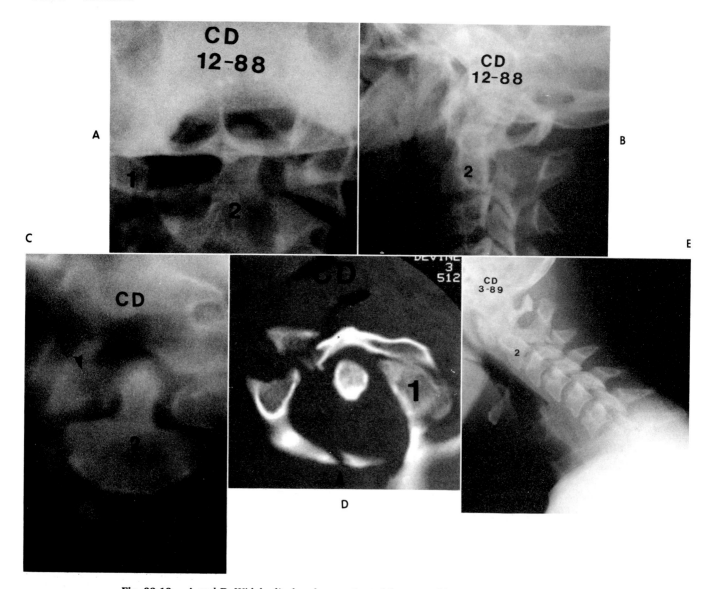

Fig. 80-19 **A** and **B,** Widely displaced, comminuted fracture of lateral mass of C1 in 22-year-old patient. Note marked asymmetry of lateral masses and extreme displacement of right lateral mass on anteroposterior open-mouth odontoid view. **C** and **D,** Anteroposterior tomogram and CT scan show associated fracture of lateral mass of C2, comminuted fracture of atlas involving right lateral mass and posterior arch. **E,** Flexion lateral view shows stability of C1-2 complex after 3 months of immobilization in halo vest.

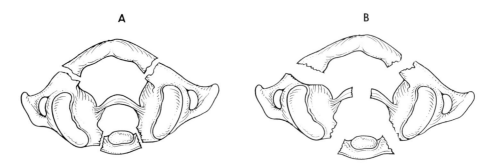

Fig. 80-20 **A,** Drawing indicating axial view of stable Jefferson's fracture (transverse ligament intact). **B,** Drawing indicating axial view of unstable Jefferson's fracture (transverse ligament ruptured). (Redrawn from Schlicke LH and Callahan R: Clin Orthop 154:18, 1981.)

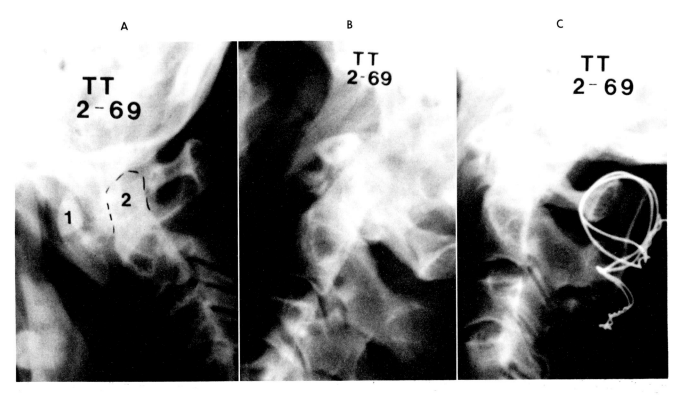

Fig. 80-21 This patient sustained a severe blow to back of head, resulting in instability of C1-2 complex because of torn transverse ligament. Note widening of atlanto-dens interval in flexion, **A,** and reduction in extension, **B. C,** After Gallie type of posterior C1-2 arthrodesis, lateral roentgenogram shows anatomic reduction of atlanto-dens interval.

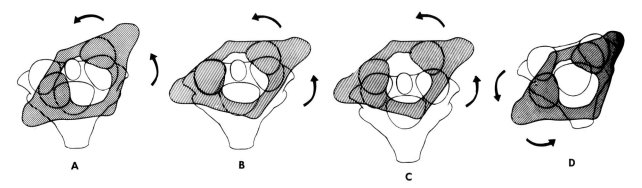

Fig. 80-22 Fielding and Hawkins classification of rotary displacement. **A,** Type I: simple rotary displacement without anterior shift; odontoid acts as pivot. **B,** Type II: rotary displacement with anterior displacement of 3 to 5 mm; lateral articular process acts as pivot. **C,** Type III: rotary displacement with anterior displacement of more than 5 mm. **D,** Type IV: rotary displacement with posterior displacement. (Redrawn from Fielding JW and Hawkins RJ: J Bone Joint Surg 59-A:37, 1977.)

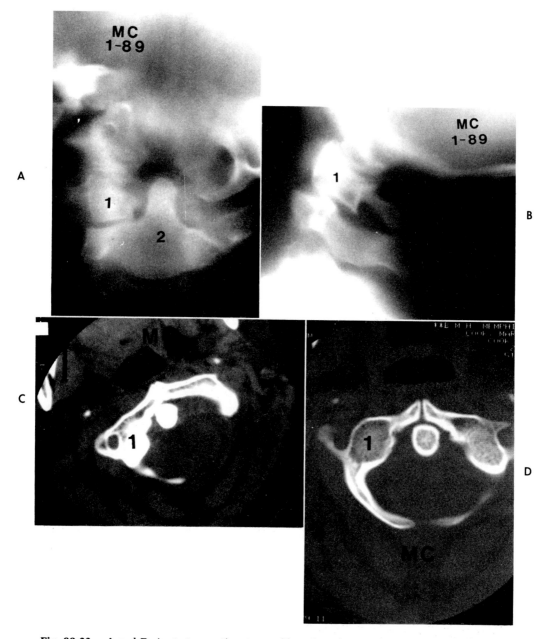

Fig. 80-23 **A** and **B,** Acute traumatic rotary subluxation of C1 on C2 sustained in motor vehicle accident. **C,** CT scan shows rotary subluxation of ring of atlas in relation to odontoid. **D,** After closed reduction, CT scan shows restoration of normal relationship of atlas and odontoid.

"wink sign" caused by overriding of the C1-2 joint on one side and a normal configuration on the other side. CT and routine anteroposterior tomography are helpful in clearly defining the osseous injury. Acute rotary dislocations of C1-2 can be reduced by closed means once the direction of the dislocation is determined (Fig. 80-23). With the patient awake and spinal cord monitoring in place, a halo ring is applied for control of the head. Using gentle traction, the halo ring is used to derotate the skull and C1 while an assistant pushes on the anteriorly displaced lateral mass through the posterior pharynx. Topical anesthesia applied to the posterior pharynx is helpful in diminishing the gag reflex. If stable reduction

is obtained and satisfactory alignment is demonstrated by roentgenogram and CT scan, the patient is immobilized in a halo vest. If closed reduction is unsuccessful, or if the injury has not been detected until late, open reduction may be attempted. With the patient prone, a midline posterior incision is made to subperiosteally expose the ring of C1 and the spinous process and lamina of C2. A wire is passed beneath the posterior arch of C1 and is used to manually derotate the ring of C1. Stabilization of the C1-2 complex can then be obtained with a posterior cervical arthrodesis using autogenous iliac bone grafting. An oblique wire from the base of the anteriorly displaced lateral mass of C1 to the spinous process

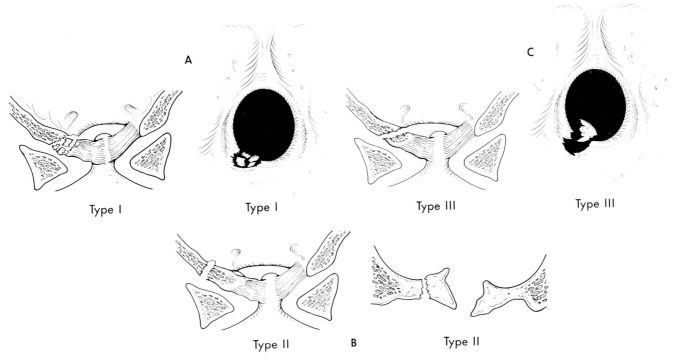

Fig. 80-24 Three types of occipital condylar fractures as described by Anderson and Montesano. **A,** Type I: impacted fracture. **B,** Type II: basilar skull fracture. **C,** Type III: avulsion fracture. (Redrawn from Anderson PA and Montesano PX: Spine 7:731, 1988.)

of C2 may be helpful in maintaining the reduction. Immobilization in a halo vest is recommended for 8 to 12 weeks to allow consolidation of the bone graft.

Fractures of the occipital condyle. Occipital condylar fractures are rare and are frequently missed on initial evaluation. These injuries usually result from axial loading and lateral bending during which force is applied to the head and neck. Recently Anderson and Montesano described three types of occipital condyle fractures (Fig. 80-24): type 1 — impaction; type 2 — associated with basilar skull fractures; and type 3 — avulsion fracture. Type 1 and 2 occipital condylar fractures are stable and can be treated in a rigid cervical orthosis or halo vest. Type 3 fractures are potentially unstable because of avulsion of the alar ligaments, and immobilization for 12 weeks in a halo vest is recommended. If instability is indicated on flexion and extension films after an adequate period of immobilization in a halo vest, then occipital to C2 fusion may be necessary. CT and routine anteroposterior and lateral tomography of the base of the skull will most likely show this fracture.

Fracture of the dens. Anderson and DeAlonzo classified odontoid fractures into three types (Fig. 80-25). Type I fractures are uncommon, and even if nonunion occurs after inadequate immobilizaton, no instability results. Type II fractures are the most common and in the study of Anderson and DeAlonzo had a 36% nonunion rate for both displaced and nondisplaced fractures. Type

III fractures have a large cancellous base and heal without surgery in 90% of patients. It also is helpful to consider the amount of displacement and angulation when determining prognosis and treatment. Clark and White, in a multicenter study of odontoid fractures, found that type II fractures united in 68% of patients treated in a halo vest and that posterior cervical fusion of the C1-2 complex was successful in 98% of patients. Treatment with orthoses was less successful. Significant displacement of more than 5 mm was evident in patients who had nonunions of type II odontoid fractures. Type III dens fracture united in 86% of patients, and the authors recommended halo vest immobilization for all displaced type III fractures because less rigid immobilization led to increased rates of nonunion and malunion. Several factors have been found to be important in union of dens fractures. The degree of initial displacement is critical: patients with displacement of more than 5 mm appear to have more nonunions. Other factors include the regional anatomy, the adequacy of reduction, the age of the patient, and type of immobilization.

The reported rates of fusion between the atlas and the axis vary widely in the literature. Schatzker, Roebeck, and Waddell reported union in 13 of 15 patients treated with primary wiring and fusion, and McGraw and Rusch reported union in 14 of 15 fractures. Because most reports have similarly good results, surgical stabilization seems a more reliable means of treating displaced fractures through the base of the odontoid.

In type II fractures of the dens, it is important to deter-

Type I

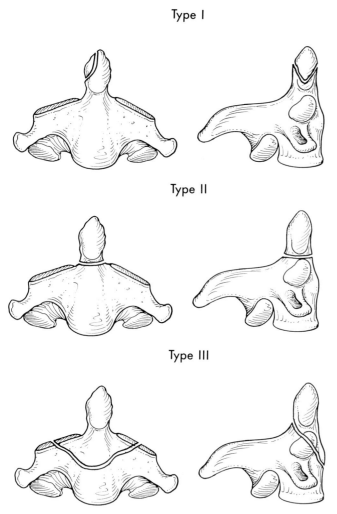

Type II

Type III

Fig. 80-25 Three types of odontoid process fractures as seen in anteroposterior and lateral planes. Type I is oblique fracture through upper part of odontoid process. Type II is fracture at junction of odontoid process and body of second cervical vertebra. Type III is fracture through upper body of vertebra. (Redrawn from Anderson LD and D'Alonzo RT: J Bone Joint Surg 56-A:1663, 1974.)

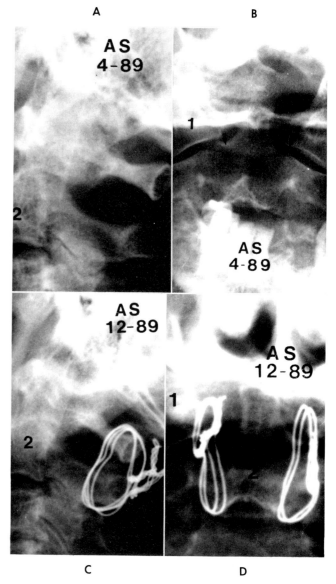

Fig. 80-26 **A** and **B**, Posteriorly displaced type II odontoid fracture in 50-year-old man. **C** and **D**, After stabilization of C1-2 complex by Brooks-Jenkins type of fusion.

mine if the displacement is anterior or posterior. Patients with posteriorly displaced dens fractures are more likely to also have fractures of the ring of C1. If a fracture in the posterior arch of C1 is not recognized, reduction may be lost after surgery or the fusion may have to be extended to include the occipitocervical joint, increasing morbidity and resulting in significant restriction of cervical motion. In addition, posteriorly displaced type II dens fractures have been found to be more unstable when treated with a Gallie type of wiring as compared to a bone block technique, such as the Brooks-Jenkins procedure. In the Gallie technique a wire passed around the ring of C1 and around the spinous process of C2 results in a posteriorly directed vector force that maintains reduction by a tension band. This posteriorly directed force may result in loss of reduction of the fracture. A bone block technique, such as the Brooks-Jenkins procedure, decreases the posterior vector force and maintains reduction

of posteriorly displaced odontoid fractures (Fig. 80-26).

Type III fractures through the body of the axis may be nondisplaced or displaced. Nondisplaced fractures are stable injuries that heal with 8 to 12 weeks of immobilization in either a halo vest or cervical collar. Levine and Edwards, in their 23 patients with displaced type III fractures through the body of the axis, found multiple combinations of angulation and translation. Although most fractures could be reduced with halo traction, continuous traction with extension was required to maintain reduction. They noted frequent loss of reduction when a halo vest was applied after only a short period of traction, but all fractures united. The goal of treatment of type III displaced dens fractures is correction of angulation in a halo vest, while allowing the fracture to settle until union occurs. No late sequelae have been demon-

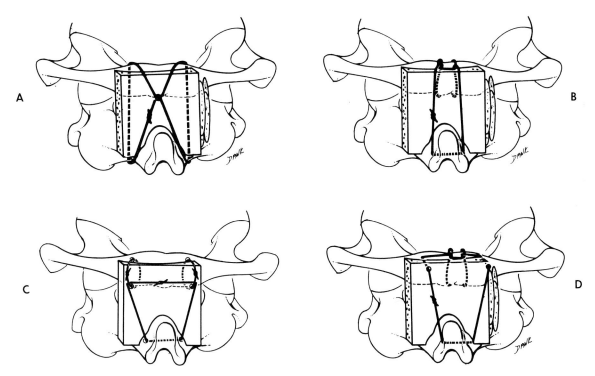

Fig. 80-27   Drawings to demonstrate various methods of using wire to hold graft in place. **A,** Wire passes under lamina of atlas and axis and is tied over graft. **B,** Wire passes through holes drilled in lamina of atlas and through spine of axis; holes are drilled through graft. **C,** Wire passes under lamina of atlas and through spine of axis and is tied over graft. This is method we use most frequently. **D,** Wire passes under lamina of atlas and through spine of axis; holes are drilled through graft. (From Fielding JW, Hawkins RJ, and Ratzan SA: J Bone Joint Surg 58-A:400, 1976.)

strated from the residual translation, although significant residual anterior angulation of the dens narrows the cervical spinal canal and may compress the spinal cord.

■ *TECHNIQUE (GALLIE).* Carefully intubate the patient in the supine position and then turn him prone on a Stryker frame with either tong or halo traction in place. In turning the patient take care to maintain the head-thoracic relationship. Then make cervical spine roentgenograms while the patient is on the operating table to be certain of the status of the fracture.

Prepare and drape the operative field in the usual fashion. Inject a 1:500,000 epinephrine solution intradermally to help with hemostasis. Then make a midline incision from the occiput to the fourth or fifth cervical vertebra. Using electrocautery and sharp dissection subperiosteally, expose the posterior arch of the atlas and the laminae of C2 and gently remove all soft tissue from the bony surfaces. The upper surface of the arch of C1 should be exposed no further laterally than 1.5 cm from the midline in adults and 1 cm in children to avoid the vertebral arteries. Decortication of C1 and C2 is generally not needed. Now pass a No. 20 gauge wire loop from below upward under the arch of the atlas ei-

ther directly or with the aid of a Mersiline suture; the suture can be passed using an aneurysm needle if necessary. Pass the free ends of the wire through the loop, thus grasping the arch of C1 in the loop (Fig. 80-27). Take a corticocancellous graft from the iliac crest and place it against the lamina of C2 and the arch of C1 beneath the wire. Then pass one end of the wire through the spinous process of C2 and twist the wire on itself to secure the graft in place. Irrigate the wound and close it in layers over suction drainage tubes.

AFTERTREATMENT. The patient is mobilized as soon as possible in either a halo vest or a rigid cervicothoracic spinal orthosis. For patients with a C1-2 arthrodesis, we prefer immobilization in a halo vest for about 12 weeks to allow consolidation of the bone grafts because biomechanical studies have shown the vest superior to cervicothoracic braces in maintaining stabilization. At 12 weeks, flexion and extension cervical roentgenograms should be made to document fusion.

■ *TECHNIQUE (BROOKS AND JENKINS).* Intubate and turn the patient on the operating table as in the Gallie fusion just described. Prepare and drape the patient in the same manner. Expose the C1-2 level

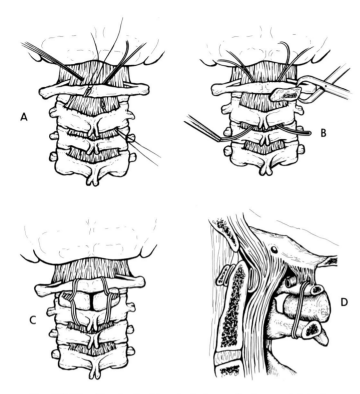

Fig. 80-28 Brooks-Jenkins technique of atlantoaxial fusion. **A,** Insertion of wires under atlas and axis. **B,** Wire in place with graft being inserted. **C** and **D,** Bone grafts secured by wires (anteroposterior and lateral views). (Redrawn from Brooks AL and Jenkins EB: J Bone Joint Surg 60-A:279, 1978.)

through a midline incision, as in the Gallie fusion. Using an aneurysm needle, pass a No. 2 Mersiline suture on each side of the midline in a cephalad-to-caudad direction, first under the arch of the atlas and then under the lamina of the axis (Fig. 80-28, *A*). These serve as guides to introduce two doubled 20-gauge stainless steel wires into place. Obtain two full-thickness rectangular bone grafts approximately 1.25 cm × 3.5 cm from the iliac crest. Bevel the grafts to fit in the interval between the arch of the atlas and each lamina of the axis (Fig. 80-28, *B*). While holding the grafts in position on each side of the midline and maintaining the width of the interlaminal space, tighten the doubled wires over them and twist and tie the wires to secure the grafts (Fig. 80-28, *C* and *D*). Irrigate and close the wound in layers over suction drains.

AFTERTREATMENT. The aftertreatment is the same as described for the Gallie fusion (see p. 3541).

Internal fixation of upper cervical spine. Recent advances in internal fixation have allowed its use in the cervical spine. Although considerable data concerning the biomechanics of internal fixation of the spine have been accumulated, indications for rigid internal fixation of specific spinal fractures are still evolving. We have lit-

tle experience with rigid internal fixation of cervical injuries at this time, but initial reports of these techniques are encouraging. With the advent of more sophisticated internal fixation techniques, however, comes an increased risk of complications. For this reason, we recommend that more aggressive internal fixation techniques be used only by experienced spinal surgeons.

Anterior screw fixation of dens fractures. Internal fixation of dens fractures with a cannulated screw system has been described by Aebi, Etter, and Coscia. This technique combines anatomic reduction of the fracture with stable internal screw fixation using the principles established by the AO/ASIF. They note that complications are frequent when this technique is not carried out properly or is used in contraindicated situations. In their series, 23 patients were treated with direct screw fixation with an overall union rate of 92.3%. They reported a 17% major complication rate from inappropriate use of the technique. Important contraindications to anterior screw fixation include an oblique fracture configuration (paralleling the direction of the intended screw fixation), an associated unstable fracture of the atlas, and pathologic fractures and nonunions of the dens in which bone stock is inadequate for internal screw fixation.

■ *TECHNIQUE (AEBI, ETTER, AND COSCIA).* After the administration of general endotracheal anesthesia, with the patient supine position on the operating table, reduce displaced fractures in skeletal traction with either Gardner-Wells tongs or a halo ring (Fig. 80-29). Anatomic reduction must be obtained before internal fixation with the cannulated screw system. Insert a large nasogastric tube to allow localization of the esophagus and to prevent perforation. Use a padded occipital ring attached to the operating table to stabilize the patient's head. The head and neck must be positioned to allow maximal access to the anterior cervical spine. A large vertical mandibular-sternal distance is required because of the size of the instrumentation and the steep inferior angle of approach necessary for screw placement. High-resolution fluoroscopic image intensification in both the anteroposterior and lateral planes is necessary for insertion of the screws. Before beginning the surgical procedure, confirm a free working path for the instrumentation by placing a long Kirschner wire along the side of the neck in the direction of the intended screw placement and viewing it with image intensification. If clearance of the sternum is not adequate, modify the patient's position. Prepare and drape the operative field in a sterile fashion with sterile draping of the image intensifier. Make an anteromedial approach to the cervical spine through a transverse skin incision approximately 6 to 7 cm long at the level of the C5-6 disc space. Because of the steep angle of inclination required relative to the anterior plane of the neck, undermine the skin and

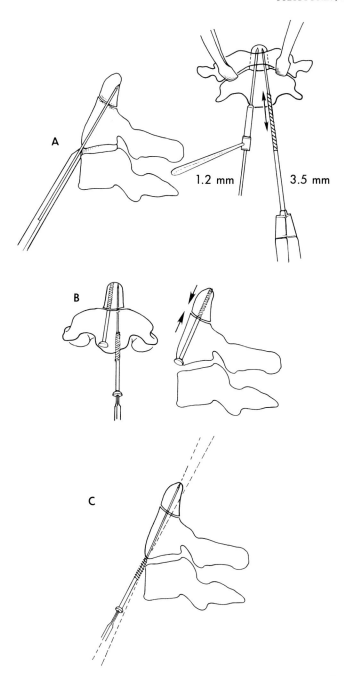

Fig. 80-29 Anterior fixation of dens fracture with cannulated screws, as described by Etter et al. **A,** Two Kirschner wires are inserted and depth is measured; 5 mm screw-starter hole is drilled. **B,** Threaded cannulated screws are inserted over wires. **C,** Screw insertion is monitored with image intensification to assure that guide wires do not bind and migrate proximally into foramen magnum. (Redrawn from Etter C, Coscis M, Jaberg H, and Aebi M: Spine 16[suppl 3]:S25, 1991.)

split the platysma muscle longitudinally in line with its fibers along the anteromedial border of the sternocleidomastoid muscle. Bluntly dissect the interval between the carotid sheath laterally and the trachea and esophagus medially. Proceed anteriorly along the front of the cervical spine until the anteroinfe-

rior margin of the C2 body is reached. Place an 8 mm–wide Hohmann retractor along the lateral mass of C2. Delineate the C2-3 intervertebral disc space and vertically incise the anterior longitudinal ligament at this level. Ligation of the superior thyroid artery may be necessary for exposure of the C2-3 level. Identify with image intensification the entry site at the anteroinferior head of the C2 body. Using a small drill sleeve, insert two 1.2 mm Kirschner wires with their sagittal orientations toward the posterior apex of the dens and their coronal orientation angled toward the midline (Fig. 80-29, *A*). Verify penetration of the dens cortex and appropriate wire alignment by image intensification in two planes. Measure directly the guide wire insertion depth. Insert the 3.5 mm cannulated drill bit over each guide wire and drill a screw starter hole to a depth of 5 mm (Fig. 80-29, *A*). Insert self-tapping 3.5 mm screws of appropriate length over each guide wire and advance them with the cannulated screwdriver until the opposing apical cortical bone is secured (Fig. 80-29, *B*). Observe the progression of each screw under image control to ensure that the guide wire does not bind and migrate proximally into the foramen magnum (Fig. 80-29, *C*). The screw heads tend to encroach on the anterior margin of the C2-3 intervertebral disc, frequently requiring removal of a small amount of anulus to create a recess. Always use tissue protection guards during drilling to avoid damage to neurovascular structures.

AFTERTREATMENT. The patient is observed closely for respiratory status in an intensive care unit for the 24 hours after surgery. Then a rigid cervical orthosis is applied and is worn for 6 weeks. The orthosis may be removed for bathing and resting. Clinical and roentgenographic evaluations are performed at 6, 12, and 24 weeks.

Traumatic spondylolisthesis of the axis (hangman's fractures). Hangman's fractures were originally those neck injuries incurred during hanging of criminals. Their most common cause now is motor vehicle accidents with hyperextension of the head on the neck. The occiput is forced down against the posterior arch of the atlas, which in turn is forced against the pedicles of C2. Levine and Edwards reviewed 52 traumatic spondylolistheses of the axis and classified these fractures into four types (Fig. 80-30). Type 1 fractures are minimally displaced and are believed to be caused by hyperextension and axial loading with failure of the neural arch in tension. Because ligamentous injury is minimal, these fractures are stable and usually heal with 12 weeks of immobilization in a rigid cervical orthosis. Type II fractures have more than 3 mm of anterior translation and significant angulation. These injuries result from hyperextension and axial loading that cause the neural arch to fail with a predom-

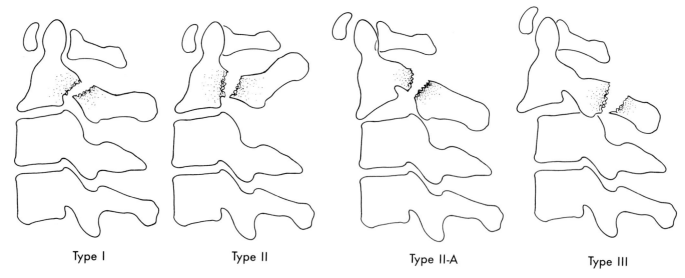

Type I   Type II   Type II-A   Type III

Fig. 80-30 Hangman's fracture.

inantly vertical fracture line, followed by significant flexion resulting in stretching of the posterior anulus of the disc and significant anterior translation and angulation. The C2-3 disc may be disrupted by the sudden flexion component involved in this injury. Treatment consists of application of skull traction through tongs or a halo ring with slight extension of the neck over a rolled-up towel. Immobilization in a halo vest does not achieve or maintain reduction, and halo traction with slight extension may be necessary for 3 to 6 weeks to maintain anatomic reduction. Then the patient can be mobilized in a halo vest for the rest of the 3-month period. These fractures usually unite with an initial gap in the neural arch and develop a spontaneous anterior fusion at C2-3. Type IIA fractures are a variant of type II fractures that demonstrate severe angulation between C2 and C3 with minimal translation. They usually have a more horizontal than vertical fracture line through the C2 arch. The mechanism of injury is predominantly flexion and distraction. It is important to identify this particular fracture pattern because application of traction can cause marked widening of the C2-3 disc space and increased displacement. The recommended treatment is application of a halo vest with slight compression applied under image intensification to achieve and maintain anatomic reduction. Once reduction is obtained, halo vest immobilization is continued for 12 weeks until union occurs. Type III injuries combine a bipedicular fracture with posterior facet injuries. They usually have both severe angulation and translation of the neural arch fracture and an associated unilateral or bilateral facet dislocation at C2-3. Type III injuries are the only type of hangman's fracture that commonly require surgical stabilization. These fractures frequently are associated with neurologic deficits. Open reduction and internal fixation usually are required because of inability to obtain or maintain reduction of the C2-3 facet dislocation. Because the lamina and spinous process of C2 are a free floating fragment, bilateral oblique wiring of C2-3 is necessary for stable reduction (Fig. 80-31). After posterior cervical fusion at the C2-3 level, halo vest immobilization for 3 months is necessary for the bipedicular fracture and for consolidation of the fusion mass.

INJURIES TO LOWER CERVICAL SPINE (C3-7). Injuries to the lower cervical spine are different from those involving the upper cervical region. Patients with these injuries may present with isolated minor compression and avulsion fractures or with severe fractures and fracture-dislocations and profound neurologic deficits. The primary goals of treatment, however, remain to realign the spine, prevent loss of function of uninjured neurologic tissue, improve neurologic recovery, obtain and maintain spinal stability, and obtain early functional recovery.

Posterior ligamentous injury. Failure of the posterior ligamentous complex is casued by distraction and flexion forces and is manifested by widening of the interspinous process space during flexion (Fig. 80-32). These injuries may be difficult to diagnose. Disruption of the posterior ligamentous complex may cause unilateral or bilateral facet dislocation and can occur with or without neurologic deficits. Because it is a purely ligamentous injury, healing is unlikely with external immobilization, and chronic pain, progressive deformity, or increasing neurologic deficit may occur. We recommend posterior cervical fusion with interspinous process wiring or oblique facet joint wiring to obtain stability, maintain alignment, prevent chronic pain or progressive deformity, and protect the neural elements.

Unilateral facet dislocation. Unilateral facet dislocations usually result from flexion and rotation of the cervical spine. They are considered stage 2 distractive flexion injuries (see p. 3524 for classification). The most

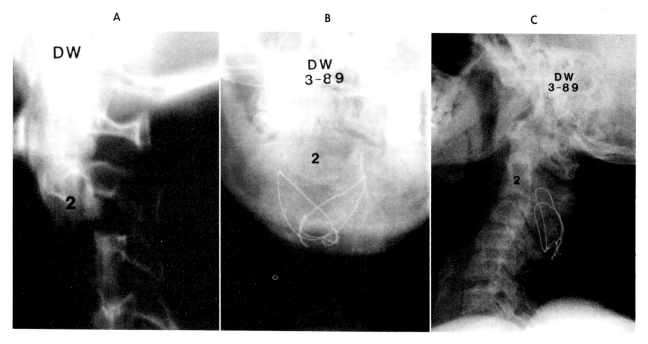

Fig. 80-31 A, Lateral tomogram of upper cervical spine demonstrating type III hangman's fracture with dislocation of C2-3 facets. **B** and **C,** After open reduction and posterior stabilization with bilateral oblique facet wires. This 18-year-old patient was a ventilator-dependent quadriplegic following this fracture.

common site of dislocation is at C5-6. Patients may present with an isolated nerve root injury or an incomplete neurologic deficit. The injury may be purely ligamentous or may involve a facet fracture in addition to the dislocation. Unilateral facet dislocations may be difficult to reduce in skeletal traction. Closed reduction may be attempted to unlock the dislocated facet joint; however, this is successful in less than 50% of patients and

we do not routinely use manipulation of the cervical spine. Rorabeck et al. reviewed 26 patients with unilateral facet dislocations and found that 12 had isolated dislocations and 14 had fractures of the facets or vertebral bodies. Closed reduction was possible in only six patients. Of the other 20, 10 fractures were left unreduced and 10 had open reduction. Those patients who underwent open reduction and fusion had better results than those whose fractures were left unreduced. In our experience, open reduction and internal fixation of unilateral facet dislocations have provided consistently good results. If a unilateral facet dislocation can be reduced in skull traction, halo vest immobilization can be used for 3 months, with the possibility that stability will be obtained by spontaneous fusion. However, if skull traction does not reduce the dislocation, we prefer to proceed with open reduction and posterior cervical fusion with either triple wiring or oblique facet wiring for additional rotational control (Fig. 80-33). Postoperative treatment consists of immobilization in a rigid cervical orthosis for 6 to 8 weeks.

Often patients present with chronic pain, limitation of rotation, and radiculopathy caused by a unilateral jump facet that was either missed initially or was allowed to heal unreduced. For these patients with nerve root impingement and chronic pain, we recommend foraminotomy with decompression of the involved nerve root and posterior cervical fusion over the involved segment. Reduction with traction may be attempted, but this usually is impossible.

Bilateral facet dislocations are flexion-rotation injuries

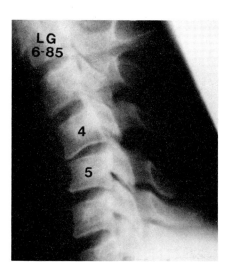

Fig. 80-32 Tearing of posterior ligamentous structures is evidenced by widening of interspinous process space, as well as widening of posterior aspect of C4-5 disc space. This patient was neurologically intact and complained only of neck pain after a motor vehicle accident.

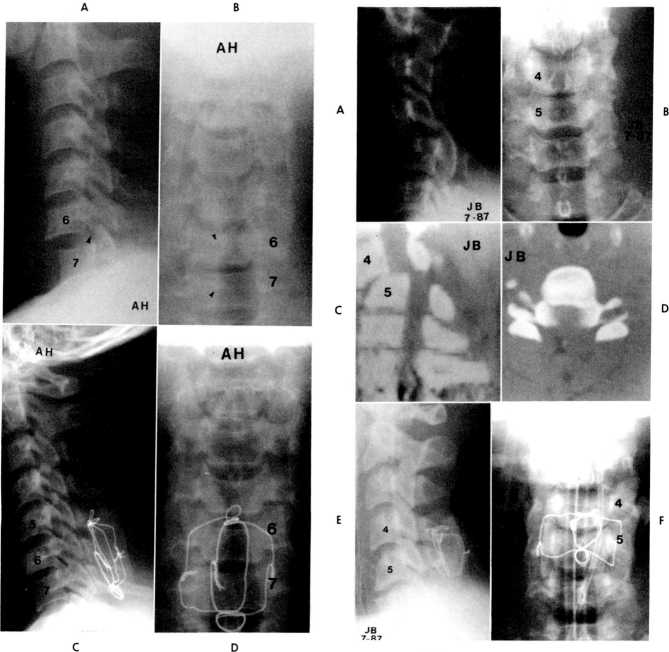

Fig. 80-33 **A** and **B,** Mild anterior subluxation of C6 on C7; spinous process fracture of C6 is visible on lateral view and malrotation of spinous process on anteroposterior view. **C** and **D,** Realignment of cervical spine after open reduction and posterior fusion from C5 to C7 with triple-wire technique.

Fig. 80-34 **A** and **B,** 20-year-old patient with distractive flexion injury of C4-5 (bilateral facet dislocation) and complete spinal cord injury. **C** and **D,** CT scans confirm facet dislocation with marked canal stenosis. **E** and **F,** Realignment of spine after posterior cervical arthrodesis with triple-wire technique.

and are considered stage 3 distractive flexion lesions (p. 3524). These injuries produce approximately 50% anterior subluxation of one vertebral body on the vertebra below. Usually both facet capsules, the posterior longitudinal ligament, and the posterior anulus fibrosus and disc are disrupted. These injuries are more frequently associated with neurologic deficits than are unilateral facet dislocations. These dislocations are more easily reduced with closed traction methods than are unilateral disloca-

tions, but because they are so unstable, redislocation is frequent when they are treated with prolonged skeletal traction or even in a halo vest. Some bilateral facet dislocations heal with spontaneous anterior interbody fusions, but this is unpredictable and we prefer open reduction and internal fixation with an interspinous process wiring technique, such as the Bohlman triple-wire technique, or oblique wiring from the inferior facet of the upper level to the spinous process of the lower level (Fig. 80-34).

Studies by Arena et al. have demonstrated the association of disc herniation with unilateral and bilateral facet dislocations. Disc herniations occurred in 6 of 68 patients (8.8%) in their series, and most were identified by myelography, postmyelography CT scanning, or MRI. One roentgenographic indication of disc herniation is marked narrowing of intervertebral disc space on the plain lateral view. Failure to recognize a herniated disc associated with unilateral or bilateral facet injuries may result in increased neurologic deficit when realignment of the spine with skull traction is attempted. Arena et al. recommend anterior discectomy for removal of extruded disc material before posterior interspinous wiring and fusion.

Fractures of vertebral body. Vertebral body fractures may range from stable compression fractures without neurologic involvement to highly unstable burst fractures with significant neurologic injury. Many mechanisms of injury are possible, but most vertebral body fractures result from axial loading and flexion. Eisemont et al. have shown that the sagittal dimension of the cervical spinal canal plays an important role in determining the degree of neurologic deficit with these injuries. Mild compression fractures with minimal displacement and without posterior element fracture, ligament disruption, facet dislocation, or neurologic injury are stable fractures that will heal with 8 to 12 weeks of external cervical orthotic immobilization. The stability of the posterior ligamentous structures should be verified by the criteria of White and Panjabi (p. 3525) or by the stretch test previously described (p. 3526). More significant body fractures, such as burst fractures with posterior element disruption and incompetent posterior ligaments, are unstable injuries and usually result in displacement of posterior fragments into the spinal canal causing spinal cord injury. The initial treatment of these injuries is application of longitudinal skull traction to realign the spinal canal, using intact soft tissue structures to pull the retropulsed bone fragments into more acceptable alignment and decrease cord compression. Care must be taken, however, not to overdistract the cervical spine, and lateral cervical roentgenograms are mandatory after application of skeletal traction. After the patient's condition has stabilized, a decision should be made as to whether the spinal cord should be decompressed through an anterior approach and whether posterior stabilization is required. Stauffer has emphasized the problems that may be encountered in anterior vertebral body excision and strut grafting when the posterior ligaments are disrupted. If decompression is indicated and the posterior interspinous ligaments are intact, anterior vertebral body excision and grafting with an iliac bone strut can be performed and has proven useful in the management of patients with incomplete quadriplegia or those who have failure of root recovery at the level of injury (see Fig. 80-15). In patients with documented compression of the neural elements from retropulsed bone fragments and

incompetent posterior elements and ligamentous structures, anterior strut grafting alone usually is inadequate. Recent studies, especially from the AO/ASIF, have indicated that anterior plate fixation is successful in the management of these injuries, but the indications for rigid internal fixation of the cervical spine are still evolving. To date, we have little experience with anterior internal fixation for traumatic cervical spine injuries. Clearly, increased complications may occur from the use of such fixation, including iatrogenic neurologic deficits and loss of reduction with loosening of the implants. More biomechanical data are necessary to define the indications for their use. For fractures that combine posterior instability with anterior compression of the cord or nerve roots, we prefer a combined procedure consisting of anterior decompression and strut grafting with posterior stabilization by interspinous wiring (see Fig. 80-16). These procedures may be carried out simultaneously or in stages. In general, we prefer to obtain posterior stabilization first and then proceed with anterior decompression and strut graft fusion. Postoperative immobilization consists of 12 weeks in a halo vest or a rigid cervical thoracic brace.

Other isolated fractures of the cervical spine may occur, including fractures of the lamina, lateral masses, spinous processes, and pedicles, as well as small avulsion fractures off of the anterior, inferior, or superior margins of the vertebral bodies. The stability of these fractures should be determined before treatment. In general, these isolated fractures are stable injuries and require only immobilization in a rigid cervical orthosis or halo vest until union occurs.

Triple-wire procedure of posterior fusion (Bohlman). This procedure may be done safely with the patient under general or local anesthesia. In patients with high cervical quadriplegia, local anesthesia may be preferred to avoid the respiratory complications that may be encountered with general anesthesia. Usually, the patient is intubated with an atraumatic, fiberoptic intubation technique and is then positioned prone on a Stryker turning frame. Longitudinal traction is applied to the shoulders and is maintained with tape. A permanent lateral roentgenogram is obtained in the operating room to document alignment of the cervical spine.

■ *TECHNIQUE.* With the patient prone on the Stryker frame, prepare and drape the posterior neck and the iliac crest. Make a midline posterior incision, usually extending one spinous process above and one below the segment to be fused. Infiltration of the skin, subcutaneous tissue, and erector spinae muscle down to the lamina with a 1:500,000 epinephrine solution is helpful in obtaining hemostasis. Carry subperiosteal exposure down to the lamina with electrocautery. Dissect laterally on either side of the lateral margin of the facet joint. With a marker on a spinous process, obtain a lateral roentgenogram to confirm accurate location.

Using either a small high-speed burr or a towel

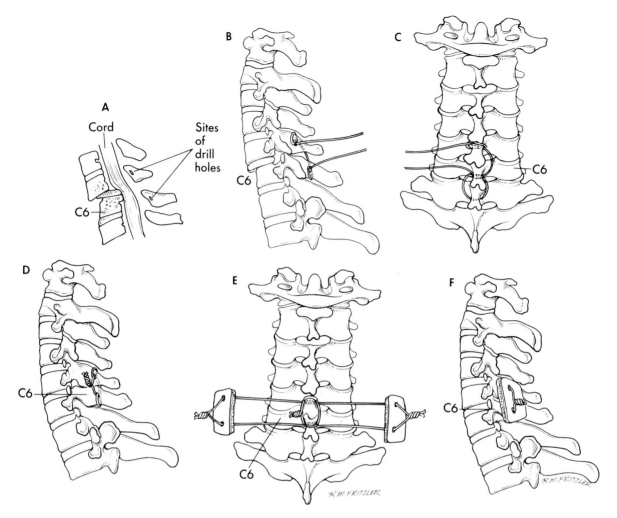

Fig. 80-35 Bohlman triple-wire technique of cervical arthrodesis. **A,** Holes are drilled above spinolaminar fusion line. **B** to **D,** Midline 20-gauge tethering wire is wrapped through and around spinous processes above and below. **E,** Two 22-gauge wires are added to secure thick unicortical cancellous bone grafts against posterior elements. **F,** Final position of graft.

clip, drill holes in the bases of the spinous processes to be wired (Fig. 80-35, *A*). To avoid passage of the wire into the spinal canal, take care to place the holes posterior to the spinal laminar fusion line. Pass a 20-gauge wire through the hole in the superior spinous process, loop it over the top of the superior edge, pass it through and around the inferior spinous process, and carefully twist its ends together (Fig. 80-35, *B* to *D*). Then pass 22-gauge wires through and around the holes in the spinous process of the superior and inferior vertebrae to be fused, in preparation for securing a thick unicortical cancellous bone graft. Measure the length of the area to be fused and harvest a bone graft from the posterior iliac crest of sufficient size that it can be divided into two pieces for placement on each side of the fusion. Harvest strips of cancellous bone from the pelvis and place them beneath the thick unicor-

tical cancellous bone grafts. Make holes in the superior and inferior ends of the grafts, pass the 22-gauge wires through them, and tighten the wires to hold the grafts in place against the lamina and spinous processes. Cut off the wires and bend them to prevent protrusion into the soft tissues (Fig. 80-35, *E*). Grasp the spinous process of one vertebra and pick it up to test stability: the wired levels should move as one unit. Confirm the position of the wires and fusion of the proper segments with a lateral roentgenogram. Thoroughly irrigate the wound with an antibiotic solution and close it in layers over a suction drain.

AFTERTREATMENT. In most patients, skeletal traction can be discontinued and a cervical orthosis can be applied immediately after surgery. If preferred, the patient may be kept supine with light cervical traction for 24 to 48 hours before the orthosis is al-

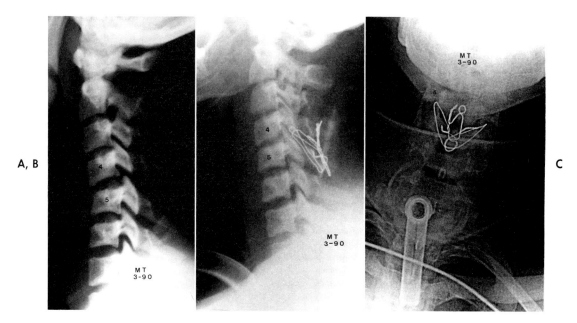

Fig. 80-36   Distraction flexion injury at C4-5 caused complete C5-level quadriplegia in 22-year-old patient. **A,** On lateral view, note widening of interspinous process space, mild anterior subluxation, and disruption of facet joints. **B** and **C,** After restoration of anatomic alignment with use of oblique facet wires and traditional midline wiring. Patient was mobilized in cervical orthosis, and early rehabilitation was begun.

lowed. Prophylactic antibiotics are recommended for 48 hours. The cervical orthosis is worn for 8 to 12 weeks, and then lateral flexion and extension roentgenograms are made. The brace is discontinued when fusion is evident and stability is documented on lateral flexion and extension views.

Oblique facet wiring. This technique is a modification of the procedure described by Robinson and Southwick. It is indicated when the posterior elements are insufficient for spinous process wiring or additional rotational stability is needed (Fig. 80-36). The procedure may be performed when there are fractures of the lamina or spinous processes or after previous laminectomy.

■ *TECHNIQUE.* Position the patient prone on a Stryker frame with cervical alignment maintained in skeletal traction with either a halo ring or Gardner-Wells tongs. Using electrocautery, expose the posterior elements in the midline as described for the triple-wire technique. Be sure to expose the lateral margins of the facet joints to allow adequate access. After roentgenographic verification of the level to be fused, use a ⁷⁄₆₄-inch bit to drill a hole in the lateral mass at 45 degrees off the horizontal through the inferior facet (Fig. 80-37, *A*). The facet joint can be pried open with a small Freer or a Penfield elevator. Pass a 20-gauge or 22-gauge stainless steel wire through the hole in the facet joint and grasp it with a small hemostat. Repeat this procedure on each facet bilaterally (Fig. 80-37, *B*). Tighten the wires

down and around an intact spinous process inferiorly (Fig. 80-37, *C* and *D*) or pass them through a thick, unicortical, cancellous bone graft. Close the wound in layers over a suction drain.

AFTERTREATMENT. A halo vest or rigid cervical orthosis is worn for 8 to 12 weeks, or until stability is confirmed by lateral flexion and extension roentgenograms.

Anterior decompression and fusion. The middle and lower cervical spine is most commonly exposed through an anterior approach medial to the carotid sheath. A thorough knowledge of anatomic fascial planes, as described by Robinson and Southwick, allows a safe, direct approach to this area.

■ *TECHNIQUE.* Place the patient supine with skeletal traction maintained through tongs or a halo ring. Exposure may be through either a transverse or longitudinal incision, depending on the surgeon's preference. We usually prefer a left-sided transverse incision (Fig. 80-38) because of the more constant anatomy of the recurrent laryngeal nerve and less risk of inadvertent injury. In general, make an incision 3 to 5 fingerbreadths above the clavicle to expose from C3-5 and 2 to 3 fingerbreadths above the clavicle to expose from C5-7. Center the transverse incision over the medial border of the sternocleidomastoid muscle. Infiltration of the skin and subcutaneous tissues with a 1:500,000 epinephrine solution aids hemostasis. Incise the platysma muscle in line

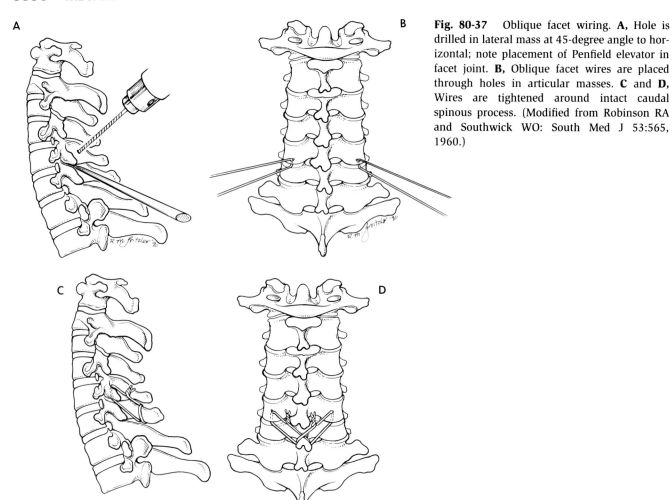

Fig. 80-37 Oblique facet wiring. **A,** Hole is drilled in lateral mass at 45-degree angle to horizontal; note placement of Penfield elevator in facet joint. **B,** Oblique facet wires are placed through holes in articular masses. **C** and **D,** Wires are tightened around intact caudal spinous process. (Modified from Robinson RA and Southwick WO: South Med J 53:565, 1960.)

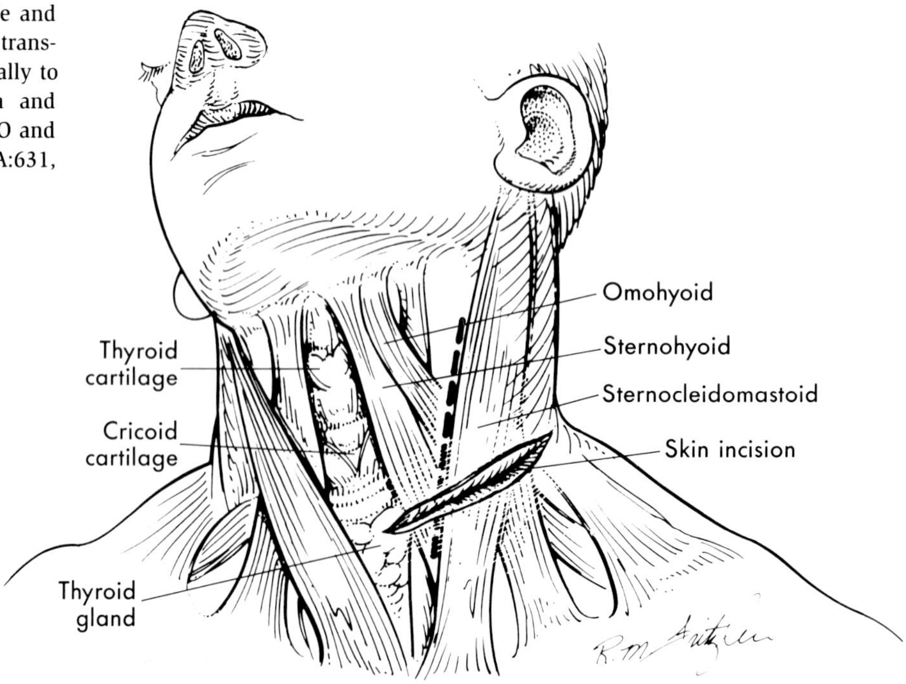

Fig. 80-38 Anterior approach to middle and lower cervical spine through left-sided transverse incision. Dissection is carried medially to carotid sheath and laterally to trachea and esophagus. (Redrawn from Southwick WO and Robinson RA: J Bone Joint Surg 39-A:631, 1957.)

Thyroid cartilage

Cricoid cartilage

Thyroid gland

Omohyoid

Sternohyoid

Sternocleidomastoid

Skin incision

with the skin incision. Identify the anterior border of the sternocleidomastoid muscle, and incise longitudinally the superficial layer of the deep cervical fascia while localizing the carotid pulse with finger palpation. Carefully divide the middle layer of the deep cervical fascia that encloses the omohyoid medial to the carotid sheath. Retract the sternocleidomastoid muscle and carotid sheath laterally and palpate the anterior aspect of the cervical spine. Identify the esophagus posterior to the trachea, and retract medially the trachea, esophagus, and thyroid. Bluntly divide the deep layers of the deep cervical fascia, consisting of the pretracheal and prevertebral fasciae overlying the musculi longus colli. Reflect the musculi longus colli subperiosteally from the anterior aspect of the spine laterally to the level of the uncovertebral joints (Fig. 80-39) to provide exposure for wide decompression and bone grafting. Usually the fractured vertebra can be readily identified; however, to accurately locate the area of decompression, place a needle into a disc space and obtain a lateral roentgenogram. After identification of the level of decompression, incise the anterior longitudinal ligament and anulus overlying the adjacent disc and remove this material with curets. Using hand-held rongeurs or a high-speed drill, remove the anterior portion of the fractured vertebral body (Fig. 80-40, *A* and *B*). Remove disc material back to the posterior longitudinal ligament. Com-

pletely remove the intervertebral disc to allow identification of the posterior longitudinal ligament and to help determine the extent of the carpectomy. Next, using power burrs and hand-held curets, carefully remove the posterior aspect of the vertebral body; use pituitary forceps as the posterior cortical wall of the vertebra is approached (Fig. 80-40, *C* and *D*). Carefully remove retropulsed bone and disc fragments from the spinal canal.

Define the lateral margin of dissection by the uncovertebral joints. Take care not to extend the dissection too far laterally because of the risk of injury to the vertebral bodies. After completion of the anterior carpectomy, expose the end plates of the superior and inferior vertebrae, and make seating holes with an angled curet or small burr in preparation for placement of the tricortical iliac crest of fibular graft (Fig. 80-40, *E*). Center these seating holes in the end plate and make them large enough to allow placement of approximately half the length of the distal phalanx of the little finger. Once the holes are made, Gelfoam can be placed over the exposed dura mater, which should expand anteriorly after complete decompression. Harvest the iliac strut graft and fashion it into a T-shape, with the cancellous portion facing anteriorly. Increase longitudinal traction and lock the graft into the seating holes. Trim the anterior aspect of the graft flush with the front of the vertebral bodies to prevent erosion into the

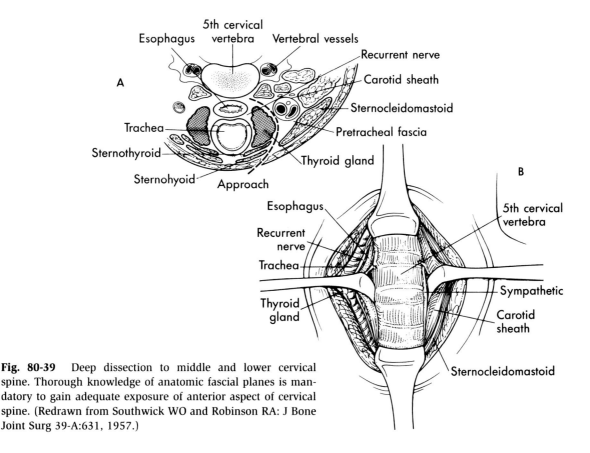

Fig. 80-39 Deep dissection to middle and lower cervical spine. Thorough knowledge of anatomic fascial planes is mandatory to gain adequate exposure of anterior aspect of cervical spine. (Redrawn from Southwick WO and Robinson RA: J Bone Joint Surg 39-A:631, 1957.)

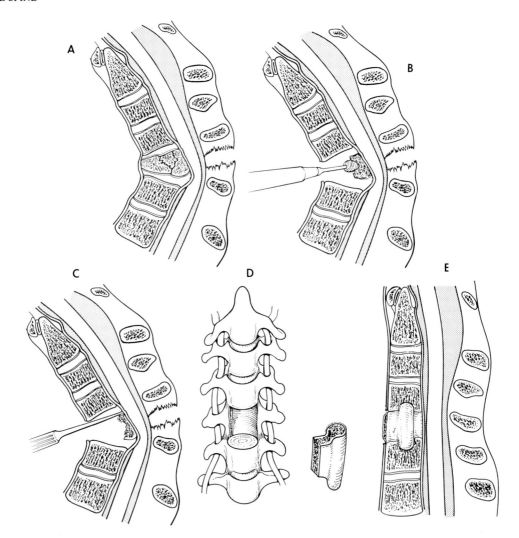

Fig. 80-40 **A,** Typical burst fracture at C5 with retropulsed bone and disc fragments in spinal canal compressing neural elements. **B,** Material above and below fractured vertebra has been removed, and high-speed power burr is used to remove bone back to level of posterior longitudinal ligament. **C,** Residual posterior vertebral margin is removed with small curet to decompress neural elements. **D,** Extent of anterior cervical corpectomy. **E,** Placement of tricortical iliac crest graft after adequate cervical decompression. (**A,** Redrawn from Bohlman HH: J Bone Joint Surg 61-A:1119, 1979; **B** through **E,** redrawn from Bohlman HH and Eismont FJ: Clin Orthop 154:57, 1981.)

esophagus. Obtain a lateral roentgenogram to confirm proper position of the graft. Place a drain along the anterior aspect of the spine to prevent postoperative respiratory compromise from a hematoma in the prevertebral space. Close the platysma muscle, the subcutaneous tissues, and the skin in layers.

Recent reports have suggested that stability is improved by the use of anterior plates and screws, but these also increase the risk of iatrogenic neurologic deficits. In our experience, anterior decompression and placement of the strut graft are safe and effective without internal fixation.

AFTERTREATMENT. Depending on the degree of stability, a rigid cervical orthosis or halo vest is worn for 8 to 12 weeks while the bone graft incorporates.

Posterior cervical fusion with rigid internal fixation. Posterior stabilization of the cervical spine with rigid internal fixation devices has been described by several authors, including Roy-Camille et al.; Magerl and Seemann; Louis; Anderson and Montesano; and Hadley et al. These implants consist of posterior plates and screws or hook plates and offer the advantage of rigid fixation of a single motion segment, therefore minimizing the fusion extent and increasing postoperative mobility of the cervical spine. In addition, Harrington and Luque instrumentation has been modified by segmental wiring of the facet joints to obtain stability of certain fractures and dislocations. Each of these techniques has advantages and disadvantages, and good results with few complications have been reported with each. Rigid internal fixation of the cervical spine was developed because of certain inherent limitations of interspinous wiring when instability is severe or the posterior elements are deficient. We have limited experience with rigid internal fixation of the cervical spine, but agree that these techniques offer advantages over conventional wiring techniques in certain high-risk groups of patients.

THORACIC AND LUMBOSACRAL FRACTURES

The treatment of unstable fractures and fracture-dislocations of the thoracic and lumbar spine has long been controversial. Many authors, such as Guttmann and Bedbrook, have advised nonoperative treatment, but more recent reports, such as those by Levine and Edwards; Bohlman; Bradford et al.; McAfee, Bohlman, and Yuan; Luque, Cassis, and Ramirez-Wiella; Eisemont et al.; and Cotrel, Dubousset, and Guillaumat have emphasized the advantages of open reduction and rigid internal fixation with posterior instrumentation. Paul of Aegina (625 to 690 AD) first introduced laminectomy for spinal cord injury, unaware of the controversy this would cause. The seventeenth century saw an increase in its use, and its use has continued to the present. Munro, in the late 1930s, advised that laminectomy be delayed and reserved for selective patients. Guttmann condemned the routine use of early laminectomy and certain forms of internal fixation and advocated a conservative program of postural reduction by extension of the spine. Holdsworth and Hardy agreed about the dangers of a routine laminectomy and preferred early open reduction and internal fixation for certain injuries of the thoracolumbar and lumbar spine. Morgan, Whartman, and Austin pointed out that laminectomy offers little benefit in these injuries and is not without morbidity and mortality. We also believe that laminectomy alone is contraindicated in fracture-dislocations because it fails to relieve the anterior compression and increases spinal instability.

Classification of Thoracolumbar Fractures

The classification of thoracolumbar fractures has evolved over the last 40 years. Nicoll described these fractures as having stable or unstable patterns. Holdsworth modified and expanded Nicoll's classification, and this modification is the basis of all subsequent classification schemes. Holdsworth classified thoracolumbar fractures into five groups according to the mechanism of injury: (1) *pure flexion,* which causes a stable wedge compression fracture; (2) *flexion and rotation,* which produce an unstable fracture-dislocation with rupture of the posterior ligament complex, separation of the spinous processes, a slice fracture near the upper border of the lower vertebra, and dislocation of the lower articular processes of the upper vertebra; (3) *extension,*

which causes rupture of the intervertebral disc and the anterior longitudinal ligament and avulsion of a small bone fragment from the anterior border of the dislocated vertebra; this dislocation almost always reduces spontaneously and is stable in flexion; (4) *vertebral compression,* which causes a fracture of the end plate as the nucleus of the intervertebral disc is forced into the intervertebral body and causes it to burst with outward displacement of fragments of the body; because the ligaments remain intact, this comminuted fracture is stable; (5) *shearing,* which results in displacement of the whole vertebra and an unstable fracture of the articular processes or pedicles. This classification system does not consider the "unstable burst fracture" described by McAfee et al.

Kelly and Whitesides described the thoracolumbar spine as consisting of two weight-bearing columns: the hollow column of the spinal canal and the solid column of the vertebral bodies. Denis developed a three-column concept of spinal injury using a series of more than 400 CAT scans of thoracolumbar injuries (Fig. 80-41). The

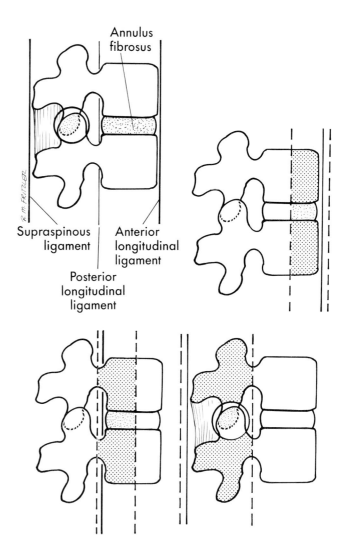

Fig. 80-41 Three-column classification of spinal instability. Illustrations of anterior, middle, and posterior columns (see text). (Redrawn from Denis F: Spine 8:817, 1983.)

anterior column contains the anterior longitudinal ligament, the anterior half of the vertebral body, and the anterior portion of the anulus fibrosus. The middle column consists of the posterior longitudinal ligament, the posterior half of the vertebral body, and the posterior aspect of the anulus fibrosus. The posterior column includes the neural arch, the ligamentum flavum, the facet capsules, and the interspinous ligaments. Denis noted that one or more of the three columns predictably failed in axial compression, axial distraction, or translation from combinations of forces in different planes. In a CT study of 100 consecutive patients with potentially unstable fractures and fracture-dislocations, McAfee et al. determined the mechanisms of failure of the middle osteoligamentous complex and developed a new system based on these mechanisms. We have found their simplified system useful in classifying injuries to the thoracolumbar spine.

1. *Wedge compression fractures* cause isolated failure of the anterior column and result from forward flexion. They rarely are associated with neurologic deficit except when in multiple adjacent vertebral levels.
2. In *stable burst fractures* the anterior and middle columns fail because of a compressive load, with no loss of integrity of the posterior elements.
3. In *unstable burst fractures* the anterior and middle columns fail in compression and the posterior column is disrupted. The posterior column can fail in compression, lateral flexion, or rotation. There is a tendency for posttraumatic kyphosis and progressive neural symptoms because of instability. If the anterior and middle columns fail in compression, the posterior column cannot fail in distraction.
4. *Chance fractures* are horizontal avulsion injuries of the vertebral bodies caused by flexion about an axis anterior to the anterior longitudinal ligament. The entire vertebra is pulled apart by a strong tensile force.
5. In *flexion distraction injuries* the flexion axis is posterior to the anterior longitudinal ligament. The anterior column fails in compression while the middle and posterior columns fail in tension. This injury is unstable because the ligamentum flavum, interspinous ligaments, and supraspinous ligaments usually are disrupted.
6. *Translational injuries* are characterized by malalignment of the neural canal, which has been totally disrupted. Usually all three columns have failed in shear. At the affected level, one part of the spinal canal has been displaced in the transverse plane.

We believe the three-column classification of McAfee et al. is the best classification scheme available at present; however, not all injuries to the thoracolumbar spine can be assigned to one of the six categories. Plain roentgenograms and CT scanning provide only static images and do not demonstrate maximal displacement. Occult ligamentous injuries are not readily identified on plain films or CT scans, and flexion and extension views of the thoracolumbar spine are risky. Recent reports, such as that by Kulkarni et al., suggest that MRI is helpful in detecting occult ligamentous injuries and hemorrhage into surrounding soft tissue structures and in determining the extent of neural damage and the degree of cord edema. They also suggest that MRI may be of value in determining the prognosis for recovery after spinal cord injuries.

Finally, many authors have noted the lack of direct correlation between the severity of neurologic deficit and the degree of spinal canal compromise. Retropulsion of bone and disc fragments into the spinal canal clearly is more significant at the thoracolumbar junction than in the lumbar spine because the spinal cord and conus medullaris have a poor prognosis for recovery while the cauda equina, which behaves as a peripheral nerve root lesion, carries a better prognosis for neural recovery. Numerous examples of nearly complete canal compromise in patients with normal neurologic function have been reported.

Timing of Surgery

The timing of surgery for spinal cord injuries is controversial. Most authors agree that in the presence of a progressive neurologic deficit emergency decompression is indicated. In patients with complete spinal cord injuries or static incomplete spinal cord injuries, some authors advocate delaying surgery for several days to allow resolution of cord edema, whereas others favor early surgical stabilization. There is no conclusive evidence in the literature that early surgical decompression and stabilization improve neurologic recovery or that neurologic recovery is compromised by a delay of several days. Studies by Bohlman, Transfeld et al., Bradford et al., and others have documented return of neurologic function after anterior decompression done more than a year after the initial injury. For neurologically normal patients with unstable spinal injuries and those with nonprogressive neurologic injuries, we believe that open reduction and internal fixation should be carried out as soon as possible.

Decompression

The role of decompression also is controversial. Compression of the neural elements by retropulsed bone fragments can be relieved indirectly by the insertion of posterior instrumentation or directly by exploration of the spinal canal through a posterolateral or anterior approach. There is no universal agreement as to indications for each of these. The indirect approach to decompression of the spinal canal generally involves insertion of posterior instrumentation (Harrington, Edwards, Cotrell-Dubousset, or Texas Scottish Rite Hospital implants). These techniques use the distraction instrumentation and the intact posterior longitudinal ligament to reduce the retropulsed bone from the spinal canal. Excellent results with this technique have been documented by numerous authors, and it is a familiar technique to most orthopaedic surgeons. Problems with this technique occur if surgery is delayed for several weeks or more because then indirect reduction of the spinal canal cannot be achieved with posterior instrumentation alone. In addition, severely comminuted fractures with multiple pieces of bone pushed into the spinal canal may not be completely reduced by distraction instrumentation. Intraoperative myelographic documentation of reduction of the retropulsed bone fragments may be inadequate and ultrasonography requires creation of a laminotomy defect to allow insertion of the transducer head; removal of excessive bone may increase instability.

The posterolateral technique for decompression of the spinal canal is effective at the thoracolumbar junction and in the lumbar spine. This procedure involves hemilaminectomy and removal of a pedicle with a high-speed burr to allow posterolateral decompression of the dura along its anterior aspect (Fig. 80-42). In the thoracic spine, where less room is available for the cord, this technique involves increased risk to the neural elements. The anterior approach allows direct decompression of the thecal sac but is an unfamiliar approach to many surgeons. Visceral and vascular structures may be injured, and this approach carries the greatest risk of potential morbidity. In addition, anterior decompression and placement of an iliac strut graft provide no immediate stability to the fracture unless anterior internal fixation is used. The role of anterior internal fixation devices is still evolving, and their use is limited to a few centers at this time. When anterior decompression and strut grafting are performed in the face of posterior instability, posterior instrumentation and fusion may be performed to improve stability. At this time, we favor early posterior instrumentation in an attempt to achieve anatomic reduction of the fracture. Decompression of the spinal canal is confirmed by intraoperative myelography or ultrasonography. If residual neural compression exists, a posterolateral decompression is carried out. Postoperatively a CT scan of the spine with sagittal reconstructions is obtained through the injured segment to further evaluate the patency of the spinal canal. If an incomplete neurologic deficit exists and significant residual neural compression is documented, we prefer to perform anterior decompression and fusion as staged procedures.

Degree of Canal Stenosis

Studies by McAfee, Denis, Trafton and Boyd, and others have demonstrated no reliable correlation between the degree of compromise of the spinal canal and the severity of the neurologic deficit. Because of variations in the diameter of the spinal canal and differences in regional blood supply to the spinal cord in the thoracic and lumbar region and the cauda equina in the lumbosacral

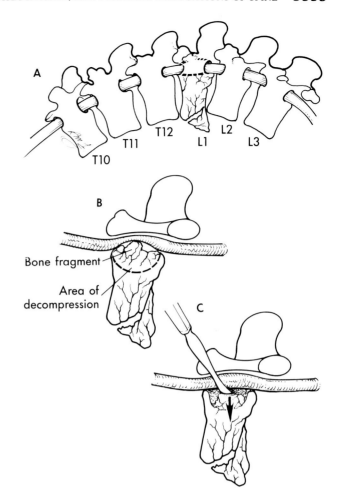

Fig. 80-42 Posterolateral decompression technique. **A,** L1 burst fracture. Pedicle, transverse process, and lateral portions of T12-L1 facet are removed after L1 root has been isolated (*dotted lines*). **B,** Area of encroachment is exposed. **C,** After fragments are undercut, they are reduced into vertebral body. (Redrawn from McAfee PC, Yuan HA, and Lasda NA: Spine 7:365, 1982.)

spine, the damage to the neural elements caused by fractures and fracture-dislocations is determined to some extent by the level of injury. The spinal canal in the thoracic area is small and the blood supply is sparse. Therefore significant neurologic injury is common with severe fractures and dislocations in the thoracic spine. Fractures or fracture-dislocations in the lumbosacral region may result in marked displacement and still cause little or no neurologic deficit. Not only is the canal large in this region, but also the spinal cord ends at approximately the first lumbar vertebra and the cauda equina is less vulnerable than the cord above. Recent experimental work in dogs by Delamarter et al. showed that the neurologic signs and symptoms after constriction of the cauda equina occurred progressively and predictably in direct proportion to the percentage of compromise of the canal.

Constriction of more than 50% of the cauda equina resulted in complete loss of cortical evoked potentials, neurologic deficits, and histologic abnormalities.

Denis et al. reported neurologic complications in 6 (21%) of 29 patients with burst fractures treated conservatively. Krompinger et al. reported that late CT analysis of patients with burst fractures treated conservatively showed significant resolution of bony canal compromise. The remodeling process appears to be age and time dependent and follows expected principles of bone remodeling to applied stress. Neurologic deficits have not developed in these patients. The treatment of thoracolumbar burst fractures must be individualized, and canal compromise from retropulsed bone fragments is not in itself an absolute indication for surgical decompression. Nonoperative treatment with canal compromise of up to 50% may be successful in selected patients, although some authors recommend surgical decompression of all burst fractures, regardless of neurologic involvement, to prevent late neurologic deterioration or progressive kyphosis. We advise patients of the risk and complications of surgery, including inadequate decompression, increased neurologic deficit, failure of internal fixation, and the need for implant removal. Our indications for surgical treatment of thoracolumbar spine injuries include burst fractures with 50% or more canal compromise and 30 degrees or more of kyphosis and clearly unstable fractures and fracture-dislocations.

The application of Harrington rods, which were initially used for scoliosis, to the treatment of thoracolumbar fractures and dislocat...

Table 80-9 Spinal instrumentation

POSTERIOR IMPLANTS

Standard fixation devices
 Harrington distraction or compression
 Edwards
 Jacobs locking hook rod
Segmental fixation devices
 Rod systems
  Luque
  Harrington-Luque
  Wisconsin (Drummond)
 Pedicle screw and plate systems
  Steffee
  Luque
  Roy-Camille
  Wiltse
 Internal fixators
  AO fixateur interne
  Vermont (Krag)
Combined fixation devices
 Edwards
 Cotrel-Dubousset
 Texas Scottish Rite Hospital
 Isola Rogozinski

ANTERIOR IMPLANTS

Anterior plate and screws
Dwyer
Zielke
Kaneda
Kostuick-Harrington

instrumented levels. Arthritic changes have been ... in the facet joints of instrumented but un... ls in animal models and in humans. Whether ... erative facet joints cause significant symptoms ... ain. It is clear from biomechanical and clinical ... hat preserving motion segments is important in ... ile lumbar spine and perhaps less important in ... racolumbar region. Extensive research is being ... further define the appropriate levels to be instru..., the length of fusion, and the rigidity of the im... used in treatment of thoracolumbar fractures.

...ific Instrumentation

... our experience, posterior instrumentation is the ...st effective treatment for instability. Numerous inter... fixation devices recently have been developed for the ...atment of thoracolumbar spinal fractures (Table ...-9). Many of these implants are investigational at this ...me, and their use is limited to specific spinal trauma ...enters. These implants have been developed because of ...he deficiencies of Harrington rods such as breakage, cutting out of hooks, and loss of fixation. Biomechanical studies suggest that these newer devices offer improved fixation, but because they may be technically more difficult to insert neurologic risks are increased. At this time, we have little experience with most of the anterior internal fixation devices and with some of the posterior segmental fixation devices, such as the AO internal fixator. The indications for use of these devices are still evolving.

HARRINGTON DISTRACTION INSTRUMENTATION. In 1958 Harrington used his instrumentation for stabilization of thoracolumbar fractures, and numerous authors, including Flesch et al.; Dixon, Harrington, and Erwin; and Bradford et al., reported satisfactory results with the use of these implants in the treatment of unstable thoracolumbar fractures. Harrington rods achieved wide acceptance but in their initial application failed to take into account the sagittal contour of the spine, especially in the lumbar spine, and they were biomechanically insufficient for unstable translational injuries. As clinical and biomechanical data were obtained, the inadequacies of conventional straight Harrington rods were documented. The most common complication was hook cut-out, which was estimated to have an incidence of 10%. McAfee et al. provided valuable data for determining the biomechanical advantages and disadvantages of various internal fixation devices. They determined that the location of ultimate failure in Harrington distraction systems was at the metal-bone interface, and they recommended segmentally wired Harrington distraction instrumentation for injuries in which resistance to axial compression was necessary and for translational injuries, including fracture-dislocations. Luque segmental spinal instrumentation more effectively stabilized the injured spinal segment against shear and torsion without risk of overdistraction. McAfee and Bohlman showed that technical problems or the improper use of Harrington instrumentation systems complicated the management of thoracolumbar fractures. They noted that serious complications can occur when decompression of the neural canal by excessive distraction force is attempted. Overdistraction, failure of fixation, and iatrogenic neurologic deficits can occur if excessive posterior distraction is used in an attempt to reduce anterior fragments of bone or disc from the spinal canal. The most common complication in their series was failure of the Harrington distraction rods to decompress the spinal canal after stabilization. Ultimately, the original straight Harrington rods were modified. Contouring of the rods and the use of square-ended rods and hooks allowed successful use of the implant for reduction and stabilization of thoracolumbar injuries. For successful use of the Harrington distraction system, the anterior longitudinal ligament should be intact. This system requires a three-point fixation principle for reduction of the fracture, and proper contouring of the rods, especially in the lumbar spine, is necessary to maintain the normal lumbar lordosis. We have the most experience with Harrington rods in the treatment of thoracolumbar injuries and, in general, these implants are

the most familiar to spinal surgeons. We have found that early stabilization (within 48 hours) allows restoration of anatomic alignment in most patients (Fig. 80-43). When surgery is delayed between 48 hours and 10 days, less than anatomic alignment usually is obtained, but results remain quite good. If surgery is delayed for more than 2 weeks, we have found little improvement in the canal area. In some burst fractures that have remained untreated for longer than 2 weeks, satisfactory reduction cannot be obtained by posterior Harrington distraction rods alone, and anterior decompression and strut grafting are necessary for decompression (Fig. 80-44). As a secondary procedure, Harrington instrumentation may be applied posteriorly.

■ *TECHNIQUE.* **Place the patient prone on a padded spinal frame or operating table with chest rolls. Perform routine, sterile skin preparation and draping. Make a midline skin incision centered over the spinous process at the level of injury. Infiltrate the skin, subcutaneous tissues, and erector spinae muscle down to the level of the lamina with a 1:500,000 epinephrine solution to minimize bleeding. Deepen the incision to expose posterior elements three levels above and three below the level of injury. Carry the dissection laterally to the tips of the transverse processes, maintaining meticulous hemostasis in a dry field. Confirm the level of injury with roentgenograms. Identify the facet joints of three intact lamina above the level of injury and remove the facet joint capsules. Prepare the site for insertion of the upper hooks and be certain that the inferior articular mass of the cephalic vertebra is not split with insertion of the Harrington hooks. Then insert two No. 1252 hooks in the facet joints. Alternatively, use two bifid hooks or keeled hooks to improve stability. Identify the interlaminar space of the lamina two below the level of injury and prepare the hook sites by removing the ligamentum flavum from the superior edge of the inferior lamina and performing small laminotomies to allow seating of the inferior hooks against the lamina. Then place two No. 1254 hooks beneath the lamina. If one side of the lamina or one side of the vertebral body seems to be more involved, place the first distraction rod on the opposite side. Reduce the fracture as the Harrington rod is inserted. Insert the opposite rod, taking care not to overdistract the fracture. We recommend distracting the rods until they are snug. Somatosensory evoked potential monitoring is currently recommended during insertion of posterior instrumentation in patients who are neurologically normal or have incomplete neurologic lesions. This allows physiologic monitoring of the spinal cord as the fracture is reduced and distraction is applied to the spine. Obtain a cross-table lateral roentgenogram to evaluate alignment and reduction. We prefer to introduce water-soluble contrast material into the**

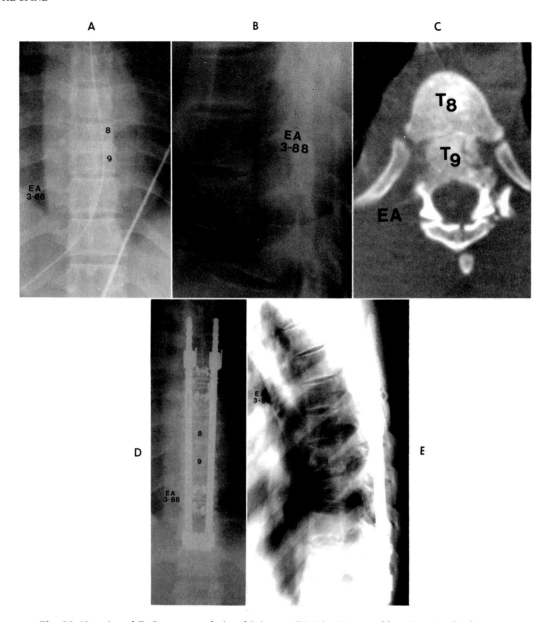

Fig. 80-43 **A** and **B,** Severe translational injury at T8-9 in 20-year-old patient involved in motor vehicle accident. This patient had complete spinal cord injury at T8 level. **C,** CT scan shows complete disruption of normal spinal alignment, with "double margin" sign at T8-9. **D** and **E,** Alignment of spine after posterior instrumentation with dual Harrington distraction rods, augmented with Wisconsin wires. This patient was mobilized in external orthosis and made rapid recovery in spinal rehabilitation program.

subarachnoid space and obtain a myelogram or to create a small laminotomy defect, fill it with saline, and confirm decompression by ultrasonography. Complete reduction of the retropulsed bone fragments with insertion of Harrington distraction rods alone is not reliable. If the reduction is incomplete, as documented by intraoperative myelography or ultrasonography, and the lesion is neurologically incomplete, proceed with a posterolateral decompression, using a high-speed drill to remove a portion of the lamina and pedicle and reverse angled curets to remove retropulsed bone fragments from the ante-

rior aspect of the dura (see Fig. 80-42). If, however, anatomic reduction is obtained or the residual compression is minimal and the patient is neurologically normal, proceed with posterior and posterolateral fusions spanning the entire length of the instrumentation in patients with a complete spinal cord injury or limited to one vertebra above and one vertebra below the injury in patients who are neurologically normal or have an incomplete spinal cord injury. We prefer autogenous iliac bone grafting, which may be supplemented with allografts if necessary.

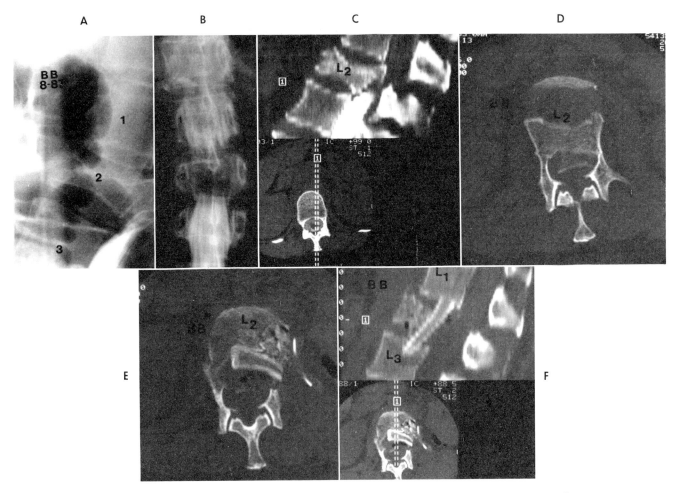

Fig. 80-44   Burst fracture of L2 in 42-year-old woman, with incomplete paraparesis, 3 weeks after injury. **A** and **B,** Myelograms show significant extradural compression at L2 level from bone retropulsed into spinal canal. **C** and **D,** Tomograms show degree of canal compromise at L2 level. **E** and **F,** CT scans show adequate decompression of spinal canal and proper placement of iliac strut graft from L1 to L3. This patient made excellent neurologic recovery and regained ambulatory status with return of bowel and bladder function.

Apply C-washers to the rachet end of the rods beneath the cephalic hooks to prevent loss of reduction. Try to minimize the number of rachets exposed below the upper hooks to decrease the chance of fracture at the junction of the rod and rachet as a late complication. Thoroughly irrigate the wound with antibiotic solution, insert closed suction drainage, and close the wound in routine fashion.

If instrumentation is used in the lower lumbar spine, we prefer the square-ended Harrington rods, contoured into lordosis, with modified square-ended hooks. This maintains the normal lumbar lordosis and improves stability. In the thoracic region and at the thoracolumbar junction, either the traditional round-ended Harrington rods or the square-ended rods may be used.

AFTERTREATMENT. The patient is kept at bed rest initially and is fitted with a molded bivalved thoracolumbosacral orthosis. The orthosis is worn for 12 to 16 weeks except during bed rest. Early ambulation and rehabilitation are encouraged.

HARRINGTON COMPRESSION INSTRUMENTATION. Harrington compression instrumentation may be indicated for thoracolumbar fractures, especially when the posterior column has failed in a tension mode. Small (⅛-inch) and large (³/₁₆-inch) threaded compression rods are available and provide rigid stabilization during fracture healing and fusion of the posterolateral arthrodesis. We have found them most useful for stabilizing flexion-distraction injuries and Chance fractures. When used in the thoracic spine, Harrington compression rods should be coupled to hooks that are placed around the base of the transverse processes. In the lumbar spine, the hook should be placed beneath the lamina to provide rigid fixation. Modifications of the Harrington compression instrumentation to include Keene hooks and bushings have made the use of this implant simpler and less time consuming. Studies have suggested that sublaminar wiring to compression rods should not be done because the wiring may pull the sublaminar hook into the underlying neural structures, resulting in iatrogenic neurologic deficits. Placing hooks in the transverse processes gives less strength than hook placement beneath the lamina; however, there is less danger of damage to the neural structures with the former technique. Biomechanical studies by Stauffer and Neil and by Pinzar et al. found compression rods to be stronger than distraction rods when subjected to a combination of flexion and rotation. Compression rods tend to fail by fracture of the transverse process during flexion and lateral bending and by hooks slipping off in extension. Recently we have favored the Edwards reversed racheted compression rods over traditional Harrington compression rods. We have found them to be technically easier to insert and equally effective (Fig. 80-45).

EDWARDS INSTRUMENTATION. Edwards and Levine developed a rod-sleeve fixation technique that appears to offer improved reduction and biomechancial fixation. The rod-sleeve reduction of spinal fractures produces indirect compression through a relatively low-risk posterior approach (Fig. 80-46). Edwards and Levine reported 135 consecutive spinal injuries and noted that in 91% of patients treated within 3 weeks anatomic correction was obtained in all planes; however, if surgery was delayed more than 3 weeks, anatomic alignment was obtained in only 20%. In addition, in 98% of patients with an intact anterior ligamentous complex, rod-sleeve fixation alone was sufficiently rigid to limit total motion across the instrumented segments to less than 2 mm in any plane. In patients treated within 48 hours of injury, reduction with the rod-sleeve technique restored 32% of the canal area; when surgery was delayed between 3 and 14 days, 23% of the canal area was restored; and if surgery was delayed for more than 2 weeks, there was little improvement in the canal area. In addition to increasing the canal area, the rod-sleeve technique was designed to create a relative lordosis at the level of injury and allow the cord to shift posteriorly in the canal, away from the remaining anterior fragments. They noted that relative lordosis averaged 3 degrees for patients treated with the bridging sleeve construct, 2.5 degrees for with a single pair of sleeves, distraction rods, and anatomic hooks, and 0 degrees with compression rods.

The Edwards instrumentation is a modification of the Harrington instrumentation. Distraction rods, polyethylene sleeves, and anatomic hook design provide simultaneous hyperextension and distraction forces that eliminate kyphotic deformity and restore vertebral height. The sleeves come in various sizes to accommodate the upper and lower thoracic regions, the thoracolumbar junction, and the lumbar spine. They wedge between the facets and spinous processes to correct translational deformity and provide rotational stability. Edwards and Levine rec-

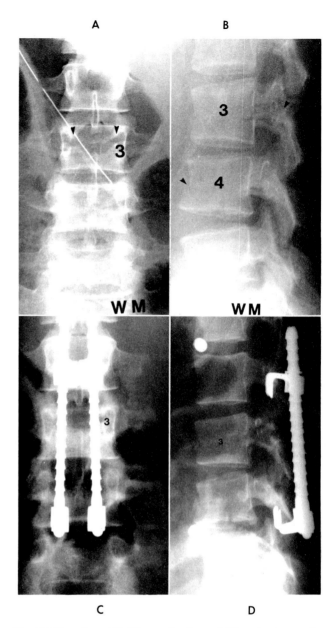

Fig. 80-45 **A** and **B,** Chance fracture of L3 and compression fracture of L4 in 20-year-old polytrauma patient without neurologic deficit. **C** and **D,** After internal fixation with dual Edwards' reverse rachet compression rods and anatomic hooks. Bilateral intertransverse process fusion from L2 to L4 was performed, and patient was mobilized in external orthosis.

ommend that the polyethylene sleeve be centered over the superior facet of the most apical fractured vertebra. If an unstable lamina or a comminuted pedicle fracture is present, they recommend a bridging sleeve construct. Care should be taken not to place the polyethylene sleeve directly over an unstable lamina or pedicle to prevent injury to the neural elements. Anatomic hooks should be inserted between 3 and 5 cm on either side of the edges of the sleeves to allow sufficient corrective moments yet keep the instrumentation relatively short. Usu-

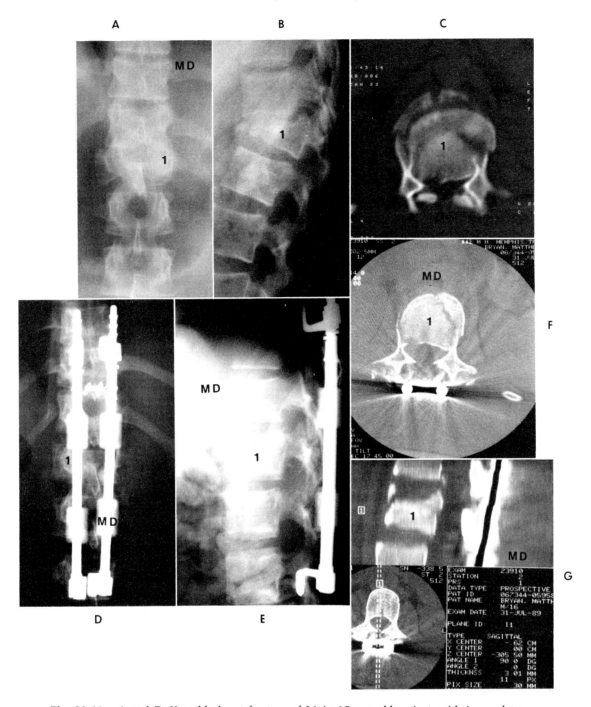

Fig. 80-46 **A** and **B**, Unstable burst fracture of L1 in 17-year-old patient, with incomplete paraparesis. **C**, CT scan shows significant canal compromise from retropulsed bone at L1 level. **D** and **E**, Realignment of spinal canal after posterior instrumentation with dual Harrington distraction rods and Edwards' sleeves in bridging construct. **F** and **G**, CT scans show nearly anatomic reduction of bone fragments from spinal canal after posterior instrumentation. This patient was immobilized in a thoracolumbosacral orthosis for 3 months and had complete neurologic recovery.

ally upper hooks are placed in the second interspace proximal to the sleeve and the first or second interspace distal to the sleeve. It is important to select the proper-sized rod sleeve to achieve anatomic alignment. The sleeves generate corrective moments to provide simulta-neous lordosis and distraction. To oppose the normal loss of rigidity caused by the gradual stretching of the anterior ligamentous structures, this method takes advantage of the normal elasticity of the stainless steel Harrington rods. A bow can be made in the rod by pressure on the sleeve between the rod and lamina. Thus, as the anterior ligamentous structures relax, the posterior rods straighten, helping to provide continuous correction (Fig. 80-47, *A*). The polyethylene sleeves and the L-shaped anatomic hooks provide increased contact surface with the lamina and minimize bone resorption, late loosening, and hook dislodgement (Fig. 80-47, *B*). With the Edwards system, the number of instrumented segments can be reduced, especially in the lumbar spine where preservation of motion segments is important. We have found this system to be effective and relatively simple to use.

■ *TECHNIQUE.* **Place the patient prone on a padded spinal frame and expose the thoracolumbar spine as described for the Harrington technique (p. 3557; Fig. 80-47). Confirm the level of injury with a lateral**

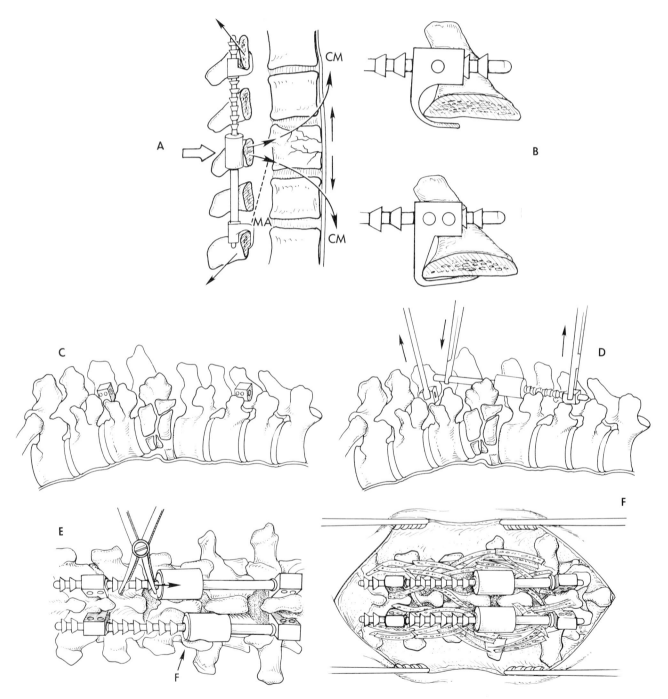

Fig. 80-47 Rod-sleeve reduction technique (see text). **A,** Sleeves generate corrective moments to provide simultaneous lordosis and distraction. **B,** C-shaped hooks provide edge contact only, anatomic hooks contact edge and undersurface. **C,** Hook placement. **D,** Reduction maneuver. **E,** Sleeve positioning. **F,** Fusion. (Redrawn from Edwards CC: Orthopaedics Today, December 15, 1985, Slack, Inc.)

roentgenogram and remove any depressed laminar fragments. Select the correct sleeve position over the superior facets of the apical vertebra or over adjacent facets if the pedicle or lamina is comminuted. Place anatomic hooks in the interspace that lies 3 to 5 cm on either side of the intended sleeve position. Use low-profile hooks in the thoracic facets and lamina and high-profile hooks to accommodate the thicker lumbar lamina. Place a trial sleeve between the apical facet and spinous process. In general, the small (2 mm) sleeve is appropriate for the midthoracic spine, the medium (4 mm) sleeve for the distal thoracic spine, the large (6 mm) sleeve for the upper lumbar spine, and the elliptical (8 mm) sleeve for the midlumbar spine. If necessary, the polyethylene sleeves can be trimmed with a high-speed burr or scalpel to assure a snug fit between the facet and spinous processes. Slide the sleeve over a distraction rod of sufficient length to allow at least 1 cm above the upper hook after final distraction. Pass the rod through the upper hook and then position the sleeve near the middle of the rod. Reduce the spine by pushing down on the distal end of the rod while pulling up on the lower hooks until the nipple of the rod engages the lower hook. To make reduction easier, a long rod on the opposite side can be used as a reduction lever. Place a large sleeve on the rod and position it over the apical lamina to serve as a fulcrum. Perform the reduction maneuver with a permanent rod while having an assistant push the end of the reduction lever in an anterocephalad direction. Once the rods and hooks are coupled, complete the reduction by refining the sleeve position. Use a rod clamp and Harrington spreader to push the sleeve into position over the superior facet of the fractured vertebral body, being sure it is wedged against the proximal spinous process. The correct size rod sleeve should fully reduce kyphosis and leave a slight but definite bow in the rods. Apply this distraction in stages for at least 20 minutes, and limit the distraction force at any one time to no more than 1 fingerbreadth on each side of the arm of the Harrington spreader. Obtain a lateral roentgenogram before final distraction to confirm the reduction and sleeve position.

For patients with incomplete paraplegia, we perform an intraoperative myelogram to confirm sufficient canal decompression to permit passage of dye anterior to the cord (Fig. 80-48). Inject water-soluble contrast dye distal to the injury with a spinal needle. Tilt the patient approximately 25 degrees with the head down and obtain a lateral roentgenogram. If residual compression of the thecal sac is present, perform a posterolateral decompression, as described by Erickson, Leider, and Brown and by and Garfin et al. Place two C-washers under each upper hook to prevent loss of distraction. Harvest a generous corticocancellous bone graft from the posterior ilium, lightly decorticate the posterior elements, and place posterior and posterolateral bone grafts over the instrumented segments. Thoroughly irrigate the wound with antibiotic solution, insert a closed suction drain, and close the wound in routine fashion.

AFTERTREATMENT. Patients are mobilized in a polypropylene orthosis. We recommend a postoperative CT scan to evaluate the adequacy of decompression. If decompression is inadequate, a staged anterior decompression should be considered in selected patients to improve neurologic recovery.

JACOBS LOCKING HOOK INSTRUMENTATION. This posterior instrumentation device (Fig. 80-49) was devised by Jacobs in conjunction with the AO group in an attempt to correct some of the deficiencies associated with traditional Harrington rod instrumentation. Recently Gertzbein et al. reviewed 95 consecutive thoracolumbar injuries treated with the locking hook spinal rod and found a 38% improvement in the initial kyphotic deformity and restoration of 37% of vertebral body height. In addition, 84% of patients with incomplete neurologic deficits improved by one or more grades. An instrument complication rate of 8.4% was noted. Possible disadvantages of this device are that it spans at least five motion segments, it may not provide adequate fixation for severely comminuted burst fractures because of insufficiency of the anterior and middle columns, and it is not recommended for fractures of the lower lumbar spine. This implant includes several modifications of the Harrington instrumentation. Instead of notches, both ends of the rods are threaded so that linear distraction of any distance is possible and weakening of the rod because of the narrow cross-section at the notches is avoided. The hooks are fixed with locking nuts and can be freely rotated on the rod. The rod can be contoured to the shape of the spine, even in lordosis, since rotation cannot occur. The rod maintains contact against the vertebral arch. The diameter of the rod is increased to 7 mm, and the lip of the cranial hook is tilted 15 degrees away from its axis, thus shaping the rod precisely to the anatomic shape of the anterior part of the proximal vertebral arch. In addition, the upper hook is fitted with a cover that can be pushed forward and is secured by corresponding grooves on the upper part of the hook. This allows the hook to grip firmly around the upper edge of the lamina. Jacobs et al. recommend that the implant be inserted in accordance with the three vertebrae above and three vertebrae below rule. They showed a 50% increase in the detachment force of the upper hook and a threefold increase in stiffness in flexion of the instrumented lumbar spine using this fixation. We have little experience with this implant but believe that it does offer improved stability over traditional Harrington rods.

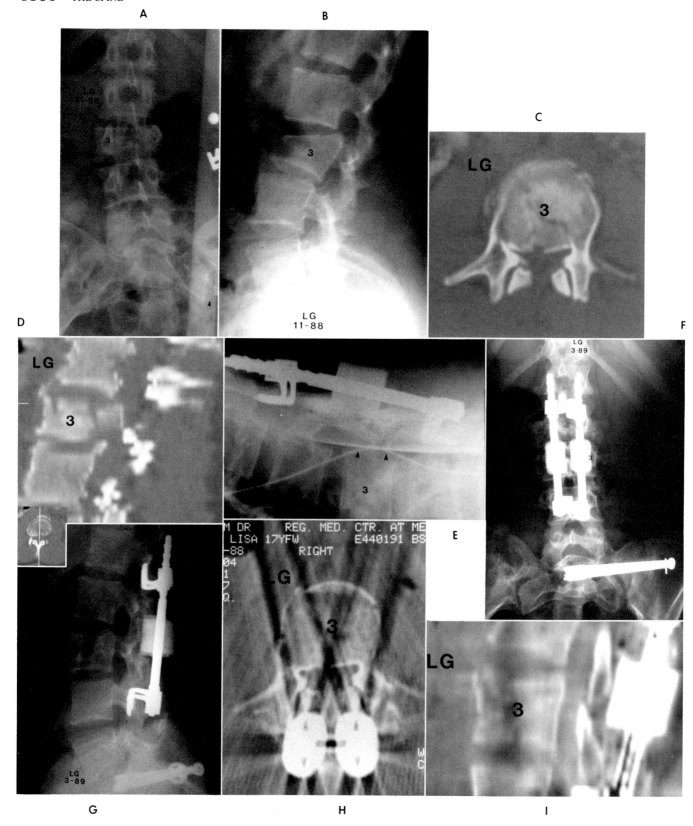

Fig. 80-48   **A** and **B**, Burst fracture of L3 in 17-year-old patient involved in motor vehicle accident. Despite significant canal compromise, patient had no neurologic deficits. **C** and **D**, CT scans show canal compromise from retropulsed bone at L3 level. **E**, Intraoperative myelogram shows excellent reduction of burst fracture with dye flowing freely past L3 level after posterior Edwards' instrumentation. **F** and **G**, Restoration of spinal alignment after posterior instrumentation with elliptical sleeves to maintain lordosis. Note internal fixation of sacroiliac joint injury with multiple cannulated screws. **H** and **I**, CT scans show restoration of spinal canal.

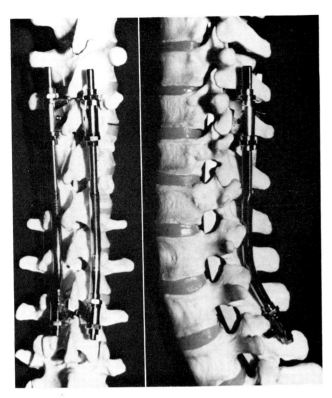

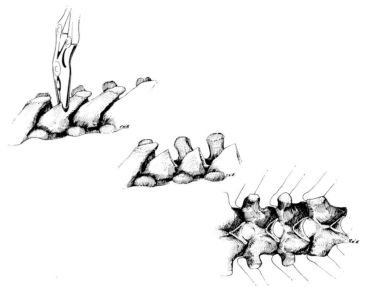

Fig. 80-50 Segmental spinal instrumentation (see text). Removal of caudally slanting spinous processes to expose ligamentum flavum. (From Segmental spinal fixation and correction using Richards L-rod instrumentation, Memphis, Smith & Nephew Richards, Inc.)

Fig. 80-49 Jacobs' posterior instrumentation. Rods are thick, are threaded on upper end, and have locking device at upper end to provide rigid fixation to lamina. (From Meyer PR Jr: Surgery of spine trauma, New York, 1989, Churchill Livingstone.)

LUQUE INSTRUMENTATION. The Luque instrumentation system provides more rigid internal fixation and resistance to rotational forces than does traditional Harrington instrumentation. This instrumentation has been used for correction of scoliotic deformities, as well as for stabilization of thoracolumbar fractures and dislocations. McAfee has shown that the ability to resist torsion is less in the Harrington distraction rods and that the system absorbing the highest energy is the Luque segmental system. Biomechanical testing found that the Luque segmental spinal instrumentation failed by fracture-dislocation, either above or below the instrumented segment. Ferguson and Allen reported one failure at the metal-bone interface and seven losses of correction in a series of 54 fractures and dislocations treated with Luque instrumentation. Loss of translational stability or malrotation did not occur. As biomechanical testing suggests, the weak point in the Luque system is a failure to counteract axial loading; thus it does not provide rigid fixation for unstable burst fractures. This system appears to be best suited for treatment of translational injuries of the thoracic or lumbar spine with complete neurologic injuries. When used in neurologically normal patients or those with incomplete neurologic lesions, care must be taken in passing the sublaminar wires to avoid neurologic injury. Wilber et al. reported transient sensory changes in 3 of 20 patients with Luque instrumentation

and a major sensory deficit in one. They listed as factors related to increased risk for spinal cord injury the passage of sublaminar wires in the thoracic and thoracolumbar spine. We have limited experience with Luque rod instrumentation in the treatment of thoracolumbar fractures but favor either a double Luque rod or a solid Luque rectangle, segmentally wired at each level with 16-gauge wire.

■ *TECHNIQUE.* With the patient prone, expose the segment of spine to be instrumented (p. 3557). For fracture-dislocations of the thoracolumbar spine, we recommend instrumentation three levels above and three levels below, using either a solid Luque rectangle or double rods. Expose the ligamentum flavum at each level to be instrumented using a needle-nose rongeur to remove soft tissue overlying the interspace (Fig. 80-50). In the lumbar spine because of the lordosis, there is often shingling of the lamina over the interspace. Excise this bone with rongeurs. Incise the ligamentum flavum with the rongeur and excise it with a small Kerrison punch (Figs. 80-51 and 80-52). The ligamentum flavum must be excised at every interspace to be instrumented. Pass wires beneath each lamina by forming a loop of 16-gauge wire and bending the loop to two right angles. The distance between the two bends should equal the width of the lamina to be instrumented. Pass the wires from a caudal to a cephalad direction (Fig. 80-53). At the upper and lower levels of instrumentation use double loops of wire (Fig. 80-54) and

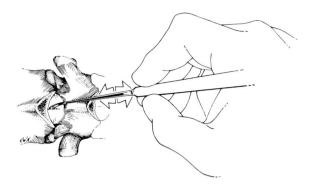

Fig. 80-51 Segmental spinal instrumentation (see text). Penfield No. 4 dissector is used to free deep surfaces of ligamentum flavum. (From Segmental spinal fixation and correction using Richards L-rod instrumentation, Memphis, Smith & Nephew Richards, Inc.)

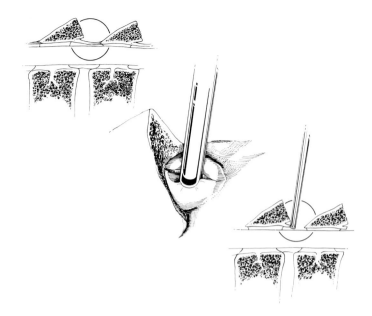

Fig. 80-52 Segmental spinal instrumentation (see text). Kerrison punch is used to remove remainder of ligamentum flavum. (From Segmental spinal fixation and correction using Richards L-rod instrumentation, Memphis, Smith & Nephew Richards, Inc.)

Fig. 80-53 Segmental spinal instrumentation (see text). Shape of double wire before it passes under lamina. (From Segmental spinal fixation and correction using Richards L-rod instrumentation, Memphis, Smith & Nephew Richards, Inc.)

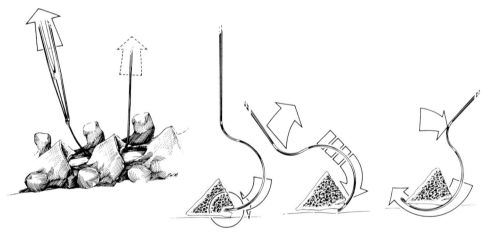

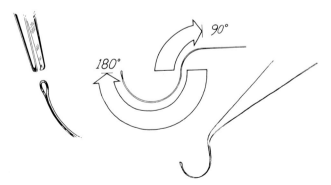

Fig. 80-54 Segmental spinal instrumentation (see text). Passage of segmental wire beneath lamina. (From Segmental spinal fixation and correction using Richards L-rod instrumentation, Memphis, Smith & Nephew Richards, Inc.)

at the intervening levels, one loop of wire. Divide the single loop of wire in the intervening levels so that two wires lie beneath each lamina and retract these to each side of the wound. Take care not to force the wires against the thecal sac during passage. Excise the facet joints bilaterally and pack bone graft around the facet joints while the laminae are decorticated. Insert the Luque rods, taking care to place the short arm or transverse limb of each rod beneath the longitudinal or long arm to prevent rotation and subsequent migration of the implant; and carefully tighten the wires around the rod to fix the spine to the rods. We usually begin tightening in the middle of the rod and proceed towards either end. Burst fractures can be reduced by applying a Har-

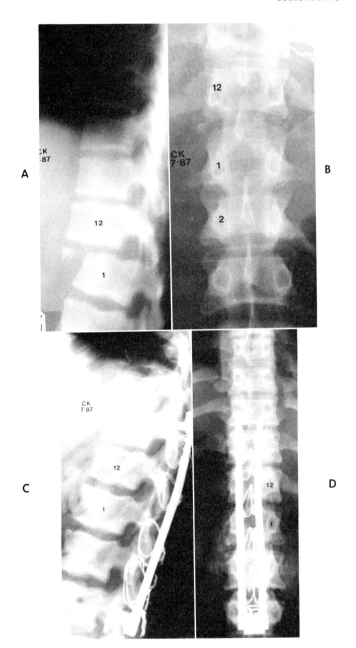

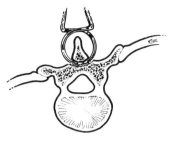

Fig. 80-56 Interspinous wiring technique (see text). Lewen clamp is used to make hole in base of spinous process for passage of wires.

Fig. 80-55 **A** and **B,** Translational injury of T12 on L1 in 19-year-old patient with complete paraplegia. **C** and **D,** Realignment of spinal canal after internal fixation with dual Harrington distraction rods augmented with sublaminar wires. This patient was mobilized early without an external orthosis.

rington outrigger and securely fixing them with a double **C**-rod to prevent collapse. Perform a routine posterolateral arthrodesis (Chapter 81), and close the wound in layers over a suction drain.

AFTERTREATMENT. Postoperative immobilization usually is not necessary, and rehabilitation can begin soon after surgery without the use of an external orthosis.

It must be emphasized that we have little experience with this technique in neurologically normal patients or in those with incomplete neurological le-

sions and have limited its use to patients with neurologically complete lesions and unstable translational injuries.

SUBLAMINAR WIRING WITH HARRINGTON DISTRACTION INSTRUMENTATION. This technique, which combines the advantages of the Harrington and Luque systems by sublaminar wiring of Harrington distraction rods, is reported to increase stability and resistance to pull-out, and it has proven effective in managing unstable thoracolumbar fractures (Fig. 80-55). Wenger et al. demonstrated that resistance to failure is greatest in intact lamina, followed in decreasing order by decorticated lamina, the transverse processes, and the spinous processes. Twist suggests that the intact lamina provides the strongest means of internal fixation. Stability of Harrington rods can therefore be increased by sublaminar wiring at multiple sites. Sullivan noted a decreased incidence of distraction rod failure and a reduction in postoperative immobilization time. Studies suggest that sublaminar wiring to compression rods should not be done because of the risk of driving the sublaminar hook into the underlying spinal canal. We have found that sublaminar wiring increases the stability of Harrington distraction rods in those patients with neurologically complete lesions and unstable thoracolumbar spine fractures. Considerable care must be taken when passing sublaminar wires, and the risk of neurologic injury must be considered when using this technique in neurologically normal patients or those with incomplete spinal cord injuries.

WISCONSIN (DRUMMOND) INTERSPINOUS SEGMENTAL SPINAL INSTRUMENTATION. Drummond, Keene, and Breed developed interspinous segmental spinal instrumentation to provide the stability of Luque instrumentation without the passage of sublaminar wires. This technique has been for the correction of scoliotic deformities and in the treatment of unstable thoracolumbar spine fractures. The base of the spinous process is readily accessible and easy to instrument and it provides a broad base of insertion for this particular implant (Fig. 80-56). The best purchase site for instrumentation with the Wisconsin system is the base of the spinous process, not the middle or tip. The anchoring hole must be created deep enough to obtain purchase in good bone stock but superficial enough to avoid penetrating the spinal canal. The button-wire implant is made of stainless steel that is 8 mm in diameter and 0.8 mm thick. The attached wire is 16- or 18-gauge stainless steel and is welded at the free end to form a smooth round bead, which eases passage of the wire through the base of the spinous process. The button has a hole in the surface large enough to allow passage of the beaded wires. Buttons are inserted on each side of the spinous processes, and a bead from each implant passes through the hole in the spinous process and then through the hole in the opposite button (Fig. 80-57). In the treatment of thoracolumbar fractures, we have used paired wires to increase stability when intact spinous processes are available in the intervening levels between the cephalad and caudal hooks (Fig. 80-58). This technique is safe and simple and the risk of neurologic injury is low if the hole is correctly placed in the base of the spinous process.

PEDICLE SCREW INSTRUMENTATION. Fixation of thoracolumbar fractures with pedicle screws and plates has been done routinely by Roy-Camille and others since 1961. Pedicle screw and plate implants for spinal fractures have been developed by Steffee and Sitkowski, Luque, Roy-Camille, and others and are presently being investigated in various centers. At present these implants have not been approved by the U.S. Food and Drug Administration (FDA) for use in thoracolumbar spinal trauma. We have found pedicle screw instrumentation to be very effective in the treatment of fractures of the lower lumbar spine (L3 to sacrum).

Luque pedicle screw

■ *TECHNIQUE.* We prefer to use a pedicle probe or a hand-held curet to enter the pedicle. Preoperative anteroposterior and lateral roentgenograms and CT scans through the pedicles of the vertebral body to be instrumented are studied to determine the correct angle of entry in both the coronal and sagittal planes. Insert blunt Kirschner wires into the pedicles and confirm their position with anteroposterior and lateral roentgenograms. Probe the pedicle in all four quadrants to be sure that a solid tube of bone exists and that violation into the spinal canal or inferiorly into the neuroforamen has not occurred. Once the Kirschner wires are in place, as confirmed by roentgenograms, introduce a cannulated screw tap over each wire and through the pedicle. If a wire bends or deforms in any way replace it to prevent inadvertent advancement of the wire as the tap is passed over it. The tapping depth should be no more than the depth of the pedicle, and the tap should not enter the vertebral body so that screw purchase is maximized. In tapping the sacral pedicles, penetrate only the posterior cortex. When all wires are in

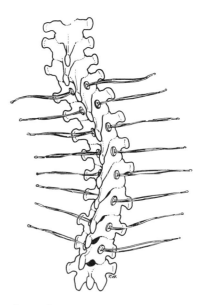

Fig. 80-57 Interspinous wiring technique (see text) with placement of buttons and wires.

proper position, select a plate of the appropriate size and contour it to maintain normal lumbar lordosis. When three or more screws are used, pass a plate ring over the plate before placing the plate over the wires. Select a cannulated screw of appropriate length so that penetration into the vertebral body is approximately 50%. Before seating the bone screws in the plate, "joy sticks" may be used to apply compression or distraction as necessary. When the screws are seated in the corresponding concavity of the plate, remove the wires at each level. Harvest a generous corticocancellous bone graft from the posterior ilium and perform a posterolateral fusion in the usual fashion. After insertion of the pedicle screws and plate, the cauda equina can be decompressed by laminectomy (Fig. 80-59). Thoroughly irrigate the wound with antibiotic solution, insert closed suction drainage, and close the wound in layers.

AFTERTREATMENT. Patients are mobilized rapidly in a lightweight lumbosacral orthosis. Routine follow-up is recommended at 3 weeks, 6 weeks, 3 months, 6 months, and 1 year.

AO SPINAL INTERNAL FIXATION SYSTEM. The AO spinal internal fixation system has been used successfully in many European centers. Magerl and Dick developed and modified the instrumentation. Presently this implant system is undergoing clinical trials in the United States. The AO spinal internal fixation system uses 5 mm transpedicular Schanz screws with 7 mm fully threaded stainless steel rods (Fig. 80-60). The screws are self-tapping, and the standard size is 35 mm of threaded length. The threaded rods are flattened on two sides and come in

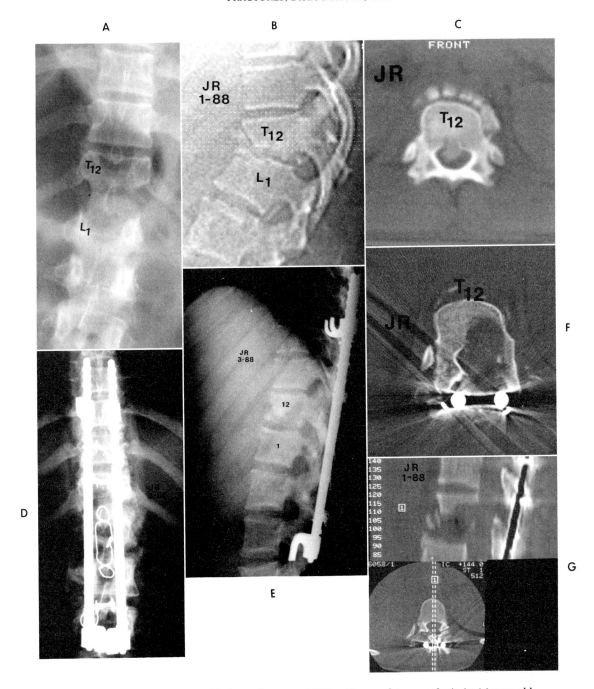

Fig. 80-58 **A** and **B,** Unstable burst fracture of T12 with complete paraplegia in 16-year-old female. **C,** CT scan shows comminution of fracture and nearly complete obliteration of spinal canal at T12 level. **D** and **E,** Realignment of spinal canal after posterior instrumentation with dual Harrington distraction rods augmented with wires. **F** and **G,** CT scans show decompression of spinal canal after removal of bone fragment through posterolateral approach.

a variety of lengths ranging from 70 to 300 mm. The coupling device is mobile in the sagittal plane and allows angulation of the Schanz screws before securing them to the rods. The nuts have a lug that can be crimped to secure them to the flattened threads. This system allows axial, angular, and rotational adjustability and permits segmental fixation of injured spinal segments. The AO internal fixator combines the advantages of the external spinal skeletal fixation device developed by Magerl and Dick with the advantage of being completely implantable. It appears to be effective in obtaining decompression of the spinal canal in burst fractures while, in most instances, limiting instrumentation to only two spinal motion segments. At this time, we have no experience with this implant but it appears to be promising for the treatment of thoracolumbar injuries.

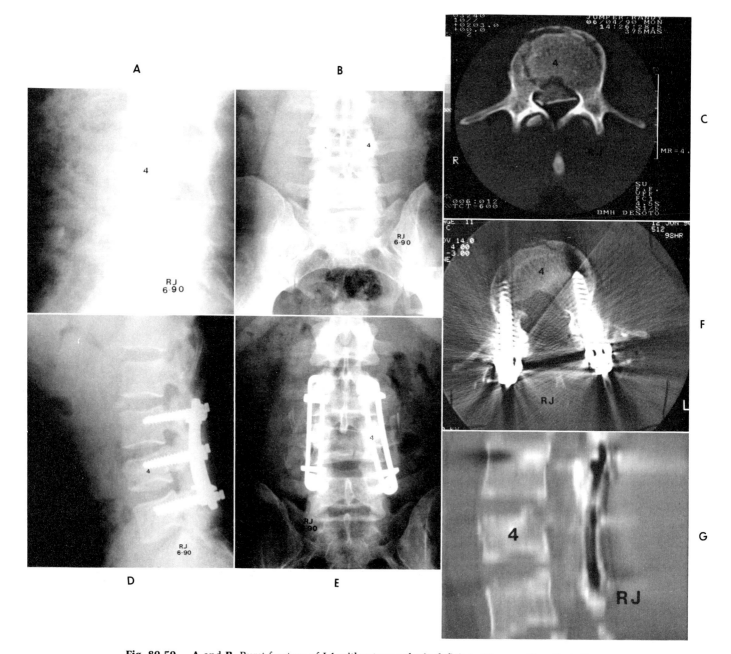

Fig. 80-59   **A** and **B,** Burst fracture of L4 without neurologic deficit in 20-year-old patient. **C,** CT scan shows significant canal compromise from retropulsed bone fragment at L4 level. **D** and **E,** After internal fixation with pedicle screws and plates; midline laminectomy defect at L4. **F** and **G,** CT scans show proper placement of pedicle screws and adequate decompression of spinal canal after total laminectomy. Bilateral intertransverse fusion from L3 to L5 was performed at time of internal fixation.

COMBINED FIXATION DEVICES. These recent instrumentation systems offer considerable flexibility in obtaining an extremely stable construct for thoracolumbar spine fractures. The Cotrel-Dubousset spinal instrumentation system was initially designed for scoliosis correction but has been used in the management of thoracolumbar spine injuries. Recently the Texas Scottish Rite Hospital implant system also has been used to obtain stability and correct deformity in spinal injuries. These systems offer advantages in that multiple hooks can be inserted and segmental fixation can be obtained. In some systems, pedicle screws can be coupled to the rods for use in the lower lumbar spine and for improved sacral fixation. Spinal injuries can be stabilized as necessary by placement of pedicle hooks, transverse process hooks, or sublaminar hooks in either a distraction or compression mode (Fig. 80-61). Proponents of these instrumentation systems suggest that another advantage is that the stabil-

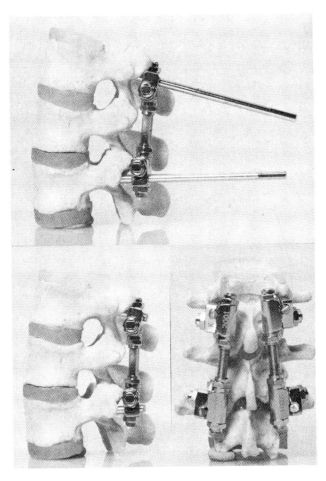

Fig. 80-60 AO spinal internal fixation system.

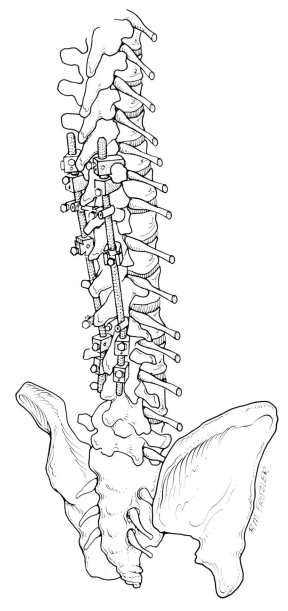

Fig. 80-61 Cotrel-Dubousset instrumentation. Type I configuration is most commonly used design and is recommended for fracture-dislocations and unstable burst fractures. (From McBride GG: Semin Spine Surg 2:24, 1990.)

ity obtained makes any form of postoperative external immobilization unnecessary, but further studies are necessary to document this. These instrumentation systems are complex and have higher incidences of neurologic injury than traditional Harrington or Edwards posterior instrumentation. Insertion is technically more difficult than with traditional Harrington or Edwards instrumentation, and there appears to be a significant learning curve in their use.

Biomechanical studies suggest that cross-linking of the rods, that is, either the device for transverse traction with the Cotrel-Dubousset system or the cross-linking plates with the Texas Scottish Rite Hospital system converts the entire construct into a stable rectangle with improved rotational stability. High fusion rates with low rates of pseudarthrosis and rod breakage have been reported in early series of scoliosis corrections. Recently McBride reported various configurations for hook placement in the treatment of unstable spinal injuries (Fig. 80-62). The basic pattern is a claw configuration at the most cephalad vertebra with various placement of intermediate and caudal hooks either in a distraction or compression mode (Fig. 80-63). In McBride's report of 48 patients, 20

were not braced after surgery. Two patients had early lower hook loosening with loss of reduction and required revision of instrumentation. Overall there was a 4% major medical complication rate and a 6% surgical complication rate. As more experience is gained with these systems and more long-term follow-up is obtained, the indications for their use will be further defined.

ANTERIOR INTERNAL FIXATION DEVICES. As stated earlier, anterior decompression of the spinal cord or cauda equina can be safely and directly obtained through an anterior approach. Placement of an iliac strut

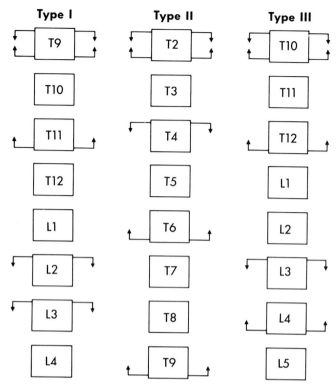

Type I	Type II	Type III
T9	T2	T10
T10	T3	T11
T11	T4	T12
T12	T5	L1
L1	T6	L2
L2	T7	L3
L3	T8	L4
L4	T9	L5

Fig. 80-62 Three configurations of Cotrel-Dubousset instrumentation for reduction and fixation of unstable spinal injuries. Type I is used for fracture-dislocations and burst fractures, type II for flexion-distraction injuries, and type III for injuries of lumbar spine where maintenance of lordosis is important. (Redrawn from McBride GG: Semin Spine Surg 2:24, 1990.)

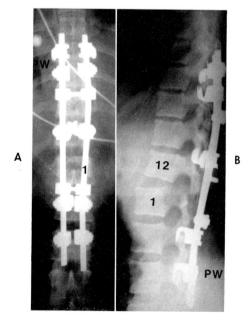

Fig. 80-63 **A** and **B**, Postoperative roentgenograms of patient shown in Fig. 80-5 with translational injury at T12-L1 level. Posterior instrumentation with Texas Scottish Rite implants with type A configuration and posterior cervical arthrodesis with triple-wire technique were performed.

graft provides no immediate stability if the posterior ligamentous or osseous structures are incompetent. Numerous anterior internal fixation devices have been developed, including the Dunn device, Dwyer instrumentation, Zeilke instrumentation, modified Kostuik-Harrington instrumentation, the Kaneda device, and anterior plates and screws. Many studies are currently underway to evaluate the stability of anterior instrumentation without additional posterior stabilization. The disadvantages of anterior instrumentation include the increased morbidity of the surgical approach and potential vascular injuries caused by large anterior implants. If complications occur, the operation to remove implants from the anterior aspect of the spine is more difficult than for posterior implants, and adequate correction of kyphosis may be impossible with anterior instrumentation alone if the posterior supporting structures are incompetent.

Anterior Vertebral Body Excision for Burst Fractures

Anterior vertebral body excision and grafting, as already mentioned, may be necessary in certain burst fractures untreated for more than 2 weeks and not believed to be candidates for posterior instrumentation and indirect decompression of the spinal canal. McAfee and Bohlman reported 70 patients with spinal cord injury secondary to thoracolumbar fractures treated by anterior decompression through a retroperitoneal approach. All had incomplete neurologic deficits caused by retropulsed bone or disc material in the spinal canal. Motor deficits in 88% of patients improved by at least one class, and nearly 50% of patients whose quadriceps and hamstrings were impaired enough to prevent walking regained independent walking ability. Of the patients with a conus medullaris injury, 37% demonstrated recovery of neurogenic bowel and bladder function. McAfee and Bohlman concluded that the degree of neurologic recovery after anterior decompression of thoracolumbar fractures was greater than after other techniques that do not decompress the spinal canal. We have limited anterior decompression and strut-graft fusion to patients with incomplete neurologic deficits and residual neural compression following posterior instrumentation and to patients whose surgery has been delayed for more than 2 weeks when indirect decompression through posterior instrumentation cannot be expected to produce satisfactory reduction of retropulsed bone and disc fragments.

■ *TECHNIQUE.* Approach the spine anteriorly through a retroperitoneal or retropleural approach (Fig. 80-64, *A* and *B*). Identify the fractured vertebra and excise the intervertebral discs above and below. Next remove the bulk of the fractured vertebral body using a rongeur and osteotome or if necessary a small power burr (Fig. 80-64, *C*). It is best to remove most of the vertebral body before removing the posterior cortex, which exposes the dura. If decompression of

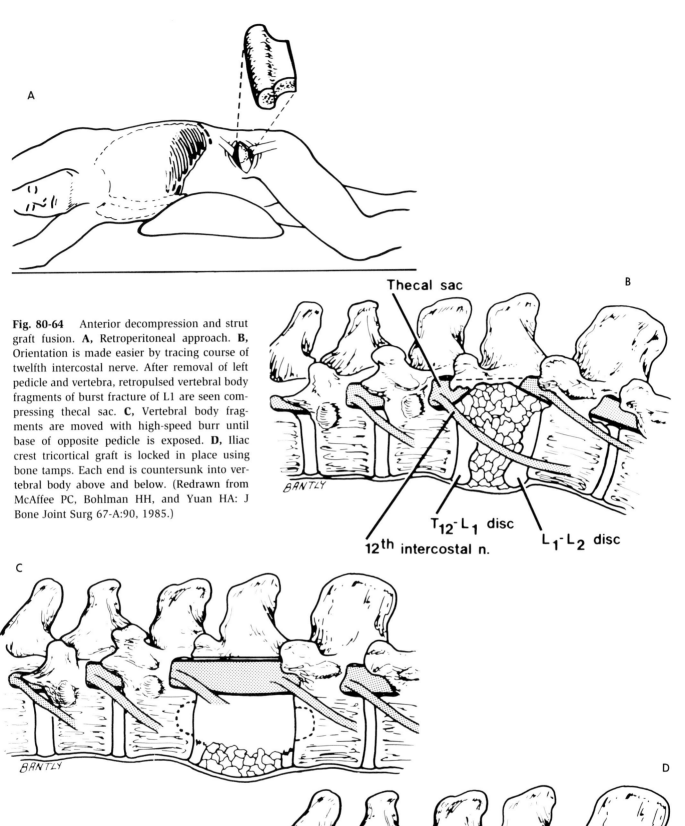

Fig. 80-64 Anterior decompression and strut graft fusion. **A,** Retroperitoneal approach. **B,** Orientation is made easier by tracing course of twelfth intercostal nerve. After removal of left pedicle and vertebra, retropulsed vertebral body fragments of burst fracture of L1 are seen compressing thecal sac. **C,** Vertebral body fragments are moved with high-speed burr until base of opposite pedicle is exposed. **D,** Iliac crest tricortical graft is locked in place using bone tamps. Each end is countersunk into vertebral body above and below. (Redrawn from McAffee PC, Bohlman HH, and Yuan HA: J Bone Joint Surg 67-A:90, 1985.)

Thecal sac

T_{12}-L_1 disc

12th intercostal n.

L_1-L_2 disc

BANTLY

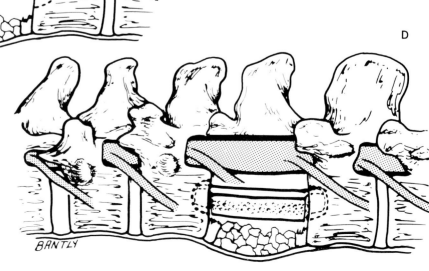

BANTLY

the posterior cortex is begun on the side of the body opposite the surgeon, troublesome bulging of the dura into the space created by removing the vertebral body will be minimized and the surgeon's view will be less obstructed. Control bleeding from the bone with bone wax and epidural bleeding with Gelfoam. After the decompression has been completed, cut slots into the end plates of the vertebral bodies above and below the defect: undercut the ends of the slots about 1 cm to allow the graft to be keyed in place. Place Gelfoam over the dura for protection and keep all bone grafts anterior and away from the dura itself. Next obtain a tricortical iliac graft or a fibular graft. Undercut the ends of the graft and key it into place to prevent it from dislodging (Fig. 80-64, *D*). Do not place any bone deep to the graft in the area of decompression. Finally obtain hemostasis and close the wound in a routine manner over suction drains.

AFTERTREATMENT. The patient is kept at bed rest until it is certain that wound infection or other complications are absent; then he is mobilized in a molded thoracolumbosacral orthosis. The orthosis is worn for 12 to 16 weeks. If posterior stability is questionable, posterior instrumentation is indicated.

SACRAL FRACTURES AND LUMBOSACRAL DISLOCATION

Sacral fractures and lumbosacral dislocation constitute approximately 1% of all spinal fractures. They are frequently associated with pelvic fractures and often are overlooked. The most common causes of these fractures are motor vehicle accidents and falls. Lafollette, Levine, and McNiesh noted that 60% of sacral fractures are missed initially. A high index of suspicioun is necessary to diagnose sacral fractures in patients with multiple trauma. These patients should be carefully examined for sacral root dysfunction suggested by decreased perianal sensation and rectal sphincter disturbance. Decreased ankle jerk reflexes and absence of a bulbocavernosus reflex also may suggest sacral root injury. Denis devised a classification system that divides the sacrum into three zones: (1) the region of the ala, (2) the region of the sacral foramina, and (3) the region of the central sacral canal (Fig. 80-65). In his series of 236 patients, he reported a 32% incidence of neurologic deficits. Nerve root damage was present in 5.9% when fractures were in zone 1, 28% in zone 2, and 87% in zone 3.

Treatment of sacral fractures and lumbosacral dislocation may be difficult, and both nonoperative management and operative management have been used with satisfactory results. Conservative treatment includes bed rest for 8 to 12 weeks, and the successful use of a hip spica cast has been reported. Sacral fractures with unsta-

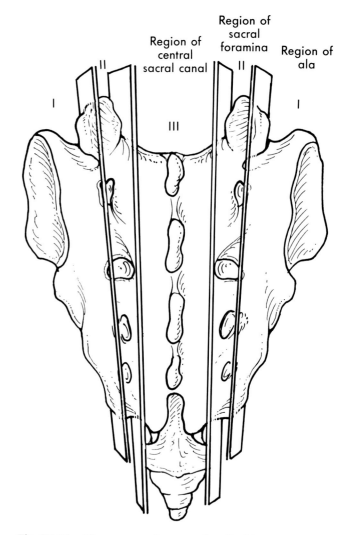

Fig. 80-65   Three zones of sacrum described by Denis: region of ala, region of sacral foramina, and region of central sacral canal. (Redrawn from Carl A: Sacral spine fractures. In Errico TJ, Bauer RD, and Waugh T, editors: Spinal trauma, Philadelphia, 1990, JB Lippincott Co.)

ble pelvic injuries may be successfully treated with external or internal fixation of the pelvic fracture. Delayed neurologic injury from entrapment of sacral nerve roots and fracture deformity and callus are not infrequent. Surgery is indicated for patients with neurologic impairment and confirmed neural compression from fracture fragments or sacral deformity. Sacral laminectomy allows nerve root exploration and decompression. The prognosis for return of bowel and bladder function is uncertain. Instrumentation and fusion with Harrington rods and pedicle screws also have been reported. We have had little experience with open reduction and internal fixation of displaced sacral fractures; however, lumbosacral dislocation may be effectively stabilized with pedicle screws (Fig. 80-66). We recommend that treatment be individualized for these infrequent injuries.

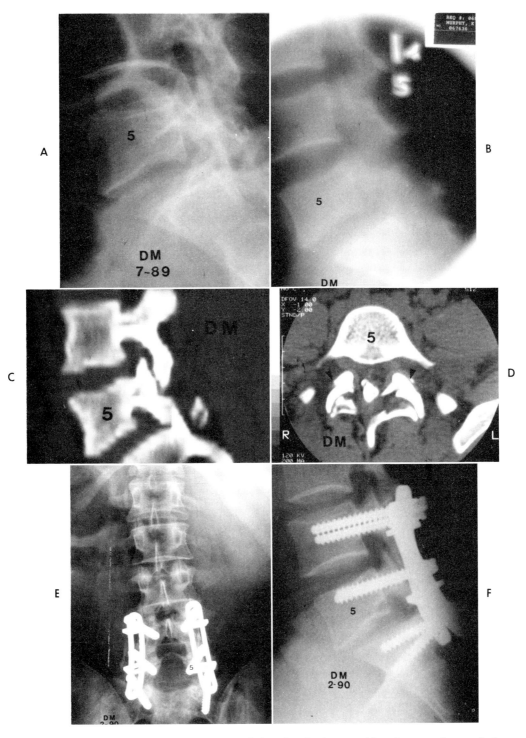

Fig. 80-66   Acute traumatic lumbosacral dislocation in 27-year-old patient causing grade 1 spondylolisthesis of L5 on sacrum. Patient had isolated left S1 nerve root injury. **A** and **B**, Lateral roentgenogram and tomogram of lumbosacral joint shows spondylolisthesis and fracture of spinous process of L5. **B**, Lateral CT scan after lumbar myelogram shows spondylolisthesis and fracture. **C** and **D**, CT scans show dislocated inferior articular masses of L5 in relationship to superior articular facets of sacrum and compression of S1 nerve root by left paracentral L5-S1 disc herniation. **E** and **F**, After internal fixation with pedicle screws and plates and midline decompressive laminectomy of L5. This patient was left with only residual decreased ankle jerk reflex on left and mild back pain that did not prevent return to work.

REFERENCES

General

Allen WE III, D'Angelo CM, and Kies EL: Correlation of microangiographic and electrophysiologic changes in experimental spinal cord trauma, Radiology 111:107, 1974.

Aufdermaur M: Spinal injuries in juveniles: necropsy findings in twelve cases, J Bone Joint Surg 56-B:513, 1974.

Bick EM: Source book of orthopaedics, Baltimore, 1948, Williams & Wilkins.

Blount WP: Fractures in children, Baltimore, 1954, Williams & Wilkins.

Bohlman HH: Pathology and current treatment concepts of acute spine injuries, AAOS Instr Course Lect 21:108, 1972.

Bors E: Phantom limbs of patients with spinal cord injury, Arch Neurol Psychiat 66:610, 1951.

Bosch A, Stauffer ES, and Nickel VL: Incomplete traumatic quadriplegia: a ten-year review, JAMA 216:473, 1971.

Brown MD, Eismont FJ, and Quencer RM: Symposium: intraoperative ultrasonography in spinal surgery, Contemp Orthop 11:47, 1985.

Burke DC: Hyperextension injuries of the spine, J Bone Joint Surg 53-B:3, 1971.

Campbell J and Bonnett C: Spinal cord injury in children, Clin Orthop 112:114, 1975.

Clark WK: Spinal cord decompression in spinal cord injury, Clin Orthop 154:9, 1981.

Convery FR, Minteer MA, Smith RW, and Emerson SM: Fracture-dislocation of the dorsal-lumbar spine, Spine 3:160, 1978.

Conwell HE and Reynolds FC: Key and Conwell's management of fractures, dislocations, and sprains, ed 7, St Louis, 1961, Mosby–Year Book, Inc.

Davis L: Treatment of spinal cord injuries, Arch Surg 69:488, 1954.

Davis L and Martin J: Studies upon spinal cord injuries. II. The nature and treatment of pain, J Neurosurg 4:483, 1947.

Davis R: Spasticity following spinal cord injury, Clin Orthop 112:66, 1975.

Davis R: Pain and suffering following spinal cord injury, Clin Orthop 112:76, 1975.

De La Torre JC: Spinal cord injury: review of basic and applied research, Spine 6:315, 1981.

Dorr LD, Harvey JP, and Nickel VL: Clinical review of the early stability of spine injuries, Spine 7:545, 1982.

Frankel HL et al: The value of postural reduction in the initial management of closed injuries of the spine with paraplegia and tetraplegia, Part I, Paraplegia 7:179, 1969.

Freeman LW and Heimburger RF: Surgical relief of pain in paraplegic patients, Arch Surg 55:433, 1947.

Garfin SR, editor: Complications of spine surgery, Baltimore, 1989, Williams & Wilkins.

Gertzbein SD, Court-Brown CM, Marks P, et al: The neurological outcome following surgery for spinal fractures, Spine 13:641, 1988.

Green BA, Callahan RA, Klore KJ, and De La Torre J: Acute spinal cord injury: current concepts, Clin Orthop 154:125, 1981.

Guttmann L: The treatment and rehabilitation of patients with injuries of the spinal cord. In Cope Z, editor: Medical history of the second world war: surgery, London, 1953, His Majesty's Stationery Office.

Guttmann L: A new turning-tilting bed, Paraplegia 3:193, 1965.

Guttmann L: Spinal deformities in traumatic paraplegics and tetraplegics following surgical procedures, Paraplegia 7:38, 1969.

Heyl HL: Some practical aspects in the rehabilitation of paraplegics, J Neurosurg 13:184, 1956.

Holdsworth FW: Traumatic paraplegia. In Platt H, editor: Modern trends in orthopaedics (second series), New York, 1956, Paul B Hoeber, Inc.

Holdsworth FW: Fractures, dislocations, and fracture-dislocations of the spine, J Bone Joint Surg 45-B:6, 1963.

Holdsworth FW: Fractures, dislocations, and fracture-dislocations of the spine, J Bone Joint Surg 52-A:1534, 1970.

Holdsworth SF: Review article: fractures, dislocations, and fracture-dislocations of the spine, J Bone Joint Surg 52-B:1534, 1970.

Holmes G: Pain of central origin. In Contributions to medical and biological research, vol 1, New York, 1919, Paul B Hoeber Medical Books.

Horal J, Nachemson A, and Scheller S: Clinical and radiological long term follow-up of vertebral fractures in children, Acta Orthop Scand 43:491, 1972.

Horwitz MT: Structural deformities of the spine following bilateral laminectomy, Am J Roentgen 46:836, 1941.

Hubbard DD: Injuries of the spine in children and adolescents, Clin Orthop 100:56, 1974.

Jelsma RK, Rice JF, Jelsma LF, and Kirsch PT: The demonstration and significance of neural compression after spinal injury, Surg Neurol 18:79, 1982.

Kahn EA: On spinal-cord injuries, J Bone Joint Surg 41-A:6, 1959 (editorial).

Kahnovitz N, Bullough P, and Jacobs RR: The effect of internal fixation without arthrodesis on human facet joint cartilage, Clin Orthop 189:204, 1984.

Kraus JF, Franti CE, Riggins RS, et al: Incidence of traumatic spinal cord lesions, J Chronic Dis 28:471, 1975.

Laborde JM, Bahniuk E, Bohlman HH, and Samson B: Comparison of fixation of spinal fractures, Clin Orthop 152:303, 1980.

McPhee IB: Spinal fractures and dislocations in children and adolescents, Spine 6:533, 1981.

Meyer PR Jr: Emergency room assessment: management of spinal cord and associated injuries. In Meyer PR Jr, editor: Surgery of spine trauma, New York, 1989, Churchill Livingstone.

Quencer RM: Intraoperative ultrasound of the spine, Surg Rounds, p 17, October 1987.

Ramsey R and Doppman JL: The effect of epidural masses on spinal cord blood flow: an experimental study in monkeys, Radiology 107:99, 1973.

Ransohoff J: Discussion of relief of myelopathic pain by percutaneous cervical cordotomy. In Proceedings of the Spinal Cord Injury Conference, vol 17, New York, 1969, Bronx Veterans Administration Hospital.

Schneider RC and Kahn EA: Chronic neurologic sequelae of acute trauma to the spine and spinal cord. II. The syndrome of chronic anterior spinal cord injury or compression, J Bone Joint Surg 41-A:449, 1959.

Sobel JW, Bohlman HH, and Freehafer AA: Charcot's arthropathy of the spine following spinal cord injury: a report of five cases, J Bone Joint Surg 67-A:771, 1985.

Southwick WO: Management of fractures of the dens (odontoid process), J Bone Joint Surg 62-A:482, 1980.

Speed K: A textbook of fractures and dislocations, Philadelphia, 1928, Lea & Febiger.

Stauffer ES: Spinal injuries in the multiply injured patient. II. Post-acute care and rehabilitation, Orthop Clin North Am 1:137, 1970.

Stauffer ES, Wood RW, and Kelly EG: Gunshot wounds of the spine: the effects of laminectomy, J Bone Joint Surg 61-A:389, 1979.

Watson-Jones R: Fractures and joint injuries, ed 4, Baltimore, vol 1, 1952, and vol 2, 1955, Williams & Wilkins.

Cervical spine

Allen BL Jr, Ferguson RL, Lehmann R, and O'Brian RP: Mechanistic classification of closed indirect fractures and dislocations of the lower cervical spine, Spine 7:1, 1982.

Anderson LD and D'Alonzo RT: Fractures of the odontoid process of the axis, J Bone Joint Surg 56-A:1663, 1974.

Anderson PA and Montesano PX: Morphology and treatment of occipital condyle fractures, Spine 13:731, 1988.

Arena MJ, Eismont FJ, and Green BA: Intervertebral disc extrusion associated with cervical facet subluxation and dislocation. Presented at the Cervical Spine Research Society 15th Annual Meeting, Washington DC, December 2-5, 1987.

Aronson N, Feltzer DL, and Bagan M: Anterior cervical fusion by Smith-Robinson approach, J Neurosurg 29:397, 1968.

Bailey RW and Badgley CE: Stabilization of the cervical spine by anterior fusion, J Bone Joint Surg 42-A:565, 1960.

Ballock RT, Botte MJ, and Garfin SR: Complications of halo immobilization. In Garfin SR, editer: Complications of spine surgery, Baltimore, 1989, Williams & Wilkins.

Beatson TR: Fractures and dislocations of the cervical spine, J Bone Joint Surg 45-B:21, 1963.

Bohlman HH: The pathology and current treatment concepts of cervical spine injuries: a critical reviw of 300 cases, J Bone Joint Surg 54-A:1353, 1972.

Bohlman HH: Pathology and current treatment concepts of cervical spine injuries, AAOS Instr Course Lect 21:108, 1972.

Bohlman HH: Complications of treatment of fractures and dislocations of the cervical spine. In Epps CH, editor: Complications in orthopaedic surgery, Philadelphia, 1978, JB Lippincott Co.

Bohlman HH: Acute fractures and dislocations of the cervical spine, J Bone Joint Surg 61-A:1119, 1979.

Bohlman HH: Complications and pitfalls in the treatment of acute cervical spinal cord injuries. In Tator CH, editor: Early management of acute spinal cord injury, New York, 1982, Raven Press.

Bohlman HH: Indications for late anterior decompression and fusion for cervical spinal cord injuries. In Tator CH, editor: Early management of acute spinal cord injury, New York, 1982, Raven Press.

Bohlman HH, Anderson PA, and Freehafer A: Anterior decompression and arthrodesis in patients with motor incomplete cervical spinal cord injury: long-term results of neurologic recovery in 58 patients, Unpublished data.

Bohlman HH, Bahnuik E, Gield G, and Raskulinecz G: Spinal cord monitoring of experimental incomplete cervical spinal cord injury, Spine 6:428, 1981.

Bohlman HH, Bahnuik E, Raskulinecz G, and Field G: Mechanical factors affecting recovery from incomplete cervical spine injury: a preliminary report, Johns Hopkins Med J 145:115, 1979.

Bosch A, Stauffer ES, and Nickel VL: Incomplete traumatic quadriplegia: a ten-year reviw, JAMA 216:473, 1967.

Braakman R and Vinken PJ: Old luxations of the lower cervical spine, J Bone Joint Surg 50-B:52, 1968.

Brashear HR Jr, Venters GC, and Preston ET: Fractures of the neural arch of the axis: a report of 29 cases, J Bone Joint Surg 59-A:879, 1975.

Brav EA, Miller JA, and Bouzard WC: Traumatic dislocation of the cervical spine: army experience and results, J Trauma 3:569, 1963.

Brooks AL and Jenkins EB: Atlanto-axial arthrodesis by the wedge compression method, J Bone Joint Surg 60-A:279, 1978.

Callahan RA et al: Cervical facet fusion for control of instability following laminectomy, J Bone Joint Surg 59-A:991, 1977.

Capen D, Zigler J, and Garland D: Surgical stabilization in cervical spine trauma, Contemp Orthop 14:25, 1987.

Capen DA, Nelson RW, Zigler JE, et al: Decompressive laminectomy in cervical spine trauma: a review of early and late complications, Contemp Orthop 17:21, 1988.

Carroll C, McAfee PC, and Riley LH Jr: Objective findings for diagnosis of "whiplash," J Musculoskel Med, p 57, March 1986.

Cattell HS and Filtzer DL: Pseudosubluxation and other normal variations of the cervical spine in children: a study of 160 children, J Bone Joint Surg 47-A:1295, 1965.

Clark CR: Dens fractures, Semin Spine Surg 3:39, 1991.

Clark CR and Whitehill R: Two views of the use of methylmethacrylate for stabilization of the cervical spine, Orthopedics 12:589, 1989.

Cloward RB: New method of diagnosis and treatment of cervical disc disease, Clin Neurosurg 8:93, 1962.

Cone W and Turner WG: The treatment of fracture-dislocation of the cervical vertebrae by skeletal traction and fusion, J Bone Joint Surg 19:584, 1937.

Cornish BL: Traumatic spondylolisthesis of the axis, J Bone Joint Surg 50-B:31, 1968.

Crenshaw AH Jr, Wood GW, Wood MW Jr, and Ray MW: Fracture and dislocation of the fourth and fifth cervical vertebral bodies with transection of the spinal cord, Clin Orthop 248:158, 1989.

Crutchfield WG: Skeletal traction for dislocation of the cervical spine, South Surgeon 2:156, 1933.

Crutchfield WG: Fracture-dislocations of the cervical spine, Am J Surg 38:592, 1937.

Crutchfield WG: Treatment of injuries of the cervical spine, J Bone Joint Surg 20:696, 1938.

Crutchfield WG: Skeletal traction in the treatment of injuries to the cervical spine, JAMA 155:29, 1954.

Davis D, Bohlman H, Walker E, et al: The pathological findings in fatal craniospinal injuries, J Neurol 34:603, 1971.

Delamarter RB: The cervical spine III: management of cervical spine injuries. Instructional course lecture presented at the 57th Annual Meeting of the American Academy of Orthopaedic Surgeons, New Orleans, February 12, 1990.

Ducker TB, Bellegarrigue R, Salcman M, and Walleck C: Timing of operative care in cervical spinal cord injury, Spine 9:525, 1984.

Dunbar HS and Ray BS: Chronic atlanto-axial dislocations with late neurologic manifestations, Surg Gynecol Obstet 113:757, 1961.

Durbin FC: Fracture-dislocations of the cervical spine, J Bone Joint Surg 39-B:23, 1957.

Eastwood WJ and Jefferson G: Discussion on fractures and dislocation of the cervical vertebrae, Proc R Soc Med 33:651, 1939.

Eismont FJ and Bohlman HH: Posterior atlanto-occipital dislocation with fractures of the atlas and odontoid process, J Bone Joint Surg 60-A:397, 1978.

Eismont FJ and Bohlman HH: Posterior methylmechacrylate fixation for cervical trauma, Spine 6:347, 1981.

Eismont FJ, Bora F, and Bohlman HH: Complete dislocations at two adjacent levels of the cervical spine, Spine 9:319, 1984.

El-Khoury GY and Kathol MH: Radiographic evaluation of cervical spine trauma, Semin Spine Surg 3:3, 1991.

Evans DK: Reduction of cervical dislocations, J Bone Joint Surg 43-B:552, 1961.

Evans DK: Anterior cervical subluxation, J Bone Joint Surg 58-B:318, 1976.

Fielding JW: Selected observations on the cervical spine in the child. In Ahstrom JP Jr, editor: Current practice in orthopaedic surgery, vol 5, St Louis, 1973, Mosby–Year Book, Inc.

Fielding JW and Griffin PP: Os odontoideum: an acquired lesion, J Bone Joint Surg 56-A:187, 1974.

Fielding JW and Hawkins RJ: Atlanto-axial rotatory fixation: fixed rotatory subluxation of the atlanto-axial joint, J Bone Joint Surg 59-A:37, 1977.

Fielding JW and Hensinger RN: Cervical spine surgery: past, present, and future potential, Orthopedics 10:1701, 1987.

Fielding JW, Hawkins RJ, and Ratzan SA: Spine fusion for atlanto-axial instability, J Bone Joint Surg 58-A:400, 1976.

Fielding JW, Rubin BD, and Stillwell WT: Cervical spine trauma, J Cont Ed Orthop 7:19, 1978.

Fielding JW, Cochran GVB, Lawsing JF III, and Hohl M: Tears of the transverse ligament of the atlas: a clinical and biomechanical study, J Bone Joint Surg 56-A:1683, 1974.

Fielding JW, Francis WR, Hawkins RJ, and Hensinger RN: Atlanto-axial rotary deformity, Semin Spine Surg 3:33, 1991.

Finerman GAM, Sakai D, and Weingarten S: Atlanto-axial dislocation with spinal cord compression in a mongoloid child: a case report, J Bone Joint Surg 58-A:408, 1976.

Forsyth HF, Alexander E Jr, Davis D Jr, and Underdal R: The advantages of early spine fusion in the treatment of fracture-dislocation of the cervical spine, J Bone Joint Surg 41-A:17, 1959.

Freehafer AA, Vonhaam E, and Allen V: Tendon transfers to improve grasp after injuries of the cervical spinal cord, J Bone Joint Surg 56-A:951, 1974.

Freiberger RH, Wilson PD Jr, and Nicholas JA: Acquired absence of the odontoid process: a case report, J Bone Joint Surg 47-A:1231, 1965.

Fried LC: Atlanto-axial fracture-dislocations: failure of posterior C1 to C2 fusion, J Bone Joint Surg 55-B:490, 1973.

Gallie WE: Fractures and dislocations of the cervical spine, Am J Surg 46:495, 1939.

Griswold DM, Albright JA, Schiffman E, et al: Atlanto-axial fusion for instability, J Bone Joint Surg 60-A:285, 1978.

Grogono BJS: Injuries of the atlas and axis, J Bone Joint Surg 36-A:397, 1954.

Hadley MN, Dickman CA, Browner CM, and Sonntag VKH: Acute traumatic atlas fractures: management and long-term outcome, Adv Orthop Surg 12:234, 1989.

Hanssen AD, Cabanela ME, and Cass JR: Fractures of the dens (odontoid process), Adv Orthop Surg 10:170, 1987.

Haralson RH and Boyd HB: Posterior dislocation of the atlas on the axis without fracture: report of a case, J Bone Joint Surg 51-A:561, 1969.

Hawkins RJ, Fielding JW, and Thompson WJ: Os odontoideum: congenital or acquired: a case report, J Bone Joint Surg 58-A:413, 1976.

Herkowitz HN and Rothman RH: Subacute instability of the cervical spine, Spine 9:348, 1984.

Herzeberger EE et al: Anterior interbody fusion in the treatment of certain disorders of the cervical spine, Clin Orthop 24:83, 1962.

Hohl M: Soft-tissue injuries of the neck in automobile accidents, J Bone Joint Surg 56-A:1675, 1974.

Holmes JC and Hall JE: Fusion for instability and potential instability of the cervical spine in children and adolescents, Orthop Clin North Am 9:923, 1978.

Holness RO, Huestis WS, Howes WJ, and Langille RA: Posterior stabilization with an interlaminar clamp in cervical injuries: technical note and review of the long-term experience with the method, Neurosurgery 14:318, 1984.

Jacobs B: Cervical fractures and dislocations (C3-7), Clin Orthop 109:18, 1975.

Jefferson G: Fracture of the atlas vertebra: report of four cases and a review of those previously recorded, Br J Surg 7:407, 1920.

Johnson RM, Owen JR, Hart DL, and Callahan RA: Cervical orthoses: a guide to their selection and use, Clin Orthop 154:34, 1981.

Johnson RM, Hart DL, Simmons EF, et al: Cervical orthoses: a study comparing their effectiveness in restricting cervical motion in normal subjects, J Bone Joint Surg 59-A:332, 1977.

Jones ET and Haid R Jr: Injuries to the pediatric subaxial cervical spine, Semin Spine Surg 3:61, 1991.

Kahn EA and Yglesias L: Progressive atlantoaxial dislocation, JAMA 105:348, 1935.

Kostuik JP: Indications of the use of halo immobilization, Clin Orthop 154:46, 1981.

Kraus DR and Stauffer ES: Spinal cord injury as a complication of elective anterior cervical fusion, Clin Orthop 112:130, 1975.

Lesoin F, Pellerin P, Villette L, and Jomin M: Anterior approach and osteosynthesis for recent fractures of the pedicles of the axis, Adv Orthop Surg 10:130, 1987.

Levine AM and Rhyne AL: Traumatic spondylolisthesis of the axis, Semin Spine Surg 3:47, 1991.

Lipscomb PR: Cervico-occipital fusion for congenital and post-traumatic anomalies of the atlas and axis, J Bone Joint Surg 39-A:1289, 1957.

Lipson SJ: Fractures of the atlas associated with fracture of the odontoid process and transverse ligament ruptures, J Bone Joint Surg 59-A:940, 1977.

Louis R: Surgery of the spine: surgical anatomy and operative approaches, New York, 1983, Springer Verlag.

Macnab I: Acceleration injuries of the cervical spine, J Bone Joint Surg 36-A:1797, 1964.

Magerl F and Seemann P-S: Stable posterior fusion of the atlas and axis by transarticular scrw fixation. In Kehr P and Weidner A, editors: Cervical spine, New York, 1987, Springer Verlag.

Marar BC: Hyperextension injuries of the cervical spine: the pathogenesis of damage to the spinal cord, J Bone Joint Surg 56-A:1655, 1974.

Marar BC: Fracture of the axis arch: "hangman's fracture" of the cervical spine, Clin Orthop 106:155, 1975.

Marar BC and Balachandran N: Non-traumatic atlanto-axial dislocation in children, Clin Orthop 92:220, 1973.

Mazur JM and Stauffr ES: Unrecognized spinal instability associated with seemingly "simple" cervical compression fractures, Spine 8:687, 1983.

McClelland SH, James RL, Jarenwattananon A, and Shelton ML: Traumatic spondylolisthesis of the axis in a patient presenting with torticollis, Clin Orthop 218:195, 1987.

McGraw RW and Rusch RM: Atlanto-axial arthrodesis, J Bone Joint Surg 55-B:482, 1973.

Meijers KAE, van Beusekom GT, Luyendijk W, and Duijfjes F: Dislocation of the cervical spine with cord compression in rheumatoid arthritis, J Bone Joint Surg 56-B:668, 1974.

Munro D: Treatment of fractures and dislocations of the cervical spine, complicated by cervical-cord and root injuries: a comparative study of fusion vs nonfusion therapy, N Engl J Med 264:573, 1961.

Nickel VL, Perry J, Garrett A, and Heppenstall M: The halo: a spinal skeletal traction fixation device, J Bone Joint Surg 50-A:1400, 1968.

Norton WL: Fractures and dislocations of the cervical spine, J Bone Joint Surg 44-A:115, 1962.

O'Brien PJ, Schweigel JF, and Thompson WJ: Dislocation of the lower cervical spine, J Trauma 22:710, 1982.

Osti OL, Fraser RD, and Griffiths ER: Reduction and stabilization of cervical dislocations, J Bone Joint Surg 71-B:275, 1989.

Perret G and Greene J: Anterior interbody fusion in the treatment of cervical fracture dislocation, Arch Surg 96:530, 1968.

Perry J and Nickels VL: Total cervical-spine fusion for neck paralysis, J Bone Joint Surg 41-A:37, 1959.

Phillips WA and Hensinger RN: The management of rotatory atlanto-axial subluxation in children, J Bone Joint Surg 71-A:664, 1989.

Pierce DS: Surgery of the cervical spine, AAOS Instr Course Lect 21:116, 1972.

Pizzutillo PD: Pediatric occipitoatlantal injuries, Semin Spine Surg 3:24, 1991.

Reid DC and Leung P: A study of the odontoid process, Adv Orthop Surg 12:147, 1989.

Reich RS: Posterior dislocation of the first cervical vertebra with fracture of the odontoid process, Surgery 3:416, 1938.

Ricciardi JE, Kaufer H, and Louis DS: Acquired os odontoideum following acute ligament injury: report of a case, J Bone Joint Surg 58-A:410, 1976.

Riggins RS and Kraus JF: The risk of neurologic damage with fractures of the vertebrae, J Trauma 17:126, 1977.

Roberts A and Wickstrom J: Prognosis of odontoid fractures, Acta Orthop Scand 44:21, 1973.

Robinson RA: Fusions of the cervical spine, J Bone Joint Surg 41-A:1, 1959 (editorial).

Robinson RA: Anterior and posterior cervical spine fusions, Clin Orthop 35:34, 1964.

Robinson RA and Southwick WO: Indications and technics for early stabilization of the neck in some fracture dislocations of the cervical spine, South Med J 53:565, 1960.

Robinson RA and Southwick WO: Surgical approaches to the cervical spine, AAOS Instr Course Lect 17:299, 1960.

Robinson RA, Walker AE, Ferlic DC, and Wiecking DK: The results of anterior interbody fusion of the cervical spine, J Bone Joint Surg 44-A:1569, 1962.

Rogers WA: Treatment of fracture-dislocation of the cervical spine, J Bone Joint Surg 24:245, 1942.

Rogers WA: Fractures and dislocations of the cervical spine: an end-result study, J Bone Joint Surg 39-A:341, 1957.

Rorabeck CH, Rock MG, Hawkins AJ, and Bourne RB: Unilateral facet dislocation of the cervical spine: an analysis of the results of treatment in 26 patients, Spine 12:23, 1987.

Rosomoff HL: Discussion of relief of myelopathic pain by percutaneous cervical cordotomy. In Proceedings of the Spinal Cord Injury Conference, vol 17, New York, 1969, Bronx Veterans Administration Hospital.

Rosomoff HL: Percutaneous radiofrequency cervical cordotomy for intractable pain. In Bonica JJ, editor: International symposium on pain. In Advances in neurology, vol 4, New York, 1974, Raven Press.

Roth DA: Cervical analgesic discography: a new test for the definitive diagnosis of the painful-disk syndrome, JAMA 235:1713, 1976.

Schatzker J, Rorabeck CH, and Waddell JP: Fractures of the dens [odontoid process]: an analysis of thirty-seven cases, J Bone Joint Surg 53-B:392, 1971.

Schlesinger EB and Taveras JM: Lesions of the odontoid and their management, Am J Surg 95:641, 1958.

Schlicke LH and Callahan RA: A rational approach to burst fractures of the atlas, Clin Orthop 154:18, 1981.

Schneider RC and Kahn EA: Chronic neurological sequelae of acute trauma to the spine and spinal cord. I. The significance of the acute-flexion or "tear-drop" fracture-dislocation of the cervical spine, J Bone Joint Surg 38-A:985, 1956.

Schneider RC and Kahn EA: Chronic neurological sequelae of acute trauma to the spine and spinal cord. II. The syndrome of chronic anterior spinal cord injury or compression: herniated intervertebral discs, J Bone Joint surg 41-A:449, 1959.

Seimon LP: Fracture of the odontoid process in young children, J Bone Joint Surg 59-A:943, 1977.

Sherk HH, Schut L, and Lane JM: Fractures and dislocations of the cervical spine in children, Orthop Clin North Am 7:593, 1976.

Spence KF Jr, Decker S, and Sell KW: Bursting atlantal fracture associated with rupture of the transverse ligament, J Bone Joint Surg 52-A:543, 1970.

Stauffer ES: Diagnosis and prognosis of acute cervical spinal cord injury, Clin Orthop 112:9, 1975.

Stauffer ES: Wiring techniques of the posterior cervical spine for the treatment of trauma, Orthopedics 11:1543, 1988.

Stauffer ES and Kelly EG: Fracture-dislocations of the cervical spine: instability and recurrent deformity following treatment by anterior interbody fusion, J Bone Joint Surg 59-A:45, 1977.

Torg JS et al: Spinal injury at the level of the third and fourth cervical vertebrae from football, J Bone Joint Surg 59-A:1015, 1977.

Waters RL, Adkins RH, Nelson R, and Garland D: Cervical spinal cord trauma: evaluation and nonoperative tratment with halo-vest immobilization, Contemp Orthop 14:35, 1987.

Watson D and Maguire WB: Cervical facets locked unilaterally, Med J Aust 1:444, 1964.

Webb JK, Broughton RBK, McSweeney T, and Park WM: Hidden flexion injury of the cervical spine, J Bone Joint Surg 58-B:322, 1976.

Weir DC: Roentgenographic signs of cervical injury, Clin Orthop 109:9, 1975.

Wertheim SB and Bohlman HH: Occipitocervical fusion: indications, technique, and long-term results in 13 patients, J Bone Joint Surg 69-A:833, 1987.

White AA III and Panjabi MM: The role of stabilization in the treatment of cervical spine injuries, Spine 9:512, 1984.

White AA III, Southwick WO, and Panjabi MM: Clinical instability in the lower cervical spine: a review of past and current concepts, Spine 1:15, 1976.

White AA III, Johnson RM, Panjabi MM, and Southwick WO: Biomechanical analysis of clinical stability in the cervical spine, Clin Orthop 109:89, 1975.

White AA III, Panjabi MM, Posner I, et al: Spine stability: evaluation and treatment, AAOS Instr Course Lect 30:457, 1981.

Whitecloud TS and LaRocca H: Fibular strut graft in reconstructive surgery of the cervical spine, Spine 1:33, 1976.

Whitehill R: Fractures of the lower cervical spine: subaxial fractures in the adult, Semin Spine Surg 3:71, 1991.

Willard D and Nicholson JT: Dislocation of the first cervical vertebra, Ann Surg 113:464, 1941.

Young R and Thomasson EH: Step-by-step procedure for applying halo ring, Orthop Rev 3(6): 62, 1974.

Thoracic and lumbar spine and sacrum

Aebi M, Etter C, Kehl T, and Thalgott J: Stabilization of the lower thoracic and lumbar spine with internal spinal skeletal fixation system: indications, techniques, and the first results of treatment, Spine 12:544, 1987.

Akbarnia BA, Fogarth JP, and Tayob AA: Contoured Harrington instrumentation in the treatment of unstable spinal fractures (the effect of supplementary sublaminar wires), Clin Orthop 189:186, 1984.

Akbarnia BA, Gaines R Jr, Keppler L, et al: Surgical treatment of fractures and fracture-dislocations of thoracolumbar and lumbar spine using pedicular screw and plate fixation. Paper presented at the 23rd Annual Meeting of the Scoliosis Research Society, Baltimore, 1988.

Allen BL and Ferguson RL: A pictorial guide to the Galveston LRI pelvic fixation technique, Contemp Orthop 7:51, 1983.

Allen BL Jr and Ferguson RL: The Galveston technique of pelvic fixation with L-rod instrumentation of the spine, Spine 9:388, 1984.

Anden U, Lake A, and Norwall A: The role of the anterior longitudinal ligament and Harrington rod fixation of unstable thoracolumbar spinal fractures, Spine 5:23, 1980.

Angtuaco EJC and Binet EF: Radiology of thoracic and lumbar fractures, Clin Orthop 189:43, 1984.

Bedbrook GM: Treatment of thoracolumbar dislocation and fractures with paraplegia, Clin Orthop 112:27, 1975.

Berry JL, Moran JM, Berg WS, and Steffee AD: A morphometric study of human lumbar and selected thoracic vertebrae, Spine 12:362, 1987.

Blauth M, Tscherne H, and Haas N: Therapeutic concept and results of operative treatment in acute trauma of the thoracic and lumbar spine: the Hanover experience, J Orthop Trauma 1:240, 1987.

Bohlman HH: Current concepts review: treatment of fractures and dislocations of the thoracic and lumbar spine, J Bone Joint Surg 67-A:165, 1985.

Bohlman HH, Freehafer A, and Dejak J: The results of acute injuries of the upper thoracic spine with paralysis, J Bone Joint Surg 67-A:360, 1985.

Bordurant FJ, Cotler HB, Kulkarni MV, et al: Acute spinal cord injury: a study using physical examination and magnetic resonance imaging, Spine 15:161, 1990.

Bostman OM, Myllynen PJ, and Riska EB: Unstable fracture of the thoracic and lumbar spine: the audit of an 8-year series with early reduction using Harrington instrumentation, Injury 18:190, 1987.

Bracken MB, Shepard MJ, Collins WF, et al: A randomized, controlled trial of methylprednisolone or naloxone in the treatment of acute spinal cord injury, N Engl J Med 322:1405, 1990.

Bradford DS, Akbarnia BA, Winter RD, and Seljeskog EC: Surgical stabilization of fractures and fracture-dislocations of the thoracic spine, Spine 2:185, 1977.

Broom MJ and Jacobs RR: Update 1988: current status of internal fixation of thoracolumbar fractures, J Orthop Trauma 3:148, 1989.

Bryant CE and Sullivan JA: Management of thoracic and lumbar spine fractures with Harrington distraction rods supplemented with segmental wiring, Spine 8:532, 1983.

Burke DC and Murray DD: The management of thoracic and thoracolumbar injuries of the spine with neurological involvement, J Bone Joint Surg 58-B:72, 1976.

Calenoff L, Geimer PC, and Rosen JS: Lumbar fracture-dislocation related to range-of-motion exercises, Arch Phys Med Rehabil 60:183, 1979.

Carl A: Sacral spine fractures. In Errico TJ, Bauer RD, and Waugh T, editors: Spinal trauma, Philadelphia, 1990, JB Lippincott Co.

Cotrel Y and Dubousset J: Universal instrumentation (CD) for spinal surgery, Technique manual, Greensburg, Penn, 1985, Stuart Inc.

Cotrel Y, Dubousset J, and Guillaumat M: New universal instrumentation for spinal surgery, Clin Orthop 227:10, 1988.

Court-Brown CM and Gertzbein SD: The management of burst fractures of the fifth lumbar vertebra, Spine 12:308, 1987.

Davies WE, Morris JH, and Hill V: An analysis of conservative (nonsurgical) management of thoracolumbar fractures and fracture dislocations with neural damage, J Bone Joint Surg 62-A:1324, 1980.

Del Bigio MR and Johnson GE: Clinical presentation of spinal cord concussion, Spine 14:37, 1989.

Delamarter RB, Bohlman HH, Dodge LD, and Biro C: Experimental lumbar spinal stenosis: analysis of the cortical evoked potentials, microvasculature, and histopathology, J Bone Joint Surg 72-A:110, 1990.

Denis F, Davis S, and Comfort T: Sacral fractures: an important problem, though frequently undiagnosed and untreated: retrospective analysis of two hundred and three consecutive cases, Orthop Trans 11:118, 1987.

Denis F, Fuiz H, and Searls K: Comparison between square-ended distraction rods and standard round-ended distraction rods in the treatment of thoracolumbar spinal injuries: a statistical analysis, Clin Orthop 189:162, 1984.

Denis F, Armstrong GWD, Searls K, and Matta L: Acute thoracolumbar burst fractures in the absence of neurologic deficit (a comparison between operative and nonoperative treatment), Clin Orthop 189:142, 1984.

DeWald RL: Burst fractures of the thoracic and lumbar spine, Clin Orthop 189:150, 1984.

Dewey P and Browne PSH: Fracture-dislocation of the lumbo-sacral spine with cauda equina lesion, J Bone Joint Surg 50-A:635, 1968.

Dick W: The "fixateur interne" as a versatile implant for spine surgery, Spine 12:882, 1987.

Dickson JH, Harrington PR, and Erwin WD: Harrington instrumentation in the fractured, unstable thoracic and lumbar spine, Texas Med 69:91, 1973.

Dickson JH, Harrington PR, and Erwin WD: Results of reduction and stabilization of the severely fractured thoracic and lumbar spine, J Bone Joint Surg 60-A:799, 1978.

Dietemann JL, Runge M, Dosh JC, et al: Radiology of posterior lumbar apophyseal ring fractures: report of 13 cases, Neuroradiology 30:337, 1988.

Drummond D and Keene J: A technique of segmental spinal instrumentation without the passing of sublaminar wires, Mediguide Orthop 6:1, 1985.

Drummond DS, Keene JS, and Breed A: The Wisconsin system: a technique of interspinous segmental spinal instrumentation, Contemp Orthop 8:29, 1984.

Drummond D, Gaudagni J, Keene JS, et al: Interspinous process segmental spinal instrumentation, J Pediatr Orthop 4:397, 1984.

Edwards CC and Levine AM: Early rod-sleeve stabilization of the injured thoracic and lumbar spine, Orthop Clin North Am 17:327, 1986.

Eismont FJ, Green BA, Berkowitz BM, et al: The role of interaoperative ultrasonography in the treatment of thoracic and lumbar spine fractures, Spine 9:782, 1984.

Erickson DL, Leider LC Jr, and Brown WE: One-stage decompression-stabilization for thoraco-lumbar fractures, Spine 2:53, 1977.

Esses SI: The placement and treatment of thoracolumbar spine fractures: an algorithmic approach, Orthop Rev 17:571, 1988.

Esses SI: The AO spinal internal fixator, Spine 14:373, 1989.

Faden AI, Jacobs TP, Patrick DH, and Smith MT: Megadose corticosteroid therapy following experimental traumatic spinal injury, J Neurosurg 60:712, 1984.

Faden DF: Displaced fracture of the lumbosacral spine with delayed cauda equina deficit, Clin Orthop 120:155, 1976.

Ferguson RL and Allen BL Jr: A mechanistic classification of thoracolumbar spine fractures, Clin Orthop 189:77, 1984.

Flesch JR, Leider LL, Erickson D, Chou SN, and Bradford DS: Harrington instrumentation and spine fusion for unstable fractures and fracture dislocations of the thoracic and lumbar spine, J Bone Joint Surg 59-A:143, 1977.

Fountain SS, Hamilton RD, and Jameson RM: Transverse fractures of the sacrum; a report of six cases, J Bone Joint Surg 59-A:486, 1977.

Fredrickson BE, Yuan HA, and Miller H: Burst fractures of the fifth lumbar vertebra, J Bone Joint Surg 64-A:1088, 1982.

Gaines RW and Humphreys WG: A plea for judgment in management of thoracolumbar fractures and fracture-dislocations: a reassessment of surgical indications, Clin Orthop 189:36, 1984.

Gaines RW, Breedlove RF, and Munson G: Stabilization of thoracic and thoracolumbar fracture-dislocations with Harrington rods and sublaminar wires, Clin Orthop 189:195, 1984.

Garfin SD, Jacobs RR, Stoll J, et al: Results of a locking-hook spinal rod for fractures of the thoracic and lumbar spine, Spine 15:275, 1990.

Garfin SR, Mowery CA, Guerra J Jr, and Marshall LF: Confirmation of the posterolateral technique to decompress and fuse thoracolumbar spine burst fractures, Spine 10:218, 1985.

Gurr KR, McAfee PC, and Shih C: Biomechanical analysis of posterior instrumentation systems following decompressive laminectomy (an unstable calf spine model), NIH Grant, Johns Hopkins University School of Medicine, May 8, 1987.

Hack HP, Zielke K, and Harms J: Spinal instrumentation and monitoring, Technique manual, Greensburg, Penn, Stuart Inc.

Hanley EN Jr and Eskay ML: Thoracic spine fractures, Orthopedics 12:689, 1989.

Harkonen M, Kataja M, Keski-Nisula L, et al: Fractures of the lumbar spine: clinical and radiological results in 94 patients, Orthop Trauma Surg 94:43, 1979.

Heinig CF, Chapman TM, Chewning SJ Jr, et al: Preliminary report on VSP spine fixation system, Unpublished data, 1988.

Herring JA and Wenger DR: Segmental spine instrumentation, Spine 7:285, 1982.

Holdsworth FW and Hardy A: Early treatment of paraplegia from fractures of the thoraco-lumbar spine, J Bone Joint Surg 35-B:540, 1953.

Jacobs RR and Casey MP: Surgical management of thoracolumbar spinal injuries (general principles and controversial considerations), Clin Orthop 189:22, 1984.

Jacobs RR, Asher MA, and Snider RK: Thoracolumbar spinal injuries: a comparative study of recumbent and operative treatment in 100 patients, Spine 5:463, 1980.

Jacobs RR, Nordwall A, and Nachemson A: Reduction, stability and strength provided by internal fixation systems for thoracolumbar spinal injuries, Clin Orthop 171:300, 1982.

Jacobs RR, Schlaepfer F, Mathys R Jr, et al: A locking-hook spinal rod system for stabilization of fracture-dislocations and correction of deformities of the dorsolumbar spine: a biomechanical evaluation, Clin Orthop 189:168, 1984.

Jane MJ, Freehafer AA, Hazel C, et al: Autonomic dysreflexia: a cause of morbidity and mortality in orthopedic patients with spinal cord injury, Clin Orthop 169:151, 1982.

Jelsma RK, Kirsch PT, Jelsma LF, et al: Surgical treatment of thoracolumbar fractures, Surg Neurol 3:156, 1982.

Johnson JR, Leatherman KD, and Holt RT: Anterior decompression of the spinal cord for neurologic deficit, Spine 8:396, 1983.

Johnson KD, Dadambis A, and Seibert GB: Incidence of adult respiratory distress syndrome in patients with multiple musculoskeletal injuries: effect of early operative stabilization of fractures, J Trauma 25:375, 1985.

Johnson LP, Nasca RJ, and Bonnin JM: Pathoanatomy of a burst fracture, Surg Rounds Orthop p 43, January 1988.

Johnston CE II, Ashman RB, Sherman MC, et al: Mechanical consequences of rod contouring and residual scoliosis in sublaminar segmental instrumentation, J Orthop Res 5:206, 1987.

Kahanovitz N, Bullough P, and Jacobs RR: The effect of internal fixation without arthrodesis on human facet joint cartilage, Clin Orthop 189:204, 1984.

Kaneda K, Abumi K, and Fujiya M: Burst fractures with neurologic deficits of the thoracolumbar-lumbar spine: results of anterior decompression and stabilization with anterior instrumentation, Spine 9:788, 1984.

Kaufer H and Hayes JT: Lumbar fracture-dislocation: a study of twenty-one cases, J Bone Joint Surg 48-A:712, 1966.

Kelly RP and Whitesides TE Jr: Treatment of lumbodorsal fracture-dislocations, Ann Surg 167:705, 1968.

King AG: Burst compression fractures of the thoracolumbar spine: pathologic anatomy and surgical management, Orthopedics 10:1711, 1987.

Kostuik JP: Anterior spinal cord decompression for lesions of the thoracic and lumbar spine: techniques, new methods of internal fixation, results, Spine 8:512, 1983.

Krag MH, Weaver DL, Beynnon BD, and Haugh LD: Morphometry of the thoracic and lumbar spine related to transpedicular screw placement for surgical spinal fixation, Spine 13:27, 1988.

Krompinger WJ, Frederickson BE, Mino DE, and Yuan HA: Conservative treatment of fractures of the thoracic and lumbar spine, Orthop Clin North Am 17:161, 1986.

Kulkarni MB, McArdle CB, Kopaniky D, et al: Acute spinal cord injury: MR imaging at 115 T1, Neuroradiology 164:837, 1987.

Kupferschmid JP, Weaver ML, Raves JJ, and Diamond DL: Thoracic spine injuries in victims of motorcycle accidents, J Trauma 29:593, 1989.

Laborde JM, Bahniuk E, Bohlman HH, and Samson B: Comparison of fixation of spinal fractures, Clin Orthop 152:305, 1980.

Lafollete BF, Levine MI, and McNiesh LM: Bilateral fracture-dislocation of the sacrum, J Bone Joint Surg 68-A:1099, 1986.

Levine AM and Edwards CC: Low lumbar burst fractures: reduction and stabilization using the modular spine fixation system, Orthopedics 1:9, 1988.

Levine AM, Bosse M, and Edwards CC: Bilateral facet dislocations in the thoracolumbar spine, Spine 13:630, 1988.

Lewis J and McKibbin B: The treatment of unstable fracture-dislocations of the thoraco-lumbar spine accompanied by paraplegia, J Bone Joint Surg 56-B:603, 1974.

Lindahl S, Willen J, Nordwall A, and Irstam I: The crush-cleavage fracture: a "new" thoracolumbar unstable fracture, Spine 8:559, 1983.

Louis R: Fusion of the lumbar and sacral spine by internal fixation with screw plates, Clin Orthop 203:18, 1986.

Luque ER, Cassis N, and Ramirez-Weilla G: Segmental spinal instrumentation in the treatment of fractures of the thoracolumbar spine, Spine 7:312, 1982.

Magerl FP: Stabilization of the lower thoracic and lumbar spine with external skeletal fixation, Clin Orthop 189:125, 1984.

McAfee PC: Biomechanical approach to instrumentation of the thoracolumbar spine: a review article, Adv Orthop Surg 8:313, 1985.

McAfee PC and Bohlman HH: Anterior decompression of traumatic thoracolumbar fractures with incomplete paralysis through the retroperitoneal approach, Orthop Trans 8:392, 1984.

McAfee PC and Bohlman HH: Complications following Harrington instrumentation for fractures of the thoracolumbar spine, J Bone Joint Surg 67-A:672, 1985.

McAfee PC, Bohlman HH, and Yuan HA: Anterior decompression of traumatic thoracolumbar fractures with incomplete neurological deficit using a retroperitoneal approach, J Bone Joint Surg 67-A:89, 1985.

McAfee PC, Werner FW, and Glisson RR: A biomechanical analysis of spinal instrumentation systems in thoracolumbar fractures: comparison of traditional Harrington side traction instrumentation with segmental spinal instrumentation, Spine 10:204, 1985.

McAfee PC, Yuan HA, and Lasada NA: The unstable burst fracture, Spine 7:365, 1982.

McAfee PC, Yuan HA, Frederickson BE, and Lubicky JP: The value of computed tomography in thoracolumbar fractures, J Bone Joint Surg 64-A:461, 1983.

McBride GG: Surgical stabilization of thoracolumbar fractures using Cotrel-Dubousset rods, Semin Spine Surg 2:24, 1990.

Meyer PR: Complications of treatment of fractures and dislocations of the dorsolumbar spine. In Epps CH, editor: Complications in orthopaedic surgery, Philadelphia, 1978, JB Lippincott Co.

Morgan FH, Wharton W, and Austin GN: The results of laminectomy in patients with incomplete spinal cord injuries, Paraplegia 9:14, 1971.

Munro AHG and Irwin CG: Interlocked articular processes complicating fracture-dislocation of the spine, Br J Surg 25:621, 1938.

Myllynen P, Bostman O, and Riska E: Recurrence of deformity after removal of Harrington's fixation of spine fractures (seventy-six cases followed for 2 years), Acta Orthop Scand 59:497, 1988.

Nagel DA, Koogle TA, Piziali RL, and Perkash I: Stability of the upper lumbar spine following progressive disruptions in the application of individual internal and external fixation devices, J Bone Joint Surg 63-A:62, 1981.

Nicoll EA: Fractures of the dorso-lumbar spine, J Bone Joint Surg 31-B:376, 1949.

Osebold WR, Weinstein SL, and Sprague BL: Thoracolumbar spine fractures: results of treatment, Spine 6:13, 1981.

Pattee GA, Bohlman HH, and McAfee PC: Compression of a sacral nerve as a complication of screw fixation of the sacro-iliac joint, J Bone Joint Surg 68-A:769, 1986.

Pearch M, Protek I, and Shepherd J: Three-dimensional x-ray analysis of normal movement in the lumbar spine, Spine 9:294, 1984.

Pinzar MS et al: Measurement of internal fixation device, a report in experimentally produced fractures of the dorsolumbar spine, Orthopaedics 2:28, 1979.

Pollock LJ et al: Pain below the level of injury of the spinal cord, Arch Neurol Psychiat 65:319, 1951.

Post MJD et al: Value of computed tomography in spinal trauma, Spine 7:417, 1982.

Pringle RG: The conservative management of the spinal injured patients, Semin Orthop 4:34, 1989.

Purcell GA, Markolf KL, and Dawson EG: Twelfth thoracic-first lumbar vertebral mechanical stability of fractures after Harrington rod instrumentation, J Bone Joint Surg 63-A:71, 1981.

Riska EB: Antero-lateral decompression as a treatment of paraplegia following vertebral fracture in the thoraco-lumbar spine, Int Orthop 1:22, 1977.

Roberts JB and Curtiss PH Jr: Stability of the thoracic and lumbar spine in traumatic paraplegia following fracture or fracture-dislocation, J Bone Joint Surg 52-A:1115, 1970.

Rogers WA: Cord injury during reduction of thoracic and lumbar vertebral-body fracture and dislocation, J Bone Joint Surg 20:689, 1938.

Roy-Camille R, Saillant G, and Mazel C: Plating of thoracic, thoracolumbar, and lumbar injuries with pedicel screw plates, Orthop Clin North Am 17:147, 1986.

Roy-Camille R, Saillant G, Mazel C, and Lapresle Ph: Posterior spinal fixation with transpedicular screws and plates, Groupe Hospitalier, La Pitié Salpêtrière, Paris, France.

Sacsh BL, Makley JT, Carter JR, et al: Primary osseous neoplasms of the thoracic and lumbar spine, Orthop Trans 8:422, 1984.

Samberg LC: Fracture-dislocation of the lumbosacral spine, J Bone Joint Surg 57-A:1107, 1975.

Saraste H: The etiology of spondylolysis: a retrospective radiographic study, Acta Orthop Scand 56:253, 1985.

Schnaid E, Eisenstein SM, and Drummond-Webb J: Delayed posttraumatic cauda equina compression syndrome, J Trauma 25:1099, 1985.

Seibel R, La Duca J, Hassett JM, et al: Blunt multiple trauma (ISS36), femur traction, and the pulmonary failure-septic state, Ann Surg 202:283, 1985.

Smith WS and Kaufer H: Patterns and mechanisms of lumbar injuries associated with lap seat belts, J Bone Joint Surg 51-A:239, 1969.

Soref J, Axdorph G, Bylund P, et al: Treatment of patients with unstable fractures of the thoracic and lumbar spine: a follow-up of surgical and conservative treatment, Acta Orthop Scand 53:369, 1982.

Soumalainen O and Pääkkönen M: Fracture-dislocation of the lumbar spine without paraplegia: a case report, Acta Orthop Scand 55:466, 1984.

Stanger JK: Fracture-dislocation of the thoracolumbar spine, J Bone Joint Surg 29:107, 1947.

Stauffer ES: Spinal cord injury syndromes, Semin Spine Surg 3:87, 1991.

Stauffer ES and Neil JL: Biomechanical analysis of structural stability of internal fixation in fractures of the thoracolumbar spine, Clin Orthop 112:159, 1975.

Steffee AD and Sitkowski DJ: Posterior lumbar interbody fusion and plates, Clin Orthop 227:99, 1988.

Sullivan JA: Sublaminar wiring of Harrington distraction rods for unstable thoracolumbar spine fractures, Clin Orthop 189:178, 1984.

Thomas JC Jr: The Wiltse system of pedicle screw fixation, Unpublished data.

Trafton PG and Boyd CA: Computed tomography of thoracic and lumbar spine injuries, J Trauma 24:506, 1984.

Trammell TR, Rapp G, Maxwell KM, et al: Luque interpeduncular segmental fixation of the lumbosacral spine, Orthop Rev 20:57, 1991.

Transfeldt EE, White D, Bradford DS, and Roche B: Delayed anterior decompression in patients with spinal cord and cauda equina injuries of the thoracolumbar spine, Spine 15:953, 1990.

Vincent KA, Benson DR, and McGahan JP: Intraoperative ultrasonography fro reduction of thoracolumbar burst fractures, Spine 14:387, 1989.

Weinstein JN, Collalto P, and Lehmann TR: Long-term follow-up of nonoperatively treated thoracolumbar spine fractures, J Orthop Trauma 1:152, 1987.

Wenger DR and Carollo JJ: The mechanics of thoracolumbar fractures stabilized by segmental fixation, Clin Orthop 189:89, 1984.

Wenger DR, Carollo JJ, Wilkerson JA, et al: Laboratory testing of segmental spinal instrumentation vs traditional Harrington instrumentation for scoliosis treatment, Spine 7:265, 1982.

Wenger D, Miller S, and Wilkerson J: Evaluation of fixation sites for segmental instrumentation of human vertebrae. Paper presented at the 16th Annual Meeting of the Scoliosis Research Society, Montreal, Canada, September 1981.

White RR, Newberg A, and Seligson D: Computerized tomographic assessment of the traumatized dorsolumbar spine before and after Harrington instrumentation, Clin Orthop 146:149, 1980.

Whitesides TE Jr and Shah SGA: On the management of unstable fractures of the thoracolumbar spine: rationale for use of anterior decompression and fusion and posterior stabilization, Spine 1:99, 1976.

Wilber RG, Thompson GH, Shaffer JW, et al: Postoperative neurological deficits in segmental spinal instrumentation, J Bone Joint Surg 66-A:1178, 1984.

Willen J, Dahiiof AG, and Nordwall A: Paraplegia in unstable thoracolumbar injuries: a study of conservative and operative treatment regarding neurological improvement and rehabilitation, J Rehab Med 9:195, 1983.

York DH, Watts C, Raffensberger M, et al: Utilization of somatosensory evoked cortical potentials in spinal cord injury, Spine 8:832, 1983.

Yosipovitch Z, Robin GC, and Makin M: Open reduction of unstable thoracolumbar spinal injuries and fixation with Harrington rods, J Bone Joint Surg 59-A:1003, 1977.

Zindrick MR, Wiltse LL, Doornik A, et al: Analysis of the morphometric characteristics of the thoracic and lumbar pedicles, Spine 12:160, 1987.

Zoltan JD, Gilula LA, and Murphy WA: Unilateral facet dislocation between the fifth lumar and first sacral vertebrae: case report, J Bone Joint Surg 61-A:767, 1979.

Arthrodesis of Spine

ALLEN S. EDMONSON

Since the descriptions of spinal fusion by Hibbs and by Albee, arthrodesis of the spine has been performed for many spinal conditions, including tuberculosis and other infections, fractures, congenital and developmental deformities, arthritic and other degenerative diseases, and disc lesions. Although it is difficult to separate discussions of arthrodesis and the conditions for which is it performed, this section discusses various techniques of arthrodesis useful in both traumatic and nontraumatic disorders of the spine. Techniques of spinal arthrodesis using instrumentation, such as rods, plates and screws, and wires, are described in Chapters 80, 83, and 84.

CERVICAL SPINE
Anterior Arthrodesis

Anterior cervical discectomy and interbody fusion have gained wide acceptance by both neurosurgeons and orthopaedic surgeons in the management of refractory symptoms of cervical disc disease. The literature attests to a low incidence of major complications and postoperative morbidity and a high degree of success in relieving these symptoms. The fundamental difference in the many techniques is whether surgery is limited to simple discectomy and interbody fusion or whether an attempt is made to enter the spinal canal to remove osteophytes or otherwise decompress the spinal cord and nerve roots. The procedures of Robinson and Smith, Bailey and Badgley, and Dereymaeker and Mulier are similar in that they limit surgery to simple discectomy and interbody fusion. The technique is thus reserved for discogenic and radicular pain syndromes that are not accompanied by significant objective signs of neurologic involvement. These

authors also performed a posterior decompression if the patient had definite cervical nerve root or cord compression signs.

Extreme care must be exercised in anterior fusion of the cervical spine. Kraus and E.S. Stauffer reported on 10 patients with spinal cord injury as a result of surgery. An incomplete spinal cord injury was present in three patients, including two incomplete quadriplegias of the anterior cervical cord type and one incomplete quadriplegia of the Brown-Séquard type. The cases of seven patients were reviewed from the literature and personal communications. The causes were identified in four of the last six patients as (1) operation of a drill without the protection of the drill guard, which allowed the drill to enter the spinal canal, and (2) displacement of a dowel bone graft into the spinal canal, either during surgery or postoperatively, which damaged the cervical cord. One of the other two patients sustained a transient postoperative transverse myelitis attributed to the use of electrocoagulation on the posterior longitudinal ligament. The cause of injury of the final patient, mentioned in a medical liability report, was not definite, but posterior displacement of the bone plug was implicated. All of these fusions had been performed by the drill and dowel method. We no longer use this technique and strongly recommend rectangular tricortical grafts.

Aronson, Bagan, and Feltzer have shown that anterior discectomy and interbody fusion have a much wider application, producing excellent results in virtually all forms of cervical disc disease and spondylosis, regardless of the objective neurologic signs. Despite subtle differences in surgical technique, the intent of their surgery is still discectomy and interbody fusion with no attempt to remove osteophytes. The extent to which the posterior and posterolateral osteophytes with spondylosis contribute to the symptoms of cervical disc disease and the indications for removing them have not been determined. One is always impressed with the frequent discrepancy between the degree of bony spurring or other roentgenographic changes and the symptoms present. Also, the level of neurologic involvement does not always coincide with the site of the greatest roentgenographic findings. Because plain roentgenograms cannot provide the necessary information for identifying the level or levels of neural compression, either computed tomographic myelography or magnetic resonance imaging is strongly recommended in operative planning — both provide the detailed diagnostic information necessary. The symptoms of the degenerative processes are related to the interplay of multiple aspects of the disease process and not solely to the amount of bony spurs present. Observation of patients who have had fusions shows that a significant percentage of the osteophytes will be spontaneously absorbed postoperatively in the presence of a stable interbody fusion. DePalma and Rothman concurred with this observation and noted that in the presence of a stable fusion the results were not influenced by the subsequent fate of these osteophytes. Aronson et al. have therefore demonstrated an important factor, namely, stabilization of the disc space as the sole procedure, thereby avoiding the hazard of entering the spinal canal routinely.

In our experience, simple discectomy and interbody fusion have been adequate in the absence of clinical evidence of neural compression, either on examination or diagnostic studies. When compression is present, as is true in most patients who are surgical candidates, direct operative decompression has given superior results and is recommended. In the hands of skilled surgeons, the use of an operating microscope and monitoring of somatosensory evoked potentials during surgery have allowed reasonably safe anterior excision of osteophytes and other offending structures from the spinal canal before grafting and stabilization.

GENERAL COMPLICATIONS. Macnab has summarized the complications of anterior cervical fusion extremely well. For every anatomic structure present in the neck, there is a possibility of a surgical error; however, he points out that poor results also occur because of poor indications and surgical technique. The following points are Macnab's, with occasional observations from our experience.

1. The *wrong patient* may be operated on, since the neck is a common target for psychogenic pain. Careful preoperative evaluation is essential to rule out a hysterical personality or a chronic anxiety state. A careful pain study is essential, including thiopental (Pentothal) narcosis or discography. In recent years we have not routinely performed discography. Disc degeneration may be a multifocal disease as in the cervical and lumbar spine. Even if an examination seems to point to a single level, it

is possible that within a short time other segments will become symptomatic and surgery will be of no long-term benefit. With multicentric disc degeneration, results have not been gratifying. Best results are obtained with a single-segment discectomy and fusion for definite nerve root impairment or for localized disc disease without root compression. Fusions of more than two segments performed for pain relief alone produce fair or poor results; improvement, not cure, is the best possible result.

2. The operation can be done at the *wrong level* if an incorrect vertebral count is made at surgery. Use of a check film with a metal marker is mandatory, and the first or second cervical vertebra must always be shown on this check film. The marker needle should be directed cranially so that the tip butts the vertebra above and avoids the theca. Roentgenographic analysis of the level may be insufficient, and the true level may only be found clinically by reproducing the pain on discography, which is more accurate than myelography. Reproduction of the clinical pain pattern on discography is best achieved by injecting a small quantity of local anesthetic. If computed tomographic myelography or magnetic resonance imaging is not available, discography may be the only way to localize the proper level for surgical treatment.

3. The operation may be performed in the *wrong way;* for example, the recurrent laryngeal nerve, esophagus, or pharynx may be injured by retractors. Sympathetic nervous system injuries are avoided by dissecting in the correct planes. Keeping the dissection medial to the carotid avoids the sympathetic nervous system. An approach from the left is less likely to damage the recurrent laryngeal nerve. In an approach from the right, the recurrent laryngeal nerve is in jeopardy from C6 downward, and it should be specifically identified and protected. This nerve enters the groove between the trachea and the esophagus at the point where the inferior thyroid artery enters the lower pole of the thyroid.

Instruments may tear the dura and must be used with extreme caution in removing the posterior disc fragments.

Osteotomes must be very sharp or have a shoulder guard to prevent injury to the cervical cord. Blunt osteotomes are more likely to cause injury. Grafts must be accurately measured and tightly fitted under compression.

4. The operation may be done at the *wrong time*. Timing of an operation is important; surgery should not be delayed if root conduction is significantly impaired. In patients in whom the clinical findings are purely subjective, consideration is usually given to delaying surgery until any possible litigation is settled. However, this may lead to chronic pain patterns difficult to eradicate. If such a patient has been significantly disabled for more than a year and has shown no improvement over the past 6 months, Macnab advises a thiopental pain study and discography. If a significant physiogenic basis for the pain is demonstrated, prompt anterior cervical fusion should be

carried out without awaiting the results of litigation. We rarely treat surgically patients who do not have objectively demonstrated neural compression or deficits. Results seem, at best, unpredictable.

POSTOPERATIVE COMPLICATIONS. All anterior surgical wounds are best drained to avoid the hazards of a retropharyngeal hematoma, which can produce obstruction of the airway with its subsequent complications. A closed suction drainage system usually is inserted deep into the wound.

Extrusion of a graft is most commonly seen in the treatment of fracture-dislocations of the neck with posterior instability. This is not as commonly seen in fusions for disc degeneration when posterior stability of the ligamentous structures is not impaired. At this clinic posterior internal fixation is a routine adjunct when posterior ligamentous stability is lost for any reason and the anterior approach for arthrodesis is necessary. Halo-vest external fixation frequently can be substituted for posterior internal fixation until the anterior arthrodesis has healed. Anteriorly placed internal fixation devices for the cervical spine have been used in some centers in attempts to provide sufficient stability for the anterior surgery. We have not used these devices, but strongly emphasize that anterior grafting alone provides undependable stability. A rectangular graft has more firm fixation than a circular Cloward graft. Unless the graft extrudes more than 50% of its width or unless it causes dysphagia, another operation usually is not indicated. The extruded portion will be absorbed and the graft will ossify, if the arthrodesis heals. Healing time is protracted. External immobilization time should be adjusted accordingly. Whitehill et al. reported a late esophageal perforation from a corticocancellous strut graft from the iliac crest. The first symptoms of dsyphagia occurred 2½ months after the surgery, and an "inferior osseous spike" on the graft apparently eroded into the esophagus.

Postoperative collapse of a vertebral body is seen on occasion with the dowel technique, which jeopardizes the vertebral blood supply. This is caused by excessive thinning of the vertebral body at its midpoint where adjacent dowel holes are closest.

Nonunion of an anterior cervical fusion is an unusual situation. It is most likely to occur in a three-segment fusion and is best treated by posterior cervical fusion.

When anterior cervical arthrodesis is being performed for traumatic disorders with resultant instability from ligamentous tears or posterior element fractures, postoperative treatment must be planned to accommodate this added factor. The aftertreatment described here usually applies to arthrodesis for "stable" degenerative or other nontraumatic conditions. When cervical instability is present, or when three or more levels are fused, a halo-vest routinely is used for up to 3 months and the patient remains ambulatory.

TYPES OF ANTERIOR ARTHRODESIS OF CERVICAL SPINE. Of the three commonly used techniques for anterior cervical spine fusion — those of Robinson and Smith, Bailey and Badgley, and Cloward — White and Hirsch found the Robinson and Smith configuration to be the strongest in compressive loading. This was followed by the Bailey and Badgley and the Cloward configurations in that order. These grafts could all bear loads of 2½ to 5 times the body weight, much more than the loads the cervical spine is normally expected to bear. Thus the limiting factor was not the graft itself but the graft vertebral construction (Fig. 81-1). The major load on the vertebrae in vivo is that of axial compression, but Simmons, Bhalla, and Butt have directed attention to the rotary displacement taking place in the spine and its relationship to the various constructions of the bone grafts. The strong configuration of the Robinson and Smith arthrodesis is the result of leaving intact the cortical shell of the vertebral body. Since it has been shown that 40% to 75% of the strength of the vertebra comes from the cortical bone, preserving the end plate is of great importance, as it prevents collapse into the cancellous portion of the body with subsequent displacement.

In our experience, removal of the adjacent vertebral end plates to accomplish more complete anterior decompression when the offending osteophyte is large has not created a serious problem unless the bone was very osteoporotic. Even then, only a partial collapse of the interspace has occurred during healing. We believe that thorough decompression is more important to relief of neural symptoms than strict preservation of the end plates, especially posteriorly. When wider than usual resection is necessary, our technique becomes more like the Simmons "keystone" graft and less like the Smith-Robinson technique. Bailey and Badgley, Robinson et al., Simmons et al., Macnab, and others have fused the cervical spine anteriorly for instability after extensive laminectomy, fractured posterior arch elements, certain fracture-dislocations, and destructive lesions. Robinson et al.; Williams, Allen, and Harkess; and many others have combined excision of cervical intervertebral discs with anterior fusion. The various approaches to the anterior aspect of the cervical spine are described beginning on p. 3497.

■ **TECHNIQUE (BAILEY AND BADGLEY).** This technique is altered as the specific pathologic problem demands. The operation is done with the patient on a Stryker frame, Foster bed, or operating table with skull-tong traction in place. Endotracheal anesthesia is used.

Place a folded towel beneath the interscapular region to hold the neck in moderate extension. Rotate the patient's head about 15 degrees to the left and approach the cervical spine anteriorly from the right. When the prevertebral fascia is reached but before it is incised, insert a drill as a marker in one of the vertebral bodies and identify it with a lateral

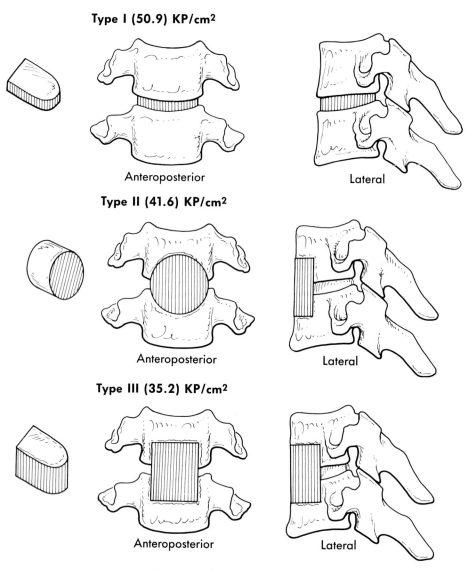

Type I (50.9) KP/cm²

Anteroposterior   Lateral

Type II (41.6) KP/cm²

Anteroposterior   Lateral

Type III (35.2) KP/cm²

Anteroposterior   Lateral

Fig. 81-1   Types (configurations) of grafts used in anterior arthrodesis of cervical spine. *Type I*, Robinson and Smith; *Type II*, Cloward; *Type III*, Bailey and Badgley. Numbers are means for load-bearing capacity for each. (Redrawn from White AA III et al: Clin Orthop 91:21, 1973.)

roentgenogram. After this orientation, incise the prevertebral fascia longitudinally in the exact midline. Place heavy silk sutures in the fascia to facilitate retraction and later to use in closure. Mobilize the fascia from the anterior surfaces of the vertebral bodies and control bleeding from the bone with electrocautery or bone wax. Identify the vertebrae to be fused and cut a trough in the anterior aspect of the vertebral bodies about 1.2 cm wide and 4.7 mm deep from near the top of the upper vertebra to near the bottom of the lower one. Use of a small power saw or drill is less traumatic than use of an osteotome and a mallet. Clean out the intervertebral disc spaces with a rongeur and remove the cartilaginous plates on the inferior and superior aspects of the bodies to be fused. Obtain and gently pack chips of cancellous iliac bone into the cleaned interverte-

bral disc spaces, trim an iliac graft to fit, and mortise it into the trough in the vertebrae (Fig. 81-2). Now decrease the extension of the cervical spine by raising the line of pull of the traction, thus wedging the graft more securely in the trough. The graft must not project further anteriorly than the anterior surface of the vertebral bodies.

When the graft is properly seated, tie the sutures previously placed in the prevertebral fascia; the fascia maintains the graft in its bed. Place a large Penrose drain or suction drainage tube in the retropharyngeal space and bring it out through the lower portion of the incision. Close the wound in layers with interrupted sutures.

AFTERTREATMENT. Traction is maintained on a Stryker frame or Foster bed. The drain is advanced in 24 hours and is removed after 48 hours. After 6

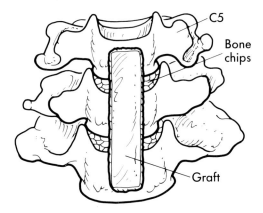

Fig. 81-2 Anterior fusion of cervical spine. Trough has been cut in anterior aspect of vertebral bodies, intervertebral disc spaces have been cleared and filled with iliac bone chips, and iliac graft has been mortised into trough. (Redrawn from Bailey RW and Badgley CE: J Bone Joint Surg 42-A:565, 1960.)

weeks in traction, the patient is allowed to get up with the neck immobilized in a Taylor back brace with an attached Forrester collar. The brace is worn until fusion is complete, usually for 4 to 6 months.

A halo-vest is almost always used rather than 6 weeks of traction. This allows much earlier ambulation and consequently much earlier hospital discharge. With proper supervision and maintenance of the halo-vest, the results should be equally satisfactory. We usually keep a halo-vest in place for about 3 months, using a cervical collar during the next 4 to 6 weeks as immobilization is gradually decreased and as rehabilitation progresses. Serial roentgenographic evaluations and support are continued until healing is complete.

• • •

Fielding, Lusskin, and Batista have found the method of Bailey and Badgley satisfactory in fusing several segments for instability after multiple laminectomies; in this situation in children, Cattell and Clark have used a strut graft of tibial bone as described by Robinson.

Robinson et al. have arthrodesed the cervical spine anteriorly for intervertebral disc degeneration by excising the disc and the cartilaginous plates from the selected disc space or spaces and inserting blocks of iliac bone.

Smith-Robinson fusions are made easier by using a system of retractors and instrumentation developed by Caspar and bearing his name. Accurate measurements for graft fitting and excellent exposure of the posterior disc space and dura are possible with this technique.

■ *TECHNIQUE (ROBINSON ET AL.).* Place the patient on the operating table and replace part of the mattress with a cassette holder that extends from the spines of the scapulae to above the head and with a pneumatic roll between the neck and the cassette

holder. Adjust the roll to permit moderate extension of the neck. When anesthesia is well established by the endotracheal method, apply a head halter and, by means of an outrigger at the head of the table, apply 5 pounds (2.2 kg) of traction.

Rotate the patient's head to the right and approach the cervical spine anteriorly from the left. Continue the approach until the exact midline of the spine has been reached. Then in the midline incise vertically and retract the alar and prevertebral fasciae. The anterior longitudinal ligament and any osteoarthritic spurs are then visible. Insert a needle into one disc and identify its level by a lateral roentgenogram. Test the resiliency of the various discs by palpating them with a finger or the tip of a forceps; also test their consistency by penetrating each with a needle. Then examine each suspicious disc by discography.

Having selected the disc space or spaces to be cleared and replaced by bone, proceed with the fusion. At the front of the disc space make a rectangular window about 1.5 cm wide in the anterior longitudinal ligament and the anulus. Then with a small curet loosen the disc material and remove it with a pituitary rongeur. Also remove the cartilaginous plate from the subchondral bone above and below the space back to the posterior part of the anulus and the posterior longitudinal ligament. After proper preparation the space created measures about 1.5 × 1.5 × 0.6 to 0.8 cm. Trim sparingly any bony spurs along the superior and inferior edges of the space but never enough to remove the normal ridge of cortical bone from the anterior part of the vertebral bodies. Now drill a few holes into the underlying cancellous bone of the vertebrae if there is no bleeding after excision of the cartilaginous plates.

Shape a 1.5 cm long iliac graft so that its cancellous part will lie against the subchondral bone above and below the space while its cortical part forms the support between the vertebrae (Fig. 81-3). Then apply 15 additional pounds (6.7 kg) of traction and hyperextend the head and neck. Insert the graft and carefully tamp it into place with a bone punch and mallet. Countersink the graft just posterior to the anterior margins of the vertebral bodies; it should be firmly fixed even before the traction is removed. Repeat the procedure at each disc space as necessary. Now suture the alar and prevertebral fasciae and close the wound.

AFTERTREATMENT. The patient is placed supine in bed with sandbags on each side of the head for about 24 hours and in 1 or 2 days is allowed out of bed. In about 4 days a neck brace is fitted and is worn during the day for 3 months. We usually use a Philadelphia collar worn day and night for 6 weeks and then a soft collar worn during the day only for 6

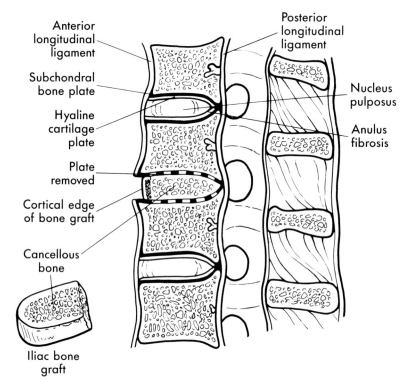

Anterior longitudinal ligament

Subchondral bone plate

Hyaline cartilage plate

Plate removed

Cortical edge of bone graft

Cancellous bone

Iliac bone graft

Posterior longitudinal ligament

Nucleus pulposus

Anulus fibrosis

Fig. 81-3 Technique of Robinson et al. for anterior fusion of cervical spine (see text). (Modified from Robinson RA, Walker EA, Ferlic DC, and Wiecking DK: J Bone Joint Surg 44-A:1569, 1962.)

more weeks. A mature arthrodesis and absence of motion on flexion and extension lateral roentgenograms are required before all mobilization is removed.

• • •

Bloom and Raney have recommended reversing the orientation of the iliac graft as it is inserted so that the rounded cortical edge of the iliac cortex is placed posteriorly and the cancellous edge is anterior. They claim that protruding portions of the graft can be trimmed off easily with a rongeur without sacrificing the cortical portion and decreasing the strength of the graft. We have experienced collapse of the anterior noncortical edge of the graft and a resulting slight kyphotic deformity at the fused level when the graft is "reversed." This has been noted especially in older female patients whose pelvic bone cortices were thinned from osteoporosis.

The cervical arthrodesis with discectomy described by Simmons et al. has produced excellent results in 80.8% of their patients. Our major experience with this technique has been with trauma, but it does provide a stable configuration.

■ *TECHNIQUE (SIMMONS ET AL.).* Use endotracheal anesthesia. Place the patient on the operating table and strap the ankles to the table. Apply a sterile head halter and drape the patient. Using a right-sided approach, make a transverse skin incision along the line of the skin creases. Divide the

platysma transversely, retract the strap muscles and viscera medially, and retract the sternocleidomastoid muscle and great vessels laterally. Insert a needle in the exposed disc and obtain roentgenographic proof of the exact level. Remove a keystone square or rectangle of tissue, beveling it upward into the vertebra above and downward into the vertebra below using special osteotomes and chisels of Simmons' design, with a depth of 1.2 cm each and with widths of 1.27, 1.1, and 0.95 cm. Exercise care to avoid outward progression of the chisel while keeping the cut in the true anteroposterior plane. Remove a 1.27 cm square of tissue for the one-level fusion in most patients. When this material is completely removed with rongeurs and by curettage, remove the disc from posteriorly to anteriorly. At the final stage of cleansing of this space, ask the anesthetist to apply strong head halter traction, which opens the disc space and allows cleaning to be carried out well to the neurocentral joints. Deepen the trough to the posterior cortex of the vertebrae. Next carefully cut the corners squarely. Measure the length of the rectangle while forceful traction is placed on the head halter to allow opening of the space at least 3 mm. Obtain a rectangular graft from the iliac crest and shape it to fit the trough. Bevel the ends upward and downward to approximately 14 to 18 degrees. Now distract the neck fully by forceful traction and place the graft into the defect.

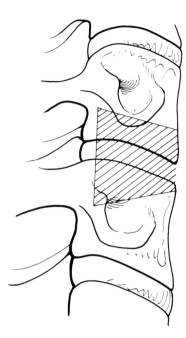

Fig. 81-4   Placement of keystone graft shown in lined area. (Redrawn from Simmons EH, Bhalla SK, and Butt WP: J Bone Joint Surg 51-B:225, 1969.)

Release the traction; the graft is thus locked firmly into position, maintaining fixed distraction and immobilization (Fig. 81-4). In a two-level fusion extend the trough and graft through the intervening vertebra into the one above and below.

AFTERTREATMENT. Early mobilization is allowed in a brace until union is achieved. Since grafting under distraction is quite stable, postoperative pain is much less than pain after other types of cervical spine arthrodesis.

Anterior Occipitocervical Arthrodesis by Extrapharyngeal Exposure

Rarely an anterior occipitocervical fusion is required for a grossly unstable cervical spine when posterior fusion is not feasible. It was used by de Andrade and Macnab in patients who had had extensive laminectomies for rheumatoid arthritis, traumatic quadriparesis, neoplastic metastasis to the spine, and congenital abnormalities. This operation is a cranial extension of the approach described by Robinson and Smith and by Bailey and Badgley; it permits access to the base of the occiput and the anterior aspect of all the cervical vertebrae.

■ *TECHNIQUE (DE ANDRADE AND MACNAB).* Maintain initial spinal stability by applying a cranial halo with the patient on a turning frame. Keep the patient on the frame and maintain the traction throughout the operation. Make the exposure from the right side with an incision coursing along the anterior border of the sternocleidomastoid muscle from above the angle of the mandible to below the cricoid cartilage (Fig. 81-5). Divide the platysma and deep cervical fascia in line with the incision and expose the anterior border of the sternocleidomastoid. Take care not to injure the spinal accessory nerve as it enters the anterior aspect of the sternocleidomastoid at the level of the transverse process of the atlas. Retract the sternocleidomastoid laterally and the pretracheal strap muscles anteriorly, and palpate the carotid artery in its sheath. Expose the latter. Divide the omohyoid muscle as it crosses at the level of the cricoid cartilage. Identify the digastric muscle and hypoglossal nerve at the cranial end of the wound. Bluntly dissect the retropharyngeal space and enter it at the level of the thyroid cartilage. Now divide the superior thyroid, lingual, and facial arteries and veins to gain access to the retropharyngeal space in the upper part of the wound. Continue blunt dissection in the retropharyngeal space and palpate the anterior arch of the atlas and the anterior tubercle in the midline. Continue above this area with the exploring finger and enter the hollow at the base of the occiput. Dissection cannot be carried further cephalad because of the pharyngeal tubercle, to which the pharynx is attached. Insert a broad right-angled retractor under the pharynx and displace it anterosuperiorly. Use intermittent traction on the pharyngeal and laryngeal branches of the vagus nerve during this maneuver to minimize temporary hoarseness and inability to sing high notes. The anterior aspect of the upper cervical spine and the base of the occiput are now exposed. Coagulate the profuse plexus of veins under the anterior border of the longus colli. Separate the muscles from the anterior aspect of the spine by incising the anterior longitudinal ligament vertically and transversely, and expose the anterior arch of C1 and the bodies of C2 and C3. The working space is approximately 4 cm, since the hypoglossal nerve exits from the skull through the anterior condyloid foramen about 2 cm lateral to the midline. Roughen the anterior surface of the base of the occiput and upper cervical vertebrae with a curet. Obtain from the iliac crest slivers of fresh autogenous cancellous bone and place them on the anterior surface of the vertebrae to be fused. Make the slivers no thicker than 4.2 mm to prevent excessive bulging into the pharynx. Close the wound by suturing the platysma and skin only with a suction drain left in the retropharyngeal space for 48 hours.

AFTERTREATMENT. The patient is kept on a turning frame and traction is maintained for 6 weeks. A tracheostomy set must be kept by the bedside in case upper airway obstruction occurs. For earlier ambulation a halo-vest may be applied; the halo is removed 16 weeks after the operation. Consolidation of the graft should occur by this time.

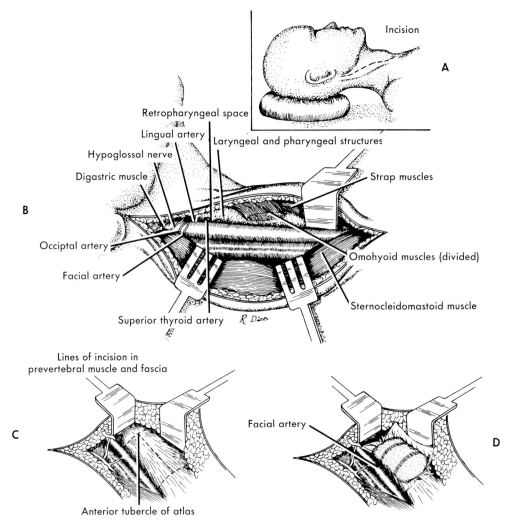

Fig. 81-5 Technique of de Andrade and Macnab for anterior occipitocervical arthrodesis (see text). (Redrawn from de Andrade JR and Macnab I: J Bone Joint Surg 51-A:1621, 1969.)

Anterior Upper Cervical Arthrodesis

■ *TECHNIQUE (ROBINSON AND RILEY).* Perform a tracheostomy and maintain anesthesia via this route. Begin the incision just to the left of the midline in the submandibular region. Carry it posteriorly to the angle of the mandible, then gently curve it lateral to the posterior border of the sternocleidomastoid muscle to the base of the neck, finally curve it anteriorly and inferiorly across the clavicle, and end it in the suprasternal space (Fig. 81-6). Develop the incision through the platysma muscle and retract the muscle flap so outlined medially to expose the sternocleidomastoid and strap muscles, the pharynx, the thyroid gland, the edge of the mandible, and the submaxillary triangle. Identify the anterior surface of the lower cervical spine by retracting the sternocleidomastoid muscle and carotid sheath laterally and transecting the tendinous portion of the omohyoid muscle. Incise the prevertebral fascia in the midline and retract the thyroid gland, esopha-

gus, and trachea medially. Now note that the continuation of this plane superiorly is impeded by the superior thyroid artery, the superior laryngeal neurovascular bundle, the hypoglossal nerve, the stylohyoid muscle, and the digastric muscle. Ligate and divide the superior thyroid artery. Divide and reflect the stylohyoid muscle and digastric muscle; identify and protect the superior laryngeal and hypoglossal nerves. Retract the larynx and the pharynx medially and the external carotid artery laterally, and identify the floor of the submaxillary triangle. Maintain superior retraction so that the base of the skull and the anterior arch of the first cervical vertebra are visible. To gain additional exposure, excise the submaxillary gland and dislocate the temporomandibular joint anteriorly by rotating the mandible superiorly and toward the right. The anterior arch of the first cervical vertebra, the odontoid process, and both vertebral arteries are now visible. Cut a trough in the anterior aspect of the second and third verte-

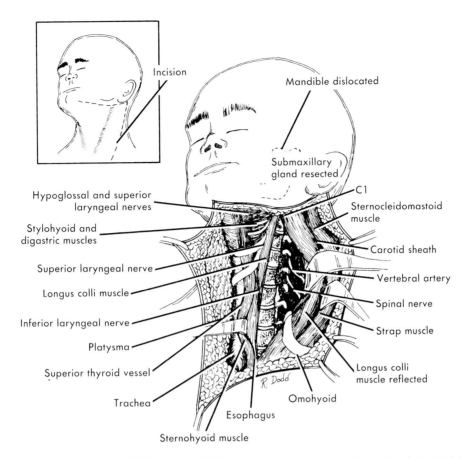

Incision

Mandible dislocated

Submaxillary
gland resected

C1

Hypoglossal and superior
laryngeal nerves

Sternocleidomastoid
muscle

Stylohyoid and
digastric muscles

Carotid sheath

Superior laryngeal nerve

Vertebral artery

Longus colli muscle

Spinal nerve

Inferior laryngeal nerve

Strap muscle

Platysma

Superior thyroid vessel

Longus colli
muscle reflected

R. Dodd

Trachea

Omohyoid

Esophagus

Sternohyoid muscle

Fig. 81-6   Technique of Robinson and Riley for anterior upper cervical arthrodesis. Incision and exposure of cervical spine. (Redrawn from Robinson RA and Riley LH Jr: Clin Orthop 109:78, 1975.)

bral bodies to the level of the posterior cortex of the odontoid process. Remove cancellous bone from the odontoid process with a small curet and convert it to a hollow shell. Shape a bone graft removed from the anterior iliac crest to the dimensions of the previously constructed trough. Shape the superior end of the graft to resemble a saddle, and fit one protrusion into the odontoid process and leave the other protrusion abutting the anterior arch of the first cervical vertebra. With the saddle supporting the anterior cortex of the odontoid and the inferior portion of the anterior arch of the first cervical vertebra, secure the inferior end of the graft with a loop of wire or heavy suture material through the cortex of the inferior vertebral body. If a twisted wire loop has been placed, use a small amount of methylmethacrylate bone cement to cover its sharp edges and avoid wire protrusion into the posterior pharynx.

AFTERTREATMENT. The aftertreatment is the same

as that described for the Bailey and Badgley technique (p. 3585).

Fibular Strut Graft in Cervical Spine Arthrodesis

■ *TECHNIQUE (WHITECLOUD AND LAROCCA).* Use the surgical approach of Robinson. Make a trough in the anterior aspect of the vertebral column, initially with a rongeur and then with a dental burr. Perform a partial vertebrectomy when long tract signs call for decompression. Use a full segment of the fibula, placing it into prepared notches in the vertebrae at both ends of the segment to be spanned. Make notches of equal length in the superior end, but make the posterior extension of the inferior notch slightly shorter than the anterior one to allow for easier graft insertion. Prepare the end plates of the superior and inferior vertebrae to accept the graft, which produces a hole within the body itself. Preserve the anterior portion of the vertebral cortex to prevent graft displacement. Increase the traction weight on the head and insert the graft into the superior vertebra. Use an impactor to sink the inferior portion of the graft into the trough and pull distally, locking it into place. Two thirds of the graft then comes to lie posterior to the anterior aspect of the vertebral column. Check the graft position by roentgenogram and close the wound over the drains.

AFTERTREATMENT. Initial immobilization is continued by skeletal traction, a plastic collar, a Philadelphia brace, or a cervicodorsal brace. The time required for fusion will understandably be longer with cortical bone than with a corticocancellous bone graft. Whitecloud and LaRocca kept their patients immobilized in a hard cervical collar, Philadelphia brace, or cervicodorsal brace for an average of 15 weeks. They concluded that this is too short a time; perhaps, like the canine fibular transplantation studied by Enneking et al., the graft may require a year for incorporation in humans. Therefore prolonged immobilization is necessary. We usually use anterior iliac crest grafts and a halo vest for postoperative immobilization.

Posterior Arthrodesis

The techniques of posterior arthrodesis of the cervical spine are discussed in the section on fractures, dislocations, and fracture-dislocations of the cervical spine (Chapter 80).

DORSAL AND LUMBAR SPINE

The indications for arthrodesis of the spine are now considerably different from in the days of Hibbs and Albee. Fusion of the lumbosacral region for degenerative, traumatic, and congenital lesions is now more common. Indications for and techniques of spinal fusion and care after surgery vary from one orthopaedic center to another. Many orthopaedists prefer posterior arthrodesis, usually some modification of the Hibbs procedure with the addition of a large quantity of autogenous iliac bone. Internal fixation is frequently used with posterior arthrodesis. Posterolateral or intertransverse process fusions are used frequently, either alone or in combination with a posterior fusion and with or without posterior internal fixation. Interbody fusions from an anterior or a posterolateral approach are preferred by other orthopaedic surgeons. For routine spinal fusion we usually prefer (1) a modified Hibbs procedure, usually combined in the thoracic and thoracolumbar spines with internal fixation and always supplemented with a great deal of autogenous iliac bone; (2) a modified Hibbs posterior fusion combined with a posterolateral fusion; or (3) a bilateral posterolateral fusion. Anterior interbody fusions are usu-

ally reserved for patients who do not have sufficient bone structure remaining for posterior fusion or who have some other unusual problem. Winter frequently adds anterior grafting in the lumbar spine to speed healing and to improve the rate of successful arthrodesis.

Posterior Arthrodesis

Posterior arthrodeses of the spine are generally based on the principles originated by Hibbs in 1911. In the Hibbs operation fusion of the neural arches is induced by overlapping numerous small osseous flaps from contiguous laminae, spinous processes, and articular facets. In the thoracic spine the arthrodesis is generally extended laterally out to the tips of the transverse processes so that the posterior cortex and cancellous bone of these portions of the vertebrae are used to widen the fusion mass. Accurate identification of a specific vertebral level is always difficult except when the sacrum can be exposed and thus identified. At any other level, despite the fact that identification of a given vertebra is frequently possible because of the anatomic peculiarities of spinous processes, laminae, and articular facets, it is almost always advisable to make marker roentgenograms at surgery. Marker films are occasionally made before surgery using a metal marker on the skin or a scratch on the skin to identify the level. We recommend a much better method consisting of the roentgenographic identification of a marker of adequate size clamped to or inserted into a spinous process within the operative field. The closer to the base of the spinous process the marker can be inserted, the more accurate and easier is the identification. Anteroposterior roentgenograms taken on the operating table to compare with good-quality preoperative roentgenograms are usually sufficient to allow accurate identification of the vertebral level.

BONE GRAFTS IN POSTERIOR FUSION OF SPINE. Autogenous bone grafts from the ilium are generally preferable to other types of grafts. Cancellous iliac bone will be incorporated into the fusion mass more rapidly than cortical tibial bone. Fresh autogenous grafts are preferable to bone bank grafts. The technique for obtaining iliac grafts is discussed on p. 18.

HIBBS FUSION OF SPINE. With the Hibbs technique fusion is attempted at four different points — the laminae and articular processes on each side. The procedure has been modified slightly over the years; at the New York Orthopaedic Hospital it is performed as follows.

■ *TECHNIQUE (HIBBS*).* Incise the skin and subcutaneous tissues in the midline along the spinous processes, and attach towels to the skin edges with Michel clips or use an adhesive plastic drape. Divide the deep fascia and supraspinous ligament in line

---

*As described by Howorth.

with the skin incision. With a Kermission or Cobb elevator remove the supraspinous ligament from the tips of the spines. Next strip the periosteum from the sides of the spines and the dorsal surface of the laminae with a curved elevator. Control bleeding with long thin sponge packs (Hibbs sponges). Incise the interspinous ligaments in the direction of their length, making a continuous longitidunal exposure. Now elevate the muscles from the ligamentum flavum and expose the fossa distal to the lateral articulation. Excise the fat pad in the fossa with a scalpel or curet. Thoroughly denude the spinous processes of periosteum and ligament with an elevator and curet, split them longitudinally and transversely with an osteotome, and remove them with the Hibbs biting forceps. Using a thick chisel elevator, strip away the capsules of the lateral articulations. Free with a curet the posterior layer (about two thirds) of the ligamentum flavum from the margins of the distal and proximal laminae in succession and peel it off the anterior layer; leave the latter to cover the dura. Excise the articular cartilage and cortical bone from the lateral articulations with special thin osteotomes, either straight or angled at 30, 45, or 60 degrees as required. (A.D. Smith emphasized that the lateral articulations of the vertebra above the area of fusion must not be disturbed, since this may cause pain later. However, it is important to include the lateral articulations within the fusion area, because if they are not obliterated, the entire fusion is jeopardized. After curetting the lateral articulations in the fusion area, he narrowed the remaining defect by making small cuts into the articular processes parallel with the joint line so that these thin slices of bone separate slightly and fill the space. This, he believed, is preferable to packing the joint spaces with cancellous bone chips.)

Using a gouge, cut chips from the fossa below each lateral articulation and turn them into the gap left by the removal of the articular cartilage or insert a fragment of spinous process into the gap. Denude the fossa of cortical bone and pack it fully with chips. Also with a gouge remove chips from the laminae and place them in the interlaminal space in contact with raw bone on each side. Use fragments from the spinous processes to bridge the laminae. Also use additional bone from the ilium near the posterosuperior spine or from the spinous processes beyond the fusion area. When large or extensive grafts are taken from the posterior ilium, postoperative pain or sensitivity of the area may be marked. Care should be taken to avoid injury to the cluneal nerves with subsequent neuroma formation. Bone from the bone bank may be used, especially if the bone available locally is scant because of spina bifida. The bone grafts should not extend beyond the laminae of the end vertebrae, because the projecting ends of the grafts may cause irritation and pain. If the nucleus pulposus is to be removed, the chips are cut before exposure of the nucleus and are kept until needed. The remaining layer of the ligamentum flavum is freed as a flap with its base at the midline, is retracted for exposure of the nerve root and nucleus, and after removal of the nucleus is replaced to protect the dura.

Suture the periosteum, ligaments, and muscles snugly over the chips with interrupted sutures. Then suture the subcutaneous tissue carefully to eliminate dead space, and close the skin either with a subcuticular suture or nonabsorbable skin suture technique.

At this clinic we routinely use an adhesive plastic film material to isolate the skin surface from the wound rather than attaching towels to skin edges with Michel clips. Michel clips have an unfortunate tendency to become displaced and may get lost within the wound. We also routinely use modified Cobb elevators, which when sharp are quite efficient in stripping away the capsules of the lateral articulations. The most important single project at the time of surgery is the preparation of an extensive fresh cancellous bed to receive the grafts. This means denuding the facets, pars interarticulares, laminae, and spinous processes completely.

AFTERTREATMENT. We routinely use closed wound suction for 12 to 36 hours, with removal mandatory by 48 hours. Depending on the level of the arthrodesis, the age of the patient, and the presence or absence of internal fixation, walking is allowed in a few days when pain permits. Skin sutures may be removed early—after several days—and replaced with adhesive strips if a Risser type of well-molded cast is to be applied. If not, they remain in place for up to 2 weeks. More appropriate means of postoperative immobilization for older adults include lower back braces, prefabricated plastic jackets, and custom-made, bivalved, plastic jackets. For obese patients all types of external fixation or support will likely be inadequate, and limitation of activity may be the only reasonable alternative.

INTERNAL FIXATION IN SPINAL FUSION. Many surgeons have used various types of internal fixation in spinal fusion. The object is to immobilize the joints during fusion and thus hasten consolidation and reduce pain and disability after surgery. For many years several surgeons fixed the spinous processes of the lumbar spine with heavy wire loops as described by Rogers for fracture-dislocation of the cervical spine (Chapter 80).

In 1949 McBride reported a method of fixing the articular facets with bone blocks. Later he used cylindrical bone grafts to transfix the facets, particularly at the lumbosacral joint. Still later he elevated subperiosteally the soft tissue attachments to the spinous processes and laminae, removed the spinous processes of L4, L5, and S1 at their bases, and with special trephine cutting tools cut mortise bone grafts from them. The laminae are then spread forcibly with laminae distractors, and, again with the use of special trephine cutting tools, a round hole is made across each facet joint into the underlying pedicle. The bone grafts are then impacted firmly across each joint into the pedicle, and the distractors are removed.

Overton has also fixed the articular facets with bone grafts, but in addition he uses H grafts between the spinous processes and adds bone chips about the fusion area. Of 187 patients treated by his method, 174 (or 93%) obtained solid fusion as judged by roentgenograms. This technique is not used at this clinic.

Internal fixation (such as pedicle screws and plates) are described in Chapter 80.

TREATMENT AFTER POSTERIOR ARTHRODESIS. Opinions vary as to the proper treatment after spinal fusion. Usually the patient is placed on a firm bed with a soft mattress pad. No one knows for sure how long bed rest or the use of any external support should be continued; certainly this will vary somewhat with the pathologic condition and the location and extent of the fusion. We once believed that absolute bed rest should be maintained for at least 6 and preferably 8 weeks after lumbosacral fusion. Many others have allowed walking in a light support soon after surgery. At this clinic, treatment now depends somewhat on the pathologic condition and the technique of fusion, but more on the preference of the various surgeons. Most of our surgeons now allow the patient to walk in a few days. If the lumbosacral area is fused, the postoperative immobilization should be in a well-molded body cast or plastic jacket applied a few days after fusion. Some of our surgeons use an extension of the cast down to the knee on one side. At 2 to 4 months most surgeons apply a rigid lower back brace that is worn until consolidation of the fusion mass is complete as seen in roentgenograms.

Anteroposterior roentgenograms made with the patient supine in right and left bending positions and lateral roentgengrams made with the patient in flexion and extension are necessary between 6 and 12 months postoperatively to confirm consolidation of the fusion mass.

PSEUDARTHROSIS AFTER SPINAL FUSION. The frequency of pseudarthrosis after spinal arthrodesis should be remembered from the time the operation is proposed until the fusion mass is solid. A frank discussion of this problem with each patient before operation is important.

In a study of lumbosacral spine fusions performed on 594 patients, Cleveland et al. found pseudarthrosis in 119, an incidence of 20%. When calculated on the basis of the number of intervertebral spaces fused, the incidence was 12.1%. There was a definite relationship between the extent of fusion and the incidence of pseudarthrosis. When the fifth lumbar vertebra was fused to the

sacrum, the pseudarthrosis rate was 3.4%; when the fourth lumbar vertebra was included, the rate was 17.4%; and when the fusion extended up to the third or second lumbar vertebra, one third of the patients showed one or more pseudarthroses. Bosworth, as a matter of fact, recommended that in the lumbosacral region arthrodesis should extend only from the fourth lumbar vertebra to the sacrum as a maximum at one stage, unless the situation at the time of surgery requires more extensive fusion. Other segments to be included in the final fusion area are added later. Ralston and W.A.L. Thompson, in a study of 1096 patients after spinal fusion, found an overall pseudarthrosis rate of 16.6%. Prothero, Parkes, and Stinchfield, in a review of 430 fusions, found a rate of 15.1%; as in the study of Cleveland et al., the rate varied with the extent of the fusion: when the fifth lumbar vertebra was fused to the sacrum, the rate was 8.3%; when the fourth lumbar vertebra was included, the rate was 15.8%; and when the fusion extended to the third lumbar vertebra, the rate was 26.6%. In contrast, DePalma and Rothman, in a review of 448 patients 5 to 17 years after spinal fusion, found an overall pseudarthrosis rate of only 8.7%.

It has been estimated that 50% of patients with pseudarthrosis have no symptoms. Bosworth, in a review of 101 patients with pseudarthrosis, found 43 who had no pain. DePalma and Rothman matched 39 patients with pseudarthrosis against 39 otherwise similar patients without pseudarthrosis. The results were a little better when the fusions were solid, but the difference was not marked. In each group some patients had pain and some did not. We have presumed that any persistent pain after spinal fusion is caused by pseudarthrosis when this condition is present. Yet, in some instances pain has continued after a successful repair. Even so, repair of any pseudarthrosis is indicated when disabling pain persists; certainly repair is contraindicated when pain is slight or absent.

The following findings are helpful in making a diagnosis of pseudarthrosis: (1) sharply localized pain and tenderness over the fusion area, (2) progression of the deformity or disease, (3) localized motion in the fusion mass, as found in biplane bending roentgenograms, and (4) motion in the fusion mass found on exploration. Cobb and others have pointed out that exploration is the only way one can be absolutely certain that a fusion mass is completely solid. Technetium bone scanning may show increased uptake over a pseudarthrosis.

Pseudarthrosis repair

■ *TECHNIQUE (RALSTON AND W.A.L. THOMPSON).* Expose the entire fusion plate subperiosteally through the old incision; should the defect be wide and filled with dense fibrous tissue, subperiosteal stripping in that area may be difficult. On the other hand, a narrow defect is often difficult to locate, since the surface of the plate is usually irregular, and the line of pseudarthrosis may be sinuous in both coronal and sagittal planes. In our experience, adherence of the overlying fibrous tissue has been the key factor. The characteristic smooth cortical surface and easily stripped fibrous "periosteum" of a solid, mature fusion mass are quite different. Thoroughly clean the fibrous tissue from the fusion mass in the vicinity of the pseudarthrosis. The adjacent superior and inferior borders of the fusion mass on either side of the pseudarthrosis will usually be seen to move when pressure is applied with a blunt instrument. As the defect is followed across the fusion mass, it will be found to extend into the lateral articulations on each side. Carefully explore these articulations and excise all fibrous tissue and any remaining articular cartilage down to bleeding bone. Should the defect be wide, excise the fibrous tissue that fills it to a depth of 3 to 6 mm across the entire mass and protect the underlying spinal dura. Thoroughly freshen the exposed edges of the defect. When the defect is narrow and motion is minimal, limit the excision of the interposed soft tissue to avoid loss of fixation. Now fashion a trough 6 mm wide and 6 mm deep on each side of the midline, extending longitudinally both well above and well below the defect. "Fish scale" the entire fusion mass on both sides of the defect, the bases of the bone chips raised being away from the defect. Now obtain both strip and chip bone grafts either from the fusion mass above or below or from the ilium, preferably the latter. Pack these grafts tightly into the lateral articulations, into the pseudarthrosis defect, and into the longitudinal troughs. Then place small grafts across the pseudarthrosis line and wedge the edge of each transplant beneath the fish-scaled cortical bone chips. Use all remaining graft material to pack neatly in and about the grafts.

Internal fixation (Chapter 80) often is used to improve the rate of healing after pseudarthrosis repair.

Posterolateral or intertransverse fusions. In 1948 Cleveland, Bosworth, and F.R. Thompson described a technique for repair of pseudarthrosis after spinal fusion in which grafts are placed posteriorly on one side over the laminae, lateral margins of the articular facets, and base of the transverse processes. In 1953, 1959, and 1964 Watkins described what he called a posterolateral fusion of the lumbar and lumbosacral spine in which the facets, pars interarticularis, and bases of the transverse processes are fused with chip grafts and a large graft is placed posteriorly on the transverse processes. When the lumbosacral joint is included, the grafts extend to the posterior aspect of the first sacral segment.

We, like many others, use this operation and its modifications in patients with pseudarthrosis, laminal defects either congenital or surgical, or spondylolisthesis, and in postlaminectomy patients with chronic pain from insta-

bility. The operation may be unilateral or bilateral, but usually is bilateral, covering one or more joints depending on the stability of the area to be fused. The large instruments designed by McElroy are useful here.

■ *TECHNIQUE (WATKINS).* Make a longitudinal skin incision along the lateral border of the paraspinal muscles, curving it medially at the distal end across the posterior crest of the ilium (Fig. 81-7, *A*). Divide the lumbothoracic fascia and establish the plane of cleavage between the border of the paraspinal muscles and the fascia overlying the transversus abdominis muscle. The tips of the transverse processes can now be palpated in the depths of the wound (Fig. 81-7, *B*). Release the iliac attachment of the muscles with an osteotome, taking a thin layer of ilium. Continue the exposure of the posterior crest of the ilium by subperiosteal dissection and remove the crest almost flush with the sacroiliac joint, taking enough bone to provide one or two grafts. Removal of the iliac crest increases exposure of the spine. Retract the sacrospinalis muscle toward the midline and denude the transverse processes of the dorsal muscle and ligamentous attachments; expose the articular facets by excising the joint capsule. Remove the cartilage from the facets with an osteotome and level the area down to allow the graft to fit snugly against the facets, pars interarticularis, and base of the transverse process at each level. Comminute the facets with a small gouge or osteotome and turn bone chips up and down from the facet area, upper sacral area, and transverse processes. Now split the resected iliac crest longitudinally into two grafts. Shape one to fit into the prepared bed and impact it firmly in place with its cut surface against the spine (Fig. 81-7, *C*). Preserve the remaining graft for use on the opposite side with or without additional bone from the other iliac crest. Now pack additional ribbons and chips of cancellous bone from the ilium about the graft. Allow the paraspinal muscles to fall in position over the fusion area, and close the wound.

AFTERTREATMENT. Aftertreatment is the same as that described for posterior arthrodesis (p. 3594).

• • •

Wiltse in 1961, Truchly and Thompson in 1962, Rombold in 1966, and Wiltse et al. in 1968 described modifications of the Watkins technique. Wiltse et al. split the sacrospinalis muscle longitudinally and include the laminae, as well as the articular facets and transverse processes, in the fusion (Figs. 81-8 and 81-9). Some members of our staff combine a modified Hibbs fusion with a posterolateral fusion using a midline approach in routine lumbar and lumbosacral fusions (Fig. 81-10); they add many chip grafts obtained from the ilium. DePalma and Prabhakar also have combined posterior and posterolateral fusions.

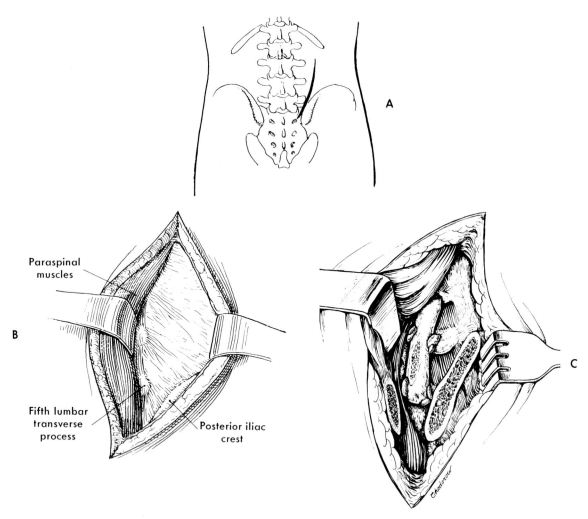

Paraspinal
muscles

B

Fifth lumbar
transverse
process

Posterior iliac
crest

C

Fig. 81-7 Watkins posterolateral fusion. **A,** Incision. **B,** Lumbothoracic fascia has been incised, paraspinal muscles have been retracted medially, and tips of transverse processes are now palpable. **C,** Split iliac crest and smaller grafts have been placed against spine. (**A** and **B,** From Watkins MB: J Bone Joint Surg 35-A:1004, 1953; **C,** from Watkins MB: Clin Orthop 35:80, 1964.)

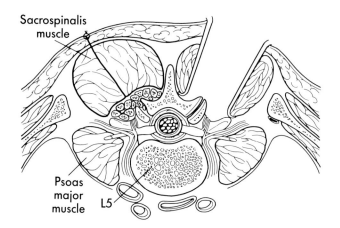

Sacrospinalis
muscle

Psoas
major
muscle

L5

Fig. 81-8 Technique of posterolateral fusion in which sacrospinalis muscle is split longitudinally and laminae, articular facets, and transverse processes are all included in fusion. (Modified from Wiltse LL, Bateman JG, Hutchinson RH, and Nelson WE: J Bone Joint Surg 50-A:919, 1968.)

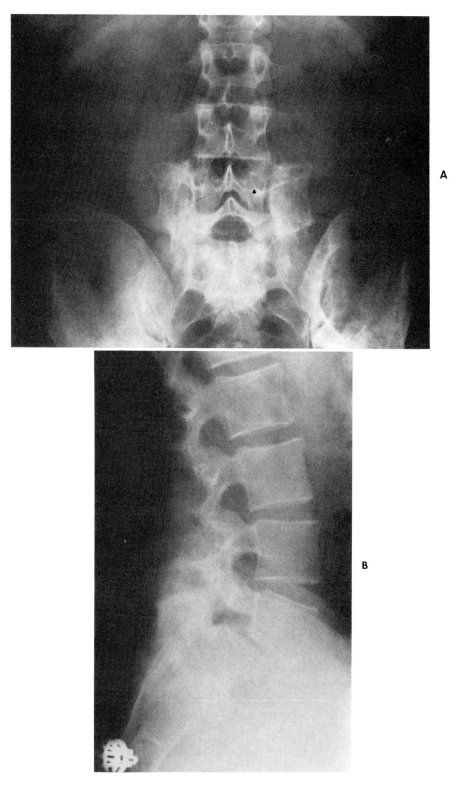

Fig. 81-9 Bilateral posterolateral fusion for spondylolisthesis in adult. **A,** Anteroposterior and, **B,** lateral roentgenograms 6 months after surgery.

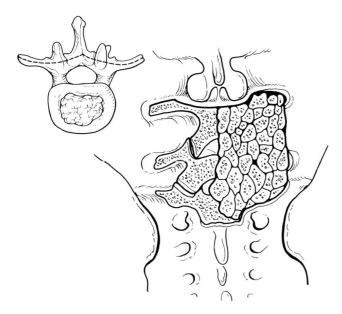

Fig. 81-10 Slocum technique combining posterior (modified Hibbs) and posterolateral fusions. Midline incision is used. *Inset,* All bone posterior to broken line is removed. (Redrawn from Wiltse LL: Clin Orthop 21:156, 1961.)

Adkins has used an intertransverse or alar transverse fusion in which tibial grafts are inserted between the transverse processes of L4 and L5 and between that of L5 and the ala of the sacrum on one or both sides.

■ *TECHNIQUE (ADKINS).* **Dissect the erector spinae muscles laterally from the pedicles, exposing the transverse processes and ala of the sacrum. This is easier when the facets have been removed, but if these are intact, exposure can be obtained without disturbing them. Cut a groove in the upper or lower border of each transverse process with a sharp gouge or forceps. Take care not to fracture the transverse process. In the ala of the sacrum, first make parallel cuts in its posterosuperior border with an osteotome, then drive a gouge across the ends of these cuts, and lever the intervening bone out of the slot so made. For fusions of the fourth to the fifth lumbar vertebrae, cut a tibial graft with V-shaped ends; insert it obliquely between the transverse processes and then rotate it into position so that it causes slight distraction of the processes and becomes firmly impacted between them. For the lumbosacral joint cut the graft so that it is V-shaped at its upper end and straight but slightly oblique at its lower end. Insert one arm of the V in front of the transverse process and punch the lower end into the slot in the sacrum. If only one side is grafted, arrange the patient so that there is a slight convex curve of the spine on the operated side; thus firm impaction occurs when the spine is straightened. Bilateral grafts are preferred. The grafts should be placed as far laterally as possible to avoid the nerve roots and to gain maximum stability.**

Currently, strips of iliac wing cortex no more than 2 mm thick are placed anterior to the transverse processes of L4 and L5 to bridge the gap and lie on the intertransverse fascia. Similarly, another strip is placed between the ala of the sacrum and L5 by wedging it into the space after the ala has been slotted and decorticated. Care must be taken that these grafts do not protrude anterior to the plane of the transverse processes. This modification does not require a tibial graft and is recommended.
AFTERTREATMENT. **Aftertreatment is the same as that described for posterior arthrodesis (p. 3594).**

Anterior Arthrodesis

Sacks, Wiltberger, Harmon, Hoover, Hodgson and Wong, and others have arthrodesed the lumbar and lumbosacral areas anteriorly for spondylolisthesis, deranged intervertebral discs, and other affections. Except in tuberculosis, tumors, kyphosis, scoliosis, or some problem such as a difficult, failed posterior arthrodesis or gross instability after extensive laminectomy, we rarely arthrodese the dorsal and lumbar areas in this manner. The approaches and techniques used in tuberculosis by Hodgson et al. (Chapter 8) should be applicable in most instances.

ANTERIOR DISC EXCISION AND INTERBODY FUSION. The rationale of management of lower back pain must depend on accurate diagnosis. The pain syndromes in this area are many, and diagnostic pitfalls are ever present. Treatment varies according to the physical and emotional profile of the patient and the experience of the surgeon involved. Hemilaminectomy and decompression of nerve roots still constitute the most widely used surgical procedure for unremitting lower back pain. With continued instability of the anterior and posterior elements, supplemental posterior or posterolateral fusion usually proves satisfactory. Rothman found only a 5% decrease in residual back pain and sciatica when disc excision is combined with spinal fusion, but this was not statistically significant. There was also no difference in postoperative evaluation between patients with solid fusion and those with pseudarthrosis.

There remains a group of patients for whom the aforementioned standard surgical procedures have been unsuccessful. R.N. Stauffer and Coventry have emphasized the causes of persistent symptoms following disc surgery:

1. Mistaken original diagnosis
2. Recurrent herniation of disc material (incomplete removal)
3. Herniation of disc at another level
4. Bony compression of nerve root
5. Perineural adhesions

6. Instability of vertebral segments

7. Psychoneurosis

In this group improved diagnostic accuracy currently can be obtained with the use of electromyography, discography, a psychologic profile assessment, computed tomographic myelographic scanning, and magnetic resonance imaging with and without gadolinium contrast. Finally, differential spinal anesthesia is helpful in discriminating between the various types of pain.

As a rule, failure of the usual posterior methods of fusion dictates consideration of anterior intervertebral disc excision and interbody spinal fusion. Goldner, Urbaniak, and McCollum used this criterion and found moderate or complete relief of lower back pain in 78% of patients and complete or moderate relief of lower extremity pain in 85%; no patients had pain worse than before surgery. The Mayo Clinic, on the other hand, reported an overall satisfactory result incidence of 36%, the difference being attributed chiefly to interpretation of clinical factors and patient type. They also recommended its use primarily as a salvage procedure.

Sacks, polling 15 surgeons in nine different countries, found variations of opinion, no adequate follow-up, and therefore inconclusive long-term results. Conversely, Freebody, Bendall, and Taylor have performed 466 operations, the first 243 (1956 to 1967) showing satisfactory results in 90% of the cases. Their indications include (1) instability causing backache and sciatica, (2) spondylolisthesis of all types, (3) pain following multiple posterior explorations, and (4) failed posterior fusions. They

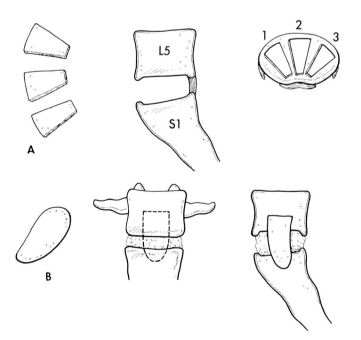

Fig. 81-11 Freebody technique for anterior interbody fusion in lower lumbar spine. **A,** Technique for degenerative disease. **B,** Technique for spondylolisthesis. (Redrawn from Sacks S: Orthop Clin North Am 6:272, 1975.)

use three iliac wedge grafts for degenerative disease and a block graft for spondylolisthesis (Fig. 81-11).

Flynn and Hoque in Florida; Fujimake, Crock, and Bedbrook in Australia; and van Rens and van Horn in the Netherlands have reported on a total of 435 patients on whom anterior interbody fusion was done. Flynn and Hoque and van Rens and van Horn had no male patients with retrograde ejaculation, and in both studies the authors suggested that the incidence of this complication may be exaggerated.

■ *TECHNIQUE (GOLDNER ET AL.).* Administer general anesthesia and place the patient in the Trendelenburg position. Develop the retroperitoneal approach to the vertebral bodies and identify the psoas muscle, the iliac artery and vein, and the left ureter. If more than three interspaces are to be fused, retract the ureter toward the left. Identify the sacral promontory by palpation. Inject saline solution under the prevertebral fascia over the lumbar vertebra and lift the sympathetic chain for easier dissection. Expose the lumbosacral disc space by retracting the left iliac artery and vein to the left. In exposure of the fourth lumbar interspace, displace the left artery and vein and ureter to the right side. Elevate the anterior longitudinal ligament as a flap with the base toward the left. Tag the flap with sutures and retract it to give additional protection to the vessels. Separate the intervertebral disc and anulus from the cartilaginous end plates of the vertebrae with a thin osteotome and remove them with pituitary rongeurs and large curets. Clean the space thoroughly back to the posterior longitudinal ligament without removing bone, thereby keeping bleeding to a minimum until the site is ready for grafting. Finally, remove the end plates from the vertebral bodies with an osteotome until bleeding bone is encountered. Cut shallow notches in the opposing surfaces of the vertebrae and measure the dimensions of the notches carefully with a caliper. Cut grafts from the iliac wing, making them larger than the notches for later firm impaction (Fig. 81-12). Hyperextend the spine, insert multiple grafts, and relieve the hyperextension. Electrocautery is useful in obtaining hemostasis, but take care not to coagulate the sympathetic fibers over the anterior aspect of the lumbosacral joint. Use of silver clips in this area is preferred. After completion of the fusion, close all layers with absorbable sutures. Estimate the amount of blood lost and replace it.

AFTERTREATMENT. Nasogastric suction may be necessary for gastric decompression for about 36 hours. Attention must be paid to mobilization of the lower extremities to prevent dependency and blood pooling. In-bed exercises with straight leg raising are started on the third postoperative day and continued indefinitely. By the fifth postoperative day the patient is allowed to sit and walk with a low

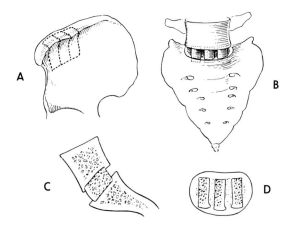

Fig. 81-12 Technique of Goldner et al. for anterior interbody fusion of lumbosacral joint. (From Goldner JL, Urbaniak JR, and McCollum DE: Orthop Clin North Am 2:543, 1971.)

back corset used for postoperative immobilization. Postoperative roentgenograms are made before discharge from the hospital to serve as a baseline for judging graft appearance. Three months later flexion and extension roentgenograms are made in the standing position to provide information about the success of arthrodesis. Roentgenograms are then repeated at 6 and 12 months after surgery, with the solid fusion not confirmed until 1 year after surgery. Laminagrams may be useful in evaluating suspected pseudarthrosis.

• • •

We have used a retroperitoneal approach to L2, L3, and L4 discs. For the L5 or lumbosacral disc, some prefer a transperitoneal approach if good anterior access is needed. The incidence of deep venous thrombosis after these approaches, especially the midline transperitoneal approach, is much higher than after ordinary spinal surgery. Suitable prophylaxis probably is indicated, even though it frequently is not successful in preventing this complication.

REFERENCES

Adkins EWO: Lumbo-sacral arthrodesis after laminectomy, J Bone Joint Surg 37-B:208, 1955.

Albee FH: Transplantation of a portion of the tibia into the spine for Pott's disease: a preliminary report, JAMA 57:885, 1911.

Albee FH: A report of bone transplantation and osteoplasty in the treatment of Pott's disease of spine, NY Med J 95:469, 1912.

Allison N: Fusion of the spinal column, Surg Gynecol Obstet 46:826, 1928.

Aronson N, Bagan M, and Feltzer DL: Results of using the Smith-Robinson approach for herniated and extruded cervical discs, J Neurosurg 32:721, 1970.

Aronson N, Feltzer DL, and Bagan M: Anterior fusion by Smith-Robinson approach, J Neurosurg 29:397, 1968.

Bailey RW and Badgley CE: Stabilization of the cervical spine by anterior fusion, J Bone Joint Surg 42-A:565, 1960.

Baker LD and Hoyt WA Jr: The use of interfacet Vitallium screws in the Hibbs fusion, South Med J 41:419, 1948.

Barr JS: Pseudarthrosis in the lumbosacral spine (discussion of paper by Cleveland M, Bosworth DM, and Thompson FR, J Bone Joint Surg 30-A:302, 1948), J Bone Joint Surg 30-A:311, 1948.

Beller HE and Kirsh D: Spondylolysis and spondylolisthesis following low back fusions, South Med J 57:783, 1964.

Bloom MH and Raney FL Jr: Anterior intervertebral fusion of the cervical spine: a technical note, J Bone Joint Surg 63-A:842, 1981.

Bosworth DM: Clothespin graft of the spine for spondylolisthesis and laminal defects, Am J Surg 67:61, 1945.

Bosworth DM: Techniques of spinal fusion: pseudarthrosis and method of repair, AAOS Instr Course Lect 5:295, 1948.

Bosworth DM: Technique of spinal fusion in the lumbosacral region by the double clothespin graft (distraction graft; "H" graft) and results, AAOS Instr Course Lect 9:44, 1952.

Bosworth DM: Circumduction fusion of the spine, J Bone Joint Surg 38-A:263, 1956.

Bosworth DM: Surgery of the spine, AAOS Instr Course Lect 14:39, 1957.

Bosworth DM, Wright HA, Fielding JW, and Goodrich ER: A study in the use of bank bone for spine fusion in tuberculosis, J Bone Joint Surg 35-A:329, 1953.

Boucher HH: A method of spinal fusion, J Bone Joint Surg 41-B:248, 1959.

Breck LW and Basom WC: The flexion treatment for low-back pain: indications, outline of conservative management, and a new spine-fusion procedure, J Bone Joint Surg 25:58, 1943.

Briggs JR and Freehafer AA: Fusion of the Charcot spine: report of 3 cases, Clin Orthop 53:83, 1967.

Brooks AL and Jenkins EB: Atlanto-axial arthrodesis by the wedge compression method, J Bone Joint Surg 60-A:279, 1978.

Callahan RA et al: Cervical facet fusion for control of instability following laminectomy, J Bone Joint Surg 59-A:991, 1977.

Campbell WC: Operative measures in the treatment of affections of the lumbosacral and sacroiliac articulation, Surg Gynecol Obstet 51:381, 1930.

Cattell HS and Clark GL Jr: Cervical kyphosis and instability following multiple laminectomies in children, J Bone Joint Surg 49-A:713, 1967.

Cleveland M: Technique of spine fusion for tuberculosis involving vertebrae, AAOS Instr Course Lect 9:58, 1952.

Cleveland M, Bosworth DM, Fielding JW, and Smyrnis P: Fusion of the spine for tuberculosis in children: a long-range follow-up study, J Bone Joint Surg 40-A:91, 1958.

Cleveland M, Bosworth DM, and Thompson FR: Pseudarthrosis in the lumbosacral spine, J Bone Joint Surg 30-A:302, 1948.

Cloward RB: The treatment of ruptured lumbar intervertebral discs by vertebral body fusion. I. Indications, operative technique, after care, J Neurosurg 10:154, 1953.

Cloward RB: Vertebral body fusion for ruptured cervical discs: description of instruments and operative technic, Am J Surg 98:722, 1959.

Cloward RB: Lesions of the intervertebral disks and their treatment by interbody fusion methods: the painful disk, Clin Orthop 27:51, 1963.

Cobb JR: Technique, after-treatment, and results of spine fusion for scoliosis, AAOS 9:65, 1952.

Connor AC, Rooney JA, and Carroll JP: Anterior lumbar fusion: a technique combining intervertebral and intravertebral body fixation, Surg Clin North Am 47:231, 1967.

Crock HV: Observations on the management of failed spinal operations, J Bone Joint Surg 58-B:193, 1976.

Curran JP and McGaw WH: Posterolateral spinal fusion with pedicle grafts, Clin Orthop 59:125, 1968.

de Andrade JR and Macnab I: Anterior occipito-cervical fusion using an extra-pharyngeal exposure, J Bone Joint Surg 51-A:1621, 1969.

DePalma AF and Prabhakar M: Posterior-posterobilateral fusion of the lumbosacral spine, Clin Orthop 47:165, 1966.

DePalma AF and Rothman RH: The nature of pseudarthrosis, Clin Orthop 59:113, 1968.

DePalma AF and Rothman RH: The intervertebral disc, Philadelphia, 1970, WB Saunders Co.

DePalma AF, Rothman RH, Lewinnek GE, and Canale ST: Anterior interbody fusion for severe cervical disc degeneration, Surg Gynecol Obstet 134:755, 1972.

Dereymaeker A and Mulier J: La fusion vertebrale par voie ventrale dans la discopathie cervicale, Rev Neurol 19:597, 1958.

Dommisse GF: Lumbo-sacral interbody spinal fusion, J Bone Joint Surg 41-B:87, 1959.

Dunn EJ: Techniques of fusion in treatment of fractures and dislocations of cervical spine, Orthop Rev 2:17, April 1973.

Enneking WF, Burchardt H, Puhl J, and Protrowski G: Physical and biological aspects of repair in dog cortical-bone transplants, J Bone Joint Surg 57-A:237, 1975.

Fang HSY, Ong GB, and Hodgson AR: Anterior spinal fusion, the operative approaches, Clin Orthop 35:16, 1964.

Farey ID, McAfee PC, Davis RF, and Long DM: Pseudarthrosis of the cervical spine after anterior arthrodesis: treatment by posterior nerve-root decompression, stabilization, and arthrodesis, J Bone Joint Surg 72-A:1171, 1990.

Fielding JW, Hawkins RJ, and Ratzan SA: Spine fusion for atlanto-axial instability, J Bone Joint Surg 58-A:400, 1976.

Fielding JW, Lusskin R, and Batista A: Multiple segment anterior cervical spinal fusion, Clin Orthop 54:29, 1967.

Flesch JR, Leider LL, Erickson DL, et al: Harrington instrumentation and spine fusion for unstable fractures and fracture-dislocations of the thoracic and lumbar spine, J Bone Joint Surg 59-A:143, 1977.

Flynn JC and Hoque A: Anterior fusion of the lumbar spine: end-result study with long-term follow-up, J Bone Joint Surg 61-A:1143, 1979.

Freebody D, Bendall R, and Taylor RD: Anterior transperitoneal lumbar fusion, J Bone Joint Surg 53-B:617, 1971.

Fujimake A, Crock HV, and Bedbrook GM: The results of 150 anterior lumbar interbody fusion operations performed by two surgeons in Australia, Clin Orthop 165:164, 1982.

Gibson A: A modified technique for spinal fusion, Surg Gynecol Obstet 53:365, 1931.

Goldner JL, Urbaniak JR, and McCollum DE: Anterior disc excision and interbody spinal fusion for chronic low back pain, Orthop Clin North Am 2:543, 1971.

Green PWB: Anterior cervical fusion: a review of thirty-three patients with cervical disc degeneration, J Bone Joint Surg 59-B:236, 1977.

Griswold DM, Albright JA, Schiffman E, et al: Atlanto-axial fusion for instability, J Bone Joint Surg 60-A:285, 1978.

Hallock H, Francis KC, and Jones JB: Spine fusion in young children: a long-term end-result study with particular reference to growth effects, J Bone Joint Surg 39-A:481, 1957.

Hallock H and Jones JB: Tuberculosis of the spine: an end-result study of the effects of the spine fusion operation in a large number of patients, J Bone Joint Surg 36-A:219, 1954.

Harmon PH: Subtotal anterior lumbar disc excision and vertebral body fusion. III. Application to complicated and recurrent multi-level degenerations, Am J Surg 97:649, 1959.

Harmon PH: Anterior extraperitoneal lumbar disc excision and vertebral body fusion, Clin Orthop 18:169, 1960.

Harmon PH: Anterior excision and vertebral body fusion operation for intervertebral disk syndromes of the lower lumbar spine: three-to-five-year results in 244 cases, Clin Orthop 26:107, 1963.

Henderson MS: Operative fusion for tuberculosis of the spine, JAMA 92:45, 1929.

Henry MO and Geist ES: Spinal fusion by simplified technique, J Bone Joint Surg 15:622, 1933.

Hibbs RA: An operation for progressive spinal deformities, NY Med J 93:1013, 1911.

Hibbs RA: A further consideration of an operation for Pott's disease of the spine, Ann Surg 55:682, 1912.

Hibbs RA: An operation for Pott's disease of the spine, JAMA 59:133, 1912.

Hibbs RA and Risser JC: Treatment of vertebral tuberculosis by the spine fusion operation: a report of 286 cases, J Bone Joint Surg 10:805, 1928.

Hodgson AR and Wong SK: A description of a technic and evaluation of results in anterior spinal fusion for deranged intervertebral disk and spondylolisthesis, Clin Orthop 56:133, 1968.

Hoover NW: Methods of lumbar fusion, J Bone Joint Surg 50-A:194, 1968.

Howorth MB: Evolution of spinal fusion, Ann Surg 117:278, 1943.

Jaslow IA: Intercorporal bone graft in spinal fusion after disc removal, Surg Gynecol Obstet 82:215, 1946.

Johnson JTH and Robinson RA: Anterior strut grafts for severe kyphosis: results of 3 cases with a preceding progressive paraplegia, Clin Orthop 56:25, 1968.

Johnson JTH and Southwick WO: Bone growth after spine fusion: a clinical survey, J Bone Joint Surg 42-A:1396, 1960.

Jones AAM, McAfee PC, Robinson RA, et al: Failed arthrodesis of the spine for severe spondylolisthesis: salvage by interbody arthrodesis, J Bone Joint Surg 70-A:25, 1988.

Kestler OC: Overgrowth (hypertrophy) of lumbosacral grafts, causing a complete block, Bull Hosp Jt Dis 27:51, 1966.

King D: Internal fixation for lumbosacral fusion, Am J Surg 66:357, 1944.

Kite JH: Nonoperative versus operative treatment of tuberculosis of the spine in children: review of 50 consecutive cases treated by each method, South Med J 26:918, 1933.

Kraus DR and Stauffer ES: Spinal cord injury as a complication of elective anterior cervical fusion, Clin Orthop 112:130, 1975.

Macnab I: The blood supply of the lumbar spine and its application to the technique of intertransverse lumbar fusion, J Bone Joint Surg 53-B:628, 1971.

Macnab I: Complications of anterior cervical fusion, Orthop Rev 1:29, September 1972.

McBride ED: A mortised transfacet bone block for lumbosacral fusion, J Bone Joint Surg 31-A:385, 1949.

McBride ED and Shorbe HB: Lumbosacral fusion: the mortised transfacet method by use of the vibrating electric saw for circular bone blocks, Clin Orthop 12:268, 1958.

Mercer W: Spondylolisthesis: with a description of a new method of operative treatment and notes of ten cases, Edinburgh Med J 43:545, 1936.

Moore AT: The unstable spine: discogenetic syndrome treatment with self-locking prop bone graft, Int Surg 8:64, 1945; correction 8:179, 1945.

Moore AT: Multiprop and interbody spinal fusion, Spectator Letter (mimeographed), September 1959.

Newman PH: Surgical treatment for derangement of the lumbar spine, J Bone Joint Surg 55-B:7, 1973.

Norrell H and Wilson CB: Early anterior fusion for injuries of the cervical portion of the spine, JAMA 214:525, 1970.

Nugent GR: Clinicopathologic correlations in cervical spondylosis, Neurology 9:273, 1959.

Overton LM: An improved technic for arthrodesis of the lumbosacral spine, Am J Surg 80:559, 1950.

Overton LM: Arthrodesis of the lumbosacral spine, Clin Orthop 5:97, 1955.

Overton LM: Lumbosacral arthrodesis: an evaluation of its present status, Am Surg 25:771, 1959.

Pennal GF, McDonald GA, and Dale GG: A method of spinal fusion using internal fixation, Clin Orthop 35:86, 1964.

Petter CK: Rib-splinter graft in spinal fusion for vertebral tuberculosis, J Bone Joint Surg 19:413, 1937.

Pierce DS: Long-term management of thoracolumbar fractures and fracture dislocations, AAOS Instr Course Lect 21:102, 1972.

Prothero SR, Parkes JC, and Stinchfield FE: Complications after low-back fusion in 1000 patients: a comparison of two series one decade apart, J Bone Joint Surg 48-A:57, 1966.

Ralston EL and Thompson WAL: The diagnosis and repair of pseudarthrosis of the spine, Surg Gynecol Obstet 89:37, 1949.

Regen EM: Pseudarthrosis in the lumbosacral spine (discussion of paper by Cleveland M, Bosworth DM, and Thompson FR, J Bone Joint Surg 30-A:302, 1948), J Bone Joint Surg 30-A:311, 1948.

Rennie W and Mitchell N: Flexion distraction fractures of the thoracolumbar spine, J Bone Joint Surgery 55-A:386, 1973.

Riley LH Jr: Cervical disc surgery: its role and indications, Orthop Clin North Am 2:443, 1971.

Roaf R, Kirkaldy-Willis WH, and Cathro AJM: Surgical treatment of bone and joint tuberculosis, Edinburgh, 1959, E & S Livingstone, Ltd.

Robinson RA: Anterior and posterior cervical spine fusions, Clin Orthop 35:34, 1964.

Robinson RA and Riley LH Jr: Techniques of exposure and fusion of the cervical spine, Clip Orthop 109:78, 1975.

Robinson RA and Smith GW: Anterolateral cervical disc removal and interbody fusion for cervical disc syndrome (abstract), Bull Johns Hopkins Hosp 96:223, 1955.

Robinson RA, Walker EA, Ferlic DC, and Wiecking DK: The results of anterior interbody fusion of the cervical spine, J Bone Joint Surg 44-A:1569, 1962.

Rombold C: Treatment of spondylolisthesis by posterolateral fusion, resection of the pars interarticularis, and prompt mobilization of the patient: an end-result study of seventy-three patients, J Bone Joint Surg 48-A:1282, 1966.

Rothman RH: New developments in lumbar disk surgery, Orthop Rev 4:23, March 1975.

Rothman RH and Booth R: Failures of spinal fusion, Orthop Clin North Am 6:299, 1975.

Roy L and Gibson DA: Cervical spine fusions in children, Clin Orthop 73:146, 1970.

Sacks S: Anterior interbody fusion of the lumbar spine, J Bone Joint Surg 47-B:211, 1965.

Sacks S: Anterior interbody fusion of the lumbar spine: indications and results in 200 cases, Clin Orthop 44:163, 1966.

Sacks S: Present status of anterior interbody fusion in the lower lumbar spine, Orthop Clin North Am 6:275, 1975.

Schmidt AC, Flatley TJ, and Place JS: Lumbar fusion using facet inlay grafts, South Med J 68:209, 1975.

Sim FH, Svien HJ, Bickel WH, and Janes JM: Swan-neck deformity following extensive cervical laminectomy: a review of twenty-one cases, J Bone Joint Surg 56-A:564, 1974.

Simeone FA: The modern treatment of thoracic disc disease, Orthop Clin North Am 2:453, 1971.

Simmons EH, Bhalla SK, and Butt WP: Anterior cervical discectomy and fusion: a clinical and biomechanical study with eight-year follow-up, J Bone Joint Surg 51-B:225, 1969.

Smith AD: Lumbosacral fusion by the Hibbs technique, AAOS Instr Course Lect 9:41, 1952.

Smith AD: Tuberculosis of the spine: results in 70 cases treated at the New York Orthopaedic Hospital from 1945 to 1960, Clin Orthop 58:171, 1968.

Smith GW and Robinson RA: The treatment of certain cervical-spine disorders by anterior removal of the intervertebral disc and interbody fusion, J Bone Joint Surg 40-A:607, 1958.

Sorrel E: The indications for, and results of, osteosynthesis in the treatment of Pott's disease, Int Abstr Surg 50:357, 1930. (Abstracted from J Chir 34:439, 1929.)

Speed K: Spondylolisthesis: treatment by anterior bone graft, Arch Surg 37:175, 1938.

Stauffer RN and Coventry MB: A rational approach to failures of lumbar disc surgery: the orthopedist's approach, Orthop Clin North Am 2:533, 1971.

Stauffer RN and Coventry MB: Anterior interbody lumbar spine fusion: analysis of Mayo Clinic Series, J Bone Joint Surg 54-A:756, 1972.

Stauffer RN and Coventry MB: Posterolateral lumbar-spine fusion: analysis of Mayo Clinic series, J Bone Joint Surg 54-A:1195, 1972.

Stinchfield FE and Sinton WA: Criteria for spine fusion with use of "H" bone graft following disc removal: results in 100 cases, Arch Surg 65:542, 1952.

Thompson WAL and Ralson EL: Pseudarthrosis following spine fusion, J Bone Joint Surg 31-A:400, 1949.

Toumey JW: Internal fixation in fusion of the lumbosacral joint, Lahey Clin Bull 3:188, 1943.

Truchly G and Thompson WAL: Posterolateral fusion of the lumbosacral spine, J Bone Joint Surg 44-A:505, 1962.

van Rens TJG and van Horn JR: Long-term results in lumbosacral interbody fusion for spondylolisthesis, Acta Orthop Scand 53:383, 1982.

Verbiest H: Anterolateral operations for fractures and dislocations in the middle and lower parts of the cervical spine: report of a series of forty-seven cases, J Bone Joint Surg 51-A:1489, 1969.

Wagoner G: A technique for lessening hemorrhage in operations on the spine, J Bone Joint Surg 19:469, 1937.

Watkins MB: Posterolateral fusion of the lumbar and lumbosacral spine, J Bone Joint Surg 35-A:1004, 1953.

Watkins MB: Posterolateral bone-grafting for fusion of the lumbar and lumbosacral spine, J Bone Joint Surg 41-A:388, 1959.

Watkins MB: Posterolateral fusion in pseudarthrosis and posterior element defects of the lumbosacral spine, Clin Orthop 35:80, 1964.

Webb JK et al: Hidden flexion injury of the cervical spine, J Bone Joint Surg 58-B:322, 1976.

Weiss M: Dynamic spine alloplasty (spring-loading corrective devices) after fracture and spinal cord injury, Clin Orthop 112:150, 1975.

Weiss M and Bentkowski Z: Biomechanical study in dynamic spondylodesis of the spine, Clin Orthop 103:199, 1974.

White AA III and Hirsch C: An experimental study of the immediate load bearing capacity of some commonly used iliac bone grafts, Acta Orthop Scand 42:482, 1971.

White AA III, Southwich WO, Deponte RJ, et al: Relief of pain by anterior cervical-spine fusion for spondylosis: a report of sixty-five patients, J Bone Joint Surg 55-A:525, 1973.

White AA III et al: An experimental study of the immediate load bearing capacity of three surgical constructions for anterior spine fusions, Clin Orthop 91:21, 1973.

Whitecloud TS III and LaRocca H: Fibular strut graft in reconstructive surgery of the cervical spine, Spine 1:33, 1976.

Whitehill R, Sirna EC, Young DC, and Cantrell RW: Late esophageal perforation from an autogenous bone graft: report of a case, J Bone Joint Surg 67-A:644, 1985.

Williams JL, Allen MB Jr, and Harkess JW: Late results of cervical discectomy and interbody fusion: some factors influencing the results, J Bone Joint Surg 50-A:277, 1968.

Williams PC: Lesions of the lumbosacral spine: chronic traumatic (postural) destruction of the lumbosacral intervertebral disc, J Bone Joint Surg 19:690, 1937.

Wilson PD and Straub LR: Lumbosacral fusion with metallic plate fixation, AAOS Instr Course Lect 9:53, 1952.

Wiltberger BR: The dowel intervertebral-body fusion as used in lumbar-disc surgery, J Bone Joint Surg 39-A:284, 1957.

Wiltberger BR: Intervertebral body fusion by the use of posterior bone dowel, Clin Orthop 35:69, 1964.

Wiltse LL: Spondylolisthesis in children, Clin Orthop 21:156, 1961.

Wiltse LL, Bateman JG, Hutchinson RH, and Nelson WE: The paraspinal sacrospinalis-splitting approach to the lumbar spine, J Bone Joint Surg 50-A:919, 1968.

Winter RB, Moe JH, and Wang JF: Congenital kyphosis, its natural history and treatment as observed in a study of one hundred and thirty patients, J Bone Joint Surg 55-A:223, 1973.

Young MH: Long-term consequences of stable fractures of the thoracic and lumbar vertebral bodies, J Bone Joint Surg 55-B:295, 1973.

Yosipovitch Z, Robin GC, and Makin M: Open reduction of unstable thoracolumbar spinal injuries and fixation with Harrington rods, J Bone Joint Surg 59-A:1003, 1977.

Scoliosis

ALLEN S. EDMONSON

Scoliosis is a lateral curvature of the spine. Structural curves are those in which lateral bending of the spine is asymmetric or the involved vertebrae are fixed in a rotated position, or both. These, then, are curves that the patient either cannot correct or can but cannot keep corrected. Lateral bending is asymmetric when the long gentle curve formed by the entire spine on bending to each side is asymmetric in some way, either in regard to the areas that bend or to the degree of bending (Fig. 82-1). Nonstructural curves, in contrast, are those in which intrinsic changes in the spine or its supporting structures are absent. In these curves, then, lateral bending is symmetric and the involved vertebrae are not fixed in a rotated position. Generally a nonstructural curve requires no treatment or any necessary treatment is directed toward its cause, which is not located in the spine itself.

According to its cause, scoliosis is of two main types: (1) that of unknown cause (idiopathic), and (2) that of known cause. Several genealogic studies with emphasis on heredity or genetic transmission of scoliosis made in both Great Britain and the United States support the hypothesis that idiopathic scoliosis is multifactorial. Recent studies suggest a neurologic developmental delay in the brain stem. In about 75% to 80% of patients scoliosis is idiopathic. In the remainder it is caused by such conditions as congenital skeletal abnormalities, both vertebral and extravertebral, neuromuscular diseases, neurofibromatosis, arthrogryposis, trauma, irritative phenomena caused by nerve root compression or spinal cord tumors, and miscellaneous affections. Obviously the prognosis and treatment of scoliosis vary with the cause.

IDIOPATHIC SCOLIOSIS

Idiopathic scoliosis is the most common of all types and is divided into infantile, juvenile, and adolescent according to the age of the patient when it is first diagnosed. Research and the accumulation of more clinical information now make it more than probable that scoliosis is a genetic disease. The inheritance pattern has not been established, but studies have confirmed the long suspected fact that many of the predecessors of patients with scoliosis seeking treatment have had unrecognized scoliosis. Just how the variation in the age of onset of the curve (any time from infancy to adolescence) can be explained genetically is another problem under study. Metabolic abnormalities have not been discovered in the many studies of children with scoliosis. Vanderpool, James, and Wynne-Davies of Edinburgh studied scoliosis developing in patients over 50 years of age and attributed it to metabolic diseases such as osteoporosis and os-

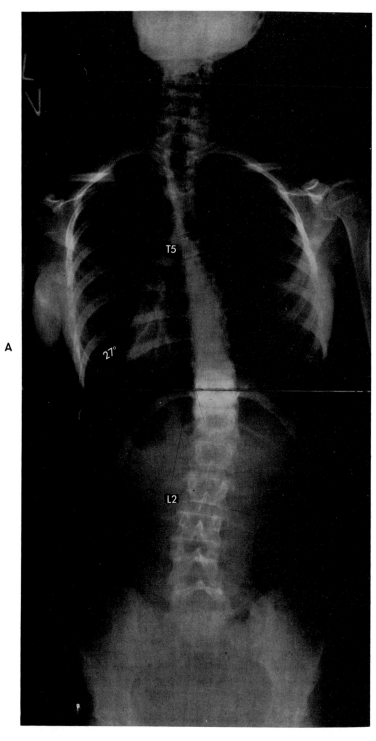

Fig. 82-1   Use of lateral bending roentgenograms to determine whether curve is structural (primary). **A,** Idiopathic thoracolumbar curve in girl 14 years of age, extending from T5 through L2 and measuring 27 degrees while standing. Rotation is minimal.

teomalacia; scoliosis of this type is in no way related to idiopathic scoliosis of childhood. Enneking and Harrington in studying several hundred specimens of articular processes in normal and scoliotic children found that impaired chondrogenesis, premature cessation of osteogenesis, increased subchondral maturation, and degenerative changes in the articular surfaces were not related to the severity of the deformity and were seen more often on the convex side of the curve rather than on the concave side. They concluded that the deformities seen in the posterior elements of the spine in scoliosis are not caused by asymmetric enchondral growth; further, they postulated that idiopathic scoliosis is produced by an extraosseous cause and that the changes in bone and cartilage are secondary adaptations. It seems apparent at present that while the exact mechanism of the production of the curves is unknown, idiopathic scoliosis is most likely of genetic origin.

Infantile Idiopathic Scoliosis

Infantile idiopathic scoliosis is a structural, lateral curvature of the spine with its onset occurring before the age of 3 years. There are two types of infantile idiopathic scoliosis: progressive, which usually increases rapidly, and resolving (or structural resolving), which resolves spontaneously within a few years with or without treatment. The resolving type occurs in 70% to 90% of patients with infantile idiopathic scoliosis. Unfortunately, when a curve is mild, no absolute criteria are available for differentiating the two types. According to James, when compensatory or secondary curves develop or when the curve measures more than 37 degrees by the Cobb method when first seen, the scoliosis probably is progressive. Conversely, if the curve measures only 10 to 15 degrees when first seen, it probably is resolving scoliosis. Mehta developed a method for differentiating re-

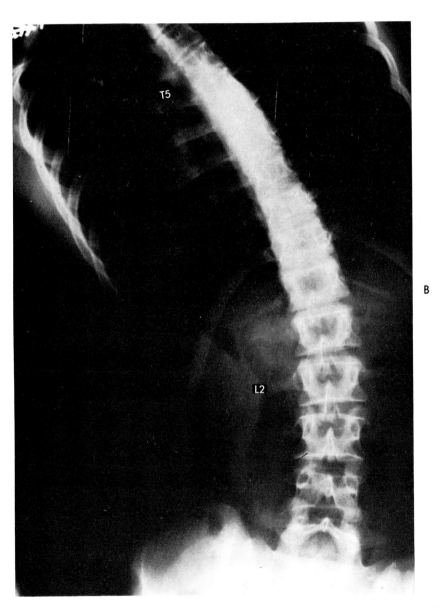

Fig. 82-1, cont'd   **B,** On bending to left there is long smooth continuous curve from T1 through L5.

Continued.

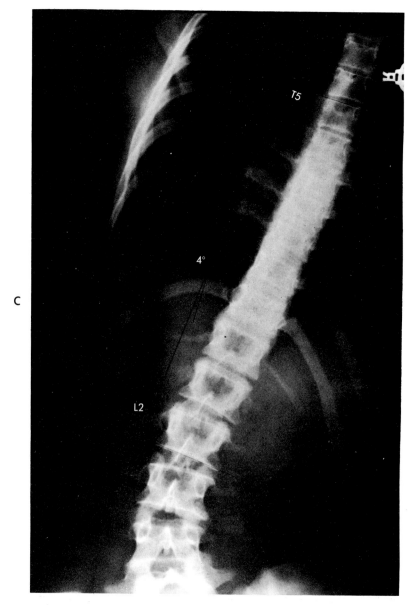

Fig. 82-1, cont'd **C,** On bending to right there is a residual curve of 4 degrees. Therefore lateral bending is asymmetric. Use of lateral bending roentgenograms is most reliable way to demonstrate whether scoliotic curves are structural.

solving from progressive curves in infantile idiopathic scoliosis. Her method is based on the development of the rib-vertebral angle (RVA). The RVA is measured by drawing a line perpendicular to the apical vertebral end plate and another line from the midneck to the midhead of the corresponding rib. The angle formed by the intersection of these two lines is the RVA (Fig. 82-2). The RVA difference (RVAD) is the difference between the values of the angles on the concave and convex sides of the curve. Mehta found that the RVAD was consistently greater in progressive curves. A curve with an initial RVAD of 20 degrees or more is considered progressive until proven otherwise. Thus whether or not a given curve is progressive can be determined by observing it for only a few months.

Treatment of infantile idiopathic scoliosis is determined by the type of curve. Resolving and flexible curves (with RVADs of less than 20 degrees) require observation only, with examination and roentgenograms every 4 to 6 months until the curve resolves. If the RVAD is greater than 20 degrees and the curve is not flexible on examination, it is considered progressive until proved otherwise. If a brace can be fitted satisfactorily in a child under 3 years of age, progression of curves may be prevented and improvement sometimes may be obtained during the early period of skeletal growth. If the curve is severe or increases despite the use of the brace, a relatively short fusion including only the structural or primary curve probably is the best treatment. Because of the "crankshaft phenomenon" described by Dubousset

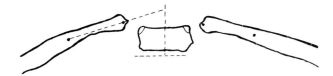

Fig. 82-2 Construction of rib-vertebral angle (RVA). (From Mehta MH: J Bone Joint Surg 54-B:232, 1972.)

(p. 3616), anterior fusion or hemiepiphysiodesis should be considered in addition to posterior fusion. The spine still must be controlled by a Milwaukee brace until growth is complete. For certain flexible curves in growing children, Moe et al. described the use of a subcutaneous Harrington rod without fusion followed by full-time wear of an external orthosis. Using the "shortening formula" (0.07 times the number of segments fused times the number of years of growth), the average shortening in their patients would have been 4.5 cm had fusion been performed. They noted an average length gain in the instrumented area of 3.8 cm for nine patients who ultimately underwent fusion. Complications, most frequently hook dislocation and rod breakage, occurred in 50% of patients.

Juvenile Idiopathic Scoliosis

Juvenile idiopathic scoliosis appears between the ages of 4 and 10 years and affects approximately 15% of all patients with idiopathic scoliosis. Multiple curve patterns can occur, but the convexity of the thoracic curve usually is to the right. The treatment of juvenile idiopathic scoliosis follows guidelines similar to those for adolescent idiopathic scoliosis. For curves of less than 20 degrees, observation is indicated with examination and standing posteroanterior roentgenograms every 4 to 6 months. The success of nonoperative treatment is variable. Figueiredo and James reported that 56% of patients require spinal fusion, and Tolo and Gillespie reported 27% required fusion. They found that it was not possible to predict which curves would increase from the curve pattern, the degree of curvature, or the patient's age at the time of diagnosis. From their experience they formulated the following guidelines.

1. If the RVAD does not go below more than 10 degrees during brace wear, progression can be expected.
2. If the RVAD values decline as treatment continues, part-time Milwaukee brace wear should be adequate.
3. Curves with RVAD values near or below 0 at the time of diagnosis require only a relatively short period of full-time brace wear before part-time brace wear is begun.
4. Unless the curve is quite advanced at the time of diagnosis, a Milwaukee brace should be applied because some curves, even in the range of 20 to 30 degrees, do not progress over a period of several months.

If orthotic treatment does not halt curve progression, surgical stabilization is indicated. If the curve progresses past 60 degrees despite brace wear, fusion of the major curve should be performed. The area of fusion is selected as for adolescent idiopathic scoliosis, and a posterior fusion with instrumentation usually is performed. In addition, because of the "crankshaft phenomenon" (p. 3616), anterior fusion or hemiepiphysiodesis should be considered.

Adolescent Idiopathic Scoliosis

Idiopathic scoliotic curves of more than 10 degrees are estimated to occur in from 2% to 3% of children younger than 16 years. The overall female-to-male prevalence is 3.6 to 1, but with increasing curve severity the female predominance increases to 10 to 1 for curves of 30 degrees or more. Fewer than 10% of children with curves of 10 degrees or more will require treatment. Brace treatment regardless of the brace type is usually effective only in preventing increases in spinal curvatures. Their main value remains in small curves detected early.

Natural History

In deciding if and when the spine should be fused, a knowledge of the natural history of idiopathic scoliosis is important. Ponseti and Friedman in 1950 and James in 1954 made extensive studies that are helpful; the conclusions from these two studies are essentially the same. Collis and Ponseti in 1969 increased this knowledge by studying a second time about one half of the patients included in the 1950 study. More recent studies by Nachemson, Lonstein, and Weinstein, and by Lonstein and Carlson have shown that the risk of curve progression decreases with increasing skeletal maturity; however, with larger curves the risk of progression remains past maturity.

The generally accepted pattern of change in idiopathic scoliosis is that while relatively mild curves seem to increase little with growth, most do increase considerably. Some curves increase steadily but in most the increase varies with growth; they often increase markedly during spurts of growth, especially in adolescents. For many years the most common treatment consisted of the periodic observation of patients until the curves became severe enough to justify surgery and then correction of the curves and spinal fusion. However, spontaneous improvement occurs in only 3% of adolescents with idiopathic scoliosis, most of whom have curves of less than 11 degrees. Progression is more likely in girls than in boys. In Bunnell's series of 123 patients with curves averaging 33 degrees, the risk of progression of more than 5 degrees is 77% for patients with thoracic curves, 67%

for those with thoracolumbar curves, 30% for those with lumbar curves, and 66% for those with double curves. The larger the curve when first seen, the more likely its progression.

The most significant prognosticators of curve progression are related to the patient's growth potential: the age at onset, the occurrence of menarche in girls, and skeletal age as determined by the Risser sign. Curves diagnosed in patients younger than 10 years of age have an 88% risk of progression, whereas those diagnosed in patients older than 15 years of age have a 29% risk. Of curves diagnosed in girls before the onset of menses, 53% progress 10 degrees or more, whereas only 11% of those diagnosed after menarche progress 10 degrees or more. A patient with a Risser sign of 0 at the time of diagnosis has a 68% risk of curve progression of 10 degrees or more; this risk is decreased to 18% for those with a Risser sign of 3 or 4.

Dickson et al. and Pedriolle and Vidal also have demonstrated the importance of loss of kyphosis in idiopathic scoliosis. Loss of thoracic kyphosis may require alterations in surgical treatment and may decrease pulmonary function in patients with severe curves.

Ponseti and Friedman reviewed 394 patients with idiopathic scoliosis in whom surgery had not been performed; of these, 335 were observed to maturity. Patients with mild scoliosis were excluded. Collis and Ponseti about 20 years later reported a long-term study of 195 of these same patients. They found that these patients had been living what they described as relatively normal lives with little difficulty caused by the scoliosis. More than 50%, however, believed that their deformity was apparent to others even when they were dressed. The most common symptom was dull backache after unusual activity. The frequency of backache was as follows: about one third never or very rarely had it, about one third had it occasionally, and about one third had it frequently or daily. They could find no correlation between the severity of any backache and the type or severity of the scoliosis. Forty-five percent had vital capacities of less than 85% of the predicted normal. Collis and Ponseti found an average increase in the curves of 15 degrees between the time of complete ossification of the epiphyses of the iliac crests and the time of the study more than 20 years later. The increase was 15 degrees or more in 26% and more than 25 degrees in 8% of 61 patients even after fusion of the epiphyses of the iliac crests. They considered this as evidence against the hypothesis that idiopathic scoliosis results from asymmetric growth of the vertebrae. They found some correlation between the type and severity of the curves and whether the curves tended to increase after maturity.

Nilsonne and Lundgren studied untreated scoliosis as much as 50 years after diagnosis. They found that most patients had a reduced work capacity: 76% were unmarried; 90% had pain in the back, and many used back supports; and 47% of those living were disabled. The mean age at death was 46.6 years. Nachemson reported on 130 untreated scoliotic adults and found mortality twice that of normal adults, a decreased ability for ordinary work, and pain as a relatively constant symptom.

Weinstein, Zavala, and Ponseti found at an average follow-up of 40 years that 80% of their 161 patients complained of backache, ranging from mild to severe. The location of pain was variable and generally unrelated to the location of the curve or its magnitude. Weinstein reported that 38% of his patients had roentgenographic evidence of degenerative joint disease, ranging from minimal osteophyte formation and mild narrowing of the intervertebral disc space to moderate facet joint sclerosis; in a few patients, spontaneous fusion on the concave curve surface had occurred. Weinstein et al., however, found that pain was unrelated to the severity of osteoarthritic changes, except in areas of translatory shifts in thoracolumbar and lumbar curves.

Examination of Patient

The original examination of the patient should include a thorough general physical examination, a neurologic examination, an examination of the back, and roentgenograms of the spine.

After the general physical examination the back should be examined carefully, and the characteristics of the deformity should be recorded. Further, the height of the patient while standing and while sitting should be measured and recorded; in observing the patient later these measurements are used to determine clinically whether the total height increases or decreases and whether any change is due principally to growth of the lower extremities or to an increase or decrease in the height of the trunk. It is encouraging to find that the patient's height while sitting has increased during a period when roentgenograms of the spine show no increase in the scoliosis. Next a thorough neurologic examination should be performed because occasionally an intraspinal neoplasm or other neurologic disorder may be the cause of scoliosis. An intraspinal neoplasm usually produces detectable neurologic signs and frequently an increase in the distances between the pedicles or erosion of one or more pedicles; thus the anteroposterior roentgenograms should be examined carefully for these changes. However, Bucy and Heimburger have pointed out that for an intraspinal neoplasm to produce a deformity of the spine, the patient must be young and the tumor must grow slowly; obviously these criteria are rarely fulfilled. We have seen scoliosis in adolescents caused by benign tumors of the vertebrae such as osteoid osteomas or eosinophilic granulomas. Both of these lesions are painful and can be discovered by careful study.

Posteroanterior roentgenograms of the spine, including distally the iliac crests and proximally most of the cervical spine, should be made with the patient standing. Supine or horizontal posteroanterior roentgenograms may be made. Usually we prefer instead right and left bending films of the spine, but as a rule, make these only when evaluation for surgery is appropriate. A standing lateral roentgenogram of the spine and a spot lateral roentgenogram of the lumbosacral joint, if necessary, also should be made during the initial examination. Any spondylolisthesis in the lumbosacral area should not be overlooked because it may be the cause of any symptoms and may determine the treatment necessary. In the posteroanterior roentgenogram made with the patient standing, any significant discrepancy in the leg length can be determined by observing the comparative levels of the iliac crests and the femoral heads. The angle of the primary or structural curve or curves on the right and left lateral bending films gives a reasonably accurate estimate of the flexibility or correctability of the curves, important also in selecting treatment. In the standing lateral roentgenogram a search should be made for anomalies such as epiphysitis, neoplastic or infectious lesions, and congenital anomalies such as hemivertebrae or fusion between vertebrae that can be seen only in this view. Because posteroanterior roentgenograms do not show the true magnitude of the deformity in larger curves with severe spinal rotation, a Stagnara derotation view (Fig. 82-3) may be indicated. In this technique, an oblique roentgenogram is made with the cassette parallel to the medial aspect of the rotational rib prominence and the roentgen beam positioned at right angles to the cassette. This view is reported to allow a more accurate measurement of curve size and better evaluation of vertebral anatomy.

We believe that one roentgenogram made with the patient standing and no oftener than every 4 to 6 months is sufficient for most clinical follow-up evaluations. Gonad shielding for all roentgenograms is the rule. Posteroanterior views reduce radiation to breast areas. Complete breast shielding has been difficult to accomplish routinely without blocking out the spinal image. Certainly if

the scoliosis is increasing or if for any other reason a change in treatment is being considered, then any additional roentgenograms should be made as indicated. It is important to avoid making several roentgenograms routinely as a "scoliosis series" and to order only the individual film or films actually necessary for reevaluation of the patient.

An anteroposterior roentgenogram of the hand and wrist should be made and used with one of the standard atlases to determine the skeletal age. Because the skeletal age may deviate considerably from the chronologic age, the skeletal age should be used in evaluating the patient for treatment. Additional signs of maturation to be used are ossification of the vertebral ring epiphyses, iliac epiphysis excursion, physiologic signs of breast development or pubic hair appearance, cessation of increasing height, and chronologic age.

Finally photographs of the patient may be made to provide an objective record of the posture and deformity and can be repeated at intervals later to record any increase in deformity or any decrease in deformity after treatment. They should be made of the front and back while standing and, because asymmetry or deformity of the thorax is usually most apparent when the spine is flexed, also of the back and side while the patient is bending forward.

Measurement of Curves

The methods of measuring curves attributed to Cobb and to Ferguson have both been widely used. They are fundamentally different and cannot be used interchangeably. For this reason a single method, the one attributed to Cobb, has been recommended by the Terminology Committee of the Scoliosis Research Society to permit comparison of patients and results of treatment of different surgeons. Consequently we have used the Cobb method, employing usually as references the end plates of the end vertebrae, but when these are not visible on the roentgenograms, employing instead the pedicles of these vertebrae.

COBB METHOD. This method consists of three steps: (1) locating the superior end vertebra, (2) locating the inferior end vertebra, and (3) drawing intersecting perpendiculars from the superior surface of the superior end vertebra and from the inferior surface of the inferior end vertebra (Fig. 82-4). The angle of deviation of these perpendiculars from a straight line is the angle of the curve. The end vertebrae of the curve are the ones that tilt the most into the concavity of the curve being measured. Generally, as one moves away from the apex of the curve being measured, the next intervertebral space inferior to the inferior end vertebra or superior to the superior end vertebra is wider on the concave side of the curve being measured. Within the curve being measured the intervertebral spaces are usually wider on the convex side and

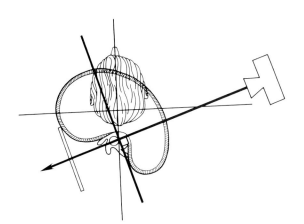

Fig. 82-3 Diagrammatic representation of Stagnara derotation view. (From Bradford DS et al: Moe's textbook of scoliosis and other spinal deformities, ed 2, Philadelphia, 1987, WB Saunders Co.)

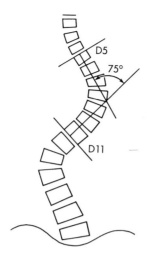

Fig. 82-4 Diagram of Cobb method of measurement. (Redrawn from Cobb JR: AAOS Instr Course Lect 5:261, 1948.)

narrower on the concave side. When significantly wedged, the vertebrae themselves rather than the intervertebral spaces may be wider on the convex side of the curve and narrower on the concave side. Some recent articles have noted interobserver and intraobserver measurement discrepancies with the Cobb method, but most differences reported are less than 4 degrees, and this method remains the most widely used.

Appelgren and Willner described a modification of the Cobb method for measuring the "end vertebra angle" to determine lateral deviation of a scoliotic curve. They divide the Cobb angle into two parts, the angles between each end vertebra and the horizontal plane. They reported that this method allows determination of the symmetry of the curve and is a better indicator of the success of brace treatment.

FERGUSON METHOD. Some recent articles have noted interobserver and intraobserver measurement discrepancies with the Cobb method, but most differences reported are less than 4 degrees, and this method remains the most widely used.

Measurement of Vertebral Rotation

The position of the pedicles on the initial posteroanterior roentgenogram indicates the degree of vertebral rotation, which Nash and Moe divided into five grades (Fig. 82-5). If the pedicles are equidistant from the sides of the vertebral bodies, there is no vertebral rotation (grade 0). The grades then increase up to grade IV rotation, which indicates that the pedicle is past the center of the vertebral body. Pedriolle's method of measuring vertebral rotation involves the use of his "torsiometer." The measurement is made from the pedicle at the convexity of the apical vertebra. The greatest diameter of the pedicle and the waists of the lateral borders of the vertebra are marked. The torsiometer is placed over the vertebra and

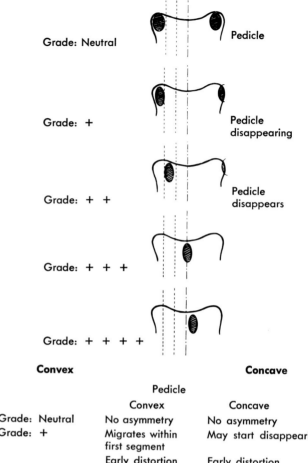

	Pedicle	
	Convex	Concave
Grade: Neutral	No asymmetry	No asymmetry
Grade: +	Migrates within first segment	May start disappearing
Grade: + +	Early distortion Migrates to second segment	Early distortion Gradually disappears
Grade: + + +	Migrates to middle segment	Not visible
Grade: + + + +	Migrates past midline to concave side of vertebral body	Not visible

Fig. 82-5 Pedicle method of determining vertebral rotation. Vertebral body is divided into six segments and grades from 0 to 4+ are assigned, depending on location of pedicle within segments. Because pedicle on concave side disappears early in rotation, pedicle on convex side easily visible through wide range of rotation is used as standard. (From Nash CL Jr and Moe JH: J Bone Joint Surg 51-A:223, 1969.)

the amount of rotation of the pedicle line is read from the rotation scale.

Several authors have described computerized, three-dimensional measurements, but these have not yet been standardized to allow their routine use. Ultrasonography also has been reported to more accurately depict the curve.

Curve Patterns

In idiopathic scoliosis most of the characteristic features of the primary curve or curves are present at the onset of deformity and rarely change. As a primary curve

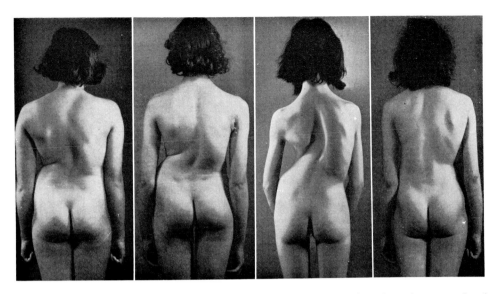

Fig. 82-6   Scoliosis deformity varies with pattern of curve. In each patient shown, angle of primary curve or curves is 70 degrees, but pattern of curve is different. *Left to right:* lumbar, thoracolumbar, thoracic, and combined thoracic and lumbar curves. (From James JIP: J Bone Joint Surg 36-B:36, 1954.)

increases, one or two vertebrae may be added to it, but its apex, its location, and the direction of rotation of the vertebrae it includes remain unchanged. The curves were found by Ponseti and Friedman to form five main patterns that behaved differently. A sixth curve pattern was described by Moe.

SINGLE MAJOR LUMBAR CURVE. In the study of Ponseti and Friedman 23.6% of the patients had this curve, which was described as the most benign and the least deforming of all curves (Fig. 82-6). It can, however, cause marked distortion of the waistline. It usually contained five vertebrae, T11 to L3, with the apex at L1 or L2; its average angle at maturity while standing was 36.8 degrees. In the study of Collis and Ponseti the average increase in this curve was 9 degrees after skeletal maturity, with curves greater than 31 degrees increasing an average of 18 degrees, but curves of less than 31 degrees not increasing. Mild degenerative arthritic changes were found in about 20% of the patients, but no correlation between the severity of the curve and the frequency of back symptoms was found. Eight of 52 patients had daily backache, but patients with lumbar curves noted no more backache than patients of the group as a whole.

SINGLE MAJOR THORACOLUMBAR CURVE. In the study of Ponseti and Friedman this curve was found in 16% of patients, usually included six to eight vertebrae, and extended from T6 or T7 to L1 or L2. Its apex was at T11 or T12. The study of Collis and Ponseti included 24 patients with such curves, many of which were severe. The curves had increased an average of 17 degrees after skeletal maturity. Only five patients had decreased vital capacities, and four of these had curves greater than 60 degrees. In our experience curves of this type produce

more cosmetically objectionable deformities than thoracic or lumbar curves of the same magnitude, especially when the curves are long.

COMBINED THORACIC AND LUMBAR CURVES (DOUBLE MAJOR CURVE). In the study of Ponseti and Friedman this pattern was found in 37% of patients, the two curves being present from onset and essentially equal. The thoracic curve was usually to the right and included five or six vertebrae from T5 or T6 to T10 or T11. Its apex was at T7 or T8. The lumbar curve was usually to the left and included five or six vertebrae from T10 or T11 to L3 or L4. Its apex was at L1 or L2. Often a neutral or unrotated vertebra was common to the adjacent ends of the curves. The prognosis as to cosmesis in this pattern, first noticed at the average age of 12.3 years, was good, since the trunk usually remained well aligned when the curves increased simultaneously. The study of Collis and Ponseti more than 20 years after skeletal maturity supported this favorable cosmetic prognosis. After ossification of the epiphyses of the iliac crests was complete, the lumbar curves increased an average of only 9 degrees and the thoracic curves only 11 degrees; after fusion of these epiphyses, the lumbar curves increased an average of only 7 degrees and the thoracic curves only 9 degrees. Deformity of the back and decrease in the vital capacity were less severe than in single thoracic curves.

SINGLE MAJOR THORACIC CURVE. In the study of Ponseti and Friedman this curve was found in 22% of patients and its onset was earlier than that of any other curve (average age of 11.1 years). It usually included six vertebrae from T5 or T6 to T11 or T12 and had its apex at T8 or T9. Because of the thoracic location of this curve, rotation of the involved vertebrae was usually marked. The curve produced prominence of the ribs on its convex side and depression of the ribs on its concave side and elevation of one shoulder, resulting in an unpleasant deformity (Fig. 82-6). The prognosis was poor when the curve was first noticed before the age of 12 years, presumably because the remaining growth potential was great. In the study of Collis and Ponseti made about 20 years later, curves measuring 60 to 80 degrees when ossification of the epiphyses of the iliac crests was complete were found to increase an average of 28 degrees. Curves of less than 60 degrees or of more than 80 degrees tended to increase less. Only 27% of the curves were less than 75 degrees. Backache was less common in patients with this curve than in the group as a whole. Mild osteoarthritic changes were seen in the roentgenograms in 71% of the patients, and the most severe cardiopulmonary symptoms were found in patients with this curve. The severity of the pulmonary symptoms and of the decrease in vital capacity correlated well with the severity of the curves, especially in curves greater than 80 degrees.

CERVICOTHORACIC CURVE. There were only five patients with this curve in the entire series of Ponseti and Friedman. Although the curve never seemed to become large, the deformity was unsightly because of the elevated shoulder and deformed thorax, which could be but poorly disguised by clothing. The apex usually was at T3 with the curve extending from C7 or T1 to T4 or T5. The curve was usually less flexible. Correction and fusion of this curve when indicated are usually for cosmetic reasons and are usually indicated early for severe deformity.

DOUBLE MAJOR THORACIC CURVES. This pattern was described by Moe. It consists of a short upper thoracic curve often extending from T1 to T5 or T6 with considerable rotation of the vertebrae and other structural changes in combination with a lower thoracic curve extending from T6 to T12 or L1. The upper curve is usually to the left, and the lower is usually to the right (Fig. 82-7). The appearance of patients with this curve is usually better than when a single thoracic curve is present, but because of asymmetry of the neckline produced by the upper curve, this pattern is more deforming than combined dorsal and lumbar curves. In double thoracic curves the fact that the upper curve is highly structural can be overlooked if the roentgenograms, especially the bending films, do not include the lower part of the cervical spine. If only the lower thoracic curve is corrected and fused using the Harrington instruments, the upper curve may not be flexible enough to allow an erect posture. Consequently both curves should usually be corrected and fused.

Winter et al. reported a rare group of patients who appeared emaciated, whose histories indicated a normal appetite but failure to gain weight, and who were found to have scoliosis with an exaggerated thoracic lordosis.

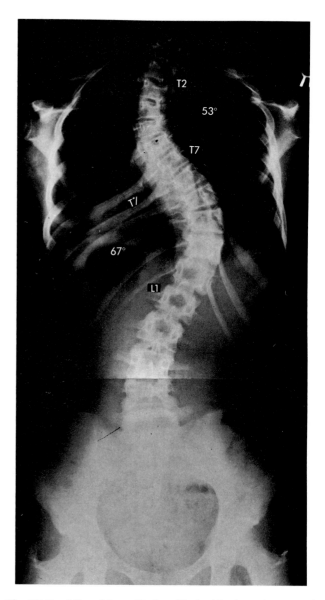

Fig. 82-7 Idiopathic scoliosis with double thoracic curves in girl 14 years of age. Primary or structural upper thoracic curve extends from T2 through T7 and measures 53 degrees, and primary or structural lower thoracic curve extends from T7 through L1 and measures 67 degrees. Shoulders and pelvis are level, and patient is less deformed than in single thoracic curve.

These rare patients do not benefit from brace treatment but should undergo posterior instrumentation and fusion. Harrington instrumentation using contoured rods combined with segmental wiring can be beneficial in reducing or reversing the lordotic thoracic spine. We usually use the Drummond type of segmental wiring with Harrington instrumentation to minimize risks. Cotrel-Dubousset or Texas Scottish Rite Hospital instrumentation can be even more effective in treating this deformity. A direct relationship can be found between the amount of correction of the lordosis and the improvement in respiratory function. Rapid mobilization of these patients with an active pulmonary exercise program yields good results.

CONSIDERATIONS FOR TREATMENT
Structural and Secondary Curves in Scoliosis

In scoliosis structural and secondary curves are different in several ways. In all patients an attempt should be made to identify the structural curve or curves because they are important in prognosis, and when indicated, in deciding in which area of the spine the curve or curves should be treated.

Characteristically structural curves deform and develop structural changes simultaneously and do not tend to correct themselves spontaneously or to retain any correction secured mechanically. On the other hand, secondary curves develop structural changes more slowly, tend to retain much longer the ability to correct themselves spontaneously, and can retain correction secured mechanically. Because secondary curves of long duration do develop structural changes, they may be difficult to distinguish from original structural curves. According to Cobb, any abnormal wedging, angulation, rotation, or position of vertebrae in a lateral spinal curve is a sign of structural change.

As a rule, an original structural curve or curves may be distinguished from secondary ones by the following criteria:

1. The vertebrae in the structural curve are usually displaced from the midline to the side of the convexity of this curve, whereas in a secondary curve they are usually displaced to the side of the concavity of the secondary curve.
2. When there are three curves, the middle one is usually structural.
3. When there are four curves, the two middle ones are usually structural.
4. The greater curve, or the one toward which the trunk is shifted, is the structural curve.
5. The curve that is least flexible and thus least correctable is the structural curve; this is determined by the lateral bending test described by Schmidt. In this test anteroposterior roentgenograms of the spine are made to show how much the structural and secondary curves can be passively corrected before spinal fusion, as is discussed later; in other words, they show the severity of structural change in each curve. The roentgenograms are made with the patient supine and the trunk bent laterally with maximum force, even to the point of discomfort, first to the right and then to the left (see Fig. 82-1). It is important that the pelvis and shoulders be kept flat on the cassette or table. The roentgenograms should include the spine from the first sacral vertebra and the iliac crests inferiorly to and including most of the cervical spine superiorly, even if two

large roentgenograms must be made while the trunk is bent in each direction.

If the head is to be balanced above the pelvis when the patient is erect, any curve or curves of the spine in one direction require a curve or curves in the opposite direction. The formation of this curve or curves in the opposite direction is called compensation. Thus in a structural thoracolumbar curve of 40 degrees convex to the right there must be secondary curves convex to the left the sum of whose angles totals 40 degrees if compensation is to be complete. If the angles of the secondary curves total less than 40 degrees, the curve is called decompensated, and if the total is more than 40 degrees, the curve is said to be overcompensated. These secondary curves develop both above and below the structural curve or curves. However, because the lumbar spine is more mobile and more efficient mechanically, it always provides a maximum secondary curve that is as low in the lumbar spine as possible.

Nonsurgical Treatment

Because there is no reliable method for accurately predicting which curves will progress, observation is the primary treatment of all curves. At present a roentgenogram of the spine is the only definitive documentation of curve size and progression. Attempts have been made to monitor external contours with measurement of the rib hump, measurement of the trunk rotation angle with a "scoliometer," and use of contour devices such as moiré topography and computer-generated images. These methods may be useful in certain small curves in low-risk patients, but periodic evaluation of the spine with roentgenograms still is necessary. In general, young patients with mild curves can be examined every 6 to 12 months. Adolescents with larger degrees of curvature should be examined every 3 to 4 months. Generally accepted guidelines for observation of scoliotic curves are as follows:

1. Curves of less than 20 degrees in skeletally immature patients should be examined roentgenographically every 6 months. Periods between examinations frequently are lengthened when curves are small and are not progressing.
2. Curves of less than 20 degrees in skeletally mature patients usually do not require further evaluation.
3. Curves of more than 20 degrees in skeletally immature patients should be examined every 3 to 4 months with standing posteroanterior roentgenograms. Orthotic treatment is considered for curve progression beyond 25 degrees or for smaller curves (20 degrees) when cosmetic deformity already is present.
4. Curves of 30 to 40 degrees in skeletally mature patients usually do not require treatment, but in view of recent studies indicating the potential for progression in adulthood, these patients should be ob-

served with standing posteroanterior roentgenograms for 2 to 3 years after skeletal maturity.

Orthotic Treatment

The use of bracing for the nonsurgical treatment of idiopathic scoliosis by Blount, by Moe, and by others has been effective enough to alter the treatment in skeletally immature patients. We have found that an efficient Milwaukee brace, conscientiously worn, will halt the increase in most mild or moderate curves. We believe that treatment consisting only of observation of an increasing curve until the patient is mature or the curve becomes severe enough to justify fusion is rarely if ever realistic.

Employing the guides formulated by Lonstein et al., we have attempted to apply brace treatment appropriately, using such factors as skeletal age, menstrual history, and iliac epiphyses, along with an evaluation of cosmetic deformity or structural change that is both subjective and objective. The "probability of progression" factors from Lonstein et al. provide numeric values to add to commonsense judgments on which we have relied in the past. We still use the 20-degree level as a rule to consider bracing. Surface electrical stimulation to replace bracing has been largely abandoned because of ineffectiveness. Milwaukee or Boston types of underarm braces are more reliable and predictable. Despite the reports of Ponseti and Nachemson, our experience agrees with that of Moe et al. in that we see many adults with painful scoliosis in whom operative treatment has resulted in relief. Adults with curves of 60 degrees or more stand a greater risk of an increasing curvature. Kostiuk, Israel, and Hall found that of 107 adults with scoliosis that was treated surgically 63% sought help because of pain and 55% because of progressive deformity.

Various methods of decreasing or correcting the curves in scoliosis have been devised, and some are discussed later in this chapter. We know of no surgical treatment of scoliosis in which permanent correction has been demonstrated unless spinal fusion of some type has been included in the operation. Posterior instrumentation and segmental instrumentation are established methods of assisting in the correction of curves and of providing internal fixation, but they must be combined with spinal fusion. Recently anterior release and interbody fusion at multiple levels have been combined with posterior surgery to improve correction and decrease the incidence of pseudoarthrosis.

There is little if any evidence that structural scoliosis can be decreased or its increase halted by exercises alone.

In 1973, Dubousset noted growth-related progression of curves after solid posterior fusion in young patients with paralytic scoliosis. He termed this the "crankshaft phenomenon" because the entire spine and trunk gradually rotated and deformed as the scoliosis progressed. In 1989, Dubousset, Herring, and Schufflebarger reported

40 spinal fusions done before Risser stage 1 for idiopathic and paralytic scoliosis in children younger than 12 years of age. Thirty-nine patients who had posterior fusions alone had progressive angulation and rotation of the spine; none had a pseudarthrosis or hardware failure. The more immature the patient at the time of fusion, the greater the progression of the deformity. The one patient who had anterior and posterior arthrodesis for lordoscoliosis had no progression. These authors attribute postoperative bending of a fusion to asymmetry of remaining growth and suggest that anterior fusion or hemiepiphysiodesis may be required to achieve stable correction in younger patients.

Surgical Treatment

CONSIDERATIONS FOR CORRECTION OF CURVES AND FOR SPINAL FUSION. The normal thoracic spine is relatively inflexible, and in scoliosis it is even more so because of secondary changes in the ribs and other supporting structures. Casts used in correcting curves were less efficient in the thoracic spine than in the lumbar. Significant correction of a high thoracic curve was often complicated by traction neuritis of the cervical or brachial plexus if a turnbuckle cast was used. High thoracic curves cause severe deformities such as elevation of the shoulder, prominence of the scapula, and projection of the ribs or razorback deformity, all on the convex side of the curve (see Fig. 82-6). Therefore surgery is indicated earlier than in lower thoracic curves, although the fundamental indications for surgery must be considered in each specific patient. In general then, the higher the curve in the thoracic spine, the more severe is the deformity, the more difficult it is to correct, and the earlier surgery is indicated. Conversely the lower the curve in the thoracic spine, the greater is the compensation by secondary curves, the less is the deformity, the more easily the curve can be corrected, and the later surgery is indicated.

In lumbar scoliosis usually there is less deformity. Although rotation of the spine may cause the lumbar muscles to bulge unilaterally, this bulge never approaches the severe prominence (razorback deformity) produced by the same amount of rotation of the thoracic spine. The lumbar spine is much more flexible and from a mechanical standpoint more easily controlled by apparatus designed to correct the scoliosis. Tilting of the fifth lumbar vertebra, whether developmental or paralytic, exerts either an exaggerative or corrective influence on the primary lumbar curve and must always be considered in treatment.

CONSIDERATIONS OF CARDIOPULMONARY FUNCTION. Patients with severe deformity of the thorax have a high incidence of chronic pulmonary disease, have frequent late cardiac failure, and tend to die prematurely. Many studies have been made of the cardiopulmonary function of patients with idiopathic and paralytic scoliosis. Although the findings of many of the studies do not necessarily reinforce those of the others, several general statements can be made from these findings. Using ordinary pulmonary function studies with spirometry, a measurable decrease in pulmonary function can be found in almost all patients with significant scoliosis. According to pulmonary physiologists, most of this decrease in function is caused by restrictive lung disease and is most readily demonstrated in the vital capacity. Although the severity of the curve or of the thoracic deformity does not correlate exactly with the decrease in the vital capacity, it is generally agreed that the more severe the curve or deformity, the more severe is the decrease in the vital capacity. Opinions vary concerning the effect on the vital capacity of the usual methods of treating scoliosis. The application of a Risser localizer or any other type of corrective cast decreases the vital capacity immediately. The Milwaukee brace is said to be less harmful in this respect, and the halo traction device is said not to decrease significantly the vital capacity. This harmful effect of immobilization with casts is only temporary, however, because in the reports of Gazioglu et al. and of Makley et al. the vital capacity definitely improved above the level present before surgery when the patient was examined several months after having resumed normal activities without any restrictive or corrective devices. In the study of Makley et al. the vital capacity definitely increased, but since vital capacity is often measured as a percent of normal related to the height of the patient, when the height increases after surgery the expected normal also increases and any actual increase in the vital capacity may be lost in the computation. Johnson and Westgate demonstrated that the vital capacity was best estimated on the nondeformed height, especially with curves greater than 60 degrees. The nondeformed height was obtained by dividing the arm span by 1.03 in men and 1.01 in women. Using the regression equations of Cook et al., the predicted vital capacity of preoperative patients could be obtained. A vital capacity of 100% to 80% was considered normal; 80% to 60% mild restriction; 60% to 40% moderate restriction; and less than 40% severe restriction. Westgate, Fisch, and Langer, as well as Moe, reported that correction and fusion using the Harrington instrumentation did not improve the average vital capacity or maximum breathing capacity but might improve arterial oxygen saturation. Even if the importance of these findings is minimized, it does seem obvious that correction and fusion of a spinal curve, either idiopathic or paralytic, at least prevent further deterioration of pulmonary function because they decrease the thoracic deformity or prevent it from increasing.

In the evaluation before surgery, pulmonary function studies are usually indicated in patients with paralytic scoliosis or with idiopathic or congenital scoliosis when the curves are severe or are associated with a significant kyphosis. All adults should have thorough cardiopulmonary function studies before surgery. We do not routinely obtain special pulmonary function studies in patients with idiopathic curves of less than 50 or 60 degrees as measured by the Cobb method unless warranted by some special circumstance. Garrett, Perry, and Nickel advocated a policy requiring a tracheostomy before surgery in any patient with paralytic scoliosis whose vital capacity is less than 30% of the predicted normal. We have in general used this policy but have found that the indications for tracheostomy can be safely narrowed if the patient spends several days after surgery in an adequately staffed intensive care unit in which respiratory functions can be constantly supervised and in which mechanical aids for respiration are readily available.

INDICATIONS FOR CORRECTION OF CURVES AND FOR SPINAL FUSION. Nonsurgical treatment of scoliosis is possibly more important than surgical treatment, but one must be able during nonsurgical treatment to recognize the indications for surgery so that treatment may be changed accordingly. The indications are not always definite, but the following are the chief ones:

1. *An increasing curve in a growing child.* The spine can be safely fused in a young child. Solid fusion of the spine causes longitudinal growth in the fused area to cease or at least to be severely retarded. But the lengthening of the spine brought about by correcting the curve or curves usually exceeds the loss of longitudinal growth caused by any fusion. And as Blount has said, a moderately short but straight trunk is better than a very short and crooked one. When the scoliosis is not severe and is either not increasing or is being controlled by bracing or other conservative means, consideration may be given to postponing surgical treatment in the young child possibly up to adolescence in deference to trunk growth. This suggestion must not be used to justify withholding surgery when deformity is increasing. It is highly preferable, however, to postpone fusion as long as possible, with the important provision that the scoliosis is not increasing or is increasing very slowly and is being controlled by bracing or other conservative means. It has been generally believed that when growth of the spine is complete, the scoliosis almost always ceases to increase. Risser pointed out a valuable sign in determining when growth of the spine has ceased in an individual patient. He found that the epiphyses of the iliac crests gradually ossify from anteriorly to posteriorly and that growth of the spine continues until this ossification reaches the posterosuperior iliac spines and turns medially and inferiorly toward the sacroiliac joints. He and others have stated that growth of the spine then usually ceases, and an increase in idiopathic scoliosis is unlikely. But more recently in many patients with idiopathic scoliosis being treated conservatively, curves have been found to increase for a year or more after ossification of the epiphyses of the iliac crests is complete. Therefore some surgeons have proposed that the time of fusion rather than the time of completion

of ossification of these epiphyses is a more reliable sign. There are indications that the time of fusion of the ring epiphyses to the vertebral bodies is more significant in this regard. Establishing the skeletal age by studying roentgenograms of the hand and wrist is another method of determining when the skeleton is mature. A skeletal age of 16 years in a female and 18 years in a male is a reasonably conservative indication of skeletal maturity. The relationship between the time when curves cease to increase and the appearance of the several signs used in determining skeletal maturation seems to vary considerably. Although completion of ossification of the ring epiphyses of the vertebral bodies is probably the most important single sign of the maturing skeleton, no one sign can be used alone as a definite indication that a curve will not increase in an individual patient.

2. *A severe deformity with asymmetry of the trunk in an adolescent, regardless of whether growth of the spine has ceased.*

3. *In older patients pain that cannot be controlled by conservative measures.* The amount of correction obtainable is often small, and the chief aim of treatment should be to produce a solid fusion. Pain in young children or adolescents with scoliosis requires extensive investigation for a cause of pain and curvature other than idiopathic scoliosis.

PATIENT ORIENTATION. An essential part of a successful spinal fusion and instrumentation is patient orientation. We agree with Harrington that successful surgery includes (1) spending time with patients to gain their confidence and allay hidden fears, (2) showing patients examples of the expected results or introducing them to other patients with whom they may confer, and (3) explaining to patients the surgery and its limitations, as well as its benefits and risks.

CORRECTION OF CURVES. The first aim in the treatment of scoliosis is to restore the symmetry of the trunk by centering the first thoracic vertebra above the sacrum and at the same time keeping the pelvis and shoulders level. The second and equally important aim is to straighten the structural curves enough, primarily in the thoracic area, to halt the deterioration in pulmonary function and to minimize the unsightly deformity of the thorax. Right and left bending roentgenograms and a standing posteroanterior roentgenogram of the entire spine are made to determine which curves are structural, which are secondary, and which should be included in the fusion. As already stated, any structural changes in a curve produce asymmetry in the side bending roentgenograms. As a general rule, unless the curves are relatively mild, all thoracic structural curves should be included in the fusion. In combined double major curves of equal size on the standing roentgenogram and involving the dorsal and lumbar areas, the thoracic curve is often highly structural and the lumbar curve is only mildly

so and will correct almost completely on side bending against the curve. In these instances, especially with posterior instrumentation, fusing only the thoracic curve usually is preferable because the lumbar curve usually will accommodate itself to the angle of the residual thoracic curve after fusion. King et al. found that selective thoracic fusion gave excellent results in their type II curves when the inferior fusion level was the stable vertebra. If the patient is immature, and therefore it is known that growth will continue, one must continue to observe the lumbar curve for any increase until maturity.

Localizer cast. The correction is obtained by applying pressure localized posterolaterally at a point level with the apex of the curve while traction is exerted on the head and pelvis. Thus the apex of the curve is forced laterally between the ends of the curve, which are relatively fixed by the traction. Risser used this jacket almost exclusively because it corrects the curve as well as the turnbuckle cast did and corrects angulation of the ribs even better. There are several advantages of this type of cast. The patient can walk. The patient's position in the cast is not changed by manipulation of the cast as in a turnbuckle or other sectioned cast. The secondary curves are not immobilized in increased angulation, and the spine is "in more or less compensation." When the cast has been applied and does not satisfactorily correct the curve, both Risser and Moe recommended that it be wedged, while fresh, level with the apex of the curve. When the alignment of the body and compensation of the spine are carefully watched, this cast can be used in the long fusion usually recommended for the collapsing type of neuromuscular scoliosis caused by poliomyelitis. Instrumentation, including segmental fixation, has largely replaced cast correction and immobilization in the treatment of neuromuscular scoliosis. Molded plastic jackets now are used widely instead of casts for external support.

Modified Cotrel (EDF) cast. Moe used the Risser table or the Risser attachments for the Bell table to apply casts patterned after those used by Cotrel in France. The cast is applied in one piece using two fabric slings looped around the waist superior to the iliac crests and crossed anteriorly and posteriorly so that as distal traction is applied to the slings and thus to the pelvis, the waistline is molded well proximal to the iliac crests. A disposable halter is used for head traction. The fabric slings are placed between the two layers of stockinette so that they will not adhere to the plaster and can be removed after the cast is applied. Cotrel applied the cast over the two layers of stockinette only. Moe usually applied in addition thin felt padding around the neck, shoulder, and pelvis. When the cast was used to correct curves before surgery, Moe recommended that a heavy layer of felt or other padding be applied to the entire anterior aspect of the pelvic and shoulder girdles so that pressure on localized areas of the skin will be minimal during the several hours the patient is prone on the operating table.

■ *TECHNIQUE (MOE).* Place the patient supine on a Risser or Bell table. Apply the two layers of stockinette, the fabric slings for pelvic traction, a halter for head traction, and any padding desired. Then apply strong pelvic and head traction and apply rapidly a cast similar to the Risser localizer cast. Next place a canvas strap 15 to 20 cm wide transversely across the table beneath the patient's back at the level of the axillae; attach it to the table frame on the side of the body opposite the rib prominence, apply it smoothly around the thorax over the rib prominence, and turn it 90 degrees to rise vertically to the overhead winch of the Bell table or to the overhead attachment of the Risser table. Just before the plaster dries tighten the strap securely against the outside of the cast for corrective molding. After the cast has dried remove the halter and the pelvic traction straps and trim the cast as desired over the abdomen and chest, and window it posteriorly if it is to be left in place during surgery. This cast also may be applied after surgery to protect spinal instrumentation.

DISTRACTION TECHNIQUES

The early assumption that the spinal cord moved up and down with vertebral motion has been replaced by evidence that the cord actually changes length as it accommodates the difference in vertebral positions. These length changes have been shown to be an accordion-like response of the fibers within the spinal cord. The neural canal, being posterior to the vertebral body mass, is therefore lengthened when the spine flexes and shortened when it extends. In the lengthened position the fibers of the spinal cord were shown to be in a linear pattern with long and slender blood vessels. When the spine is extended and the cord shortens, the fibers assume a parallel, wavy form with the blood vessels tortuous and broad. The cervical portion of the spinal cord lengthens 25 mm between the extremes of full flexion and extension with an average of 3.6 mm per segment. In the lumbar area the length changes average 15 mm, or 3 mm per segment. The least extensible portion of the spine, which is of greatest concern to the surgeon in the treatment of scoliosis, is the thoracic region. Here there is only a 10 mm difference in length of the cord, or an average of 0.8 mm per segment. The studies of Brieg have shown that as the cord is stretched over a mass, such as a protruding disc, the fluidity of the spinal cord tends to distribute the tension so that the degree of damage is not as great as would otherwise be anticipated. These findings, then, dictate a caution to the surgeon treating scoliosis to take care in altering the length of the thoracic portion of the spine.

Halo-femoral Distraction

Perry and Nickel in 1959 introduced a halo device that provides stable fixation while remaining quite comfortable. Moe reported his results of the combination of this device with femoral pins for correcting spinal deformity.

Halo-femoral distraction has been rarely used since spinal instrumentation and spinal cord monitoring have been developed more extensively. The need for supplemental correction of severe stiff curves and for functional monitoring of an unanesthetized patient has greatly diminished.

The halo may be used as follows:
1. Cervical spine stabilization
   a. Severe cervical muscle paralysis
   b. Cervical fractures
   c. Cervical spine deformity in rheumatoid arthritis
   d. Extensive cervical laminectomy
2. Correction of more distal spine deformities
   a. Halo-femoral traction
   b. Halo-pelvic traction

HALO APPLICATION

■ *TECHNIQUE.* The halo and pins are sterilized. A thorough shampoo of the hair is all that is needed before application. With the hair wet, pin insertion is easier without entangling the hair. Skin preparation can include shaving only in the immediate areas of pin insertion. Smaller children usually require general anesthesia, but local anesthesia is used routinely in older patients. Not only the skin but also the periosteum must be infiltrated thoroughly with the local anesthetic when this means is chosen. Preselecting the pin sites through the halo will keep the area of infiltration to a small skin wheal.

The halo must be at or below the maximum diameter of the skull. The front pins should be centered in the groove at the upper margin of the eyebrows between the supraciliary ridge and the frontal prominences. The halo then extends about ⅛ inch (3.2 mm) above the ear, care being taken not to allow the halo to touch the pinnae, which may result in skin necrosis. A bit more distance is allowed between the skull and halo posteriorly and anteriorly. Although some prefer keeping the pin insertions within the hairline, this requires a more posterior location in the temporalis muscle, a site more likely to produce a pin reaction from the action of the temporalis muscle during chewing and also more likely to be painful. The bone is also thinner in this area. Involvement of the temporalis artery also must be avoided.

With an assistant or positioning device holding the halo in the appropriate position, introduce the pins and tighten two diagonally opposed pins simultaneously. Continue this until the four pins just engage the bone. Then continue tightening diagonally located pairs of pins with a torque screwdriver to about 5½ inch-pounds for adults. Using only the fingertips and not the palm on a short screwdriver will give a final tension of about 5½ inch-pounds. We have used 3.5 to 4 inch-pounds for halos on small children. Alternate tightening of the pins prevents migration of the halo to an asymmetric position. After all pins are tightened to 5½ inch-pounds, unscrew each about one-quarter turn. This will allow the rotary stretch of the skin to return to a relaxed position, preventing any skin necrosis. Finally secure the pins to the halo with a locknut. Currently we recommend 8 to 10 inch-pounds of torque on the pins for adults with normal bone density. We have found loosening to be less of a problem with tighter pins.

AFTERTREATMENT. The halo pins may be cleansed at the pin-skin interface with hydrogen peroxide daily, but we usually recommend only daily inspection and application of a small amount of Betadine ointment. They should not be tightened daily as has been the habit with the use of tongs because the pins rarely enter the skull more than 2 mm, but rather act as a wedge forcing the halo from the skull. In more muscular patients attempts to move the head within the halo may result in pin loosening caused by erosion and accompanied by an inflammatory process. When used with a cast that extends down around the pelvis, apparently little stress on the pins occurs and loosening is rarely a problem. When attached to one of the commercially available plastic halo-vests, loosening of the skull pins is more frequent, and we usually check these every 2 to 3 weeks for tension. The indications for changing the pins are serous drainage, inflammation, or a clicking sensation. The pins should otherwise be undisturbed. If a pin must be replaced, this is achieved by inserting a new sterilized pin into an adjacent hole before removal of the offending pin. Three pins alone will not long hold a halo. O'Brien, Yau, and Hodgson recommend (1) that slipping of the skull halo be prevented by routine tightening of the skull pins 1 week after their fitting and (2) that six pins be used when treatment is to be prolonged.

Halo removal is painless if performed carefully. All traction should be removed from the halo and the pins removed in reverse of the order in which they were applied. External nuts are removed, and then diagonal pairs of pins are loosened and removed. It is important than an assistant stabilize the halo while the pins are removed to prevent pain as the number of holding pins decreases. The pin sites usually promptly close and heal with small scars that are usually cosmetically acceptable.

FEMORAL PIN INSERTION

■ *TECHNIQUE.* Prepare both knee areas thoroughly and drape them in a sterile field. Introduce a large,

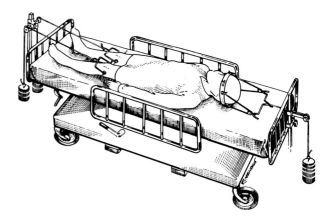

Fig. 82-8 Halo-femoral traction for severe scoliosis curvatures.

smooth Steinmann pin through a stab wound into each distal diaphyseal area well above the epiphysis. The addition of a plaster cuff incorporating the pin will prevent medial or lateral migration and decrease pin tract infections.

AFTERTREATMENT. Traction is begun with about 6 kg on the head and 3 kg on each leg (Fig. 82-8). Weights are gradually and equally added to a total of 12 kg on each end. Periods of traction exceeding 10 days have not added improved angular corrections. In pelvic obliquity most of the lower extremity weight can be placed on the high-side limb.

Rather than confine the patient to bed, a halo wheelchair may be substituted as designed by Stagnara. Winter has used this technique with the patient spending days in the chair and nights back in halo-femoral traction in bed.

Letts, Palakar, and Bobechko studied 10 patients with an average curve of 81 degrees. Halo-femoral traction was used over a 2- to 3-week period with 1.8 kg added per day to a maximum total of 18.1 kg. They showed an average improvement of 34 degrees (41%), mostly within the first week. Subsequent Harrington instrumentation added 13.5 degrees (16%) for a total of 47 degrees (57%) correction. They recommend preliminary traction for curves greater than 65 degrees, but not for more than 10 days. Nachemson and Nordwall believe that only the more severe but still flexible curves greater than 90 degrees in patients over 20 years of age need treatment by their two-stage procedure; rigid curves of more than 90 degrees would be treated with halo-pelvic or halo-femoral traction preoperatively. Again, halo-femoral traction *rarely* is indicated.

Halo-pelvic Distraction

DeWald and Ray first reported the pelvic halo in 1970; it was designed for use in patients with severe pulmonary restriction, pressure sores from a cast, soft tissue contractures, or inability to control pelvic tilt and rota-

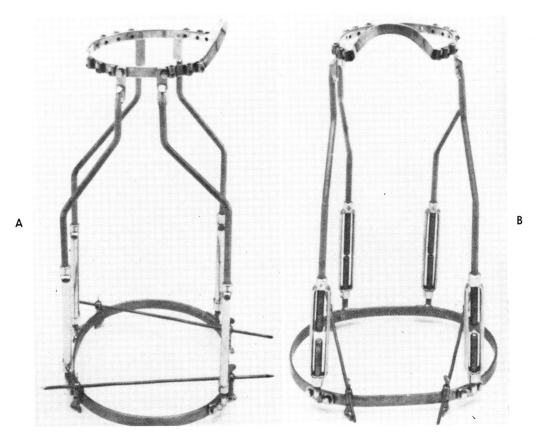

Fig. 82-9 Halo-pelvic distraction apparatus. **A,** Lateral view. **B,** Anterior view. (From Dewald RL and Ray RD: J Bone Joint Surg 52-A:233, 1970.)

tion (Fig. 82-9). Halo-pelvic distraction is now used rarely, if ever. Segmental spinal instrumentation and other internal spinal fixation devices largely have displaced it. The pelvic halo provides gradual and controlled forces that are excellent in treating severe, rigid spinal deformities, and it allows unrestricted respiratory excursions, ambulation, and easy access for spinal surgery. The complications include skin intolerance with pin tract infections, bowel perforation, nerve palsy and paraplegia, hip subluxation, and degenerative cervical arthritis. Further, the areas for obtaining grafts are poorly accessible.

Clark, Hsu, and Yau have emphasized that the deformed spine is a nonhomogenous, viscoelastic structure composed of many component parts and exhibiting the biomechanical properties of elasticity and plasticity. Biologic materials have a complex behavior under load. Under consideration are the duration of the applied load, the deformation of strain rate, the rate of application of the load, and yielding that produces permanent deformation or plastic strain. As pointed out by Nachemson and Elfström, these factors have a bearing on the application of externally applied means for correction of deformity. These biomechanical properties are further affected by the cause of the spine deformity, its clinical behavior, and any surgical intervention. During the creep phase of distraction there is a time-dependent relaxation of struc-

tures resisting correction of deformity during distraction (Fig. 82-10). The gradient and length of this creep phase are a function of the rigidity of the curve, the angle, and the level of deformity. This explains the great variation from deformity to deformity. Collagen fibers are the extension limiting constituent, with the ligaments stiffening abruptly after 30% to 60% strain. The stress-strain relationship in nerves is influenced greatly by the rate of application of the load, with slow stretching producing a greater increase in length without disturbance of function. The turnbuckles originally used on the four uprights have been modified by other investigators and in the system of O'Brien et al. have been replaced by a spring scale to measure distraction forces.

Kalamchi et al. reported on 150 consecutive patients treated with the halo-pelvic device and emphasized that it must be reserved for spinal deformity in which all other means of surgical correction will not yield a satisfactory result. Their indications for use of the device are about the same as those of O'Brien et al. listed below.

O'Brien et al. have also had extensive experience with the use of halo-pelvic traction in Hong Kong. Their indications for halo-pelvic traction include (1) kyphosis; (2) severe scoliosis (over 100 degrees and rigid) with associated problems such as pelvic obliquity, respiratory insufficiency, or marked kyphotic elements; (3) salvage procedure following failed spinal surgery; and (4) unstable

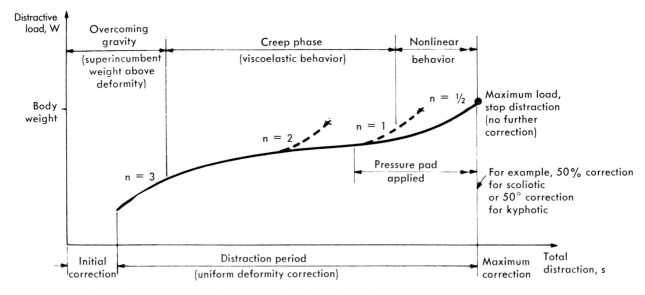

Fig. 82-10 Halo-pelvic distraction divided into three phases: overcoming gravity, creep phase, and nonlinear behavior. *n,* Rate of distraction in terms per day; *t,* time in days from beginning of distraction period; *W,* applied distractive force; *s,* total increase in length between skull and pelvis. (From Clark JA et al: Clin Orthop 110:90, 1975.)

spine secondary to laminectomy, malignancy, or trauma.

They have recommended the following procedures for preoperative assessment:

1. Myelography in all patients to rule out any intraspinal pathologic condition causing cord compression such as in kyphotic deformities of any cause or diastematomyelia
2. Tomograms of the deformity to show the presence of any spontaneous fusion, which would require osteotomies before any traction
3. Lateral roentgenograms of the cervical spine to provide a baseline for comparison with subsequent films of the neck during distraction
4. Intravenous pyelograms to discover any urinary tract abnormalities, which are present in 20% of patients with congenital deformities
5. Bending films to define the flexibility of the curve
6. Respiratory function studies to be used as a baseline for evaluation

O'Brien et al. emphasize that following application of the halo and pelvic hoop for a kyphotic deformity, a primary anterior osteotomy or excision of a vertebral body should be accomplished. If the spine is not "springy" at the conclusion of this procedure or if a spontaneous fusion is present in this area, a posterior osteotomy must be done. Distraction then can begin with maximum protection of neural structures. Following the period of distraction, when the maximum correction has been reached, the chest is reopened and anterior strut grafting is carried out. Following recovery from this stage of the procedure a posterior fusion is also added as the final stage. The halo-pelvic distraction apparatus can then be maintained for a time and is finally replaced by a properly applied and fitted plaster cast.

O'Brien et al. also recommend that psychologic aspects of treatment be given consideration by letting prospective patients see and talk with those presently under treatment. This demonstrates that they may be ambulatory and that their deformities can be helped by the treatment.

APPLICATION OF PELVIC HALO

■ *TECHNIQUE.* General anesthesia is used. They emphasize that the pelvic pins should enter a point on the iliac crest anteriorly opposite the rough gluteal tubercle and emerge posteriorly just medial to the posterosuperior iliac spine (Fig. 82-11, *A*); they believe that this placement is responsible for the few pin tract infections in a large group of patients so treated. Fitting of the drilling jig is likewise important to ensure the proper path of the penetrating and self-tapping pelvic pin introduced with a carpenter's brace (Fig. 82-11, *B*).

AFTERTREATMENT. Postoperatively the patient should have no more than minor discomfort from either the skull halo or the pelvic halo. Continuing severe pain indicates something wrong, especially in regard to the pelvic halo. After several days the extension bars are fitted between the cranial halo and the pelvic halo with the patient awake (Fig. 82-11, *C*). O'Brien et al. use large spring balances with an upward distracting force of 20 to 30 pounds (9 to 13.5 kg) (Fig. 82-12). The protruding pins in the pelvic region are covered with dry dressings; if drainage begins, appropriate antibiotics are given. Distraction is increased at the rate of 2 or 3 mm per day. If neck pain develops, the distraction is discontinued for several days. A daily neurologic examina-

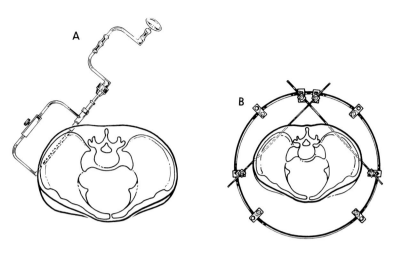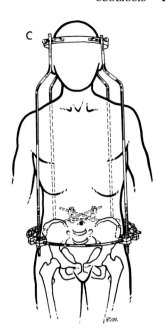

Fig. 82-11 Halo-pelvic distraction device. **A** and **B,** Pelvic pin insertion. **C,** Extension bars fitted between cranial and pelvic halos.

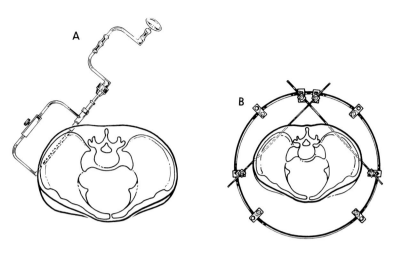

Fig. 82-12 Compression spring at base of extension bar for measuring forces. (From O'Brien JP: Acta Orthop Scand Suppl, No 163, 1975.)

tion of the patient is essential, and a clinical examination of those nerves most prone to injury is carefully performed each day. This evaluation includes not only the lower extremities but the upper extremities and cranial nerves as well. To evaluate any overdistraction of the neck, especially at the occipital and atlantoaxial joints, a lateral view of the cervical spine is included each time roentgenograms of the deformed spine are made.

• • •

In a study of 104 patients treated by O'Brien et al. the average time in the halo-pelvic apparatus was 7½ months. The average correction of deformity included tuberculous kyphosis, 31%; paralytic scoliosis, 51%; idiopathic scoliosis, 42%; congenital kyphoscoliosis, 26%; and neurofibromatous kyphoscoliosis, 43%. The most common significant complication of halo-pelvic distraction is in the cervical spine; degenerative changes in the posterior joints were found in 34% and avascular necrosis of the upper pole of the odontoid in 17% of patients. Cranial nerve neurapraxias occurred in 7% of the patients and brachial plexus palsy in 3%. The halo-pelvic apparatus is therefore not a casual alternative treatment for spinal deformities but rather must always be a part of a carefully planned approach in the management of severe spinal curvatures when other treatment methods are not acceptable.

Halo Cast

Combining the cranial halo with a Risser cast has provided ambulatory treatment of cervical fractures and after cervicothoracic fusions. The neck piece of the cast is replaced by well-padded shoulder straps that support the halo uprights (Fig. 82-13, *A*). A halo yoke described by Houtkin and Levine was a major modification over the original large overhead assembly present on the halo cast assemblies. Anderson and Bradford presented a low-profile halo assembly, which was simple in design and had a wide margin of adjustability, an improved cosmetic acceptance, and a low cost (Fig. 82-13, *B*). Several modifications are now available.

Halo Vest

Semirigid plastic vests with shoulder straps and attachments for a skull halo are commercially available from several sources. They are fitted from measurements and are usually lined with synthetic plastic "sheepskin." Indications include cervicothoracic and cervical fusion and injuries. They do not provide immobilization as secure as a halo cast that includes the pelvis for support and potentially they are only as secure as the patient allows. All straps and adjustments are accessible and can be loosened.

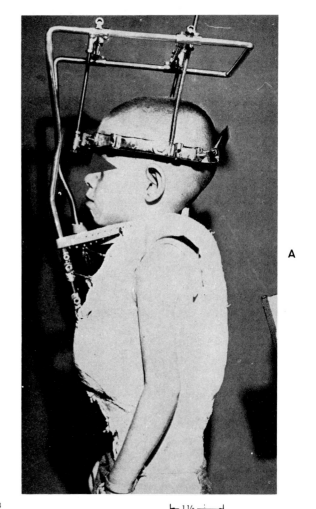

Fig. 82-13 **A**, Halo attached to patient and to body cast. **B,** Low-profile halo assembly. (**A,** From Garrett AL et al: J Bone Joint Surg 43-A:474, 1961; **B,** from Anderson S and Bradford DS: Clin Orthop 103:72, 1974.)

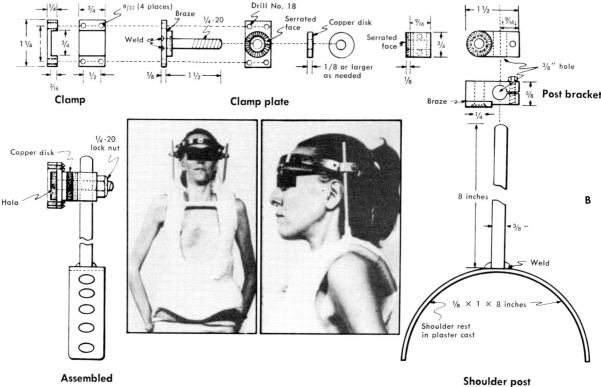

SPINAL FUSION
Determination of Fusion Area

The minimum fusion area is said to include every vertebra in the primary curve. In idiopathic scoliosis the minimum fusion area should also include all vertebrae that are rotated in the same direction as those in the primary curve (see Fig. 82-5). Even with this additional stipulation, fusing only the minimum fusion area is rarely recommended. Such a fusion might be satisfactory in a congenital curve or in a progressive idiopathic curve in a very young child in whom keeping the length of the fusion as short as possible is desirable to minimize the loss in height of the trunk. But even then, a brace will probably be necessary to control the unfused areas of the spine. The maximum fusion area has traditionally been described as the area of the spine that includes the one or more structural curves with the addition of enough vertebrae at each end so that the end vertebrae will be parallel to each other and transverse to the long axis of the trunk. A fusion area of this type is usually best suited for paralytic scoliosis in which both stabilizing the trunk and treating the deformity are desirable. When one considers the minimum and maximum fusion areas as just described, the area of fusion usually recommended includes the minimum area (all the primary curves plus the vertebrae at each end that are rotated in the same direction as those in the curve) with the addition of at least one vertebra at each end.

Side bending roentgenograms are especially important in selection of the fusion area (see Fig. 82-1). For example, in a right thoracic, left lumbar pattern there is usually a large structural thoracic component with the lumbar curve having a large flexible component. In this case thoracic fusion alone is often possible because the lumbar flexibility will allow it to balance and compensate for a surgically corrected curve.

Vertebral rotation, as already mentioned, must be analyzed and the basic principle followed that fusion must extend from neutral to neutral vertebrae. The exceptions to this must be determined from cast-corrected films or bending films. Also, in the lumbar region fusion need not extend to the sacrum if L4 and L5 are rotated. One segment below the end vertebra is sufficient at this lower level, since the extended rotation is less important as the curve approaches the sacrum. The penalty for lack of careful evaluation of the extent of fusion will be lengthening of the curve with loss of correction and usually an unacceptable cosmetic effect.

General Considerations

The most careful study of roentgenograms to determine the exact location and extent of the fusion area is obviously of little value unless during the operation the vertebrae in the operative field can be identified precisely. The sacrum is an unmistakable anatomic landmark, but the contour of the various individual vertebrae is not sufficiently characteristic for exact identification. A method frequently used to identify vertebrae is to make a marker film. The use of superficial marks or scratches on the skin or the injection of dye into the soft tissues before making a marker film has not been reliable in identifying vertebrae. The simplest and most reliable method of establishing a landmark and the one we use consists of pausing briefly to make a marker roentgenogram when the spine has been exposed enough that the spinous processes are accessible. Before the patient is placed on the table, a cassette holder is properly positioned beneath him. Then during the operation a metal marker, usually an instrument, is attached to the spinous process of a vertebra in the fusion area, the operative field is covered by a sterile drape, and a posteroanterior roentgenogram is made. In identifying the vertebra it must be remembered that the spinous processes, especially in the thoracic area, droop inferiorly, usually as far as the body of the next vertebra inferior to the one in question.

The skin incision is best made in a straight line from a level one vertebra superior to the proposed fusion area to a level one vertebra inferior to it. A straight scar improves the appearance of the back, but a curved one over the spinous processes draws attention to any residual curve. When autogenous iliac bone is to be added to the fusion area, it is usually obtained through a vertical incision made just lateral to the posterosuperior iliac spine, avoiding cluneal nerve injury. It need not be made when the level of fusion is in the lower lumbar or in the lumbosacral area because the posterior part of the ilium can be reached by dissecting from the midline incision laterally just superficial to the fascia and deep to the subcutaneous tissue.

The exact techniques of fusion used by various orthopaedic surgeons experienced in the surgical treatment of scoliosis vary in detail, but all aim at forming a fusion plate that is as substantial as possible. Harrington and Dickson made a thorough study of 578 patients with idiopathic scoliosis treated by one of eight methods. Differences among the methods included varying the instrumentation, the use or nonuse of extra autogenous iliac bone grafts, varying the type of cast, and varying the time of ambulation. During this 11-year study, each of the eight groups illustrated a step in the evolution of the design of instrumentation and the change in spinal fusion procedure or postoperative management. They concluded that (1) the spine can be satisfactorily corrected with the Harrington distraction and compression systems providing the maximum correction; (2) the correction is maintained, with a loss of 6% (2.5 degrees); (3) a robust well-developed fusion results from a facet block fusion in the thoracic region with a lateral gutter extension widening the base of the fusion mass in the lumbar region and using autogenous iliac supplemental bone grafts; and (4) external immobilization with a well-molded body cast is necessary for a minimum of 9 months after surgery. Gradual ambulation within days of the fusion, reaching a near normal level by 3 months, promotes early fusion and a robust fusion mass. Other instrumentation systems are successful without external immobilization or with plastic jackets.

Most surgeons, in addition to using all bone available in the fusion area, add other grafts, preferably of autogenous bone and usually from the posterior ilium. When the spinal fusion is performed through a window in the cast, now rarely done, autogenous iliac grafts usually can be obtained satisfactorily if the window is enlarged over the ilium on the convex side of the curve to be fused. When necessary, additional grafts may be obtained by resecting one or more segments of any prominent ribs. We dislike removing grafts from the patient's tibia and believe this is rarely indicated. A large defect in the bone and the osteoporosis of disuse may cause the tibia to be fractured, especially since when the patient is first allowed up, the lack of normal agility and the weight of the plaster cast increase the stresses that the bone must withstand.

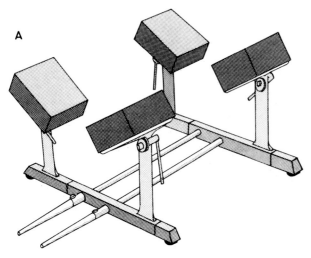

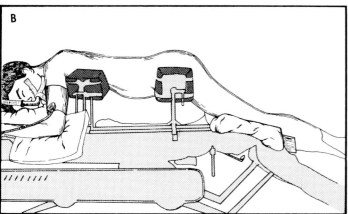

Fig. 82-14   A, Scoliosis operating frame. **B,** Patient in position on frame. (Redrawn from Relton JES and Hall JE: J Bone Joint Surg 49-B:327, 1967.)

With modern techniques of anesthesia and blood replacement, carrying out spinal fusions in two or more stages as was so often done in the past is now rarely, if ever, necessary. If such a staged procedure is necessary, the principle of fusing the apex of the curve during the first stage and then both ends of the curve during the second stage should be followed so that the fusion areas do not overlap at the point of maximum stress. Endotracheal anesthesia, usually with either controlled or assisted respiration, is essential. Equipment for warming blood before transfusion should be used so that rapid replacement of lost blood with refrigerated blood is unnecessary. Access to one or preferably two veins large enough for intravenous infusions should be maintained throughout the operation and the period immediately after surgery. In larger children and adolescents we avoid the veins of the legs for infusions because of the risk of thrombophlebitis in these age groups. All sponges should be weighed and all liquid blood removed by suction from the operative field should be carefully measured. By using appropriate self-retaining retractors, an electrocautery, and wound packing, spinal fusions can be carried out quite satisfactorily with one assistant. Meticulous attention to details of hemostasis will reduce blood loss to less than 1000 ml in most uncomplicated cases.

Autotransfusions of stored blood or of washed red cells obtained from wound suction should be used routinely to help avoid or minimize the use of homologous blood transfusions.

Spinal surgery requires extensive dissection and the possibility of severe blood loss. Relton and Hall first emphasized the role of intraabdominal pressure and designed an apparatus to reduce blood loss (Fig. 82-14). The use of this frame has been beneficial for us as well as other spine surgeons. Modifications of this frame have been reported by Mouradian and Simmons.

The gouges, osteotomes, curets, and other instruments used in the operations should have large long handles so that they may be controlled with both hands. Their edges should be sharp so that forceful use of a mallet can be minimized. A few very small gouges should be available for use in children below the age of 6 years.

Techniques of Fusion

The importance of the technique of fusion in scoliosis is difficult to evaluate because many different techniques have been successful. The classic Hibbs technique was replaced at our clinic by a modification of the intraarticular fusion of the lateral articulations described by Moe and the meticulous dissection around the transverse processes recommended by Goldstein. The fusion techniques of Moe and of Hall are described in Chapter 83. Other techniques are described here for historical interest. When facilities and instrumentation are not available for more modern techniques, these historical techniques may still be useful.

Cobb preferred and used most often the Hibbs technique, which is essentially an extraarticular fusion to which autogenous iliac grafts are added. He described his method in great detail (1958), and his description is recommended. The operation is performed through a window cut in the back of the turnbuckle cast; a marker film made before surgery is essential. After the spine has been exposed, turn long spicules of bone from the spinous processes, laminae, and pedicles across the adjacent intervertebral spaces to lock under laterally bent spicules on the laminae and pedicles of the adjacent vertebrae. Use all bone available in the area to create as many spicules as possible still attached at their bases. However, Cobb recommended leaving intact the superior half of the spinous process of the superior vertebra of the fusion area and the inferior half of the spinous process of the inferior one so that the interspinous ligaments can become attached better, thus resulting in a more normal relationship between the superior and inferior ends of the fusion mass and the adjacent vertebrae. Cobb believed that the time necessary to carry out intraarticular fusion can be better used in obtaining more spicules of bone for bridging the intervertebral spaces. However, he stated that intraarticular fusion may be preferable in the lumbar area but not in the cervical area. He often used cancellous homogenous bone to shorten the operating time and to minimize shock. His results were excellent.

■ *TECHNIQUE (GOLDSTEIN).* At the sites of incision,

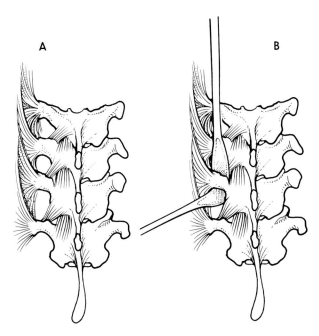

Fig. 82-15 In Goldstein technique muscles and ligaments are stripped from transverse processes in thoracic area with Cobb elevator. **A,** Muscle attachments and ligaments usually seen during exposure of thoracic spine for fusion. **B,** After reflection of all soft tissue structures from laminae, lateral articulations, and transverse processes. (Modified from Goldstein LA and Dickerson RB: Atlas of orthopedic surgery, St Louis, 1969, Mosby–Year Book, Inc.)

infiltrate the skin and subcutaneous tissue with a 1:500,000 solution of epinephrine in saline unless this is contraindicated by the anesthetic agent being used. Next expose the ilium widely through an incision parallel to the posterior two thirds of the iliac crest and obtain cortical and cancellous bone for grafting. Remove the cortex in strips with a gouge or an osteotome and the cancellous bone in strips from the entire exposed surface with a sharp hand gouge. Cut the cortical strips into thin slivers and save the cancellous strips intact. Close the incision over the ilium in layers. Then expose the spine subperiosteally, including the transverse processes in the thoracic area and the lateral articulations in the lumbar area. In the thoracic area carefully strip with a Cobb elevator all of the ligamentous attachments from the transverse processes, including the posterior costotransverse ligaments on the concave side of the curve (Fig. 82-15). In the lumbar area meticulously clean the posterior cortical surface of the spine and remove the capsules of the lateral articulations. Control bleeding with electrocautery and with self-retaining retractors. Thus the operative field is widely exposed with the soft tissues under tension. Using a sharp gouge with both hands, apply firm pressure to the spine and with a twisting motion carefully decorticate it (Fig. 82-16). Have several sharp gouges available and use a mallet only in older adolescents or adults with harder bone. In the lumbar area resect the posterior part of the lateral articulations while decorticating the laminae. In the thoracic area remove the inferior edges of the inferior articular processes, the adjacent bases of

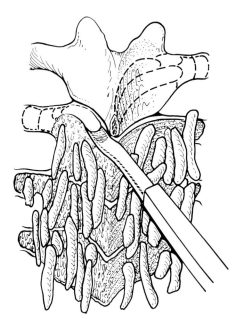

Fig. 82-16 Goldstein technique of spinal fusion (see text). (Redrawn from Goldstein LA: J Bone Joint Surg 41-A:321, 1959.)

the superior articular processes, and the exposed cartilaginous surfaces while decorticating the laminae. Lay the strips of bone thus obtained and some of the bone grafts obtained from the ilium along the lateral edges of the spine, covering the intertransverse spaces, the lateral articulations, and the interlaminar areas. Then distribute the rest of the grafts along the fusion area, making the fusion mass slightly thicker on the concave than on the convex side of the curve. Insert the cancellous grafts first and the cortical grafts last. When using the Harrington instruments, prepare the insertion sites for the distraction hooks before starting the decortication. Then remove the spinous processes from the vertebrae and decorticate the laminae and transverse processes on the concave side of the curve only, but lay the bone chips aside. Next insert the distraction hooks, attach the distraction rod, and correct the curve as much as possible. If a compression rod assembly is also used, attach it and then decorticate the medial part of the laminae on the convex side of the curve and all of the laminae and transverse processes that are not used for hook attachments. For rib hump reduction when not using the compression system, perform an osteotomy of the convex transverse processes (Fig. 82-17). Finally insert the bone grafts. The fusion must include all vertebrae on which a purchase has been made by either distraction or compression hooks.

AFTERTREATMENT. If the curves have been corrected by a cast only, a new localizer cast is applied

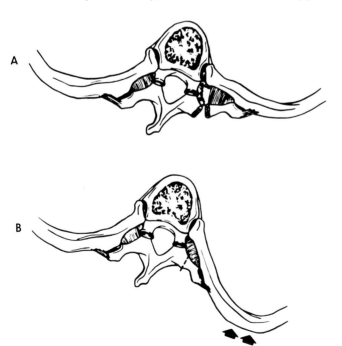

Fig. 82-17   Osteotomy for convex rib hump through transverse process. **A,** Correction after osteotomy and cast application. **B,** Deformity before surgery. (From Goldstein LA: Clin Orthop 93:131, 1973.)

12 to 20 days after surgery and the patient is discharged home to remain in bed for a total of 6 months. If the correction obtained is not being lost and an anteroposterior and two oblique roentgenograms of the fusion area show no evidence of a pseudarthrosis, then a new Risser localizer cast is applied and the patient is allowed to walk. This cast is worn for 3 or 4 months. Thus the average total time a cast is worn is 9 or 10 months. Originally, if Harrington instrumentation was used, patients with thoracic fusions were kept in bed for 3 months and patients with both thoracic and lumbar curves or thoracolumbar curves were kept in bed for 4 months. The localizer cast was worn for an additional month while the patient began to walk. Then a "double shoulder strap cast" was applied and was worn for 2 to 4 months. Thus the average total time of cast immobilization was about 8 months. Early ambulation can produce results equal to or better than those obtained with 3 to 6 months of bed rest. This is the result of secure spinal instrumentation combined with a well-fitted cast. Loss of as little as 5 degrees of correction can be achieved, and the arthrodesis appears to be stronger with vertical loading. The psychologic benefits for the child are immeasurable.

• • •

Leider, Moe, and Winter, in a study of 106 consecutive patients 12 to 20 years old, found that early ambulation after posterior instrumentation and fusion decreased the morbidity and was quite beneficial psychologically. These patients had fusion in an adequately prepared preoperative cast using Harrington instrumentation and autogenous iliac bone grafting. In 7 to 10 days a Risser-Cotrel cast was applied over double stockinette, emphasizing proper molding about the iliac crests and over the apex of the curve. The patients were allowed to walk within 10 days and had a cast change in 4 to 5 months, with a total cast time of 9 months. The loss of correction compared favorably with earlier methods, with a loss of only 5 degrees and a pseudarthrosis rate of 4.7%. A loss greater than 5 degrees indicates poor casting methods, and a change into a new, good cast is mandatory.

■ *TECHNIQUE (RISSER).* Correct the scoliosis by a localizer cast. Bivalve the cast and perform the fusion with the patient out of it. Expose the fusion area subperiosteally. In the dorsal area elevate the posterior half of the lateral facet, curet the lateral joint, and raise a flap of bone from the base of the transverse process and turn it into the joint. In the lumbar area carefully curet the articular facets, make longitudinal and transverse cuts across the facets into the joints, and then impact the resulting fragments of bone into the joints (Fig. 82-18). Next, carry out a Hibbs fusion and add to the fusion area autogenous iliac bone.

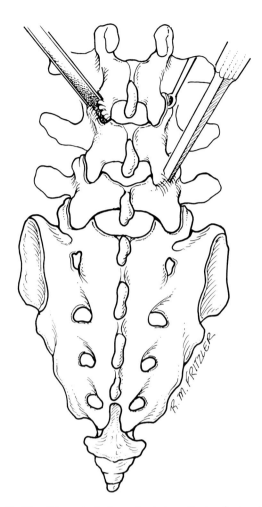

Fig. 82-18 Risser technique for intraarticular fusion in lumbar area (see text). (Redrawn from Moe JH: South Med J 50:79, 1957.)

AFTERTREATMENT. **When the patient has recovered from the anesthetic, the bivalved localizer cast is reapplied. At 7 to 10 days the cast and sutures are removed, and a new localizer cast is applied. The patient is then allowed to be up and to walk. According to Risser, a loss of 2 to 3 degrees of correction with the patient standing and in the cast is acceptable; if greater loss occurs, the cast is inadequate. The cast is changed at intervals of 3 to 4 months until the fusion is mature. According to Risser, because each localizer cast is a corrective one, the correction is less frequently lost than when other casts are used.**

• • •

Risser and Norquist report that of 177 patients treated with a turnbuckle cast and fusion, the correction was maintained in 41%, and of 62 treated with a localizer cast and fusion, the correction was maintained in 68% even though walking was allowed early. We have adopted early ambulation following spinal fusion in uncomplicated idiopathic curves; results have been equal to those reported, and we have found the psychophysiologic benefits tremendous.

Partial Discectomy

Schultz and Hirsch have shown experimentally that in cadaver spines the stiffness in lateral bending of a typical thoracic spine motion segment is in the order of 20 kpcm per degree. This would mean that a curve of 60 degrees over six vertebral levels would require a corrective moment on the order of 200 kpcm. The present methods of correction do not produce moments of this magnitude. It further has been shown that the intervertebral disc and longitudinal ligaments contribute 80% to 90% of the stiffness of the motion segment in lateral bending. The surgical attack on intervertebral discs does significantly decrease resistance to correction as exemplified by the Dwyer and Zielke procedures. Similarly, partial discectomy allows better correction with posterior instrumentation when lateral deviations are great or enables one to improve correction when lateral corrective forces are used such as in casting. Moreover, greater derotations are possible with partial discectomy in conjunction with lateral force correcting procedures.

Fusion with Instrumentation

More complete discussions of various devices are given and techniques of spinal fusion with instrumentation are described in Chapter 83.

HARRINGTON INSTRUMENTATION. In 1972 Harrington reviewed 1055 patients with curves ranging from 35 to 170 degrees; there were 37 different causes, and ages of the patients ranged from 4 to 63 years. The minimum follow-up was 3 years. He drew the following conclusions:

1. The scoliotic spine is structurally unsound in a growing child when the factor is 3 or more, and curvature will progress at an unpredictable rate. The factor is obtained by dividing the number of degrees of curvature by the Cobb method by the number of vertebrae in the curve.
2. The scoliotic spine in the mature patient is structurally unsound when the curve has reached a factor of 5. After maturity progression can be expected in all patients when the factor is 7. Progression or degeneration of the spine proceeds at an unpredictable rate but generally follows that rate cited by Risser of 1 degree per year.
3. When the major curve is located in the thoracic segment of the spine, the structurally unsound and deformed spine will cause cardiopulmonary compromise and can lead to shortening of the expected life span.
4. When the major curve is in the lower segment of the spine, the symptoms are primarily pain and fa-

THE SPINE

tigue with a diminished work capacity. Terminal disabilities may be moderate or severe, with the possibility of paraplegia.

5. A structurally unsound, deformed spine with a kyphotic component will lead to increased deformity and with the passage of time may produce a paraplegia.

6. The cosmetic effects to be gained by instrumentation of the scoliotic spine must be considered to be secondary, for although they are gratifying to both the patient and the surgeon, this aspect should not take precedence in the surgeon's judgment.

Instrumentation is a metallic system designed to apply forces of distraction and compression over several segments of the spine in the area of the posterior elements. The instruments hold the correction obtained for a reasonable length of time until the fusion can develop and take over stabilization of the original correction. Although the major force is provided by the distraction system, the contribution of the compression system is integral to the effectiveness of the total system. To dispense with the compression mechanism altogether amounts to an infraction on the correcting and holding potential of the total system. From 80 to 100 pounds (36.3 to 45.4 kg) is the safe range of force applied to a distraction hook; force on the compression hook is rarely more than 25 pounds (11.3 kg).

SEGMENTAL SPINAL INSTRUMENTATION. Eduardo Luque of Mexico City in 1974 reported the use of multiple wires passed beneath the laminae on each side of each spinous process to mechanically straighten or contour the spine by twisting the wires around long round rods laid along each posterior laminar surface. Contouring the two rods allows the spine to be pulled over to the corrected position as the wires are tightened. Internal fixation is more rigid than with the Harrington instrumentation, and arthrodesis seems to be enhanced. The internal fixation provided has been efficient enough to convince many spine surgeons that external immobilization is not needed postoperatively. Neurologic complications, apparently from passage or manipulation of the wires in the spinal canal, have been reported frequently enough that the procedure should be used in neurologically normal patients only by experienced spine surgeons in medical centers where spinal cord monitoring can be carried out. This system is now rarely used for idiopathic scoliosis because of the potential complications, and its primary application is in patients with neuromuscular scoliosis.

Drummond, Keene, and Breed in 1984 reported segmental spinal instrumentation or wiring in which the wires are passed transversely through a small steel button and then through the base of the spinous process to be twisted and tightened around rods laid on the laminae as with the Luque technique. Thus the spinal canal is not invaded by the wires, and neurologic complications are minimal. As a rule we use Drummond wiring for neurologically intact patients and Luque wiring for patients with neuromuscular scoliosis and for patients with complete neurologic deficits when these techniques are determined to be appropriate.

Cotrel and Dubousset introduced the concept of three-dimensional segmental instrumentation. Its primary advantages are the three-dimensional correction of deformity and the less frequent need for postoperative immobilization. The Texas Scottish Rite Hospital implant system is a modification of the Cotrel-Dubousset system. Advantages and disadvantages of these systems are discussed in Chapter 83.

DWYER INSTRUMENTATION. For most patients with spinal deformity surgery from the posterior approach is preferred, but for some patients posterior surgery is impossible or alone is insufficient. In 1964 Dwyer, in cooperation with Newton, developed instrumentation for correction and fixation through an anterior approach. Dwyer instrumentation uses large metal staples of several sizes that fit over the vertebral bodies and are attached to each body with a large screw. The screws have a large head with a hole for passage of a cable that is tightened at each level and then fixed by crimping the screw head.

By placing the staples more anteriorly, lordosis can be corrected. By placing the staples and screws in the same location in each vertebral body regardless of the position of the body, rotation can also be corrected as the curve straightens. Kyphosis will be made worse by Dwyer instrumentation.

The indications for the Dwyer procedure are limited. The Dwyer procedure is a valuable adjunct to treatment of selected spinal deformities, but most deformities can be treated adequately with posterior instrumentation. At present, the indications for the Dwyer procedure are (1) lumbar curves in patients with deficient posterior elements such as in myelomeningocele, (2) thoracolumbar curves with extreme lordosis, and (3) rigid thoracolumbar paralytic curves for which a combined anteroposterior fusion in two stages is required. An absolute contraindication to the Dwyer procedure is kyphosis in the area to be treated. The Dwyer apparatus is not recommended for children less than 10 years of age because of the small size of the vertebral bodies. It is also not recommended for adults with extremely osteoporotic bone. There are several advantages of Dwyer instrumentation, anterior correction, and fusion:

1. Because the discs are large, their removal results in marked mobilization with increased correction and sound fixation of the curve obtained at every level.

2. Excellent correction of lordosis is obtained.

3. Correction of rotation along with the curve is possible by placing the screw and staple in the same relative position in each vertebral body.

The Dwyer procedure also has disadvantages:

1. The procedure is time consuming.

2. Instrumentation of the sacrum is difficult, and therefore correction of pelvic obliquity is difficult.

3. Instrumentation above the T6 level is difficult.

Complications of the Dwyer procedure include those common to any major anterior surgical exposure of the spine: pneumothorax, hemothorax, aspiration pneumonia, and paralytic ileus. In addition to these there is the possibility of mechanical damage to the spinal cord by a screw or vascular damage to the cord from the extensive exposure with division of multiple segmental arteries. The latter, while possible theoretically, may or may not have occurred clinically. In addition, cable breakage and loss of fixation at one level are common, and even with an intact apparatus, solid interbody fusion does not always occur. With the Dwyer procedure alone for rigid paralytic curves, the group at Rancho Los Amigos Hospital has noted a pseudarthrosis rate of over 50% and consequently recommends that the anterior Dwyer fusion be supplemented by a posterior fusion.

ZIELKE INSTRUMENTATION. Zielke of Germany modified Dwyer's principles by using a solid, flexible rod instead of a cable. Experienced spine surgeons in medical centers have successfully used this type of anterior instrumentation, which can be used in kyphotic areas of the spine and is recommended for its derotating ability.

COMPLICATIONS OF TREATMENT

The operative treatment of scoliosis is formidable, and many significant complications are possible during this treatment. These complications may occur in any stage of treatment. They should be prevented, of course, if at all possible. Complications of instrumentation in scoliosis are discussed in Chapter 83.

Complications in Cast

Because casts are no longer a routine part of many treatment protocols, special diligence is necessary when they are used. Pressure sores may develop over any improperly padded bony prominence. Any complaint of localized pain under the cast should be investigated immediately, and usually a part of the cast should be removed and repadded or the entire cast should be removed and reapplied. Moe recommends making a cruciate cut in the cast over the painful area and carefully bending out the plaster at the edges. Brachial plexus palsies were much more common when turnbuckle casts were used than when the Risser or similar casts were used. Single nerve palsies are still occasionally produced by localized pressure at the edge of the cast. Meticulous technique in applying casts will minimize pressure sores and nerve palsies.

Compression of the duodenum in its third portion by the superior mesenteric artery was described by Rokitan-

sky more than 100 years ago. This condition may appear in two forms: the acute form and the chronic form, designated Wilkie's syndrome. The condition has been observed in various pathologic states. The cast syndrome described by Dorph in 1950 is an acute form of this syndrome. The syndrome consists of vascular compression of the duodenum leading to acute duodenal obstruction and gastric dilatation. Pernicious and often projectile vomiting ensue and a potentially dangerous situation exists. A high index of suspicion must be maintained in those individuals with vomiting, abdominal distention, and mild pain. Since this is a partial obstruction, flatus will continue to be passed and symptoms may be intermittent. Diagnosis is based on the radiologic findings of a dilated duodenum. Contrast studies will show a linear obstruction at the level where the superior mesenteric vessels cross the duodenum. A lateral decubitus examination of the abdomen with the patient's right side up will reveal a dilated duodenal loop with a long air-fluid level. When combined with the appropriate history and physical findings, this is virtually a pathognomonic sign. The treatment should consist of prompt removal of the cast if present, combined with early nasogastric suction. Other measures should be position changes, particularly to a prone position, restriction to a liquid diet, and ambulation if possible. General surgical consultation should be sought because surgery may be required if these measures are not successful.

Evarts, Winter, and Hall reported on 30 patients from the literature and from their own experience with vascular compression of the duodenum, properly termed a "superior mesenteric artery syndrome." Eighteen of these cases had occurred with correction of the scoliosis operatively; 12 occurred with the application of body casts only. It is emphasized that with correction of the curvature an increase in the angle of the superior mesenteric artery with the aorta results in compression of the duodenum and symptoms of partial intestinal obstruction.

Years ago we saw this syndrome develop in a patient in whom the course had been uneventful during the correction of scoliosis by a cast followed by Harrington instrumentation and rest in bed in a Risser cast for 6 months. Yet 2 years later after a spica cast was applied after reconstructive surgery on a hip, the typical syndrome developed.

Complications of Skeletal Traction

Skeletal traction is a safe method for correcting many types of spinal curves when carefully supervised. Halo-femoral traction is not recommended for congenital kyphosis, and for any other type of pure kyphosis it must be considered dangerous. Moe was a pioneer in the use of this traction and has stated that forces of more than 25 to 35 pounds (11.3 to 15.9 kg) are not helpful even in older patients and that probably a force of 20 pounds (9 kg) is sufficient. We used 15 to 25 pounds (16.8 to 11.3

kg) without neurologic complications. Temporary palsies of the extraocular muscles and of the brachial plexus have been reported when the traction was too forceful. One patient of ours, a male 18 years of age, developed severe hypertension while in halo-femoral traction. When the traction was discontinued, the hypertension subsided and we were unable to find any other cause for the hypertension. When the weights are added in small increments and the patient is observed carefully, skeletal traction is probaby a safe method for correcting congenital scoliosis and very stiff curves of any type. Infections around the halo pins are rare and usually can be avoided by meticulous skin care and by moving pins to new locations when necessary. Skeletal traction, both the halo-femoral and halo-pelvic types, are now rarely used as internal corrective devices become more efficient.

Complications after Surgery

Complications after surgery are discussed in Chapter 83.

PARAPLEGIA SECONDARY TO SCOLIOSIS

The spontaneous development of paraplegia in a patient with scoliosis is rarely if ever caused by the scoliotic deformity alone. A progressive neurologic deficit or paraplegia is most common in congenital scoliosis but is usually caused by some other anomaly such as diastematomyelia, and treating the scoliosis alone will probably not be helpful. Further, measures to correct the curve may be extremely dangerous and may cause a marked increase in the neurologic deficit. In congenital scoliosis associated with congenital kyphosis, paraplegia may be caused by pressure on the anterior aspect of the cord by the vertebral body or fragment of a body at the apex of the curve. Laminectomy is not beneficial and usually should not be attempted. Rather, anterior decompression by removing the offending bone and anterior interbody fusion are indicated. Then a posterior fusion in which attempts are made to correct the deformity superior and inferior to the apex of the curve may be necessary later. The same combination of scoliosis and kyphosis is common in neurofibromatosis and is treated similarly. We have not seen paraplegia in progressive idiopathic or progressive paralytic scoliosis unless either an angular kyphosis or some other pathologic condition is present in addition to the scoliosis.

ADULT SCOLIOSIS

Idiopathic curves not only may progress into adulthood, but also may cause significant clinical symptoms. The incidence of scoliosis in adults has been reported by various investigators to range from 1.9% to 3.9% of the population. Weinstein and Ponseti reviewed 102 patients at an average follow-up of 40.5 years and found that 68% of the curves progressed after skeletal maturity. In general, curves of less than 30 degrees at skeletal maturity tended not to progress, regardless of curve pattern. Progression of curves of more than 30 degrees appeared related to the amount of vertebral rotation. The most marked progression occurred in thoracic curves between 50 and 75 degrees at skeletal maturity; these progressed almost 1 degree per year. The progression of lumbar curves was related to vertebral rotation, the direction of the curve, and the position of the fifth lumbar vertebra relative to the intercrest line.

Pain is the most common complaint of adult patients with scoliosis. Kostuik and Bentivoglio found that 60% of adult patients with lumbar and thoracolumbar scoliosis reported pain. Jackson, Simmons, and Stripinis reported that 51% of their adult scoliosis patients had significant pain. Nachemson and Nilsonne reported similar findings but noted that the pain rarely was clinically significant. Weinstein, Zavala, and Ponseti reported that 80% of 161 patients complained of some backache; however, of a control group of 100 age- and sex-matched patients without scoliosis, 86% reported backache. Jackson, Simmons, and Stripinis reported that pain increased with age and the degree of the curve. Pain is most common in patients with curves of more than 45 degrees at skeletal maturity and in patients between the ages of 40 and 60 years. Pain in an adult patient with scoliosis, however, is not always caused by the spinal deformity. A careful history and physical examination, routine roentenograms and if necessary CT, myelography, discography, MRI, or facet joint injection should be used to determine that the pain is caused by the scoliosis. When pain is associated with the scoliosis, it may be caused by muscle fatigue or strain, disc pathologic conditions, nerve root entrapment, or facet joint pathologic conditions, and the exact source of the pain must be identified.

For many years, conservative care was recommended by most authors, including Nachemson, who reported high risks with scoliosis surgery in adults. With the development of spinal instrumentation, advances in anesthetic and intraoperative monitoring techniques, and improvements in postoperative care, a more aggressive surgical approach to scoliosis in adults has become possible. Operative treatment, however, may not be indicated for all adult patients with scoliosis, especially elderly patients and those with mild pain. Pain from muscle fatigue and strain often can be managed with the use of non-narcotic analgesics, nonsteroidal anti-inflammatory drugs, and proper back care. Immobilization in a custom-made plastic orthosis and the use of anti-inflammatory medications often ease pain from facet arthrosis. For facet arthrosis isolated to one or two levels, injection of an anesthetic agent and a long-acting steroid in and around the joint can provide long-lasting relief.

According to Kostuik, surgery is indicated in adults

with scoliosis to (1) relieve pain, (2) prevent further progression of the curve, (3) manage significant neurologic dysfunction or prevent such dysfunction, and (4) improve cosmetic appearance. Complications are more frequent in adult patients than in adolescents, and the degree of curve correction is less. Sponseller et al. reported minor complications in 40% and major complications in 20% of 45 adult patients after surgical treatment of scoliosis, and Swank et al. reported complications in 53%. Complications can be minimized by careful preoperative evaluation and meticulous surgical technique.

The surgical techniques used for correction of adult scoliosis are the same as used for adolescent scoliosis (see Chapter 83); however, posterior instrumentation alone in adults may require external support postoperatively. With instrumentation of lumbar or thoracolumbar curves, lumbar lordosis may be lost if the rods are not properly contoured (Fig. 82-19), and segmental wiring is necessary. Although 79% of their patients had relief of pain, van Dam et al. reported a 15% incidence of pseudarthrosis after Harrington instrumentation and hook dislodgement in 5%. Ponder et al. reported similar results, with significant improvements in symptoms but

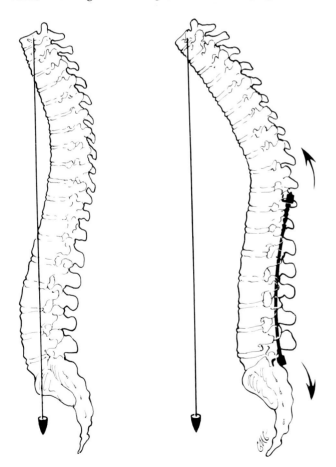

Fig. 82-19   Effects of distraction rod in lumbar spine. If contouring for lordosis is inadequate, lumbar spine can be flattened by distracting force. Also note kyphotic deformity just superior to distraction rod. (From La Grone MO: Orthop Clin North Am 19:383, 1988.)

early complications in 24% of patients and late complications in 52%, most often pseudarthrosis.

Johnson and Holt recommend a two-stage procedure, anterior fusion followed by posterior fusion and instrumentation. They cite the following advantages to this approach: (1) more correction, (2) fewer operative failures, (3) shorter lumbar fusion for double major curves, and (4) better correction of rigid thoracolumbar curves that increases maximum ventilatory volume. Kostuik recommends anterior Zielke instrumentation for thoracolumbar or lumbar curves that do not require extension of the fusion to the sacrum and are mobile on bending roentgenograms. For kyphoscoliotic deformities, he recommends a two-stage approach, with anterior multiple-level discectomies and fusion, followed in 2 weeks by posterior Cotrel-Dubousset instrumentation. Kostuik and Hall emphasized that fusion to the sacrum should be performed only if the lumbosacral disc is clearly a source of pain or the degree of pelvic obliquity requires sacral fusion; every effort must be made to preserve lumbar lordosis.

SCOLIOSIS OF KNOWN CAUSE
Neuromuscular Scoliosis

Neuromuscular scoliosis may be secondary to an array of underlying disorders, and patients have varying sensory abnormalities, asymmetric or symmetric paralysis, and progressive or nonprogressive disease. However, common to all is a paralytic state resulting in limb and spinal deformities. An abbreviated classification is as follows:

1. Neuropathic
   a. Spinal cord injury
   b. Poliomyelitis
   c. Progressive neurologic disorders
   d. Syringomyelia
   e. Myelomeningocele
   f. Cerebral palsy
2. Myopathic
   a. Arthrogryposis
   b. Muscular dystrophy
3. Neurofibromatosis
4. Miscellaneous

O'Brien and Yau and others emphasize the different problems in paralytic and idiopathic scoliosis. First, as J.I.P. James indicates, paralytic curves are longer. Second, pelvic obliquity often exists with muscle imbalance affecting the ultimate fusion mass. Third, the pseudarthrosis rate is higher and approaches 20% as reported by Winter or 50% as reported by Bonnett. Pelvic obliquity results in pressure sores on the ischium on the low side of the pelvis with hip subluxation on the high side as the severity of the deformity increases. Regular follow-up is essential to prevent these severe sequelae and should be combined with appropriately timed treatment.

In paralytic scoliosis the aim of surgery is not only correction of the curves and prevention of their recurrence but also secure stabilization of the weakened trunk. Consequently the indications for fusion and the determination of the fusion area are different from those in idiopathic scoliosis.

Blount et al. once advised fusion from D1 to L3 or L4 in two or three posterior stages for severe paralysis of the trunk. Bonnett et al., reporting the Rancho Los Amigos experience with paralytic scoliosis in 351 patients, provided the following indications for surgery:

1. A collapsing and unstable paralytic deformity
2. Progressive increase in the scoliosis
3. Decreasing cardiorespiratory function
4. Decreased independence necessitating the use of hands for more stable sitting
5. Back pain or loss of sitting balance coincident with increasing pelvic obliquity

As experience at Rancho Los Amigos and elsewhere increased and technologic advances appeared, the results improved. This occurred because of improved skeletal fixation. It has been found that the Dwyer anterior operation is excellent for improving the percentage of correction but is inadequate in that the fusion mass is too short. The Harrington posterior distraction rod allows greater correction above and below the apex of the curve. The combined anterior and posterior approach therefore permits improved correction and a decrease in the rate of pseudarthrosis. Posterior segmental instrumentation (p. 3630) generally and with extension to the pelvis as performed by Allen and Ferguson became the most widely used method of stabilization and correction for neuromuscular deformity before the introduction of Cotrel-Dubousset instrumentation.

An unacceptable curve that increases despite conservative treatment should be corrected and fused regardless of the patient's age. However, if an increase in the curve can be prevented with an orthosis, it is preferable to wait until the patient is 10 years of age or older. Moe has stated that high cervicodorsal curves should not be treated conservatively but should be fused early because in them irreversible structural changes soon develop, and because even when moderate they produce severe deformity. Garrett, Perry, and Nickel have had much experience in treating severe instability of the neck and trunk caused by paralysis of the muscles that control them. To them, even in the absence of scoliosis, instability itself is an indication for fusion. They devised a halo (see Fig. 82-11) that is attached to a body cast (see Fig. 82-13, *A*) to stabilize the head and neck during and after fusion of the cervical spine. They point out that the ease with which a patient can balance his head and trunk determines to a great extent how much he can develop the muscles of his extremities. If less energy is required to maintain erect posture, the demands of respiratory function are decreased, fatigue is decreased, and the patient's efforts can be better directed toward productive activity.

Therefore stabilizing the paralyzed trunk is the first consideration in treatment. They also recommended that tracheotomy be made routinely before any fusion operation in patients with severe respiratory embarrassment and that often respiratory aids be used afterward. With better pulmonary medicine and critical care units, tracheotomies are rarely mandatory.

To stabilize the trunk effectively in a patient with paralytic scoliosis or with an unstable spine, a much longer fusion is necessary than is usually indicated in one with idiopathic scoliosis. While in idiopathic scoliosis only the primary curve need necessarily be fused, in paralytic scoliosis the area including the primary and both secondary curves must often be fused. This area generally extends from a horizontal vertebra in the upper spine to a horizontal vertebra in the lower. As already mentioned, Blount et al. have recommended that a severely paralyzed trunk be stabilized by fusion from D1 to L3 or L4. Of course, the spine must be compensated (the head centered over the pelvis) by the fusion or the instrumentation procedure.

The paralytic patient presents additional problems to the unwary such as (1) significant pulmonary function deficits caused by intercostal paralysis, (2) more osteoporotic bone and the possibility of instrument failure, (3) atrophic pelvis with insufficient bone for grafting, (4) an increased blood loss in a patient with an initially smaller blood volume, (5) prolonged postoperative immobilization, (6) more postoperative pulmonary complications, and (7) immobilization pressure sores, especially in those with altered skin sensation. Suffice it to say that a more complicated course is to be expected and appropriate measures must be taken to prepare for and manage any eventuality.

The consensus is therefore that nonoperative treatment may be entirely futile and that superior results occur with operative management. Procedures that provide segmental instrumentation, such as Luque instrumentation with intralaminar wiring and Cotrel-Dubousset instrumentation, usually are efficient in correction and fusion of neuromuscular scoliosis (Chapter 83). Surgery most often is performed later than is ideal.

A progressive kyphosis is managed as discussed in the section on kyphosis (Chapter 86).

SPINAL CORD INJURY. Of 104 children with spinal cord injury reviewed by Kilfoyle, Foley, and Norton, 97 developed spinal curvature and pelvic obliquity; lordosis was most common, scoliosis second, and kyphosis least common. Early surgical treatment was "considered an expression of conservatism." Bonnett, Perry, and Brown reported 57 of 123 patients with significant spinal deformity and stressed the progression of deformity in the growing child. Total care of the cord-injured child was emphasized. Lancourt, Dickson, and Carter reported that scoliotic curves of more than 20 degrees developed in 31 of 50 patients and, more significantly, that scoliosis de-

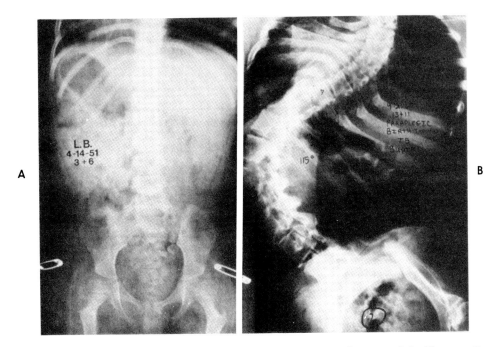

Fig. 82-20   A, Spine of paraplegic infant with T5 lesion. **B,** Development of significant scoliosis at age 14. (From Mayfield JK et al: J Bone Joint Surg 63-A:1401, 1981.)

veloped in all paitents who were younger than 10 years of age at the time of injury. In a study of 40 children with spinal cord injury, Mayfield, Erkkila, and Winter found that paralytic spinal deformity developed in all 25 patients who were injured before the adolescent growth spurt (Fig. 82-20). Milwaukee braces and plastic orthoses are of limited value in the presence of anesthetic skin. Some authors suggest that, although orthotic treatment is difficult, it can be effective in delaying progression of the curvature and allowing further spinal growth before fusion is necessary. Surgical stabilization is needed in virtually all children before the growth spurt. Internal stabilization is of utmost importance, and segmental fixation techniques that allow mobilization without external support are highly suitable for these patients with anesthetic skin and frequently diminished respiratory ability. Combined anterior and posterior procedures are effective.

POLIOMYELITIS. Curves in poliomyelitis may affect any part of the spine including the neck, may resemble the idiopathic type or be the long C type, and may have the many features of other paralytic curves. Nonoperative treatment is primarily for delaying fusion during growth. The surgical management follows the same principles as for scoliosis in other neuromuscular diseases, but it must be emphasized that a *long* fusion is necessary to result in a balanced spine. Segmental instrumentation or Cotrel-Dubousset type instrumentation is most often indicated. Halo-femoral traction may produce additional osteoporosis and has vew indications. Postoperative immobilization may include a Risser-Cotrel cast, halo cast,

or plastic orthosis as the stability of the instrumentation and other factors dictate.

PROGRESSIVE NEUROLOGIC DISORDERS. Hensinger and MacEwen point out that these conditions carry a significant risk of serious spinal deformity as with paralytic scoliosis following poliomyelitis. The curves are difficult to control with bracing and do not cease progression at maturation. Increasing spinal curvature leads to loss of ambulation, or for the wheelchair-bound patient, loss of sitting balance. Hardy noted scoliosis in 19% of patients under age 5 years, 58% between 6 and 11 years, and 84% at 12 years and older. Spinal muscular atrophy is a genetically determined neuromuscular disorder characterized by widespread weakness secondary to degeneration of the anterior horn cells of the spinal cord (see also Chapter 48). This disease has been given many names, including Werdnig-Hoffman's disease, Kugelberg-Welander's disease, Oppenheim's disease, amyotonia congenita, proximal spinal muscular atrophy, juvenile spinal muscular atrophy, and anterior horn cell disease. Phillips et al. reported a 60% incidence of scoliosis in 34 patients with infantile spinal muscular atrophy. The average age of diagnosis of scoliosis was 9 years, with a range from 5 months to 14 years. Brown et al. noted scoliosis in all of their patients before puberty, and Daher et al. reported diagnosis at an average age of 7 years in a group of surgically treated patients.

Because of the clinical variations in the condition, infantile spinal muscular atrophy (Werdnig-Hoffmann's disease) has been divided into three groups, depending on the extent of involvement and the time within the first

2 years of life when the diagnosis becomes apparent. Group I patients are diagnosed within the first 2 months of life, remain severely hypotonic, and often die within the first year or two of life. Group II patients are diagnosed between the ages of 2 and 12 months, and group III patients are diagnosed between the ages of 1 and 2 years. As noted by Schwentker and Gibson and by Evans, Drennan, and Russman, scoliosis develops in almost all patients with this condition. The onset often is in childhood, and most curves are progressive. In patients who survive childhood, the scoliosis often is the most severe problem. Bracing may slow the progression of curves and also allow sitting for longer periods of time. When the curve approaches 40 to 50 degrees, posterior spinal fusion with posterior instrumentation and bone grafting is recommended. Because fusion to the sacrum is necessary for many of these patients, Luque-rod fixation with sublaminar wires and fixation to the pelvis (see Chapter 83) provides the best internal fixation. If the curve has progressed to more than 100 degrees with a severe fixed lumbar curve and pelvic obliquity, the addition of an anterior fusion may be necessary, but this adds considerably to the risks of the operation. Complications are frequent in this group of patients, especially pulmonary complications. Bradford discourages routine use of traction and encourages early mobilization.

The juvenile form (Kugelberg-Welander's disease) begins between the ages of 2 and 12 years with the patient surviving into adult life. In the report of Hensinger and MacEwen 29 of 50 patients evaluated had a significant scoliosis. They recommended surgery with emphasis on proper preoperative management, including an intensive physical therapy program for general muscle strengthening initially. Special attention must be paid to cardiorespiratory problems, and instructions in pulmonary exercises should also be included. Fusion was by a standard posterior approach with Harrington instrumentation and bone grafting. The children were of small stature with reduced blood volume, and blood loss was of major proportions. This requires that surgery be accomplished with speed and skill. Dorr, Brown, and Perry fused an average of 18 levels and used postoperative support for 17 months.

Friedreich's ataxia usually has its clinical onset between the ages of 6 and 20 years, and affected children frequently are wheelchair bound in the first and second decades of life. Labelle et al. found that all of their patients with Friedreich's ataxia had scoliosis. Most authors have found bracing for progressive curvatures in these patients to be ineffective. Treatment of patients with Friedreich's ataxia is influenced by the degree of cardiac involvement since this is the most common cause of death in these patients. Since the mean age of death in Friedreich's ataxia is 36 years, evaluation of a teenager with progressive scoliosis must consider this factor. In Friedreich's ataxia, as in spinal muscular atrophy, bed rest in preoperative traction or during the postoperative period must be kept to a minimum; otherwise a rapid increase in weakness will occur. For this reason, the best instrumentation for these patients is segmental spinal instrumentation by the Luque technique with early postoperative ambulation without external support.

Studies by Hensinger and MacEwen and by Daher et al. indicate that patients with Charcot-Marie-Tooth disease and spinal deformity may be managed with the same techniques used for idiopathic scoliosis, including bracing and surgery. Brace wear usually is well tolerated without any special problems.

Patients with familial dysautonomia (Riley-Day syndrome) present many problems in management. Vasomotor and thermal instability and dysphagia are frequent features of the syndrome and can cause troublesome and sometimes fatal complications. Experience in surgery with these patients is quite limited. Bradford has performed few spine fusions in these patients, and he emphasizes that the risks and complications are high and should be well appreciated before any surgical correction is undertaken.

SYRINGOMYELIA. Huebert and MacKinnon reported the presence of scoliosis in 63% of 43 children with syringomyelia. Scoliosis was found in 82% when symptoms of the disease had been noted before the age of 16 years. Syringomyelia is discussed here for two reasons. First, in patients with scoliosis and a neurologic deficit, syringomyelia should be considered in the differential diagnosis. Second, of two patients with severe curves reported by Huebert and MacKinnon, the curve was corrected and fused using the Harrington instruments in one, but a spinal fusion after a laminectomy was fatal in the other when a large cyst in the cord ruptured. Obviously, the rate of progression of the neurologic deficit and the prognosis of life should be considered before any extensive operations are considered for patients with this disease. Experience with this condition is limited, but the curve patterns resemble idiopathic and not paralytic scoliosis and hence may be misdiagnosed. In a study by Weber 19 of 51 patients with syringomyelia had scoliosis; the curves were usually thoracic, were more common in males, and correlated with the neurologic level. Bradford advocates initial treatment of this condition with drainage of the cyst followed by observation to determine the subsequent curve status. If the curve progresses, surgical stabilization and fusion should be carried out. He believes that sublaminar wiring poses additional risks to the dilated spinal cord and favors the use of Harrington instrumentation alone, with intraoperative spinal cord monitoring and the wake-up test. Phillips, Hensinger, and Kling also recommend drainage of the cyst, noting that while this did not prevent curve progression, it did have several benefits: it stabilized or improved neurologic function, it appeared to make surgical correction of the scoliosis less dangerous, and it temporarily arrested progression of the curve in immature patients.

MYELOMENINGOCELE. Since advances in neurosurgical and urologic skills have enabled more children with myelomeningocele to survive, there are now more patients with a type of scoliosis that has been the most severe and most difficult form to treat. In response to this challenge, capabilities to handle severe deformities have increased; however, the spinal problem cannot be handled in isolation and the total child must be cared for in a multidisciplinary setting. (See discussion of myelomeningocele in Chapter 47.)

Raycroft and Curtis reported an incidence of spine deformity in 52% of 103 patients without vertebral body abnormalities with myelomeningocele; 41 patients had scoliosis, 30 had lordosis, and 12 had kyphosis; of the 27 with vertebral body abnormalities, all had a congenital spine deformity. Mackel and Lindseth report a 66% incidence in 82 patients; Banta and Hamada pointed out an increase in deformity in the higher level lesions in 268 patients, and Shurtleff et al. showed an increased incidence with advancing age.

Plain posteroanterior and lateral roentgenograms should be made with the patient upright and supine. The upright films allow better evaluation of the actual deformity when the patient is functioning, and the supine films show better detail of various associated spinal deformities. The flexibility of the curves can be determined with traction films. Myelography and MRI may be useful for evaluating such conditions as hydromyelia, tethered cord, diastematomyelia, and Arnold-Chiari malformation.

Nonoperative bracing is difficult but can be effective for several years until fusion is indicated. If the curve fails to respond to bracing, or if bracing become impossible because of presure sores or noncompliance, surgery is indicated.

Sriram, Bobechko, and Hall reported 33 patients with spina bifida undergoing operative fusion. They had 16 good results, 8 fair, and 9 poor. The surgical procedures varied considerably, but the following observations could be made. Posterior spinal fusion is fraught with many difficulties, primarily because of densely scarred and adherent soft tissue. Spinal exposure is often lengthy and hemorrhagic. The deformity is often rigid and proper correction impossible. The quality of the bone often provides poor seating for Harrington hooks, and the inadequacy of the posterior bone mass provides a poor bed for grafting. Segmental spinal instrumentation and fusion probably are used most commonly now. The infection rate is quite high. Pseudarthrosis can possibly be best managed by anterior procedures such as Dwyer instrumentation and fusion.

Hall et al. reported 14 patients with communicating hydrosyringomyelia. They found a compensated hydrocephalus in all of their myelodysplastic patients with developmental scoliosis. The hydrosyringomyelia produced progressive extremity paresis, often with spasticity. After the initial detection of a developmental scoliosis in patients with myelodysplasia, an investigation for hydrosyringomyelia should be instituted. This can be studied with computerized axial tomography, positive contrast shuntogram under fluoroscopy, or radioisotope ventriculography. Treatment of the hydrosyringomyelia is accomplished by ventricular drainage using a standard shunt procedure. This resulted in short-term stabilization in six of their patients; two patients with advanced curves continued to progress. Even advanced neurologic deficits were improved. Arrested hydrocephalus was present in all 14 patients.

Many techniques of surgery have been recommended for correction of scoliosis in patients with myelomeningocele. There is no one best system, and correction often requires a combination of techniques. Bone-bank bone usually is necessary because of hypoplasia of the iliac crest. The area to be fused should be determined from preoperative sitting, supine, and traction roentgenograms. Almost all patients with myelomeningocele require fusion from the upper portion of the thoracic region to the sacrum. A combined anterior and posterior fusion, if possible, is desirable. The lack of posterior bony elements makes the reliability of a posterior fusion uncertain even with newer systems of segmental instrumentation.

CEREBRAL PALSY. Scoliosis often is overlooked in patients with cerebral palsy. Rosenthal, Levene, and McCarver examined 50 adolescents and found a 38% incidence, Robson found an incidence of 23% in 152 patients, and Samilson and Bechard found an incidence of 25.6% in 906 patients. The average age in the latter group was 22 years. Of the 232 patients with scoliosis, only 22 were ambulatory, 41 were sitters, and 169 were bed care patients. There were 58 primary lumbar curves, 104 thoracolumbar curves, 37 thoracic curves, and 33 double primary curves. The most severe curves were thoracolumbar in location. MacEwen reported 100 cerebral palsy patients, most of whom were ambulatory, with a 21% incidence of scoliosis.

Of 294 patients with cerebral palsy seen at Rancho Los Amigos Hospital by Bonnett, Brown, and Brooks, 42 were considered to have clinically significant lumbar and thoracolumbar scoliosis (31 to 135 degrees). Of these 42 patients 33 were treated by spine surgery, 10 by Harrington instrumentation and posterior spinal fusion, 18 by the Dwyer procedure and anterior fusion, and 5 by a two-stage combined anterior and posterior fusion. They concluded that only the combined procedure appeared to give adequate correction and a low incidence of pseudarthrosis; this was also recommended by Moe et al. They concluded that for severe spastic and progressive scoliosis in a patient with the potential for rehabilitation, surgical treatment is indicated. Improved results are seen in curves of less than 60 degrees at the time of surgery. MacEwen reported 10 patients with severe and progressive curves treated surgically; two required repair of

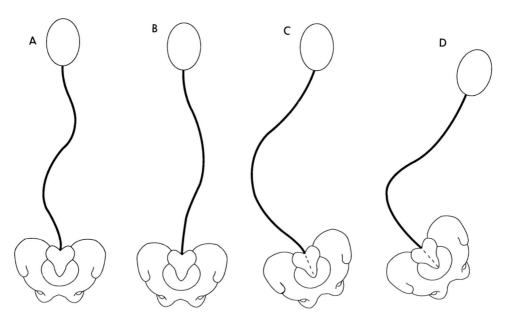

Fig. 82-21 Scoliosis in cerebral palsy. **A** and **B,** Group I double curves with thoracic and lumbar component and little pelvic obliquity. **C** and **D,** Group II large lumbar or thoracolumbar curves with marked pelvic obliquity. (Redrawn from Lonstein JE and Akbrania BA: J Bone Joint Surg 65-A:43, 1983.)

pseudarthroses before a successful fusion was accomplished. Our experience with this type of surgery in cerebral palsy has also been favorable and we agree that to avoid surgery for scoliosis in these patients who already have serious problems in walking and in trunk stability is unreasonable.

When surgery is indicated, the type of surgery and instrumentation must be determined. Lonstein and Akbrania classified scoliotic curves in patients with cerebral palsy into two groups (Fig. 82-21). Group I curves, double curves with both a thoracic and a lumbar component, occurred in 40% of patients, were similar to curves of idiopathic scoliosis, and occurred more commonly in patients who were ambulatory. Group I curves usually require only a posterior fusion; fusion to the sacrum rarely is needed. Group II curves are more severe lumbar or thoracolumbar curves that extend into the sacrum with marked pelvic obliquity. These were present in 58% of patients, usually patients who were nonambulatory and had spastic quadriplegia. Group II curves usually require a long fusion to the sacrum (Fig. 82-22). Lonstein and Akbrania found that a combined approach gave better correction of the scoliosis, slightly better correction of the pelvic obliquity, and a lower rate of pseudarthrosis. Gersoff and Renshaw and Allen and Ferguson found superior results with Luque-rod segmental instrumentation. Lonstein and Renshaw recommend traction roentgenograms made with the patient on a Risser-Cotrel frame and with the use of a head halter, pelvic straps, and a lateral convex Cotrel strap. If a level pelvis and balanced spine can be obtained, a one-stage posterior approach is indicated. If the traction roentgenogram shows residual pelvic obliquity or if the torso is not balanced

over the pelvis, a two-stage approach is best. In general, the larger the lumbar curve, the more severe the pelvic obliquity, and the more rigid the curve, the more likely a two-stage procedure will be needed.

Gersoff and Renshaw listed several important technical points in use of the Luque-rod instrumentation: (1) 0.25-inch rods are used if the patient is large enough to accept them (usually a weight of 80 pounds or more); (2) when possible, two doubled 16-gauge wires are passed under each lamina; (3) facet joints are excised before the wires are passed; (4) the spinous processes are morcellized and the transverse processes are decorticated; and (5) bone-bank bone is necessary. Allen and Ferguson reported good results without decortication and facet excision. They also use the 0.25-inch rods only in patients with athetosis, large body mass, seizure disorders, or unusual activity demands and in patients whose condition cannot be corrected to a compensated position after anterior release. They prefer the 3/16-inch rods made of MP-35-N alloy rather than stainless steel for flexible curves.

Most authors report that traction does not aid in the treatment of these curves either before surgery or between the anterior and posterior procedures. Postoperative immobilization depends on the activity level of the child and the stability of the internal fixation. If a child can tolerate external support without any detrimental effect on function, it is used no matter how secure the fixation, usually for 9 to 12 months or until the fusion is solid.

Complications have been reported to occur in as many as 81% of cerebral patients undergoing spinal fusion. However, with improved techniques of instrumentation

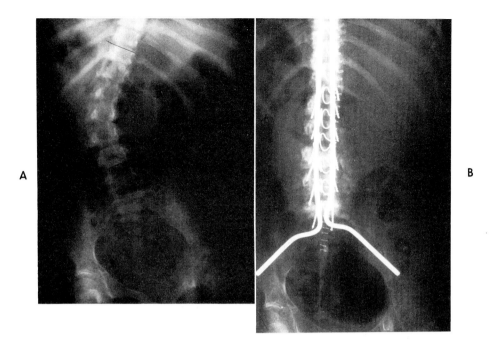

Fig. 82-22 **A,** Group II 49-degree thoracolumbar curve in child with cerebral palsy. **B,** After Luque instrumentation with fixation to pelvis by Galveston technique.

and preoperative and postoperative management, this rate is decreasing. The most common complications include infection, pseudarthrosis, pulmonary difficulties, and development of kyphosis. Although complications are frequent in patients with cerebral palsy, functional improvement or prevention of deterioration of function is well worth the efforts and risks of surgery.

ARTHROGRYPOSIS MULTIPLEX CONGENITA. In arthrogryposis multiplex congenita any scoliosis is secondary to the abnormality of the muscles and ligaments rather than to any abnormality of bone. That scoliosis may develop should be anticipated from birth, and the spine should be included in each examination. In 1978 Herron, Westin, and Dawson reported 88 patients with arthrogryposis multiplex congenita, finding scoliosis in 18 patients (20%). The predominant pattern was a thoracolumbar curve associated with pelvic obliquity and lumbar hyperlordosis. The curves were mostly progressive, becoming rigid and fixed at an early age. Significant associated contractures of the hips, dislocation of the hips, or both were present in all but one patient. Boys were affected three times as often as girls. If scoliosis was detected at birth or within the first few years of life, progression of a pelvic obliquity always meant progression of the curve and demanded aggressive treatment. Correction of hip contractures must often be followed by spinal fusion to the sacrum to halt progression of the curve. The postoperative complication rate is high in this group, and appropriate intraoperative and postoperative measures are mandatory. Daher et al. reported the average blood loss to be 2000 ml. Herron, Westin, and Dawson

obtained a maximum correction of only 25%. Siebold, Winter, and Moe observed that the scoliosis in this condition is usually of a neuromuscular pattern. They found the Milwaukee brace to be a valuable treatment for mild curves. In larger curves for which surgery is necessary halo-femoral traction can be effective, but it is complicated by associated osteoporosis and halo pin slippage. Spinal fusion was as effective as in idiopathic scoliosis, but the complications included excessive blood loss, infection, and instrument failure. If surgery becomes necessary, it must be remembered that respiratory problems are common in patients with this disease and segmental instrumentation may be best.

MUSCULAR DYSTROPHY. According to Bunch, in muscular dystrophy spinal deformity seldom occurs in ambulatory patients but rather develops after 1 to 3 years of wheelchair existence. Robin and Brief analyzed 27 patients averaging 14.8 years (6 to 26 years) of age and found 24 with spine deformity. The curves were predominantly long thoracolumbar curves with pelvic obliquity, the collapse caused by absence of muscles and not asymmetric muscle activity or contracture. The curves increased with advancing age to a severe deformity. Dubowitz found no scoliosis in patients who were ambulatory or had been in a wheelchair less than 1 year. Beyond 1 year 32 of 50 had scoliosis.

Wilkins and Gibson studied 62 patients with Duchenne muscular dystrophy ranging in age from 7 to 24 years. They identified five major groups each composed of basically the same number of patients. Group I patients had essentially straight spines averaging a curve of about 7 degrees and an average age of 9.9 years. Group II patients had kyphotic spines with average curves of 14.5 degrees and an average age of 11.1 years. Group III patients had kyphoscoliotic spines with average curves of 65 degrees and an average age of 14.6 years. Group IV patients had scoliotic spines without kyphosis with average curves of 82 degrees and with an average age of 16.1 years. Group V patients had extended spines with lateral curves averaging 20 degrees and an average age of 19.3 years. The severity of the deformity increased as the age increased in groups I to IV, but the unique group V patients all had extended spines with little scoliotic deformity. Wilkins and Gibson thought that perhaps an extended spine maintained the facet joints in a locked position and was therefore less prone to develop a scoliotic deformity. They recommended early spinal support to stabilize the pelvis in a level position, providing some extension moment to prevent kyphosis and ultimately severe scoliosis.

Nonoperative treatment is best accomplished using bivalved plastic orthoses when curves exceed 20%. However, Renshaw found that 77% of patients continued to show curve progression in spite of orthotic treatment. In patients with Duchenne muscular dystrophy, pulmonary function deteriorates approximately 4% each year after the age of 12 years, and if orthotic treatment is continued until pulmonary function deteriorates significantly, surgical stabilization may become impossible. Lonstein and Renshaw emphasize that orthotic treatment of scoliosis in patient with muscular dystrophy must not delay surgery until the patient is at greater operative and postoperative risk. Their indications for spinal fusion in these patients are curves of more than 30 degrees, a forced vital capacity of more than 30% of normal, and prognosis of at least 2 years of life remaining. Luque-rod instrumentation with sublaminar wires is the best technique for patients with Duchenne muscular dystrophy (Fig. 82-23). If there is no fixed pelvic obliquity, the fusion and instrumentation can be stopped at L5. If fixed pelvic obliquity is present, fusion to the pelvis with a Galveston-type technique is indicated. The fusion must extend into the high upper thoracic spine at T2 or T3. The sagittal contours of the spine, especially lumbar lordosis, should be maintained for good sitting balance. Because of pulmonary compromise, these patients cannot tolerate any postoperative external immobilization, and rapid mobilization is important.

NEUROFIBROMATOSIS. The patterns of the curves in patients with neurofibromatosis vary. Long gentle curves that develop slowly and fail to increase significantly are occasionally seen. Perhaps these unusual curves are caused by involvement of the soft tissues by the disease or by asymmetry of the arms or legs. For these, conservative treatment is usually sufficient but the patient must be observed carefully. Roentgenologic findings were delineated by Hunt and Pugh and included the following:

1. The classic sharply angulated curve has five to eight vertebrae with an acute kyphosis in the same area; these vertebrae are typically dystrophic, whereas those in nonkyphotic curves are less so.
2. Ribs at the apical portion of the curve show "penciling."
3. Vertebrae are scalloped, with invaginations on myelography probably caused by meningoceles.

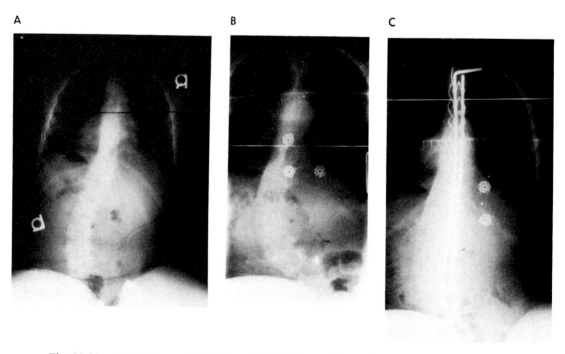

A   B   C

Fig. 82-23 Progressive scoliosis (from 35 to 79 degrees) in patient with muscular dystrophy. Luque instrumentation and fusion corrected curve to 45 degrees.

4. Dystrophic vertebrae are less common in patients with more skin manifestations.

5. An idiopathic-type curve or congenital vertebral abnormalities may occur.

6. Enlarged intervertebral foramina may be present.

Chaglassian, Riseborough, and Hall, reporting on 141 patients, found the incidence of scoliosis to be 26%. Other reported series range from 10% reported by James to as high as 58%. Chaglassian et al. found no standard pattern of spinal deformity in neurofibromatosis, but single right thoracic curves were the most common. The traditional short curve considered indicative of neurofibromatosis was not as common as long curves (more than five vertebrae) in this series. These curves showed a higher incidence of progression, but both types did progress. Kyphosis occurred in 19%. The most effective treatment was posterior Harrington instrumentation and fusion. Postoperative complications ran as high as 36%. Severity of progression of the scoliosis was not necessarily related to the severity of the systemic neurofibromatosis and did not depend on the curve length.

Even though actual neurofibromas of the intraspinal, extraspinal, or combined or dumbbell type have been described, biopsies of the spine both anteriorly and posteriorly usually are completely negative. Further, no visible neurofibromatous tissue in or around the spine has been reported even in extremely severe kyphoscoliosis. Many methods of correction and fusion have been used in this disease. The idiopathic type of curve can be managed like any other idiopathic curve and the congenital form like any other congenital curve. In patients without a significant kyphotic deformity, posterior fusion alone produces satisfactory results. Unless contraindicated because of young age, osteoporotic bone, or peculiar anatomic configurations, Harrington instrumentation provides greater correction and permits ambulation with a well-fitted Risser-Cotrel cast without significant loss of correction. When the kyphosis is severe, anterior spinal fusion with grafts bridging the apex of the kyphos combined with a posterior fusion is necessary. Myelographic studies may be indicated before treatment because intraspinal tumor masses and congenital anomalies have been reported in patients with neurofibromatosis. Even though skeletal traction for correcting a purely kyphotic deformity of the spine is extremely dangerous, we have, as have Moe et al., decreased considerably a severe kyphosis associated with a severe scoliosis without producing neurologic complications.

MISCELLANEOUS CAUSES OF SCOLIOSIS. Hilal, Marton, and Pollack reported 34 patients with diastematomyelia. Fifteen patients had no scoliosis and had an average age of 4 years, 5 months; seven patients had moderate scoliosis with an average age of 7 years, 7 months; and twelve patients had severe scoliosis and an average age of 11 years, 1 month. This suggests that the natural history of the condition is an increasing tendency for sco-

liosis to develop with age. Scoliosis was also more common in patients with a higher location of the septa within the spinal canal. Guthkelch supports the observation that scoliosis is more frequently associated with spurs in the thoracic region.

Herring has reported a case of rapidly progressive scoliosis in multiple epiphyseal dysplasia necessitating spinal instrumentation and fusion. Micheli, Hall, and Watts have reported spinal instability in Larson's syndrome, which consists of multiple congenital anomalies including anterior dislocation of the knees, dislocation of the elbows and hips, and equinovarus deformities of the feet. Associated shortened metacarpals and long, cylindric fingers characterize the hands; the facial features include hypertelorism, prominent forehead, and depressed nasal bridge. Significant spinal anomalies were found in the cervical and thoracic regions. These were characterized by cervical vertebrae that were flattened and hypoplastic, resulting in a midcervical kyphosis. Thoracolumbar scoliosis has also been reported. Sudden deaths that have been reported may have resulted from this cervical instability. It is recommended therefore that careful evaluation of the cervical spine be made and appropriate bracing or early surgical stabilization be considered.

Scoliosis often occurs in patients with osteogenesis imperfecta, especially those with severe involvement. Bauze, Smith, and Francis reported that 16 of 17 severely involved patients had scoliosis. Benson and Donaldson found a high incidence of progressive scoliosis in patients older than 8 years of age with severe osteogenesis imperfecta. Hanscom and Bloom reported 45 patients with osteogenesis imperfecta and spinal deformity and divided them into four groups. They recommend bracing for scoliosis between 20 and 40 degrees in patients with mild disease (type A) and fusion for curves of more than 45 degrees. For more severely involved patients (type B), fusion and segmental instrumentation are recommended for kyphosis and scoliosis of more than 45 degrees uncontrolled by bracing. For type C patients fusion with segmental instrumentation is recommended for curves of 35 degrees. In the most severely involved patients (type D), with osteoporotic bones and limited life spans, bracing is contraindicated and surgery has not been reported.

Congenital Scoliosis

Congenital scoliosis is a lateral curvature of the spine caused by congenital anomalies of the vertebrae and the adjacent supporting structures. Some type of anomaly must be visible on the roentgenograms of the spine before a diagnosis of congenital scoliosis can be made. Scoliotic curves in the presence of fused ribs are said to be congenital unless proved otherwise. Fused ribs in the absence of scoliosis are rarely of clinical significance. Many patients with congenital scoliosis have other congenital anomalies. The most serious anomalies of the spine are those involving the neural elements such as diastemato-

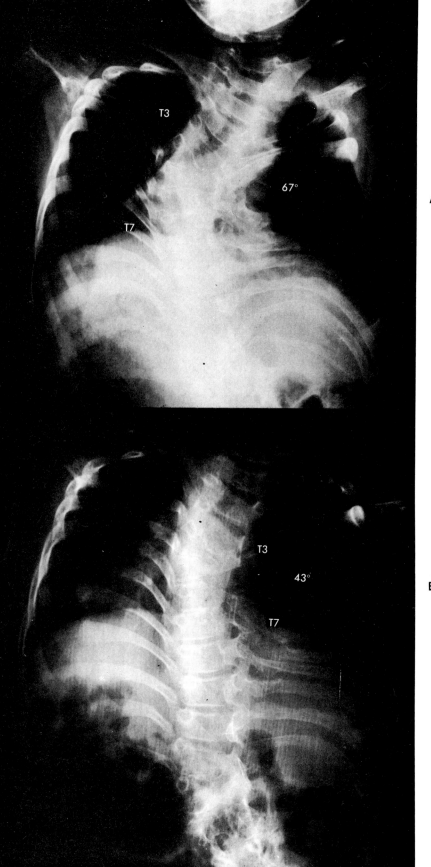

Fig. 82-24   Congenital scoliosis with unilateral bar treated by osteotomy and halofemoral distraction. **A,** Curve in boy 9 years of age extending from T3 through T7 and measuring 67 degrees; bar is on right. At surgery, bar was osteotomized across its center and fusion from T2 through T8 was performed. Halo-femoral distraction was applied in operating room after surgery. **B,** After patient had been in traction 2 weeks, curve had been corrected to 43 degrees. Additional surgery will be necessary to stabilize congenital kyphosis in lumbar spine.

myelia and the many types of spinal dysraphism. Spina bifida with meningomyelocele is often accompanied by other congenital anomalies of the spine such as errors in segmentation and often either congenital scoliosis or congenital kyphosis. Any neurologic abnormality associated with congenital scoliosis makes vigorous treatment of the scoliosis potentially dangerous.

In a study by Winter, Moe, and Eilers of 234 patients with congenital scoliosis, the type of spinal anomaly, except for the unilateral bar, was not found to be significant in the prognosis. They again emphasized that observing patients with congenital scoliosis throughout the period of growth is absolutely essential; neurologic examinations and roentgenograms of the spine are necessary periodically. Characteristically the curves in their patients that progressed did so gradually and continuously during periods of slow growth, frequently no more than 5 degrees per year, and then increased rapidly during spurts of rapid growth, usually in preadolescence. All roentgenograms must be measured carefully and must be compared not only with the most recent roentgenograms but also with the earliest ones available so that very slow increases in the curves can be detected. The unilateral bar (Fig. 82-24), usually caused by failure of segmentation of the posterior elements of two or more

vertebrae on one side, is the type of anomaly most likely to cause significant progressive scoliosis. This unilateral failure of segmentation may also involve the vertebral bodies. The study by Winter et al. indicated that the area in which the spine is anomalous is of prognostic significance. All of the thoracic curves observed to maturity increased. Usually thoracic and thoracolumbar curves increased more than cervicothoracic, lumbar, or miscellaneous curves with multiple anomalies.

Winter in 1973 emphasized the unique nature of congenital scoliosis. The classification of MacEwen has been well accepted:

1. Failure of formation (Fig. 82-25)
   a. Partial failure of formation (wedge vertebra)
   b. Complete failure of formation (hemivertebra)
2. Failure of segmentation (Fig. 82-26)
   a. Unilateral failure of segmentation (unilateral unsegmented bar)
   b. Bilateral failure of segmentation (block vertebra)
3. Miscellaneous

If one thinks of the balance of growth potentials in the spine, it is clear that if one side is unsegmented and has no growth potential, the opposite side with growth potential will produce a progressive curve. On the other hand, if the spine has a group of miscellaneous anomalies, the growth potential may be approximately the same on the two sides. Therefore the most malicious anomaly is the unilateral unsegmented bar. The second most malicious is multiple hemivertebrae adjacent to one another on the same side of the spine. Single hemivertebrae are less predictable. The greater the curve in terms of degrees and the longer the curve in terms of the number of vertebral segments involved, the more likely is progression to take place.

Careful measurements and comparison of spine films at 6-month intervals must be made, using the Cobb system of measurement. It is then determined whether the curve is progressive; Winter has shown progression to occur at about 5 degrees per year. If the curve is proved to be progressive, prompt treatment must be instituted.

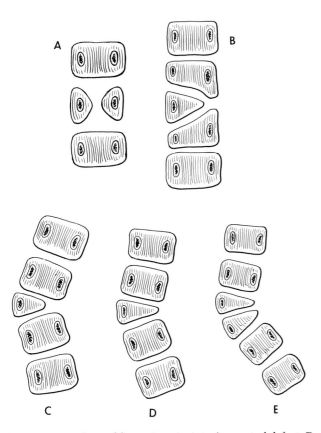

Fig. 82-25 Defects of formation. **A,** Anterior central defect. **B,** Incarcerated hemivertebra. **C,** Free hemivertebra. **D,** Wedge vertebra. **E,** Multiple hemivertebrae. (Redrawn from Bradford DS and Hensinger RM: The pediatric spine, New York, 1985, Thieme Medical Publishers, Inc.)

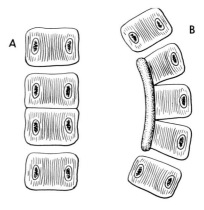

Fig. 82-26 **A,** Block vertebra. **B,** Unilateral unsegmented bar. (Redrawn from Bradford DS and Hensinger RM: The pediatric spine, New York, 1985, Thieme Medical Publishers, Inc.)

All curves must be measured, including the compensatory or secondary ones in the seemingly normal parts of the spine. We measure from each end of the anomalous area as well as from each end of the entire curve generally considered in treatment, that is, from the vertebra maximally tilted at each end. We believe that measuring the anomalous area separately is possibly a more accurate way of determining whether growth is asymmetric or the curve is increasing because more vertebrae are being added to it. Because a congenital kyphosis is often produced by a posterior or posterolateral hemivertebra or other errors in segmentation, lateral roentgenograms of the spine should be made at intervals to detect a kyphos. When a congenital kyphosis increases, an early posterior fusion is mandatory and while the deformity is relatively mild this treatment is usually sufficient. A more severe kyphosis, however, is more difficult to control. Winter, Moe, and Eilers have been unable to obtain a solid fusion or stablize a congenital kyphosis with an angle of more than 60 degrees without combining posterior and anterior fusions.

The physical examination must be thorough, looking for other congenital anomalies and the state of the nervous system. There is a 20% incidence of associated genitourinary anomalies and a 7% incidence of congenital heart disease. Diastematomyelia may occur in approximately 5% of patients. Appropriate evaluation of any associated abnormality must precede definitive care of the spine. Myelography or magnetic resonance imaging (MRI) may be used routinely and must be used if there is a suspicion of a diastematomyelia or if any neurologic abnormality exists in the lower extremities. Gillespie et al. reported their experience with 31 patients with congenital scoliosis and intraspinal anomalies, 17 with diastematomyelia, and 14 with a miscellaneous group of developmental tumors. They emphasized the probable high risk of congenital intraspinal anomalies with congenital scoliosis. A significant number of these may have no cutaneous manifestations. Preoperative myelography or MRI is clearly advisable in these patients, with neurosurgical management preceding spinal fusion.

NONOPERATIVE TREATMENT. The Milwaukee brace is the most effective of the usually ineffective methods of nonoperative treatment. It is used primarily for the compensatory curves above and below the congenital one. If the brace maintains the curves in an acceptable position, it can be continued. If, however, any curve begins to progress despite faithful brace wearing, fusion is indicated. No attempt should be made to brace curves exceeding 50 degrees.

OPERATIVE TREATMENT. Surgery remains the fundamental treatment for congenital scoliosis since 75% of the curves are progressive and the Milwaukee brace is relatively ineffective. Fusion for congenital scoliosis may be done at very young ages since it is far better to take away the growth on the convex side and prevent progression. We do not routinely use a Milwaukee brace after scoliosis fusions in young patients. The brace may be required, however, in a patient with congenital scoliosis in which the primary curve is not increasing but the secondary curves in the normal part of the spine must be controlled until growth is complete. Without this type of treatment the curves in the previously normal area of the spine sometimes become structural and more than double the angle of the congenital curve.

Fusion in situ. Fusion in situ is appropriate for those curves detected at an early stage with minor deformity. A wide exposure of the area to be fused is gained to the tips of the transverse processes bilaterally by careful subperiosteal dissection. The facet joints are then excised, and the cartilage is removed. Preferably autogenous iliac bone should be placed in the facet joints with the entire area decorticated and additional bone added. The top and bottom of the fused area can be marked with a wire suture or metal clip for postoperative observation. Postoperative immobilization is in a Risser cast and the patient is continued ambulatory. Some surgeons add anterior interbody fusion and hemiepiphysiodeses at multiple levels to the posterior fusion.

Cast correction and fusion. Cast correction and fusion are useful in curves flexible enough to allow cast correction but in which instrumentation is impractical or is considered dangerous. Casting can be done either preoperatively or postoperatively. The fusion should always encompass the measured curve with at least one vertebra above and one below, and all vertebrae rotated in the same direction as those in the apex of the curve should be included. The surgical technique is the same as for fusion in situ. Cast application is by maximal correction using longitudinal traction and localizer force. Formerly the patient was kept in bed for 6 months, and then an ambulatory cast was applied and worn for an additional 4 months. Recently most children have been ambulated immediately even though some correction may be lost. A brace sometimes is used until about 12 years of age in an attempt to prevent bending of the fusion mass and lengthening of the curve and to control the secondary curves. Pseudarthroses are repaired early if identified on roentgenograms 6 and 9 months after surgery.

Halo-femoral traction and fusion. Halo-femoral traction and fusion *rarely are used in congenital curves* and are reserved for more rigid curves for which cast correction is inadequate and a greater degree of correction is desired. As a general rule, the amount of weight used in the traction should not exceed 50% of the total body weight. Weights are added slowly and gradually each day with careful monitoring of the neurologic status. An inability to void would be the first sign of neurologic dysfunction of the cord. Cranial nerve function should be evaluated as well as peripheral nerve function. Any sudden pain, numbness, or weakness should result in all weights being discontinued and only gradually restarted after symptoms have disappeared. Usually a period up to 3 weeks is necessary to gain maximum correction with the slow addition of weights. The patient is operated on in traction with the weights reduced 50%. The weights are gradually brought back up to the preoperative level between 24 and 72 hours postoperatively. Harrington instrumentation should be added only as a stabilizing strut to prevent collapse when the traction is removed and at the time of casting. Any attempt at further correction with Harrington instrumentation may result in paraplegia. Alternatively, a halo cast can be used postoperatively.

Harrington instrumentation and fusion. Harrington instrumentation and fusion are far more dangerous in congenital scoliosis than idiopathic and should be used with spinal cord monitoring. Instrumentation is inserted sometimes as a stabilizing strut only, relying on all correction to have been achieved by halo-femoral or cast correction.

Combined anterior and posterior convex fusion. In 1981 Winter reported 10 patients with progressive con-genital scoliosis treated by convex anterior and posterior epiphysiodesis and arthrodesis. The technique is not new, but interest in it has been revived by reports from authors such as Roaf, Andrew and Piggott, and Winter. All authors list as criteria for patient selection: (1) a documented progressive curve, (2) a curve of less than 60 degrees, (3) a curve of six segments or less, and (4) a child aged 5 years or less. Winter's criteria for effective correction with this procedure are (1) epiphysiodesis of the entire curve, not merely the apical segments; (2) both anterior and posterior fusion; (3) arthrodesis of the involved segment, which accompanies the epiphysiodesis; (4) rigid immobilization of the spine until the arthrodesis is solid; and (5) performance of the procedure at an early age. He reported excellent early results but stated that several more years of follow-up are necessary before conclusions can be reached.

- ■ *TECHNIQUE (WINTER).* Position the patient on the concave side in the straight lateral position, and prepare and drape the back and side in the same field. Make two incisions, a midline posterior and a second one along the rib to be removed (the rib leading to the upper end of the curve). Expose the vertebrae anteriorly by a transpleural, retropleural, or retroperitoneal approach, depending on the area involved. Identify the proper levels by a roentgeno-

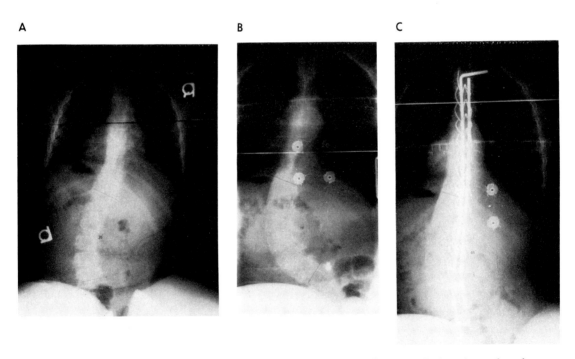

Fig. 82-27   A, Thoracolumbar scoliosis secondary to hemivertebra at L5. **B,** Anterior wedge of bone removed through left retroperitoneal exposure. **C,** Posterior Harrington compression rod closing wedge on convex side. (From Bradford DS et al: Moe's textbook of scoliosis and other spinal deformities, ed 2, Philadelphia, 1987, WB Saunders Co.)

---

gram. Ligate segmental vessels. Remove the lateral half of the growth plate and the bony end plate. Insert an autogenous bone graft (usually the rib), and close the wound. Posteriorly, expose only the convexity of the curve. Excise the facet joints, decorticate the lamina and transverse process, and insert an autogenous graft. Apply a corrective cast, which is worn for 6 months and followed by 6 more months of brace wear.

Wedge resection (hemivertebra excision). Wedge resection is used infrequently since it is far better to perform an early fusion to prevent progression. This must be reserved for those with pelvic obliquity uncorrectable by other means or with a fixed lateral translation of the thorax that cannot be corrected by other means (Fig. 82-27). The safest level to perform such excision is at the L3 and L4 level below the conus medullaris. Wedge resection in the T4 to T9 area should be viewed with alarm since this is the area of the narrowest spinal canal and the least blood supply to the cord. Hemivertebra excision is best performed as a two-stage procedure as described by Leatherman and Dickson in which the vertebral body is removed by an anterior exposure initially. Two weeks later a posterior approach and excision of the remainder of the hemivertebra are carried out. The defect can then be closed with a Harrington compression rod or other appropriate instrumentation. This procedure must always be accompanied by a fusion of the appropriate length. Postoperative care consists of cast immobilization in a supine position for 6 months, followed by an ambulatory cast for another 4 months or until fusion is completely solid.

REFERENCES

Infantile idiopathic scoliosis

Ceballos T et al: Prognosis in infantile idiopathic scoliosis, J Bone Joint Surg 62-A:863, 1980.

Conner AN: Developmental anomalies and prognosis in infantile idiopathic scoliosis, J Bone Joint Surg 51-B:711, 1969.

Ferriera JH and James JR: Progressive and resolving infantile idiopathic scoliosis: differential diagnosis, J Bone Joint Surg 54-B:648, 1972.

James JIP, Lloyd-Roberts GC, and Pilcher MF: Infantile structural scoliosis, J Bone Joint Surg 41-B:719, 1959.

James JIP: Infantile idiopathic scoliosis, Clin Orthop 21:106, 1961.

James JIP: The management of infants with scoliosis, J Bone Joint Surg 57-B:422, 1975.

McMaster MJ and Macnicol MF: The management of progressive infantile idiopathic scoliosis, J Bone Joint Surg 61-B:36, 1979.

Mehta MH: The rib-vertebra angle in the early diagnosis between resolving and progressive infantile scoliosis, J Bone Joint Surg 54-B:230, 1972.

Mehta MH: Radiographic estimation of vertebral rotation in scoliosis, J Bone Joint Surg 55-B:513, 1973.

Moe JH et al: Harrington instrumentation without fusion plus external orthotic support for treatment of difficult curvature problems in young children, Clin Orthop 185:34, 1985.

Morgan TH and Scott JC: Treatment of infantile idiopathic scoliosis, J Bone Joint Surg 38-B:450, 1956.

Scott JC and Morgan TH: The natural history and prognosis of infantile idiopathic scoliosis, J Bone Joint Surg 37-B:400, 1955.

Thompson SK and Bentley G: Prognosis in infantile idiopathic scoliosis, J Bone Joint Surg 62-B:151, 1980.

Walker GF: An evaluation of an external splint for idiopathic structural scoliosis in infancy, J Bone Joint Surg 47-B:524, 1965.

Wynne-Davies R: Infantile idiopathic scoliosis: causative factors, particularly in the first six months of life, J Bone Joint Surg 57-B:138, 1975.

Juvenile idiopathic scoliosis

Figueiredo UM and James JIP: Juvenile idiopathic scoliosis, J Bone Joint Surg 63-B:61, 1981.

Koop SE: Infantile and juvenile idiopathic scoliosis before skeletal maturity, Orthop Clin North Am 19:331, 1988.

Tolo VT and Gillespie R: The characteristics of juvenile idiopathic scoliosis and results of its treatment, J Bone Joint Surg 60-B:181, 1978.

Adolescent idiopathic scoliosis

General; natural history; patient evaluation

Aaro S and Adhlborn M: Vertebral rotation: estimation of vertebral rotation and spinal and rib cage deformity in scoliosis by computerized tomography, Spine 6:460, 1981.

Abbott EG: Correction of lateral curvature of the spine, NY Med J 95:833, 1912.

Appelgren G and Willner S: End vertebra angle-a roentgenographic method to describe a scoliosis: a follow up study of idiopathic scoliosis treated with the Boston brace, Spine 15:71, 1990.

Ascani E, Bartolozzi P, Logroscino T, et al: Natural history of untreated idiopathic scoliosis after skeletal maturity, Spine 11:784, 1986.

Binstadt DH, Lonstein JE, and Winter RB: Radiographic evaluation of the scoliotic patient, Minn Med 61:478, 1978.

Bjure J and Nachemson A: Non-treated scoliosis, Clin Orthop 93:44, 1973.

Brooks HL, Azen SP, Gerberg E, et al: Scoliosis: a perspective epidemiological study, J Bone Joint Surg 57-A:968, 1975.

Bunnell WP: Vertebral rotation: a simple method of measurement in routine radiographs, Orthop Trans 9:114, 1985 (abstract).

Bunnell WP: The natural history of idiopathic scoliosis before skeletal maturity, Spine 11:773, 1986.

Cobb JR: The treatment of scoliosis, Conn Med J 7:467, 1943.

Cobb JR: Observations on the treatment of idiopathic scoliosis, 1948 (unpublished).

Cobb JR: Outline for the study of scoliosis, AAOS Instr Course Lect 5:261, 1948.

Cobb JR: Correction of scoliosis. In Poliomyelitis, Second International Poliomyelitis Congress, Philadelphia, 1952, JB Lippincott Co.

Cobb JR: The problem of the primary curve, J Bone Joint Surg 42-A:1413, 1960.

Collis DK, and Ponseti IV: Long-term follow-up of patients with idiopathic scoliosis not treated surgically, J Bone Joint Surg 51-A:425, 1969.

DeSmet A, Fritz SL, and Ahser MA: A method for minimizing the radiation exposure from scoliosis radiographs, J Bone Joint Surg 61-A:156, 1981.

Enneking WF and Harrington P: Pathological changes in scoliosis, J Bone Joint Surg 51-A:165, 1969.

Ferguson AB: The study and treatment of scoliosis, South Med J 23:116, 1930.

Ferguson AB: Roentgen interpretations and decisions in scoliosis, AAOS Instr Course Lect 7:214, 1950.

Galeazzi R: The treatment of scoliosis, J Bone Joint Surg 11:81, 1929.

Gazioglu K, Goldstein LA, Femi-Pearse D, and Yu PN: Pulmonary function in idiopathic scoliosis: comparative evaluation before and after orthopaedic correction, J Bone Joint Surg 50-A:1391, 1968.

Gray JE, Hoffman AE, and Peterson HA: Reduction of radiation exposure during radiography for scoliosis, J Bone Joint Surg 65-A:5, 1983.

James JIP: Two curve patterns in idiopathic structural scoliosis, J Bone Joint Surg 33-B:399, 1951.

James JIP: Idiopathic scoliosis: the prognosis, diagnosis, and operative indications related to curve patterns and the age at onset, J Bone Joint Surg 36-B:36, 1954.

Johnson BE and Westgate HD: Methods of predicting vital capacity in patients with thoracic scoliosis, J Bone Joint Surg 52-A:1433, 1970.

Kleinberg S: A survey of structural scoliosis: the principles of treatment and their application, AAOS Instr Course Lect 7:130, 1950.

Kleinberg S: Scoliosis: pathology, etiology, and treatment, Baltimore, 1951, The Williams & Wilkins Co.

Kleinman RE, Csongradi JJ, Rinsky LA, et al: The radiographic assessment of spinal flexibility in scoliosis: a study of the efficacy of the prone push film, Clin Orthop 162:47, 1982.

Lonstein JE: Natural history and school screening for scoliosis, Orthop Clin North Am 19:227, 1988.

Lonstein JE and Carlson JM: The prediction of curve progression in untreated idiopathic scoliosis during growth, J Bone Joint Surg 66-A:1061, 1984.

Mankin HJ, Graham JJ, and Schack J: Cardiopulmonary function in mild and moderate idiopathic scoliosis, J Bone Joint Surg 46-A:53, 1964.

Nachemson A: A long term follow-up study of nontreated scoliosis, Acta Orthop Scand 39:466, 1968.

Nachemson A: A long term follow-up study of nontreated scoliosis, J Bone Joint Surg 50-A:203, 1969.

Nilsonne U and Lundgren KD: Long-term prognosis in idiopathic scoliosis, Acta Orthop Scand 39:456, 1968.

Perdriolle R: La scoliose, Paris, 1979, Maloine.

Perdriolle R and Vidal J: Morphology of scoliosis: three-dimensional evolution, Orthopedics 10:909, 1987.

Ponseti IV and Friedman B: Prognosis in idiopathic scoliosis, J Bone Joint Surg 32-A:381, 1950.

Riseborough EJ and Wynne-Davies R: A genetic study of idiopathic scoliosis in Boston, Massachusetts, J Bone Joint Surg 55-A:974, 1973.

Risser JC: Acquired scoliosis. In: The cyclopedia of medicine, vol 11, Philadelphia, 1933, FA Davis Co.

Risser JC: Important practical facts in the treatment of scoliosis, AAOS Instr Course Lect 5:248, 1948.

Risser JC: Scoliosis, AAOS Instr Course Lect 14:91, 1957.

Risser JC: The iliac apophysis: an invaluable sign in the management of scoliosis, Clin Orthop 11:111, 1958.

Risser JC: Modern trends in scoliosis, Bull Hosp J Dis Ortho Inst 19:166, 1958.

Risser JC: Scoliosis: past and present, J Bone Joint Surg 46-A:167, 1964.

Risser JC and Ferguson AB: Scoliosis: its prognosis, J Bone Joint Surg 18:667, 1936.

Risser JC and Norquist DM: A follow-up study of the treatment of scoliosis, J Bone Joint Surg 40-A:555, 1958.

Roaf R: Scoliosis, Baltimore, 1966, The Williams & Wilkins Co.

Rogala EJ, Drummond DS, and Gurr J: Scoliosis: incidence and natural history; a prospective epidemiological study, J Bone Joint Surg 60-A:173, 1978.

Schmidt AC: Fundamental principles and treatment of scoliosis, AAOS Instr Course Lect 16:184, 1959.

Shands AR Jr, Barr JS, Colonna PC, and Noall L: End-result study of the treatment of idiopathic scoliosis: report of the research committee of the American Orthopaedic Association, J Bone Joint Surg 23:963, 1941.

Weinstein SL: Idiopathic scoliosis: natural history, Spine 11:780, 1986.

Weinstein SL and Ponseti IV: Curve progression in idiopathic scoliosis: long-term follow-up, J Bone Joint Surg 65-A:447, 1983.

Weinstein SL, Zaval DC, and Ponseti IV: Idiopathic scoliosis: long-term follow-up and prognosis in untreated patients, J Bone Joint Surg 63-A:702, 1981.

Winter RB: Scoliosis and other spinal deformities, Acta Orthop Scand 46:400, 1975.

Winter RB, Lovell WW, and Moe JH: Excessive thoracic lordosis and loss of pulmonary function in patients with idiopathic scoliosis, J Bone Joint Surg 57-A:972, 1974.

Wynne-Davies R: Familial (idiopathic) scoliosis: a family survery, J Bone Joint Surg 50-B;24, 1968.

Wynne-Davies R: Genetic and other factors in the etiology of scoliosis, PhD Thesis, University of Edinburgh.

Nonsurgical treatment

Aaro S, Brustrom R, and Dahlborn M: The derotating affect of the Boston brace: a comparison between computer tomography and a conventional method, Spine 6:477, 1981.

Anderson S, and Bradford DS: Low-profile halo, Clin Orthop 103:72, 1974.

Andriacchi TP, Schultz AB, Belytschko TB, et al: Milwaukee brace correction of idiopathic scoliosis: a biomechanical analysis and a retrospective study, J Bone Joint Surg 58-A:806, 1976.

Arkin AM: Correction of structural changes in scoliosis by corrective plaster jackets and prolonged recumbency, J Bone Joint Surg 46-A:33, 1964.

Blount WP and Schmidt AC: The Milwaukee brace, 1953, (mimeographed privately).

Blount WP, Schmidt AC, and Bidwell RG: Making the Milwaukee brace, J Bone Joint Surg 40-A:526, 1958.

Blount WP, Schmidt AC, Keever ED, and Leonard ET: The Milwaukee brace in the operative treatment of scoliosis, J Bone Joint Surg 40-A:511, 1958.

Bunnell WP: Nonoperative treatment of spinal deformity: the case for observation, AAOS Instr Course Lect 34:106, 1985.

Carr WA, Moe JH, Winter RB, et al: Treatment of idiopathic scoliosis in the Milwaukee brace, J Bone Joint Surg 62-A:599, 1980.

Clark JA, Hsu LCS, and Yau ACMC: Viscoelastic behaviour of deformed spines under correction with halo pelvic distraction, Clin Orthop 110:90, 1975.

Cook CD, Barrie H, Deforest SA, and Helliesen PJ: Pulmonary physiology in children. III. Lung volumes, mechanics of respiration and respiratory muscle strength in scoliosis, J Pediatr 25:766, 1960.

Cotrel Y: Le corset de platre E.D.F dans le traitement de la scoliose idiopathique, Med Hyg 28:1032, 1970.

DeWald RL and Ray RD: Skeletal traction for the treatment of severe scoliosis: the University of Illinois halo-loop apparatus, J Bone Joint Surg 52-A:233, 1970.

DeWald RL, Mulcahy TM, and Schultz AB: Force measurement studies with the halo-loop apparatus in scoliosis, Orthop Rev 2:17, December 1973.

Dove J, Hsu LC, and Yau AC: The cervical spine after halo-pelvic traction: an analysis of the complications of 83 patients, J Bone Joint Surg 62-B:158, 1980.

Edmonson AS and Morris JT: Follow-up study of Milwaukee brace treatment in patients with idiopathic scoliosis, Clin Orthop 126:58, 1977.

Hall JE, Emans JB, Kaelin A, et al: Boston brace system treatment of idiopathic scoliosis: follow-up in 400 patients finished treatment, Orthop Trans 8:148, 1983 (abstract).

Hassan J and Bjerkreim I: Progression in idiopathic scoliosis after conservative treatment, Acta Orthop Scand 54:88, 1983.

Houtkin S, and Levine DB: The halo yoke: a simplified device for attachment of the halo to a body cast, J Bone Joint Surg 54-A:881, 1972.

Humbyrd DE, Latimer RF, Lonstein JE, et al: Brain abscess as a complication of halo traction, Spine 6:364, 1981.

Kahanovitz N, Levine DB, and Lardone J: The part-time Milwaukee brace treatment of juvenile idiopathic scoliosis, Clin Orthop 167:145, 1982.

Kalamchi A, Yau ACMC, O'Brien JP, and Hodgson AR: Halo-pelvic distraction apparatus: an analysis of one hundred and fifty consecutive patients, J Bone Joint Surg 58-A:1119, 1976.

Kehl OK and Morrissy RT: Brace treatment in adolescent idiopathic scoliosis: an update on concepts and technique, Clin Orthop 229:34, 1988.

Kuhn RA and Garrett A: The halo in the management of cervical spine lesions, Orthop Rev 1:25 December, 1972.

Lindth M: The effect of sagittal curve changes on brace correction of idiopathic scoliosis, Spine 5:26, 1980.

Lonstein JE and Winter RB: Adolsecent idiopathic scoliosis: nonoperative treatment, Orthop Clin North Am 19.239, 1988.

McCullough NC, Schultz M, Javech H, and Latta L: Miami TLSO in the management of scoliosis: preliminary results from 100 cases, J Pediatr Orthop 1:141, 1981.

Miller JAA, Nachemson AL, and Schultz AB: Effectiveness of braces in mild idiopathic scoliosis, Spine 9:632, 1984.

Montgomery F, Willner S, and Appelgren G: Long-term follow-up of patients with adolescent idiopathic scoliosis treated conservatively: an analysis of the clinical value of progression, J Pediatr Orthop 10:48, 1990.

Nash CL: Current concepts review: scoliosis bracing, J Bone Joint Surg 62-A:848, 1980.

Nickel VL, Perry J, Garrett A, and Heppenstall M: The halo: a spinal skeletal traction fixation device, J Bone Joint Surg 50-A:1400, 1968.

O'Brien JP: The halo-pelvic apparatus: a clinical, bio-engineering and anatomical study, Acta Orthop Scand, suppl 163, 1975.

O'Brien JP, Yau ACMC, and Hodgson AR: Halo pelvic traction: a technic for severe spinal deformities, Clin Orthop 93:179, 1973.

O'Brien JP, Yau ACMC, Smith TK, and Hodgson AR: Halo pelvic traction: a preliminary report on a method of external skeletal fixation for correcting deformities and maintaining fixation of the spine, J Bone Joint Surg 53-B:217, 1971.

Perry J: The halo in spinal abnormalities: practical factors and avoidance of complications, Orthop Clin North Am 3:69, 1972.

Perry J and Nickel VL: Total cervical-spine fusion for neck paralysis, J Bone Joint Surg 41-A:37, 1959.

Pieron AP and Welply WR: Halo traction, J Bone Joint Surg 52-B:119, 1970.

Ransford AO, and Manning CWSF: Complications of halo-pelvic distraction for scoliosis, J Bone Joint Surg 57-B:131, 1975.

Renshaw TS: Orthotic treatment of idiopathic scoliosis and kyphosis, AAOS Instr Course Lect 34:110, 1985.

Risser JC: Plaster body-jackets, Am J Orthop 3:19, 1961.

Risser JC, Lauder CH, Norquist DM, and Craig WA: Three types of body casts, AAOS Instr Course Lect 10:131, 1953.

Rudel S and Renshaw TS: The effect of the Milwaukee brace on spinal decompensation in idiopathic scoliosis, Spine 8:385, 1983.

Schmidt AC: Halo-tibial traction combined with the Milwaukee brace, Clin Orthop 77:73, 1971.

Toledo LC, Toledo CH, and MacEwen GD: Halo traction with the Circolectric bed in the treatment of severe spinal deformities: a preliminary report, J Pediatr Orthop 2:554, 1982.

Uden A and Willner S: The effect of lumbar flexion and Boston thoracic brace on the curves in idiopathic scoliosis, Spine 8:846, 1983.

Watts HG: Bracing spinal deformities, Orthop Clin North Am 10:769, 1979.

Weisl H: Unusual complications of skull caliper traction, J Bone Joint Surg 54-B:143, 1972.

Wilkins C and MacEwen GD: Halo-traction affecting cranial nerves, J Bone Joint Surg 56-A:1540, 1974.

Willner S: Effect of the Boston thoracic brace on the frontal and sagittal curves of the spine, Acta Orthop Scand 55:457, 1984.

Winter RB, Moe JH, MacEwen GD, and Peon-Vidales H: The Milwaukee brace in the non-operative treatment of congenital scoliosis, Spine 1:33, 1976.

Young R and Thomassen EH: Step-by-step procedure by applying halo ring, Orthop Rev 3:62, June 1974.

Surgical treatment

Akbarnia BA: Selection of methodology in surgical treatment of adolescent idiopathic scoliosis, Orthop Clin North Am 19:319, 1988.

Bieber E, Tolo V, and Uematsu S: Spinal cord monitoring during posterior spinal instrumentation and fusion, Clin Orthop 229:121, 1988.

Bradshaw K, Webb JK, and Fraser AM: Clinical evaluation of spinal cord monitoring in scoliosis surgery, Spine 9:636, 1984.

Breig A: Biomechanics of the central nervous system: some basic normal and pathologic phenomena concerning spine, discs, and cord, Stockholm, 1960, Almquist and Wiksell (translated by Victor Braxton, Chicago, 1960, Year Book Medical Publishers).

Brown RH and Nash CL Jr: Current status of spinal cord monitoring Spine, 4:466, 1979.

Butte FL: Scoliosis treated by the wedging jacket: selection of the area to be fused, J Bone Joint Surg 20:1, 1938.

Cobb JR: Technique, after-treatment, and results of spine fusion for scoliosis, AAOS Instr Course Lect 9:65, 1952.

Cobb JR: Spine arthrodesis in the treatment of scoliosis, Bull Hosp J Dis Ortho Inst 19:187, 1958.

Cotrel Y and Dubousset J: New segmental posterior instrumentation of the spine, Orthop Trans 9:118, 1985.

Cotrel Y, Dubousset J, and Guillaunat M: New universal instrumentation and spinal surgery, Clin Orthop 227:10, 1988.

Cowell HR and Swickard JW: Autotransfusion in children's orthopaedics, J Bone Joint Surg 56-A:908, 1974.

Dickson JH: Spinal instrumentation and fusion in adolescent idiopathic scoliosis: indications and surgical techniques, Contemp Orthop 4:397, 1982.

Dolan JA and MacEwen GD: Surgical treatment of scoliosis, Clin Orthop 76:125, 1971.

Donaldson WF Jr and Wissinger HA: The results of surgical exploration of spine fusion performed for scoliosis, Western J Surg Obstet Gynecol 72:195, 1964.

Dorang LA, Klebanoff G, and Kemmerer WT: Autotransfusion in long-segment spinal fusion: an experimental model to demonstrate the efficacy of salvaging blood contaminated with bone fragments and marrow, Am J Surg 123:686, 1972.

Dorph MH: The cast syndrome, N Engl J Med 243:440, 1950.

Dorr J, Brown J, and Perry J: Results of posterior spine fusion in patients with spinal muscle atrophy: a review of 34 cases. Paper presented at the Scoliosis Research Society, 1972.

Drummond DS, Keene JS, and Breed A: The Wisconsin system: a technique of interspinous segmental spinal instrumentation, Contemp Orthop 8:29, 1984.

Drummond DS, Guadagni J, Keene JS, et al: Interspinous process segmental spinal instrumentation, J Pediatr Orthop 4:397, 1984.

Dubousset J: Recidive dune scoliose lombaire et dun bassin oblique apres fusion precoce: le phenomene due ville brequin. Proc Group Etud de la Scoliose, Paris, 1973.

Dubousset J, Herring JA, and Shufflebarger H: The crankshaft phenomenon, J Pediatr Orthop 9:541, 1989.

Dwyer AF: Experience of anterior correction of scoliosis, Clin Orthop 93:191, 1973.

Dwyer AF, Newton NC, and Sherwood AA: An anterior approach to scoliosis: a preliminary report, Clin Orthop 62:192, 1969.

Engler GL, Spielholz NJ, Bernhard WN, et al: Somatosensory evoked potentials during Harrington instrumentation for scoliosis, J Bone Joint Surg 60-A:528, 1978.

Evarts CM: The cast syndrome: report of a case after spinal fusion for scoliosis, Clin Orthop 75:164, 1971.

Evarts CM, Winter RB, and Hall JE: Vascular compression of the duodenum associated with the treatment of scoliosis: review of the literature and report of eighteen cases, J Bone Joint Surg 53-A:431, 1971.

Fielding JW and Waugh T: Postoperative correction of scoliosis, JAMA 182:541, 1962.

Goldstein LA: Results in the treatment of scoliosis with turnbuckle plaster cast correction and fusion, J Bone Joint Surg 41-A:321, 1959.

Goldstein LA: The surgical management of scoliosis, Clin Orthop 35:95, 1964.

Goldstein LA: Surgical management of scoliosis, J Bone Joint Surg 48-A:167, 1966.

Goldstein LA: Treatment of idiopathic scoliosis by Harrington instrumentation and fusion with fresh autogenous iliac bone grafts: results in eighty patients, J Bone Joint Surg 51-A:209, 1969.

Goldstein LA: The surgical management of scoliosis, Clin Orthop 77:32, 1971.

Goldstein LA: The surgical treatment of idiopathic scoliosis, Clin Orthop 93:131, 1973.

Goldstein LA and Evarts CM: Further experiences with the treatment of scoliosis by cast correction and spine fusion with fresh autogenous iliac-bone grafts, J Bone Joint Surg 48-A:962, 1966.

Gollehon D, Kahanovitz N, and Happel LT: Temperature effects on feline cortical and spinal evoked potentials, Spine 8:443, 1983.

Hall JE: The place of the anterior approach to the spine in scoliosis surgery. In Keim HA, editor: Postgraduate course on the management and care of the scoliosis patient, November 5-7, 1970, pp 32-34.

Hall JE: Pre-operative assessment of the patient with a spinal deformity, AAOS Instr Course Lect 34:127, 1985.

Hall JE, Levine CR, and Sudhir KG: Intraoperative awakening to monitor spinal cord function during Harrington instrumentation and spine fusion: descriptions of procedure and report of three cases, J Bone Joint Surg 60-A:533, 1978.

Hardy JH and Gossling HR: Combined halo and sacral bar fixation: a method for immobilization and early ambulation following extensive spine fusion, Clin Orthop 75:205, 1971.

Harrington PR: Treatment of scoliosis: correction and internal fixation by spine instrumentation, J Bone Joint Surg 44-A:591, 1962.

Harrington PR: The management of scoliosis by spine instrumentation: an evaluation of more than 200 cases, South Med J 56:1367, 1963.

Harrington PR: Technical details in relation to the successful use of instrumentation in scoliosis, Orthop Clin North Am 3:49, 1972.

Harrington PR: The history and development of Harrington instrumenation, Clin Orthop 93:110, 1973.

Harrington PR and Dickson JH: An eleven-year clinical investigation of Harrington instrumentation: a preliminary report of 578 cases, Clin Orthop 93:113, 1973.

Hibbs RA: A report of fifty-nine cases of scoliosis treated by the fusion operation, J Bone Joint Surg 6:3, 1924.

Hibbs RA, Risser JC, and Ferguson AB: Scoliosis treated by the fusion operation, J Bone Joint Surg 13:91, 1931.

Jones SJ, Edgar MA, Ransford AO, and Thomas NP: A system for the electrophysiological monitoring of the spinal cord during operations for scoliosis, J Bone Joint Surg 65-B:134, 1983.

King HA, Moe JH, Bradford DS, and Winter RB: The selection of fusion levels in thoracic idiopathic scoliosis, J Bone Joint Surg 65-A:1302, 1983.

Kojima Y, Yamamoto T, Ogino H, et al: Evoked spinal potentials as a monitor of spinal cord viability, Spine 4:471, 1979.

Larson SJ, Walsh PR, Sances A Jr, et al: Evoked potentials in experimental myelopathy, Spine 5:299, 1980.

Leatherman KD: The management of rigid spinal curves, Clin Orthop 93:215, 1973.

Leider LL Jr, Moe JH, and Winter RB: Early ambulation after the surgical treatment of idiopathic scoliosis, J Bone Joint Surg 55-A:1003, 1973.

Letts RM, Palakar G, and Bobechko WP: Preoperative skeletal traction in scoliosis, J Bone Joint Surg 57-A:616, 1975.

Levy WJ, and York DH: Evoked potentials from motor tracts in humans, Neurosurgery 12:422, 1983.

Lindseth RE: Posterior iliac osteotomy for fixed pelvic obliquity, J Bone Joint Surg 60-A:17, 1978.

Lueders H, Gurd A, Hahn J, et al: A new technique for intraoperative monitoring of spinal cord function: multichannel recording of spinal cord and subcortical evoked potentials, Spine 7:110, 1982.

Luque ER: Anatomy of scoliosis and its correction, Clin Orthop 105:298, 1974.

Luque ER: Segmental spinal instrumentation for correction of scoliosis, Clin Orthop 163:192, 1982.

Machida M, Weinstein SL, Yamada T, and Kimura J: Spinal cord monitoring: electrophysiological measures of sensory and motor function during spinal surgery, Spine 10:407, 1985.

McCarroll HR, and Costen W: Attempted treatment of scoliosis by unilateral vertebral epiphyseal arrest, J Bone Joint Surg 42-A:965, 1960.

McKittrick JE: Banked autologous blood in elective surgery, Am J Surg 128:137, 1974.

Moe JH: A critical analysis of methods of fusion for scoliosis: an evaluation in two hundred and sixty-six patients, J Bone Joint Surg 40-A:529, 1958.

Moe JH: Complications of scoliosis treatment, Clin Orthop 53:21, 1967.

Moe JH and Gustilo RB: Treatment of scoliosis: results in 196 patients treated with cast correction and fusion, J Bone Joint Surg 46-A:293, 1964.

Morgenstern JM, Hassmann GC, and Keim HA: Modifying post-transfusion hepatitis by gamma globulin in spinal surgery, Orthop Rev 4:29, June 1975.

Mouradian WH and Simmons EH: A frame for spinal surgery to reduce intra-abdominal pressure while continuous traction is applied, J Bone Joint Surg 59-A:1098, 1977.

Nach CD and Keim HA: Prophylactic antibiotics in spinal surgery, Orthop Rev 2:27, June 1973.

Nachemson AL and Elfström G: Intravital wireless telemetry of axial forces in Harrington distraction rods in patients with idiopathic scoliosis, J Bone Joint Surg 53-A:445, 1971.

Nachemson A and Nordwall A: Effectiveness of preoperative Cotrel traction for correction of idiopathic scoliosis, J Bone Joint Surg 59-A:504, 1977.

Nachlas IW and Borden JN: The cure of experimental scoliosis by directed growth control, J Bone Joint Surg 33-A:24, 1951.

Nash CL Jr, Lorig RA, Schatzinger LA, and Brown RH: Spinal cord monitoring during operative treatment of the spine, Clin Orthop 126:100, 1977.

Nash CL, Schatzinger L, and Lorig R: Intraoperative monitoring of spinal cord function during scoliosis spine surgery, J Bone Joint Surg 56-A:1765, 1974 (abstract).

Nordwall A, Axelgaard J, Harada Y, et al: Spinal cord monitoring using evoked potentials recorded from vertebral bone in cat, Spine 4:486, 1979.

O'Brien JP, Dwyer AP, and Hodgson AR: Paralytic pelvic obliquity: its prognosis and management and the development of a technique for full correction of the deformity, J Bone Joint Surg 57-A:626, 1975.

O'Brien JP and Yau ACMC: Anterior and posterior correction and fusion for paralytic scoliosis, Clin Orthop 86:151, 1972.

Puranik SR, Keiser RP, and Gilbert MG: Arteriomesenteric duodenal compression in children, Am J Surg 124:334, 1972.

Rappaport M, Hall K, Hopkins K, et al: Effects of corrective scoliosis surgery on somatosensory evoked potentials, Spine 7:404, 1982.

Reger SI, Henry DT, Whitehill R, et al: Spinal evoked potentials from the cervical spine, Spine 4:495, 1979.

Reid RL and Gamon RS Jr: The cast syndrome, Clin Orthop 79:85, 1971.

Relton JES and Hall JE: An operation frame for spinal fusion: a new apparatus designed to reduce haemorrhage during operation, J Bone Joint Surg 49-B:327, 1967.

Renshaw TS: Spinal fusion with segmental instrumentation, Contemp Orthop 4:413, 1982.

Resina J and Alves AF: A technique for correction and internal fixation for scoliosis, J Bone Joint Surg 59-B:159, 1977.

Rieth PL, Hopkins WA, and Dunlap EB Jr: A new surgical procedure in scoliosis therapy: unilateral vertebral body growth arrest by transpleural approach, Southern Surg 16:368, 1950.

Riseborough EJ: The anterior approach to the spine for the correction of deformities of the axial skeleton, Clin Orthop 93:207, 1973.

Risser JC: Scoliosis treated by cast correction and spine fusion: a long term follow-up study, Clin Orthop 116:86, 1976.

Roaf R: Vertebral growth and its mechanical control, J Bone Joint Surg 42-B:40, 1960.

Roaf R: The treatment of progressive scoliosis by unilateral growth-arrest, J Bone Joint Surg 45-B:637, 1963.

Roaf R: Wedge resection for scoliosis, J Bone Joint Surg 46-B:798, 1964.

Schultz AB and Hirsch C: Mechanical analysis of techniques for improved correction of idiopathic scoliosis, Clin Orthop 100:66, 1974.

Smith A, DeF Butte FL, and Ferguson AB: Treatment of scoliosis by the wedging jacket and spine fusion: a review of 265 cases, J Bone Joint Surg 20:825, 1938.

Smith A deF, von Lackum WH, and Wylie R: An operation for stapling vertebral bodies in congenital scoliosis, J Bone Joint Surg 36-A:342, 1954.

Spielholz NI, Benjamin MV, Engler GL, and Ransohoff J: Somatosensory evoked potentials during decompression and stabilization of the spine: methods and findings, Spine 4:500, 1979.

Steel HH: Rib resection and spine fusion in correction of convex deformity in scoliosis, J Bone Joint Surg 65-A:920, 1983.

Ulrich HF: The operative treatment of scoliosis, Am J Surg 45:235, 1939.

Van Rens TJG and Van Horn JR: Long-term results in lumbosacral interbody fusion for spondylolisthesis, Acta Orthop Scand 53:383, 1982.

Vauzelle C, Stagnara P, and Jouvinroux P: Functional monitoring of spinal cord activity during spinal surgery, Clin Orthop 93:173, 1973.

Vauzelle C, Stagnara P, and Jouvinroux P: Functional monitoring of spinal activity during spinal surgery, J Bone Joint Surg 55-A:441, 1973.

Von Lackum WH: The surgical treatment of scoliosis, AAOS Instr Course Lect 5:236, 1948.

Von Lackum WH: Surgical scoliosis, Surg Clin North Am 31:345, 1951.

Von Lackum WH: The surgical treatment of scoliosis. In Bancroft FW and Marble HC: Surgical treatment of the motor-skeletal system, ed 2, Philadelphia, 1951, JB Lippincott Co.

Von Lackum WH and Miller JP: Critical observations of the results in the operative treatment of scoliosis, J Bone Joint Surg 31-A:102, 1949.

Westgate HD, Fisch RO, and Langer LO: Pulmonary function in kyphoscoliosis before and after correction by the Harrington instrumentation method, J Bone Joint Surg 51-A:935, 1969.

White AA III, Southwick WO, DePonte RJ, et al: Relief of pain by anterior cervical-spine fusion for spondylosis: a report of sixty-five patients, J Bone Joint Surg 55-A:525, 1973.

Whitehill R, Sirna EC, Young DC, and Cantrell RW: Late esophageal perforation from an autogenous bone graft: report of a case, J Bone Joint Surg 67-A:644, 1985.

Wilson RL, Levine DB, and Doherty JH: Surgical treatment of idiopathic scoliosis, Clin Orthop 81:34, 1971.

Zielke K: Ventral derotation spondylodesis: preliminary report on 58 cases, Beitr Orthop Traumatol 25:85, 1978.

Zuege RC, Blount WP, and Dicus WT: Indications for operative treatment of spinal deformities, Wis Med J 74:S33, 1975.

Adult scoliosis

Balderston RA, Winter RB, Moe JH, et al: Fusion to the sacrum for nonparalytic scoliosis in the adult, Spine 11:824, 1986.

Bradford DS: Adult scoliosis: current concepts of treatment, Clin Orthop 229:70, 1988.

Byrd JA III, Scoles PV, Winter RB, et al: Adult idiopathic scoliosis treated by anterior and posterior spinal fusion, J Bone Joint Surg 69-A:843, 1987.

Dawson EG, Moe JH, and Caron A: Surgical measurement of scoliosis in the adult, Scoliosis Research Society, 1972, J Bone Joint Surg 55-A:437, 1973.

Devlin VJ, Boachie-Adjei O, Bradford DS, et al: Treatment of adult spinal deformity with fusion to the sacrum using CD instrumentation, J Spinal Disorders 4:1, 1991.

Grubb SA, Lipscomb HJ, and Coonrad RW: Degenerative adult onset scoliosis, Spine 13:241, 1988.

Jackson RP, Simmons EH, and Stripinis D: Incidence and severity of back pain in adult idiopathic scoliosis, Spine 8:749, 1983.

Johnson JR and Holt RT: Combined use of anterior and posterior surgery for adult scoliosis, Orthop Clin North Am 18:361, 1988.

Kostuik JP: Treatment of scoliosis in the adult thoracolumbar spine with special reference to fusion to the sacrum, Orthop Clin North Am 19:371, 1988.

Kostuik JP and Bentiviglio J: The incidence of low back pain in adult scoliosis, Spine 6:268, 1981.

Kostuik JP and Hall BB: Spinal fusions to the sacrum in adults with scoliosis, Spine 8:489, 1983.

Kostuik JP, Carl A, and Ferron S: Anterior Zielke instrumentation for spinal deformity in adults, J Bone Joint Surg 71-A:898, 1989.

Kostuik JP, Israel J, and Hall JE: Scoliosis surgery in adults, Clin Orthop 93:225, 1973.

Ponder RC, Dickson JH, Harrington PR, and Erwin WD: Results of Harrington instrumentation and fusion in the adult idiopathic scoliosis patient, J Bone Joint Surg 57-A:797, 1975.

Robin GC, Span Y, Steinberg R, et al: Scoliosis in the elderly: a follow-up study, Spine 7:355, 1982.

Saer EH III, Winter RB, and Lonstein JE: Long scoliosis fusion to the sacrum in adults with nonparalytic scoliosis: an improved method, Spine 15:650, 1990.

Sicard A, Lavarde G, and Chaleil B: La greffe vertébrale dans les scolioses de l'adulte, J Chir (Paris) 93:517, 1967.

Sicard A, Lavarde G, and Chaleil B: Seventy instances of adult scoliosis treated with spinal fusion, Surg Gynecol Obstet 126:682, 1968.

Sponseller PD, Cohen MS, Nachemson AL, et al: Results of surgical treatment of adults with idiopathic scoliosis, J Bone Joint Surg 69-A:667, 1987.

Stagnara P: Scoliosis in adults: surgical treatment of severe forms, Excerpta Med Found Int Congress Series No 192, 1969.

Stagnara P: Utilization of Harrington's device in the treatment of adult kyphoscoliosis above 100 degrees. Fourth International Symposium, 1971, Nijmegen, Stuttgart, 1973, Georg Thieme Verlag.

Stagnara P, Fleury D, Pauchet R, et al: Scolioses majeures de l'adulte superieures a 100° -183 castraites chirurgicalement, Rev Chir Orthop 61:101, 1975.

Stagnara P, Jouvinroux P, Peloux J, et al: Cyphoscolioses essentielles de l'adulte: formes sévères de plus de 100°: redressement partial et arthordése, XI SICOT Congress, 206, Mexico City, 1969.

Swank S, Lonstein JE, Moe JH, et al: Surgical treatment of adult scoliosis: a review of two hundred and twenty-two cases, J Bone Joint Surg 63-A:268, 1981.

van Dam BE: Nonoperative treatment of adult scoliosis, Orthop Clin North Am 19:347, 1988.

van Dam BE: Operative treatment of adult scoliosis with posterior fusion and instrumentation, Orthop Clin North Am 19:353, 1988.

van Dam BE, Bradford DS, Lonstein JE, et al: Adult idiopathic scoliosis treated by posterior spinal fusion and Harrington instrumentation, Spine 12:32, 1987.

Vanderpool DW, James JIP, and Wynne-Davies R: Scoliosis in the elderly, J Bone Joint Surg 51-A:446, 1969.

Winter RB, Lonstein JE, and Denis F: Pain patterns in adult scoliosis, Orthop Clin North Am 19:339, 1988.

Neuromuscular scoliosis, general

Bonnett C, Brown JC, Perry J, et al: Evolution of treatment of paralytic scoliosis at Rancho Los Amigos Hospital, J Bone Joint Surg 57-A:206, 1975.

Brown JC, Swank SM, Matta J, and Barras DM: Late spinal deformity in quadriplegic children and adolescents, J Pediatr Orthop 4:456, 1984.

Bucy PC, and Heimburger RF: The neurological aspects of deformities of the spine, Surg Clin North Am 29:163, 1949.

DeWald RL and Faut MM: Anterior and posterior spinal fusion for paralytic scoliosis, Spine 4:401, 1979.

Ferguson RL and Allen BL: Staged correction of neuromuscular scoliosis, J Pediatr Orthop 3:555, 1983.

Fisk JR and Bunch WH: Scoliosis in neuromuscular disease, Orthop Clin North Am 10:863, 1979.

Garrett AL, Perry J, and Nickel VL: Paralytic scoliosis, Clin Orthop 21:117, 1961.

Garrett AL, Perry J, and Nickel VL: Stabilization of the collapsing spine, J Bone Joint Surg 43-A:474, 1961.

Hamel AL and Moe JH: The collapsing spine, Surgery 56:364, 1964.

Hardy J: Neuromuscular scoliosis, J Bone Joint Surg 52-A:407, 1970.

Kilfoyle RM, Foley JJ, and Norton PL: Spine and pelvic deformity in childhood and adolescent paraplegia: a study of 104 cases, J Bone Joint Surg 47-A:659, 1965.

Kleinberg S: Scoliosis with paraplegia, J Bone Joint Surg 33-A:225, 1951.

Kleinberg S and Kaplan A: Scoliosis complicated by paraplegia, J Bone Joint Surg. 34-A:162, 1952.

Lonstein JE and Renshaw TS: Neuromuscular spine deformities, AAOS Instr Course Lect 36:285, 1987.

Luque ER: Paralytic scoliosis in growing children, Clin Orthop 163:202, 1982.

Makley JT, Herndon CH, Inkley S, et al: Pulmonary function in paralytic and non-paralytic scoliosis before and after treatment: a study of sixty-three cases, J Bone Joint Surg 50-A:1379, 1968.

McCarthy RE et al: Allograft bone in spinal fusion for paralytic scoliosis, J Bone Joint Surg 68-A:370, 1986.

McKenzie KG and Dewar FT: Scoliosis with paraplegia, J Bone Joint Surg 31-B:162, 1949.

Meiss WC: Spinal osteotomy following fusion for paralytic scoliosis, J Bone Joint Surg 37-A:73, 1955.

Moe JH: The management of paralytic scoliosis, South Med J 50:67, 1957.

O'Brien JP and Yau AC: Anterior and posterior correction and fusion for paralytic scoliosis, Clin Orthop 86:151, 1972.

Sullivan JA and Conner SB: Comparison of Harrington instrumentation and segmental spinal instrumentation in the management of neuromuscular spinal deformity, Spine 7:299, 1982.

Taddonio RG: Segmental spinal instrumentation in the management of neuromuscular spinal deformity, Spine 7:305, 1982.

Spinal cord injuries

Bonnett CA: The cord injured child. In Lovell, WW, and Winter, RB, editors: Children's orthopaedics, Philadelphia, 1978, JB Lippincott Co.

Bonnett C, Perry J, and Brown J: Cord injury and spine deformity in children, Presented at the Scoliosis Research Society, 1972.

Johnston CE II, Hakaka MW, and Rosenberger R: Paralytic spine deformity: orthotic treatment in spinal discontinuity syndromes, J Pediatr Orthop 2:233, 1982.

Lancourt JC, Dickson JH, and Carter RE: Paralytic spinal deformities following traumatic spinal cord injury in children and adolescents, J Bone Joint Surg 63-A:47, 1981.

Mayfield JK, Erkkila JD, and Winter RB: Spine deformity subsequent to acquired childhood spinal injury, J Bone Joint Surg 63-A:1401, 1981.

McSweeney T: Spinal deformity after spinal cord injury, Paraplegia 6:212, 1969.

Prolo DJ, Runnels JB, and Jameson RM: The injured cervical spine: immediate and long-term immobilization with the halo, JAMA 224:591, 1973.

Ruhlin CW, and Albert S: Scoliosis complicated by spinal cord involvement, J Bone Joint Surg 23:877, 1941.

Progressive neurologic disorders

Aprin H, Bowen JR, MacEwen GD, et al: Spine fusion in patients with spinal muscle atrophy, J Bone Joint Surg 64-A:1179, 1982.

Bethea JS III and Doherty JH: Scoliosis and dysautonomia, J Bone Joint Surg 52-A:409, 1971.

Cady RB and Bobechko WP: Incidence, natural history, and treatment of scoliosis in Friedrich's ataxis, J Pediatr Orthop 4:673, 1984.

Daher YH, Lonstein JE, Winter RB, and Bradford DS: Spinal surgery in spinal muscle atrophy, J Pediatr Orthop 5:391, 1985.

Daher YH, Lonstein JE, Winter RB, and Bradford DS: Spinal deformities in patients with Friedreich's ataxia: a review of 19 patients, J Pediatr Orthop 5:553, 1985.

Daher YH, Lonstein JE, Winter RB, and Bradford DS: Spinal deformities in patients with Charcot-Marie-Tooth: a review of 12 patients, Clin Orthop 202:219, 1986.

Dorr J, Brown J, and Perry J: Results of posterior spine fusion in patients with spinal muscle atrophy: a review of 25 cases, J Bone Joint Surg 55-A:436, 1973.

Evans GA, Drennan JC, and Russman BS: Functional classification and orthopaedic management of spinal muscle atrophy, J Bone Joint Surg 63-B:516, 1981.

Hensinger RN and MacEwen GD: Spinal deformity associated with heritable neurological conditions: spinal muscular atrophy, Friedreich's ataxia, familial dysautonomia, and Charcot-Marie-Tooth disease, J Bone Joint Surg 58-A:13, 1976.

LaBelle H, Tohmé S, DuLaime M, and Allard D: Natural history of scoliosis in Friedreich's ataxia, J Bone Joint Surg 68-A:564, 1986.

Riddick M, Winter RB, and Lutter L: Spinal deformities in patients with spinal muscle atrophy, Spine 8:476, 1982.

Robin GC: Scoliosis in familial dysautonomia, Bull Hosp Jt Dis Orthop Inst 44:16, 1984.

Schwentker EP and Gibson DA: The orthopaedic aspects of spinal muscular atrophy, J Bone Joint Surg 58-A:32, 1976.

Shapiro F and Bresnan MJ: Current concepts review: management of childhood neuromuscular disease. I. Spinal muscle arthropathy, J Bone Joint Surg 64-A:785, 1982.

Shapiro F and Bresnan MJ: Current concepts review: management of childhood neuromuscular disease. II. Peripheral neuropathies, Friedreich's ataxia, and arthrogryposis multiplex congenita, J Bone Joint Surg 64-A:949, 1982.

Siebold RM, Winter RB, and Moe JH: The treatment of scoliosis in arthrogryposis multiplex congenita, Clin Orthop 103:191, 1974.

Syringomyelia

Huebert HT and MacKinnon WB: Syringomyelia and scoliosis, J Bone Joint Surg 51-B:338, 1969.

Phillips WA, Hensinger RN, and Kling TF Jr: Management of scoliosis due to syringomyelia in childhood and adolescence, J Pediatr Orthop 10:351, 1990

Weber FA: The association of syringomyelia and scoliosis, J Bone Joint Surg 56-B:589, 1974.

Myelomeningocele

Allen B and Ferguson R: Operative treatment of myelomeningocele spinal deformities, Orthop Clin North Am 10:845, 1979.

Banta JV: Combined anterior and posterior fusion for spinal deformity in myelomeningocele, Spine 15:946, 1990.

Banta JV and Hamada JS: Natural history of the kyphotic deformity in myelomeningocele, J Bone Joint Surg 58-A:279, 1960.

Banta JV and Park SM: Improvement in pulmonary function in patients having combined anterior and posterior spine fusion for myelomeningocele scoliosis, Spine 8:766, 1983.

Drummond DS, Morear M, and Cruess RL: The results and complications of surgery for the paralytic hip and spine in myelomeningocele, J Bone Joint Surg 62-B:49, 1980.

Hall PV, Lindseth RE, Campbell RL, and Kalsbeck JE: Myelodysplasia and developmental scoliosis: a manifestation of syringomyelia, Spine 1:48, 1976.

Hull WJ, Moe JH, and Winter RB: Spinal deformity in myelomeningocele: natural history, evaluation, and treatment, J Bone Joint Surg 56-A:1767, 1974.

Kahanovitz N and Duncan JW: The role of scoliosis and pelvic obliquity on functional disability in myelomeningocele, Spine 6:494, 1981.

Mackel JL and Lindseth RE: Scoliosis in myelodysplasia, J Bone Joint Surg 57-A:1031, 1975.

Mayfield JK: Severe spine deformity and myelodysplasia and sacral agenesis: an aggressive surgical approach, Spine 6:489, 1981.

McMaster MJ: Anterior and posterior instrumentation and fusion of thoracolumbar scoliosis due to myelomeningocele, J Bone Joint Surg 69-B:20, 1987.

Osebold WR, Mayfield JK, Winter RB, et al: Surgical treatment of paralytic scoliosis associated with myelomeningocele, J Bone Joint Surg 64-A:841, 1982.

Piggott H: The natural history of scoliosis in myelomeningocele, J Bone Joint Surg 61-B:122, 1979.

Raycroft JF and Curtis BH: Spinal curvature in myelomeningocele: natural history and etiology. In American Academy of Orthopaedic Surgeons: Symposium on myelomeningocele, St Louis, 1972, Mosby–Year Book, Inc.

Shurtleff DB et al: Myelodysplasia: the natural history of kyphosis and scoliosis: a preliminary report, Dev Med Child Neurol 37(suppl):126, 1976.

Sriram K, Bobechko WP, and Hall JE: Surgical management of spinal deformities in spina bifida, J Bone Joint Surg 54-B:666, 1972.

Cerebral palsy

Allen BL and Ferguson RL: L-rod instrumentation for scoliosis in cerebral palsy, J Pediatr Orthop 2:87, 1982.

Balmer GA and MacEwen GD: The incidence and treatment of scoliosis in cerebral palsy, J Bone Joint Surg 52-B:134, 1970.

Bonnett C, Brown J, and Brooks HL: Anterior spine fusion with Dwyer instrumentation for lumbar scoliosis in cerebral palsy, J Bone Joint Surg 55-A:425, 1973.

Bonnett C, Brown JC, and Grow T: Thoracolumbar scoliosis in cerebral palsy: results of surgical treatment, J Bone Joint Surg 58-A:328, 1976.

Brown JC, Swank SM, and Specht L: Combined anterior and posterior spine fusion in cerebral palsy, Spine 7:570, 1982.

Bunnell WP and MacEwen GD: Non-operative treatment in scoliosis in cerebral palsy: preliminary report on the use of a plastic jacket, Dev Med Child Neurol 19:45, 1977.

Ferguson RL and Allen BL: Considerations in the treament of cerebral palsy patients with spinal deformities, Orthop Clin North Am 19:419, 1988.

Gersoff WK and Renshaw JS: The treatment of scoliosis in cerebral palsy by posterior spinal fusion with Luque-rod segmental instrumentation, J Bone Joint Surg 70-A:41, 1988.

Lonstein JE and Akbrania BA: Operative treatment of spinal deformities in patients with cerebral palsy or mental retardation: an analysis of 107 cases, J Bone Joint Surg 65-A:43, 1983.

MacEwen GD: Operative treatment of scoliosis in cerebral palsy, Reconstr Surg Traumatol 13:58, 1972.

Madigan RR and Wallace SL: Scoliosis in the institutionalized cerebral palsy population, Spine 6:583, 1981.

Rinsky LA: Surgery of spinal deformity in cerebral palsy: twelve years in the evolution of scoliosis management, Clin Orthop 253:100, 1990.

Robson P: The prevalence of scoliosis in adolescents and young adults with cerebral palsy, Dev Med Child Neurol 10:447, 1968.

Rosenthal RK, Levine DB, and McCarver CL: The occurence of scoliosis in cerebral palsy, Dev Med Child Neurol 16:664, 1974.

Samilson RL, and Bechard R: Scoliosis in cerebral palsy: incidence, distribution of curve patterns, natural history, and thoughts on etiology. In Ahstrom JP Jr, editor: Current practice in orthopaedic surgery, vol 5, St Louis, 1973, Mosby–Year Book, Inc.

Stanitski CL et al: Surgical correction of spinal deformity in cerebral palsy, Spine 7:563, 1982.

Arthrogryposis multiplex congenita

Brown LM and Robson MJ: The pathophysiology of arthrogryposis multiplex congenita neurologica, J Bone Joint Surg 62-B:291, 1980.

Daher YH, Lonstein JE, Winter RB, et al: Spinal deformities in patients with arthrogryposis: a review of 16 patients, Spine 10:609, 1985.

Drummond D and McKenzie DA: Scoliosis in arthrogryposis multiplex congenita, Spine 3:146, 1978.

Herron LD, Westin GW, and Dawson EG: Scoliosis in arthrogryposis multiplex congenita, J Bone Joint Surg 60-A:293, 1978.

Siebold RM, Winter RB, and Moe JH: The treatment of scoliosis in arthrogryposis multiplex congenita, Clin Orthop 103:191, 1974.

Muscular dystrophy

Bunch WH: Muscular dystrophy. In Hardy JH, editor: Spinal deformity in neurological and muscular disorders, St Louis, 1974, Mosby–Year Book, Inc.

Cambridge W and Drennan JC: Scoliosis associated with Duchenne muscular dystrophy, J Pediatr Orthop 7:436, 1987.

Daher YH, Lonstein JE, Winter RB, et al: Spinal deformities in patients with muscular dystrophy other than Duchenne: review of 11 patients having surgical treatment, Spine 10:614, 1984.

Dubowitz V: Some clinical observations on childhood muscular dystrophy, Br J Clin Pract 17:283, 1963.

Gibson DA, Koreska J, Robertson D, et al: The management of spinal deformity in Duchenne's muscular dystrophy, Orthop Clin North Am 9:437, 1978.

Hsu JD: The natural history of spine curvature progression in the nonambulator Duchenne muscular dystrophy patient, Spine 8:771, 1983.

Kurz LT, Mubarak SH, Schultz P, et al: Correlation of scoliosis and pulmonary function in Duchenne muscular dystrophy, J Pediatr Orthop 3:347, 1983.

Renshaw TS: Treatment of Duchenne's muscular dystrophy, JAMA 248:922, 1982.

Rideau Y et al: The treatment of scoliosis in Duchenne muscular dystrophy, Muscle Nerve 7:281, 1984.

Robin GC and Brief LP: Scoliosis in childhood muscular dystrophy, J Bone Joint Surg 53-A:466, 1971.

Sakai DN, Hsu JD, Bonnett CA, et al: Stabilization of the collapsing spine in Duchenne muscular dystrophy, Clin Orthop 128:256, 1977.

Seeger BR, Sutherland AD, and Clard MS: Orthotic management of scoliosis in Duchenne muscular dystrophy, Arch Phys Med Rehabil 65:83, 1984.

Shapiro F and Bresnan MJ: Current concepts review: orthopaedic management of childhood neuromuscular disease. III. Diseases of muscle, J Bone Joint Surg 64-A:1102, 1982.

Siegel IM: Scoliosis in muscular dystrophy: some comments about diagnosis, observations on prognosis, and suggestions for therapy, Clin Orthop 93:235, 1973.

Siegel IM: Spinal stabilization in Duchenne muscular dystrophy: rationale and method, Muscle Nerve 5:417, 1982.

Swank SM, Brown JC, and Perry RE: Spinal fusion in Duchenne's muscular dystrophy, Spine 7:484, 1982.

Wilkins KE and Gibson DA: The patterns of spinal deformity in Duchenne muscular dystrophy, J Bone Joint Surg 58-A:24, 1976.

Neurofibromatosis

Casselman E and Mandell G: Vertebral scalloping in neurofibromatosis, Radiology 131:89, 1979.

Chaglassian JH, Riseborough EJ, and Hall JE: Neurofibromatous scoliosis: natural history and results of treatment in thirty-seven cases, J Bone Joint Surg 58-A:695, 1976.

Chaglassian J, Riseborough E, and Hall J: Neurofibromatosis, J Bone Joint Surg 58-A:695, 1976.

Hsu L, Lee P, and Leong J: Dystrophic spinal deformities in neurofibromatosis J Bone Joint Surg 66-B:495, 1984.

Hunt J and Pugh D: Skeletal lesions in neurofibromatosis, Radiology 76:1, 1961.

Lonstein J, Winter RB, Moe JH, et al: Neurologic deficits secondary to spinal deformity: a review of the literature and report of 43 cases, Spine 5:331, 1980.

McCarroll H: Clinical manifestations of congenital neurofibromatosis, J Bone Joint Surg 32-A:601, 1950.

Rezaian S: The incidence of scoliosis due to neurofibromatosis, Acta Orthop Scand 47:534, 1976.

Savini R, Parisini P, Cervellati S, et al: Surgical treatment of vertebral deformities in neurofibromatosis, Ital J Orthop Traumatol 9:13, 1983.

Winter RB and Edwards W: Neurofibromatosis with lumbosacral spondylolisthesis, J Pediatr Orthop 1:91, 1981.

Winter RB, Moe JH, Bradford DS, et al: Spine deformity in neurofibromatosis, J Bone Joint Surg 61-A:677, 1979.

Miscellaneous causes

Amis J and Herring J: Iatrogenic kyphosis: complication of Harrington instrumentation in Marfan's syndrome, J Bone Joint Surg 66-A:460, 1984.

Bauze RJ, Smith R, and Francis MJO: A new look at osteogenesis imperfecta: a clinical, radiological and biochemical study of 42 patients, J Bone Joint Surg 57-B:1, 1975.

Benson DR and Donaldson DH: The spine in osteogenesis imperfecta, J Bone Joint Surg 60-A:925, 1978.

Benson DR and Newman DC: The spine and surgical treatment in osteogenesis imperfecta, Clin Orthop 159:147, 1981.

Bethem B, Winter RB, and Lutter L: Disorders of the spine in diastrophic dwarfism: a discussion of 9 patients and review of the literature, J Bone Joint Surg 62-A:529, 1980.

Birch JG and Herring JA: Spinal deformity in Marfan's syndrome, J Pediatr Orthop 7:546, 1987.

Cristofaro RL, Hoek KJ, Bonnett CA, et al: Operative treatment of spine deformity in osteogenesis imperfecta, Clin Orthop 139:40, 1979.

Gitelis S, Whiffen J, and DeWald RL: The treatment of severe scoliosis in osteogenesis imperfecta, Clin Orthop 175:56, 1983.

Guthkelch AN: Diastematomyelia with median septum, Brain 97:729, 1974.

Hanscom DA and Bloom BA: The spine in osteogenesis imperfecta, Orthop Clin North Am 19:449, 1988.

Herring JA: Rapidly progressive scoliosis in multiple epiphyseal dysplasia: a case report, J Bone Joint Surg 58-A:703, 1976.

Herring JA: The spinal disorders in diastrophic dwarfism, J Bone Joint Surg 60-A:177, 1978.

Jacobsen S, Rosenklint A, and Halkier E: Post-pneumonectomy scoliosis, Acta Orthop Scand 45:867, 1974.

Loynes RD: Scoliosis after thoracoplasty, J Bone Joint Surg 54-B:484, 1972.

Micheli LJ, Hall JE, and Watts HG: Spinal instability in Larsen's syndrome: report of three cases, J Bone Joint Surg 58-A:562, 1976.

Phillips DA, Roye DP Jr, Farcy J-P C, et al: Surgical treatment of scoliosis in a spinal muscular atrophy population, Spine 15:942, 1990.

Robins PR, Moe JH, and Winter RB: Scoliosis in Marfan's syndrome: its characteristics and results of treatment in thirty-five patients, J Bone Joint Surg 57-A:358, 1975.

Stauffer ES and Mankin HJ: Scoliosis after thoracoplasty: a study of thirty patients, J Bone Joint Surg 48-A:339, 1966.

Williams JM and Stevens H: Recognition of surgically treatable neurologic disorders of childhood JAMA 151:455, 1953.

Winter RB, Haven JJ, Moe JH, and Lagaard SM: Diastematomyelia and congenital spine deformities, J Bone Joint Surg 56-A:27, 1974.

Yong-Hing K and MacEwen GD: Scoliosis associated with osteogenesis imperfecta: results of treatment, J Bone Joint Surg 64-B:36, 1982.

Congenital scoliosis

Akbrania BA and Moe JH: Familial congenital scoliosis with unilateral unsegmented bar: case report of two siblings, J Bone Joint Surg 60-A:259, 1978.

Andrew T and Piggott H: Growth arrest for progressive scoliosis: combined anterior and posterior fusion of the convexity, J Bone Joint Surg 67-B:193, 1985.

Bernard TN Jr, Bueke SW, Johnston CE III, and Roberts JM: Congenital spine deformities: a review of 47 cases, Orthopedics 8:777, 1985.

Bradford DS: Partial epiphyseal arrest and supplemental fixation for progressive correction of congenital spine deformity, J Bone Joint Surg 64-A:610, 1982.

Gillespie R et al: Intraspinal anomalies in congenital scoliosis, Clin Orthop 93:103, 1973.

Hall JE, Herndon WA, and Levine CR: Surgical treatment of congenital scoliosis with or without Harrington instrumentation, J Bone Joint Surg 63-A:608, 1981.

Hilal SK, Marton D, and Pollack E: Diastematomyelia in children: radiographic study of 34 cases, Radiology 112:609, 1974.

Leatherman KD and Dickson RA: Two-stage corrective surgery for congenital deformities of the spine, J Bone Joint Surg 61-B:324, 1979.

MacEwen GD, Conway JJ, and Miller WT: Congenital scoliosis with a unilateral bar, Radiology 40:711, 1968.

MacEwen GD, Winter RB, and Hardy JH: Evaluation of kidney anomalies in congenital scoliosis, J Bone Joint Surg 54-A:1451, 1972.

McMaster MJ: Occult intraspinal anomalies and congenital scoliosis, J Bone Joint Surg 66-A:588, 1984.

McMaster MJ and David CV: Hemivertebra as a cause of scoliosis: a study of 104 patients, J Bone Joint Surg 68-B:588, 1986.

McMaster MJ and Ohtsuka K: The natural history of congenital scoliosis: a study of 251 patients, J Bone Joint Surg 64-A:1128, 1982.

Nasca RJ, Stelling FH, and Steel HH: Progression of congenital scoliosis due to hemivertebrae and hemivertebrae with bars, J Bone Joint Surg 57-A:456, 1975.

Roaf R: Vertebral growth and its mechanical control, J Bone Joint Surg 42-B:40, 1960.

Shapiro F and Eyre D: Congenital scoliosis: a histopathologic study, Spine 6:107, 1981.

Stoll J and Bunch W: Segmental spinal instrumentation for congenital scoliosis: a report of two cases, Spine 8:43, 1983.

Tsou P, Yau A, and Hodgson A: Congenital spinal deformities: natural history, classification, and the role of anterior surgery, J Bone Joint Surg 56-A:1767, 1974.

Winter RB: Congenital scoliosis, Clin Orthop 93:75, 1973.

Winter RB: Congenital spine deformity: natural history and treatment, Isr J Med Sci 9:719, 1973.

Winter RB: Congenital kyphoscoliosis with paralysis following hemivertebra excision, Clin Orthop 119:116, 1976.

Winter RB: Convex anterior and posterior hemiarthrodesis and epiphyseodesis in young children with progressive congenital scoliosis, J Pediatr Orthop 1:361, 1981.

Winter RB: Congenital deformities of the spine, New York, 1983, Thieme-Stratton.

Winter RB: Congenital scoliosis, Orthop Clin North Am 19:395, 1988.

Winter RB and Moe JH: The results of spinal arthrodesis for congenital spine deformity in patients younger than five years old, J Bone Joint Surg 64-A:419, 1982.

Winter RB, Moe JH, and Eilers VE: Congenital scoliosis: a study of 234 patients treated and untreated. I. Natural history, J Bone Joint Surg 50-A:1, 1968.

Winter RB, Moe JH, and Eilers VE: Congenital scoliosis: a study of 234 patients treated and unteated. II. Treatment, J Bone Joint Surg 50-A:15, 1968.

Winter RB, Moe JH, and Lonstein JE: Posterior spinal arthrodesis for congenital scoliosis: an analysis of the cases of two hundred and ninety patients, five to nineteen years old, J Bone Joint Surg 66-A:1188, 1984.

Winter RB, Moe JH, and Wang JF: Congenital kyphosis, J Bone Joint Surg 55-A:223, 1973.

Winter RB, Haven JJ, Moe JH, and Lagaard SM: Diastematomyelia and congenital spine deformities, J Bone Joint Surg 56-A:27, 1974.

CHAPTER 83

Instrumentation and Techniques for Scoliosis and Kyphosis

BARNEY L. FREEMAN III

The success of any surgical procedure for scoliosis depends on the achievement of a solid arthrodesis with stability of the spine. Spinal instrumentation is a tool for obtaining fusion and stability and the variety of instrumentation available should not obscure these goals.

PREOPERATIVE PREPARATION

A thorough history and physical examination and any necessary tests are completed before surgery. In addition to the standard preoperative tests, other studies such as pulmonary function tests, bleeding studies, myelograms, computed tomography, or magnetic resonance imaging may be necessary. For most patients, we recommend the use of autologous blood to decrease or eliminate the need for bank blood with all its potential problems. In most spinal surgery, we use spinal cord monitoring. The occipital electrodes are applied preoperatively, and a baseline reading is obtained, allowing continuous spinal cord monitoring during surgery. A wake-up test often also is peformed and the patient is prepared for this preoperatively. Before any fusion of the spine, the levels to be fused must be appropriately determined by careful study of roentgenograms.

SURGICAL TECHNIQUE

Spinal surgery requires extensive dissection and may result in severe blood loss. If significant blood loss is expected, a large-bore intravenous line and an arterial line are required. Because the patient is in a prone position for many hours, Relton and Hall designed a frame to eliminate intraabdominal pressure and reduce blood loss (Fig. 83-1, A). The patient's arms are carefully supported with the elbows padded. The shoulders should not be abducted more than 90 degrees to avoid pressure or stretch on the brachial plexus. The cephalad pads of the frame rest on the chest, and not in the axilla, to relieve pressure on the brachial plexus (Fig. 83-1, B). When the patient is positioned on the frame with the hips flexed, lumbar lordosis is partially eliminated. If the fusion is to be extended into the lumbar spine, the knees and thighs should be elevated with the hip joints extended to preserve physiologic lumbar lordosis.

The patient's back is scrubbed with a surgical soap solution for 5 to 10 minutes and is then prepared with antiseptic solution. The area of the operative site is then draped and a plastic Steri-drape is used to seal off the skin.

Make the skin incision in a straight line from one or

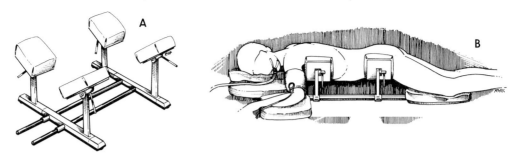

Fig. 83-1   A, Relton-Hall frame for reduction of intraabdominal pressure. **B,** Positioning of patient on Relton-Hall frame with hips in extension to maintain lumbar lordosis. (Redrawn from Relton JES and Hall JE: J Bone Joint Surg 49-B:327, 1967.)

two vertebrae superior to the proposed fusion area to one vertebra inferior to it. A straight scar improves the postoperative appearance of the back (Fig. 83-2, *A*). Make the initial incision through the dermal layer only. Infiltrate the intradermal and subcutaneous areas with an epinephrine solution (1:500,000). Deepen the incision to the level of the spinous processes, and use self-retaining Weitlaner retractors to retract the skin margins. Control bleeding with electrocautery. Identify the interspinous ligament between the spinous processes; this often appears as a white line. As the incision is deepened, keep the Weitlaner retractors tight to help with exposure and minimize bleeding. Now incise the cartilaginous cap overlying the spinous processes as close to the midline as

possible (Fig. 83-2, *B*). This midline may vary because of rotation of the spinous processes. Using a Cobb elevator, expose the spinous processes subperiosteally after the cartilaginous caps are moved to either side. After several of the spinous processes have been exposed, move the Weitlaner retractors to a deeper level and maintain tension for retraction and hemostasis. After exposure of all the spinous processes, obtain a localizing roentgenogram. While the roentgenogram is being developed, reopen the wound and continue subperiosteal exposure of the entire area to be fused, keeping the retractors tight at all times (Fig. 83-2, *C*). It is generally easier to dissect from caudad to cephalad because of the oblique attachments of the short rotator muscles and ligaments of the

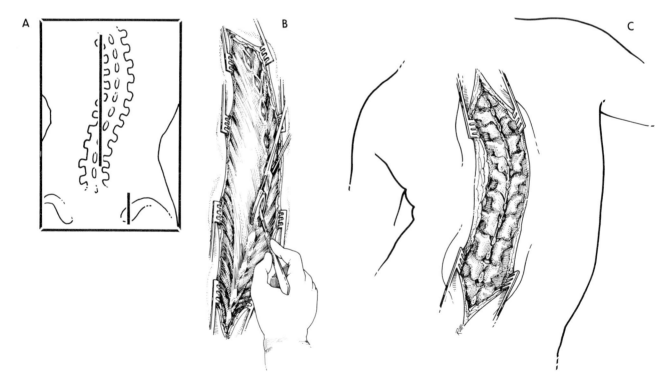

Fig. 83-2   A, Skin incisions for posterior fusion and autogenous bone graft. **B,** Incisions over spinous processes and interspinous ligaments. **C,** Weitlaner retractors used to maintain tension and exposure of spine during dissection.

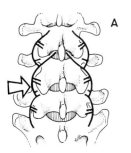
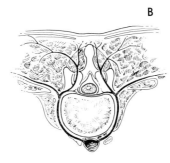
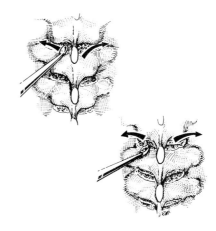

Fig. 83-3 **A,** Posterior view of segmental vessels just lateral to each facet joint. **B,** Axial view of arteries supplying posterior spinal muscles. (**A,** Redrawn from Macnab I and Dall D: J Bone Joint Surg 53-A: 628, 1971; **B,** redrawn from Wagoner G: J Bone Joint Surg 19:469, 1937.)

Fig. 83-4 Cobb curets used to clean facets of ligament attachments.

spine. Extend the subperiosteal dissection first to the facet joints on one side and then the other side, deepening the retractors as necessary. Continue the dissection laterally to the ends of the transverse processes on both sides. Coagulate the branch of the segmental vessel just lateral to each facet (Fig. 83-3). Place the self-retaining retractors deeper to hold the entire excision open and exposed. Sponges soaked in the 1:500,000 epinephrine solution can be used to help maintain hemostasis. Use a curet and a pituitary rongeur to completely clean the interspinous ligaments and the lateral facets of all ligamentous attachments and capsule, proceeding from the midline laterally (Fig. 83-4) to decrease the possibility of the curet's slipping and penetrating into the spinal canal. The entire spine is now exposed from one transverse process to another, all soft tissue is removed, and the spine is ready for instrumentation and decortication as indicated by the procedure chosen.

Although some studies indicate that the use of bone bank allograft achieves acceptable fusion rates, we believe that large amounts of autogenous bone should be used whenever possible. If autogenous bone is deficient or cannot be used for other reasons, we then supplement the graft with bone bank allograft, preferably from a femoral head.

Make an incision over the iliac crest to be used (see Fig. 83-2, *A*). If the original incision extends far enough distally into the lumbar spine, the iliac crest can be exposed through the same incision by subcutaneous dissection. Infiltrate the intradermal and subcutaneous areas with 1:500 epinephrine solution. Expose the cartilaginous apophysis overlying the posterior iliac crest and split it in the middle. Using a Cobb elevator, expose the ilium subperiosteally. The superior gluteal artery emerges from the area of the sciatic notch (Fig. 83-5, *A*) and should be carefully avoided during the bone grafting procedure. If bicortical grafts are desired, expose the posterior crest of the ilium on the inner side and obtain two or three strips of bicortical graft with a large gouge. Otherwise, take cortical and cancellous strips of bone from

the outer table of the ilium (Fig. 83-5, *B*). Place these bone grafts in a kidney basin and cover them with a sponge soaked in saline or blood. Control bleeding from the iliac crest with bone wax or Gelfoam. Approximate the cartilaginous cap of the posterior iliac crest with an absorbable stitch. Place a Hemovac drain at the donor site and connect it to a separate reservoir to monitor postoperative bleeding here and at the spinal fusion site.

FUSION TECHNIQUES

Spinal fusion may be extraarticular or intraarticular. The classic Hibbs technique is essentially an extraarticular fusion and has been replaced at our clinic by a modification of the intraarticular fusion described by Moe, along with meticulous dissection around the transverse

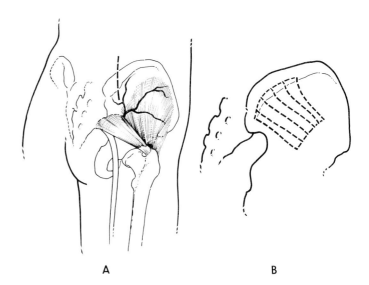

Fig. 83-5 **A,** Superior gluteal artery as it emerges from area of sciatic notch. **B,** Cortical and cancellous strips removed from outer table of ilium for autogenous bone grafts.

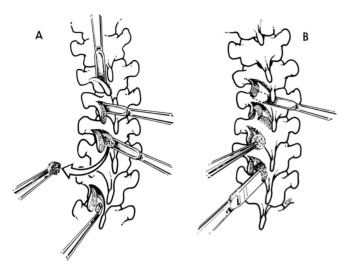

Fig. 83-6 Moe technique of thoracic facet fusion. (Redrawn from Bradford DS et al: Moe's textbook of scoliosis and other spinal deformities, ed 2, Philadelphia, 1987, WB Saunders Co.)

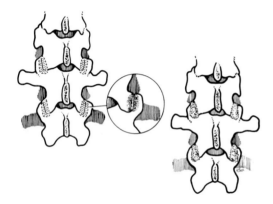

Fig. 83-7 Moe technique of lumbar facet fusion. (Redrawn from Bradford DS et al: Moe's textbook of scoliosis and other spinal deformities, ed 2, Philadelphia, 1987, WB Saunders Co.)

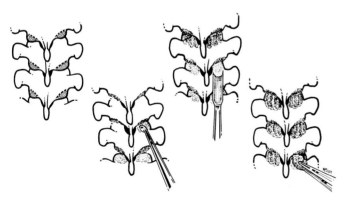

Fig. 83-8 Hall technique of facet fusion. (Redrawn in part from Bradford DS et al: Moe's textbook of scoliosis and other spinal deformities, ed 2, Philadelphia, 1987, WB Saunders Co.)

processes as recommended by Goldstein. Hall also described a technique for intraarticular fusion.

■ *TECHNIQUE (MOE).* Expose the spine to the tips of the transverse processes as previously described. Begin a cut over the cephalad lateral articular process at the base of the lamina and carry it along the transverse process almost to its tip. Bend this fragment laterally to lie between the transverse processes, leavng it hinged if possible (Fig. 83-6, *A*), to expose the superior articular process and its cartilage; thoroughly remove these. Now with the Cobb gouge make another cut in the area of the superior articular facet, beginning medially and working laterally to produce another hinged fragment. Place cancellous bone grafts in the created defect (Fig. 83-6, *B*).

In the lumbar spine, the facet joints are oriented in a more sagittal direction and fusion is best accomplished by removing the adjoining joint surfaces. This can be done with a small osteotome or a rongeur, creating a defect that is packed with cancellous bone (Fig. 83-7).

Decorticate the entire exposed spine with Cobb gouges from the midline laterally so that if the gouge were to slip, it would be moving away from the spinal canal. Then add cancellous bone grafts. If the fusion is performed for scoliosis and the amount of bone available is limited, concentrate the bone graft on the concave side of the curve because the bone will be subjected to compressive forces on this side as opposed to tension forces on the convex side.

■ *TECHNIQUE (HALL).* First, sharply cut the inferior facet with a gouge and remove this bone fragment to expose the superior facet cartilage. Remove this cartilage with a sharp curet. Create a trough by removing the outer cortex of this superior facet and add cancellous bone grafts (Fig. 83-8). Then proceed with decortication as described for the Moe technique.

At the completion of fusion, close the deep tissues with absorbable suture. Place a drain in the subcutaneous tissue or the deep layer, keeping the reservoir for this drain separate from the reservoir for the bone graft to allow monitoring of bleeding from the incision sites. Approximate the subcutaneous tissues with 2-0 absorbable sutures and the skin edges with skin staples or a running subcuticular absorbable stitch.

SPINAL INSTRUMENTATION

The role of instrumentation in scoliosis surgery is to correct the deformity as much as possible and to stabilize the spine while the fusion mass becomes solid. The fusion mass in a well-corrected spine is subjected to much lower bending moments and tensile forces than

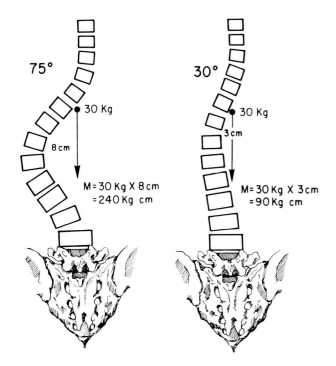

Fig. 83-9 Comparative bending forces exerted at apexes of 75-degree curve and 30-degree curve. (From Dunn HK: AAOS Instr Couse Lect 32:192, 1983.)

Table 83-1 Expectation of representative strengths of fixation

	Thoracic vertebrae	Lumbar vertebrae
Facet and lamina	70 kgf	140 kgf
Base of transverse process	35 kgf	7 kgf
Tip of transverse process	7 kgf	
Base of spinous process	15 kgf	

From Dunn HK: AAOS Instr Course Lect 32:192, 1983.

the fusion mass in an uncorrected spine (Fig. 83-9). Moe and Gustilo reported a 19.4% incidence of pseudarthrosis in patients treated with fusion after correction by casting. Other authors also have found this high incidence of pseudarthrosis after spinal arthrodesis without instrumentation. Moskowitz et al. found that patients with a solid spinal fusion rarely had progression of their scoliosis. The purpose of instrumentation, therefore, is to lower the rate of pseudarthrosis and improve the amount of correction obtained at surgery.

The ideal spinal instrumentation system has high rates of safety and reliability and low rates of instrument failure and breakage. It should be strong enough to resist loads from all directions without external support. It should be easy to use with little increase in operative time. It should restore normal spinal contours and not create new deformities. Of the currently available spinal instrumentation systems, none meets all of the criteria for an ideal system. No one device is the best choice for every surgeon or every patient.

Harrington Instrumentation

In 1962, Harrington introduced an instrumentation system for spinal deformities that applies forces of distraction and compression over several segments of the spine in the area of the posterior elements. The instruments hold the correction obtained for a reasonable length of time until the fusion can develop and stabilize the original correction. The major correcting force is pro-

vided by the distraction system, but Harrington believes the contribution of the compression system to be integral to the effectiveness of the total system. Other surgeons, including Moe, believe that the compression rod does not offer additional correction, and they use the distraction rod alone. The principal limiting factor on the amount of force that can be placed on the spine is the strength of the bone in which the instruments are inserted. Dunn outlined the relative strengths of fixation in longitudinally applied forces through the midthoracic and lumbar vertebrae (Table 83-1). It should be emphasized that these forces are for longitudinally applied forces and not posteriorly directed forces. Most hook failures we have seen consisted of cutting out of the hook posteriorly when the lamina failed with posteriorly directed forces. Many modifications of the Harrington system have evolved over the years, including the addition of a transverse traction device, sublaminar wires, and spinous process wires.

There are several disadvantages to the Harrington instrumentation system. The average curve correction in adolescent idiopathic scoliosis is approximately 50%. As the curve is corrected with distraction, the efficiency of correction is decreased. Dunn has shown that in a 90-degree scoliotic curve about 70% of the distraction forces act to correct the curve; in a 45-degree curve, only 35% of the force is corrective. With the Harrington distraction rods, the distraction force is applied only at the two laminae where the hooks are seated. If a load exceeds the strength of the laminae, fracture and loss of correction can result. As distraction is applied, elongation of the spine results in reduction of spinal curves in both the coronal and sagittal planes. The coronal plane curve (scoliosis) is pathologic, whereas the sagittal plane curve is physiologic. If the spine is instrumented to the lower lumbar region with a straight distraction rod, normal lumbar lordosis is reduced. To overcome this problem, Moe modified the Harrington rod by making the inferior end of the rod and the corresponding hole in the lower hook square. This allows the rod to be contoured to preserve lumbar lordosis while preventing unwanted rotation of the rod. In addition, as described by LaGrone, the spinous processes of the lower two vertebrae can be wired together to help maintain lordosis as distraction is

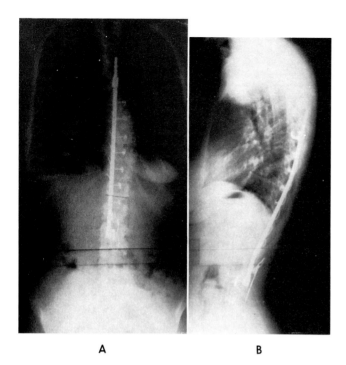

A **B**

Fig. 83-10 **A,** Postoperative posteroanterior view of instrumentation and fusion into lumbar spine for idiopathic scoliosis. **B,** Lateral view of contoured Moe rod with wiring of spinous processes of lower two vertebrae to maintain lumbar lordosis.

applied (Fig. 83-10). The use of this technique has diminished the loss of sagittal plane curves but has not completely eliminated the problem. The contoured rods are weakened and are more likely to break and the mechanical efficiency of distraction is reduced. The squared-ended contoured rods are also more difficult to insert. Because of the risk of hook dislodgment, most surgeons recommend some form of external immobilization after Harrington instrumentation (Fig. 83-11).

Despite the problems inherent in the Harrington system, it is the only system available for which long-term results are known, and the advantages of any newer system must be compared with these results.

Before using the Harrington instrumentation system, the surgeon should be aware of the implants available, as well as the instruments necessary to use these implants. The Harrington distraction rod is a stainless steel rod that is connected to the posterior elements of the spine, and distraction is adjusted by the ratchet principle (Fig. 83-12). The distraction rod is available in lengths that vary by ½ inch. Older rods have 11 ratchets and newer rods have only six ratchet ends, requiring different distractors as well as different length rods depending on the rod chosen.

A variety of hooks are available for use at the ratchet end of the Harrington rods. They all perform the same basic function of securing the ratchet end of the rod to the spine (Fig. 83-13). Collar-end hooks receive the smaller stem of the rod at the collared end. These collar-ended hooks are not large enough to receive the ratchet end of the rod (Fig. 83-14). Insertion of the distraction

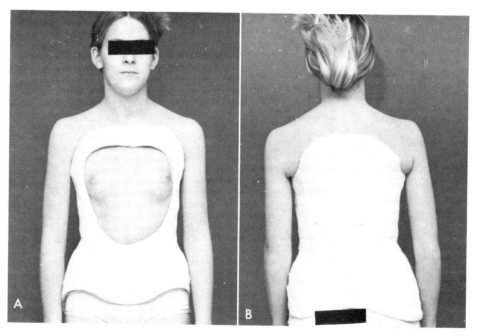

A **B**

Fig. 83-11 Underarm cast for postoperative immobilization in idiopathic scoliosis. (From Bradford DS et al: Moe's textbook of scoliosis and other spinal deformities, ed 2, Philadelphia, 1987, WB Saunders Co.)

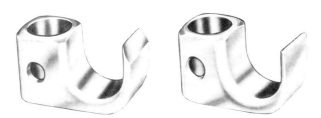

Fig. 83-12   Harrington distraction rod. (Courtesy Zimmer, Inc., Warsaw, Indiana.)

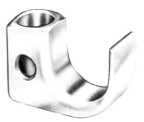

Fig. 83-13   Examples of two of many varieties of rachet-end hooks available for Harrington distraction rod. (Courtesy Zimmer, Inc., Warsaw, Indiana.)

Fig. 83-14   Example of one of many types of collar-end hooks available for Harrington distraction rod. Diameter of these hooks is smaller and will accept collar end of rod but not rachet end. (Courtesy Zimmer, Inc., Warsaw, Indiana.)

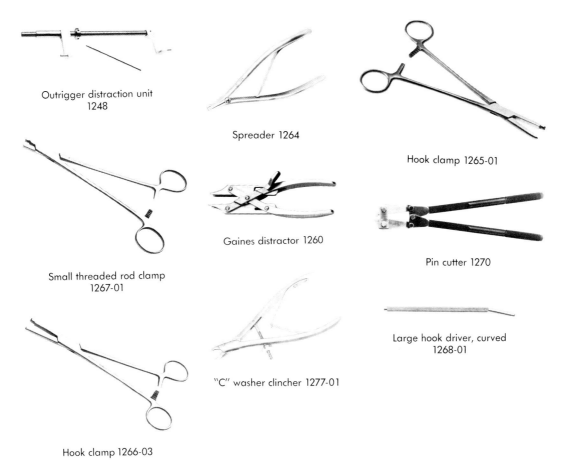

Outrigger distraction unit
1248

Spreader 1264

Hook clamp 1265-01

Small threaded rod clamp
1267-01

Gaines distractor 1260

Pin cutter 1270

Hook clamp 1266-03

"C" washer clincher 1277-01

Large hook driver, curved
1268-01

Fig. 83-15   Basic instrumentation for insertion of Harrington hooks and rods. (From Erwin WD et al: Fracture management: surgical technique — utilization of Harrington spinal instrumentation and fusion for scoliosis, Zimmer, Inc., Warsaw, Indiana.)

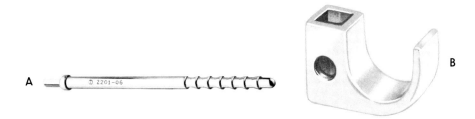

Fig. 83-16   Moe square-end rod, **A,** with corresponding square-end collar hook, **B.** (Courtesy Zimmer, Inc., Warsaw, Indiana.)

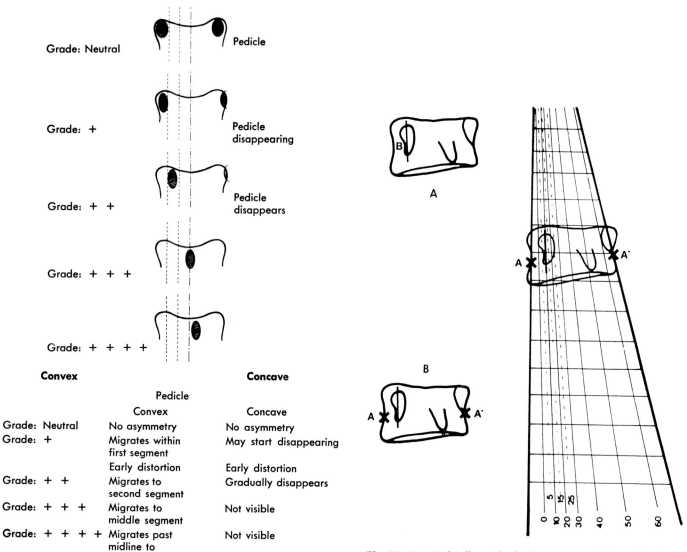

Grade	Convex	Concave
Grade: Neutral	No asymmetry	No asymmetry
Grade: +	Migrates within first segment	May start disappearing
	Early distortion	Early distortion
Grade: + +	Migrates to second segment	Gradually disappears
Grade: + + +	Migrates to middle segment	Not visible
Grade: + + + +	Migrates past midline to concave side of vertebral body	Not visible

Fig. 83-17   Pedicle method of determining vertebral rotation. Vertebral body is divided into six segments and grades from 0 to 4+ are assigned, depending on location of pedicle within segments. Because pedicle on concave side disappears early in rotation, pedicle on convex side, easily visible through wide range of rotation, is used as standard. (From Nash CL Jr and Moe JH: J Bone Joint Surg 51-A:223, 1969.)

Fig. 83-18   Pedriolle method of measurement of vertebral rotation. Measurement is made from pedicle situated at convexity of apical vertebra under consideration. **A,** Mark greatest diameter of pedicle *(B)*. **B,** Mark reference at waist of each lateral border of vertebra *(A* and *A•)*. **C,** Superimpose torsiometer on vertebra so that edges of rule are at sides of vertebral body. Amount of rotation of pedicle line is read from rotation scale, 10 degrees in this example. (From Bradford DS et al: Moe's textbook of scoliosis and other spinal deformities, ed 2, Philadelphia, 1987, WB Saunders Co.)

rod requires certain basic instruments as shown in Fig. 83-15.

For contouring of the rods, Moe modified the instrumentation with a square-collar end on the rod and a corresponding square hook (Fig. 83-16). If the square-ended rods are not used, the collared ends would allow the rod to rotate and the contouring would end up in a different plane from that which the surgeon intended.

SELECTION OF FUSION LEVELS. Before inserting the Harrington instrumentation, appropriate fusion levels must be determined. The major curve or curves must be identified, the neutrally rotated end vertebrae for each major curve must be determined, and the relationship of the curves to a vertically drawn midsacral line must be evaluated.

The major curve or curves are identified by determining curve flexibility on side-bending roentgenograms. The stiffer curves, and therefore the more structural curves, are the major curves. Two curves with nearly identical flexibility constitute a double major curve pattern. The rotation of the individual vertebrae is determined by the relationship of the pedicle and the vertebral body margins on the posteroanterior roentgenogram, as described by Nash and Moe (Fig. 83-17). The Pedrialle template also can be used to more accurately measure vertebral rotation (Fig. 83-18). Generally, the instrumented level should extend from one end vertebra to the other end vertebra as determined by neutral rotation of the vertebrae involved. Harrington recommends that the fusion extend from one vertebra above the curve to two vertebrae below the curve in primary thoracic and thoracolumbar curves. He also recommends that if the centroid of function of the lower hook does not fall within the stable zone, the instrumentation be supplemented (Fig. 83-19) by overlapping distraction rods or by using a dollar-sign rod for application to both curves.

King et al. divided the combined curve patterns into five types. Type I is an S-shaped configuration with both the thoracic and lumbar curves crossing the midline. The lumbar curve is larger than the thoracic curve on the standing roentgenogram. The thoracic curve is more flexible than the lumbar curve on side bending. (Fig. 83-20, A). Type II also is an S-shaped configuration in which the thoracic and the lumbar curves both cross the midline, but the thoracic curve is larger than the lumbar curve, and the lumbar curve is more flexible on the bending films (Fig. 83-21, A). Type III is a thoracic curve in which the compensatory lumbar curve does not cross the midline (Fig. 83-22, A). Type IV is a long thoracic curve in which L5 is centered over the sacrum, but L4 tilts into the long thoracic curve (Fig. 83-23), and type V is a double thoracic curve with T1 tilted into the convexity of the upper curve that is structural on side bending (Fig. 83-24, A).

In type I curves, fusion of both the thoracic and lumbar curves is required (Fig. 83-20, B). In type II curves, a

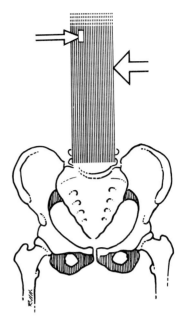

Fig. 83-19 Stable zone for inferior vertebra as described by Harrington.

selective thoracic fusion can be performed (Fig. 83-21, B), but the stable vertebra must be selected for the lower hook. The stable vertebra is that vertebra bisected or most closely bisected by a single line drawn through the center of the sacrum perpendicular to the iliac crest (Fig. 83-25). If the neutral vertebra and the stable vertebra do not correspond, fusion must be to the stable vertebra.

In type III curves, the fusion should include the measured thoracic curve but the lower end of the fusion ends at the first vertebra that is most closely bisected by the center sacral line (Fig. 83-22, B). In type IV curves, the fusion should include the measured thoracic curve and the lower level should end at the vertebra bisected by the center sacral line. Type IV curves are longer than type III curves, and the fusion generally must be carried further into the lumbar spine. Type V curves are significant in that both thoracic curves should be fused. If not, progression of the upper thoracic curve can result in a disfigured shoulder line and loss of balance. The lower level of this fusion should include the vertebra that is most closely bisected by the center sacral line (Figs. 83-24, B, and 83-26).

For single major thoracolumbar and lumbar curves, fusion above and below the end vertebrae is best. It is usually necessary to extend the fusion to L4. Continuing the fusion to the sacrum is never indicated in adolescents with idiopathic scoliosis and this curve pattern.

HARRINGTON DISTRACTION ROD

■ *TECHNIQUE.* Expose the spine as described on p. 3655. Seating of the Harrington distraction hooks requires the utmost care to prevent lateral rotation of the hook. Rotation can be prevented in three

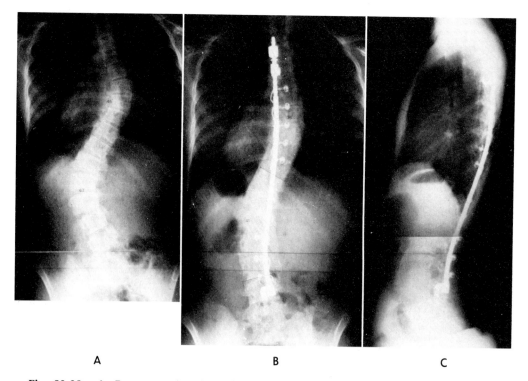

A   B   C

Fig. 83-20   **A,** Posteroanterior view of King type I idiopathic scoliosis. **B,** Postoperative posteroanterior view showing both curves instrumented and fused. **C,** Postoperative lateral view; note contoured Moe distraction rod used to maintain lumbar lordosis.

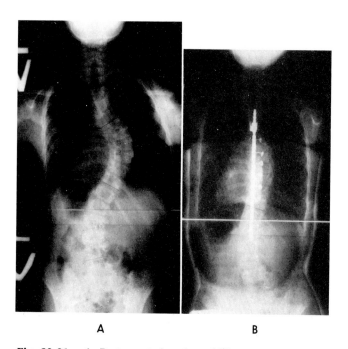

A   B

Fig. 83-21   **A,** Posteroanterior view of King type II curve. **B,** Postoperative posteroanterior view of instrumentation of thoracic curve only, with lower hook in stable vertebra.

ways: (1) seating the distraction hook in the pedicle at the described angle; (2) using a No. 1262 hook, the keel of which will prevent rotation and lateral slipping, or a bifid hook to encircle the pedicle on either side; and (3) introducing the whole shoe of a No. 1254 hook into the spinal canal distally. Prepare the site for the upper hook by removing a small piece of the inferior facet (Fig. 83-27, *A*) to allow the hook to be securely seated into the stronger portion of the facet and into the pedicle or around the pedicle. Using the hook inserter, insert a sharp-edged, plain, large Harrington hook (No. 1251) without excessive force, making sure that the blade of the hook actually goes between the two joint surfaces and not within the medulla of the lamina of the vertebra above. When the location for the hook has been established, withdraw this hook and insert a large, dull-flanged hook (No. 1262) in its place. The vertical flange is designed to prevent the blade and the hook from slipping laterally out of the joint or the unlikely possibility of its slipping medially towards the spinal canal. The proper seating for this hook is shown in Fig. 83-27, *B* and *C.* Alternatively, use a bifid hook to incorporate the pedicle and prevent lateral or medial displacement of the hook (Fig. 83-27, *D*). Once the hook is fully seated, check its stability by forcing it superiorly to be sure an adequate distractive force can be applied to it.

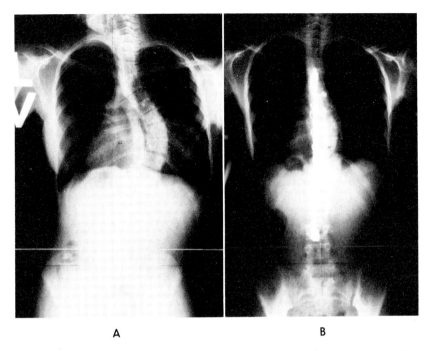

Fig. 83-22   **A,** Preoperative posteroanterior view of King type III thoracic curve. **B,** Postoperative posteroanterior view; note inferior hook in L3, which was bisected by center sacral line in preoperative roentgenograms.

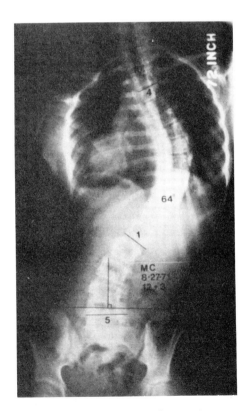

Fig. 83-23   King type IV curve. (From King HA et al: J Bone Joint Surg 65-A:1306, 1983.)

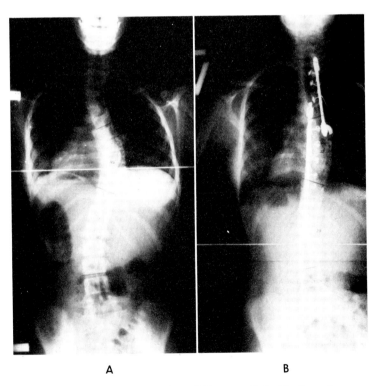

Fig. 83-24   **A,** Posteroanterior view of King type V double thoracic curve. **B,** Postoperative view of instrumentation of both thoracic curves.

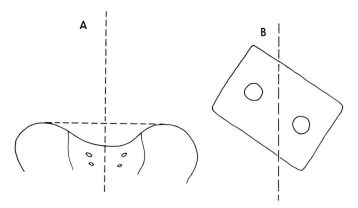

Fig. 83-25 **A,** Center sacral line as described by King et al. **B,** Vertebra most closely bisected by line is stable vertebra. (Redrawn from King HA et al: J Bone Joint Surg 65-A:1303, 1983.)

The most inferior distraction hook usually is placed in a lumbar vertebra, although we have occasionally placed this hook under lamina of T12 when the posterior elements of this vertebra were similar to those of the lumbar vertebra; do not place the hook through the lamina of a thoracic vertebra. Remove the ligamentum flavum from the superior portion of the lamina of the lumbar vertebra to be instrumented. Use a laminar spreader or hinged retractor to spread the spinous processes apart, making this portion of the procedure a little easier (Fig.

83-28). Once the ligamentum flavum has been removed, remove portions of the lateral part of the lamina with a Kerrison rongeur to allow enough room to insert a dull hook (No. 1254 or No. 1279-001). If the compression system is to be used, insert it at this time (p. 3668). If desired, now use the Harrington outrigger to allow decortication with the spine in the corrected position (Fig. 83-29). Alternatively, insert the distraction rod on the concave side of the curve and perform decortication around the distraction rod. We prefer to perform the decortication with the distraction rod in place and have not found that it prevents adequate intraarticular fusion. The advantage of not having to carry out the distraction in the face of active bleeding from decortication more than outweighs the disadvantage of having the rod in the way. Select a distraction rod of suitable length and insert its notched end through the superior hook, while holding the hook in place with a hook holder. Then, while the superior hook and hook holder are held by an assistant, grasp the inferior hook with a hook holder and feed the inferior end of the rod into the eye of that hook. If Moe's square-ended rods are used with square-ended hooks and the rod is contoured to maintain lumbar lordosis, this can be difficult. A rod-holding device (Fig. 83-30) and a pushing device can greatly assist in this portion of the procedure. Next fit the spreader between the superior hook and the notch

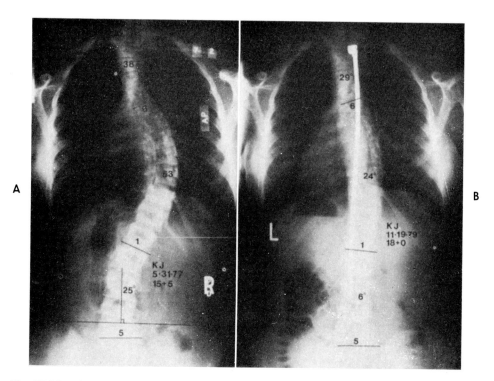

Fig. 83-26 **A,** Preoperative posteroanterior view of King type V curve. **B,** Postoperative view of instrumentation of upper thoracic curve with dollar-sign rod. (From King HA et al: J Bone Joint Surg 65-A:1303, 1983.)

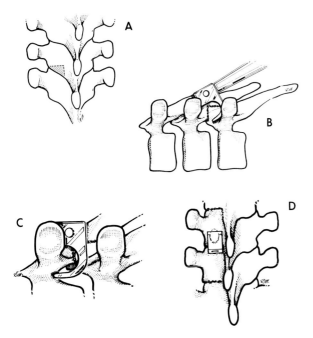

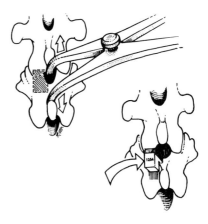

Fig. 83-28 Insertion of inferior distraction hook for Harrington distraction instrumentation. (Redrawn from Bradford DS et al: Moe's textbook of scoliosis and other spinal deformities, ed 2, Philadelphia, 1987, WB Saunders Co.)

Fig. 83-27 **A,** Removal of inferior portion of superior facet. **B,** Proper angle for insertion of upper Harrington hook. **C,** Upper hook should be in facet joint and engage pedicle above. **D,** Bifid hook incorporating pedicle.

of the rod just inferior to it. By repeated spreading of the instrument, force the superior hook up the notched part of the rod (Fig. 83-31, *A*). When the six-ratchet rods are used, a Gaines distractor must be used (Fig. 83-31, *B*). Try to keep the superior hook as close to the solid rod-to-ratchet transition region as possible; this will result in a much longer service life for the rod and much better fatigue characteristics for the system. As the distance between the hooks at each end of the rod is increased with each successive click of the instrument, distraction is applied. Proceed carefully with the distraction while observing the stability of both hooks. As the distraction becomes more difficult and the instrument is tightened, any evidence of fracture or tearing of the posterior elements indicates that the distraction should be stopped, and the correction obtained at this point should be accepted. At the completion of the distraction, apply a **C**-washer distal to the upper hook to prevent loss of distraction.

The correction obtainable varies considerably, depending on the age and maturity of the patient and the hardness of the bone. When the bone is mature, distraction usually can be continued until the rod begins to bow. It must be remembered that considerably more force can be exerted with the Harrington distractor than can be tolerated by any of the posterior elements.

After insertion of the distraction rod, complete decortication and intraarticular fusion and close the wound as described on p. 3658.

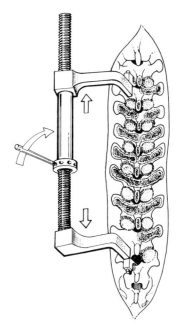

Fig. 83-29 Diagram of use of Harrington outrigger allowing distraction and correction of curve and decortication of spine in corrected position.

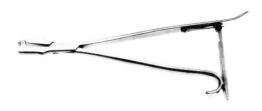

Fig. 83-30 Rod clamp used to hold and manipulate distraction rods. (Courtesy Zimmer, Inc., Warsaw, Indiana.)

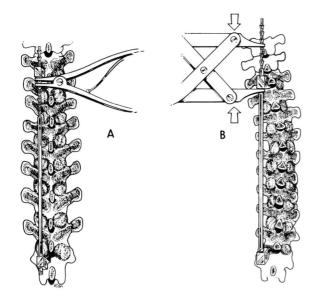

Fig. 83-31 A, Spreader used for Harrington distraction rods when rachets are proximal to upper hook. **B,** Gaines distractor useful in Harrington rods with six rachets. With this short rachet segment, there are no rachets proximal to upper hook to use ordinary distractor and Gaines distractor is necessary.

HARRINGTON DISTRACTION INSTRUMENTATION TO SACRUM

■ *TECHNIQUE.* Distraction implants to the sacrum should be avoided if at all possible. Distraction in this area produces a loss of lumbar lordosis, sacral malrotation, and high risks of pseudarthrosis, implant failure, and hook dislodgment. In idiopathic scoliosis, fusions distal to L4 rarely are needed. Fusion to the sacrum generally is necessary for neuromuscular scoliosis. If Harrington instrumentation to the sacrum is necessary, prepare the upper hook site as previously described. Expose the ala of the sacrum, and use square-ended Harrington rods and square-ended sacral alar hooks. Place the alar hook around the ala of the sacrum and insert the appropriate-length square-ended rod. Appropriate contouring for lumbar lordosis must be used when instrumenting to the sacrum. Appropriate intraarticular fusion is then carried out.

HARRINGTON COMPRESSION INSTRUMENTATION

■ *TECHNIQUE.* According to Harrington, the compression rod assembly is an integral part of the Harrington instrumentation system. The compression rod applies a significant corrective force to any kyphotic deformity, and we believe the compression rod is most useful in scoliosis in which there is a

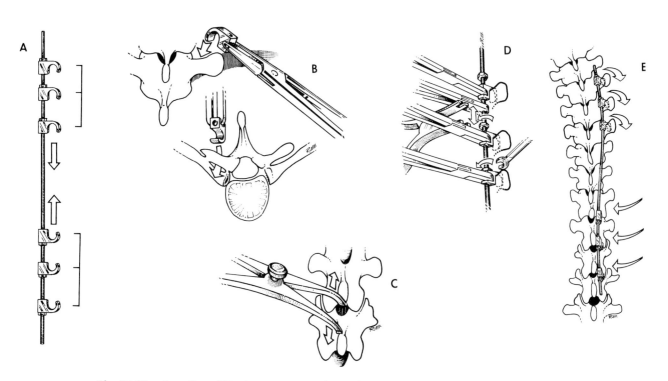

Fig. 83-32 Insertion of Harrington compression rod on convex side of thoracic spine for idiopathic scoliosis (see text). (Redrawn from Bradford DS et al: Moe's textbook of scoliosis and other spinal deformities, ed 2, Philadelphia, 1987, WB Saunders Co.)

significant kyphotic component. It also is useful in the lumbar spine to help maintain lumbar lordosis if the fusion extends lower into the spine. The insertion of the compression assembly is somewhat complex and also decreases the amount of bone available for decortication and subsequent fusion. The equipment available includes two threaded rods: a larger rod of ³⁄₁₆ inch (4.8 mm) diameter that requires a No. 1256 hook, and a smaller rod, most commonly used in conjunction with the Harrington distraction rod, of ⅛ inch (3.2 mm) diameter that requires a No. 1259 hook.

Assemble the compression rod with three hooks facing distally and three hooks facing proximally (Fig. 83-32, *A*). Cut the costotransverse ligaments around the transverse processes with the sharp No. 1259 hook introduced beneath the transverse process with the hook holder (Fig. 83-32, *B*). Alternatively, use the No. 1251 sharp distraction hook, which is a little larger and will provide a larger area for subsequent insertion of the No. 1259 hooks. Direct these hooks caudad on all vertebrae above the apex of the curve and cephalad on all vertebrae below the apex of the curve. Caudal to T10, the transverse processes are generally inadequate; place the hooks under the lamina (Fig. 83-32, *C*). Then grasp the compression assembly with hook holders. Beginning cranially, place all the hooks beneath the transverse processes. Place the caudal hooks beneath the transverse processes or lamina as indicated (Fig. 83-32, *D*). Tighten the system by using the spreader between a rod holder and a hook holder (Fig. 83-32, *E*). Similarly, use a wrench to tighten the nuts. If the compression assembly is used in conjunction with the distraction rod for ky-

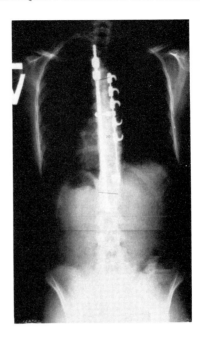

Fig. 83-33 Transverse loading device connecting Harrington distraction and compression rods.

phoscoliosis, the compression assembly usually is tightened before the distraction is applied.

Perform decortication, fusion, and closure as described on p. 3658.

HARRINGTON SYSTEM WITH TRANSVERSE LOADING DEVICE. The transverse loading device connects the Harrington distraction rod with the Harrington compression system (Fig. 83-33). The basic concept of this device is reduction of the distance from the apex of the curve to the midline, thereby producing a more stable spine as

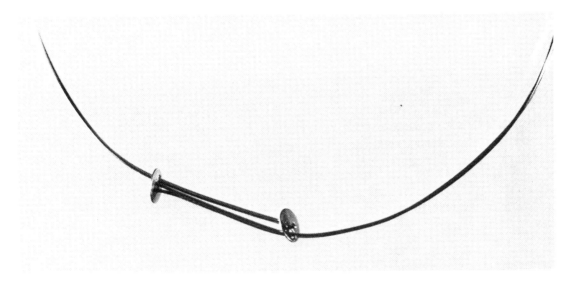

Fig. 83-34 Drummond wires. Note hole in surface of button, which allows wires from other implant to pass through. Free ends of each wire are welded together to form small round bead. (From Drummond DS: Orthop Clin North Am 19:282, 1988.)

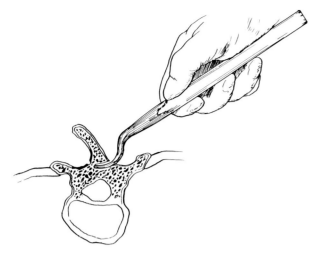

Fig. 83-35 Use of awl to produce hole at base of spinous process for passage of Drummond wires. (From Drummond DS: Orthop Clin North Am 19:282, 1988.)

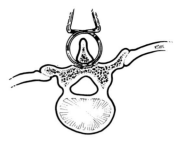

Fig. 83-36 Use of Lewin clamp to make hole in base of spinous process for Drummond wires.

well as providing additional support to the convex side of the curve at the apex through the linkage to the compression rod. Biomechanically, longitudinally applied distraction force is effective in large curves, but in smaller curves it becomes much less effective and transverse loading becomes more effective. The transverse traction device has been used successfully for many years, but one must be careful of the problem of medial hook cutout when using these devices.

DRUMMOND WIRING. Drummond modified the Harrington instrumentation system with an interspinous segmental wiring system to provide the stability afforded by segmental spinal instrumentation without the risks of passing sublaminar wires. To provide a broad purchase at the base of the spinous process, he developed a button wire implant made from ³/₁₆-inch stainless steel (Fig. 83-34). The button is 8 mm in diameter and 0.8 mm thick. The wire is 1 mm thick (18 gauge) and has its free ends welded together to form a rounded bead. Laboratory tests have shown that the base of the spinous process is an adequate area to provide a good purchase site for fixation.

■ *TECHNIQUE (DRUMMOND).* Select the fusion levels as for Harrington distraction instrumentation. After the spine has been exposed (p. 3655), insert the upper hook as described on p. 3664. The use of a bifid hook to grasp the pedicle is recommended (see Fig. 83-27, *D*). Make a hole at the base of each involved spinous process, using an awl (Fig. 83-35) or a Lewin clamp (Fig. 83-36). Then pass two wires in opposite directions through the hole in the spinous process. Pass the wires through the hole on the opposite button and pull the buttons snugly to the base of the spinous process (Fig. 83-37). Tamp the buttons into position with a mallet and tamp. Insert

only one button wire from the concave to the convex side at the uppermost and lowermost segments. Use a square-ended Harrington distraction rod (Moe), carefully contoured to preserve physiologic kyphosis and lordosis, and pass it through the open loops of wire implants on the concave side of the curve and then into the upper and lower hooks in a routine manner. Obtain initial correction by distraction. Contour a ³/₁₆-inch Luque rod (L-rod) to preserve physiologic kyphosis and lordosis, and make right-angle bends at the upper and lower ends of the rod. Pass the upper limb of the rod under the ratchet system of the distraction rod to prevent rotation of this rod. At this point, decorticate the convex side of the curve; only the posterior elements lateral to the button should be decorticated. Pass the contoured L-rod through the open wire loops of the implants on the convex side of the curve. Correction is obtained as an assistant presses the rod against the spine while each loop is tightened with the wire tightener. Tighten the apical wire first and then alternately tighten each proximal and distal level. The Harrington distraction rod can then be distracted further if possible. Place a C-clamp just below the upper hook to prevent loss of this distraction. Then tighten the wires on the Harrington rod but not so tight as to rotate the hooks on the distraction rod (Fig. 83-38). Now obtain bone grafts from the iliac crest, complete the decortication, and perform the grafting. Postoperatively, the patient is allowed to ambulate by the third or fourth day without any external immobilization (Fig. 83-39).

• • •

We have used contoured, square-ended Harrington distraction rods in combination with Drummond wires without the addition of the L-rod on the convex side of the curve. We have obtained safe segmental fixation with this technique and believe it offers the advantages of facet fusion, better decortication, and more bony area for bone graft incorporation. This technique, however, does not offer sufficient fixation to allow postoperative ambulation without external support.

■ *TECHNIQUE (DRUMMOND, MODIFIED).* Expose the spine in the routine manner and pass Drummond

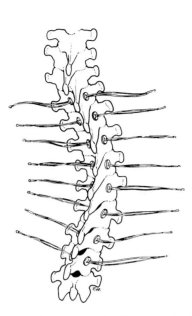

Fig. 83-37 Typical placement for Drummond wires in single thoracic curve.

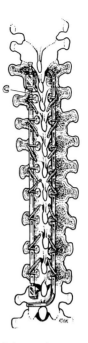

Fig. 83-38 Completed interspinous segmental instrumentation with Harrington distraction rod and L-rod with decortication of the spine.

wires from the convex to the concave side of the curve with the button on the convex side and the wire on the concave side (Fig. 83-40). Place the Moe contoured distraction rod through the concave wires. Apply enough distraction to seat the hooks, but before applying significant distraction, tighten the Drummond wires with a wire tightener to obtain some correction of the hypokyphosis that is frequently present in the thoracic spine. After the

wires are tightened, apply further distraction to the rod. Apply a **C**-clamp just below the upper hook. Then decorticate the spine, emphasizing a facet fusion as well as decortication of the laminae and transverse processes lateral to the buttons (Fig. 83-41).

AFTERTREATMENT. A Risser cast is applied at about 1 week (see Fig. 83-11) and is worn for about 4 months if the fusion is confined to the thoracic area

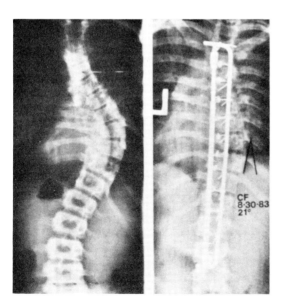

Fig. 83-39 Preoperative and postoperative roentgenograms of patient who underwent interspinous segmental instrumentation. (From Guadagni J et al: J Pediatr Orthop 4:405, 1984.)

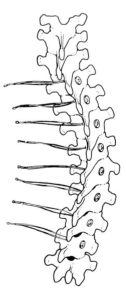

Fig. 83-40 Typical placement of Drummond wires when used in conjunction with Harrington distraction rod only. Wires are passed from convex to concave side of curve.

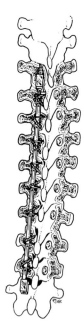

Fig. 83-41 Decortication along lamina and transverse processes lateral to Drummond buttons with Harrington distraction rod wired in place.

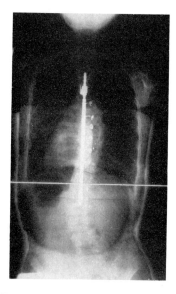

Fig. 83-42 Posteroanterior roentgenogram of patient in underarm cast after instrumentation with contoured Moe distraction rod and Drummond segmental wires.

(Fig. 83-42). If the fusion extends down into the lumbar spine, the cast is worn for 6 months.

Cotrel-Dubousset Instrumentation

The concept of segmental instrumentation for three-dimensional correction of idiopathic scoliosis was developed by Cotrel and Dubousset and was introduced in the United States in 1984. This method rapidly achieved widespread use because of its three-dimensional correction of the scoliotic deformity and the less frequent need for postoperative immobilization. Other advantages include (1) the ability to distract and compress between segments with multiple hook (the Harrington distraction system distracts only at the end hooks); (2) correction of the curve in three dimensions, accomplished by bending of the concave rod, hook placement at strategic locations, and the ability to rotate the rod; (3) a more normal sagittal contour of the spine; and (4) stability provided by multiple segmental fixation sites and the transverse traction device that forms a coupled rectangle, which greatly increases the rigidity of the system and eliminates the need for postoperative braces or casts.

Several disadvantages of the system also must be considered: (1) surgical technique is more complicated and time consuming than with the Harrington distraction system; (2) experience is necessary to apply this system because of the multiple options of hook placement; (3) increased blood loss can be expected because of the longer time interval between decortication and closure; (4) the system implants are significantly more expensive than the Harrington system; (5) although still quite low,

the neurologic complication rate is greater than with the Harrington system alone; (6) a thorough understanding of the three-dimensional nature of the spinal deformity is required; and (7) long-term studies to establish the efficacy of this procedure are not yet available.

As with any new instrumentation system, further experience and longer follow-up are needed before the definite role of this system can be determined; however, early reported results are encouraging. Many of the design problems are being corrected, and other instrumentation systems based on the same three-dimensional correction technique, such as the Texas Scottish Rite Hospital (TSRH) system, are currently being developed.

The hardware used for the Cotrel-Dubousset instrumentation is quite varied. The rods are solid, 7 mm 316-L stainless steel. Diamond-shaped surface irregularities allow secure fixation of the hooks and screws to the rod (Fig. 83-43).

There are three basic hook types: pedicle, lumbar laminar, and thoracic laminar, each of which is available in either an "open" or "closed" style (Fig. 83-44). The hook blocker allows conversion of an open hook to a closed hook. The device for transverse traction consists of a small rod and hooks (with irregularities matching the large rod) that interlock the two rods. A minimum of two of these hooks are used to convert the rods to a fixed, coupled rectangle, which greatly increases rigidity, particularly in torsion (Fig. 83-45). Set screws are provided to prevent the rod from rotating once the position has been set.

SELECTION OF FUSION LEVELS. The selection of the vertebrae to be included in the fusion with Cotrel-Dubousset instrumentation is often not as straightfor-

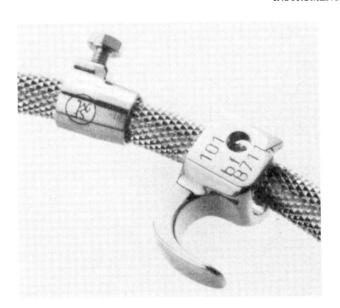

Fig. 83-43 Cotrel-Dubousset rod with diamond-shaped irregularities allows strong fixation of vertebral hooks or screws at any level, with any degree of rotation, and in distraction and compression. Rod can be bent along entire length. (From Cotrel Y, Dubousset J, and Guillaumat M: Clin Orthop 227:11, 1988.)

ward as with the Harrington system because the three-dimensional spinal pathologic condition must be appreciated. Several principles must be kept in mind: (1) distraction is required to produce kyphosis; (2) compression is required to produce lordosis; (3) to produce kyphosis (or correct lordosis), the concave rod must be inserted first; (4) to produce lordosis (or correct kyphosis), the convex rod must be inserted first; (5) at the thoracolumbar junction (T11 to L1), each vertebra should have a hook to provide rigid fixation in this transition zone from kyphosis to lordosis; and (6) the position of the proximal and distal hooks must be carefully evaluated on the lateral roentgenogram. The upper hooks should not stop at the apex of the kyphosis proximally and the inferior hook should extend well into the lordotic segment of the spine distally. Although, in general, the same guidelines apply as for the selection of the end vertebra with the Harrington system, including the concept of the "stable zone," these principles must be kept in mind when determining the upper and lower end vertebrae of the curves. Preoperative bending films are used to determine the intermediate vertebrae, generally one to two vertebral bodies on either side of the apical vertebra that show the least mobility on side bending (Fig. 83-46). The apical vertebra is the vertebral body with the most rotation on the plain standing film. Planned hook placement is marked on the preoperative

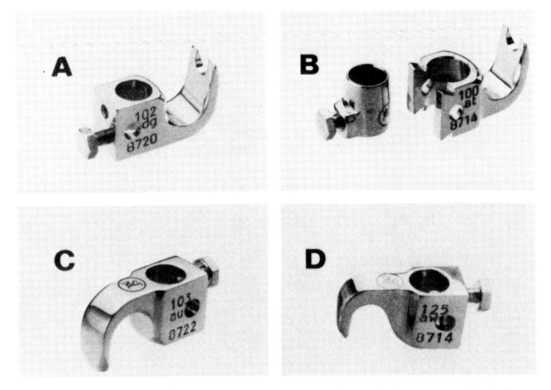

Fig. 83-44 Hooks used in Cotrel-Dubousset instrumentation. **A,** Pedicular hook with closed body. **B,** Pedicular hook with open body and cylindroconic ring. **C,** Lumbar laminar hook with closed body. **D,** Thoracic laminar hook with closed body. (From Cotrel Y, Dubousset J, and Guillaumat M: Clin Orthop 227:11, 1988.)

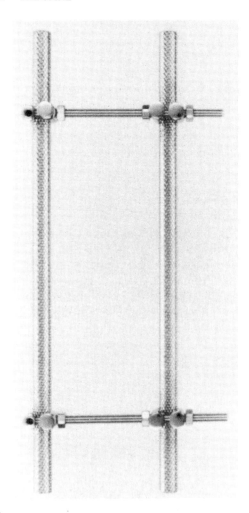

Fig. 83-45 Double rods locked by two transverse loading rods resulting in strong framelike setup. (From Cotrel Y, Dubousset J, and Guillaumat M: Clin Orthop 227:11, 1988.)

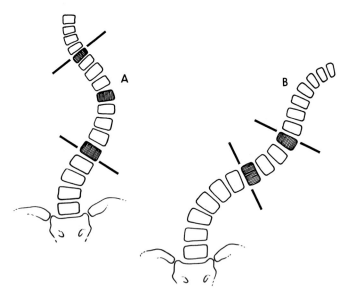

Fig. 83-46 **A,** Anteroposterior diagrams of uppermost and lowermost instrumented vertebrae. **B,** Upper and lower rigid bodies are shown on bending films.

roentgenograms (Table 83-2). To help prevent dislodgment of the lower convex hook, some have added an additional downward-facing hook to claw this area (Fig. 83-47).

In double major right thoracic and left lumbar curves, the appropriate thoracic vertebrae to be instrumented are the same as the right thoracic curve. The lower level of instrumentation is determined by vertebral neutraliza-

tion and disc space opening and closing on the bending films. The left lumbar curve is distracted through the right hemilamina of its lower end vertebra. On the convex side of the left lumbar curve, the hook on the left hemilamina of the inferior vertebra is applied facing proximally so that compression can be applied, which also helps maintain lumbar lordosis. The apical vertebra of the lumbar curve is also instrumented with a proximal facing hook. Typical hook placement for a double major curve is shown in Fig. 83-48.

Proper hook site selection is necessary for optimal results and common mistakes occur in this area. There is a significant learning curve in hook placement decisions.

Right Thoracic Curve

■ **TECHNIQUE.** Expose the spine as described on p. 3653. Prepare the concave hook sites, using a closed pedicle hook for the superior hook. Insert the hooks after excision of some of the inferior facet. Start the vertical cut in the facet at the junction of the con-

Table 83-2 Hook placement in Cotrel-Dubousset technique

Instrumented vertebra	Concave hook	Convex hook
Uppermost instrumented vertebra = Proximal		Closed laminar (transverse process)
neutral or end vertebra	Closed pedicular	Closed pedicular
Uppermost vertebra of most rigid curve	Open pedicular	
Apical vertebra		Open pedicular
Lowermost vertebra of most rigid curve	Open thoracic laminar	
Lowermost instrumented vertebra = Distal	Closed laminar	Closed laminar
Neutral or end vertebra	Facing caudally	Facing cranially

From Farcy JP, Weidenbaum M, and Roye DP, Jr: Surg Rounds Orthop, p 13, May 1987.

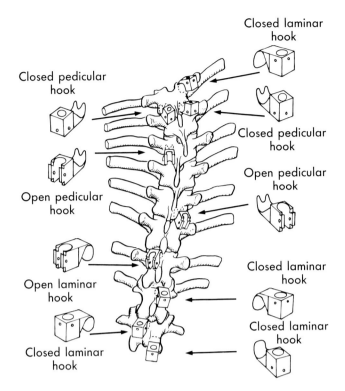

Fig. 83-47 Typical hook selection for right thoracic curve T5 to L1. (From Mubarak SJ et al: Update on Spinal Disorders 2:4, 1987.)

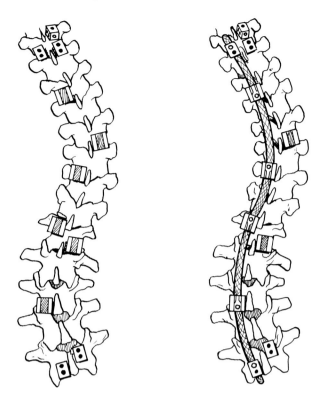

Fig. 83-48 Hook placement in double major right thoracic and left lumbar curve. (From Denis F: Orthop Clin North Am 19:307, 1988.)

vexity of the inferior facet and the concavity joining the inferior facet to the base of the spinous process. Start the horizontal cut of the inferior facet 4 mm caudad to the line joining the inferior aspects of the two transverse processes. After removal of the fragment of facet, use a curet to remove the hyaline cartilage from the facet joint. Then introduce a pedicle finder into the space and push it against the pedicle (Fig. 83-49, *A*). Gently pound it further into place with a mallet. Then insert the closed pedicle hook with a hook holder and an angled hook inserter (Fig. 83-49, *B*). Take care to be certain that the horns of the bifid hook remain in the facet joint and do not hook into the remaining bone of the inferior facet. After the pedicle hook has been inserted into place manually, tap it further against the pedicle with a mallet.

The upper intermediate hook is also a pedicle hook, but is open; it is inserted in a similar manner. The lower intermediate concave hook is the most risky hook to insert because it is placed in a relatively tight spinal canal right behind the spinal cord. Because of the curve, the spinal cord will be toward the concavity of the curve in the area where this hook is placed. Both lower concave hooks are in the spinal canal, but the canal is wider at the distalmost level and the hooks face the cauda equina rather than the spinal cord itself. Make a laminot-

omy for the insertion of this hook, keeping it as small as possible. Remove the ligamentum flavum from the superior aspect of the intermediate vertebra on the concave side and make a small laminotomy for insertion of this hook, usually an open thoracic laminar hook (Fig. 83-49, *C*). When this hook is in place, pressure over its open end should not displace the hook into the canal. Remove this hook until the remainder of the hook sites have been prepared and the rod is ready to be inserted. Place the lower end vertebra concave hook, generally a closed lumbar laminar hook, in a supralaminar position similar to placement of the No. 1254 hook in the Harrington system (p. 3666).

Next, prepare the hook sites on the convex side. The upper end vertebra on the convex side receives a transverse process hook and a pedicle hook to "claw" this vertebra. Insert the transverse process hook first. Divide the costotransverse ligaments with the transverse process elevator on the superior side of the transverse process. Then insert the transverse process hook around the transverse process. Place the upper end vertebra pedicle hook on the convex side in a manner similar to the upper hook on the concave side. Insert the apical hook (an open pedicle hook) in a manner similar to the upper end

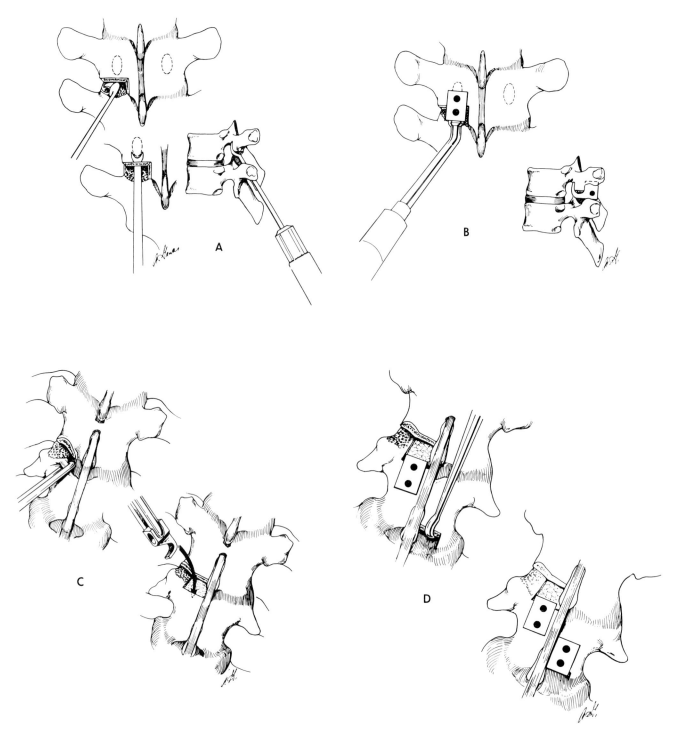

Fig. 83-49 **A,** Insertion of pedicle hook. Inferior facet is excised. Curet is used to clean carti-lage. Pedicle finder rides over pedicle and indicates whether more bone should be taken off. It is moved sideways to determine how stable the pedicle purchase is. Beware in this sideways movement of "plunging" into the spinal canal. **B,** Pedicle hook is pushed into place by closed hook inserter. Three additional pedicle hooks will be inserted in a similar manner. **C,** Supralam-inar hook insertion. This insertion applies to lower two concave hooks in single thoracic curve instrumentation. Laminotomy is kept as small as possible to minimize risk of deep penetration into spinal canal during rod insertion. Tight fit is necessary and thoracic laminar hook is used when laminar thickness is too small to allow lumbar laminar hook to be stable in anteroposte-rior plane. **D,** Infralaminar hook insertion. Lower convex hook in right thoracic curve is in-serted in this manner. Ligamentum flavum is dissected off underside of lamina. Small inferior laminotomy provides horizontal purchase site for hook. Adjacent facet capsule should be spared because it is not included in fusion.

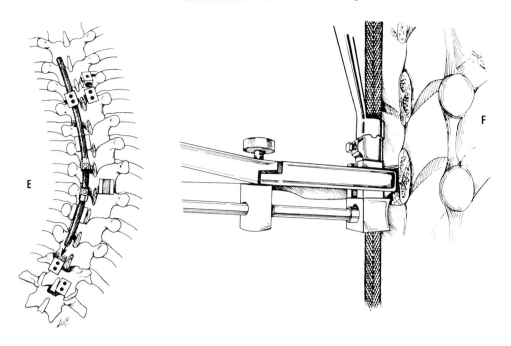

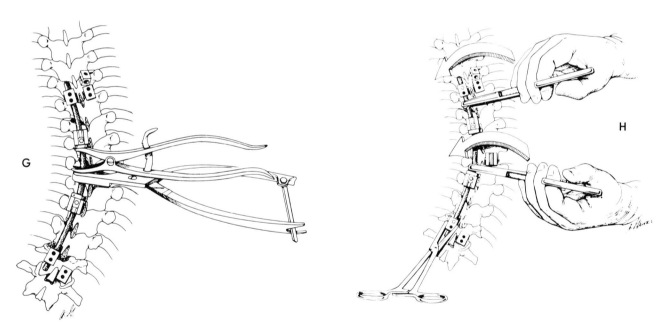

Fig. 83-49, cont'd   **E,** Concave rod bending must match scoliosis contouring observed on table as well as anticipated final kyphosis, assuming that rod will be rotated 90 degrees. When lower hook is placed on L1 or lower, rod is bent slightly in opposite direction which presents some "lordosis contouring" to more closely represent normal sagittal contour of lumbar spine. As rod is inserted, lower intermediate hook is carfully observed to avoid penetration into spinal canal. **F,** Example of rod being introduced into lower intermediate hook with rod introducer. Hook blocker is also shown. **G,** C-rings are introduced onto rod between two intermediate hooks. Hex screw is positioned as far as possible towards convexity of curve to allow removal after 90-degree rotation of rod. Distraction of this most structural part of curve is performed and held by C-rings. At this point, hex screws on open hooks are still loose, allowing rod rotation. **H,** Rotation of rod is done very carefully. Observation of all concave hooks is important because of risk of sudden fracture of lamina or hook displacement. Special attention is given to lower intermediate hook. If there are no apparent problems, rod is rotated 90 degrees where its initial scoliotic configuration is then replaced by kyphotic configuration.

Continued.

vertebra pedicle hook. Place the lower end vertebra hook on the convex side (a closed lumbar laminar hook) in an infralaminar position (Fig. 83-49, *D*). Do not remove the ligamentum flavum from the interspace but simply lift it with an elevator to allow insertion of the inferior hook. Try to preserve the adjacent capsule of the facet joint that is not included in the fusion. Pay careful attention to this inferior convex hook, being sure it is well seated beneath the lamina. This hook is frequently knocked out of place when hooks proximal to it are seated. A claw configuration of this hook can be obtained by placing a distally facing open laminar hook in the supralaminar position of the vertebra above.

Once the hook sites are prepared, contour the concave rod, using a malleable rod as a template. Determine the length of the concave rod from this malleable rod and contour it to conform to the scoliotic curve in the anteroposterior plane. Perform concave facet joint decortication and fusion just before inserting the concave rod. Facet fusions are done wherever accessible, provided they do not compromise hook purchase. Reinsert the intermediate inferior hook and insert the concave rod into the upper closed pedicle hook first. Then insert the rod into the lower closed hook (Fig. 83-49, *E*). If the rod has been contoured appropriately, it should go into the open box of the intermediate vertebra hooks. As the rod is pushed into the lower hook, carefully observe the inferior intermediate hook because it is close to the spinal cord and can be quite easily pushed into the canal. Push the hook blockers into the open pedicle and laminar hooks of the intermediate vertebra. The rod introducer (Fig. 83-49, *F*) often is required to insert the rod into the lower intermediate hook. Place two C-rings over the rods between the intermediate hooks (Fig. 83-49, *G*). Then distract the intermediate hooks and hold them in position by temporarily tightening the C-rings but not tightening the set screws of the bushings within the open hooks. If these set screws are tightened, rotation of the rod will not be possible. Segmental distraction is accomplished at the intermediate open hooks, using a spreader between appropriate open rings and locally applied rod grippers. This distraction affords some correction but mainly assures that the intermediate hooks are well seated. Check the upper and lower end hooks for position and seat them if necessary. Use two rod holders to rotate the rod 90 degrees from its scoliotic configuration to a kyphotic configuration (Fig. 83-49, *H*). As this occurs, the scoliotic deformity is corrected and the sagittal contours are improved (Fig. 83-49, *I*). This maneuver may be easy in supple curves but can be quite difficult in more severe or more rigid curves. During this procedure, the length of the spine is increased slightly, and the intermediate hooks may become

slightly loose. Seat these hooks more snugly if needed. Also examine the upper and lower hooks to be certain they are seated snugly and tighten the set screws to prevent derotation of the rod. Remove the two C-rings from the intermediate hook sites.

Now contour the convex rod, producing less kyphosis than the patient's to push the convexity forward during instrumentation. Contour the bottom of the rod into slight lordosis as seen physiologically at the thoracolumbar junction. Then perform a facet decortication and fusion on the convex side. Insert the convex rod in its upper claw first and push it

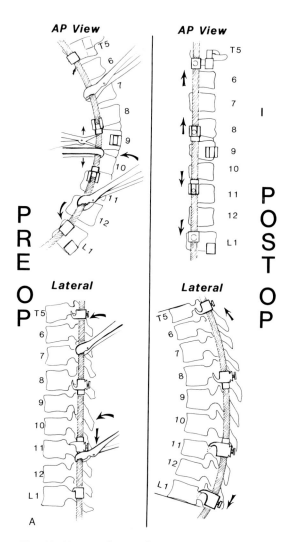

Fig. 83-49, cont'd For legend see opposite page.

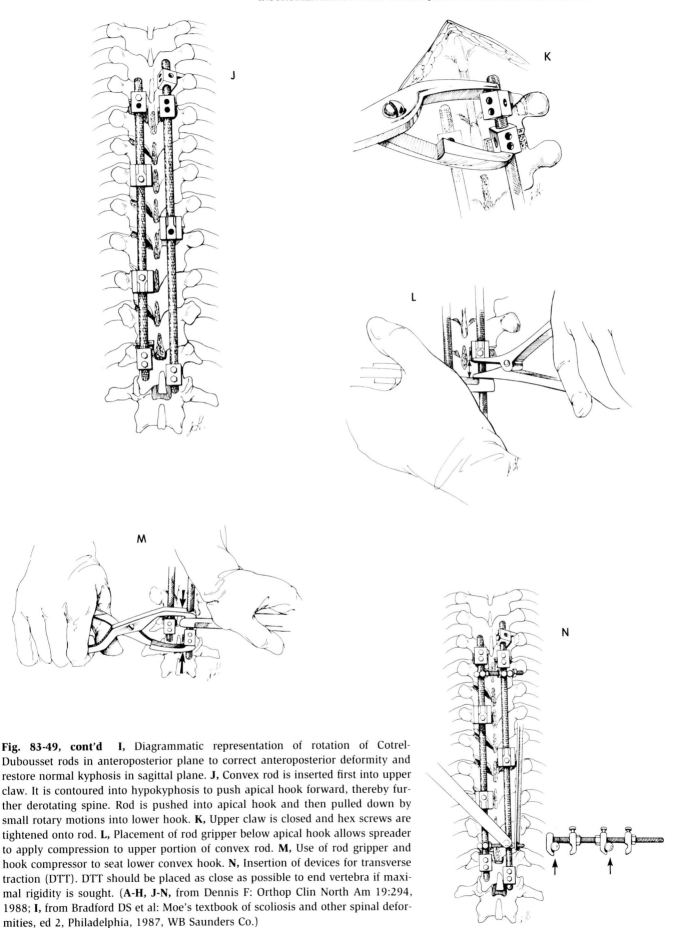

Fig. 83-49, cont'd   **I,** Diagrammatic representation of rotation of Cotrel-Dubousset rods in anteroposterior plane to correct anteroposterior deformity and restore normal kyphosis in sagittal plane. **J,** Convex rod is inserted first into upper claw. It is contoured into hypokyphosis to push apical hook forward, thereby further derotating spine. Rod is pushed into apical hook and then pulled down by small rotary motions into lower hook. **K,** Upper claw is closed and hex screws are tightened onto rod. **L,** Placement of rod gripper below apical hook allows spreader to apply compression to upper portion of convex rod. **M,** Use of rod gripper and hook compressor to seat lower convex hook. **N,** Insertion of devices for transverse traction (DTT). DTT should be placed as close as possible to end vertebra if maximal rigidity is sought. (**A-H, J-N,** from Dennis F: Orthop Clin North Am 19:294, 1988; **I,** from Bradford DS et al: Moe's textbook of scoliosis and other spinal deformities, ed 2, Philadelphia, 1987, WB Saunders Co.)

down into the apical open hook. Move the blocker cephalad into the apical hook. Place the rod holder approximately 3 to 5 cm from the lower end, allowing the rod to slip into the lower hook (Fig. 83-49, *J*). This inferior hook may have to be repositioned and care must be taken that the hook is well seated; otherwise, it will pull out posteriorly. Tighten the upper claw against itself (Fig. 83-49, *K*) and compress the convex apical hook against the upper claw (Fig. 83-49, *L*). Then compress the lower hook against the rod gripper with a hook compressor (Fig. 83-49, *M*). Check all the hex bolts to be certain that they are tight and that the rods are stable within the hooks. Now further decorticate all of the available parts of the posterior arches throughout the length of the instrumented curve. Insert two transverse traction devices, one at each end just below the upper hooks and just above the lower hooks (Fig. 83-49, *N*). If desired, perform a wake-up test at this point. Apply the autogenous iliac bone graft and tighten all hex screws all the way to shearing. Insert second hex screws and shear them on all closed hooks. Close the incision over drains in a routine manner.

AFTERTREATMENT. The patient is logrolled in bed for 2 to 3 days, and mobilization and ambulation are begun when the drains are removed. No postoperative immobilization is needed. Most patients are dismissed from the hospital on the sixth or seventh day. The patient's activities are gradually increased, but full release to normal activities is not allowed for 1 year while the bone graft matures (Fig. 83-50).

Double Major Right Thoracic and Left Lumbar Curves

■ *TECHNIQUE.* Expose the spine in routine fashion. Instrument the right thoracic curve as described on p. 3674, but use open hooks for both of the thoracic curve lower end hooks. On the concave side of the lumbar curve, place a closed laminar hook in the supralaminar position. On the convex side of the lumbar curve, use an infralaminar closed lumbar laminar hook to apply compression and lordotic forces in the lumbar spine. On the lumbar side use an open lumbar laminar hook as the convex apical hook, placing it in an infralaminar position. After preparation of the hook sites and insertion of the hooks, contour the left rod into an S-shape to match the scoliosis. On rotation, this rod will provide kyphosis in the thoracic spine and lordosis in the lumbar spine (Fig. 83-51). After contouring of the rod, perform facet decortication and fusion. Then insert the left rod first through the proximal closed pedicle hook, then into the open intermediate hooks, and finally into the closed laminar hook on the left side of

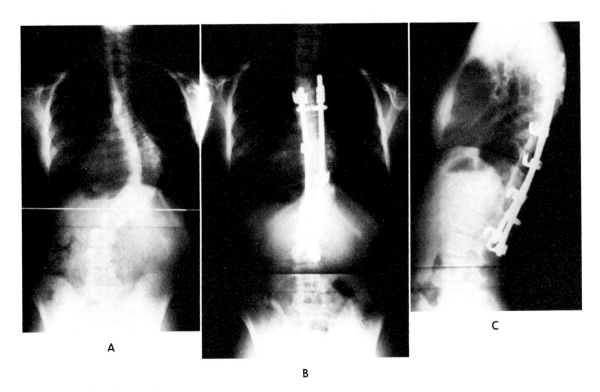

A

B

C

Fig. 83-50   **A,** Preoperative posteroanterior roentgenogram of patient undergoing Cotrel-Dubousset instrumentation. **B** and **C,** Posteroanterior and lateral views after Cotrel-Dubousset instrumentation.

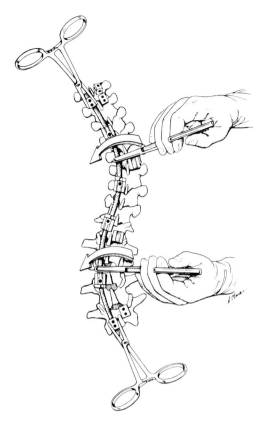

Fig. 83-51 Rotation of rod in double major scoliosis producing kyphosis in thoracic spine and lordosis in lumbar spine while correcting scoliosis deformity. (From Dennis F: Orthop Clin North Am 19:294, 1988.)

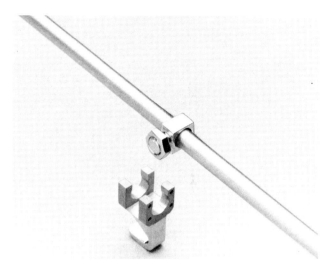

Fig. 83-52 Expanded of three-point shear clamp. (Courtesy Danek Medical, Memphis, Tennessee.)

the lumbar curve. Apply distraction between the intermediate hooks in the thoracic spine and hold it with the **C**-rings. Check all hook sites to be certain that the hooks are well seated. Using two rod holders, perform a derotation maneuver to convert the scoliosis in the thoracic spine to a kyphosis and the scoliosis in the lumbar spine to a lordosis. Further seat the hooks and tighten the hex nuts. Then contour the right-side rod. This rod will be straighter than the left-side rod, with a hypokyphotic configuration in the thoracic spine and the lordosis in the lumbar area. Perform facet decortication on the right side of the spine and insert the right rod through the superior claw configuration, into the intermediate hooks, and into the closed lumbar laminar hook distally. Apply compression across the convex side of the thoracic curve as described for the thoracic curve. Apply distraction across the lumbar spine. Tighten the hex nuts. Three transverse traction devices are usually needed to provide maximum rigidity in this double major curve. Place one in the middle and two as close as possible to the end vertebrae proximally and distally. Aftertreatment is the same as after instrumentation of a single right thoracic curve (p. 3680).

TEXAS SCOTTISH RITE HOSPITAL SPINAL IMPLANT SYSTEM. Surgeons at the Texas Scottish Rite Hospital (TSRH) in Dallas modified the Cotrel-Dubousset Universal spinal system. The primary difference between this system and other systems is that all TSRH attachments to the spinal rods are made with a single mechanism, a three-point shear clamp (nut and eyebolt), reducing the number of different connectors to one and eliminating ratchets, collars, and blockers. The surgical techniques, however, as far as hook placement selection, surgical exposure, fusion, and derotation of the spinal column, are similar.

All hooks, screws, and cross-links use the same three-point shear clamp locking mechanism to attach to the spinal rods (Fig. 83-52). This mechanism provides significant resistance to axial, torsional, and shear forces as long as 150 inch-pounds of torque are applied to the nut during assembly (Fig. 83-53). Three rod diameters are available: $\frac{3}{16}$ inch, $\frac{1}{4}$ inch, and 7 mm. All rods are shot-peened to enhance fatigue resistance (Fig. 83-54).

To accommodate the different rod diameters, three eyebolt assemblies are available ($\frac{3}{16}$ inch, $\frac{1}{4}$ inch, and 7 mm). To ensure a proper fit of the locking mechanism, the appropriate size eyebolt must be used to accommodate the rod size.

There are four basic shoe shapes: large laminar, small laminar, thoracic laminar, and pedicle (Fig. 83-55). There are three hook tops for these shoe shapes: full top, half top, and closed top (Fig. 83-56). All hooks, regardless of shoe shape (offset or top) use the same eyebolt for connection to the rod. In addition to the different shoe shapes and hook tops, hook shoes can be offset from the hook top. In general, the following considerations should be given to hook choice and placement: (1) the smallest possible shoe should be used to mini-

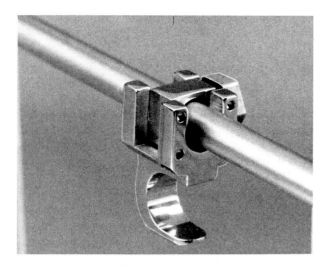

Fig. 83-53 Average maximum forces necessary to move hook on rod (nut tightened to 150 inch-pounds). (Courtesy Danek Medical, Memphis, Tennessee.)

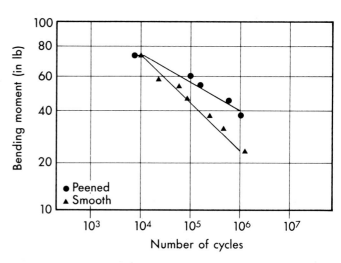

Fig. 83-54 Effect of shot peening on fatigue resistance of Harrington rods. (Courtesy Danek Medical, Memphis, Tennessee.)

mize encroachment into the spinal canal, and (2) the hook tops of adjacent hooks should be of the same height to allow the rod to maintain a smooth contour.

■ *TECHNIQUE (TSRH).* Position, prepare, and drape the patient as described on p. 3655 and make a routine posterior exposure of the spine (p. 3655). The hook sites are determined preoperatively in the same manner as for the Cotrel-Dubousset instru-

mentation (p. 3672). The cranially facing hooks in the thoracic spine generally receive a pedicle hook. Insert these hooks after excision of some of the inferior facet. Using an osteotome, make a horizontal cut in the inferior facet, beginning approximately 4 mm caudad to the line joining the inferior aspects of the two spinous processes. This cut ensures that the hook engages both the pedicle and the lamina (Fig.

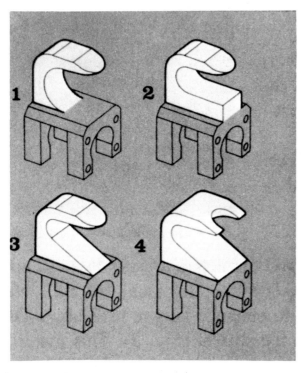

Fig. 83-55 Four basic shoe shapes: (1) large laminar, (2) small laminar, (3) thoracic laminar, and (4) pedicle. (Courtesy Danek Medical, Memphis, Tennessee.)

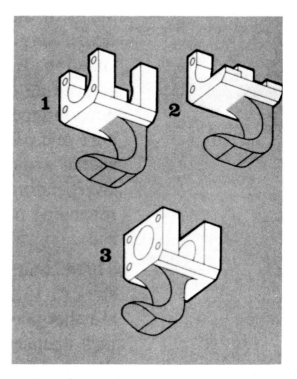

Fig. 83-56 Three hook tops: (1) full top, (2) half top, and (3) closed top. (Courtesy Danek Medical, Memphis, Tennessee.)

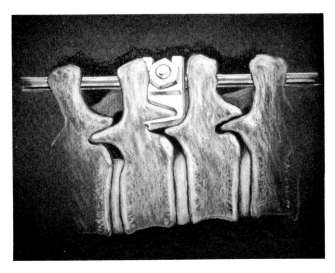

Fig. 83-57 Laminae must be cut so that pedicle hook engages both pedicle and back of laminae. (Courtesy Danek Medical, Memphis, Tennessee.)

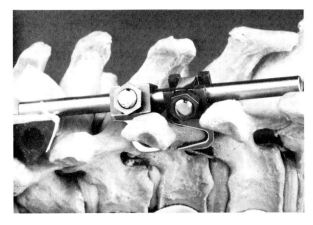

Fig. 83-58 Claw construct of upper hook. (Courtesy Danek Medical, Memphis, Tennessee.)

83-57). The pedicle hook has a bifid shoe that resists rotation.

The caudal-facing hooks in the thoracic spine generally receive thoracic laminar hooks. Make a small laminotomy on the supralaminar side of the lamina to be instrumented. Insert the hook into this laminotomy, resting it securely on the thoracic lamina to prevent migration into the spinal canal. The caudal-facing hook on the transverse process is a transverse process hook. The shoe shape is exactly the equivalent of the large laminar hook. The transverse process hook has a closed hook top and is used to form a "claw" construct in conjunction with a cranial-facing pedicle hook (Fig. 83-58). Separate

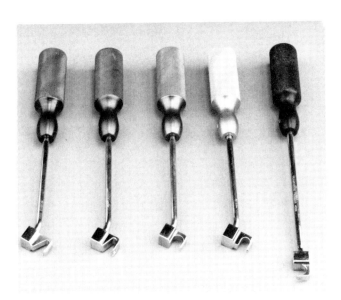

Fig. 83-59 Trial hooks to prepare hook sites and determine proper hook size. (Courtesy Danek Medical, Memphis, Tennessee.)

the costotransverse ligaments using the transverse process hook trial and then place the transverse process hook around the superior border of the transverse process. Cranial-facing hooks in the lumbar spine are generally large or small lumbar laminar hooks with an offset. The decision about large or small lumbar laminar hooks depends on the individual anatomy. Using the trial hooks (Fig. 83-59), lift the ligamentum flavum from the inferior aspect of the lamina but do not remove it from this interspace. Insert the hook under the lamina. If necessary, for proper hook fit, make a small inferior laminotomy to provide a horizontal purchase site for the hook. The caudal facing hooks in the lumbar spine are generally large or small lumbar laminar hooks, with or without offset, depending on the individual anatomy. Make a small laminotomy in the supralaminar portion of the vertebra to be instrumented. Again, keep the laminotomy as small as possible to minimize the risk of deep penetration of the hook during rod insertion. Use a trial laminar hook to determine the size of hook needed and then insert the appropriate hook. Once the hooks have been positioned, contour the appropriate-sized rod to the shape of the scoliosis and to the shape of the anticipated sagittal contour. At this point, place on the rod the appropriate-sized eyebolts corresponding to each hook. Also place appropriate-sized eyebolts for the cross-link apparatus in their appropriate positions relative to the hooks (Fig. 83-60). Now perform facet decortication and fusion. Engage the contoured rod in the individual hooks, all of which have an open top on the concave side allowing the rod to be laid into the appropriate hooks. Firmly engage the eyebolts in the hooks; it is the undercut in the hook together with the eyebolt that captures the rod (Fig. 83-61).

Three different instruments are used to engage the eyebolt into the hook top. The more closely the rod is contoured to the set of the hooks, the easier this portion of the procedure. For very short distances requiring little force, the eyebolt spreader provides a quick method of inserting the eyebolt

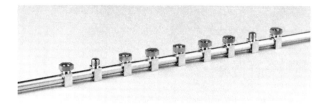

Fig. 83-60 Eyebolts positioned on rod. Eyebolts for hooks have nuts "staked" on. Cross-link eyebolts do not have nuts. (Courtesy Danek Medical, Memphis, Tennessee.)

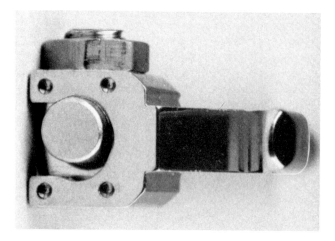

Fig. 83-61 View of hook showing undercut in hook that captures rod. (Courtesy Danek Medical, Memphis, Tennessee.)

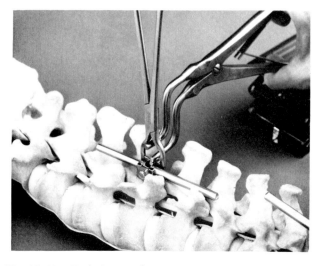

Fig. 83-62 Eyebolt spreader in position to insert eyebolt into hook. (Courtesy Danek Medical, Memphis, Tennessee.)

into the hook (Fig. 83-62). When the fit is not quite as good, the minicorkscrew can be used to provide the rod-moving action. To use this device, screw the pivot block to the end of the threaded rod. Then wedge the pivot between the jaws of the hook holder and place the block on the eyebolt (Fig. 83-63). In using this system, carefully insert all four pins of the hook holder into the hook or the system will pull loose. For long distances and stiff curves, the hook holder with rod mover should be used (Fig. 83-64). Again, take care that the four pins on the jaws are properly engaged into the four holes on the hook top before applying the corkscrew mechanism. Also, back the nut off enough to allow the eyebolt to easily engage the hook top and enter properly.

Once the rod is inserted, accomplish distraction

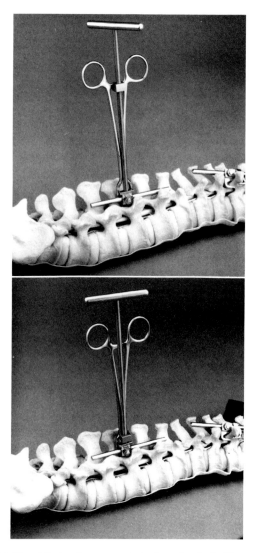

Fig. 83-63 Minicorkscrew attached to hook holder, rod in hook. (Courtesy Danek Medical, Memphis, Tennessee.)

and compression of the hooks before the nut is torqued down completely. Tighten the nut only to the point where it starts to bind to hold compression and distraction without additional instruments. Set the intermediate hooks in distraction as described for the Cotrel-Dubousset instrumentation (p. 3678); this distraction can be held without additional instrumentation. Once the hooks are set and the appropriate distraction and compression are applied, rotate the rod. Once the nut starts to bind, the hook can withstand forces directed transversely to the rod while still allowing rotation, compression, and distraction. Use the longer, 9-inch, open-ended wrench to firmly tighten the nut to 150 inch-pounds. A rod pusher or vise grip can be used to secure the rods during this final tightening stage. It is difficult to overtighten the nut, and exceeding 150 inch-pounds of tightening torque is more desirable than under-tightening the nut.

Now contour the convex rod. As in the Cotrel-Dubousset system, contour the thoracic portion of the convex rod with less kyphosis to push the convexity forward during instrumentation. Contour the bottom portion of the rod to match the patient's physiologic lordosis at the thoracolumbar junction. Apply to the rod appropriately placed eyebolts for the hooks, as well as the cross-link plates. The eyebolts for the cross-link plates should correspond to the position between the hooks where the cross-link is to span. Perform a convex facet fusion. Since the upper transverse process hook is a closed hook, first insert the rod into this hook. Then insert the rod with eyebolts into the remaining hooks, using either the eyebolt spreader, minicorkscrew, or hook holder with rod mover as indicated. Tighten the nuts until they begin to bind. The convex apical hook is compressed against the upper claw and the nut is tightened. Compress the lower hook against the upper hooks as described for Cotrel-Dubousset instrumentation (p. 3680). Tighten all these nuts to 150 inch-pounds of torque.

Now apply the cross-link plates. The cross-link plates are available in widths from ⅝ inches to ⅗ inches (Fig. 83-65) and use the same eyebolt locking mechanism as the hook and screws; however, the ½ inch nuts used with the cross-links are larger. Also, the nuts are not preassembled or staked onto the cross-link eyebolts. Again, the eyebolt sizes are designed to fit different rod diameters and care must be taken to ensure the appropriate-sized eyebolt is used for the rod. Place one cross-link at the superior end of the construct, caudal to the top hook. Place the other cross-link at the lower end of the construct just superior to the bottom hook. Avoid cross-linking at the primary curve apex because of the high rod stress at this location. Determine the size of the cross-link needed with a template (Fig. 83-66). Ap-

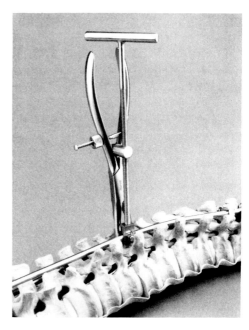

Fig. 83-64 Hook holder with rod mover showing attachment to rod and hook. (Courtesy Danek Medical, Memphis, Tennessee.)

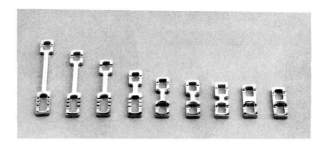

Fig. 83-65 Cross-link plates are available in sizes that connect rods out to 2¾ inches. (Courtesy Danek Medical, Memphis, Tennessee.)

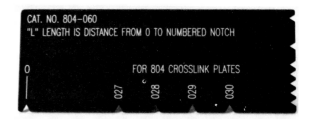

Fig. 83-66 Template used for selecting cross-link plate size. (Courtesy Danek Medical, Memphis, Tennessee.)

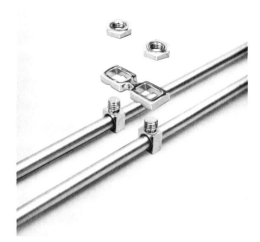

Fig. 83-67 Appropriate-sized plates connect to rods using previously applied eye-bolts and ½-inch nuts. Rounded surface of nut should be up. (Courtesy Danek Medical, Memphis, Tennessee.)

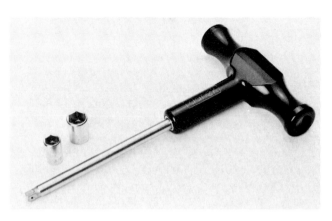

Fig. 83-68 Torque wrench and ½-inch socket used to tighten nuts on cross-link plates to 150 inch-pounds. (Courtesy Danek Medical, Memphis, Tennessee.)

ply the appropriate-sized cross-link plate over the eyebolts and attach it with the ½-inch nuts (Fig. 83-67). Note that the nut has a rounded and a flat surface; place the flat surface of the nut toward the plate and the rounded surface superiorly (the rounded surface has "up" etched on it). Make sure the rod lies exactly in the groove of the plate or the nut may loosen. Use a T-handle torque wrench with a ½-inch socket to tighten the nuts to 150 inch-

pounds (Fig. 83-68). Perform a wake-up test at this point, if desired. Further decorticate the exposed posterior arches and add the remainder of the bone graft. Close the wound over suction drains.

AFTERTREATMENT. The patient is log rolled in bed for 2 to 3 days, and mobilization and ambulation are begun when the drains are removed. No postoperative immobilization is needed. Most patients are dismissed from the hospital on the sixth or seventh

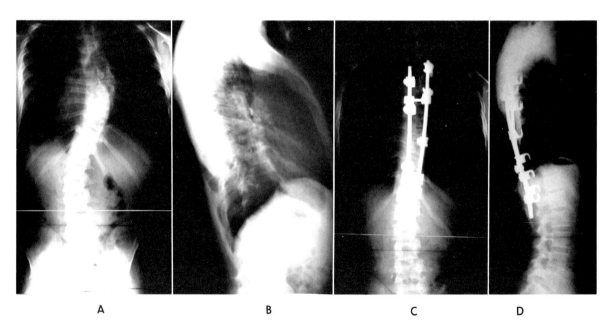

A   B   C   D

Fig. 83-69   **A** and **B,** Preoperative posteroanterior and lateral roentgenograms of patient undergoing TSRH instrumentation for idiopathic scoliosis. **C** and **D,** Postoperative roentgenograms showing correction of the scoliosis in anteroposterior plane and restoration of some thoracic kyphosis in lateral plane.

day. The patient's activities are gradually increased, but full return to normal activities is not allowed for approximately 1 year while the bone graft matures (Fig. 83-69).

Luque Instrumentation

The use of L-shaped rods and sublaminar wires to accomplish segmental spinal instrumentation was introduced by Luque of Mexico City in 1973 and was developed and standardized in the United States by Allen and Ferguson. This instrumentation system offers more rigid fixation than the Harrington distraction system, superior correction of sagittal plane deformities of the spine, and improved instrumentation of the lumbosacral joint when combined with the Galveston technique of pelvic fixation. Allen and Ferguson reported excellent results using this type of instrumentation for adolescent idiopathic scoliosis. Most centers, however, rarely use this system for idiopathic scoliosis because of the potential complications.

The principal use of Luque instrumentation and fusion at this time is in the treatment of neuromuscular scoliosis. Studies by Boachie-Adjei et al., Gersoff and Renshaw, Stevens and Beard, Herndon et al., and Broom, Banta, and Renshaw have shown that this system can offer rigid fixation and good results in patients with neuromuscular scoliosis.

The major disadvantage of the system is the potential for neurologic complications. Zindrick et al. have shown that the sublaminar wire will almost always contact the dural sac as it passes underneath the lamina. The space that is occupied by the wire at the time of insertion is created by forcefully moving the dural sac and its contents anteriorly. Although neurologic injury usually does not occur, the potential for injury is certainly present. The potential for injury is increased in patients who have had previous surgery or an injury at the site because local scarring, edema, or adhesions might limit the ability of the dural sac and neural structures to move during sublaminar passage of the wire. Thompson et al. used somatosensory evoked potentials to monitor function of the spinal cord and described a 16% incidence of neurologic complications. Other authors have reported fewer complications, but there is universal agreement that experience is necessary to use this system successfully.

The long-term effects of sublaminar wires are unknown. Animal models by Schrader, Bethem, and Scerbin have demonstrated epidural fibrosis, dural perforation, loss of the vascular pattern of the spinal cord, dorsal spinal cord indentations, distortion of spinal cord shape, and microscopic evidence of cellular destruction without any correlation with the length of time the wires were implanted. Nicastro et al. and Schrader et al. have also demonstrated significant indentation of the cord during extraction of the wires. In the clinical situation, however, Olson and Gaines have found no changes in neurologic function after removal of sublaminar wires.

Any metallic device implanted may ultimately fail. Bernard et al. and Johnston et al. reported neurologic symptoms related to the breakage of sublaminar wires and progression of the spinal deformity. Other potential disadvantages of the Luque technique include a longer operating time, increased blood loss, and a significant "learning curve" as the surgeon becomes familiar with the technique.

At our clinic, this procedure is used mainly for the neuromuscular type of scoliosis in individuals in whom external immobilization must be limited or eliminated entirely. In these particular curves, the fixation is very secure. If, however, the curve is quite rigid, anterior release is often required. Johnston et al. found the stiffness of the L-rod construct to decrease rapidly in spines with a residual deformity of more than 38 degrees. Cross-linking of the rods greatly increases the stiffness and rigidity of the system (see Fig. 83-65). The basic instrumentation for the Luque system consists of smooth ¼-inch and ³⁄₁₆-inch L-shaped rods and 16- or 18-gauge wire loops. The original system was made of stainless steel, but because of difficulties with fatigue failure, especially in the wires, Allen and Ferguson developed a system made of a nickel chrome alloy (MP 35 N). This is available only in ³⁄₁₆-inch diameter rods. It is important to note that if the alloy type of rod is used, a compatible alloy type of wire should be used, also.

■ *TECHNIQUE.* **Expose the spine in the routine manner (p. 3655) and excise the ligamentum flavum. Using a needle-nose rongeur, gradually thin the ligamentum flavum until the midline cleavage plane is visible. In the thoracic spine, the spinous processes slant distally and must be removed before the ligamentum flavum can be adequately exposed (Fig. 83-70, *A*). Once the midline cleavage plane is visible, carefully sweep a Penfield No. 4 dissector across the deep surface of the ligamentum flavum on both sides (Fig. 83-70, *B*). Then use a Kerrison punch to remove the remainder of the ligamentum flavum (Fig. 83-70, *C*), taking care to avoid damaging the dura or the epidural vessels. Shape the sublaminar wire as shown in Fig. 83-70, *D,* with the major diameter of the bend larger than the lamina. The wire passage is the most critical and dangerous part of the operation in terms of neurologic injury, and the surgeon and assistant must be completely prepared for each step before the passage of the wire and even more careful about sudden movement and inadvertent touching of the wires that have already been passed. Gently place the tip of the wire into the neural canal at the inferior edge of the lamina in the midline. Hold the long end of the doubled wire in one hand and advance the tip with the other. Rest the hand advancing the tip firmly on the patient's back. Lift the tails of the wire slightly, pulling them to keep the wires snugly against the undersurface of**

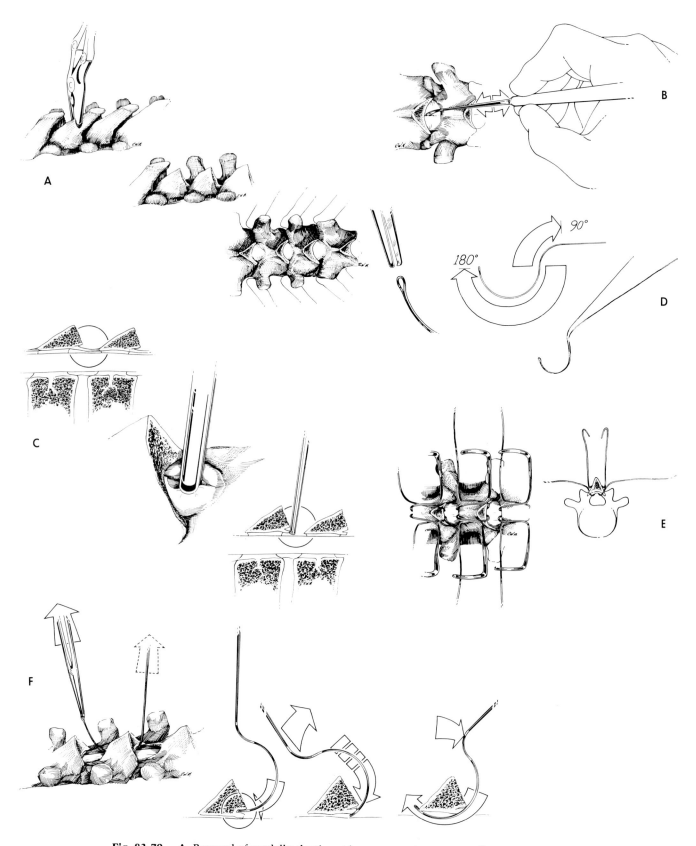

Fig. 83-70 **A,** Removal of caudally slanting spinous processes to expose ligamentum flavum. **B,** Penfield No. 4 dissector for freeing deep surfaces of ligamentum flavum. **C,** Kerrison punch for removing remainder of ligamentum flavum. **D,** Shape of double wire before it passes under lamina. **E,** After division of wire, wire is crimped on laminar surface of each side of spinous process. **F,** Passage of segmental wire beneath lamina. (From Segmental spinal fixation and correction using Richards L-rod instrumentation, Memphis, Smith & Nephew Richards, Inc.)

the lamina, and roll the tip so that it emerges on the upper end of the lamina (Fig. 83-70, *E*). As the tip of the wire presents itself, have an assistant grasp it with a needle holder or wire holder that will not spring off the loop. Take the clamp from the assistant and pull the wire with the clamp until it is positioned beneath the lamina with half its length protruding above and half below. As the clamp is pulled, gently feed from the long end of the wire. Now, cut off the tip of the wire and place one length on the right side and the other on the left side. As an alternative, leave double wires on one side and pass another wire to leave double wires on both sides. Then crimp each wire onto the surface of the lamina to prevent them from accidently being pushed into the neural canal (Fig. 83-70, *F*).

As more wires are passed, it is easy to accidently hit wires already in place. When the wires are crimped, crimp the superior wire towards the midline and the inferior wire laterally. Use double wires at the cephalad and caudal laminae of the instrumented segment.

• • •

Two rods are used for most scoliosis operations, and there are two techniques for applying these rods. The first rod may be applied to the convex side of the curve or to the concave side.

CONVEX ROD

■ *TECHNIQUE.* The convex rod technique is useful in correction of thoracic curves. Contour the appropriate lordosis or kyphosis into the L-rod with a rod bender. Fasten the initial rod to the upper region of the scoliotic curve with the short limb placed transversely across the lamina of the upper vertebra to be fused. Tighten the second and third wires on the convex side, and then sequentially tighten the wires from proximal to distal as the rod is levered toward the spine (Fig. 83-71, *A*). After about half of the convex wires have been tightened, apply the concave rod. Pass the L-portion of this rod through a hole in the spinous process of the lamina of the distal vertebra to be instrumented and underneath the convex rod distally. Then tie this rod down over the distal lamina, working distally to proximally. Sequentially tighten the remaining wires. At the proximal end, the long end of the concave rod (Fig. 83-71, *B*) should lie over the short L-leg of the convex rod. Cut the ends of the wire and bend them toward the midline. Perform appropriate fusion.

CONCAVE ROD

■ *TECHNIQUE.* The concave technique is preferable for lumbar scoliosis. Contour the appropriate amount of lordosis or kyphosis into the rods with a rod bender. Place the initial rod with its short limb passing transversely across the lamina of the lowermost vertebra to be instrumented. Pass it through a hole at the base of the spinous process. Tighten the inferior double-end wire on the concave side to apply

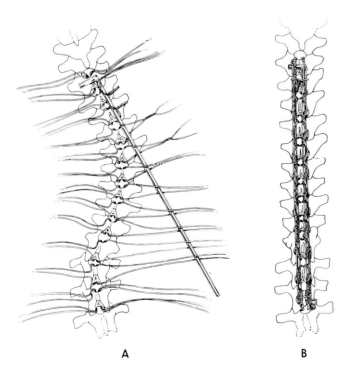

A   B

Fig. 83-71   A, Convex rod technique for correction of thoracic scoliosis. **B,** Completed L-rod instrumentation for thoracic scoliosis. (From Segmental spinal fixation and correction using Richards L-rod instrumentation, Memphis, Smith & Nephew Richards, Inc.)

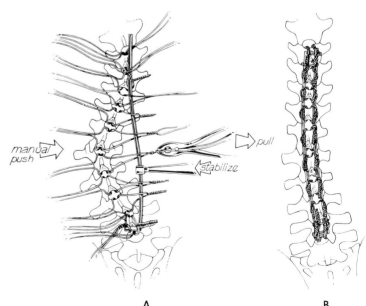

A   B

Fig. 83-72   A, Concave rod technique for correction of lumbar scoliosis. **B,** Completed L-rod instrumentation for lumbar scoliosis. (From Segmental spinal fixation and correction using Richards L-rod instrumentation, Memphis, Smith & Nephew Richards, Inc.)

firm fixation of the distal level. Tighten the wires to the laminae above the vertebra of the curve. Loosely attach the convex rod proximally after the short L-end of the rod is placed loosely under the long limb of the concave rod. Once the concave rod is completely tightened, it is difficult to pass this short limb under the long limb of the concave rod. Reduce the spine to the rod, using either manual correction or a wire tightener. Have an assistant apply appropriate manual correction by pressure on the trunk as the wires beneath the apex of the curvature are tightened (Fig. 83-72, *A*). Then securely fasten the convex rod, tightening wires from cephalad to caudad. Once in position, both rods usually can be brought into firm contact with the lamina by squeezing them together with a rod approximator. As the rods are approximated, the concave wires will loosen and must be tightened again. Trim the wires to about 1 cm and bend them toward the midline (Fig. 83-72, *B*).

GALVESTON PELVIC FIXATION

■ *TECHNIQUE (ALLEN AND FERGUSON)*. At our clinic, the Luque system generally is used for neuromuscular scoliosis and many of these curves include the sacrum with significant pelvic obliquity, making pelvic fixation an important part of the system. This technique provides long lever arms for pelvic fixation to gain leverage for reducing both lateral bending and flexion extension moments. It has the theoretical disadvantage of spanning the sacroiliac joints, which are not included in the fusion. It also limits availability of autogenous bone graft in the area where the pin is inserted.

Expose both iliac crests to the sciatic notches. Drill a Steinmann pin, the same diameter as the rod, along the transverse bar of the ilium, entering just posterior to the sacroiliac joint at the posterosuperior iliac spine. Drill this pin to a depth of 6 to 9 cm (Fig. 83-73). Then contour the rod in three different planes. Using two sleeve benders, make the first bend at a 90-degree angle, leaving the short arm approximately 12 cm long. Make the second bend about 2 cm lateral to the first bend, using the pelvic rod-bending clamp and a sleeve bender in combination; this angle is generally between 50 and 75 degrees but basically is contoured to fit the angle of the ilium with the midsagittal plane of the patient. Using a French rod bender, bend lordosis into the long limb of the rod. As this lordosis is applied to the rod, the short limb of the rod will accommodate the angle of the pin as concerns its caudal tilt (Fig. 83-74). Remove the pelvic pin and drive the iliac portion of the rod into the prepared hole (Fig. 83-75). Tighten the sublaminar wires and perform appropriate fusion.

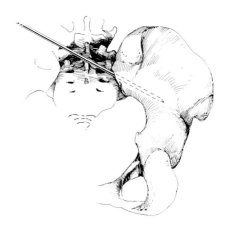

Fig. 83-73 Insertion of guide pin just posterior to sacroiliac joint at level of posterosuperior iliac spine. (From Segmental spinal fixation and correction using Richards L-rod instrumentation, Memphis, Smith & Nephew Richards, Inc.)

Anterior Instrumentation

The anterior approach was not commonly used in spinal surgery until the 1950s. Leaders in the anterior approach to the cervical and lumbar areas have been Cloward, Southwick and Robinson, Bailey and Badgley, Harmon, and Wiltberger. Nachlas and Borden, and Smith, Von Lackum, and Wylie were among the first to report their experiences with the transthoracic approach to the thoracic spine. Major proponents of the anterior surgical technique were Hodgson et al. of Hong Kong. The advent of Dwyer and Zielke instrumentation has improved management of various deformities of the thoracic and lumbar spine.

Most spine deformities can still be treated from the posterior approach. The principal uses of anterior spinal instrumentation and fusion in scoliosis treatment are instrumentation of a flexible thoracolumbar or lumbar curve and as the initial stage of a two-stage anterior and posterior spinal instrumentation and fusion. The primary potential problem of anterior systems is a localized kyphosis at the site of the fusion resulting from disc removal and subsequent shortening of the spinal column. Retroperitoneal fibrosis and ureteral obstruction have also been reported.

In anterior approaches to the spine, we routinely have the assistance of a thoracic or general surgeon during both the intraoperative exposure and the postoperative management. The orthopaedic surgeon, however, must be aware of the basic anatomy and should guide the thoracic surgeon as to the exposure needed for the spinal portion of the procedure. The various anterior approaches to the spine at different levels are described in Chapter 79.

Just as in posterior surgery, fusion is essential to the long-term success of anterior spinal instrumentation. Once the anterior portion of the spine has been exposed,

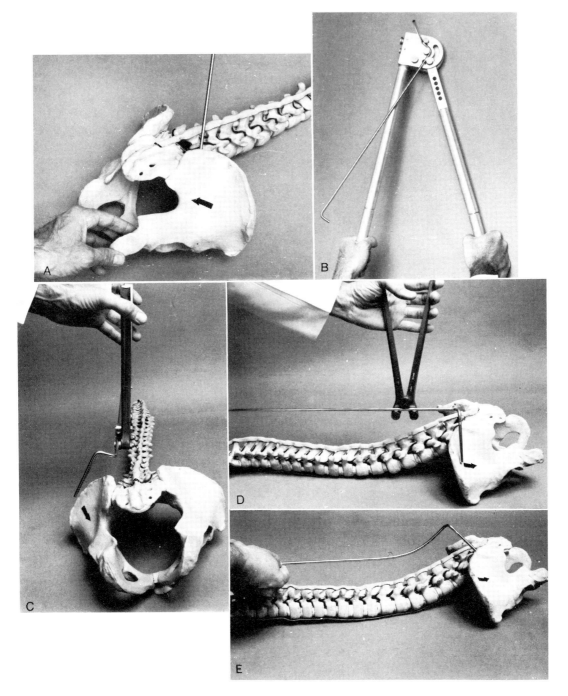

Fig. 83-74 Contouring to L-rod to maintain lumbar lordosis. (From Bradford DS, et al: Moe's textbook of scoliosis and other spinal deformities, ed 2, Philadelphia, 1987, WB Saunders Co.)

various techniques are available for anterior arthrodesis. One can simply remove the discs and obtain a fusion with an interbody technique (Fig. 83-76) or an anterior strut type of fusion can be performed (Fig. 83-77). The type of fusion depends on the condition for which the surgery is performed.

ANTERIOR ARTHRODESIS

Disc excision and interbody fusion

■ *TECHNIQUE.* This method of disc excision and interbody fusion is the type of fusion usually performed in the Dwyer or Zielke instrumentation techniques. Expose the desired levels of the spine and identify

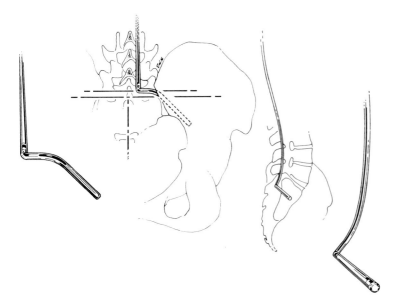

Fig. 83-75 Insertion of └-rod into previously prepared hole in ilium. (From Segmental spinal fixation and correction using Richards └-rod instrumentation, Memphis, Smith & Nephew Richards, Inc.)

the discs, which can be felt as rounded protuberant areas of the spine rather than the concave surfaces of the vertebral body. Sharply divide the annulus, and remove the annulus and nucleus pulposus with rongeurs and curets. Once the disc has been excised, remove the cartilage end plates with an osteotome or a sharp periosteal elevator (Fig. 83-76, *A*). The posterior aspects of the cartilage end plates are more easily removed with angled curets. At this point, control hemostasis with Gelfoam soaked in thrombin. If a rib has been removed for the exposure, cut it into small pieces. Then insert the bone grafts into the disc spaces (Fig. 83-76, *B*). It usually is not necessary with this approach to remove the posterior annulus of the disc, which lessens the chance of injury to the spinal cord. Suture the parietal pleura over the vertebral bodies, and close the wound in the routine manner.

Inlay graft

■ *TECHNIQUE.* Expose the spine in the routine manner, and cut a trough into the lateral aspect of the

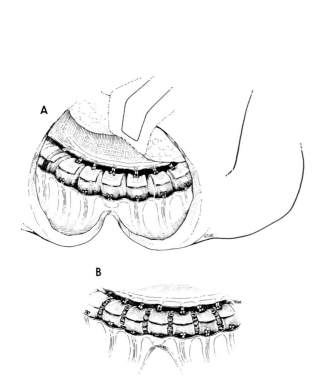

Fig. 83-76 **A,** Exposure of anterior spine and removal of discs and end plates before insertion of bone graft. **B,** Insertion of cancellous bone and rib struts in disc space anteriorly. (Redrawn in part from Bradford DS et al: Moe's textbook of scoliosis and other spinal deformities, ed 2, Philadelphia, 1987, WB Saunders Co.)

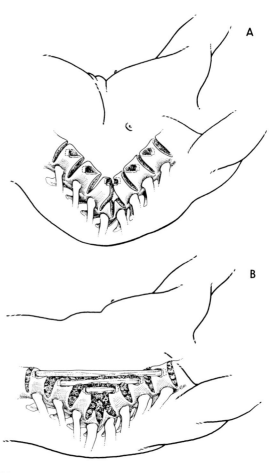

Fig. 83-77 **A,** Preparation of tunnels for anterior strut grafts. **B,** Insertion of strut grafts into pre-prepared tunnels with cancellous bone grafts in disc spaces. (Redrawn from Bradford DS et al: Moe's textbook of scoliosis and other spinal deformities, ed 2, Philadelphia, 1987, WB Saunders Co.)

vertebral bodies to be fused. Place complete rib strut grafts into the trough to act as supporting bone. Undercut the trough posteriorly back towards the subchondral bone to better lock the strut grafts in place. If necessary, add iliac bone grafts to provide additional cancellous bone along the strut graft and also in the disc spaces.

Strut graft

■ *TECHNIQUE.* For severe, uncorrectable angular kyphosis, inlay grafts may not be possible and the strut grafts must be placed well anterior to the vertebral bodies. Make this exposure subperiosteal because the bone grafts must be placed against the vertebral body rather than within the axis of the vertebral bodies themselves. Fashion tunnels proximally and distally (Fig. 83-77, *A*) and place the struts in position (Fig. 83-77, *B*). Significant kyphosis may require greater strength than a rib can pro-

vide, and a fibula may be used instead. Place pressure over the apex of the kyphos to obtain some correction, and place the strut in position. Pack the space between the strut grafts and the vertebral bodies with bone graft. Place Gelfoam over the lateral aspect of the grafts at the completion of the procedure to prevent bone chips from dislodging into the thoracic or retroperitoneal space.

SELECTION OF FUSION LEVELS. Anterior instrumentation systems should be reserved for flexible primary thoracolumbar or lumbar curves in idiopathic scoliosis. The levels for instrumentation are determined from preoperative roentgenograms. The superior instrumented vertebra is the neutral vertebra at the upper end of the curve on the bending roentgenogram. The inferior vertebra demonstrates less than 10 degrees of rotation and 15 degrees of obliquity with respect to the intercrestal line as seen on appropriate side-bending films (Fig. 83-78). It is im-

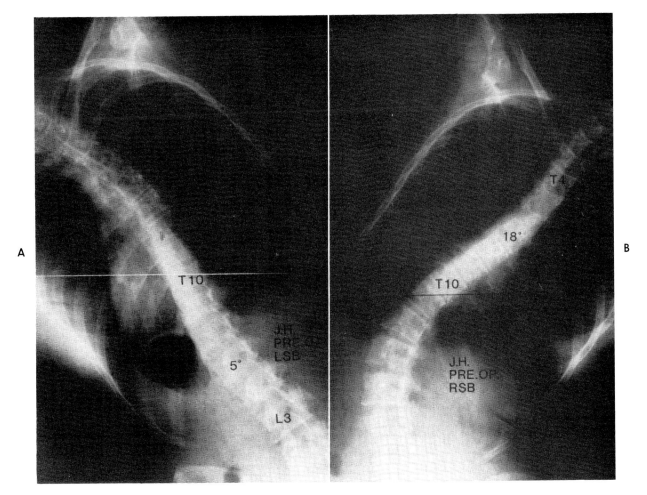

Fig. 83-78 **A,** Preoperative lateral bending roentgenogram of thoracolumbar curve. This demonstrates flexibility of major curve. T10 is lowest neutral vertebra and is selected as superior instrumented vertebra. **B,** Opposite bending roentgenogram demonstrates minor curve above. L3 almost comes to horizontal with minimal rotation and is selected as inferior instrumented vertebra. (From Hammerberg KW et al: Orthopedics 11:1365, 1988.)

portant that the compensatory curve not present unacceptable cosmetic deformity and that it have little rotation on the preoperative standing film. Extension of the fusion beyond the neutral vertebra into the compensatory curve proximally may result in unacceptable decompensation of the trunk and an increased cosmetic deformity of the thorax and shoulder level.

CONTRAINDICATIONS. Anterior instrumentation should not be used in patients with a pre-existing kyphotic deformity. The presence of an oblique lumbosacral takeoff that does not correct with side bending can lead to decompensation of the spine.

DWYER INSTRUMENTATION. In 1964 Dwyer, in cooperation with Newton, developed instrumentation for correction and fixation of spinal deformity through an anterior approach. Dwyer instrumentation uses large metal staples of several sizes that are attached to each vertebral body with a large screw. The screws have a large head with a hole for passage of a cable that is tightened at each level and then fixed by crimping the screw heads (Fig. 83-79).

By placing the staples more anteriorly, lordosis can be corrected. By placing the staples and screws in the same location in each vertebral body, regardless of the position of the body, rotation can also be corrected to some extent. The Dwyer instrumentation is contraindicated in kyphosis.

The strength of the internal fixation provided by the Dwyer system is limited because the strength of fixation is directly dependent on the strength of the bone-screw interface. The flexible braided titanium cable can resist forces only in tension. Flexion, extension, lateral bending toward the cable, and rotation are not resisted by anything other than the impacted vertebral end plates. Dwyer instrumentation is not recommended for children younger than 10 years of age because of the small size of the vertebral bodies.

■ *TECHNIQUE (DWYER).* Position the patient in the lateral decubitus position with the convex aspect of the curve uppermost. Approach the spine anteriorly (Fig 83-80, *A*). Excise the discs as described for the interbody fusion technique (p. 3658).

Instrumentation proceeds from above downward on the convex side of the curve. Incise the annulus of the intact disc of the uppermost body to allow the flange of the staple to grip just over the end plate. During placement of the screws, check and recheck the direction to avoid penetration of the posterior

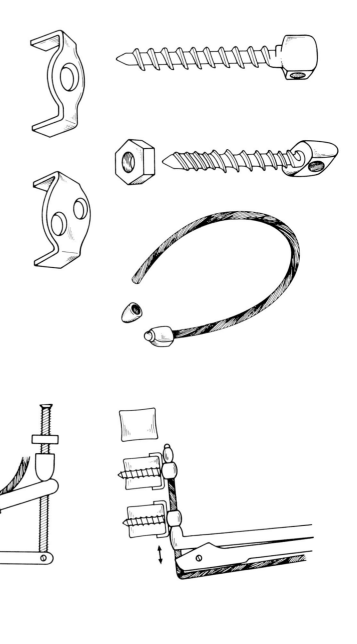

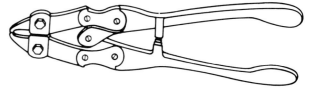

Fig. 83-79 Instrumentation and implants for Dwyer procedure. (From Laurin CA, Riley LH Jr, and Roy-Camille R: Atlas of orthopaedic surgery, vol 1. General principles — spine, Chicago, 1989, Mosby – Year Book, Inc.)

cortex of the vertebral body into the spinal canal. The ideally placed screw runs horizontally across the body, just engaging the opposite cortex and lying safely in front of the neural foramen. Measure the width of the vertebral body, select a staple of the same width, and place it onto the staple holder. Then place the staple holder along the convex aspect of the vertebra using a mallet (Fig. 83-80, *B*). Remove the staple holder; a hole will be seen in the vertebral body made by the spike of the staple holder. Insert an appropriate-length screw through the staple and into the vertebral body, trying to engage the opposite cortex but avoiding the neural canal (Fig. 83-80, *C*). After the first two staples and screws have been placed, insert rib chips into the disc space. By placing these anteriorly in the excised disc beds, local kyphosis can be minimized. Introduce a cable through the two screws and apply a tensioner. Obtain correction by pressure on the convex side of the curve rather than by tension on the cable (Fig. 83-80, *D*). Use the tensioner only to take up slack in the cable; if it is used for correction, the screws can pull out. When correction is ob-

tained, crimp the screw head onto the cable (Fig. 83-80, *E*). Prepare each succeeding disc space in the same manner (Fig. 83-80, *F*). Apply a collar over the cable before the cable is cut and crimp it onto the cable below the final screw. Cover the cables and screws, with the pleura or the psoas muscle if possible in the thoracic or lumbar areas, respectively. Close the wound in a routine manner.

AFTERTREATMENT. When a thoracotomy is performed, a chest tube is needed for 2 to 3 days after surgery. Once the patient's condition is stabilized, he can ambulate with the protection of a brace or cast. This brace or cast is needed for approximately 6 months.

ZIELKE INSTRUMENTATION. Zielke modified the Dwyer instrumentation by substituting a semirigid, threaded rod for the flexible cable and first reported use of the ventral derotation spondylodesis (VDS) instrumentation in 1978. A derotation device has also been developed that provides simultaneous corrective forces for both rotation and lordosis. The implants are made of stainless steel rather than titanium. The screw heads are

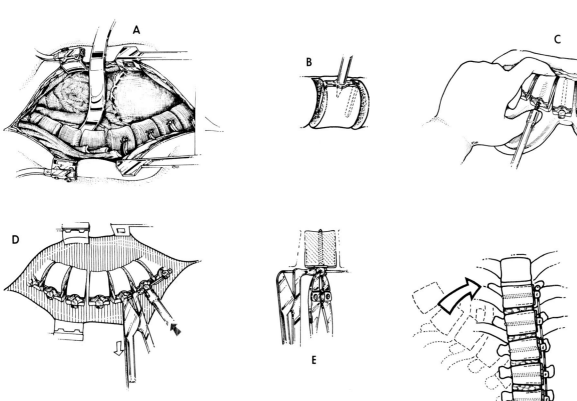

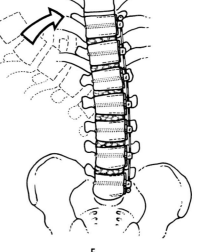

Fig. 83-80 **A,** Exposure of thoracolumbar spine for insertion of Dwyer apparatus. **B,** Insertion of staple around vertebral body. **C,** Appropriately sized Dwyer screw inserted through staple and into vertebral body, engaging opposite cortex. **D,** Correction obtained with pressure on screwdriver; tensioner used to remove slack and tighten cable between vertebral screws. **E,** Crimper to fix shortened cable in screw head. **F,** Diagrammatic representation of correction obtained at each instrumented level with Dwyer instrumentation.

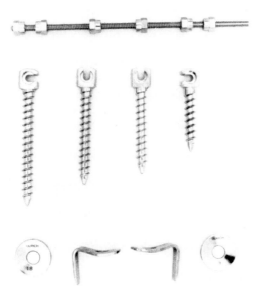

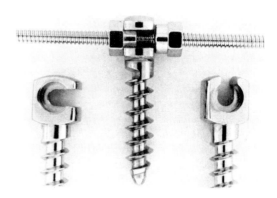

Fig. 83-82 Detail of screw heads. Cylindrical process of left nut is inserted to corresponding part of screw head to prevent displacement. (From Bradford DS and Hensinger RN: The pediatric spine, New York, 1985, Theime, Inc.)

Fig. 83-81 Compression rod fitted with ventral-derotation-spondylodesis hex nuts. Insertion slits for rod in screws point upward or laterally. Shorter screws have deep thread. Sharp-angled blade plates are used for end vertebra and washers are used in intermediate vertebrae. (From Bradford DS and Hensinger RN: The pediatric spine, New York, 1985, Theime, Inc.)

slotted instead of cannulated, and the slots have either a top opening or a side opening (Fig. 83-81). The screws are implanted into the vertebral bodies through convex circular washers or angled plates. Collared hex nuts are used to lock the rod in the screw heads and provide compression and fixation (Fig. 83-82).

■ *TECHNIQUE (ZIELKE).* Expose the convexity of the curvature by a standard thoracoabdominal or abdominal retroperitoneal approach (Chapter 79). After the desired levels of the spine are exposed, perform a thorough discectomy at each interspace within the area of instrumentation. Clean out the intervertebral disc posteriorly to the posterior longitudinal ligament to reduce the tendency for kyphosis. Release the anulus in the posterior convex corner to allow for derotation. At this point, control bleeding with thrombin-soaked Gelfoam in the intervertebral spaces. Moe has suggested leaving the outer fibers of the annulus on the concave side intact to act as a hinge and prevent overcorrection. Measure the transverse diameter of the vertebral body with a caliper and use an awl to make a hole in the side of the body at its midlateral portion. Select a Zielke screw of the appropriate length. Impact a staple just below the subchondral end plate of the end vertebra. Use a washer on the intermediate vertebrae, convex side up for better presentation of the screw head (Fig. 83-83, *A*). The end screws have a lateral opening that is dorsally directed to prevent dislodgment during derotation. The intermediate screws are top opening to facilitate placement of the threaded rod.

Select a screw 5 mm longer than the measured depth to accommodate the washer. As the screw is inserted, use the index finger of the opposite hand as a guide and to feel the tip of the screw penetrating the opposite cortex. Moe has emphasized the proper placement of the screws. Place the screws as far posteriorly in the vertebral body as is prudent to lessen the tendency for instrumentation kyphosis. Direct the screws in a slightly posteroanterior direction across the midportion of the vertebra to enhance the derotation effect (Fig. 83-83, *B*). Place the screw in the apical vertebral body more posterior than adjacent screws, producing a gentle **C**-shaped curve when the rod is viewed laterally (Fig. 83-83, *C*). When the spine is derotated and the rod assumes a straighter position, the maximum derotational effect is obtained at the apical vertebra where it is most needed. Insert a flexible stainless steel threaded rod of appropriate length into the screw heads (Fig. 83-83, *D*).

On the most proximal and distal screws use double nuts, one facing the other; intervening screws need only have one locking nut facing the apex of the deformity. When seating the nuts, place a rod holder tightly against the opposite side of the screw head. Then force the nut sleeve into the recessed screw head rather than pushing the screw over. Apply the derotation instrument with the bar engaging the rod at both ends by movable couplings and secured in the middle by a lordosing spanner to create three-point fixation (Fig. 83-83, *E*). With the attached handle, derotate the spine and produce lordosis. At this stage, cut the rib into 1 cm to 2 cm pieces and wedge them anteriorly between each vertebral body at its most anterior lip to help prevent instrumentation kyphosis and help produce lumbar lordosis. Further roughen the vertebral end plates if necessary, and loosely pack the remaining portion of rib bone into the intervertebral disc space. With

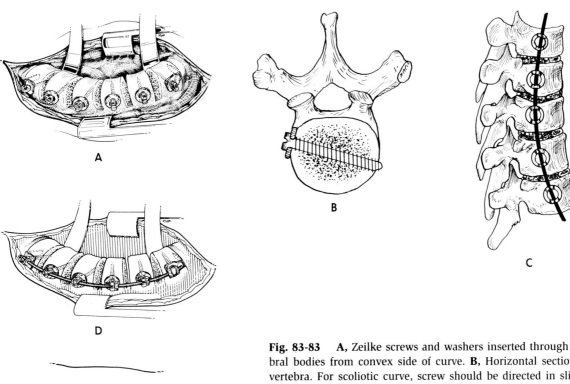

Fig. 83-83 **A,** Zeilke screws and washers inserted through appropriate vertebral bodies from convex side of curve. **B,** Horizontal section of instrumented vertebra. For scoliotic curve, screw should be directed in slightly posteroanterior direction across vertebral body from convex to concave side of curve. This increases derotation effect and helps prevent instrumentation kyphosis. **C,** Lateral view of spine with Zielke instrumentation. Screw in apical vertebral body is more posterior than adjacent screws, thus producing maximal derotation effect at apical vertebra when spine is derotated. Anterior wedge grafts and bone chips are placed into intervertebral disc spaces over instrumented segment of spine. **D,** Threaded rod applied through screw heads; note C-shaped curve of rod. **E,** Derotation and lordosis forces applied to spine. (**B** and **C** from Moe JH et al: Clin Orthop 180:136, 1983.)

the spine held in the derotated position, sequentially tighten the locking nuts, approximating the vertebral bodies on the convex side and correcting the curve. Remove the derotation instrumentation. Destroy the threads of the compression rod to prevent the nuts from unwinding. Approximate the soft tissues over the instrumentation, making certain that the great vessels are not lying over the implant. Close the wound in a routine manner.

AFTERTREATMENT. Prophylactic antibiotic coverage is continued for 48 hours. The patient is kept at bed rest until a polypropylene orthosis is ready. The chest tube usually is removed at 72 hours if drainage is minimal. The orthosis is worn full-time for approximately 6 months. The patient is restricted to light activity for 1 year and to moderate activity for another year.

Posterior Instrumentation for Kyphosis

Moe in 1965 presented his early experience with posterior fusion alone for the management of kyphosis.

Bradford et al. reported 22 patients with Scheuermann's kyphosis who underwent posterior Harrington compression instrumentation and fusion (Fig. 83-84). Loss of correction occurred in 16 of these patients; these failures were caused by the presence of severe initial deformity, inadequate length of the fusion, severe wedging of the vertebral bodies, and probably a contracted anterior longitudinal ligament. They noted the problems of obtaining a solid posterior arthrodesis over a kyphosis because the fusion mass posteriorly is placed under tension rather than compression. Kostuik and Lorenz in 1983 also noted a high percentage of pseudarthrosis after posterior arthrodesis alone.

In a later report, Bradford et al. reported 24 patients with an average age of 21 years who underwent combined anterior and posterior fusion for Scheuermann's disease. Their indications for the combined fusion include kyphosis of more than 70 degrees in a patient who is skeletally mature and who has pain that cannot be controlled by conservative means. They also consider as good surgical candidates patients who are physiologically immature but in whom the kyphosis has not been

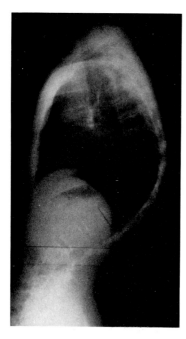

Fig. 83-84 Kyphosis of 81 degrees in patient with Scheuermann's disease.

controlled by a brace and patients with early spastic paraparesis caused by the kyphosis. Their recommendations do not include patients with neurologic changes secondary to a sharply angular kyphotic component or localized anterior cord compression. Bradford et al. and Taylor et al. reported loss of correction when the posterior fusion and instrumentation were not extended to the lowermost and uppermost vertebrae of the kyphosis. The end vertebra should be the last vertebra from the apex that is tilted maximally into the concavity of the curve. We add at least one vertebra above and one vertebra below this recommended level. Anteriorly, the fusion should include the most rigid apical segment of the curve as identified by comparison of the standing lateral roentgenogram with a supine hyperextension roentgenogram. This usually involves six or seven apical vertebrae that can be conveniently exposed through a single thoracotomy incision with the removal of a single rib. Using a combined anterior and posterior approach, Bradford et al. obtained over 50% correction (Fig. 83-85). We reserve posterior instrumentation alone for the more flexible degrees of kyphosis or for adolescent patients with growth remaining in the magnitude of the deformity of less than 70 degrees.

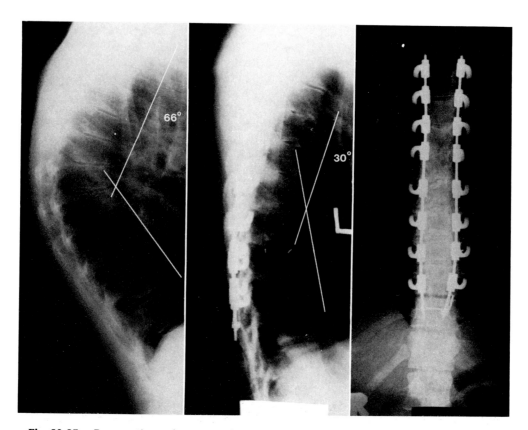

Fig. 83-85 Preoperative and postoperative roentgenograms of 24-year-old patient undergoing anterior discectomy and posterior compression instrumentation for Scheuermann's disease. (From Bradford DS et al: J Bone Joint Surg 57-A:439, 1975.)

ANTERIOR AND POSTERIOR FUSION

■ *TECHNIQUE (BRADFORD)*. Place the patient prone on the Hall frame. Prepare the skin and drape the patient in a routine sterile manner. Make a midline incision over the area to be fused, and expose the spine subperiosteally (p. 3655). Use two Harrington compression rods posteriorly (Fig. 83-86). Prepare the hook sites for the No. 1259 hooks in the routine manner around the transverse processes (p. 3666). The upper hook will extend as high as T2 or T3. Place the compression hooks distal to the apex of the kyphosis beneath the lamina. The more levels instrumented above and below the kyphosis, the

more stable will be the construct of the system. Use autogenous cancellous bone grafts to supplement the fusion. Apply compression of the hooks towards the apex of the kyphosis.

AFTERTREATMENT. External immobilization in an underarm Risser cast or a molded plastic jacket is used for 9 to 12 months or until the fusion is solid.

■ *TECHNIQUE.* Perform disc excision and interbody fusion as described on p. 3658. Do not remove the bony end plate. At approximately 1 week after anterior fusion, perform posterior compression instrumentation as described above.

AFTERTREATMENT. External mobilization by an underarm Risser cast or a molded plastic jacket is used for 9 to 12 months until the fusion is solid.

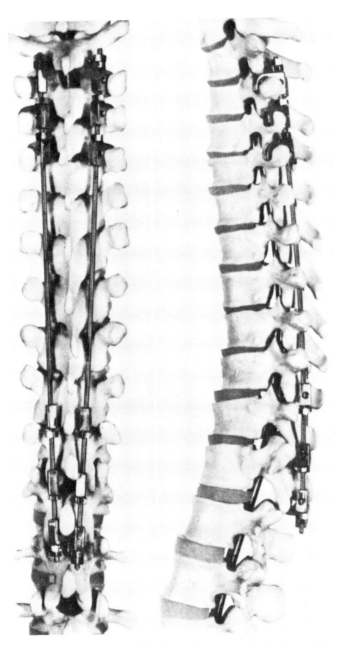

Fig. 83-86   Spinal model of use of compression instrumentation posteriorly in treatment of Scheuermann's disease. (From Bradford DS et al: J Bone Joint Surg 57-A:439, 1975.)

INSTRUMENTATION IN MYELOMENINGOCELE

Instrumentation of the spine in patients with myelomeningocele is one of the most challenging aspects of the surgery of spinal deformities. Generally, there is no one best system for treating these curves; instead, various combinations of different techniques are required. The surgeon must be familiar with all types of spinal instrumentation to determine the best treatment for these complex deformities.

Sriram, Bobechko, and Hall emphasized the problems with posterior spinal fusion in these patients. The spinal exposure is often lengthy and hemorrhagic, primarily because of densely scarred and adherent soft tissue. The deformity is often rigid, and proper correction is impossible. The quality of the bone often provides poor seating for the Harrington hooks, and the inadequacy of the posterior bone mass provides a poor bed for grafting. Osebold et al. reported superior results combining anterior fusion with either the Dwyer or Zielke instrumentation and posterior instrumentation to the sacrum. Our experience also has been that combined anterior and posterior fusion, if possible, is the best treatment of these deformities.

Preoperative Evaluation

In the myelomeningocele patient, careful preoperative evaluation is critical. Every report of surgery for this condition emphasizes the problems and complications that make these deformities so difficult to treat. Thorough evaluations by the orthopaedist, neurosurgeon, urologist, pediatrician, plastic surgeon, and anesthesiologist are required. The patient should be evaluated for hydrocephalus, shunt function, hydromyelia, tethered cord, diastematomyelia, and Arnold-Chiari malformation. Ideally, the urine should be sterile, but if this is not possible, the infecting organism should be identified, and appropriate prophylactic antibiotics should be begun be-

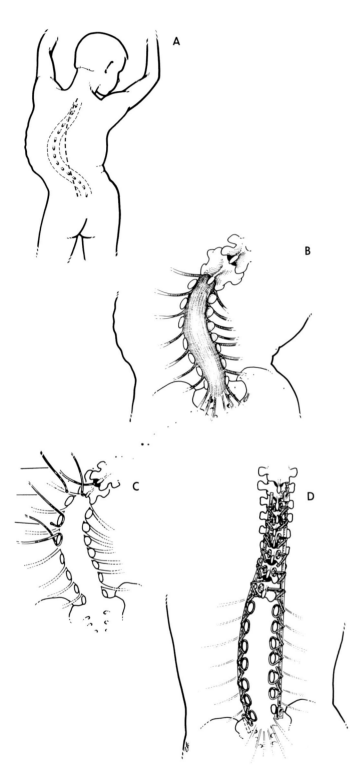

Fig. 83-87   **A,** Skin incision. **B,** Spinal exposure; dural sac is not dissected. **C,** Sublaminar wires placed in normal spine; in area of spina bifida, wires encircle pedicle for segmental fixation. **D,** Contoured Harrington distraction rod inserted on concave side of spine. L-rod applied to convex side of curve and instrumented to sacrum with Dunn technique; segmental wires are tightened to provide more correction and stability.

fore surgery. Prophylactic antibiotics are essential because the infection rate in these patients is quite high. If skin coverage is inadequate, a plastic surgeon should be consulted preoperatively for evaluation of appropriate skin coverage, to be done either before or at the time of spinal fusion.

The area to be fused is determined from preoperative sitting, supine, and traction films. Almost all meningomyelocele patients require fusion from the upper thoracic region to the sacrum. Pelvic obliquity is a major deformity, causing seating problems and pressure sores, in these patients, and this cannot be corrected without including the sacrum in the fusion. The instrumentation of the lumbosacral area presently is the most difficult problem in instrumentation.

Posterior Instrumentation and Fusion

■ *TECHNIQUE.* The technique described is a combined technique using Harrington distraction instrumentation and segmental wires combined with an L-rod and segmental wires. Either of these systems may be used in the myelomeningocele patient. Many will require this combined technique, but some may require only bilateral L-rod fixation with segmental wiring. The surgeon should be capable of modifying either of these posterior instrumentation systems to fit the anatomy at the time of surgery.

Place the patient prone on the Hall frame. Prepare and drape the back in a sterile manner. Make a midline incision from the area of the superior vertebra to be instrumented down to the sacrum (Fig. 83-87, *A*). In the area of the normal spine, carry out subperiosteal dissection as described on p. 3655. In the area of the sac, avoid the midline area; there are no useful bony elements for fusion in this area. Carry the dissection laterally over the facet areas on both the convex and concave sides and down to the ala of the sacrum (Fig. 83-87, *B*). The area of normal spine to be fused and the bony elements of the abnormal sac area are now exposed. Usually, the fusion should extend to the sacrum, so lumbar lordosis must be contoured into the posterior instrumentation. If Harrington rods are used, use the square-ended rods and square-ended distal hooks (p. 3663). Apply the square-ended sacral alar hook over the ala on the concave side of the lumbar curve. Prepare the upper Harrington distraction hook site in the routine manner and insert the upper hook (p. 3664). Pass wires beneath the lamina of the normal vertebra above the sac area (p. 3670). In the area of the defect, try to achieve segmental fixation. Pass the wire around the pedicle and twist it on itself to secure fixation (Fig. 83-87, *C*). Pass wires on both the concave and convex sides of the curve. Contour the square-ended Harrington distraction rod to maintain lumbar lordosis. Insert the rod, perform

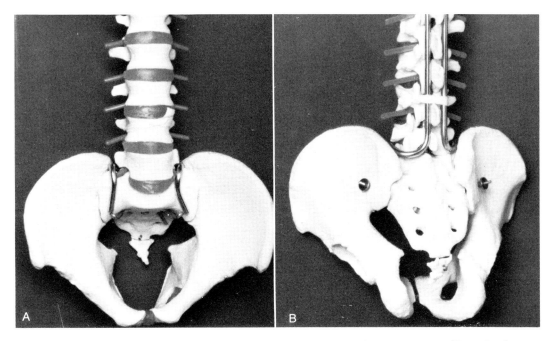

Fig. 83-88   Dunn technique for contouring L-rod for alar purchase on sacrum. (From Bradford DS et al: Moe's textbook of scoliosis and other spinal deformities, ed 2, Philadelphia, 1987, WB Saunders Co.)

distraction, and secure the rod in place by tightening the segmental wires. On the convex side, contour an L-rod to fit the sagittal curves of the spine (Fig. 83-87, *D*). Alternatively, use two L-rods instead of a Harrington distraction rod on the concave side.

Fixation to the pelvis is difficult in the meningomyelocele patient. Allen and Ferguson reported no difficulty with small hypoplastic iliac crests in their use of the Galveston technique (p. 3690). We have

had more difficulty with this technique in the meningomyelocele patient and have generally achieved fixation of the L-rods to the sacrum with the technique described by Dunn (Fig. 83-88). Prebend the L-rod to curve over the sacral ala and past, anterior to the sacrum. Hold the rod in place with segmental wires. Decorticate any areas of exposed bone that can be decorticated without compromising the fixation device. Cut bone-bank bone into small pieces

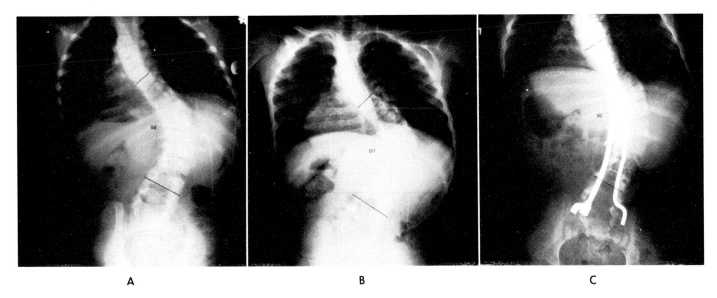

A   B   C

Fig. 83-89   **A** and **B,** Progression of paralytic scoliosis from 68 to 80 degrees in patient with myelomeningocele. **C,** Posterior instrumentation and fusion to sacrum using combined Harrington and L-rod instrumentation with segmental wires.

and place them along the entire area of the spine, emphasizing the lateral gutters. The lateral bone grafts are especially important in the lumbar spine, as the only areas with bone available for fusion are out laterally (Fig. 83-89).

AFTERTREATMENT. The patient is managed in a bivalved plastic body jacket and a standard wheelchair for 12 months. Although not ideal, if fixation to the pelvis is extremely tenuous, this bivalved jacket can be extended down one thigh. The thigh portion is then removed at 3 months and the patient is allowed to sit in a plastic thoracolumbosacral orthosis (TLSO) in an inclined wheelchair for another 3 months. At 6 months, the patient is allowed to sit upright with the bivalved body jacket. External immobilization is continued for 1 year.

Anterior and Posterior Fusion

■ *TECHNIQUE.* If at all possible, anterior and posterior instrumentation and fusion should be considered. If bone strength is sufficient and the spine is large enough to accept it, we recommend anterior Dwyer (p. 3694) or Zielke (p. 3695) instrumentation. A posterior fusion should be performed about 1 week after the anterior fusion (Fig. 83-90). Anterior instrumentation should be performed to the sacrum, if possible; in our experience, however, this is often difficult, especially in the face of a severe lordotic curve.

AFTERTREATMENT. Postoperative care is the same as after posterior instrumentation. Generally speaking, however, if the patient's bones are strong

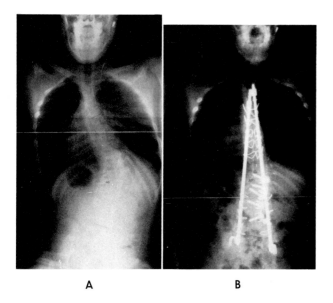

A   **B**

Fig. 83-90   **A,** Paralytic scoliosis in patient with myelomeningocele. **B,** After anterior Dwyer instrumentation and posterior instrumentation with dual Harrington distraction rods and segmental wires.

enough to accept anterior instrumentation, external immobilization will not need to include the hips.

Kyphosis in Myelomeningocele Patient

Kyphosis in the myelomeningocele patient may be either developmental or congenital. Developmental kyphosis is not present at birth, progresses slowly, and is a paralytic kyphosis, aggravated by the lack of posterior stability. Congenital kyphosis usually occurs in patients with a T12 lesion with total paraplegia. The kyphosis is rigid, progresses rapidly during infancy, and causes difficulty in wearing braces, skin problems over the prominent kyphos, possible deterioration of respiration because of crowding of the abdominal contents and upward pressure on the diaphragm, and interference with urinary drainage if urinary diversion becomes needed.

The surgical correction of kyphosis is difficult and demanding. Apical vertebral osteotomy was proposed by Sharrard. This technique facilitates closure of the skin in the newborn but provides only short-term improvement. Lindseth and Selzer found their most consistent satisfactory results followed partial resection of the apical vertebra and of the proximal lordotic curve. They outlined the goals of treatment of kyphosis: (1) straighten and stabilize the spine to allow balance in sitting, (2) decrease the prominence of the bone, and (3) allow an increase in the height of the abdominal wall. They emphasized that the operation is a major undertaking and is technically difficult. A considerable loss of blood and frequent complications are to be expected.

KYPHECTOMY

■ *TECHNIQUE.* With the patient prone (Fig. 83-91, *A*), make a midline, posterior incision, adapting it to the nature of the local skin conditions. Expose subperiosteally the more normal vertebrae superiorly. In the area of the abnormality, continue the exposure past the lateral bony ridges. Continue dissection inside the lamina until the foramina are exposed on each side of the spine. Expose the nerve, artery, and vein within each foramen, and divide and coagulate them to expose the dural sac distally where it is scarred and thinned. At the distal level of this sac, cross clamp it with Kelly clamps and divide the sac between the clamps (Fig. 83-91, *B*). Close the scarred ends with a running stitch. Dissect the sac proximally. As this proximal dissection is performed, large venous channels connecting the sac to the posterior vertebral body will be encountered. Control the bleeding from the bone with bone wax and from the soft tissues with electrocautery. Then dissect the sac up to the level of more normal-appearing dura (Fig. 83-91, *C*). At this point the sac can be transected. If this is done, close the dura with a purse-string suture. Do not suture the cord itself but leave it open so that spinal fluid can escape

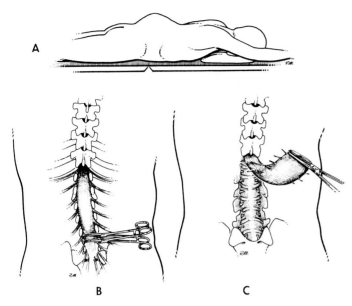

Fig. 83-91 **A,** Patient positioned on table for kyphectomy. **B,** Exposure of area of kyphosis and dural sac. **C,** Sac is divided distally and is dissected proximally.

from the central canal of the cord into the arachnoid space. We prefer not to remove the sac, but to use the sac at the completion of the procedure to further cover the area of the resected vertebrae. Now continue the dissection around the vertebral bodies. We prefer to expose only the area to be removed. If the entire area of the spine is exposed subperiosteally, there is the potential for avascular necrosis of these vertebral bodies. At this point, remove the vertebrae between the apex of the lordosis and the apex of the kyphosis (Fig. 83-92, *A*). We generally remove the vertebra at the apex of the kyphosis first by remov-

ing the intervertebral disc with a Cobb elevator and curets. Try to leave the anterior longitudinal ligament intact to act as a stabilizing hinge. Once this vertebra is removed, the spine can be preliminarily corrected, giving an indication as to how many more vertebrae must be removed. Remove enough vertebrae to correct the kyphosis as much as possible but do not remove so many that reapproximation of the spine is impossible (Fig. 83-92, *B*). Morsel the removed vertebral bodies to be used as additional bone grafts.

Of the many techniques for internal fixation, we have been most satisfied with L-rod instrumentation to the pelvis (Fig. 83-92, *C*) using the technique of Dunn or the technique described by Fackler, Warner, and Vander Woude. For the latter technique, contour the rod with the L-portion distally and pass this L-portion through the foramina of the S1 vertebral body anterior to the sacrum. After fixation to the pelvis, move the distal segment to the proximal segment. Tighten the segmental wires and apply additional allograft bone graft. Irrigate the wound and close it over suction drains. Antibiotics are given intravenously for several days before and after surgery.

AFTERTREATMENT. The postoperative care of these patients requires close observation by all subspecialties involved. When the patient is stabilized after surgery, a bivalved body jacket is applied. If good pelvic fixation is obtained, immobilization of the hips is unnecessary. If the pelvic fixation is tenuous, we extend the body jacket down one or both thighs and keep the patient in a supine position for 3 months. The body jacket is worn until the fusion is solid, generally in 9 to 12 months. High incidences of postoperative infections, urinary tract problems, skin problems, and pseudarthrosis can be expected. The improved function of these patients and the prevention of further progression and loss of functional abilities make the benefits of the surgery worth the risks (Fig. 83-93).

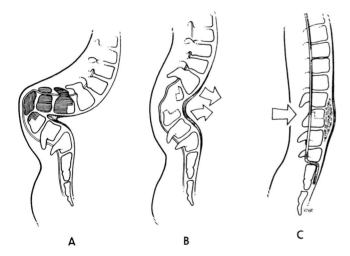

Fig. 83-92 **A,** Vertebrae between apex of lordosis and apex of kyphosis are removed. **B,** Kyphosis is reduced. **C,** Reduction is maintained with stable internal fixation (in this instance with L-rods and segmental wires).

COMPLICATIONS OF INSTRUMENTATION IN SCOLIOSIS

The operative treatment of scoliosis is formidable, and significant complications are possible. Complications may occur at any stage of treatment.

Complications during Surgery

Neurologic injury at the time of surgery remains the most devastating complication. Neurologic injury may result from direct injury to the cord or nerves or from excessive traction during correction. In a 1973 report of 124 patients, Stagnara described a method of anesthesia

A   B   C

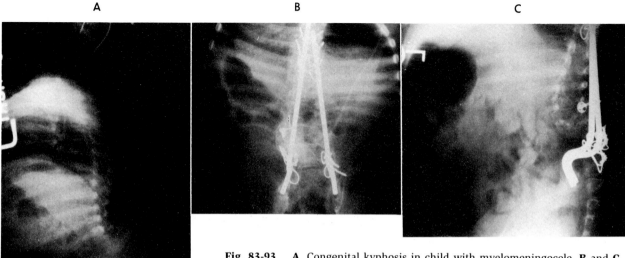

Fig. 83-93 **A,** Congenital kyphosis in child with myelomeningocele. **B** and **C,** After kyphectomy and instrumentation with L-rods and segmental wires. Fixation to pelvis was accomplished with Dunn technique.

to sufficiently disassociate pain and consciousness while permitting spontaneous motion on command after instrumentation. By observing motion of the hands and feet, the neurologic function distal to the spinal surgery can be determined. If motor power does not clearly appear in the lower extremities but does so in the hands, instrumentation is immediately removed and the request repeated. The success of this method depends on careful and controlled anesthesia. On the other hand, Engler et al. pointed out the real hazards in arousing a prone, intubated patient from anesthesia: (1) raising the head may cause accidental extubation; (2) a sudden deep inhalation while awakening could lead to air embolism; and (3) a violent movement could dislodge the spinal instrumentation or intravenous tubings. As Brown and Nash also have pointed out, this test documents only that spinal cord function has not suffered a major compromise at the time the test is performed. Because of this, multiple wake-up tests are used by some surgeons to increase the safety factor.

To enhance the safety of spinal surgery, electrical monitoring of spinal cord function has evolved as researchers have approached the problem from at least three slightly different directions. Stimulation of a peripheral nerve produces an evoked response or electrical potential that with sophisticated electronic equipment can be detected proximally in the spinal cord itself, in the vertebrae, or from the cerebral cortex. The spinal evoked potentials from the cord and cortical evoked potentials from the brain are frequently referred to as somatosensory evoked potentials. It is generally accepted that these potentials and their transmissions effectively reflect function of the dorsal columns only.

If, while performing surgery, the somatosensory evoked potentials change suddenly, especially with an increase in latency, a wake-up test should be performed. If neurological injury is confirmed, the internal fixation should be removed. An intravenous bolus of dexamethasone can be given if neurologic injury is confirmed.

Dural tears can occur at the time of surgery as the ligamentum flavum is removed or as a hook or wire is manipulated into the spinal canal. Repair of all dural tears should be attempted, if possible. If an adequate, watertight repair is obtained, the patient should not exhibit any ill effects from these tears.

Complications Immediately after Surgery

Ileus is a common complication after spinal fusion in scoliosis. We prefer to withhold oral feedings until the bowel sounds return, usually within 36 to 72 hours after surgery. Until then, intravenous fluids are administered.

Atelectasis is a common cause of fever after surgery. Frequent turning of the patient and deep breathing and coughing usually will control or prevent serious atelectasis. The use of inhalation therapy with intermittent positive pressure breathing may be beneficial in cooperative patients, but inflation of the stomach at the time of forced breathing must be avoided. Incentive spirometry is now commonly used instead.

Prophylactic antibiotics generally are given at the start of the operation and are used for 48 hours postoperatively. In spite of this, deep wound infections can occur. The tissues in the area of fusion are generally vascular, and the autogenous cancellous bone grafts seem extremely resistant to most infections. The extensive operative dissection, the lengthy time required for the operation, the use of metallic implants, and the closure of the wound over freely bleeding bone are all factors common to most surgery for scoliosis and theoretically make infection more likely. Infection rates also are high in patients with myelomeningocele or urinary tract infections and when traffic is increased in the operating room.

Moe reported two types of wound infections after surgery. The first is obvious in that sepsis with high fever develops, usually within 2 to 5 days after surgery, and the wound almost always appears infected. In the second type, the temperature is elevated only slightly or moderately, and the wound appears relatively normal. In this case, diagnosis of wound sepsis may be difficult. Patients often have a postoperative temperature elevation of up to 102° Fahrenheit, but this should gradually decline over the first 4 days. Any spike of temperature above 102° Fahrenheit should raise strong suspicion of a deep wound infection, especially if a steady improvement in the general condition is not seen. The appearance of the wound usually is deceiving, with no significant swelling, erythema, or tenderness. Moe recommends prompt aspiration of the wound in several sites. Cultures should be submitted, but the results should not be awaited and reoperation should be planned immediately. If a wound infection is diagnosed, the wound is opened widely and is thoroughly irrigated and debrided. The bone grafts and instrumentation are left in place, and the wound is closed over two plastic ingress-egress tubes. According to Tolo, suction irrigation is unnecessary and he simply closes the wound over subfascial and subcutaneous suction drains. If ingress and egress tubes are used, antibiotic irrigation is carried out for about 5 days and is discontinued when the patient is afebrile and laboratory evidence of an infection is decreasing. Intravenous antibiotics are administered for approximately 10 days and oral administration is continued for approximately 6 weeks.

Most fusion masses become solid even after an infection, but occasionally a draining sinus persists until the instruments are removed. After removal of the instrumentation, the wound should be closed over suction drains or suction irrigation drains.

Another treatment for deep wound infections after Harrington instruments or other devices have been implanted is the time-honored technique of opening the wound widely and allowing it to close secondarily. This technique is satisfactory if a single Harrington distraction rod is used. If, however, one of the segmental spinal instrumentation systems such as the Cotrel-Dubousset or Luque systems has been used, the wound may be quite difficult to pack well because the implants impede the dressing contact needed to promote granulation tissue and therefore secondary wound closure. This treatment may be satisfactory, but the morbidity is much greater than the first treatment described, and the cosmetic result is less desirable. We believe, therefore, that this technique should probably be used only in patients in whom the first technique was unsuccessful.

Many patients undergoing spinal instrumentation for adolescent idiopathic scoliosis develop the syndrome of inappropriate anti-diuretic hormone (ADH). In these cases a decline in urinary output is noted with maximal diminution noted on the evening after surgery. Serum and urine osmolality should be checked before these patients are treated with large volumes of fluid replacement. If both are elevated, the patient is likely to be hypovolemic. The inappropriate ADH syndrome is present if the serum osmolality is diminished and the urine osmolality is elevated. Fluid overload should be avoided under these circumstances. Urinary output gradually increases over the next 2 to 3 days.

Late Complications

The most common late complications are pseudarthrosis and recurrence of the deformity. Pseudarthrosis indicates a failure of the operation to accomplish its purpose. Recurrence of the deformity is usually caused by one or more pseudarthroses but can be caused instead by bending of the fusion mass, traumatic fracture of the fusion mass, or the addition to the curve of one or more adjacent vertebrae superior or inferior to the fusion so that the curve is lengthened.

Improvements in instrumentation and fusion techniques have produced a steady decrease in the rate of pseudarthrosis. In the adolescent with idiopathic scoliosis, the pseudarthrosis rate is approximately 1%. This percentage is, however, higher in adults and in children with neuromuscular scoliosis.

Spinal fusion for scoliosis is usually considered successful if the correction obtained is not lost. Loss of correction then is the only indication for repair of a suspected pseudarthrosis. Late breakage of internal fixation devices usually is presumptive evidence that the fusion is not solid. In the absence of significant loss of correction, however, this is not a definite indication for reoperation. Pain or other symptoms of the pseudarthrosis in the absence of demonstrable loss of correction in our experience are quite rare.

Pseudarthrosis can be demonstrated on anteroposterior and right and left oblique roentgenograms of good quality. The finding roentgenographically of a wedged or "open" interspace, an unfused lateral articulation, or a defect in the fusion mass is helpful in locating the pseudarthrosis. Bone scans and computed tomography may be useful adjuncts, but they are not always completely accurate in predicting the presence of a pseudarthrosis.

At surgical exploration of a pseudarthrosis, the cortex usually is smooth and firm over the mature and intact areas of the fusion mass, and the soft tissues strip away easily. Conversely, at a pseudarthrosis, the soft tissues are usually adherent and are continuous into the defect. Then, locating the pseudarthrosis is usually easy. However, a narrow pseudarthrosis may be extremely difficult to locate, especially if its motion is only slight. In this instance, decorticating the fusion in a suspicious area is indicated. Further, a search should always be made for several pseudarthroses. When the one or more have been identified, they are cleared of fibrous tissue, and the curves are again corrected by instrumentation. When the loss of correction is significant, osteotomy of one or more intact areas of the fusion mass is sometimes justified to obtain additional correction. When most or all of the correction has been lost and the spine is explored late, a solid fusion mass is often found and several osteotomies may be indicated to permit correction of the curves. These osteotomies and any pseudarthroses are treated as ordinary joints to be fused, and their edges are freshened and decorticated. If the fusion mass is thick and of good quality, it may be decorticated throughout to obtain additional bone for grafting. If necessary, fresh autogenous iliac bone is added. According to most reports, pseudarthroses are most common at the thoracolumbar junction, in the lumbar area, and at the extreme ends of the fusion mass.

As previously mentioned, instrument breakage generally indicates that fusion over the entire instrumented area has not become solid. If a rod breaks, the patient generally complains of pain that resolves over a few days. The instrumentation is removed only if pain persists or if loss of correction is noted, the same indications as for the repair of a pseudarthrosis. Tolo reported that over half of the broken Harrington rods do not have as-

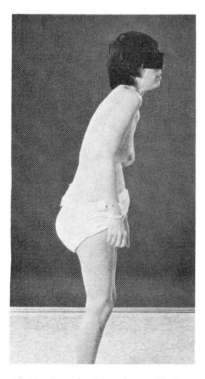

Fig. 83-94 Thirty-six-year-old patient with flattening of normal lumbar lordosis secondary to Harrington rod instrumentation from T4 to sacrum. (From Bradford DS et al: Moe's textbook of scoliosis and other spinal deformities, ed 2, Philadelphia, 1987, WB Saunders Co.)

sociated pseudarthroses, but at the time of rod removal the entire spinal fusion should be explored and re-fused if a nonunion is found. If a rod breaks and the patient remains without pain or further curve progression, the broken rod need not be removed.

If the spinal instrumentation and fusion eliminates the physiologic lumbar lordosis, disability and unsightly posture can result (Fig. 83-94). This condition has been called the lumbar "flat-back" syndrome. The most common cause of a painful flat-back syndrome in our experience is the presence of a pseudarthrosis. Prevention of this syndrome is most important in the initial surgical care. Care should be taken to preserve the lumbar lordosis as much as possible at the time of the original operation. If the syndrome presents late and is painful, the pseudarthrosis should be repaired and if possible the fusion mass should be osteotomized to allow some correction of the deformity.

Complications in Cast

With newer forms of instrumentation, postoperative cast immobilization is needed less frequently. There are still, however, certain conditions in which casting is necessary and cast complications can occur. Pressure sores may develop over any improperly padded bony prominence. Any complaint of localized pain under the cast should be investigated immediately and usually a portion of the cast should be removed and repadded.

Compression of the duodenum in its third portion by the superior mesenteric artery was described by Rokitansky more than 100 years ago. This condition may appear in two forms: the acute form and the chronic form, designated Wilkie's syndrome. The cast syndrome described by Dorph in 1950 is an acute form of this syndrome, consisting of vascular compression of the duodenum leading to acute duodenal obstruction and gastric dilatation. A high index of suspicion must be maintained in those patients with vomiting, abdominal distention, and mild pain. Since this is a partial obstruction, flatus will continue to be passed and symptoms may be intermittent. Diagnosis is based on the radiologic finding of a dilated duodenum. A lateral decubitus roentgenogram of the abdomen, with the patient's right side up, will reveal a dilated duodenal loop and a long air fluid level. Evarts, Winter, and Hall reported 30 patients from the literature and from their own experience with vascular compression of the duodenum. Eighteen cases occurred with correction of the scoliosis operatively; 12 occurred with the application of the body cast only. They emphasized that with correction of the curvature and an increase in the angle of the superior mesenteric artery with the aorta, compression of the duodenum and symptoms of partial intestinal obstruction can occur. Treatment of this syndrome consists of prompt removal of the cast if present, combined with early nasogastric suction. Other measures include position changes, particularly to a prone position, restriction to a liquid diet, and ambulation if possible. General surgical consultation should be sought early since those facing prolonged immobilization may require surgery.

REFERENCES
Idiopathic scoliosis

Aaro S and Dahlborn M: The effect of Harrington instrumentation on the longitudinal axis rotation of the apical vertebra and on the spinal and rib-cage deformity in idiopathic scoliosis studied by computed tomography, Spine 7:456, 1982.

Aaro S and Ohlen G: The effect of Harrington instrumentation on the sagittal configuration and mobility of the spine in scoliosis, Spine 8:570, 1983.

Abbott EG: Correction of lateral curvature of the spine, NY Med J 95:833, 1912.

Akbarnia BA: Selection of methodology in surgical treatment of adolescent idiopathic scoliosis, Orthop Clin North Am 19:319, 1988.

Akbarnia BA and Moe JH: Familial congenital scoliosis with unilateral unsegmented bar: case report of two siblings, J Bone Joint Surg 60-A:259, 1978.

Alexander J: Postoperative management of thoracoplasty patients, Am Rev Tuberc 61:57, 1950.

Allen BL Jr: The place for segmental instrumentation in the treatment of spinal deformity, Orthop Trans 6:21, 1982 (abstract).

Allen BL Jr: Segmental spinal instrumentation with L-rods, AAOS Instr Course Lect 32:202, 1983.

Allen BL Jr and Ferguson RL: The Galveston technique for L-rod instrumentation of the scoliotic spine, Spine 7:276, 1982.

Allen BL Jr and Ferguson RL: Neurologic injuries with the Galveston technique of L-rod instrumentation for scoliosis, Spine 11:14, 1986.

Allen BL Jr and Ferguson RL: The Galveston experience with L-rod instrumentation for adolescent idiopathic scoliosis, Clin Orthop 229:59, 1988.

Allen BL Jr and Ferguson RL: A 1988 perspective on the Galveston technique of pelvic fixation, Orthop Clin North Am 19:409, 1988.

Arkin AM: Correction of structural changes in scoliosis by corrective plaster jackets and prolonged recumbency, J Bone Joint Surg 46-A:33, 1964.

Armstrong GWD and Connock SHG: A transverse loading system applied to a modified Harrington instrumentation, Clin Orthop 108:70, 1975.

Ashman RB, Birch JG, Bone LB, et al: Mechanical testing of spinal instrumentation, Clin Orthop 227:113, 1988.

Aurori BF, Weierman RJ, Lowell HA, et al: Pseudarthrosis after spinal fusion for scoliosis: a comparison of autogeneic and allogeneic bone grafts, Clin Orthop 199:153, 1985.

Bailey RW and Badgley CE: Stabilization of the cervical spine by anterior fusion, J Bone Joint Surg 42-A:565, 1960.

Bailey TE and Mahoney OM: The use of banked autologous blood in patients undergoing surgery for spinal deformity, J Bone Joint Surg 69-A:329, 1987.

Barnes J: Rib resection in infantile idiopathic scoliosis, J Bone Joint Surg 61-B:31, 1979.

Ben-David B: Spinal cord monitoring, Orthop Clin North Am 19:427, 1988.

Bennett SH, Hoye RC, and Riggle GC: Intraoperative autotransfusion: preliminary report of a new blood suction device for anticoagulation of autologous blood, Am J Surg 123:257, 1972.

Bernard TN, Johnston CE, Roberts JM, and Burke SW: Late complications due to wire breakage in segmental spinal instrumentation, J Bone Joint Surg 65-A:1339, 1983.

Bieber E, Tolo V, and Uematsu S: Spinal cord monitoring during posterior spinal instrumentation and fusion, Clin Orthop 229:121, 1988.

Birch JG, Herring JA, Roach JW, and Johnston CE: Cotrel-Dubousset instrumentation in idiopathic scoliosis: a preliminary report, Clin Orthop 227:24, 1988.

Boachie-Adjei O, Lonstein JE, Winter RB, et al: Management of neuromuscular spinal deformities with Luque segmental instrumentation, J Bone Joint Surg. 71-A:548, 1989.

Bradford DS: Anterior spinal surgery in the management of scoliosis: indications, techniques, results, Orthop Clin North Am 10:801, 1979.

Bradford DS: Anterior vascular pedicle bone grafting for the treatment of kyphosis, Spine 5:318, 1980.

Bradford DS, Ganjavian S, Antonious D, et al: Anterior strut grafting for the treatment of kyphosis, Spine 5:318, 1980.

Bradford DS, Lonstein JE, Ogilvie JW, and Winter RB, editors: Moe's textbook of scoliosis and other spinal deformities, ed 2, Philadelphia, 1987, WB Saunders Co.

Bradford DS, Winter RB, Lonstein JE, and Moe JH: Techniques of anterior spine surgery for the management of kyphosis, Clin Orthop 128:129, 1977.

Bradshaw K, Webb JK, and Fraser AM: Clinical evaluation of spinal cord monitoring in scoliosis surgery, Spine 9:636, 1984.

Broadstone T: Consider postoperative immobilization of double L-rod SSI patients, Orthop Trans 8:171, 1984 (abstract).

Broom MJ, Banta JV, and Renshaw TS: Spinal fusion augmented by Luque rod segmental instrumentation for neuromuscular scoliosis, J Bone Joint Surg 71-A:32, 1989.

Brown RH and Nash CL Jr: Current status of spinal cord monitoring, Spine 4:466, 1979.

Burrington JD, Brown C, Wayner ER, and Odom J: Anterior approach to the thoracolumbar spine: technical considerations, Arch Surg 111:456, 1976.

Butte FL: Scoliosis treated by the wedging jacket: selection of the area to be fused, J Bone Joint Surg 20:1, 1938.

Cloward RB: The treatment of ruptured lumbar intervertebral discs by vertebral body fusion. I. Indications, operative technique, after care, J Neurosurg 10:154, 1953.

Cobb JR: The treatment of scoliosis, Conn Med J 7:467, 1943.

Cobb JR: Correction of scoliosis. In Poliomyelitis, Second International Poliomyelitis Congress, Philadelphia, 1952, JB Lippincott Co.

Cobb JR: Technique, after-treatment, and results of spine fusion for scoliosis, AAOS Instr Course Lect 9:65, 1952.

Cobb JR: Spine arthrodesis in the treatment of scoliosis, Bull Hosp Jt Dis Ortho Inst 19:187, 1958.

Cobb JR: The problem of the primary curve, J Bone Joint Surg 42-A:1413, 1960.

Cochran T, Irstam L, and Nachemson A: Long-term anatomic and functional changes in patients with adolescent idiopathic scoliosis treated by Harrington rod fusions, Spine 8:576, 1983.

Collis DK and Ponseti IV: Long-term follow-up of patients with idiopathic scoliosis not treated surgically, J Bone Joint Surg 51-A:425, 1969.

Conner AN: Developmental anomalies and prognosis in infantile idiopathic scoliosis, J Bone Joint Surg 51-B:711, 1969.

Cook CD, Barrie H, Deforest SA, and Helliesen PJ: Pulmonary physiology in children. III. Lung volumes, mechanics of respiration and respiratory muscle strength in scoliosis, J Pediatr 25:766, 1960.

Cook WA: Transthoracic vertebral surgery, Ann Thorac Surg 12:54, 1971.

Cotrel Y and Dubousset J: New segmental posterior instrumentation of the spine, Orthop Trans 9:118, 1985.

Cotrel Y, Dubousset J, and Guillaumat M: New universal instrumentation and spinal surgery, Clin Orthop 227:10, 1988.

Cowell HR and Swickard JW: Autotransfusion in children's orthopaedics, J Bone Joint Surg 56-A:908, 1974.

Dabney KW, Salzman SK, Wakabayashi T, et al: Experimental scoliosis in the rat. II. Biomechanical analysis of the forces during Harrington distraction, Spine 13:472, 1988.

Dawson EG, Moe JH, and Caron A: Surgical measurement of scoliosis in the adult, Scoliosis Research Society, 1972, J Bone Joint Surg 55-A:437, 1973.

Denis F: Cotrel-Dubousset instrumentation in the treatment of idiopathic scoliosis, Orthop Clin North Am 19:291, 1988.

DeWald RL: New trends in the operative treatment of scoliosis. In Ahstrom JP Jr, editor: Current practices in orthopaedic surgery, vol 5, St Louis, 1973, Mosby–Year Book, Inc.

Dickson JH: Spinal instrumentation and fusion in adolescent idiopathic scoliosis: indications and surgical techniques, Contemp Orthop 4:397, 1982.

Dickson JH and Harrington PR: The evolution of the Harrington instrumentation technique in scoliosis, J Bone Joint Surg 55-A:993, 1973.

Dolan JA and MacEwen GD: Surgical treatment of scoliosis, Clin Orthop 76:125, 1971.

Dommisse GG: The blood supply of the spinal cord J Bone Joint Surg 56-B:225, 1974.

Donaldson WF Jr and Wissinger HA: The results of surgical exploration of spine fusion performed for scoliosis, West J Surg Obstet Gynecol 72:195, 1964.

Dorang LA, Klebanoff G, and Kemmerer WT: Autotransfusion in long-segment spinal fusion: an experimental model to demonstrate the efficacy of salvaging blood contaminated with bone fragments and marrow, Am J Surg 123:686, 1972.

Dorph MH: The cast syndrome, N Engl J Med 243:440, 1950.

Dove J, Lin TY, Shen YS, and Ditmanson ML: Aortic aneurysm complicating spinal fixation with Dwyer's apparatus: report of a case, Spine 6:524, 1981.

Drummond DS: Harrington instrumentation with spinous process wiring for idiopathic scoliosis, Orthop Clin North Am 19:281, 1988.

Drummond D et al: Interspinous process segmental spinal instrumentation, J Pediatr Orthop 4:397, 1984.

Drummond DS, Keene JS, and Breed A: The Wisconsin system: a technique of interspinous segmental spinal instrumentation, Contemp Orthop 8:29, 1984.

Drummond DS and Keene S Jr: Spinous process segmental spinal instrumentation, Orthopedics 11:1403, 1988.

Drummond D, Narechania R, Wenger D, et al: Wisconsin segmental spinal instrumentation, Orthop Trans 6:22, 1982 (abstract).

Dunn HK: Spinal instrumentation. I. Principles of posterior and anterior instrumentation, AAOS Instr Course Lect 32:192, 1983.

Dunn HK and Bolstad KE: Fixation of Dwyer screws for the treatment of scoliosis: a postmortem study, J Bone Joint Surg 59-A:54, 1977.

Dwyer AF: Experience of anterior correction of scoliosis, Clin Orthop 93:191, 1973.

Dwyer AF, Newton NC, and Sherwood AA: An anterior approach to scoliosis: a preliminary report, Clin Orthop 62:192, 1969.

Dwyer AF, O'Brien JP, Seal PP, et al: The late complications after the Dwyer anterior spinal instrumentation for scoliosis, J Bone Joint Surg 59-B:117, 1977.

Engler GL: Preoperative and intraoperative considerations in adolescent idiopathic scoliosis, AAOS Instr Course Lect 38:137, 1989.

Engler GL et al: Somatosensory evoked potentials during Harrington instrumentation for scoliosis, J Bone Joint Surg 60-A:528, 1978.

Erwin WD, Dickson JH, and Gaines JH III: Utilization of Harrington spinal instrumentation and fusion for scoliosis. Technique manual, 1986, Zimmer.

Erwin WD, Dickson JH, and Harrington PR: The postoperative management of scoliosis patients treated with Harrington instrumentation and fusion, J Bone Joint Surg 58-A:479, 1976.

Evarts CM: The cast syndrome: report of a case after spinal fusion for scoliosis, Clin Orthop 75:164, 1971.

Evarts CM, Winter RB, and Hall JE: Vascular compression of the duodenum associated with the treatment of scoliosis: review of the literature and report of eighteen cases, J Bone Joint Surg 53-A:431, 1971.

Farcy J, Weidenbaum M, and Roye DP, Jr: Correction of thoracic scoliosis using the Cotrel-Dubousset technique, Surg Rounds Orthop, p 11, May, 1987.

Ferguson RL and Allen BL Jr: Segmental spinal instrumentation for routine scoliotic curve, Contemp Orthop 2:450, 1980.

Flynn JC and Hoque A: Anterior fusion of the lumbar spine: end-result study with long-term follow-up, J Bone Joint Surg 61-A:1143, 1979.

Freebody D, Bendall R, and Taylor RD: Anterior transperitoneal lumbar fusion, J Bone Joint Surg 53-B:617, 1971.

Fujimake A, Crock HV, and Bedbrook GM: The results of 150 anterior lumbar interbody fusion operations performed by two surgeons in Australia, Clin Orthop 165:164, 1982.

Gaines R, York DH, and Watts C: Identification of spinal cord pathways responsible for the peroneal-evoked response in the dog, Spine 9:810, 1984.

Gaines RW Jr and Abernathie DL: Mersilene tapes as a substitute for wire in segmental spinal instrumentation for children, Spine 11:907, 1986.

Gaines RW Jr, McKinley LM, and Leatherman KD: Effect of the Harrington compression system on the correction of the rib hump in spinal instrumentation for idiopathic scoliosis, Spine 6:489, 1981.

Galeazzi R: The treatment of scoliosis, J Bone Joint Surg 11:81, 1929.

Gardner RC: Blood loss after spinal instrumentation and fusion in scoliosis (Harrington procedure): results using a radioactive tracer and an electronic blood volume computer: a preliminary report, Clin Orthop 71:182, 1970.

Gazioglu K, Goldstein LA, Femi-Pearse D, and Yu PN: Pulmonary function in idiopathic scoliosis: comparative evaluation before and after orthopaedic correction, J Bone Joint Surg 50-A:1391, 1968.

Gersoff WK and Renshaw TS: The treatment of scoliosis in cerebral palsy by posterior spinal fusion with Luque-rod instrumentation, J Bone Joint Surg 70-A:41, 1988.

Goldstein LA: Results in the treatment of scoliosis with turnbuckle plaster cast correction and fusion, J Bone Joint Surg 41-A:321, 1959.

Goldstein LA: The surgical management of scoliosis, Clin Orthop 35:95, 1964.

Goldstein LA: Surgical management of scoliosis, J Bone Joint Surg 48-A:167, 1966.

Goldstein LA: Treatment of idiopathic scoliosis by Harrington instrumentation and fusion with fresh autogenous iliac bone grafts: results in eighty patients, J Bone Joint Surg 51-A:209, 1969.

Goldstein LA: The surgical management of scoliosis, Clin Orthop 77:32, 1971.

Goldstein LA: The surgical treatment of idiopathic scoliosis, Clin Orthop 93:131, 1973.

Goldstein LA and Evarts CM: Further experiences with the treatment of scoliosis by cast correction and spine fusion with fresh autogenous iliac-bone grafts, J Bone Joint Surg 48-A:962, 1966.

Goll SR, Balderston RA, Stambough JL, et al: Depth of intraspinal wire penetration during passage of sublaminar wires, Spine 13:503, 1988.

Gollehon D, Kahanovitz N, and Happel LT: Temperature effects on feline cortical and spinal evoked potentials, Spine 8:443, 1983.

Guadagni J, Drummond D, and Breed A: Improved postoperative course following modified segmental instrumentation and posterior spinal fusion for idiopathic scoliosis, J Pediatr Orthop 4:405, 1984.

Hall JE: The place of the anterior approach to the spine in scoliosis surgery. In Keim HA, editor: Postgraduate course on the management and care of the scoliosis patient, pp 32-34, New York November 5-7, 1970, New York Orthop. Hospital of Columbia-Presbyterian Medical Center.

Hall JE: The anterior approach to spinal deformities, Orthop Clin North Am 3:81, 1972.

Hall JE: Preoperative assessment of the patient with a spinal deformity, AAOS Instr Course Lect 34:127, 1985.

Hall JE, Levine CR, and Sudhir KG: Intraoperative awakening to monitor spinal cord function during Harrington instrumentation and spine fusion: descriptions of procedure and report of three cases, J Bone Joint Surg 60-A:533, 1978.

Hallock H, Francis KC, and Jones JB: Spine fusion in young children, J Bone Joint Surg 39-A:41, 1957.

Hamel AL and Moe JH: The collapsing spine, Surgery 56:364, 1964.

Hammerberg KW, Rodts MF, and Dewald RL: Zielke instrumentation, Orthopedics 11:1365, 1988.

Hardy JH and Gossling HR: Combined halo and sacral bar fixation: a method for immobilization and early ambulation following extensive spine fusion, Clin Orthop 75:205, 1971.

Harmon PH: Subtotal anterior lumbar disc excision and vertebral body fusion. III. Application to complicated and recurrent multilevel degenerations, Am J Surg 97:659, 1959.

Harrington PR: Surgical instrumentation for management of scoliosis, J Bone Joint Surg 42-A:1448, 1960.

Harrington PR: Treatment of scoliosis: correction and internal fixation by spine instrumentation, J Bone Joint Surg 44-A:591, 1962.

Harrington PR: The management of scoliosis by spine instrumentation: an evaluation of more than 200 cases, South Med J 56:1367, 1963.

Harrington PR: Technical details in relation to the successful use of instrumentation in scoliosis, Orthop Clin North Am 3:49, 1972.

Harrington PR: The history and development of Harrington instrumentation, Clin Orthop 93:110, 1973.

Harrington PR and Dickson JH: An eleven-year clinical investigation of Harrington instrumentation: a preliminary report of 578 cases, Clin Orthop 93:113, 1973.

Heilbronner DM and Sussman MD: Early mobilization of adolescent scoliosis patients following Wisconsin interspinous segmental instrumentation as an adjunct to Harrington distraction instrumentation, Clin Orthop 229:52, 1988.

Herndon WA, Sullivan JA, Yngeve DA, et al: Segmental spinal instrumentation with sublaminar wires: a critical appraisal, J Bone Joint Surg 69-A:851, 1987.

Herring JA and Wenger DR: Early complications of segmental spinal instrumentation, Orthop Trans 6:22, 1982 (abstract).

Herring JA and Wenger DR: Segmental spinal instrumentation: a preliminary report of 40 consecutive cases, Spine 7:285, 1982.

Herron LD and Dawson EG: Methylmethacrylate as an adjunct in spinal instrumentation, J Bone Joint Surg 59-A:866, 1977.

Herron LD, Westin GW, and Dawson EG: Scoliosis in arthrogryposis multiplex congenita, J Bone Joint Surg 60-A:293, 1978.

Hibbs RA: An operation for progressive spinal deformities, NY Med J 93:1013, 1911.

Hibbs RA: A report of fifty-nine cases of scoliosis treated by the fusion operation, J Bone Joint Surg. 6:3, 1924.

Hibbs RA, Risser JC, and Ferguson AB: Scoliosis treated by the fusion operation, J Bone Joint Surg 13:91, 1931.

Hodgson AR and Stock FE: Anterior spine fusion, Br J Surg 44:266, 1956.

Hodgson AR, Stock FE, Fang HSY, and Ong GB: Anterior spine fusion, Br J Surg 48:172, 1960.

Hsu LCS, Zucherman J, Tang SC, and Leong JCY: Dwyer instrumentation in the treatment of adolescent idiopathic scoliosis, J Bone Joint Surg 64-B:536, 1982.

Jackson JW: Surgical approaches to the anterior aspect of the spinal column, Ann Roy Coll Surg 48:83, 1971.

James JIP: Two curve patterns in idiopathic structural scoliosis, J Bone Joint Surg 33-B:399, 1951.

Johnson BE and Westgate HD: Methods of predicting vital capacity in patients with thoracic scoliosis, J Bone Joint Surg 52-A:1433, 1970.

Johnson CE, Ashman RB, and Sherman MC: Mechanical consequences of rod contouring and residual scoliosis in sublaminar pelvic segmental spinal instrumentation, Orthop Trans 10:5, 1986 (abstract).

Johnson CE II, Ashman RB, Sherman MC, et al: Mechanical consequences of rod contouring and residual scoliosis in sublaminar segmental instrumentation, J Orthop Res 5:206, 1987.

Johnson RM and McGuire EJ: Urogenital complications of anterior approaches to the lumbar spine, Clin Orthop 154:114, 1981.

Johnston CE, Happel LT, Norris R, et al: Delayed paraplegia complicating sublaminar segmental spinal instrumentation, J Bone Joint Surg 68-A:556, 1986.

Jones SJ, Edgar MA, Ransford AO, and Thomas NP: A system for the electrophysiological monitoring of the spinal cord during operations for scoliosis, J Bone Joint Surg 65-B:134, 1983.

Kaneda K, Fujiya N, and Satoh S: Results with Zielke instrumentation for idiopathic thoracolumbar and lumbar scoliosis, Clin Orthop 205:195, 1986.

Keller RB and Pappas AM: Infection after spinal fusion using internal fixation instrumentation, Orthop Clin North Am 3:99, 1972.

King HA: Selection of fusion levels for posterior instrumentation and fusion in idiopathic scoliosis, Orthop Clin North Am 19:247, 1988.

King HA, Moe JH, Bradford DS, and Winter RB: The selection of the fusion levels in thoracic idiopathic scoliosis, J Bone Joint Surg 65-A:1302, 1983.

Kleinberg S: A survey of structural scoliosis: the principles of treatment and their application, AAOS Instr Course Lect 7:130, 1950.

Knapp DR and Jones ET: Use of cortical allograft for posterior spinal fusion, Clin Orthop 229:99, 1988.

Kojima Y, Yamamoto T, Ogino H, et al: Evoked spinal potentials as a monitor of spinal cord viability, Spine 4:471, 1979.

Korovessis P: Combined VDS and Harrington instrumentation for treatment of idiopathic double major curves, Spine 12:224, 1987.

LaGrone MO: Loss of lumbar lordosis: a complication of spinal fusion for scoliosis, Orthop Clin North Am 19:393, 1988.

LaGrone MO, Bradford DS, Moe JH, et al: Treatment of symptomatic flatback after spinal fusion, J Bone Joint Surg 70-A:569, 1988.

Larson SJ, Walsh PR, Sances A, Jr, et al: Evoked potentials in experimental myelopathy, Spine 5:299, 1980.

Leatherman KD: The management of rigid spinal curves, Clin Orthop 93:215, 1973.

Leider LL Jr, Moe JH, and Winter RB: Early ambulation after the surgical treatment of idiopathic scoliosis, J Bone Joint Surg 55-A:1003, 1973.

Letts RM and Bobechko WP: Fusion of the scoliotic spine in young children: effect on prognosis and growth, Clin Orthop 101:136, 1974.

Letts RM and Hollenberg C: Delayed paresis following spinal fusion with Harrington instrumentation, Clin Orthop 125:45, 1977.

Levy WJ and York DH: Evoked potentials from motor tracts in humans, Neurosurgery 12:422, 1983.

Lieponis JV, Bunch WH, Lonser RE, et al: Spinal cord injury during segmental sublaminar spinal instrumentation: an animal model, Orthop Trans 8:173, 1984 (abstract).

Lonstein J, Winter R, Moe J, and Gaines D: Wound infection with Harrington instrumentation and spine fusion for scoliosis, Clin Orthop 96:222, 1973.

Lowe TG: Morbidity and mortality committee report. Presented at the 22nd Annual Meeting of the Scoliosis Research Society, Vancouver, British Columbia, 1987.

Lueders H, Gurd A, Hahn J, et al: A new technique for intraoperative monitoring of spinal cord function: multichannel recording of spinal cord and subcortical evoked potentials, Spine 7:110, 1982.

Luque ER: Anatomy of scoliosis and its correction, Clin Orthop 105:298, 1974.

Luque ER: Segmental spinal instrumentation: a method of rigid internal fixation of the spine to induce arthrodesis, Orthop Trans 4:391, 1980 (abstract).

Luque ER: Segmental spinal instrumentation for correction of scoliosis, Clin Orthop 163:192, 1982.

Luque ER: The anatomic basis and development of segmental spinal instrumentation, Spine 7:256, 1982.

Luque ER and Cardoso A: Segmental correction of scoliosis with rigid internal fixation, Orthop Trans 1:136, 1977 (abstract).

MacEwen GD, Bunnell WP, and Sriram K: Acute neurological complications in the treatment of scoliosis: a report of the Scoliosis Research Society, J Bone Joint Surg 57-A:404, 1975.

Machida M, Weinstein SL, Yamada T, and Kimura J: Spinal cord monitoring: electrophysiological measures of sensory and motor function during spinal surgery, Spine 10:407, 1985.

Mankin HJ, Graham JJ, and Schack J: Cardiopulmonary function in mild and moderate idiopathic scoliosis, J Bone Joint Surg 46-A:53, 1964.

Manning EW, Prime FJ, and Zorab PA: Partial costectomy as a cosmetic operation in scoliosis, J Bone Joint Surg 55-B:521, 1973.

May VR Jr and Mauck WR: Exploration of the spine for pseudarthrosis following spinal fusion in the treatment of scoliosis, Clin Orthop 53:115, 1967.

McCarroll HR and Costen W: Attempted treatment of scoliosis by unilateral vertebral epiphyseal arrest, J Bone Joint Surg 42-A:965, 1960.

McCarthy RE Dunn H, and McCullough FL: Luque fixation to the sacral ala using the Dunn-McCarthy modification, Spine 14:281, 1989.

McKittrick JE: Banked autologous blood in elective surgery, Am J Surg 128:137, 1974.

McMaster MJ and James JIP: Pseudarthrosis after spinal fusion for scoliosis, J Bone Joint Surg 58-B:305, 1976.

Michel CR and Lalain JJ: Late results of Harrington's operation: long-term evolution of the lumbar spine below the fused segments, Spine 10:414, 1985.

Mir SR et al: Early ambulation following spinal fusion and Harrington instrumentation in idiopathic scoliosis, Clin Orthop 110:54, 1975.

Moe JH: A critical analysis of methods of fusion for scoliosis: an evaluation in two hundred and sixty-six patients, J Bone Joint Surg 40-A:529, 1958.

Moe JH: Complications of scoliosis treatment, Clin Orthop 53:21, 1967.

Moe JH: Methods of correction and surgical techniques in scoliosis, Orthop Clin North Am 3:17, 1972.

Moe JH and Gustilo RB: Treatment of scoliosis: results in 196 patients treated with cast correction and fusion, J Bone Joint Surg 46-A:293, 1964.

Moe JH, Purcell GA, and Bradford DS: Zielke instrumentation (VDS) for the correction of spinal curvature: analysis of results in 66 patients, Clin Orthop 180:133, 1983.

Moore SV: Segmental spinal instrumentation: complications, correction, and indications, Orthop Trans 7:413, 1983 (abstract).

Moskowitz A, Moe JH, Winter RB, and Binner H: Long-term follow-up of scoliosis fusion, J Bone Joint Surg 62-A:364, 1980.

Mouradian WH, and Simmons EH: A frame for spinal surgery to reduce intra-abdominal pressure while continuous traction is applied, J Bone Joint Surg 59-A:1098, 1977.

Mubarak SJ, Wenger DR, and Leach J: Evaluation of Cotrel-Dubousset instrumentation for treatment of idiopathic scoliosis, Update on Spinal Disorders 2:3, 1987.

Nach CD and Keim HA: Prophylactic antibiotics in spinal surgery, Orthop Rev 2:27, June 1973.

Nachemson AL and Elfström G: Intravital wireless telemetry of axial forces in Harrington distraction rods in patients with idiopathic scoliosis, J Bone Joint Surg 53-A:445, 1971.

Nachlas IW and Borden JN: The cure of experimental scoliosis by directed growth control, J Bone Joint Surg 33-A:24, 1951.

Nasca RJ: Segmental spinal instrumentation, South Med J 78:303, 1985.

Nash CL Jr, Lorig RA, Schatzinger LA, and Brown RH: Spinal cord monitoring during operative treatment of the spine, Clin Orthop 126:100, 1977.

Nash CL and Moe JH: A study of vertebral rotation, J Bone Joint Surg 51-A:223, 1969.

Nash CL, Schatzinger L, and Lorig R: Intraoperative monitoring of spinal cord function during scoliosis spine surgery, J Bone Joint Surg 56-A:1765, 1974 (abstract).

Nicastro JF, Traina J, Lancaster M, and Hartjen C: Sublaminar segmental wire fixation: anatomic pathways during their removal, Orthop Trans 8:172, 1984 (abstract).

Nordwall A et al: Spinal cord monitoring using evoked potentials recorded from vertebral bone in cat, Spine 4:486, 1979.

Ogilvie JW: Anterior spine fusion with Zielke instrumentation for idiopathic scoliosis in adolescents, Orthop Clin North Am 19:313, 1988.

Ogilvie JW, and Millar EA: Comparison of segmental spinal instrumentation devices in the correction of scoliosis, Spine 8:416, 1983.

Olson SA and Gaines RW: Removal of sublaminar wires after spinal fusion, J Bone Joint Surg 69-A:1419, 1987.

Phillips WA and Hensinger RN: Wisconsin and other instrumentation for posterior spinal fusion, Clin Orthop 229:44, 1988.

Piggott H: Posterior rib resection in scoliosis, J Bone Joint Surg 53-B:663, 1971.

Piggott H: Treatment of scoliosis by posterior fusion, Harrington instrumentation and early walking, J Bone Joint Surg 58-B:58, 1976.

Ponder RC, Dickson JH, Harrington PR, and Erwin WD: Results of Harrington instrumentation and fusion in the adult idiopathic scoliosis patient, J Bone Joint Surg 57-A:797, 1975.

Ponseti IV and Friedman B: Changes in the scoliotic spine after fusion, J Bone Joint Surg 32-A:751, 1950.

Ponseti IV and Friedman B: Prognosis in idiopathic scoliosis, J Bone Joint Surg 32-A:381, 1950.

Rappaport M, Hall K, Hopkins K, et al: Effects of corrective scoliosis surgery on somatosensory evoked potentials, Spine 7:404, 1982.

Reger SI, Henry DT, Whitehill R, et al: Spinal evoked potentials from the cervical spine, Spine 4:495, 1979.

Reid RL and Gamon RS Jr: The cast syndrome, Clin Orthop 79:85, 1971.

Relton JES and Hall JE: An operation frame for spinal fusion: a new apparatus designed to reduce haemorrhage during operation, J Bone Joint Surg 49-B:327, 1967.

Renshaw TS: Spinal fusion with segmental instrumentation, Contemp Orthop 4:413, 1982.

Renshaw TS: The role of Harrington instrumentation and posterior spine fusion in the management of adolescent idiopathic scoliosis, Orthop Clin North Am 19:257, 1988.

Resina J and Alves AF: A technique for correction and internal fixation for scoliosis, J Bone Joint Surg 59-B:159, 1977.

Riseborough EJ: The anterior approach to the spine for the correction of deformities of the axial skeleton, Clin Orthop 93:207, 1973.

Risser JC: Scoliosis treated by cast correction and spine fusion: a long term follow-up study, Clin Orthop 116:86, 1976.

Risser JC and Norquist DM: A follow-up study of the treatment of scoliosis, J Bone Joint Surg 40-A:555, 1958.

Roaf R: Vertebral growth and its mechanical control, J Bone Joint Surg 42-B:40, 1960.

Roaf R: The treatment of progressive scoliosis by unilateral growth arrest, J Bone Joint Surg 45-B:637, 1963.

Roaf R: Wedge resection for scoliosis, J Bone Joint Surg 46-B:798, 1964.

Roth A et al: Scoliosis and congenital heart disease, Clin Orthop 93:95, 1973.

Schmidt AC: Fundamental principles and treatment of scoliosis, AAOS Instr Course Lect 16:184, 1959.

Schrader WC, Bethem D, and Scerbin V: The chronic local effects of sublaminar wires: an animal model, Spine 13:449, 1988.

Schultz AB and Hirsch C: Mechanical analysis of Harrington rod correction of idiopathic scoliosis, J Bone Joint Surg 55-A:983, 1973.

Schultz AB and Hirsch C: Mechanical analysis of techniques for improved correction of idiopathic scoliosis, Clin Orthop 100:66, 1974.

Shands AR Jr, Barr JS, Colonna PC, and Noall L: End-result study of the treatment of idiopathic scoliosis; report of the research committee of the American Orthopaedic Association, J Bone Joint Surg 23:963, 1941.

Shifrin LZ: The lateral position for spine fusion and Harrington instrumentation for scoliosis: a brief report, Clin Orthop 81:48, 1971.

Shufflebarger HL, Kahn A, Rinsky LA, and Shank M: Segmental spinal instrumentation: retrospective analysis of 234 cases, Orthop Trans 9:124, 1985 (abstract).

Silverman BJ and Greenbarg PE: Idiopathic scoliosis posterior spine fusion with Harrington rod and sublaminar wiring, Orthop Clin North Am 19:269, 1988.

Smith A DeF, von Lackum WH, and Wylie R: An operation for stapling vertebral bodies in congenital scoliosis, J Bone Joint Surg 36-A:342, 1954.

Smith A DeF, Butte FL, and Ferguson, AB: Treatment of scoliosis by the wedging jacket and spine fusion: a review of 265 cases, J Bone Joint Surg 20:825, 1938.

Southwick WO and Robinson RA: Surgical approaches to the vertebral bodies in the cervical and lumbar regions, J Bone Joint Surg 39-A:631, 1957.

Spielholz NI, Benjamin MV, Engler GL, and Ransohoff J: Somatosensory evoked potentials during decompression and stabilization of the spine: methods and findings, Spine 4:500, 1979.

Stagnara P: Scoliosis in adults: surgical treatment of severe forms, Excerpta Med Found International Congress Series, No. 192, 1969.

Stagnara P: Utilization of Harrington's device in the treatment of adult kyphoscoliosis above 100 degrees. Fourth International Symposium, 1971, Nijmegen, Stuttgart, 1973, Georg Thieme Verlag.

Steel HH: Rib resection and spine fusion in correction of convex deformity in scoliosis, J Bone Joint Surg 65-A:920, 1983.

Stevens DB and Beard C: Segmental spinal instrumentation for neuromuscular spinal deformity, Clin Orthop 242:164, 1989.

Taddonio RF: Segmental spinal instrumentation in the management of neuromuscular spinal deformity, Spine 7:305, 1982.

Taddonio RF, Weller K, and Appel M: A comparison of patients with idiopathic scoliosis managed with and without post-operative immobilization following segmental spinal instrumentation with Luque rods, Orthop Trans 8:172, 1984 (abstract).

Tambornino JM, Armbrust EN, and Moe JH: Harrington instrumentation in correction of scoliosis: a comparison with cast correction, J Bone Joint Surg 46-A:313, 1964.

Thompson GH, Wilber RG, Shaffer JW, et al: Segmental spinal instrumentation in idiopathic scoliosis: a preliminary report, Spine 10:623, 1985.

Thompson GH, Wilber RG, Shaffer JW, et al: Segmental spinal instrumentation in idiopathic spinal deformities, Orthop Trans 9:123, 1985 (abstract).

Thompson JD, Callaghan JJ, Savory CG, et al: Prior deposition of autologous blood in elective orthopaedic surgery, J Bone Joint Surg 69-A:320, 1987.

Thompson WAL and Ralston EL: Pseudarthrosis following spine fusion, J Bone Joint Surg 31-A:400, 1949.

Thulbourne T and Gillespie R: The rib hump in idiopathic scoliosis: measurement, analysis and response to treatment, J Bone Joint Surg 58-B:64, 1976.

Tolo VT: Surgical treatment of adolescent idiopathic scoliosis, AAOS Instr Course Lect 38:143, 1989.

Ulrich HF: The operative treatment of scoliosis, Am J Surg 45:235, 1939.

Van Grouw A, Nadel CI, Weierman RJ, and Lowell HA: Long-term follow-up of patients with idiopathic scoliosis treated surgically: a preliminary subjective study, Clin Orthop 117:197, 1976.

Vauzelle C, Stagnara P, and Jouvinroux P: Functional monitoring of spinal activity during spinal surgery, J Bone Joint Surg 55-A:441, 1973.

Vauzelle C, Stagnara P, and Jouvinroux P: Functional monitoring of spinal cord activity during spinal surgery, Clin Orthop 93:173, 1973.

Von Lackum WH: The surgical treatment of scoliosis, AAOS Instr Course Lect 5:236, 1948.

Von Lackum WH: Surgical scoliosis, Surg Clin North Am 31:345, 1951.

Von Lackum WH: The surgical treatment of scoliosis. In Bancroft FW and Marble HC: Surgical treatment of the motor-skeletal system, ed 2, Philadelphia, 1951, JB Lippincott Co.

Von Lackum WH and Miller JP: Critical observations of the results in the operative treatment of scoliosis, J Bone Joint Surg 31-A:102, 1949.

Weiler PJ, McNeice GM, and Medley JB: An experimental study of the buckling behavior of L-rod implants used in the surgical treatment of scoliosis, Spine 11:991, 1986.

Wenger DR, Carollo JJ, and Wilkerson JA: Biomechanics of scoliosis correction by segmental spinal instrumentation, Spine 7:260, 1982.

Wenger DR et al: Laboratory testing of segmental spinal instrumentation versus traditional Harrington instrumentation for scoliosis treatment, Spine 7:265, 1982.

Wenger DR, Miller S, and Wilkerson J: Evaluation of fixation sites for segmental instrumentation of the human vertebra, Orthop Trans 6:23, 1982 (abstract).

Westgate HD and Moe JH: Pulmonary function in kyphoscoliosis before and after correction of the Harrington instrumentation method, J Bone Joint Surg 51-A:935, 1969.

Wilber RG, Thompson GH, Shaffer JW, et al: Postoperative neurologic deficits in segmental spinal instrumentation: a study using spinal cord monitoring, J Bone Joint Surg 66-A:1178, 1984.

Wiltberger BR: The dowel intervertebral body fusion as used in lumbar-disc surgery, J Bone Joint Surg 39-A:284, 1957.

Wilson RL, Levine DB, and Doherty JH: Surgical treatment of idiopathic scoliosis, Clin Orthop 81:34, 1971.

Winter RB: Posterior spinal fusion in scoliosis: indications, techniques, and results, Orthop Clin North Am 10:787, 1979.

Winter RB: Posterior spinal arthrodesis with instrumentation and sublaminar wire: 100 consecutive cases, Orthop Trans 9:124, 1985 (abstract).

Winter RB, Lovell WW, and Moe JH: Excessive thoracic lordosis and loss of pulmonary function in patients with idiopathic scoliosis, J Bone Joint Surg 57-A:972, 1974.

Winter RB, Moe JH, and Eilers VE: Congenital scoliosis: a study of 234 patients treated and untreated. I. Natural history, J Bone Joint Surg 50-A:1, 1968.

Winter RB, Moe JH, and Eilers VE: Congenital scoliosis: a study of 234 patients treated and unteated. II. Treatment, J Bone Joint Surg 50-A:15, 1968.

Woolson ST, Marsh JS, and Tanner JB: Transfusion of previously deposited autologous blood for patients undergoing hip-replacement surgery, J Bone Joint Surg 69-A:325, 1987.

Wu Z: Posterior vertebral instrumentation for correction of scoliosis, Clin Orthop 215:40, 1987.

Zielke K: Derotation spondylodese vorlaufiger ergebnisbericht uder 26 operierte falle, Arch Orthop Unfallchir 83:257, 1976.

Zielke K: Derotation and fusion: anterior spinal instrumentation, Orthop Trans 2:270, 1978 (abstract).

Zielke K: Ventral derotation spondylodesis: preliminary report on 58 cases, Beitr Orthop Traumatol 25:85, 1978.

Zielke K: Ventrale Derotationsspondylodese, Behandlungsergenbnisse bei idiopathischen Lumbalskoliosen, Z Orthop 120:320, 1982.

Zindrick MR, Knight GW, Bunch WH, et al: Factors influencing the penetration of wires into the neural canal during segmental wiring, J Bone Joint Surg 71-A:742, 1989.

Zuege RC, Blount WP, and Dicus WT: Indications for operative treatment of spinal deformities, Wisc Med J 74:S33, 1975.

Neuromuscular scoliosis

Allen BL and Ferguson RL: L-rod instrumentation for scoliosis in cerebral palsy, J Pediatr Orthop 2:87, 1982.

Balmer GA and MacEwen GD: The incidence and treatment of scoliosis in cerebral palsy, J Bone Joint Surg 52-B:134, 1970.

Bonnet C, Brown J, and Brooks HL: Anterior spine fusion with Dwyer instrumentation for lumbar scoliosis in cerebral palsy, J Bone Joint Surg 55-A:425, 1973.

Bonnet CA, Brown JC, and Grow T: Thoracolumbar scoliosis in cerebral palsy: results of surgical treatment, J Bone Joint Surg 58-A:328, 1976.

Brown JC, Swank SM, and Specht L: Combined anterior and posterior spine fusion in cerebral palsy, Spine 7:570, 1982.

DeWald RL and Faut MM: Anterior and posterior spinal fusion for paralytic scoliosis, Spine 4:401, 1979.

Ferguson RL and Allen BL: Considerations in the treatment of cerebral palsy patients with spinal deformities, Orthop Clin North Am 19:419, 1988.

Ferguson RL and Allen BL: Staged correction of neuromuscular scoliosis, J Pediatr Orthop 3:555, 1983.

Gersoff WK and Renshaw JS: The treatment of scoliosis in cerebral palsy by posterior spinal fusion with Luque-rod segmented instrumentation, J Bone Joint Surg 70-A:41, 1988.

Lonstein JE and Akbarnia BA: Operative treatment of spinal deformities in patients with cerebral palsy or mental retardation: an analysis of 107 cases, J Bone Joint Surg 65-A:43, 1983.

McCarthy RE, Peek RD, Morrissy RT, and Hough AJ: Allograft bone in spinal fusion for paralytic scoliosis, J Bone Joint Surg 68-A:370, 1986.

Stanitski CL, Micheli LJ, Hall JD, and Rosenthal RK: Surgical correction of spinal deformity in cerebral palsy, Spine 7:563, 1982.

Sullivan JA and Conner SB: Comparison of Harrington instrumentation and segmental spinal instrumentation in the management of neuromuscular spinal deformity, Spine 7:299, 1982.

Taddonio RF: Segmental spinal instrumentation in the management of neuromuscular spinal deformity, Spine 7:305, 1982.

Myelomeningocele

Allen B and Ferguson R: Operative treatment of myelomening-ocele spinal deformities, Orthop Clin North Am 10:845, 1979.

Banta JV and Hamada JS: Natural history of the kyphotic deformity in myelomeningocele, J Bone Joint Surg 58-A:279, 1960.

Bodel JG and Stephane JP: Luque rods in the treatment of kyphosis in myelomeningocele, J Bone Joint Surg 65-B:98, 1983.

Brown HP: Management of spinal deformity in myelomeningocele, Orthop Clin North Am 9:391, 1978.

Christofersen MR and Brooks AL: Excision and wire fixation of rigid myelomeningocele kyphosis, J Pediatr Orthop 5:691, 1985.

Dunn HK: Kyphosis of myelodysplasia: operative treatment based on pathophysiology, Orthop Trans 7:19, 1983 (abstract).

Eyring EJ, Wanken JJ, and Sayers MP: Spine ostectomy for kyphosis in myelomeningocele, Clin Orthop 88:24, 1972.

Fackler CD, Warner WC Jr, and Vander Woude L: A comparison of two instrumentation techniques in the treatment of lumbar kyphosis in myelodysplasia. Presented at the 57th Annual Meeting of the American Academy of Orthopaedic Surgeons, New Orleans, February 10, 1990.

Feiwell E: Selection of appropriate treatment for patients with myelomeningocele, Orthop Clin North Am 12:101, 1981.

Gillespie R, Torode I, and van Olm RS Jr: Myelomeningocele kyphosis fixed by kyphectomy and segmental spinal instrumentation, Orthop Trans 8:162, 1984 (abstract).

Hall JE and Poitras B: The management of kyphosis in patients with myelomeningocele, Clin Orthop 128:33, 1977.

Heydemann JS and Gillespie R: Management of myelomeningocele kyphosis in the older child by kyphectomy and segmental spinal instrumentation, Spine 12:37, 1987.

Hoppenfeld S: Congenital kyphosis in myelomeningocele, J Bone Joint Surg 49-B:276, 1967.

Hull WJ, Moe JH, and Winter RB: Spinal deformity in myelomeningocele: natural history, evaluation, and treatment, J Bone Joint Surg 56-A:1767, 1974.

Jones ET: Kyphectomy in myelodysplasia, Orthop Trans 7:432, 1983, (abstract).

Kahanovitz N and Duncan JW: The role of scoliosis and pelvic obliquity on functional disability in myelomeningocele, Spine 6:494, 1981.

Leatherman KD and Dickson RA: Congenital kyphosis in myelomeningocele: vertebral body resection and posterior spinal fusion, Spine 3:222, 1978.

Lindseth RE and Selzer L: Vertebral excision of kyphosis in myelomeningocele, J Bone Joint Surg 61-A:699, 1979.

Lowe GP and Menelaus MB: The surgical management of kyphosis in older children with myelomeningocele, J Bone Joint Surg 60-B:40, 1978.

Mackel JL and Lindseth RE: Scoliosis in myelodysplasia, J Bone Joint Surg 57-A:131, 1975.

McMaster MJ: Anterior and posterior instrumentation and fusion of thoracolumbar scoliosis due to myelomeningocele, J Bone Joint Surg 69-B:20, 1987.

Osebold W, Mayfield JK, Winter RB, and Moe JH: Surgical treatment of paralytic scoliosis in myelomeningocele, J Bone Joint Surg 64-A:841, 1982.

Piggot H: The natural history of scoliosis in myelodysplasia, J Bone Joint Surg 61-B:122, 1979.

Poitras B and Hall JE: The management of kyphosis in patients with myelomeningocele, Clin Orthop 128:33, 1977.

Poitras B, Rivard C, Duhaime M, et al: Correction of the kyphosis in myelomeningocele patients by both anterior and posterior stabilization procedure, Orthop Trans 7:432, 1983 (abstract).

Raycroft JF and Curtis BH: Spinal curvature in myelomeningocele. In AAOS symposium on myelomeningocele, St Louis, 1972, Mosby–Year Book, Inc.

Sharrard WJW: Spinal osteotomy for congenital kyphosis in myelomeningocele, J Bone Joint Surg 50-B:446, 1968.

Sharrard WJW and Drennan JC: Osteo-excision of the spine for lumbar kyphosis in older children with myelomeningocele, J Bone Joint Surg 54-B:50, 1972.

Sriram K, Bobechko WP, and Hall JE: Surgical management of spinal deformities in spina bifida, J Bone Joint Surg 54-B:666, 1972.

Winston K, Hall JE, Johnson D, and Micheli L: Acute elevation of intracranial pressure following transection of non-functional spinal cord, Clin Orthop 128:41, 1977.

Scheuermann's kyphosis

Bradford DS: Juvenile kyphosis. In Bradford DS, Lonstein JE, Ogilvie JW, and Winter RB, editors: Moe's textbook of scoliosis and other spinal deformities, ed 2, Philadelphia, 1987, WB Saunders Co.

Bradford DS, Khalid BA, Moe JH, et al: The surgical management of patients with Scheuermann's disease: a review of 24 cases managed by combined anterior and posterior spine fusion, J Bone Joint Surg 62-A:705, 1980.

Bradford DS, Moe JH, Montalvo FJ, and Winter RB: Scheuermann's kyphosis: results of surgical treatment in 22 patients, J Bone Joint Surg 57-A:439, 1975.

Coscia MF, Bradford DS, and Ogilvie JW: Scheuermann's kyphosis: treatment with Luque instrumentation: a review of 19 patients. Presented at the 55th Annual Meeting of the American Academy of Orthopaedic Surgeons, Atlanta, February 4-9, 1988.

Herndon WA, Emans JB, Micheli LJ, and Hall JE: Combined anterior and posterior fusion for Scheuermann's kyphosis, Spine 6:125, 1981.

Kostuik J and Lorenz M: Long-term follow-up of surgical management in adult Scheuermann's kyphosis, Orthop Trans 7:28, 1983 (abstract).

Scheuermann H: Kyphosis dorsalis juvenile, Ztschr Orthop Chir 41:305, 1921.

Strum PF, Dobson JC, and Armstrong GWD: The surgical management of Scheuermann's disease. Presented at the 55th Annual Meeting of the American Academy of Orthopaedic Surgeons, Atlanta, February 4-9, 1988.

Taylor TC, Wenger DR, Stephen J, et al: Surgical management of thoracic kyphosis in adolescents, J Bone Joint Surg 61-A:496, 1979.

CHAPTER 84

Lower Back Pain and Disorders of Intervertebral Disc

GEORGE W. WOOD II

Humans have been plagued by back and leg pain since the beginning of recorded history. Primitive cultures attributed it to the work of demons. The early Greeks recognized the symptoms as a disease. They prescribed rest and massage for the ailment. In the fifth century AD, Aurelianus clearly described the symptoms of sciatica. He noted that sciatica arose from either hidden causes or observable causes, such as a fall, a violent blow, pulling, or straining. In the eighteenth century Cotugnio (Cotunnius) attributed the pain to the sciatic nerve. Gradually, as medicine advanced as a science, the number of specific diagnoses capable of causing back and leg pain increased dramatically.

A number of physical maneuvers were devised to isolate the true problem in each patient. The most notable of these is the Lasègue sign, or straight-leg raising test, described by Forst in 1881 but attributed to Lasègue, his teacher. This test was devised to distinguish hip disease from sciatica. Although sciatica was widespread as an ailment, little was known about it because only rarely did it result in death, allowing examination at autopsy. Virchow (1857), Kocher (1896), and Middleton and Teacher (1911) described acute traumatic ruptures of the intervertebral disc that resulted in death. The correlation between the disc rupture and sciatica was not appreciated by these examiners. Goldthwait in 1911 attributed back pain to posterior displacement of the disc. Oppenheim and Krause in 1909 performed the first successful surgical excision of a herniated intervertebral disc. Unfortunately, they did not recognize the excised tissue as disc material and interpreted it as an enchondroma. Oil contrast myelography was serendipitously introduced when iodized poppy seed oil, injected to treat sciatica in 1922, was inadvertently injected intradurally and was noted to flow freely. Dandy in 1929 and Alajouanine in the same year reported removal of a "disc tumor" or chondroma from patients with sciatica. The commonly held opinion of that time was that the disc hernia was a neoplasm. Finally in 1932 Barr attributed the source of sciatica to the herniated lumbar disc. Mixter and Barr in their classic paper published in 1934 again attributed sciatica to lumbar disc herniation. They suggested surgical treatment. The acceptance of myelography for confirmation of disc disease was resisted because of toxicity of the agents used in the years that followed.

The standard procedure for disc removal was a total laminectomy followed by a transdural approach to the disc. In 1939 Semmes presented a new procedure to remove the ruptured intervertebral disc that included subtotal laminectomy and retraction of the dural sac to expose and remove the ruptured disc with the patient under local anesthesia. Love in the same year also described this same technique independently. This procedure is now the classic approach for the removal of the intervertebral disc.

As more people were treated for herniated lumbar discs, it became obvious that surgery was not universally successful. In an attempt to identify other causes of back pain Mooney and Robertson popularized facet injections, thus resurrecting an idea proposed originally in 1911 by Goldthwait. Smith et al. in 1963 approached the problem by suggesting a radical departure in treatment—enzymatic dissolution of the disc. Finally through the anatomic dissections and clinical observations of Kirkaldy-Willis and associates, spinal aging and the development of pathologic processes associated with or complicating the process of aging have evolved as a primary theory in disc disease.

A thorough and complete history of all aspects of lumbar spinal surgery was compiled by Wiltse in 1987.

EPIDEMIOLOGY

Back pain, the ancient curse, is now appearing as a modern, international epidemic. Hult estimates that up to 80% of the population is affected by this symptom at some time in life. Impairments of the back and spine are ranked as the most frequent cause of limitation of activity in people younger than 45 years by the National Center for Health Statistics.

Although back pain as a presenting complaint may account for only 2% of the patients seen by a general practitioner, Dillane, Fry, and Kalton reported that in 79% of men and 89% of women the specific cause was unknown. Svensson and Andersson noted the lifetime incidence of low back pain to be 61% and the prevalence to be 31% in a random sample of 40- to 47-year-old men. They noted that 40% of those reporting back pain also

reported sciatica. In women 38 to 64 years of age the lifetime incidence of low back pain was 66% with a prevalence of 35%. Svensson and Anderson noted psychologic variables associated with low back pain to be dissatisfaction with the work environment and a higher degree of worry and fatigue at the end of the workday. The cost to society and the patient in the form of lost work time, compensation, and treatment is staggering. Snook reported that Liberty Mutual Insurance Company paid $247 million for compensable back pain in 1980. Because this company represents only 9% of the insured workers' compensation market, Webster and Snook estimated the compensable costs of low back pain in the United States to be $11.1 billion. Of the billions of dollars spent annually in the United States because of back complaints, it is estimated that only about one third is spent for medical treatment; the remaining costs are for disability payments. This does not include the losses from absenteeism. Although absenteeism because of back pain varies with the type of work, it rivals the common cold in total workdays lost.

Saal and Saal noted an 18% incidence of chronic back pain in 1135 adults. Eighty percent of those reporting chronic pain did not report limitation of activity, while fewer than 4% reported significant limitation of activity. Females reported back pain more freqently than males. There were no racial differences, but the lower the educational level of those interviewed the greater the proportion of those reporting back pain.

Multiple factors affect the development of back pain. Frymoyer et al. note that risk factors associated with severe lower back pain include jobs requiring heavy and repetitive lifting, the use of jackhammers and machine tools, and the operation of motor vehicles. They also note that patients with severe pain were more likely to be cigarette smokers and had a greater tobacco consumption. In an earlier study Frymoyer et al. noted that patients complaining of back pain reported more episodes of anxiety and depression. They also had more stressful occupations. Women with back pain had a greater number of pregnancies than those who did not. Jackson, Simmons, and Stripinis noted that adult patients with scoliosis are more likely to have back pain and that the pain persists and progresses. Gyntelberg reported a slightly greater incidence of back pain in patients taller than 181 cm. Individuals of normal or slightly higher body weight were more likely to report back pain than those with below or above normal body weight. Deyo and Bass noted a strong relationship between smoking and back pain in patients younger than 45 years of age. They also noted a greater tendency for back pain in those patients who were the most obese. Other investigators, however, have found no relationship between obesity and back pain. Svensson and Anderson have associated low back pain with cardiovascular risk factors, including calf pain on exertion, high physical activity at work, smoking, and frequent worry and tension.

In another report they also associated low back pain with monotonous work and less overtime work.

GENERAL DISC AND SPINE ANATOMY

The development of the spine begins in the third week of gestation and continues until the third decade of life. Formation of the primitive streak marks the beginning of spinal development, which is followed by the formation of the notochordal process. This process induces neurectodermal, ectodermal, and mesodermal differentiation.

Somites form in the mesodermal tissue adjacent to the neural tube (neurectoderm) and notochord. They number 42 to 44 in humans. The somites begin to migrate in preparation for the formation of skeletal structures. At the same time, the portion of the somites around the notochord separates into a sclerotome with loosely packed cells cephalad and densely packed cells caudally. Each sclerotome then separates at the junction of the loose and densely packed cells. The caudal dense cells migrate to the cephalad loose cells of the next more caudal sclerotome.

The space where the sclerotome separates eventually forms the intervertebral disc. Vessels that originally were positioned between the somites are now overlying the middle of the vertebral body. As the vertebral bodies form, the notochord that is in the center degenerates. The only remaining notochordal remnant forms the nucleus pulposus. Notochordal remnants usually are not distinguishable in the adult nucleus pulposus (Fig. 84-1).

In the adult the intervertebral disc is composed of the anulus fibrosus and the nucleus pulposus. The anulus fibrosus is composed of numerous concentric rings of fibrocartilaginous tissue. Fibers in each ring cross radially, and the rings attach to each other with additional diagonal fibers. The rings are thicker anteriorly (ventrally) than posteriorly (dorsally). The nucleus pulposus, a gelatinous material, forms the center of the disc. Because of the structural imbalance of the anulus, the nucleus is slightly posterior (dorsal) in relation to the disc as a whole. The discs vary in size and shape with their position in the spine.

The nucleus pulposus is composed of a loose, nonoriented, collagen fibril framework supporting a network of cells resembling fibrocytes and chondrocytes. This entire structure is embedded in a gelatinous matrix of various glucosaminoglycans, water, and salts. This material usually is under considerable pressure and is restrained by the crucible-like anulus. Inoue demonstrated that the cartilage end plate contains no fibrillar connection with the collagen of the subchondral bone of the vertebra. This lack of interconnection between the end plate and

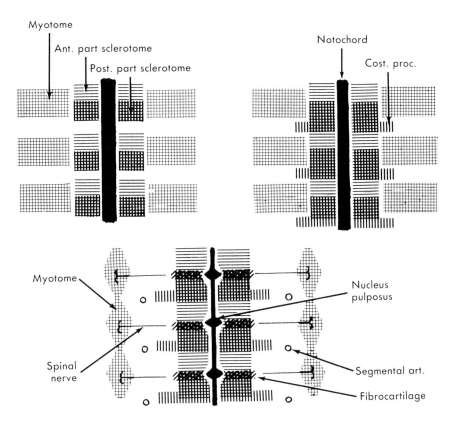

Fig. 84-1 Schematic representation of development of vertebrae and discs. (From Rothman RH and Simeone FA: The spine, vol 1, Philadelphia, 1982, WB Saunders Co.)

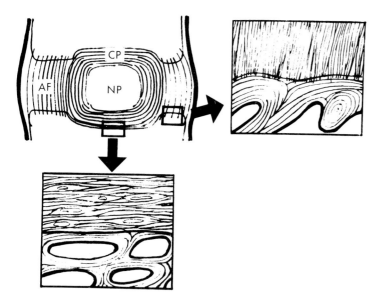

Fig. 84-2   Schematic representation of orientation of fibers in disc and end plate. *AF,* Anulus fibrosus; *NP,* nucleus pulposus; *CP,* cartilaginous plate. (From Inoue H: Spine 6:139, 1981.)

the vertebra may render the disc biomechanically weak against horizontal shearing forces. Inoue also demonstrated that the collagen fibrils in the outer two thirds of the anulus fibrosus are firmly anchored into the vertebral bodies (Fig. 84-2).

The intervertebral disc in the adult is avascular. The cells within it are sustained by diffusion of nutrients into the disc through the porous central concavity of the vertebral end plate. Histologic studies have shown regions where the marrow spaces are in direct contact with the cartilage and that the central portion of the end plate is permeable to dye. Motion and weight bearing are believed to be helpful in maintaining this diffusion. The metabolic turnover of the disc is relatively high when its avascularity is considered but slow compared with other tissues. The glycosaminoglycan turnover in the disc is quite slow, requiring 500 days. Inoue has postulated that the degeneration of the disc may be prompted by decreased permeability of the cartilage end plate, which is normally dense.

Recent studies by Bogduk and others have demonstrated neural fibers in the outer rings of the anulus. These fibers are branches of the sinu-vertebral nerve dorsally. Ventral branches arise from the sympathetic chain that courses anterolaterally over the vertebral bodies.

Neural Elements

The organization of the neural elements is strictly maintained throughout the entire neural system even at the conus medullaris and cauda equina distally. Wall et al. noted that the orientation of the nerve roots in the dural sac and at the conus medullaris follows a highly organized pattern, with the most cephalad roots lying lat-

eral and the most caudal lying centrally. The motor roots are ventral to the sensory roots at all levels. The arachnoid holds the roots in these positions.

The relational anatomy specifically with respect to the neural elements is extremely important in surgical exposure. In the lumbar spine each nerve root exits just below the pedicle and above the disc. This root is numbered for the vertebral body at which it exits. Each root crosses the disc above (cephalad) the vertebral body but not below (caudal) the vertebral body.

At the level of the intervertebral foramen is the dorsal root ganglion. The ganglion lies within the bony confines of the canal but near the outer confines of the foramen. Distal to the ganglion three distinct branches arise; the most prominent and important is the ventral ramus, which supplies all structures ventral to the neural canal. The second branch, the sinu-vertebral nerve, is a small filamentous nerve that originates from the ventral ramus and progresses medially over the posterior aspect of the disc and vertebral bodies, innervating these structures and the posterior longitudinal ligament. The third branch is the dorsal ramus. This branch courses dorsally, piercing the intertransverse ligament near the pars interarticularis. Three branches from the dorsal ramus innervate the structures dorsal to the neural canal. The lateral and intermediate branches provide innervation to the posterior musculature and skin. The medial branch separates into three branches to innervate the facet joint at that level and the adjacent levels above and below (Fig. 84-3).

Pedersen, Blunck, and Gardner noted that the clinically significant function of the sinu-vertebral nerves and the posterior rami is the transmission of pain. The proprioceptive functions of these nerves are not known but assumed.

NATURAL HISTORY OF DISC DISEASE

The natural process of spinal aging has been studied by Kirkaldy-Willis and Hill and by others through observation of clinical and anatomic data. A theory of spinal degeneration has been postulated that assumes that all spines degenerate and that our present methods of treatment are for symptomatic relief, not for a cure.

The degenerative process has been divided into three separate stages with relatively distinct findings. The first stage is dysfunction. This stage is found in the age group between 15 and 45 years. It is characterized by circumferential and radial tears in the disc anulus and localized synovitis of the facet joints. Varlotta et al. noted a familial predisposition to lumbar disc herniation in patients who had disc herniation before the age of 21 years. In this group the familial incidence was 32% compared to a matched control group of asymptomatic individuals in whom the rate was only 7%. Gibson et al. noted disc degeneration by magnetic resonance imaging (MRI) in all

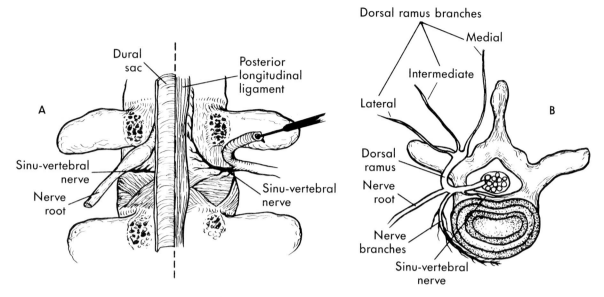

Fig. 84-3   **A,** Dorsal view of lumbar spinal segment with lamina and facets removed. On left side, dura and root exiting at that level remain. On right side, dura has been resected and root is elevated. Sinu-vertebral nerve with its course and innervation of posterior longitudinal ligament is usually obscured by nerve root, and dura. **B,** Cross-sectional view of spine at level of endplate and disc. Note that sinu-vertebral nerve innervates dorsal surface of disc and posterior longitudinal ligament. Additional nerve branches from ventral ramus innervate more ventral surface of disc and anterior longitudinal ligament. Dorsal ramus arises from root immediately on leaving foramen. This ramus divides into lateral, intermediate, and medial branches. Medial branch supplies primary innervation to facet joints dorsally.

adolescent patients who had back and leg pain and in 4 of 20 asymptomatic adolescents.

The next stage is instability. This stage, found in 35- to 70-year-old patients, is characterized by internal disruption of the disc, progressive disc resorption, degeneration of the facet joints with capsular laxity, subluxation, and joint erosion. The final stage, present in patients older than 60 years, is stabilization. In this stage the progressive development of hypertrophic bone about the disc and facet joints leads to segmental stiffening or frank ankylosis (Table 84-1).

Each spinal segment degenerates at a different rate. As one level is in the dysfunction stage, another may be entering the stabilization stage. Disc herniation in this scheme is considered a complication of disc degeneration in the dysfunction and instability stages. Spinal stenosis from degenerative arthritis in this scheme is a complication of bony overgrowth compromising neural tissue in the late instability and early stabilization stages.

The stages and progression of degeneration have been confirmed by histologic studies. Miller, Schmatz, and Schultz noted that disc degeneration progresses histologically as age increases. Males were found to have more degeneration than females. L4-5 and L3-4 disc levels showed the greatest degree of disc degeneration. Urban and McMullin noted that the hydration of disc material decreased with age. The relationship between the change

in hydration and swelling pressure was dependent on the composition of the disc rather than on the age of the patient or the degree of degeneration. In their study L1-2 and L5-S1 discs had the lowest hydration. Yasuma et al. noted progressive histologic changes in the prolapsed discs when compared to protruded discs. Urovitz and Fornasier were unable to detect any evidence of autoimmune reaction in human disc tissue, but they did detect evidence of the response to mechanical injury. Using postmyelogram computed tomography (CT) scans, Takata et al. found that the cauda equina and affected nerve roots were swollen in 17 of 28 patients studied. The affected roots returned to normal size after disc excision.

Excellent long-term studies by Hakelius in 1970 and Weber in 1983 compared disc herniations on which operations were performed with those on which no surgery was done. The prognosis in disc herniation was found to be good regardless of the treatment. These studies found that patients operated on for proven disc herniations improved more rapidly during the first year than patients who had no surgery, but within 4 to 5 years the statistical difference between the groups was negligible. Neurologic recovery was noted in both the operated and unoperated patients who had neurologic deficit at the beginning of the study. Weber correlated good results with physical activity and a slightly younger age. No other

Table 84-1   Spectrum of pathologic changes in facet joints and discs and the interaction of these changes

Phases of spinal degeneration	Facet joints		Pathologic result		Intervertebral disc
Dysfunction	Synovitis	→	Dysfunction	←	Circumferential tears
	Hypermobility		↓	↖	
	Continuing degeneration	↗	Herniation	←	Radial tears
Instability	Capsular laxity	→	Instability	←	Internal disruption
	Subluxation	→	Lateral nerve entrapment	←	Disc resorption
Stabilization	Enlargement of articular processes	→	One-level stenosis	←	Osteophytes
		↘	Multilevel spondylosis and stenosis	↙	

Modified from Kirkaldy-Willis WH, editor: Managing low back pain, New York, 1983, Churchill Livingstone.

variables were of statistical significance. In both studies some patients had such disabling symptoms that surgery was elected regardless of the predetermined treatment group. Acute sciatica in these studies ran a relatively short course (1 to 2 years) and was associated in most instances with neurologic recovery. Surgery provided symptomatic relief during this short course, but the long-term results were essentially the same regardless of treatment.

The natural history of disc disease is one of recurrent episodes of pain followed by periods of significant or complete relief. Biering-Sørensen and Hilden noted that the memory of painful low back episodes was short. At 6-month follow-up only 84% of patients answered consistently, and after 6 months only 60% of those interviewed answered consistently. They questioned the long-term analysis of data from this standpoint and noted that the clinician should be aware of the potential vagueness and unreliability of a history of previous back injury.

DIAGNOSTIC STUDIES
Roentgenography

The simplest and most readily available diagnostic tests for back or neck pain are the anteroposterior and lateral roentgenograms of the involved spinal segment. These simple roentgenograms show a relatively high incidence of abnormal findings. Ford and Goodman reported only 7.3% normal spine roentgenograms in a group of 1614 patients evaluated for back pain. Scavone, Latshaw, and Rohrer reported a 46% incidence of abnormal incidental findings in lumbar spine films taken over 1 year in a university hospital. Unfortunately, when these roentgenographic abnormalities are critically evaluated with respect to the patients' complaints and physical findings, the correlation is very low. Fullenlove and Williams clearly identified the lack of definition between the roentgenographic findings in symptomatic, asymptomatic, and operated patients. Rockey et al. and Liang and Komaroff concluded that spinal roentgenograms on the initial visit for acute low back pain do not contribute to

patient care and are not cost effective. They recommended that plain roentgenograms be taken only after the initial therapy fails.

There is insignificant correlation between back pain and the roentgenographic findings of lumbar lordosis, transitional vertebra, disc space narrowing, disc vacuum sign, and claw spurs. Additionally, the entity of disc space narrowing is extremely hard to quantitate in all but the operated backs or in obviously abnormal circumstances. Frymoyer et al. in a study of 321 patients found that only when traction spurs and obvious disc space narrowing or both were present, did the incidence of severe back and leg pain, leg weakness, and numbness increase. These positive findings had no relationship to heavy lifting, vehicular exposure, or exposure to vibrating equipment. Other studies have shown some relationship between back pain and the findings of spondylolysis, spondylolisthesis, and adult scoliosis, but these findings can also be observed in the spine roentgenograms of asymptomatic patients.

Special roentgenographic views may be helpful in further defining or disproving the initial clinical roentgenographic impression. Oblique views are useful in further defining spondylolisthesis and spondylolysis but are of limited use in facet syndrome and hypertrophic arthritis of the lumbar spine. Conversely, in the cervical spine hypertrophic changes about the foramina are easily outlined. Lateral flexion and extension roentgenograms may reveal segmental instability. Hayes et al. attempted to identify the pathologic level of abnormal lumbar spine flexion, but they found a wide range of motion in asymptomatic patients. They also found that translational movements of 2 to 3 mm were frequent. Therefore there is little correlation between abnormal motion and pathologic instability. There are no standards available to make this distinction. Unfortunately, the interpretation of these views is dependent on patient cooperation, patient positioning, and reproducible technique. Knutsson, Farfan, Kirkaldy-Willis, Stokes et al., and Macnab are excellent references on this topic. The Ferguson view (20-degree caudocephalic anteroposterior roentgenogram) has been shown by Wiltse et al. to be of value in the diagnosis of the "far out syndrome," that is, fifth root compression produced by a large transverse process of the fifth lumbar vertebra against the ala of the sacrum. Abel, Smith, and Allen note that angled caudal views localized to areas of concern may show evidence of facet or laminar pathologic conditions.

Myelography

Myelography of the lumbar spine and especially of the cervical spine should not be taken lightly. The recent development and popularity of computed tomography (CT) of the spine have made myelography optional or unnecessary in many instances. The value of this procedure is the ability to check all disc levels for abnormality and to define intraspinal lesions. It may be unnecessary when the clinical and CT findings are in complete agreement. The primary indications for the procedure are suspicion of an intraspinal lesion or questionable diagnosis resulting from conflicting clinical findings and other studies. Additionally, myelography is of value in the previously operated spine and in spinal stenosis, especially when used in conjunction with reformatted CT scans done shortly after the myelography. Bell et al. found myelography more accurate than CT scanning for identifying herniated nucleus pulposus and only slightly more accurate than CT scanning in the detection of spinal stenosis. Szypryt et al. found myelography slightly less accurate than MRI in detecting spinal abnormalities.

Several contrast agents have been used for myelography: air, oil contrast, and water-soluble (absorbable) contrast including metrizamide (Amipaque), iohexol (Omnipaque), and iopamidol (Isovue-M). The water-soluble forms of contrast are now the most popular contrast agents. Since these agents are absorbable, the discomfort of removing them and the severity of the postmyelographic headache have been minimized.

Isophendylate (Pantopaque) was the contrast agent of choice from 1944 until the late 1970s (Fig. 84-4). This agent has a relatively low toxicity and provides excellent contrast. Unlike metrizamide, it should be removed after injection, and it does not require mixing. Because it is a more viscous material, the nerve roots are not as easily defined and its flow is more easily obstructed than is the flow of metrizamide. Isophendylate is a meningeal irritant that can cause an inflammatory response. Usually this response is mild and limited to an increase in cerebrospinal fluid white cell count, but the response may be more severe. The usual response is headache, backache, generalized aching, and neck pain. Rarely the response is severe with transient paralysis, cauda equina syndrome, and focal neurologic defects.

Arachnoiditis is a severe complication that has been attributed on occasion to the combination of isophendylate and blood in the cerebrospinal fluid. Unfortunately, this diagnosis usually is confirmed only by repeat myelography. Attempts at surgical neurolysis have resulted

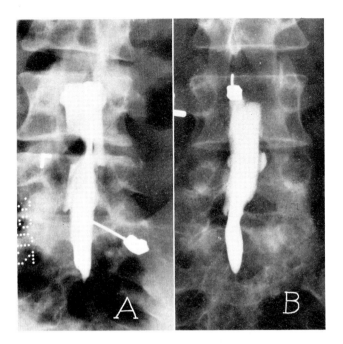

Fig. 84-4 **A,** Anteroposterior roentgenogram of iophendylate (Pantopaque) myelogram showing lumbar disc herniation. **B,** Oblique roentgenogram showing large L4-5 disc herniation.

in only short-term relief and a return of symptoms in 6 to 12 months after the procedure. Fortunately, time may decrease the effects of this serious problem in some patients, but progressive paralysis has been reported in rare instances. Arachnoiditis also may be caused by tuberculosis and other types of meningitis. Arachnoiditis has not been noted to be related to the use of water-soluble contrast, with or without injection, in the presence of a bloody tap.

Water-soluble contrast media are rapidly becoming the standard agents for myelography (Fig. 84-5). Their advantages include absorption by the body, enhanced definition of structures, tolerance, absorption from other soft tissues, and the ability to vary the dosage for different contrasts. Like isophendylate they are meningeal irritants, but they have not been associated with arachnoiditis. The complications of these agents include nausea, vomiting, confusion, and seizures. Rare complications include stroke, paralysis, and death. Iohexol and iopamidol have a significantly lower complication rate than metrizamide. The more common complications appear to be related to patient hydration, phenothiazines, tricyclics, and migration of contrast into the cranial vault. Many of the reported complications can be prevented or minimized by using the lowest possible dose to achieve the desired degree of contrast. Adequate hydration and discontinuation of phenothiazines and tricyclic drugs before, during, and after the procedure should also minimize the incidence of the more common reactions. Likewise, maintenance of at least a 30-degree elevation of the patient's head until the contrast is absorbed also should

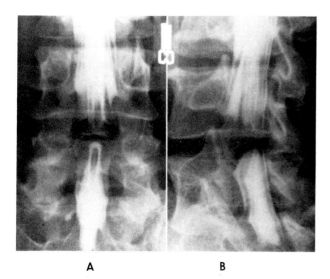

Fig. 84-5 **A,** Anteroposterior roentgenogram of metrizamide lumbar myelogram showing lumbar disc herniation. **B,** Oblique roentgenogram showing large L4-5 disc herniation.

help prevent reactions. Complete information about these agents and the dosages required is found in their package inserts.

Iohexol (Omnipaque) is a nonionic contrast medium approved for thoracic and lumbar myelography. The incidence of reactions to this medium is low. The most common reactions are headache (less than 20%), pain (8%), nausea (6%), and vomiting (3%). Serious reactions are very rare and include mental disturbances and aseptic meningitis (0.01%). Good hydration is essential to minimize the common reactions. The use of phenothiazine antinauseants is contraindicated when this medium is employed. Management before and after the procedure is the same as for metrizamide.

Air contrast is used rarely and probably should only be used in situations in which myelography is mandatory and the patient is extremely allergic to iodized materials. The resolution from such a procedure is poor. Recently air epidurography in conjunction with CT has been suggested in patients in whom further definition between postoperative scar and recurrent disc material is required.

Myelographic technique begins with a careful explanation of the procedure to the patient before its initiation. Hydration of the patient before the procedure may minimize the postmyelographic complaints. Heavy sedation rarely is needed. Proper equipment, including a fluoroscopic unit with a spot film device, image intensification, tiltable table, and television monitoring, is useful.

■ *TECHNIQUE.* Place the patient prone on the fluoroscopic table. Use of an abdominal pillow is optional. Prepare the back in the usual surgical fashion. Determine needle placement by the suspected pathologic level. Placement of the needle cephalad to L2-3

is extremely dangerous because of the chance of damage to the conus medullaris.

Infiltrate the selected area of injection with a local anesthetic. Use an 18-gauge needle for isophendylate injections and a smaller one for metrizamide injections. Midline needle placement usually minimizes lateral nerve root irritation and epidural injection. Advance the needle with the bevel parallel to the long axis of the body. Subarachnoid placement may be enhanced by tilting the patient up to increase the intraspinal pressure and minimize the epidural space.

When the dura and arachnoid have been punctured, turn the bevel of the needle cephalad. A clear continuous flow of cerebrospinal fluid should continue with the patient in the prone position. Manometric studies may be performed at this time if desired or indicated. Remove 3 to 5 ml of cerebrospinal fluid for laboratory evaluation as indicated by the clinical suspicions. In most patients a cell count, differential white cell count, and protein analysis are performed.

Inject a test dose of the contrast material under fluoroscopic control to confirm a subarachnoid injection. If a mixed subdural-subarachnoid injection is suspected, change the needle depth; occasionally a lateral roentgenogram may be required to be sure of the proper depth. If there is good flow, inject the contrast material slowly.

Be certain of continued flow by occasionally drawing back on the syringe while injecting. If isophendylate is used, 3 to 6 ml is usually injected. The usual dose of metrizamide for lumbar myelography in an adult is 10 to 15 ml with a concentration of 170 to 190 mg/ml. Higher concentrations of water-soluble contrast are required if higher areas of the spine are to be demonstrated. Consult the package insert of the contrast used. The needle may be removed if a water-soluble contrast (metrizamide) is used. The needle must remain in place and be covered with a sterile towel if isophendylate is used.

Allow the contrast material to flow caudally for the best views of the lumbar roots and distal sac. Make spot films in the anteroposterior, lateral, and oblique projections. A full examination should include thoracic evaluation to about the level of T7 because lesions at the thoracic level may mimic lumbar disc disease. Take additional spot films as the contrast proceeds cranially.

If a total or cervical myelogram is desired, allow the contrast to proceed cranially. Extend the neck and head maximally to prevent or minimize intracranial migration of the contrast medium.

If isophendylate (oil contrast) was used, then remove the contrast medium by extracting through the original needle or a multiholed stylet inserted through the original needle or by inserting another needle if extraction through the first needle is difficult. Occasionally a small amount of medium is retained, but remove as much as possible.

If blood is encountered in the initial tap, abandon the procedure if oil contrast is to be used. It may be attempted again in several days if the patient has no symptoms related to the first tap and is well hydrated. If the proper needle position is confirmed in the anteroposterior and lateral views and cerebrospinal fluid flow is minimal or absent, suspect a neoplastic process. Then place the needle at a higher or lower level as indicated by the circumstances. If failure to obtain cerebrospinal fluid continues, abandon the procedure and reevaluate the clinical picture.

The most common technical complications of myelography are significant retention of contrast medium (oil contrast only), persistent headache from a dural leak, and epidural injection. These problems usually are minor. Persistent dural leaks usually are responsive to a blood patch. With the use of a water-soluble contrast medium, the persistent abnormalities caused by retained medium and epidural injection are eliminated.

Computed Tomography

Computed tomography has revolutionized the diagnosis of spinal disease (Fig. 84-6). As with any new and revolutionary technique, the levels of technical capability vary greatly. This has resulted in conflicting reports as to the efficacy of CT scans in the diagnosis of disc herniations when compared with myelography and other techniques. Most clinicians now agree that CT is an extremely useful diagnostic tool in the evaluation of spinal disease.

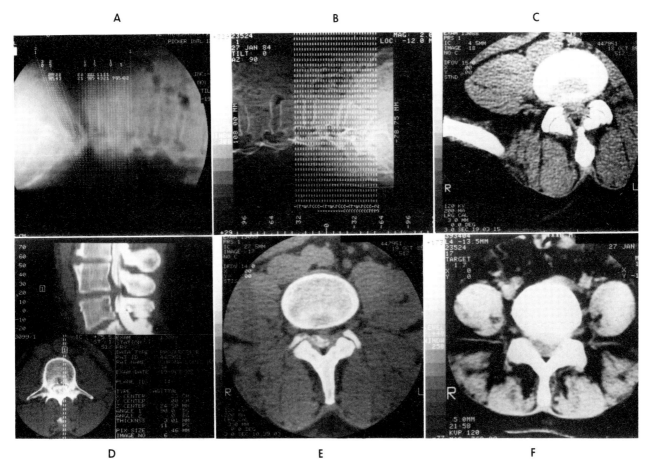

Fig. 84-6 **A,** CT scan "scout view" of lumbar disc herniation at lumbar disc level showing angled gantry technique. **B,** CT scan "scout view" of straight gantry technique. **C,** CT scan of lumbar disc herniation at L4-5 disc level showing cross-sectional anatomy with gantry straight. **D,** CT scan of L4-5 disc herniation at lumbar disc level showing cross-sectional, sagittal, and coronal anatomy using computerized reformatted technique. **E,** CT scan of L4-5 disc herniation at lumbar disc level showing cross-sectional anatomy 2 hours after metrizamide myelography. **F,** CT scan of lumbar disc herniation at L4-5 disc level showing cross-sectional anatomy after intravenous injection for greater soft tissue contrast.

The most recent advances in technology and computer software have resulted in the ability to reformat the standard axial cuts in almost any direction and magnify the images so that exact measurements of various structures can be made. Software is even available to evaluate the density of a selected vertebra and compare it with vertebrae of the normal population to give a numerically reproducible estimate of vertebral density to quantitate osteopenia.

Numerous types of CT studies for the spine are available. These studies vary from institution to institution and even within institutions. One must be careful in ordering the study to be certain that the areas of clinical concern are included.

Several basic routines are used in most institutions. The most common routine for lumbar disc disease is to take serial cuts through the last three lumbar intervertebral discs. If the equipment has a tilting gantry, an attempt is made to keep the axis of the cuts parallel with the disc. The problem with this is that frequently the gantry cannot tilt enough to allow a parallel beam through the lowest disc space. This technique does not allow demonstration of the canal at the pedicles. Another method is to make cuts through the discs without tilting the gantry. Once again, the entire canal is not demonstrated, and the lower cuts frequently have the lower and upper end plates of adjacent vertebrae superimposed in the same view.

The final and most complex method is to make multiple parallel cuts at equal intervals. This method allows the computer to reconstruct the images in different planes — usually sagittal and coronal. These reformatted views allow an almost three-dimensional view of the spine and most of its structures. The greatest benefit of this technique is the ability to see beyond the limits of the dural sac and root sleeves. Thus the diagnosis of foraminal encroachment by bone or disc material can now be made in the face of a normal myelogram. The proper procedure can be chosen that fits all of the pathologic conditions involved.

Optimum reformatted CT should include enlarged axial and sagittal views with clear notation as to laterality and sequence of cuts. Several sections of the axial cuts should include the local soft tissue and contiguous abdominal contents. Finally, darker cuts are necessary to show bony detail with reference to the facet joints. Naturally this study should be centered on the level of greatest clinical concern. The study can be further enhanced when it is done following water contrast myelography or with intravenous contrast medium. Enhancement techniques are especially useful when the spine being evaluated has been operated on previously.

This noninvasive, painless, outpatient procedure can supply more information about spinal disease than was previously available with a battery of invasive and noninvasive tests usually requiring hospitalization. Unfortunately, CT neither demonstrates intraspinal tumors and

arachnoiditis nor differentiates scar from new disc herniation. Recently Bell et al. compared myelography to CT scanning and noted that myelography was more accurate. They did not compare the results of postmyelogram CT scanning. Weiss et al. and Teplick and Haskin in separate reports have suggested that the use of intravenous contrast medium (Fig. 84-6, *E*) followed by CT can improve the definition between scar and new disc herniation. Myelography is still required to demonstrate intraspinal tumors and to "run" the spine to detect occult or unsuspected lesions. New developments with low-dose metrizamide or iohexol myelography with reformatted CT done as an outpatient procedure may allow a maximum of information to be obtained with a minimum of time, risk, discomfort, and cost.

Magnetic Resonance Imaging

MRI is the newest technologic advance in spinal imaging. This technique uses the interaction of nuclei of a selected atom with an external oscillating electromagnetic field that is changing as a function of time at a particular frequency. Energy is absorbed and subsequently released by selected nuclei at particular frequencies after irradiation with radiofrequency electromagnetic energy. This reaction is recorded and formatted by computer in a pattern similar to CT. Present MRI techniques concentrate on imaging the proton (hydrogen) distribution. The advantages of this technique include the ability to demonstrate intraspinal tumors, examine the entire spine, and identify degenerative discs. Unfortunately, the equipment

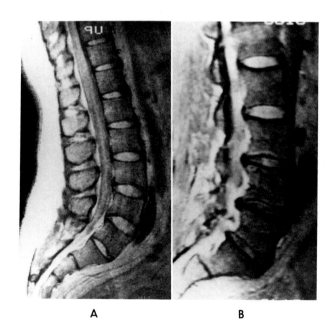

A   B

Fig. 84-7   Magnetic resonance imaging of lumbar spine. **A,** Normal T$_2$-weighted image. **B,** T$_2$-weighted image showing degenerative bulging and/or herniated discs at L3-4, L4-5, and L5-S1.

required for this procedure is costly and requires specially constructed facilities (Fig. 84-7).

Szypryt et al. found MRI slightly better than myelography in the identification of spinal lesions. The MRI accuracy in their study was 88% and the myelographic accuracy was 75%; combined accuracy was 94%. MRI is clearly superior in the detection of disc degeneration, tumors, and infections. Most MRI scans allow evaluation of a complete spinal group (such as cervical, thoracic, or lumbar) rather than three segments. They also can clearly view areas in the foramen.

MRI is so accurate that a significant number of lesions may be identified in asymptomatic patients. Gibson et al. found disc degeneration in all symptomatic adolescent patients and in 4 of 20 asymptomatic adolescents. Boden et al. found cervical spinal abnormalities in 14% of asymptomatic patients younger than 40 years of age and in 28% of asymptomatic patients over the age of 40 years. Cervical disc degeneration was found in 25% of those younger than 40 years of age and in 60% of those 60 years and older. They studied lumbar MRI scans of 67 asymptomatic patients and found that 20% of those younger than 60 years of age had herniated nuclei pulposi. Asymptomatic abnormalities were found in 57% of those 60 years of age or older. Lumbar disc degeneration was found in 35% of those from 20 to 39 years of age and in 100% of those over 50 years of age.

Positron Emission Tomography

Positron emission tomography (PET) and single-photon emission CT are other similar techniques that may offer additional diagnostic information in the near future. Collier et al. and others have recently reported that single-photon emission CT is more sensitive in the identification of symptomatic sites in spondylolisthesis than planar bone scintigraphy. PET scanners are considered experimental by most third-party payers at this time. Their use is presently limited to a few centers.

No test is perfect. Our present technical ability may exceed our clinical ability to identify the source of the pain. Roentgenography, CT, myelography, and their combinations all may frequently show numerous pathologic conditions. The question is which if any is responsible for the patient's symptoms? The incidence of lumbar disc herniation in asymptomatic patients undergoing myelography for other reasons is near 30%. The incidence of asymptomatic pathologic conditions in patients being studied with CT is presently unknown but probably is even higher. The answer lies in a meticulous clinical evaluation and comparison with studies that one hopes will be confirmatory.

Other Diagnostic Tests

Numerous diagnostic tests have been used in the diagnosis of intervertebral disc disease in addition to roent-genography, myelography, and CT. The primary advantage of these tests is to rule out diseases other than primary disc herniation, spinal stenosis, and spinal arthritis.

Electromyography is the most notable of these tests. One advantage of electromyography is in the identification of peripheral neuropathy and diffuse neurologic involvement indicative of higher or lower lesions. Macnab et al. report that denervation of the paraspinal muscles is found in 97% of previously operated spines as a result of the surgery. Therefore paraspinal muscles in the previously operated patient usually are abnormal and are not reliable for a diagnosis.

Somatosensory evoked potentials (SSEP) are another diagnostic modality that may identify the level of root involvement. Unlike electromyography this test can only indicate a problem between the cerebral cortex and the end organs. The test cannot pinpoint the level of the lesion. This procedure is of benefit during surgery to avoid neurologic damage. Both electromyography and SSEP depend on the skill of the technician and interpreter. Delamarter et al. used cortical evoked potentials to monitor experimentally induced spinal stenosis. They noted changes in the cortical response at 25% constriction. This was the only change noted in this group. Higher degrees of constriction were accompanied by much more significant changes. Somatosensory evoked potentials constitute an extremely sensitive monitoring technique.

Bone scans are another procedure in which positive findings usually are not indicative of intervertebral disc disease but can confirm neoplastic, traumatic, and arthritic problems in the spine. Various laboratory tests such as a complete blood count, differential white cell count, biochemical profile, urinalysis, and sedimentation rate are extremely good screening procedures for other causes of pain in the spine. Rheumatoid screening studies such as rheumatoid arthritis latex, antinuclear antibody, lupus erythematosus cell preparation, and HLA-B27 are also useful when indicated by the clinical picture.

Some tests that were developed to enhance the diagnosis of intervertebral disc disease have been surpassed by the more advanced technology of reformatted CT. Lumbar venography and sonographic measurement of the intervertebral canal are two such examples.

INJECTION STUDIES

Whenever the diagnosis is in doubt and the complaints appear real or the pathologic condition is diffuse, the problem is identifying the source of pain. The use of local anesthetics or contrast media in various specific anatomic areas may be useful. These agents are relatively simple, safe, and minimally painful to the patient. Contrast media such as diatrizoate meglumine (Hypague), iothalamate meglumine (Conray), iohexol, iopamidol, and metrizamide have been used for discography and

Table 84-2 Pain scale and diary

0	No pain
1	Mild pain that you are aware of but not bothered by
2	Moderate pain that you can tolerate without medication
3	Moderate pain that is discomforting and requires medication
4-5	More severe and you begin to feel antisocial
6	Severe pain
7-9	Intensely severe pain
10	Most severe pain; you might contemplate suicide over it

Activity	Comments	Location of pain	Time	Severity of pain (0 to 10)

From White AH: Back school and other conservative approaches to low back pain, St Louis, 1983, Mosby-Year Book, Inc.

blocks with no reported ill effects. Recent reports of neurologic complications with contrast media used for discography and subsequent chymopapain injection are well documented. The best choice of a contrast medium for demonstrating structures outside the subarachnoid space is an absorbable medium with low reactivity because it might be inadvertently injected into the subarachnoid space. Local anesthetics such as lidocaine (Xylocaine), tetracaine (Pontocaine), and bupivacaine (Marcaine) are used frequently both epidurally and intradurally. The use of bupivacaine should be limited to low concentrations and low volumes because of recent reports of death following epidural anesthesia using concentrations of 0.75% or higher. Steroids prepared for intramuscular injection also have been used frequently in the epidural space with few and usually transient complications. The effect of long-acting cortisone in the intrathecal space is questionable at this time. Isotonic saline is the only other injectable medium used frequently about the spine with no reported adverse reactions.

When injection techniques are used, grading the degree of the patient's pain is helpful. This can be done by asking the patient to grade the degree of pain experienced at that moment on a 0 to 10 scale (Table 84-2). This also can be incorporated into a pain diary that is continued after the injection.

Differential Spinal

The graded spinal anesthetic or differential spinal is the simplest of general screening tests for chronic, long-standing, and constant lower back and leg pain. The primary value of this test is to separate patients into specific clinical groups on the basis of placebo, physiologic, and nonphysiologic responses. This test appears to cover areas not touched by psychologic testing. The correlation between the abnormal responses and abnormal results on the Minnesota Multiphasic Personality Inventory (MMPI) is only 50%.

Our results indicate that patients who are not relieved of their pain with a full spinal anesthetic (nonphysiologic response) have not been and are not likely to be helped by spinal surgery. These patients frequently are using large doses of narcotic analgesics without relief of pain. Presently these patients are given counseling, taken off all narcotics, and encouraged to return to their previous occupations.

Patients who are relieved with a spinal anesthetic are subjected to further studies to determine the source of the pain. Patients who exhibit the placebo response are assumed to have some source for their pain, but more conservative, noninvasive treatments are used. There is no difference between the placebo group and the physiologic group with reference to the potential success of surgery. Unfortunately, this test cannot detect the patient who is feigning pain. Such a patient may be normal in all aspects of evaluation but he may show inconsistency in response during the progression of the test.

The use of the differential spinal should be limited to patients with constant, unremitting lower back or leg pain unrelieved by usual means and with equivocal clinical and roentgenographic findings. The patient is informed that a test will be performed to see if the pain can be relieved. All narcotic pain medication and, if possible, all other medications are withdrawn for 12 hours before the procedure. No preoperative medication is given. Since this is a spinal anesthetic, we prefer that it be performed by an anesthesiologist familiar with the technique. It is suggested that the treating physician be present during the procedure to monitor the results. The patient is asked to grade the pain on a 0 to 10 scale with 0 being no pain and 10 a pain so intense that if it were to continue, suicide would be contemplated (Table 84-2). The painful areas are also delineated by the patient. An examination of the lower extremities, including straight-leg raising, motor strength, deep tendon reflexes, light touch, and pinprick sensibility, is performed repeatedly during the procedure.

■ *TECHNIQUE.* Position the patient with the painful side against the table (this may vary with the anesthesiologist's choice of anesthetic agent). Surgically prepare the back as for a spinal tap. Infiltrate the skin with a local anesthetic at the chosen level of entry (usually L4-5). Advance a 22-gauge spinal needle into the subarachnoid space. A good flow of cerebrospinal fluid is mandatory, and a sample should be taken for laboratory evaluation. Then ask the patient to grade the pain. Inject the anesthetic agent at 10- to 15-minute intervals. Repeat patient questioning and examination before each injection. When the patient is completely relieved of pain and the examination does not exacerbate the pain, terminate the procedure. The initial description of this procedure by Ahlgren et al. used procaine hydrochloride. The reader is referred to the works of Ahlgren and others for further details of the procedure and anesthetic concentrations. We prefer to use lidocaine at concentrations of 0.5%, 1.0%, and 1.5%. The maximum dosage of lidocaine that we use is 100 mg.

Root Infiltration or Block

The individual areas of the spine that can produce back pain are bone, joints, nerve roots, and the outer edge of the anulus. Injection of local anesthetics into these areas for exacerbating pain has been used for some time. These procedures are invasive, are mildly uncomfortable, and require some patient preparation and cooperation to get the maximum information. The simplest technique involves the instillation of 1% lidocaine into a compressed vertebral body at the time of needle biopsy. It is only slightly more complex to inject nerve roots just distal to their exit from the intervertebral foramen, individual facet joints, and the intervertebral disc.

Nerve root block or selective nerve root infiltration has been described by Macnab as a method to identify nerve root compression at the level of the intervertebral foramen. The technique has been expanded by Tajima, Furukawa, and Kuramochi and by Krempen and Smith. The primary indications are radicular complaints or findings with inconclusive or confusing studies. This test is not of benefit in identifying patients with functional overlay. It is primarily a preoperative test to identify and confirm the area of primary pain. The test is most useful

when the nerve root is entrapped laterally as in foraminal stenosis. Complete pain relief may not be obtained in simple disc herniations because more than one root may be affected. The diagnostic usefulness of this test is minimal in the placebo-positive patient.

CERVICAL NERVE ROOT INJECTION. Cervical root injection as described by Kikuchi, Macnab, and Moreau is another technique that may identify the level of a symptomatic pathologic condition. As with lumbar root injection, the nerve root is identified with the injection of contrast material, and a local anesthetic is then injected. If the patient's symptomatic pain is abolished by the injection, then that root or level is presumed to be the site of the offending pathologic condition. Unlike lumbar roots, cervical roots emerge from the intervertebral foramen above the level of the segment (Fig. 84-8). The roots lie anterolaterally in the costotransverse canal after they emerge from the intervertebral foramen.

The roots are covered by an epiradicular sheath peripherally. This sheath is a continuation of the epidural membrane that surrounds the dura centrally. Proper identification of the epiradicular sheath is mandatory for successful cervical root injection.

■ *TECHNIQUE (KIKUCHI, MACNAB, AND MOREAU)*

Anterior approach. Position the patient supine with the neck extended and rotated to the opposite side (as in cervical discography). Pull the carotid sheath laterally by the fingers, which are placed into the sulcus between the sheath and midline structures. Insert the needle, directed under image intensification control, as far as the tip of the transverse process immediately lateral to the vertebral artery. Inject a small amount of water-soluble radiopaque dye to ensure that the needle is in the epiradicular sheath. If the needle is properly positioned, the root will be outlined by the contrast material. Then inject a small amount of local anesthetic. After a short time, question the patient to determine his pain symptoms.

Lateral approach. Place the patient in the supine position with the chin pointing upward and identify the transverse process using the fingers. Insert the needle 0.5 cm anterior to the line joining the tip of the mastoid process and the tubercle of Chassaignac, directed under image intensification control to strike the transverse process at one level above the suspected root. Then withdraw the needle and direct it caudally and medially. This avoids the inadvertent insertion of the needle into the intervertebral foramen. Inject contrast medium and anesthetic as in the anterior approach.

Posterior approach. Place the patient on his side with the affected extremity uppermost. To inject the

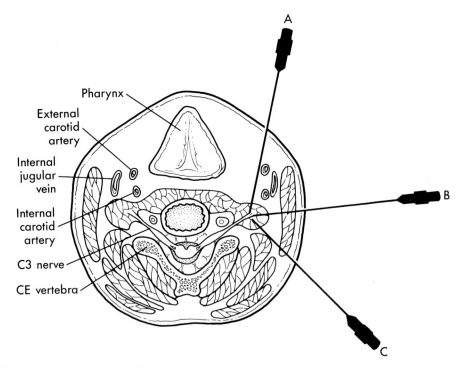

Fig. 84-8 Cross-sectional diagram of cervical spine indicating anterior *(A)*, lateral *(B)*, and posterior *(C)* approaches for cervical root infiltration. (From Kikuchi S, Macnab I, and Moreau P: J Bone Joint Surg 63-B:272, 1981.)

C3, C4, C5, and C6 nerve roots insert the needle, directed under image intensification control at an angle of 45 degrees, 5 cm from the midline and advance it until it touches the transverse process. Injection of the C7 and C8 roots by this approach is difficult because of the thickness of the tissues at the puncture site and the size of the transverse process.

Complications. Potential complications of cervical root injection include puncture of a major blood vessel, penetration of the apex of the lung with resultant pneumothorax, penetration of the dura and spinal cord injury, and injury to the root with a large cutting needle. It is not uncommon to precipitate a vagal reaction with injection. The use of atropine may minimize this reaction. Kikuchi, Macnab, and Moreau used the anterior approach in all of their 75 patients. They noted no complications from this procedure. When cervical discography reproduced the symptoms of pain in this group, the symptoms were abolished by cervical root injection.

Although this series included patients with and without obvious symptomatic levels, this technique is most helpful in the identification of a painful segment in patients with refractory cervicobrachial pain with normal or equivocal studies. We have limited experience with this technique. The use of a small-bore, blunted, 45-degree needle similar to that used with cervical discography is suggested. Metrizamide and lidocaine have been the only contrast medium and anesthetic agent reported injected with this technique.

LUMBAR NERVE ROOT INJECTION

■ *TECHNIQUE.* The procedure is carried out with the aid of an image intensifier. Equipment with the ability to take lateral roentgenograms also is desirable. Prepare the patient by explaining the technique and asking him to gauge the level of his pain on the 0 to 10 scale with 0 being no pain and 10 being a pain so intense that its persistence might result in the contemplation of suicide. Atropine may be given before the procedure to prevent a vasovagal reaction, but no other medication is given at that time.

Place the patient on the image intensification table in the prone position. Prepare the back in the standard surgical fashion. Identify the proper level of injection by placing a needle or other metallic object at about the level of the transverse process of the involved vertebra. When the proper position is identified, anesthetize the skin with a local anesthetic agent about 3 to 4 cm from the midline or spinous process. A selection of spinal needles ranging from 10.2 to 20.3 cm (4 to 8 inches) in length in sizes from 18- to 22-gauge should be available.

Advance the needle almost perpendicularly so that it skirts the inferior edge of the transverse process near the outline of the lateral border of the vertebral body (Fig. 84-9). Slight resistance will be encountered when the needle passes through the intertransverse ligament. When the nerve is pierced, the patient will usually complain of an exacerbation or appearance of radicular pain. At this point take a

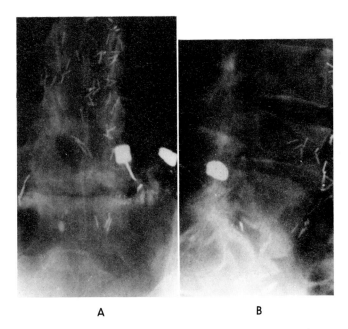

A   B

Fig. 84-9 **A,** Proper placement of needle about two finger breadths lateral to midline and inserted to level of foramen. **B,** Anteroposterior roentgenogram of L5 root injection showing metrizamide outlining root.

lateral roentgenogram to be certain that the needle point is at the level of the intervertebral foramen.

When certain that the needle point is at the proper level, inject contrast medium if desired. Only 0.2 ml of contrast medium is needed. The nerve root sleeve should be easily outlined. If only a ball of contrast medium is seen, the needle is not in the sleeve and should be redirected. Inject 2 ml of 1% lidocaine and question the patient as to the degree of pain relief using the 0 to 10 scale. An optional method is to use a larger bolus of lidocaine and omit

the contrast medium. If an 18-gauge needle is used, then a longer 22-gauge needle should be placed in it just before traversing the intertransverse ligament to avoid damage to the nerve root. We prefer to use a 22-gauge spinal needle for this technique to prevent nerve root damage.

To inject the first sacral root, place the needle through the first dorsal foramen of the sacrum on the involved side. The needle usually is placed 2 to 3 cm distal and medial to the transverse process of the fifth lumbar vertebra. The angle can vary from 90 degrees (perpendicular) to 45 degrees directed cephalad (Fig. 84-10).

LUMBAR FACET INJECTION. Lumbar facet injection is another simple technique that may establish a source of back and buttock pain. The term "facet syndrome" was coined in 1933 by Ghormley. Mooney reported extensively on the syndrome and added a technique for local injection of the joint as a therapeutic and diagnostic procedure. Others, most notably Shealy and Rees, have advocated operative denervation of the facet joints. Facet injection is best limited to the patient with primary lower back, buttock, or thigh pain with local point tenderness lateral to the midline and pain that is exacerbated by maneuvers that increase lumbar extension. Patients with radiculopathy should be excluded because they may have more pain after this procedure. Like any steroid injection into a joint, the degree and length of relief vary. Most patients should be completely relieved of pain with the injection of an anesthetic, but prolonged relief may vary from several days to months. The return of pain is usually associated with increased activity. In many patients nonsteroidal anti-inflammatory medication, a lumbar corset or brace to limit lumbar motion, and education in proper back care may be used before and after such injections to decrease the intensity of the symptoms.

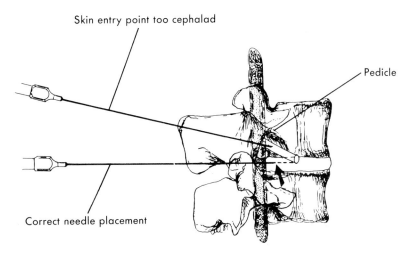

Skin entry point too cephalad

Pedicle

Correct needle placement

Fig. 84-10 Diagram contrasts correct needle placement with needle that entered from a point too high. (From Chung BU: In Brown JE, Nordby EJ, and Smith L: Chemonucleolysis, Thorofare, NJ, 1985, Slack.)

Lumbar facet injection is a simple technique that can be done as an outpatient procedure. Image intensification equipment is quite helpful, but the ability to get lateral views is unnecessary. The procedure is explained to the patient, and he is asked to rate the pain on the 0 to 10 scale before initiation of the procedure. Medication before the procedure is unnecessary unless atropine is desired to prevent a vasovagal reaction.

Murtagh reported that 54% of 194 patients injected had relief of pain for longer than 3 months. Eisenstein and Parry found distinct histologic changes in the facet joint cartilage in 12 patients who had limited lumbar fusion facet syndrome. Jackson, Jacobs, and Montesano reported only a 29% mean initial pain relief in 454 patients with nonradicular back pain who were injected by this technique. They concluded that the facet joints rarely are the sole cause of back pain. We agree with their conclusions and limit this procedure to those few patients who have specific back pain over the facet joints (two finger-breadths lateral to the spinous processes), with reproducible, isolated point tenderness in the same area on examination and exacerbation of that specific pain with the facet maneuver and passive extension in a prone position. Relief of back pain with this procedure should not be used as a predictor of the success of a spinal fusion. This procedure should be viewed in the same light as steroid injection into any other diarthrodial joint.

■ *TECHNIQUE.* Place the patient prone on a radiolucent table and prepare the back in the usual sterile fashion after first determining the levels of point tenderness. Anesthetize the skin about 2 cm lateral to the midline in a linear fashion centered about the area of point tenderness. In many patients needle placement at the point of maximal tenderness will be at the level of the facet joint. It is preferable to place the needle at the inferior corner of the joint. Advance the standard 20-gauge spinal needle until the tip strikes bone.

Once proper placement in the anteroposterior plane is achieved, ask the patient to turn toward the opposite side. When the proper oblique angle to delineate the facet joint is noted by fluoroscopy, ask the patient to hold that position. Position the needle so that it appears to enter the joint (Fig. 84-11). Frequently, the patient will complain of an exacerbation of symptoms when the capsule of the joint is entered. Occasionally in markedly arthritic joints thick, yellow synovial fluid can be aspirated. At this point inject a small amount of contrast material (0.5 ml) to verify intraarticular needle placement. Frequently two or three contiguous joints must be injected to relieve the pain. Take spot roentgenograms in the anteroposterior and oblique projections to document placement of the needles. A local anesthetic and a long-acting intramuscular steroid preparation can then be injected into and about the joint. At the completion of the procedure ask the patient to grade the pain from 0 to 10. If the patient is injected with a steroid preparation, tell him to expect some increased back soreness for the first few days. Immediate return to heavy activity is not recommended if a prolonged therapeutic response is desired.

Most patients should notice significant relief of back and buttock pain after this procedure as a result of the local anesthetic. If a patient notes increased pain after injection, primary root compression or functional overlay should be considered.

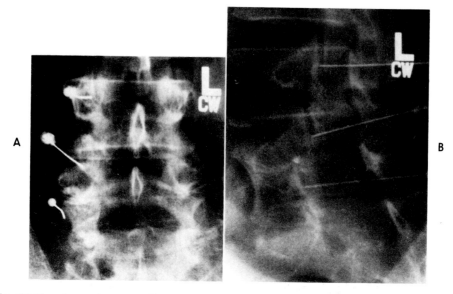

Fig. 84-11 Approximate needle position on anteroposterior, **A,** and lateral, **B,** roentgenograms of facet block. Roentgenograms also show normal facet arthrogram.

Discography

Discography has been used since the late 1940s for the experimental and clinical evaluation of disc disease in both the cervical and lumbar regions of the spine. Lindblom first described discography in 1948. Since that time, it has been used for experimental and clinical evaluation of the intervertebral disc in the cervical and lumbar spine. Discography has been and still is a technique of great controversy regarding the clinical usefulness of the data obtained.

Advocates claim that it allows the proper choice of symptomatic disc level for intervertebral fusion. Critics note the high incidence of degenerative discs in asymptomatic patients and question the reliability of pain reproduction with the technique. It is still the most exact way to determine disc degeneration. Unfortunately, asymptomatic disc degeneration is common, and the correlation with various painful conditions about the back is hard to substantiate. In addition, the technique is not superior to myelography in the detection of disc rupture.

The application of the technique should be limited to those patients in whom conservative treatment has failed and other evaluation studies are normal or conflicting. We have found the technique of more use in identifying normal discs than pathologic ones. Kikuchi, Macnab, and Moreau warn that needle placement is critical to the accurate reproduction of pain. Needle placement in the end plate may result in pain. Therefore needle placement in the nucleus is critical before injection. Interpretation of the results on the roentgenographic finding of disc degeneration alone is not recommended. The patient response to injection is critical.

The use of discography as an indication for spinal fusion has been advanced by some investigators. Colhoun et al. reported 89% improvement in 137 patients who had pain on discography and who had successful anterior or posterior fusion. They also noted that the success rate was only 52% when the pain was not re-created on discography but the disc was morphologically degenerative. Johnson and Macnab reported using discography to identify pseudarthroses. They noted re-creation of the pain at the mobile segment or the level above the fusion. Johnson performed repeat discography on 34 patients after a mean interval of 16 months and noted no changes in the previously injected discs. Only one disc was degenerative at the second procedure. Walsh et al. reported a carefully performed comparison of discography in normal volunteers and in symptomatic patients. They noted degenerative but painless discs in the volunteers. There were no false positive results, and specificity of the test was 100%. The exact implications of a positive discogram and its correlation to spinal fusion or disc excision remain to be determined.

LUMBAR DISCOGRAPHY. With the advent of chemonucleolysis, lumbar discography has reemerged as a technique to confirm needle placement. The original technique described a transdural approach to the lumbar disc. This approach is not recommended because of the potential risk of intradural leak of neurotoxic contrast medium and other agents. We have limited the indications for this technique to those rare patients in whom the needle placement in a chemonucleolysis procedure is in doubt and to those in whom all other procedures have failed to localize the source of pain or pathologic condition. The fear of disc degeneration initiated by this procedure has not been proven or disproven. Kahanovitz et al. found no evidence of gross histologic change in canine discs examined up to 10 weeks after injection with metrizamide, diatrizoate meglumine, and saline. The most common complication resulting from discography is a disc space infection. Fraser, Osti, and Vernon-Roberts noted a 2.7% rate of discitis with a single-needle technique and 0.7% with a double-needle technique. Others have reported a 0.5% rate of infection with the double-needle technique.

Lumbar discography is a simple procedure that can be done as an outpatient procedure if additional injections are not performed. The procedure is explained to the patient before its initiation. Medication is not required unless atropine is desired to prevent a vasovagal reaction. Image intensification equipment with the ability to produce anteroposterior and lateral views of the spine is necessary. A selection of spinal needles ranging from 4 to 9 inches (10 to 22.9 cm) long and 18- to 22-gauge should be available.

■ *TECHNIQUE (Fig. 84-12)*. **Place the patient on the image intensification table in the left lateral decubitus position with the hips and knees flexed at 45 degrees with needle placement on the right side. If the injection is to be at the L5-S1 disc, place a roll or inflatable balloon under the left iliac crest. Confirm exact anteroposterior and lateral positioning of the patient by image intensification. Prepare and drape the back in the standard surgical fashion.**

Using a long radiopaque object such as a steel ruler, identify the disc levels of interest. Use a marking pen to draw a line on the back parallel with and at the level of each disc to be injected. Then make marks about 8.5 cm lateral (or a distance determined by triangulation) to the midline or spinous process bisecting the disc lines. If a plastic adhesive drape is used to cover the skin it may be advisable to remove the drape over the points of needle insertion to avoid carrying bits of drape into the disc. Infiltrate the skin with a local anesthetic at each level. Make a small stab wound with a No. 11 blade. Direct a spinal needle of at least 18-gauge and 4 inches (10 cm) long parallel with the disc line at about 45 degrees to the back angling toward the spine. Inject additional anesthetic as the needle is advanced.

Monitor proper alignment in both anteroposterior and lateral projections as the needle is advanced. When the level of the lamina is reached, the needle

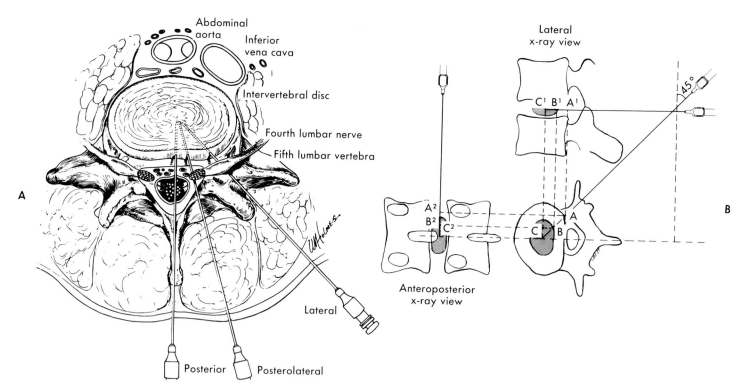

Fig. 84-12 Needle approaches used for discography. We prefer lateral approach. (**A,** From Brown JE and **B,** from Chung BU: In Brown JE, Nordby EJ, and Smith L: Chemonucleolysis, Thorofare, NJ, 1985, Slack.)

should be near the outer border of the vertebral bodies and disc in the anteroposterior view and at the lamina in the lateral view. A double-needle technique is recommended. If the larger needle (usually 18-gauge) is blunted, advance the needle as far as the disc in both anteroposterior and lateral planes. Then insert the smaller needle (usually 22-gauge and at least 2 inches longer) into the larger needle and advance it into the disc.

When the needle enters the disc, a distinct change in resistance and a gritty sensation are noted. The only pain that occurs with this maneuver is the result of nerve root irritation or penetration by the needle just lateral to the disc. Aspiration of the needle should be performed if there is any question of dural penetration by the needle. If the dura is penetrated, it is probably best to abandon the procedure (this may depend on the purpose of the procedure and the contrast medium). Proper needle placement should put the needle slightly posterior in the lateral view and dead center over the spinous process in the anteroposterior view. Then inject 1 to 2 ml of contrast medium and take roentgenograms in the anteroposterior and lateral views for documentation (Fig. 84-13).

Usually more than one disc is injected when the procedure is done for diagnostic purposes. If the L5-S1 disc is to be injected, place the needle near

the entrance for the L4-5 needle and advance it about 45 degrees to the plane of the back and 35 to 40 degrees caudally. Difficulty may be encountered in entering the disc at this angle. The use of the double-needle technique or putting a slight bend in the tip of the insertion needle may help "skive" the needle off the endplate of S1. It is common to encounter the L5 root when entering this disc. In some patients with a high iliac crest it is impossible to place a needle in this disc. If a blunt 18-gauge needle and a prebent 22-gauge needle are used, the 18-gauge needle must touch the disc. Failure to do this may result in damage to neural structures when the prebent needle is inserted. Cadaver practice with the prebent needles is suggested before attempting to use this equipment.

CERVICAL DISCOGRAPHY. The technique of cervical discography is considerably different from lumbar discography. This procedure is primarily indicated for the patient with persistent neck or arm pain without evidence of functional overlay but with normal myelography and CT in whom all conservative therapy has failed. This procedure usually is done as a preoperative test for anterior intervertebral fusion. Image intensification equipment capable of both anteroposterior and lateral exposure is required. Standard 1-inch (2.5 cm), 21-gauge needles and 3- to 4-inch (7.5 to 10 cm), 25-gauge nee-

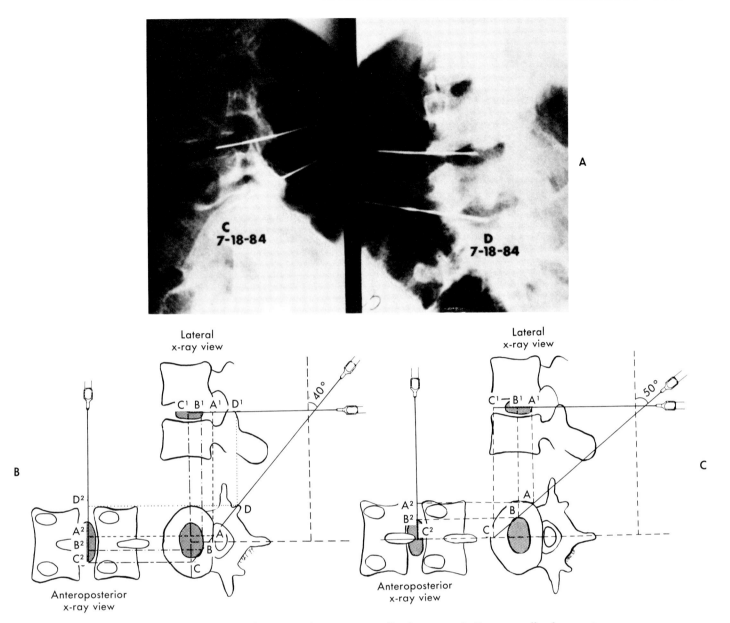

Fig. 84-13   Examples of proper and improper needle placement. **A,** Proper needle placement at center of nucleus. **B,** Needle placed too far medially. **C,** Needle placed too far laterally. (From Chung BU: In Brown JE, Nordby EJ, and Smith L: Chemonucleolysis, Thorofare, NJ, 1985, Slack.)   *Continued.*

dles are also required. Minimal patient premedication is necessary. Atropine may minimize any vasovagal reaction.

■ *TECHNIQUE.* Place the patient on the image intensification table in the supine position with the head extended. Prepare and drape the neck in the standard surgical fashion. Ask the patient to grade the degree of neck and arm pain on the 0 to 10 scale. Mark the levels of disc insertion using a thin metal object such as a ruler placed parallel with the disc. Mark the skin laterally at that point using a skin marker.

Infiltrate the skin laterally near the neurovascular

bundle. Use the fingers of the left hand to palpate and pull this bundle laterally. Insert the short, blunt-beveled needle, avoiding the neurovascular bundle. Direct the second needle through the first needle at an angle of about 35 degrees from the sagittal plane toward the disc. Once again, central placement of the needle confirmed by anteroposterior and lateral roentgenograms is mandatory.

Slowly inject the contrast medium. Excessive pressure must be avoided to prevent extrusion of any disc fragments. The patient's response to the injection is critical. The proper evaluation of this response usually requires the injection of multiple

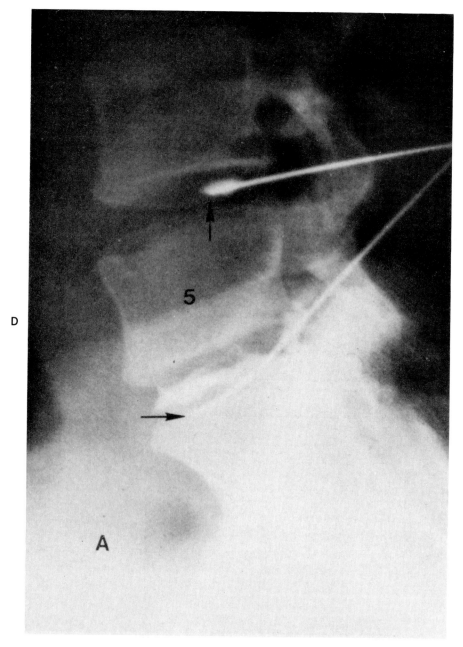

Fig. 84-13. cont'd   **D** and **E,** Upper needles show medial needle placement while lower needles show lateral placement.

discs and a comparison of the responses. Ask the patient to grade the degree of pain from 0 to 10 and localize the pain at the time of injection. Usually only one disc is painful on injection, and that disc should also be abnormal. Take great care to determine if the patient's pain pattern is re-created by the injection. The presence of a degenerative disc alone is not an indication for surgery. Pain at all levels of injection or a variable pain pattern should be interpreted as a negative response.

TRIANGULATION TECHNIQUE OF PERCUTANEOUS NEEDLE PLACEMENT. Lateral needle placement for dis-

cography, needle biopsy, or chemonucleolysis is mandatory to prevent intrathecal injection or dural injury. Because of differences in body size and iliac crest height a standard starting point for needle insertion is only a rough suggestion. Occasionally, considerable difficulty may be encountered with needle placement. Ford proposed a technique to preoperatively determine the lateral insertion distance and needle angle for lumbar chemonucleolysis and discography. This technique requires good lateral and anteroposterior roentgenograms with the skin edge visible posteriorly in the lateral view.

■ *TECHNIQUE (FORD).* Mark the center of the disc spaces to be injected on both anteroposterior and

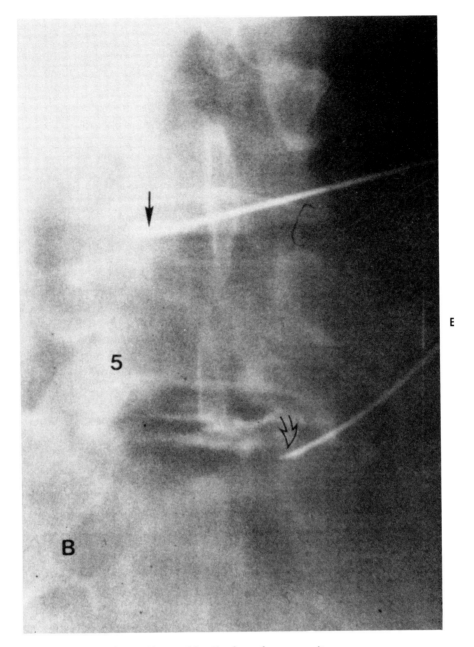

Fig. 84-13, cont'd For legend see opposite page.

lateral roentgenograms. Measure the distance in centimeters from the body surface to the apophyseal (facet) joint (*a* in Figs. 84-14 and 84-15). This is the point at which the needle should first touch the bone of, and then skid by, the apophyseal joint in its lateral approach to the anulus fibrosus and the nucleus pulposus. Then measure the distance from the apophyseal joint to the center of the disc space (*b* in Figs. 84-14 and 84-15). On the anteroposterior view of the disc space to be injected, measure the distance from the lateral edge of the apophyseal joint to the center of the nucleus pulposus (*c* in Fig. 84-15) (see also Fig. 84-16). Transfer line segments *a*,

b, and *c* in centimeters to a piece of paper, arranging them in a triangular form, as though creating a large CT scan at that vertebral level. Draw a line indicating the proper course of the needle from the skin surface and along the apophyseal joint to the center of the disc. Extend a line perpendicular to *a* at its skin-surface endpoint. The point at which the line intersects the pathway of the needle designates the approximate distance from the midline for the ideal start of the needle approach (*d* in Fig. 84-14).

If more discs are to be injected, slight modifications can be made depending on the position of the first needle. When the needle tip appears to the

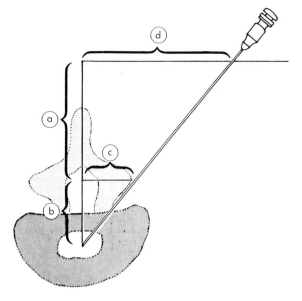

Fig. 84-14 Triangulation technique. Distances *a* and *b* are measured in centimeters from lateral view, and *c* is measured from anteroposterior view. Needle course then is sketched to produce *d*, approximate lateral distance from midline. (From Ford LT: Chemonucleolysis procedure manual no. 1. Needle placement — a triangulation approach for chemonucleolysis, 1984, Smith Laboratories.)

right of the midline and central in the lateral view, it is wise to begin needle insertion at the second disc slightly more lateral to the midline than the starting point actually derived. On the other hand, if the needle tip appears to be to the left of the midline in the first space and central in the lateral view, start the approach to the second space a little closer to the midline than indicated by triangulation.

■ *MODIFIED TRIANGULATION TECHNIQUE.* This technique uses a CT scan of the axial technique at the level to be injected with the skin edge or a sizable portion of the spinous process visible, a goniometer, ruler (metal if used for direct measurement), pencil, and paper.

Draw a line from the center of the disc or vertebral body through the spinous process to the skin line on the CT scan. Center a goniometer at the previously chosen disc center and plot a second line past the facet joint laterally. Measure the angle *x* between line *a* and line *b*. Measure the back skin to disc center as noted in Fig. 84-16, *A,* or measure the depth directly under image intensification. Using paper and pencil, draw a line equal to the length of line *ab* and construct a second line *d* at the previously calculated angle *x.* Draw a third line *e* perpendicular from the skin end of line *ab* intersecting line *d.* The distance from line *ab* to *d* along line *e* should approximate the distance the needle should be placed from the midline of the back. The angle *y* also approximates the angle of needle placement

Table 84-3   Result expectancy related to Hs and Hy T scores on the MMPI test

Hs and Hy T scores	No. of patients	Chances of good or excellent functional recovery (percent)
85 and above	10	10
75 to 84	32	16
65 to 74	31	39
55 to 64	36	72
54 and below	21	90
Prediction from base rate	63	48

From Wiltse LL and Rocchio PD: J Bone Joinnt Surg 57-A:478, 1975.

relative to the skin line *d.* Note that the curvature of the back (line *s*) may require extending the line up above the back and placing the needle at the calculated angle of insertion *z.* When the needle touches the skin, this should reasonably approximate the proper point of entry for that patient and disc level.

The lumbosacral disc always requires the most lateral starting position for injection. Midlumbar or upper lumbar discs always require a more medial starting position, sometimes even as close as 5 cm to the midline. Needle placement in patients with lateral lumbar fusions is extremely difficult.

PSYCHOLOGIC TESTING

Psychologic testing has been demonstrated to be a reasonable predictor of surgical and conservative treatment results regardless of the spinal pathologic condition. The Minnesota Multiphasic Personality Inventory (MMPI) is the most reliable and well-documented test used for this purpose. This test is predictive of preinjury susceptibility to back injury and the potential for failure of conservative and surgical treatment. Wiltse and Rocchio demonstrated that elevations of the hysteria (Hs) and hypochondriasis (Hy) T scores above 75 are indicative of a poor postoperative response (16% good results). Their study evaluated patients treated with chymopapain and their clinical results (Tables 84-3 and 84-4).

Table 84-3 indicates the rate of good to excellent results using the MMPI test Hs and Hy scores alone in the study by Wiltse and Rocchio. Table 84-4 illustrates the lack of statistical significance between the MMPI scores and the presence of the following objective findings:

1. Reflex changes
2. Motor weakness
3. Sensory deficits
4. Positive myelogram
5. Positive electromyogram
6. Elevated cerebrospinal fluid protein

Similar studies of surgically and conservatively treated patients have resulted in similar findings. Written reports are helpful, but the raw T score read on the far right or

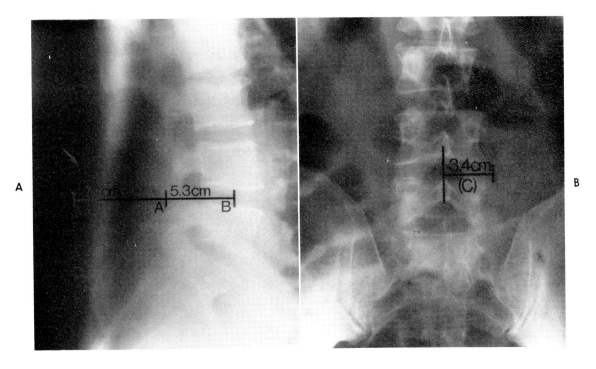

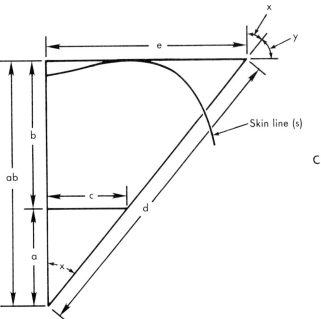

Fig. 84-15   **A,** Lateral roentgenogram of lumbar spine with metallic marker at highest point on skin of back. This point marks skin level. Draw line parallel with disc space or spaces to be injected. Measure length of lines from center of disc to skin line $(a + b)$. Divide lines by selecting point that best approximates widest portion of facet joints. Line nearest disc center is line a and other line is line b. (This point is usually ventral surface of facet as seen in lateral view.) **B,** Anteroposterior roentgenogram of lumbar spine with line drawn parallel to disc space or spaces to be injected. Line is measured from center of disc to lateralmost aspect of facet joint (c). **C,** Line drawing showing transposition of lines a, b, and c extrapolated from above roentgenograms. Draw line d from center point of line a intersecting lateral edge of line c and extending beyond to level of other end of line b. Draw line e perpendicular from outer end of line b intersecting line d. Measure length of line e. Length of line e should reasonably approximate space that needle should be placed from midline of back. Note that curvature of back (line s) may require extending line up above back and placing needle at calculated angle of insertion (y). When needle touches skin, that should reasonably approximate proper point of entry for that patient and disc level.

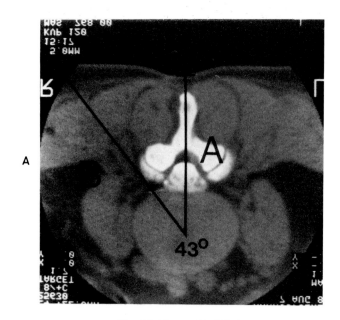

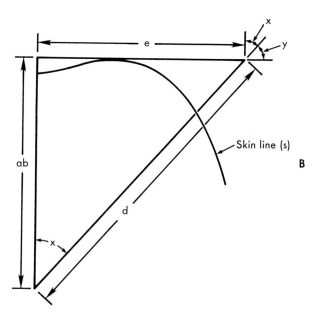

Fig. 84-16   **A,** Modified triangulation technique. CT scan of patient showing level of disc to be injected and skin level(s). Draw line from center of disc or vertebral body through spinous process to skin line. Center goniometer at previously chosen disc center and plot second line past facet joint laterally. Measure angle *x* between line *a* and line *b*. Measure back skin to disc center as previously noted in Fig. 84-15, *A,* or measure depth directly under image intensification. **B,** Draw line equal to length of line *ab* and construct second line *d* at previously calculated angle *x*. Draw third line *e* perpendicular from skin end of line *ab* intersecting line *d*. Distance from line *ab* to *d* along line *e* should approximate distance needle should be placed from midline of back. Angle *y* also approximates angle of needle placement relative to skin line *d*. Note that curvature of back (line *s*) may require extending line up above back and placing needle at calculated angle of insertion *z*. When needle touches skin, this should reasonably approximate proper point of entry for patient and disc level.

left side of the standard test result sheet is the simplest guide with regard to postoperative outcome. If surgery is necessary in a patient with an elevated Hs or Hy score, then psychiatric or psychologic assistance before and after the procedure may be helpful, but a poor result should be anticipated. Gentry observed a group of patients with objective evidence of psychologic disturbance as indicated by the MMPI. Those patients who had surgery were less likely to return to work, less likely to have a reduction in their pain, and more likely to have greater disability than similar patients who did not have surgery. Wiltse and Rocchio recommend restraint and conservative treatment in these patients. Elevation of the Hs and

Hy scores on the MMPI should be a relative contraindication to elective spinal surgery.

Additional material on this test may be obtained in the excellent articles by Dennis et al., Wiltse and Rocchio, and Southwick and White. Numerous other tests are available, but none have been shown to be as predictive of surgical outcome as the Hs and Hy scores on the MMPI. The main problem with the MMPI is that it requires the ability to read and comprehend the material. Pincus et al. also note that the MMPI questions may be in line with natural disease processes such as rheumatoid arthritis. Patients with chronic diseases may, by the nature of their disease symptoms, have MMPI elevations.

Table 84-4   Hs and Hy T scores of patients with good or excellent results versus number of preexisting objective deficits

Hs and Hy T scores	No. of patients	Percent good or excellent results	Percent with the no. of preinjection objective deficits indicated*				
			1+	2+	3+	4+	5+
75 and over	42	25	95.0	57.5	30.0	7.5	2.5
64 and below	57	87	95.2	64.4	32.6	8.7	2.2

From Wiltse LL and Rocchio PD: J Bone Joint Surg 57-A:478, 1975.
*X^2 = <0.001.

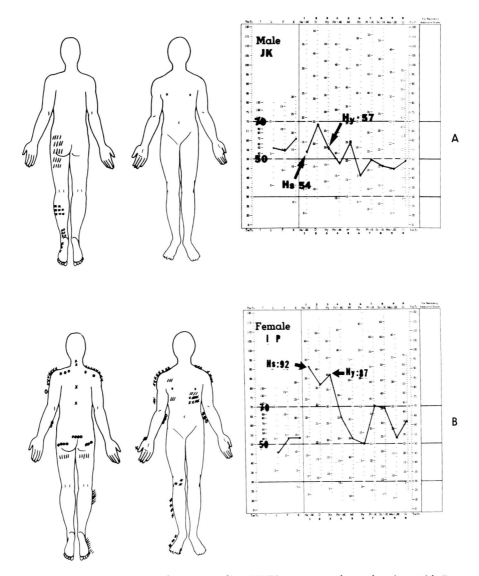

Fig. 84-17 **A,** Pain drawing and corresponding MMPI raw score sheet of patient with "conversion V" who was unrelieved of pain after disc surgery. **B,** Pain drawing and corresponding MMPI raw score sheet of patient with normal findings who was relieved of pain after disc surgery.

Chronic back pain without a specific disease association should not be considered as similar to chronic disease such as rheumatoid arthritis.

A simple test that is a good screening aid is the pain drawing. The pain drawing correlates well with the Hs and Hy scores. This test also requires some ability to follow simple directions. Additional information may be obtained in the articles by Rainsford, Cairns, and Mooney and by Dennis et al. (Fig. 84-17). Udén and Landin found that the pain drawing correlated well with the clinical results. Patients with low Rainsford scores were most likely to have definite pathologic conditions and those with high Rainsford scores were least likely to have a demonstrable pathologic condition. Cummings and Routan warn that the pain drawing should not be used to identify areas of somatic disturbance in chronic pain patients.

CERVICAL DISC DISEASE

Herniation of the cervical intervertebral disc with spinal cord compression has been identified since Key detailed the pathologic findings of two cases of cord compression by "intervertebral substance" in 1838. During the late 1800s and early 1900s there were many reports of chondromas of the cervical spine. Stookey described the clinical findings and anatomic location of cervical disc herniation in 1928 but attributed the lesion to a cervical chondroma. Finally, Mixter and Barr reported lumbar disc herniation in 1934, including four cervical disc protrusions.

The classic approach to discs in this region has been posteriorly with laminectomy. This approach had been used as a standard exposure for extradural tumors. In 1943 Semmes and Murphey reported four patients in whom cervical disc rupture simulated coronary disease and introduced the concept that cervical disc disease usually manifested itself in root symptoms and not cord compression symptoms. Bailey and Badgley, Cloward, Smith and Robinson in the 1950s popularized the anterior approach coupled with interbody fusion. Robertson in 1973, after the initial report by Hirsch in 1960, reported anterior cervical discectomy without fusion. He showed that simple anterior disc excision without fusion can give results similar to anterior cervical disc excision with anterior interbody fusion. Presently, anterior cervical fusion is the procedure of choice when the disc is removed anteriorly and hemilaminectomy is the procedure of choice when the disc fragment is removed posteriorly.

Kelsey et al. in the epidemiologic study of acute cervical disc prolapse indicated that cervical disc rupture was more common in men by a ratio of 1.4 to 1. Factors associated with the injury were frequent heavy lifting on the job, cigarette smoking, and frequent diving from a board. The use of vibrating equipment and time spent in motor vehicles were not positively associated with this

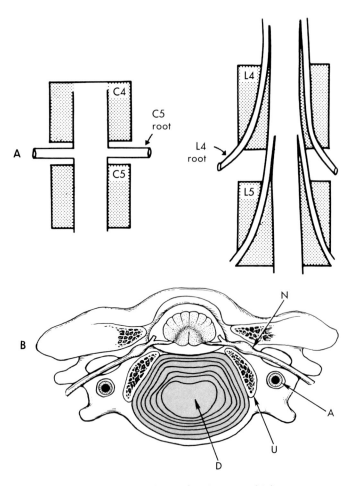

Fig. 84-18 **A,** Comparison of points at which nerve roots emerge from cervical and lumbar spine. **B,** Cross-sectional view of cervical spine at level of disc *(D).* Uncinate process *(U)* forms ventral wall of foramen. Root *(N)* exits dorsal to vertebral artery, *(A).* (**A,** From Kikuchi S, Macnab I, and Moreau P: J Bone Joint Surg 63-B:272, 1981.)

problem. Participation in sports other than diving, frequent wearing of shoes with high heels, frequent twisting of the neck on the job, time spent sitting on the job, and smoking of cigars and pipes were not associated with cervical intervertebral disc collapse. Horal reported that 40% of the population in Sweden were sometimes affected by neck pain during their lives. Patients with cervical disc disease are also likely to have lumbar disc disease. MRI studies have shown increasing cervical disc degeneration with age.

The pathophysiology of cervical disc disease is the same as degenerative disc disease in other areas of the spine. Disc swelling is followed by progressive anular degeneration. Frank extrusion of nuclear material can occur as a complication of this normal degenerative process. Cramer postulated that hydraulic pressure on the disc rather than excessive motion produced traumatic disc herniation. As the disc degeneration proceeds, hypermobility of the segment can result in instability or degenerative arthritic changes or both. Unlike in the lumbar spine, these hypertrophic changes are predominantly at the uncovertebral joint (uncinate process) (Fig. 84-18). Eventually hypertrophic changes develop about the facet joints and vertebral bodies. As in lumbar disease, progressive stiffening of the cervical spine and loss of motion are the usual result in the end stages. Occasionally hypertrophic spurring anteriorly can result in dysphagia.

Signs and Symptoms

The signs and symptoms of intervertebral disc disease are best separated into symptoms related to the spine itself, symptoms related to nerve root compression, and symptoms of myelopathy. Several authors have reported that when the disc is punctured anteriorly for the purpose of discography, pain is noted in the neck and shoulder. Complaints of neck pain, medial scapular pain, and shoulder pain are therefore probably related to primary pain about the disc and spine. Anatomic studies have indicated cervical disc and ligamentous innervations. This has been inferred to be similar in the cervical spine to that of the lumbar spine with its sinu-vertebral nerve. Tamura has noted cranial symptoms such as headache, vertigo, tinnitus, and ocular problems associated with C3-4 root sleeve defects on myelography.

Symptoms of root compression usually are associated with pain radiating into the arm or chest with numbness in the fingers and motor weakness. Cervical disc disease also can mimic cardiac disease with chest and arm pain. Usually the radicular symptoms are intermittent and combined with the more frequent neck and shoulder pain.

The signs of midline cervical compression (myelopathy) are unique and varied. The pain is poorly localized and aching in nature. Occasional sharp pain or generalized tingling may be described with neck extension. This is not unlike Lhermitte's sign in multiple sclerosis. The pain may be in both the shoulder and pelvic girdles. It is occasionally associated with a generalized feeling of weakness in the lower extremities and a feeling of instability.

In patients with predominant cervical spondylosis, symptoms of vertebral artery compression also may be found. These symptoms consist of dizziness, tinnitus, intermittent blurring of vision, and occasional episodes of retroocular pain.

The signs of lateral root pressure from a disc or osteophytes are predominantly neurologic (see boxes, p. 000). By evaluating multiple motor groups, multiple levels of deep tendon reflexes and sensory abnormalities, the level of the lesion can be localized as accurately as any other lesion in the nervous system. The multiple innervation of muscles can sometimes lead to confusion in determining the exact root involved. For this reason, myelography or other studies done for roentgenographic verification of the clinical impression usually are helpful.

Rupture of the C4-5 disc with compression of the C5 nerve root should result in weakness in the deltoid and biceps muscles. The deltoid is almost entirely innervated by C5, but the biceps is poorly innervated. The biceps reflex may be diminished with injury to this nerve root, although it also has a C6 component, and this may be considered. Sensory testing should show a patch on the lateral aspect of the arm to be diminished (Fig. 84-19).

Rupture of the C5-6 disc with compression of the C6 root may be confused with other root levels because of dual innervation of structures. Weakness may be noted in the biceps and extensor carpi radialis longus and brevis. As mentioned above, the biceps is dually innervated by C5 and C6, whereas the long extensors are du-

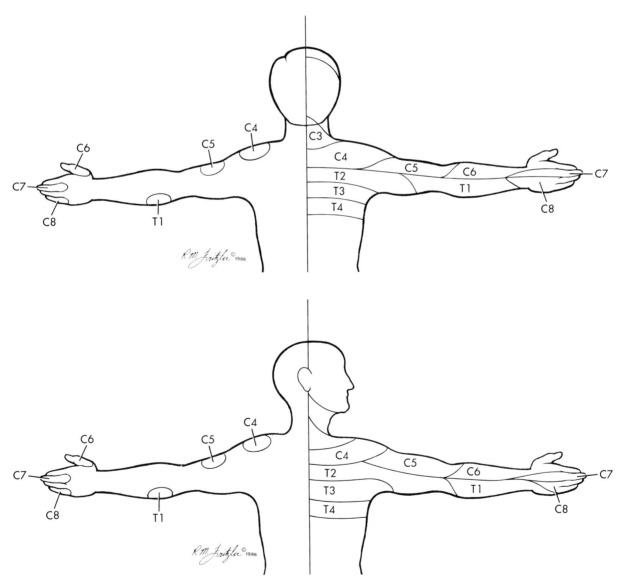

Fig. 84-19   C5 neurologic level. (After Hoppenfeld S: Physical examination of the spine and extremities, Norwalk, Conn, 1976, Appleton-Century-Crofts.)

C5 NERVE ROOT COMPRESSION

(indicative of C4-5 disc rupture or other pathologic condition at that level)

Sensory deficit
  Upper lateral arm and elbow
Motor weakness
  Deltoid
  Biceps (variable)
Reflex change
  Biceps (variable)

C6 NERVE ROOT COMPRESSION

(indicative of C5-6 disc herniation or other local pathologic condition)

Sensory deficit
  Lateral forearm, thumb, and index finger
Motor weakness
  Biceps
  Extensor carpi radialis longus and brevis
Reflex change
  Biceps
  Brachioradialis

C7 NERVE ROOT COMPRESSION

(indicative of C6-7 disc rupture or other pathologic condition at that level)

Sensory deficit
  Middle finger (variable because of overlap)
Motor weakness
  Triceps
  Wrist flexors (flexor carpi radialis)
  Finger flexors (variable)
Reflex change
  Triceps

C8 NERVE ROOT COMPRESSION

(indicative of C7-T1 disc rupture or other pathologic condition at that level)

Sensory deficit
  Ring finger, little finger, and ulnar border of palm
Motor weakness
  Interossei
  Finger flexors (variable)
  Flexor carpi ulnaris (variable)
Reflex change
  None

---

ally innervated by C6 and C7. The brachioradialis and biceps reflexes may also be diminished at this level. Sensory testing usually indicates a decreased sensibility over the lateral forearm, thumb, and index finger.

Rupture of the C6-7 disc with compression of the C7 root frequently results in weakness of the triceps. Weakness of the wrist flexors, especially the flexor carpi radialis, is also more indicative of C7 root problems. Weakness of the flexor carpi ulnaris is usually caused more by C8 lesions. As mentioned above, finger extensors may also be weakened in that they have both C7 and C8 innervation. The triceps reflex may be diminished. Sensation is lost in the middle finger. C7 sensibility is variable because it is so narrow and overlap is prominent. Strong sensibility change may be hard to document.

Rupture between C7 and T1 with compression of the C8 nerve root results in no reflex changes. Weakness may be noted in the finger flexors and in the interossei of the hand. Sensibility is lost on the ulnar border of the palm, including the ring and little fingers. Compression of T1 shows weakness of the interosseus muscles, decreased sensibility about the medial aspect of the elbow, and no reflex changes.

The clinical series of Odom, Finney, and Woodhall noted considerable variability in the level of compression and the neurologic findings. Change in the triceps reflex was the predominant reflex change with compression of the sixth cervical root (56%). It was also the predominant reflex change in seventh root compression (64%). Similarly the index finger was the predominant digit with sensory change, with evidence of hypalgesia in both sixth (68%) and seventh (70%) cervical root compression.

Care should be taken in the examination of the extremity when radicular problems are encountered to rule out more distal compression syndromes in the upper extremities such as thoracic outlet syndrome, carpal tunnel syndrome, and cubital tunnel syndrome. The lower extremities should be examined with special attention to long tract signs indicative of myelopathy.

There are no tests for the upper extremity that correspond with straight leg raising tests in the lower extremity. Recently Davidson, Dunn, and Metzmaker described a shoulder test that may be helpful in the diagnosis of

---

T1 NERVE ROOT COMPRESSION

(indicative of T1-2 disc rupture or other pathologic condition at that level)

Sensory deficit
  Medial aspect of elbow
Motor weakness
  Interossei
Reflex change
  None

cervical root compression syndromes. The test consists of shoulder abduction and elbow flexion with placement of the hand on the top of the head. This should relieve the arm pain caused by radicular compression. It is interesting to note that if this position is allowed to persist for a minute or two and pain is increased, then more distal compressive neuropathies such as a tardy ulnar nerve syndrome (cubital tunnel syndrome) or primary shoulder pathologic conditions often are the cause. Viikari-Juntura, Porras, and Laasonen note that the shoulder abduction, axial compression, and manual axial traction tests are related to disc disease but the sensitivity of these tests is low.

Cervical paraspinal spasm and limitation of neck motion are frequent findings of cervical spine disease but are not indicative of a specific pathologic process. Special maneuvers involving neck motion may be helpful in the choice of conservative treatment and identification of pathologic processes. The distraction test, which involves placing the hands on the occiput and jaw and distracting the cervical spine in the neutral position, may relieve root compression pain but may increase pain caused by ligamentous injury. Neck extension and flexion with or without traction may be helpful in selecting conservative therapies.

Patients relieved of pain with the neck extended, with or without traction, usually have hyperextension syndromes with ligamentous injury posteriorly, whereas patients relieved of pain with distraction and neck flexion are more likely to have nerve root compression caused by either a soft ruptured disc or most likely hypertrophic spurs in the neural foramina. Pain usually is increased in any condition with compression. One must be careful before applying compression or distraction to be sure no cervical instability or fracture is present. One must also be careful in interpreting the distraction test to be certain the temporomandibular joint is not diseased or injured because distraction also will increase the pain in this area.

The signs of midline disc herniation are those of spinal cord compression. If the lesion is high in the cervical region, paresthesias, weakness, atrophy, and occasionally fasciculations may occur in the hands. Most commonly, however, the first and most prominent symptoms are those of involvement of the corticospinal tract; less commonly the posterior columns are affected. The primary signs are clonus, hyperactive reflexes, and the Babinski reflex. Lesser findings are varying degrees of spasticity, weakness in the legs, and impairment of proprioception. Equilibrium may be grossly disturbed, but sense of pain and temperature sense rarely are lost and usually are of little localizing value.

Differential Diagnosis

The differential diagnosis of cervical disc disease is best separated into extrinsic and intrinsic factors. Extrinsic factors basically deal with those disease processes extrinsic to the neck resulting in symptoms similar to primary neck problems. Included in this group are tumors of the chest, nerve compression syndromes distal to the neck, degenerative processes such as shoulder and upper extremity arthritis, temporomandibular joint syndrome, and lesions about the shoulder such as acute and chronic rotator cuff tears and impingement syndromes. Intrinsic problems deal primarily with lesions directly associated with the cervical spine, the most common, of course, being cervical disc degeneration with a concomitant complication of disc herniation and later development of hypertrophic arthritis. Congenital factors such as spinal stenosis in the cervical region also may produce symptoms. Primary and secondary tumors of the cervical spine and fractures of the cervical vertebrae also should be considered as intrinsic lesions.

Cervical disc disease has been categorized by Odom et al. into four groups: (1) unilateral soft disc protrusion with nerve root compression; (2) foraminal spur, or hard disc, with nerve root compression; (3) medial soft disc protrusion with spinal cord compression; and (4) transverse ridge or cervical spondylosis with spinal cord compression. Soft disc herniations usually affect one level, whereas hard discs can be multiple. Central lesions usually result in cord compression symptoms, and lateral lesions usually result in radicular symptoms.

Odom et al. report that most of the soft disc herniations in their series occurred at the sixth cervical interspace (70%) and fifth cervical interspace (24%). Only 6% occurred at the seventh interspace. Foraminal spurs were also found predominantly at the sixth interspace (48%). The fifth interspace (39%) and seventh interspace (13%) accounted for the remaining levels where foraminal spurs were found. They also noted the incidence of medial soft disc protrusion with myelopathy to be rare (14 of 246 patients).

Disc material sometimes is extruded into the midline of the spinal canal anteriorly, with compression of the spinal cord and without nerve root involvement. Occasionally this is the result of a violent injury to the cervical spine, with or without fracture-dislocation, and at times it is associated with immediate quadriplegia. In some instances, however, the symptoms are progressive and may be suggestive of spinal cord tumor or degenerative diseases of the spinal cord, such as amyotrophic lateral sclerosis, posterolateral sclerosis, and multiple sclerosis. In most of these ailments no block of the spinal canal has been reported, and for many years the mechanism whereby the cervical cord compression was produced was not understood. However, in the rare patients whom we have observed, spinal fluid block could be produced by hyperextending the neck, although with the neck in the neutral or flexed position the canal was completely open. This finding has been previously reported. It has since been observed that during operation on such patients when the neck is hyperextended, the superior edge of the lamina compresses the cord against the herniated disc, and it is therefore probable that repeated hyperextension of the neck over a period of weeks, months, or years could gradually damage the spinal cord.

The patient with a midline herniation rarely complains of pain or stiffness of the neck. The first symptom may occasionally be a shocklike sensation in the trunk and extremities as a result of flexing or hyperextending the neck, somewhat but not exactly similar to Lhermitte's sign in multiple sclerosis. If the lesion is high in the cervical region, paresthesias, weakness, atrophy, and occasionally fasciculations may occur in the hands. Most commonly, however, the first and most prominent symptoms are those of involvement of the corticospinal tract and less commonly the posterior columns with varying degrees of spasticity, weakness in the legs, and impairment of proprioception. Equilibrium may be grossly disturbed, but sense of pain and temperature sense rarely are lost and are usually of little localizing value.

In view of the disturbances of the spinal fluid dynamics just mentioned, jugular compression should be carried out during lumbar puncture with the neck in the flexed, neutral, and hyperextended positions. Roentgenographically there is more often than not little or no alteration in the cervical curve.

We are in complete agreement with Bucy, Heimburger, and Oberhill that every patient suspected of having degenerative spinal cord disease should have a spinal puncture. All of these patients should also have a myelogram unless cranial nerve involvement is present. Neither evidence of mild cranial nerve involvement such as hypalgesia in the fifth cranial nerve distribution nor lower motor neuron abnormality in the upper or lower extremity should deter one from carrying out this procedure. However, further experience with spinal fluid dynamics with the neck in various positions may alter our opinion about the necessity of myelography in patients who do not have a block on hyperextension.

MYELOGRAPHY. Myelography is performed in the same way as for ruptured lumbar discs except that considerable attention must be paid to the flow of the column of contrast medium with the neck in hyperextended, neutral, and flexed positions. One cannot conclude that spinal cord compression is not present until one is certain that the cephalad flow of the medium is not obstructed with the neck acutely hyperextended. The neck should be hyperextended carefully because of the danger of further damage to the spinal cord.

Confirmatory Testing

Roentgenographic evaluation of the cervical spine frequently shows loss of the normal cervical lordosis. Disc space narrowing and hypertrophic changes are frequently increased with age but are not indicative of cervical disc rupture. Usually roentgenograms are most helpful to rule out other problems. Oblique roentgenograms of the cervical spine may reveal foraminal encroachment.

Cervical myelography is indicated when the clinical findings fail to localize the lesion or there is a question of the level involved. Limiting the exploration and disc excision to one disc space is highly desirable because exploration of more than one root may result in increased neurologic deficit. Cervical myelography is usually more exact than lumbar myelography regardless of the contrast medium used. Isophendylate (Pantopaque) is still the contrast medium of choice at this time for cervical myelography. This is primarily because cervical myelography involves more danger if the contrast medium metrizamide is allowed to proceed intracranially. The dose of metrizamide is also higher for good cervical myelography, thus increasing the side effects of nausea, vomiting, and headache, as well as the complications of seizures and mental changes. From a technical standpoint metrizamide does provide a greater degree of nerve root definition than does isophendylate. The use of low-dose water-soluble myelography followed by a standard or reformatted CT scan may provide more information with less risk of illness.

CT scans of the cervical spine are also helpful. In addition, reformatted CT scans in the cervical spine usually result in a much less distinct picture than in the lumbar spine.

Cervical discography is a highly controversial technique with limited benefits. It is not indicated in frank disc rupture, spondylosis, or spinal stenosis. The primary use is in patients with persistent neck pain without localized neurologic findings in whom standard myelographic and tomographic scan studies are negative. Some investigators believe that isolated painful discs can be identified in some patients by discography. Certainly a degenerative disc without pain on injection is not the source of the patient's complaint. The technique of cervical discography requires considerable care and caution. It should be considered a preoperative test in those patients in whom an anterior disc excision and interbody fusion are considered for primary neck and shoulder pain. Great care is required both in the technique and interpretation if reproducible results are desired. Cervical root blocks also have been suggested for the localization and confirmation of symptomatic root compression when used in conjunction with cervical discography.

Conservative Treatment

Many conservative treatment modalities for neck pain are used for multiple diagnoses. The primary purpose of the cervical spine and associated musculature is to support and mobilize the head while providing a conduit for the nervous system. The forces on the cervical spine are therefore much smaller than on the lower spinal levels.

The cervical spine is vulnerable to muscular tension forces, postural fatigue, and excessive motion. Most non-operative treatments focus on one or more of these factors. The best primary treatment is rest, massage, ice, and aspirin. The position of the neck for comfort is essential for relief of pain. The position of greatest relief may suggest the offending pathologic process or mechanism of injury. Patients with hyperflexion injuries are usually more comfortable with the neck in extension over a small roll under the neck. No specific position is indicative of lateral disc herniation although most tolerate the neutral position best. Patients with spondylosis (hard disc) are most comfortable with the neck in flexion.

Cervical traction may be helpful in selected patients. Care must be exercised in instructing the patient in the proper use of the traction. It should be applied to the head in the position of maximum pain relief. Traction should never be continued if it increases pain. The weights should rarely exceed 10 pounds (weight of the head). The proper head halter and duration of traction sessions should be chosen to prevent irritation of the temporomandibular joint. Traction should also allow general relaxation of the patient. "Poor man's" traction is a simple method of evaluating the efficacy of cervical traction. It uses the weight of the unsupported head for the traction weight (about 10 pounds). For extension traction, the patient is supine and the head is allowed to gently extend off the examining table or bed. For flexion the same procedure is repeated in the prone position. The patient continues the exercise in the position that is most comfortable for 5 to 10 minutes several times daily.

The postural aspects of neck pain may be treated with more frequent changes in position and changes in the work area to prevent fatigue and encourage good posture. Techniques to minimize or relieve tension are also helpful.

Cervical braces usually limit excessive motion. Like traction, they should be tailored to the most comfortable neck position. They may be most helpful in situations where the patient is quite active.

Neck and shoulder exercises are most beneficial as the acute pain subsides. Isometric exercises are helpful in the acute phase. Occasionally shoulder problems such as adhesive capsulitis may be found concomitantly with cervical spondylosis. Therefore complete immobilization of the painful extremity should be avoided.

Surgery

The primary indications for surgical treatment of cervical disc disease are (1) failure of conservative therapy, (2) increasing neurologic deficit, and (3) cervical myelopathy that is progressive. In most patients the persistence of pain is the primary indication. The choice of approach should be determined by the position and type of lesion. Soft lateral discs are easily removed from the pos-terior approach, whereas soft central or hard discs (central or lateral) are probably best treated with an anterior approach. The decision to fuse the spine at the time of anterior discectomy is controversial. Osteophytes that were not removed at surgery have been shown frequently to be absorbed at the level of fusion. The use of a graft also prevents the collapse of the disc space and possible foraminal narrowing.

REMOVAL OF POSTEROLATERAL HERNIATIONS BY POSTERIOR APPROACH

■ *TECHNIQUE*. With the patient under general endotracheal anesthesia in the prone position and the face in a cerebellar headrest that fits comfortably, the neck is flexed to obliterate the cervical lordosis as much as possible. The upright position for surgery decreases the venous bleeding, but concern regarding the possibility of air embolism and cerebral hypoxia in the event of a significant drop in blood pressure makes us reluctant to recommend its use. The shoulders are retracted inferiorly with tape if roentgenograms of the lower cervical levels are contemplated.

Appropriately prepare and drape the operative field. Make a midline incision 2.5 cm lower than the interspace to be explored (Fig. 84-20). Retract the edges of this incision and the skin will withdraw in a cephalad direction so that the wound becomes properly placed. Divide the ligamentum nuchae longitudinally to expose the tips of the spinous processes above and below the designated area. The correct position is reasonably well assured by palpation of the last bifid spine, which is usually the sixth cervical vertebra. However, it should be verified preoperatively by a marker on the lateral cervical spine roentgenogram. If still uncertain as to the proper level, count downward from the second cervical spinous process. Dissect subperiosteally the paravertebral muscles from the laminae on the side of the lesion and retract them with a self-retaining retractor such as the Hoen or with the help of an assistant using a Hibbs retractor. Mark the spine with an Oschner clamp or towel clip in a spinous process and have a lateral roentgenogram made to confirm the level of dissection if there is any question.

With a small Hudson burr, rongeur, or power drill, grind away the medial edge of the facet along with the dorsal surface of the adjacent laminae. Remove a minimal portion of the trailing edge of the lamina above and the superior edge of the lamina below with a standard rongeur and with an angulated Kerrison rongeur. Sharply excise the ligamentum flavum and identify the nerve root, which is commonly displaced posteriorly and flattened by pressure from the underlying disc fragments. Removal of additional bone along the dorsal aspect of the foramen and immediately above and below the nerve root is often beneficial at this point.

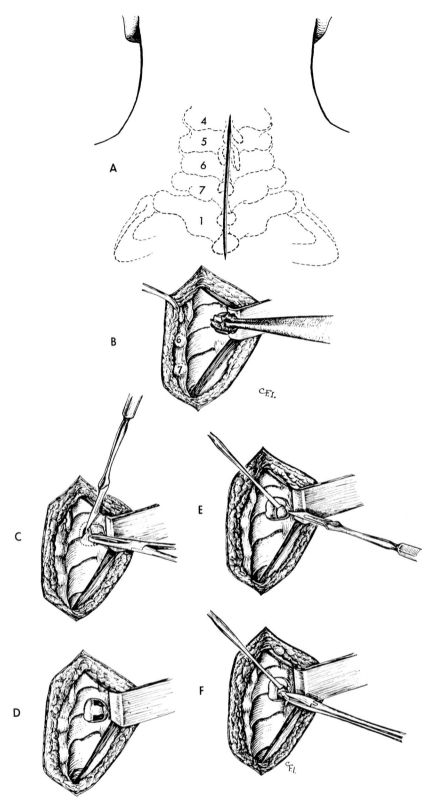

Fig. 84-20 Technique of removal of disc between fifth and sixth cervical vertebrae. **A,** Midline incision extending from spinous process of fourth cervical vertebra to that of first thoracic vertebra. **B,** Paraspinal muscles have been dissected from laminae and retracted laterally. Hole is to be drilled with Hudson burr (see text). **C,** Ligamentum flavum is being dissected. **D,** Defect measuring about 1.3 × 1.3 cm has been made (see text) to expose nerve root and lateral aspect of dura. **E,** Nerve root has been separated from nucleus and retracted superiorly to expose herniated disc. **F,** Longitudinal ligament has been incised, and loose fragment of nucleus is being removed.

The herniated nucleus pulposus most often lies slightly below the center of the nerve root but occasionally is above it. Gently retract the nerve root superiorly to expose the extruded nuclear fragments or a distended posterior longitudinal ligament. To control troublesome venous oozing at this point, place tiny pledgets of cotton above and below the nerve root. Take care not to pack the pledgets tightly around the nerve. The nerve root can then be retracted slightly to allow incision of the posterior longitudinal ligament over the herniated nucleus pulposus in a cruciate manner to permit the removal of the disc fragments.

After removal of all visible loose fragments, it is imperative to make a thorough search for additional fragments, both laterally and medially. It is equally important to be sure that the nerve root is thoroughly decompressed by inserting a probe in the intervertebral foramen. If the nerve root still seems to be tight, remove more bone from the articular facets until the nerve root is completely free. Since recurrence is so rare, do not curet the intervertebral space. Remove the cotton pledgets and control bleeding with bits of Gelfoam dipped in thrombin. Hemostasis must be complete, because postoperative hemorrhage can produce cord compression and quadriplegia. Close the wound by suturing the fascia to the supraspinous ligament with interrupted sutures and then suturing the subcutaneous layers and skin.

AFTERTREATMENT. The patient is given enough opiates to control the pain and is observed closely for evidence of spinal cord compression. Motor power and sensation in the legs are checked at hourly intervals for 24 hours. The patient is allowed out of bed the next day and is usually discharged from the hospital by the seventh day. Recovery of power is usually dramatic and prompt, although hypesthesia may persist for weeks or months. The patient is allowed to return to clerical work when comfortable and to manual labor after 2 months. As a rule neither support nor physical therapy is necessary, and the patient's future activity is not restricted. Isometric neck exercises, upper extremity range-of-motion exercises, and posterior shoulder girdle exercises may be useful for patients in whom atrophy or inactivity has been considerable.

Results. In no operation in neurosurgery are the results better than after the removal of a lateral herniated cervical disc. In the series of 250 operations reported by Simmons there were no deaths or major complications involving the brain or spinal cord. Three patients had reflex sympathetic dystrophy after operation. Two of these have completely recovered and one almost so. Two patients continued to have arm pain after operation and were reexplored during the initial hospital stay; in each,

Table 84-5   Results of removal of lateral herniated discs in cervical region (patient's estimate of percent improvement)

Relief (%)	Patients improved (%)	No. of patients
95-100	65.3	98
90-94	23.3	35
75-89	8.0	12
50-74	3.3	5
TOTAL	100.0	150

several more fragments of disc were found and removed. It is assumed that these fragments were overlooked at the initial operation. One patient had a recurrent extrusion at the same level. Two other patients have had soft extrusions on the opposite side at another level, also requiring a second operation.

Murphey, Simmons, and Brunson analyzed the results in a series of 150 patients who returned questionnaires concerning the success or failure of the operation. They were asked to state the percentage of benefit they derived from the procedure (Table 84-5), whether they were performing the same work as they had done preoperatively, and if not, whether the change of work had resulted from neck trouble. Approximately 90% had extremely good results, and there were none who were not significantly improved, as the data concerning work done confirm. Only 7 (6%) of the 125 patients who answered this part of the questionnaire found a change of work necessary because of neck trouble.

More recently Aldrich reported 53 patients with monoradiculopathy secondary to a soft posterolateral cervical disc hernia. After surgery there were no complications and all patients had relief of the radicular pain and resolution of motor weakness. Some sensory abnormalities persisted.

ANTERIOR APPROACH TO CERVICAL DISC. Smith and Robinson in 1955 were the first to recommend an anterior approach to the cervical spine in the treatment of cervical disc disease. They described an anterolateral discectomy with interbody fusion (Fig. 84-21). This procedure attained widespread acceptance and application after Cloward in 1958 modified the procedure and introduced new instrumentation.

There are three basic techniques for anterior cervical disc excision and fusion. The Cloward technique involves making a round hole centered at the disc space. A slightly larger, round iliac crest plug is then inserted into the disc space hole. The Smith-Robinson technique involves inserting a tricortical plug of iliac crest into the disc space after removing the disc and cartilaginous end plate. The graft is inserted with the cancellous side facing the cord (posterior). More recently Bloom and Raney suggested a modification of this technique by fashioning the tricortical graft to be thicker in its midportion and

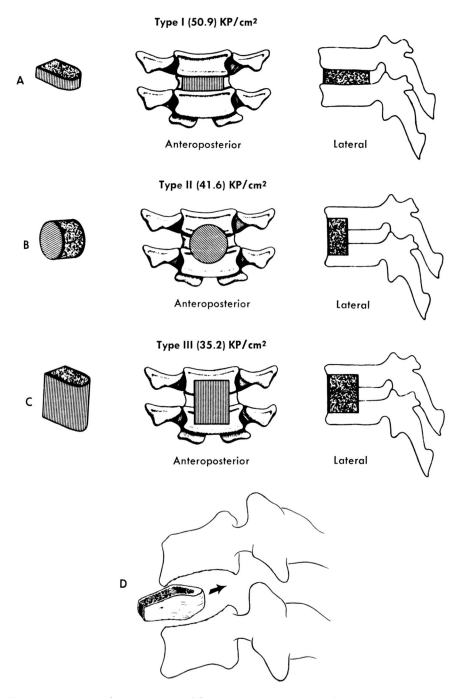

Type I (50.9) KP/cm²

A

Anteroposterior   Lateral

Type II (41.6) KP/cm²

B

Anteroposterior   Lateral

Type III (35.2) KP/cm²

C

Anteroposterior   Lateral

D

Fig. 84-21 Types of anterior cervical fusion. **A,** Smith-Robinson fusion. **B,** Cloward fusion. **C,** Bailey-Badgley fusion. **D,** Bloom-Raney modification of Smith-Robinson fusion. (**A** to **C,** From White AA III et al: Clin Orthop 91:21, 1973; **D,** from Bloom MH and Raney FL: J Bone Joint Surg 63-A:842, 1981.)

then inserting the graft with the cancellous portion facing anteriorly. The Bailey-Badgley technique involves the creation of a slot in the superior and inferior vertebral bodies. This technique is most applicable to reconstruction when one or more vertebral bodies are excised for tumor, stenosis, or other extensive pathologic conditions. Simmons and Bhalla have modfied this technique by using a keystone graft that increases the surface area of the graft by 30% and allows more complete locking of the graft. Biomechanically, the Smith-Robinson technique provides the greatest stability and least risk of extrusion.

White et al. reported relief of pain in 90% of 65 patients undergoing anterior cervical spine fusion for spondylosis with the technique of Smith and Robinson. Analysis of 90 patients with anterior cervical discectomies and fusion for cervical spondylosis with radiculopathy using the Cloward technique showed good to excellent results in 82% in the study by Jacobs, Krueger, and

The patient is allowed out of bed following surgery if he desires. When the patient begins eating, it is suggested that the physician be present to watch for signs of choking. Liquids should be started first. If the patient has no dysphagia and is able to swallow without problems, he may be slowly advanced to solid foods, but it may be several days before eating solid food is allowed. If the patient complains of any dysphagia, eating should be discontinued to prevent aspiration and respiratory problems.

MIDLINE HERNIATIONS OF CERVICAL DISCS INTO SPINAL CANAL. Once the diagnosis of midline herniation into the spinal canal is established, early operation is indicated to prevent further damage to the spinal cord. In large extrusions with immediate complete paraplegia and with block of the spinal canal, it is unlikely that any treatment will restore function, but the herniated fragments should be removed immediately. If a posterior approach is preferred, a full laminectomy should be performed, and the fragments should be removed transdurally. Commonly a midline or paracentral soft disc protrusion is difficult to differentiate from a neoplasm, and approaching the lesion posteriorly through the dura is mandatory. When the lesion is unquestionably a midline or paracentral disc protrusion, however, the anterior approach may be preferred to allow complete disc removal.

Generally the results of this operation have been disappointing because irreparable damage to the cord has occurred before operation. Should the diagnosis be made early and prompt treatment instituted, however, the results should be comparable to removal of any other mass from within the spinal canal.

THORACIC DISC DISEASE

Thoracic intervertebral disc rupture is extremely rare. Most studies place the incidence between 0.25% to 0.5% of all intervertebral disc ruptures. Arseni and Nash in 1963 were able to collect only 95 cases from the literature. The first diagnosis of a ruptured thoracic disc was probably made by Antoni in 1931. Several ruptures thereafter were misinterpreted as enchondrosis. In the late 1950s sporadic case reports and small series of thoracic intervertebral disc excisions appeared. Because of the small numbers of patients affected with this problem, the exact etiology and contributing factors have not been isolated. Trauma has been indicated in some patients, although in most the onset is somewhat insidious and intermittent as is true in disc disease in other areas of the spine. There is no clear-cut preponderance of males over females. The average age appears to be about 45 years in a collection of 102 cases from the world literature in 1965. Arseni and Nash noted that the discs between T10 and T12 are the most common areas for herniation, although herniation has been recorded at all thoracic levels.

Signs and Symptoms

The duration of symptoms appears to be relatively long, averaging approximately 2 years. This is believed to be attributable to the somewhat vague and misleading symptoms. Patients may complain of bowel or bladder incontinence. Pain is predominantly in the thoracic region, although the lower back is the next most frequent site of pain. Pain occasionally is found in the abdominal or leg region. Complaints of unilateral and bilateral numbness, unilateral or bilateral weakness, both unilateral and bilateral hyperesthesias, and unsteadiness of gait have also been recorded. Physical examination has shown occasional spinal deformity. Localized dorsal kyphosis is extremely rare. Weakness may be demonstrated in the lower abdominal muscles in addition to leg weakness, which frequently is bilateral. Proximal and distal muscle groups usually are comparably weak, but some patients may have symptoms similar to a more distal lumbar disc herniation. Occasionally the initial presentation may be a complete paraplegia or sudden onset of Brown-Séquard syndrome (unilateral paralysis with contralateral loss of sensibility). Sensory loss is common and is usually bilateral. Deep tendon reflexes usually are hyperreflexic. Plantar responses frequently are extensor, and clonus may be demonstrated.

Confirmatory Testing

Since the level of herniation cannot be determined clinically, myelography is mandatory. With present technology, CT that is performed after myelography at the area of pathologic findings may provide additional information as to the extent and location of the herniation. MRI offers the ability to identify intradural and extradural tumors, disc degenerations, nerve root impingements, and disc herniations. This procedure also may present further evidence as to the nature of the lesion because an extradural tumor also can result in findings similar to a herniated thoracic disc. In mild ruptures in which minimal findings can be identified, cystometrograms may indicate bladder dysfunction. Somatosensory testing may also be abnormal.

Treatment Results

There is no evidence to indicate the value of conservative therapy in this problem because of its low incidence of clinical detection. All patients reported in the literature have been treated surgically. The initial procedure recommended for this lesion was posterior thoracic laminectomy and disc excision. At least half of the lesions have been identified as being central, making the excision from this approach extremely difficult, and the results were somewhat disheartening. Most series reported fewer than half of the patients improving, with some becoming worse after posterior laminectomy and discectomy. Most recent studies suggest that lateral rachiotomy (modified costotransversectomy) or an anterior transthoracic approach for discectomy produces considerably better results with no evidence of worsening after the procedure. Bohlman and Zdeblick reported the results of anterior thoracic disc excision in 19 patients: 16 patients had excellent to good results and 3 had fair to poor results. Pain was relieved in 10, decreased in 8, and unchanged in 1. None had worsening of neurologic symptoms.

Surgery

COSTOTRANSVERSECTOMY. Costotransversectomy is probably best suited for thoracic disc herniations that are predominantly lateral or herniations that are suspected to be extruded or sequestered. Central disc herniations are probably best approached transthoracically. Some surgeons have recommended subsequent fusion after disc removal anteriorly or laterally.

■ *TECHNIQUE.* The operation usually is done with the patient under general anesthesia with a cuffed endotracheal tube or a Carlen tube to allow lung deflation on the side of approach. Place the patient prone and make a long midline incision or a curved incision concave to the midline centered over the level of involvement. Expose the spine in the usual manner out to the ribs. Remove a section of rib 5 to 7.5 cm long at the level of involvement, taking care to avoid damage to the intercostal nerve and artery. Carry the resection into the lateral side of the disc, exposing it for removal. Additional exposure can be made by laminectomy and excision of the pedicle and facet joint. Fusion is unnecessary unless more than one facet joint is removed. Close the wound in layers.

AFTERTREATMENT. The aftertreatment is similar to that for lumbar disc excision without fusion (p. 3761).

ANTERIOR APPROACH FOR THORACIC DISC EXCISION. Because of the relative age of patients with thoracic disc ruptures, special care must be taken to identify those with pulmonary problems. In these patients, the anterior approach may be detrimental medically, making a posterolateral approach safer. Patients with midline protrusions probably are best treated with the transthoracic approach to ensure complete disc removal. A Carlen tube may be beneficial in allowing deflation of the lung on the side of the operation.

■ *TECHNIQUE.* The operation is performed with the patient under general anesthesia, using a cuffed endotracheal tube or Carlen tube for lung deflation on the side of the approach. Place the patient in a lateral recumbent position. A left-sided anterior approach usually is preferred, making the operative procedure easier. Make a skin incision along the line of the rib that corresponds to the second thoracic vertebra *above* the involved intervertebral disc except for approaches to the upper five thoracic segments where the approach is through the third rib. Choose the skin incision by inspection of the anteroposterior roentgenogram. Cut the rib subperiosteally at its posterior and anterior ends and then insert a rib retractor. Save the rib for grafting later in the procedure. One may then decide on an extrapleural or transpleural approach depending on familiarity and ease. Exposure of the thoracic vertebrae should give adequate access to the front and opposite side. Dissect the great vessels free of the spine. Ligate the intersegmental vessels near the great vessels and not near the foramen. One should be able to insert a finger tip against the opposite side of the disc when the vascular mobilization is complete. Exposure of the intervertebral disc without disturbing more than three segmental vessels is preferable to avoid ischemic problems in the spinal cord. In the thoracolumbar region strip the diaphragm from the eleventh and twelfth ribs. The anterior longitudinal ligament usually is sectioned to allow spreading of the intervertebral disc space. Remove the disc as completely as possible. The use of the operating microscope or loupe magnification eases the removal of the disc near the posterior longitudinal ligament. Remove the disc up to the posterior longitudinal ligament using nibbling instruments. Then place a finger on the opposite side of the disc to avoid penetration when removing disc material on the more distant side. Carefully inspect the posterior longitudinal ligament for tears and extruded fragments. Remove the posterior longitudinal ligament only if necessary. Significant bleeding may occur if the venous plexus near the dura is torn. After removal of the disc, strip the end plates of their cartilage. Make a slot in one vertebral body and a hole in the body on the opposite side of the disc space to accept the graft material. Make the hole large enough to accept several sections of rib, but make the slot only large enough to accept one rib graft at a time. Then insert iliac, tibial, or rib grafts into the disc space. Tie the grafts together with heavy suture material when the maximum number of grafts have been inserted. Close the wound in the usual manner and employ standard chest drainage.

The transthoracic approach removing a rib two levels above the level of the lesion may be used up to T5. The transthoracic approach from T2 to T5 is best made by excision of the third or fourth rib and elevation of the scapula by sectioning of attachments of the serratus anterior and trapezius from the scapula. The approach to the T1-2 disc is best made from the neck with a sternal splitting incision. *AFTERTREATMENT.* Postoperative care is the same as for a thoracotomy. The patient is allowed to walk after the chest tubes are removed. Extension in any position is prohibited. A brace or body cast that limits extension should be used if the stability of the graft is questionable. The graft usually is stable without support if only one disc space is removed. Postoperative care is the same as for the anterior corpectomy and fusion if more than one disc level is removed.

LUMBAR DISC DISEASE
Signs and Symptoms

Although back pain is common from the second decade of life on, intervertebral disc disease and disc herniation are most prominent in otherwise healthy people in the third and fourth decades of life. Most people relate their back and leg pain to a traumatic incident, but close questioning frequently reveals that the patient has had intermittent episodes of back pain for many months or even years before the onset of severe leg pain. In many instances, the back pain is relatively fleeting in nature and is relieved by rest. This pain often is brought on by heavy exertion, repetitive bending, twisting, or heavy lifting. In other instances, an exacerbating incident cannot be elicited. The pain usually begins in the lower back, radiating to the sacroiliac region and buttocks. The pain can radiate down the posterior thigh. Back and posterior thigh pain of this type can be elicited from many areas of the spine, including the facet joints, longitudinal ligaments, and the periosteum of the vertebra. Radicular pain, on the other hand, usually extends below the knee and follows the dermatome of the involved nerve root.

The usual history of lumbar disc herniation is of repetitive, lower back and buttock pain, relieved by rest after a short period of time. This pain is then suddenly exacerbated by a flexion episode, with the sudden appearance of leg pain much greater than back pain. Most radicular pain from nerve root compression caused by a herniated nucleus pulposus is evidenced by leg pain equal to, or in many cases much greater than, the degree of back pain. Whenever leg pain is minimal and back pain is predominant, great care should be taken before making the diagnosis of a herniated intervertebral disc. The pain from disc herniation usually is intermittent in nature, increasing with activity, especially sitting. The pain may be relieved by rest, especially in the semi-Fowler position, and may be exacerbated by straining, sneezing, or coughing. Whenever the pattern of pain is bizarre or the pain itself is constant, a diagnosis of herniated disc should be viewed with some skepticism.

Other symptoms of disc herniation include weakness and paresthesias. In most patients the weakness is intermittent, variable with activity, and localized to the neurologic level of involvement. Paresthesias also are variable and limited to the dermatome of the involved nerve root. Whenever these complaints are generalized, the di-

agnosis of a simple unilateral disc herniation should be questioned.

Numbness and weakness in the involved leg and occasionally pain in the groin or testicle can be associated with a high or midline lumbar disc herniation. If a fragment is large or the herniation is high, symptoms of pressure on the entire cauda equina can be elicited. These include numbness and weakness in both legs, rectal pain, numbness in the perineum, and paralysis of the sphincters. This diagnosis should be the primary consideration in patients who complain of sudden loss of bowel or bladder control. Whenever the diagnosis of a cauda equina syndrome or acute midline herniation is suspected, evaluation and treatment should be aggressive.

Physical Findings

The physical findings in back pain with disc disease are variable because of the time intervals involved. Usually patients with acute pain show evidence of marked paraspinal spasm that is sustained during walking or motion. A scoliosis or a list in the lumbar spine may be present, and in many patients the normal lumbar lordosis is lost. As the acute episode subsides, the degree of spasm diminishes remarkably, and the loss of normal lumbar lordosis may be the only telltale sign. Point tenderness may be present over the spinous process at the level of the disc involved and in some patients pain may extend laterally.

If there is nerve root irritation, it centers over the length of the sciatic nerve, both in the sciatic notch and more distally in the popliteal space. In addition, stretch of the sciatic nerve at the knee should reproduce buttock and leg pain. A Lasègue sign usually is positive on the involved side. A positive Lasègue sign or straight leg raising should elicit buttock or leg pain or both on the side tested. Occasionally if leg pain is significant the patient will move back from a sitting position and assume the tripod stance to relieve the pain. Contralateral leg pain produced by straight leg raising should be regarded as pathognomonic of a herniated intervertebral disc. The absence of a positive Lasègue sign should make one skeptical of the diagnosis. Likewise, inappropriate findings and inconsistencies in the examination usually are nonorganic in origin. If the leg pain has persisted for any length of time, atrophy of the involved limb may be present as demonstrated by asymmetric girth of the thigh or calf. The neurologic examination will vary as determined by the level of root involvement (see boxes that follow).

Unilateral disc herniation between L3 and L4 usually compresses the fourth lumbar root as it crosses the disc before exiting at the L4 intervertebral foramen. Pain may be localized around the medial side of the leg. Numbness may be present over the anteromedial aspect of the leg. The quadriceps and hip adductor group, both innervated from L2, L3, and L4, may be weak and, in extended ruptures, atrophic. Reflex testing may reveal a diminished or

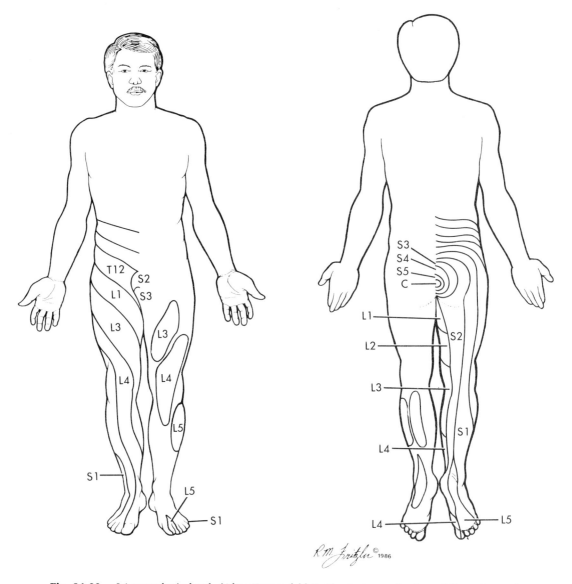

Fig. 84-22 L4 neurologic level. (After Hoppenfeld S: Physical examination of the spine and extremities, Norwalk, Conn, 1976, Appleton-Century-Crofts.)

absent patellar tendon reflex (L2, L3, and L4) or tibialis anterior tendon reflex (L4). Sensory testing may show diminished sensibility over the L4 dermatome, the isolated portion of which is the medial leg (Fig. 84-22) and the autonomous zone of which is at the level of the medial malleolus.

Unilateral disc herniation between L4 and L5 results in compression of the fifth lumbar root. Fifth lumbar root radiculopathy should produce pain in the dermatomal pattern. Numbness, when present, follows the L5 dermatome along the anterolateral aspect of the leg and the dorsum of the foot, including the great toe. The autonomous zone for this nerve is the first web of the foot and the dorsum of the third toe. Weakness may involve the extensor hallucis longus (L5), gluteus medius (L5), or extensor digitorum longus and brevis (L5). Reflex change usually is not found. A diminished tibialis posterior reflex is possible but hard to elicit.

In a unilateral ruptured disc between L5 and S1 the findings of an S1 radiculopathy are noted. Pain and numbness involve the dermatome of S1. The S1 dermatome includes the lateral malleolus and the lateral and plantar surface of the foot, occasionally including the heel. There is numbness over the lateral aspect of the leg and more importantly over the lateral aspect of the foot, including the lateral three toes. The autonomous zone for this root is the dorsum of the fifth toe. Weakness may be demonstrated in the peroneus longus and brevis (S1), gastrocnemius-soleus (S1), or gluteus maximus (S1). In general, weakness is not a usual finding in S1 radiculopathy. Occasionally mild weakness may be demonstrated by asymmetric fatigue with exercise of these motor groups. The ankle jerk usually is reduced or absent.

Massive extrusion of a disc involving the entire diameter of the lumbar canal or a large midline extrusion may

---

L4 ROOT COMPRESSION

(indicative of L3-4 disc herniation or pathologic condition localized to the L4 foramen)

Sensory deficit
Posterolateral thigh, anterior knee and medial leg
Motor weakness
Quadriceps (variable)
Hip adductors (variable)
Reflex changes
Patellar tendon
Tibialis anterior tendon (variable)

L5 ROOT COMPRESSION

(indicative of L4-5 disc herniation or pathologic condition localized to the L5 foramen)

Sensory deficit
Anterolateral leg, dorsum of the foot and great toe
Motor weakness
Extensor hallucis longus
Gluteus medius
Extensor digitorum longus and brevis
Reflex changes
Usually none
Tibialis posterior (difficult to elicit)

S1 ROOT COMPRESSION

(indicative of an L5-S1 disc herniation or pathologic condition localized to the S1 foramen)

Sensory deficit
Lateral malleolus, lateral foot, heel, and web of fourth and fifth toes
Motor weakness
Peroneus longus and brevis
Gastrocnemius-soleus complex
Gluteus maximus
Reflex changes
Tendo calcaneus (gastrocnemius-soleus complex)

---

produce pain in the back, legs, and occasionally perineum. Both legs may be paralyzed, the sphincters may be incontinent, and the ankle jerks may be absent. Tay and Chacha in 1979 reported that the combination of saddle anesthesia, bilateral ankle areflexia, and bladder symptoms constituted the most consistent symptoms of cauda equina syndrome caused by massive intervertebral

disc extrusion at any lumbar level. In these instances a cystometrogram may show bladder denervation.

More than 95% of the ruptures of the lumbar intervertebral discs occur at L4 and L5. Ruptures at higher levels in many patients are not associated with a positive straight-leg raising test. In these instances, a positive femoral stretch test may be helpful. This test is carried out by placing the patient in the prone position and acutely flexing the leg while placing the hand in the popliteal fossa. When this procedure results in anterior thigh pain, the result is positive and a high lesion should be suspected. In addition, these lesions may occur with a more diffuse neurologic complaint without significant localizing neurologic signs.

Often the neurologic signs associated with disc disease vary over time. If the patient has been up and walking for a period of time, the neurologic findings may be much more pronounced than if he has been at bed rest for several days, thus decreasing the pressure on the nerve root and allowing the nerve to resume its normal function. Additionally, various conservative treatments may change the physical signs of disc disease.

Comparative examination of a patient with back and leg pain is essential in finding a clear-cut pattern of signs and symptoms. It is not uncommon for the evaluation to change. Adverse changes in the examination may warrant more aggressive therapy, whereas improvement of the symptoms or signs should signal a resolution of the problem. Early symptoms or signs suggestive of cauda equina syndrome or severe or progressive neurologic deficit should be treated aggressively from the onset. McLaren and Bailey warn that the cauda equina syndrome is more frequent when disc excision is performed in the presence of an untreated spinal stenosis at the same level.

Differential Diagnosis

The differential diagnosis of back and leg pain is extremely lengthy and complex. It includes diseases intrinsic to the spine and those involving adjacent organs but causing pain referred to the back or leg. For simplicity, lesions can be categorized as being extrinsic or intrinsic to the spine. Extrinsic lesions include diseases of the urogenital system, gastrointestinal system, vascular system, endocrine system, nervous system not localized to the spine, and the extrinsic musculoskeletal system. These lesions may include infections, tumors, metabolic disturbances, congenital abnormalities, or the associated diseases of aging. Intrinsic lesions involve those diseases that arise primarily in the spine. They include diseases of the spinal musculoskeletal system, the local hematopoietic system, and the local neurologic system. These conditions include trauma, tumors, infections, diseases of aging, and immune diseases affecting the spine or spinal nerves.

Although the predominant cause of back and leg pain

in healthy people usually is lumbar disc disease, one must be extremely cautious to avoid a misdiagnosis. Therefore a full physical examination must be performed before making a presumptive diagnosis of herniated disc disease. Common diseases that can mimic disc disease include ankylosing spondylitis, multiple myeloma, vascular insufficiency, arthritis of the hip, osteoporosis with stress fractures, extradural tumors, peripheral neuropathy, and herpes zoster. Infrequent but reported causes of sciatica not related to disc hernia include synovial cysts, rupture of the medial head of the gastrocnemius, sacroiliac joint dysfunction, lesions in the sacrum and pelvis, and fracture of the ischial tuberosity.

Conservative Treatment

The number and variety of nonoperative therapies for back and leg pain are overwhelming. Treatments range from simple rest to expensive traction apparatus. All of these therapies are reported with glowing accounts of miraculous "cures." Unfortunately, few have been evaluated scientifically. In addition, the natural history of disc disease is characterized by exacerbations and remissions with improvement eventually regardless of treatment. Finally, several distinct symptom complexes appear to be associated with disc disease. Few if any studies have isolated the response to specific and anatomically distinct diagnoses.

The simplest treatment for acute back pain is rest. Deyo, Diehl, and Rosenthal reported that 2 days of bed rest were better than a longer period. Biomechanical studies indicate that lying in a semi-Fowler position or on the side with the hips and knees flexed with a pillow between the legs should relieve most pressure on the disc and nerve roots. Muscle spasm can be controlled by the application of ice, preferably in a massage over the muscles in spasm. Pain relief and anti-inflammatory effect can be achieved with aspirin. Most acute exacerbations of back pain respond quickly to this therapy. As the pain diminishes, the patient should be encouraged to begin isometric abdominal and lower extremity exercises. Walking within the limits of comfort also is encouraged. Sitting, especially riding in a car, is discouraged.

Education in proper posture and body mechanics is helpful in returning the patient to his usual level of activity after the acute exacerbation is eased or relieved. This education can take many forms from individual instruction to group instruction. Back education of this type is now usually referred to as "Back School." Although the concept is excellent, the quality and quantity of information provided may vary widely. The work of Bergquist-Ullman and Larsson and others indicates that patient education of this type is extremely beneficial in decreasing the amount of time from work lost initially but does little to decrease the incidence of recurrence of symptoms or length of time lost from work during recurrences. Certainly the combination of back education and combined physical therapy is superior to placebo treatment.

Numerous medications have been used with varied results in back and leg pain syndromes. The present trend appears to be away from the use of strong narcotics and muscle relaxants in the outpatient treatment of these syndromes. This is especially true in the instances of chronic back and leg pain where drug habituation and increased depression are frequent. Oral steroids used briefly also may be beneficial as strong anti-inflammatory agents. The numerous types of nonsteroidal anti-inflammatory medications also are helpful when aspirin is not tolerated or is of little help. When depression is prominent, mood elevators such as amitriptyline may be beneficial in reducing sleep disturbance and anxiety without increasing depression. In addition, the use of amitriptyline also decreases the need for narcotic medication.

Physical therapy should be used judiciously. The exercises should be fitted to the symptoms and not forced as an absolute group of activities. Patients with acute back and thigh pain eased by passive extension of the spine in the prone position may be helped by extension exercises rather than flexion exercises. Improvement in symptoms with extension is indicative of a good prognosis with conservative care. On the other hand, patients whose pain is increased by passive extension may be improved by flexion exercises. These exercises should not be forced in the face of increased pain. This may avoid further disc extrusion. Any exercise that increases pain should be discontinued. Lower extremity exercises may increase strength and relieve stress on the back, but they may also exacerbate lower extremity arthritis. The true benefit of such treatments may be in the promotion of good posture and body mechanics rather than of strength.

Numerous treatment modalities have been and will be advanced for the treatment of back pain. Some patients respond to the use of transcutaneous electrical nerve stimulation (TENS). Others do well with traction varying from skin traction in bed with 5 to 8 pounds to body inversion with forces of over 100 pounds. Back braces or corsets may be helpful to other patients. Ultrasound and diathermy are other treatments used in back pain. The scientific efficacy of many of these treatments has not been proven. In addition, all therapy for disc disease is only symptomatic.

Epidural Steroids

The epidural injection of a combination of a long-acting steroid with an epidural anesthetic is an excellent method of symptomatic treatment of back and leg pain from discogenic disease and other sources. Most studies show a 60% to 85% short-term success rate that falls to a 30% to 40% long-term (6-month) good result rate. The local effect of the steroids has been shown to last at least 3 weeks at a therapeutic level. In a well-controlled study Berman et al. found that the best results were obtained in patients with subacute or chronic leg pain with no prior surgery. They also found that the worst results were in patients with motor or reflex abnormalities (12% to 14% good results). A negative myelogram also was associated with a better result. Cuckler et al. in a double-blind randomized study of epidural steroid treatment of disc herniation and spinal stenosis found no difference in the results at 6 months between placebo and a single epidural injection. Our experience parallels that of Berman et al. We agree that epidural steroids are not a cure for disc disease, but they do offer relatively prolonged pain relief without excessive narcotic intake if conservative care is elected.

In experienced hands the complication rate from this procedure should be small. White, Derby, and Wynne have shown that the most common problem is a 25% rate of failure to place the material in the epidural space. Another technique-related problem is intrathecal injection with inadvertent spinal anesthesia. Other reported complications include transient hypotension, difficulty in voiding, severe paresthesias, cardiac angina, headache, and transient hypercorticoidism. The most serious complication reported was a bacterial meningitis. The total complication rate in most series is about 5%, and the complications are almost always transient.

This procedure is contraindicated in the presence of infection, neurologic disease (such as multiple sclerosis), hemorrhagic or bleeding diathesis, cauda equina syndrome, and a rapidly progressive neural deficit. Rapid injections of large volumes or the use of large doses of steroid also may increase the complication rate. The exact effects of intrathecal injection of steroids are not known. This technique must be used only in the low lumbar region. We prefer to abort the procedure if a bloody tap is obtained or if cerebrospinal fluid is encountered.

We prefer to perform the procedure in a room equipped for resuscitation and with the capability to monitor the patient. Experienced anesthesiologists usually perform the procedure in our institution. This procedure lends itself well to outpatient use, but the patient must be prepared to spend several hours to recover from the block. Methylprednisolone (Depo-Medrol) is the usual steroid injected. The dosage may vary from 80 to 120 mg. The anesthetics used may include lidocaine, bupivacaine, or procaine. Our present protocol is to inject the patient three times. These injections are made at 48- to 72-hour intervals. This ensures at least one good epidural injection and decreases the volume of material injected at each procedure.

■ *TECHNIQUE (BROWN)*. **The equipment needed includes material for an appropriate skin preparation, sterile rubber gloves, a 3½-inch, 20-gauge or 22-gauge disposable spinal needle (45-degree blunt- or curve-tipped epidural needles are preferred), several disposable syringes, bacteriostatic 1% lidocaine, and methylprednisolone acetate, 40 mg/ml. The injection may be performed with the patient in the sitting or lateral decubitus position. Anesthetize the skin near the midline. Advance the needle until the**

resistance of the ligamentum flavum is encountered. Then attach a syringe and slowly advance the needle while applying light pressure on the syringe. When the epidural space is encountered, the resistance is suddenly lost and the epidural space will accommodate the air. Remove the syringe and inspect the needle opening for blood or spinal fluid. If there is no flow out of the needle, then inject 3 ml of 1% lidocaine or other appropriate anesthetic. This may be preceded or followed by the chosen dosage of methylprednisolone.

Several variations also may be used. Some physicians use a sterile balloon to indicate the proper space. Others use the "disappearing drop" technique which involves placing a drop of sterile saline over the hub of the needle. When the epidural space is entered, the drop will disappear. Caudal injection is also used, but this may require larger volumes to wash the steroid up to the involved level. This method is safer but less reliable than an injection at L4-5.

Surgery

When conservative treatment for lumbar disc disease fails, the next consideration is surgical treatment. Before this step is taken, the surgeon must be sure of the diagnosis. The patient must be certain that the degree of pain and impairment warrants such a drastic step. Both the surgeon and the patient must realize that disc surgery is not a cure but may provide symptomatic relief. It neither stops the pathologic processes that allowed the herniation to occur nor restores the back to its previous state. The patient must still practice good posture and body mechanics after surgery. Activities involving repetitive bending, twisting, and lifting with the spine in flexion may have to be curtailed or eliminated. If prolonged relief is to be expected, then some permanent modification in the patient's life-style may be necessary.

The key to good results in disc surgery is appropriate patient selection. The optimum patient is one with predominant, if not only, unilateral leg pain extending below the knee that has been present for at least 6 weeks. The pain should have been decreased by rest, anti-inflammatory medication, or even epidural steroids but should have recurred to the initial levels after a minimum of 6 to 8 weeks of conservative care. Physical examination should reveal signs of sciatic irritation and possibly objective evidence of localizing neurologic impairment. CT, lumbar MRI, or myelography should confirm the level of involvement consistent with the patient's examination. Finally, psychologic testing should show a hysteria or hypochondriasis T score of 75 or less. Regardless of the technique or surgeon, one can easily predict a better than 90% chance of improvement or relief of the leg pain in this situation.

Surgical disc removal is only mandatory and urgent in cauda equina syndrome with significant neurologic def-

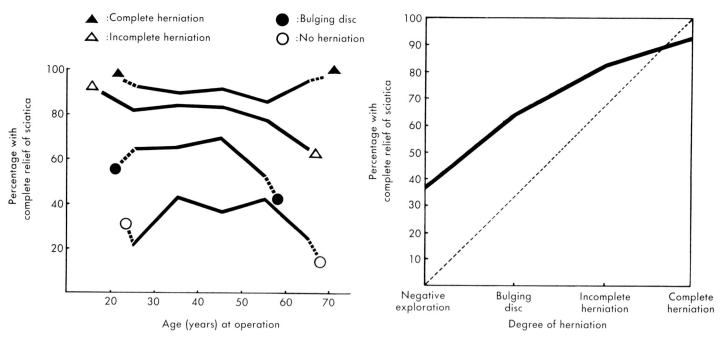

Fig. 84-23 Percent relief of sciatica with type of disc herniation. (From Spangfort E: Acta Orthop Scand Suppl 142:1, 1972.)

icit, especially bowel or bladder disturbance. All other disc excisions should be considered elective. This should allow a thorough evaluation to confirm the diagnosis, level of involvement, and the physical and psychologic status of patient. Frequently when there is a rush to the operating room to relieve pain without proper investigation both the patient and physician later regret the decision.

Regardless of the method chosen to surgically treat a disc rupture, the patient should be aware that the procedure is for the symptomatic relief of leg pain. Patients with predominant back pain may not be relieved of their major complaint — back pain. Spangfort in reviewing 2504 lumbar disc excisions found that about 30% of the patients complained of back pain after disc surgery. Failure to relieve sciatica was proportional to the degree of herniation. The best results of 99.5% complete or partial pain relief were obtained when the disc was free in the canal or sequestered. Incomplete herniation or extrusion of disc material into the canal resulted in complete relief for 82% of patients. Excision of the bulging or protruding disc that had not ruptured through the anulus resulted in complete relief in 63%, and removal of the normal or minimally bulging disc resulted in complete relief in 38% (this is near the stated level for the placebo response). Likewise, the incidence of persistent back pain after surgery was inversely proportional to the degree of herniation. In patients with complete extrusions the incidence was about 25%, but with minimal bulges or negative explorations the incidence rose to over 55% (Figs. 84-23 and 84-24).

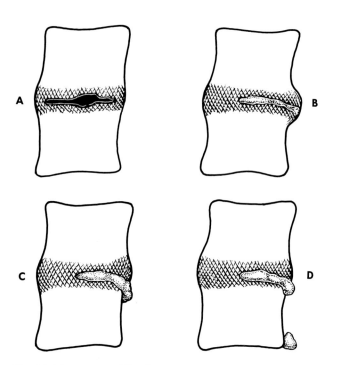

Fig. 84-24 Types of disc herniation. **A,** Normal bulge. **B,** Protrusion. **C,** Extrusion. **D,** Sequestration.

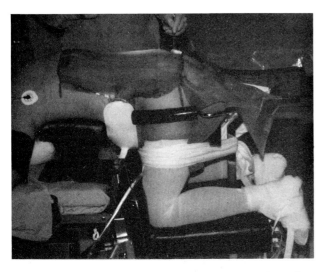

Fig. 84-25 Kneeling position for lumbar disc excision allows abdomen to be completely free of external pressure.

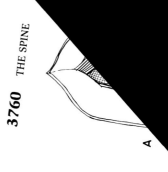

GENERAL PRINCIPLES FOR OPEN DISC SURGERY. Most disc surgery is performed with the patient under general endotracheal anesthesia, although local anesthesia has been used with minimal complications. Patient positioning varies with the operative technique and surgeon. To position the patient in a modified kneeling position, a specialized frame or custom frame modified from the design of Hastings is gaining popularity. Positioning the patient in this manner allows the abdomen to hang free, minimizing epidural venous dilation and bleeding (Fig. 84-25). A head lamp allows the surgeon to direct light into the lateral recesses where a large proportion of the surgery may be required. The addition of loupe magnification also greatly improves the identification and exposure of various structures. Some surgeons also use the operative microscope to further improve visibility. Roentgenographic confirmation of the proper level may be necessary if the exposure is small or if there is question as to the anatomic level during the dissection. Care should be taken to protect neural structures. Epidural bleeding should be controlled with bipolar electrocautery. Any sponge, pack, or cottonoid patty placed in the wound should extend to the outside. Pituitary rongeurs should be marked at a point equal to the maximum allowable disc depth to prevent accidental biopsy of viscera or aorta. Considerable research has gone into techniques to prevent epidural fibrosis. The placement of a large chunk of autogenous fat appears to be a reasonable although not foolproof or complication-free technique of minimizing postoperative epidural fibrosis.

RUPTURED LUMBAR DISC EXCISION

■ *TECHNIQUE.* After thoroughly preparing the back, identify the spinous processes of L3, L4, L5, and S1. Make a midline incision 5 to 10 cm long, in most instances from the spinous process of the fourth lumbar vertebra to the fir ploration of the third incision to the third the supraspinous lig to the first sacral sp osteal dissection sti and laminae of thes sion. Retract the m retractor or with th one interspace at sacrum by palpat mistake is made r plored. Secure hemostasis with electroc wax, and packs. Leave a portion of each pack completely outside the wound for ready identification.

Denude the laminae and ligamentum flavum with a curet (Fig. 84-26). Commonly the lumbosacral interspace is large enough to permit exposure and removal of a herniated nucleus pulposus without removal of any bone. If not, remove a small part of the inferior margin of the fifth lumbar lamina. Exposure of the disc at higher levels usually requires removal of a portion of the inferior lamina. Grasp the ligamentum flavum with an Allis or Kocher clamp and incise it with a bayonet-pointed knife where it fuses with the interspinous ligament. During dissection of the ligament keep the point of the knife in view so that the dura will not be nicked. Remove the flap of ligamentum flavum by sharp dissection. With an angulated Kerrison rongeur carefully remove the small shelving portion of ligamentum flavum left laterally. Next, retract the dura medially and identify the nerve root. If the root is compressed by a large extruded fragment, it will commonly be displaced posteriorly. Retract the nerve root, once identified, medially so that the underlying extruded fragment or bulging posterior longitudinal ligament can be seen. Occasionally the nerve root adheres to the fragment or to the underlying ligamentous structures and will require sharp dissection from these structures. If there is any question as to the position of the root, remove the lamina until the pedicle is visible. This will allow the identification of the upper and lower roots. Use cottonoid patties to tamponade the epidural veins both caudad and cephalad once the nerve root has been identified and retracted. Take care to minimize packing about the nerve root. Retract the root or dura, identify any bleeding vein, and cauterize it with a bipolar cautery. Earlier insertion of cotton patties may well displace fragments from view. The underlying disc should be clearly visible at this time.

Hold the nerve by a Love root retractor or a blunt dissector, thus exposing the herniated fragment or posterior longitudinal ligament and anulus. If an extruded fragment is not seen, carefully palpate the posterior longitudinal ligament and seek a defect or

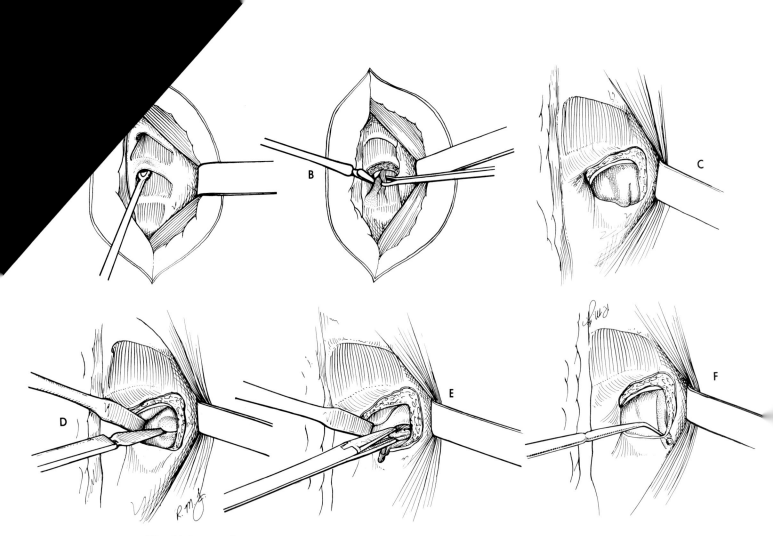

Fig. 84-26 Technique of lumbar disc excision. **A,** With lamina and ligamentum flavum exposed, use curet to remove the ligamentum flavum from inferior surface of lamina. Kerrison rongeur is used to remove bone. **B,** Elevate ligamentum flavum at upper corner and carefully dissect it back to expose dura and epidural fat below. Patties should be used to protect dura during this procedure. **C,** Expose dura and root. Remove additional bone if there is any question about adequacy of exposure. **D,** Retract nerve root and dural sac to expose disc. Inspect capsule for rent and extruded nuclear material. If obvious ligamentous defect is not visible, then carefully incise capsule of disc. If disc material does not bulge out, press on disc to try to dislodge herniated fragment. **E,** Carefully remove disc fragments. It is safest to avoid opening pituitary rongeur until it is inserted into disc space. **F,** After removing disc, carefully explore foramen, subligamentous region, and beneath dura for additional fragments of disc. Obtain meticulous hemostasis using bipolar cauterization.

hole in the ligamentous structures. If no obvious abnormality is detected, follow the root around the pedicle or even outside the canal in search of fragments that may have migrated far laterally. Additional searching in the root axilla helps ensure that fragments that have migrated inferiorly are not missed.

If the herniated fragment is especially large, it is much better to sacrifice the facet to obtain a more lateral exposure than to risk injury to the root or cauda equina by excessive medial retraction. With such a lateral exposure the nerve root usually can be elevated, and the herniated fragment can be teased from beneath the nerve root and cauda equina, even when the fragment is large enough to block the entire canal. If the disc cannot be teased from under the root, make a cruciate incision in the disc laterally. Gently remove disc fragments until the bulge has been decompressed to allow gentle retraction of the root over the defect.

If the herniation is upward or downward, further removal of bone from the lamina and facet edges may be required. The herniated nucleus pulposus may be covered by a layer of posterior longitudinal ligament or may have ruptured through this structure. In the latter event carefully lift the loose fragments out by suction, blunt hook, or pituitary forceps. If the ligament is intact, incise it in a cruciate fashion and remove the loose fragments. The tear or hole in the anulus should then be identifiable in most instances. The cavity of the disc may be entered through this hole, or occasionally the hole may need enlargement to allow insertion of the pituitary forceps. Remember that the anterior part of the anulus is adjacent to the aorta, vena cava, or iliac arteries and that one of these structures may be injured if one proceeds too deeply. Remove other loose fragments of nucleus pulposus with the pituitary forceps and curet loose and remove the additional nuclear material along with the central portion of the cartilaginous plates, both above and below.

Early in the dissection of the disc space measure or palpate the level of the anterior anulus and take care throughout this portion of the procedure not to exceed the distance to the anterior anulus. Then carry out a complete search for additional fragments of nucleus pulposus, both inside and outside the disc space. Additional fragments commonly migrate medially beneath the posterior longitudinal ligament but outside the anulus and may easily be missed. Then remove all cotton pledgets and control residual bleeding with Gelfoam or bits of muscle or fat; remove the Gelfoam or muscle after bleeding has been controlled with bipolar cautery. Close the wound routinely with absorbable sutures in the supraspinous ligament and subcutaneous tissue. Various nonabsorbable sutures or skin staples are most commonly used in routine skin closure.

AFTERTREATMENT. The patient is allowed to turn in bed at will and to select a position of comfort such as a semi-Fowler position. Opiates are used for pain control. Bladder stimulants may be used to assist voiding. The patient is allowed to stand with assistance on the evening after surgery to go to the bathroom. The patient is encouraged to walk on the first postoperative day. Isometric abdominal and lower extremity exercises are reinstituted. Sitting is minimized, but walking is progressively increased. When the patient is walking comfortably and pain medication intake is minimal, the patient is discharged. The patient is instructed to minimize sitting and riding in a vehicle. Increased walking on a daily basis is recommended. Lifting, bending, and stooping are prohibited for the first several weeks. The sutures are removed in 10 to 14 days. As the patient's strength increases, gentle isotonic leg exercises are started.

Between the fourth and sixth postoperative week Back School instruction is resumed or started provided pain is minimal. Lifting, bending, and stooping are gradually restarted after the sixth week. Increased sitting is allowed after the fourth week, but

long trips are to be avoided for at least 3 months. Lower extremity strength is increased from the eighth to twelfth postoperative weeks. Patients with jobs requiring much walking without lifting are allowed to return to work within 4 weeks. Patients with jobs requiring prolonged sitting usually are allowed to return to work within 6 to 8 weeks provided minimal lifting is required. Patients with jobs requiring heavy labor or long periods of driving are not allowed to return to work until the twelfth week and then to a modified duty. Some patients with jobs requiring exceptionally heavy manual labor may have to permanently modify their occupation or seek a lighter occupation. Keeping the patient out of work beyond 3 months rarely improves recovery or pain relief.

MICROLUMBAR DISC EXCISION. Microlumbar discectomy requires an operating microscope with a 400 mm lens; special retractors; a 1 mm, 45-degree Kerrison rongeur; a micropituitary rongeur; and a combination suction nerve root retractor. The procedure is performed with the patient prone. A vacuum pack is molded around the patient, and an inflatable pillow is positioned under the abdomen and is removed after evacuation of the vacuum pack. The microscope is used from skin incision to closure. If the proper level is in question, a lateral roentgenogram is taken to confirm placement.

■ *TECHNIQUE (WILLIAMS).* Make the incision from the spinous process of the upper vertebra to the spinous process of the lower vertebra at the involved level. This usually results in a 1-inch (2.5 cm) skin incision (Fig. 84-27). Maintain meticulous hemostasis with electrocautery as the dissection is carried to the fascia. Incise the fascia at the midline using electrocautery. Then insert a periosteal elevator in the midline incision. Using gentle lateral movements separate the deep fascia and muscle subperiosteally from the spinous processes and lamina. Meticulously cauterize all bleeding points. Then insert a finger to palpate the interlaminar space. Insert the microlumbar retractor into the wound and adjust the microscope. Identify the ligamentum flavum and lamina. Using a No. 15 blade with the microscope set at a 25× magnification, carefully incise the ligamentum flavum superficially. Then use a Penfield No. 4 dissector to perforate the ligamentum. Minimal force should be used in this maneuver to prevent penetration of the dura. Once the ligamentum is open, use a 45-degree Kerrison rongeur with a 1 mm cup to remove the ligamentum flavum toward the surgeon. The lamina, facet, and facet capsule should remain intact. Then make the extradural exploration using a blunt 90-degree hook. Gentle manipulation with the nerve hook will assist in identification of the nerve root. In large herniations the nerve root will appear as a

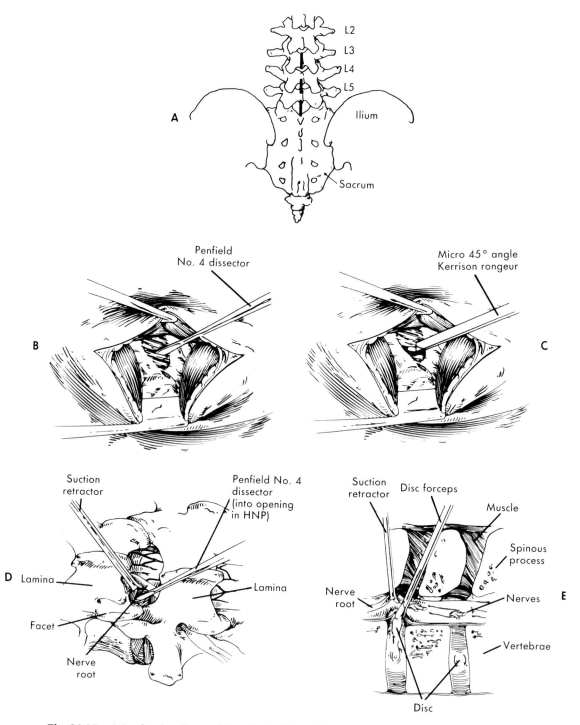

Fig. 84-27   Microlumbar disc excision. **A,** Position of skin incision for microlumbar disc excision. **B,** Entrance of epidural space by penetration of ligamentum flavum. **C,** Removal of ligamentum flavum with Kerrison rongeur. **D,** Dilation of anular defect before removal of disc fragment. **E,** Decompression of disc hernia by repeated small evacuations with discectomy forceps. (From Cauthen JC: Lumbar spine surgery, Baltimore, 1983, Williams & Wilkins.)

large, white, glistening structure and can easily be mistaken for a ruptured disc. If an epidural vein ruptures, proceed with the dissection and remove the disc.

Do not attempt to use pressure techniques or electrocautery in the limited space because severe nerve root injury may result. Epidural fat is not removed in this procedure. Insert the nerve root retractor, suction with its tip turned medially under the nerve root, and hold the manifold between the thumb and index finger. With the nerve root retracted the disc will now be visible as a white, fibrous, avascular structure. Small tears may be visible in the anulus under the magnification. Now enlarge the anular tear with a Penfield No. 4 dissector and remove the disc material with the microdisc forceps. Do not insert the instrument into the disc space beyond the angle of the jaws. Remove only exposed disc material. Do not curet the disc space. Inspect the root and adjacent dura for disc fragments. Close the fascia and skin in the usual fashion.

AFTERTREATMENT. Postoperative care is similar to that after standard open disc surgery. Those who perform this surgery indicate that a 3-day postoperative hospitalization is usual. We have no experience with this technique.

RESULTS OF OPEN SURGERY FOR DISC HERNIATION. Numerous retrospective and some prospective reviews of open disc surgery are available. The results of these series vary greatly with respect to patient selection, treatment method, evaluation method, length of follow-up, and conclusions. Good results range from 46% to 97%. Complications range from none to over 10%. The reoperation rate ranges from 4% to over 20%. The detailed studies of Spangfort, Weir, and Rish are suggested for more detailed analysis. A comparison between techniques also reveals similar reports. Few reports concerning microlumbar discectomy have appeared (Table 84-6). Two recent reports found the only statistically significant difference in microsurgical patients to be a shorter period of hospitalization. Kahanovitz, Viola, and Muculloch reported a 2-day stay for the microdiscectomy group and 7 days for the open group. This may be altered by other factors. Our average hospitalization is 2½ days for open lumbar disc surgery.

Several points do stand out in the analysis of the results of lumbar disc surgery. Patient selection appears to be extremely important. Several recent studies have noted that a low educational level is significantly related to poor results of surgery. The works of Wiltse and Rocchio, and of Gentry indicate that valid results of the Minnesota Multiphasic Personality Inventory (hysteria and hypochondriasis T scores) are extremely good indicators of surgical outcome regardless of the degree of the pathologic condition. The extremely detailed work of Weir suggests that the duration of the present episode, the age of the patient, the presence or absence of predominant back pain, the number of previous hospitalizations, and the presence or absence of compensation for a work injury are factors with regard to the final outcome. Spangfort's work also indicates that the softer the findings for disc herniation clinically and at the time of surgery, the lower the chance for a good result.

COMPLICATIONS OF OPEN DISC EXCISION. The complications associated with standard disc excision and microlumbar disc excision are similar. Spangfort's series (Table 84-7) of 2503 open disc excisions lists a postoperative mortality of 0.1%, a thromboembolism rate of 1.0%, a postoperative infection rate of 3.2%, and a deep disc space infection rate of 1.1%. Postoperative cauda equina lesions developed in five patients. Laceration of the aorta or iliac artery has also been described as a rare complica-

Table 84-6   Results of lumbar disc excision by various methods

Technique	Year	Number performed	Excellent	Partial/good	None	Worse	Complications	Reoperation	Persistent back pain
Open disc									
Semmes	1955	1440	53.6	43.3	1.7	1.4	NA*	6.3	
Spangfort	1972	2503	76.9	17.0	5.0	0.5	8.0		31.5
Weir	1979	100	73.0	22.0	3.0	1.0	NA	NA	
Rish	1984	57	74.0	17.0	9.0		4.0	18.0	
Microdiscectomy									
Williams and Hudgins	1983	200		88.0	8.0	4.0	1.5	5.0	
Anterior lumbar intervertebral fusion									
Harmon	1963	220		84.5	12.7	1.4		1.4	
Posterior lumbar intervertebral fusion									
Rish	1984	13	62.0	20.0	18.0				

*Not available.

Table 84-7 Complications of lumbar disc surgery

Complication	Incidence (percent)
1. Cauda equina syndrome	0.2
2. Thrombophlebitis	1.0
3. Pulmonary embolism	0.4
4. Wound infection	2.2
5. Pyogenic spondylitis	0.07
6. Postoperative discitis	2.0 (1122 patients)
7. Dural tears	1.6
8. Nerve root injury	0.5
9. Cerebrospinal fluid fistula	*
10. Laceration of abdominal vessels	*
11. Injury to abdominal viscera	*

Modified from Spangfort EV: Acta Orthop Scand Suppl 142:65, 1972.
*Rare occurrence (10 and 11 not identified in Spangfort's study but reported elsewhere).

tion of this operation. Rish, in a more recent report with a 5-year follow-up, noted a total complication rate of 4% in a series of 205 patients. The major complication in his series involved a worsening neuropathy postoperatively. There were one disc space infection and one wound infection. Dural tears with cerebrospinal fluid leaks, pseudomeningocele formation, cerebrospinal fluid fistula formation, and meningitis are also possible but are more likely after reoperation. Two series of microlumbar disc excisions do not note postoperative complications. Alexander reviewed patients who had sustained accidental durotomy at the time of disc surgery and found no perioperative morbidity or compromise of results if the dura was repaired. They noted a 4% incidence of this complication in 450 discectomies.

The presence of a dural tear or leak results in the potentially serious problems of pseudomeningocele, cerebrospinal fluid leak, and meningitis. Eismont, Wiesel, and Rothman have suggested five basic principles in the repair of these leaks (Fig. 84-28):

1. The operative field must be unobstructed, dry, and well exposed.
2. Dural suture of a 6-0 or 7-0 gauge with a tapered or reverse cutting needle is used in either a simple or running locking stitch. If the leak is large or inaccessible, a free fat graft or fascial graft may be sutured to the dura.
3. All repairs should be tested by using the reverse Trendelenburg position and Valsalva maneuvers.
4. Paraspinous muscles and overlying fascia should be closed in two layers with nonabsorbable suture used in a watertight fashion. Drains should not be used.
5. Bed rest in the supine position should be maintained for 4 to 7 days after the repair of lumbar dural defects.

The development of headaches on standing and a stormy postoperative period should alert one to the possibility of an undetected cerebrospinal fluid leak. This can be confirmed by myelography or radioiodinated serum albumin scans. The presence of glucose in drainage fluid is not a reliable diagnostic test. On rare occasions a pseudomeningocele has been implicated as a cause of persistent pain from pressure on a nerve root by the cystic mass.

ADDITIONAL EXPOSURE TECHNIQUES. The presence of a large disc herniation or other pathologic condition such as lateral recess stenosis or foraminal stenosis may dictate a greater exposure of the nerve root. Usually the additional pathologic condition can be identified before surgery. If the extent of the lesion is known before surgery, the proper approach can be planned. Additional exposure includes hemilaminectomy, total laminectomy, and facetectomy. Hemilaminectomy usually is required when identifying the root is a problem. This may occur with a conjoined root. Total laminectomy usually is reserved for patients with spinal stenoses that are central in nature. Facetectomy usually is reserved for foraminal stenosis or severe lateral recess stenosis. If more than one facet is removed, then a fusion should be considered in addition. This is especially true in the removal of both facets and the disc at the same interspace in a young, active person with a normal disc height at that level.

On rare occasions disc herniation has been reported to be intradural. An extremely large disc that cannot be dissected from the dura or the persistence of an intradural mass after dissection of the disc should alert one to this potential problem. Excision of an intradural disc requires a transdural approach. This approach increases the risk of complications from cerebrospinal fluid leak and intradural scarring.

FREE FAT GRAFTING. Fat grafting for the prevention of postoperative epidural scarring has been suggested by Kiviluoto; Jacobs, McClain, and Neff; and Bryant, Bremer, and Nguyen. The study by Jacobs et al. indicated that free fat grafts were superior to Gelfoam in the prevention of postoperative scarring. The present rationale for free fat grafting appears to be the possibility of making any reoperation easier. Unfortunately, the benefit of reduced scarring and its relationship to the prevention of postoperative pain have not been established; neither has the increased ease of reoperation in patients in whom fat grafting was performed. Fat grafts also are useful in the prevention of cerebrospinal fluid leaks. Caution should be taken in applying a fat graft to a large laminar defect because this has been reported to result in an acute cauda equina syndrome in the early postoperative period. We presently reserve the use of a fat graft for dural leaks and small laminar defects where the graft is supported by the bone.

The technique of free fat grafting is straightforward. At the end of the procedure, just before closing, take a large chunk of subcutaneous fat and insert it over the laminectomy defect. If the patient is thin, a separate incision over

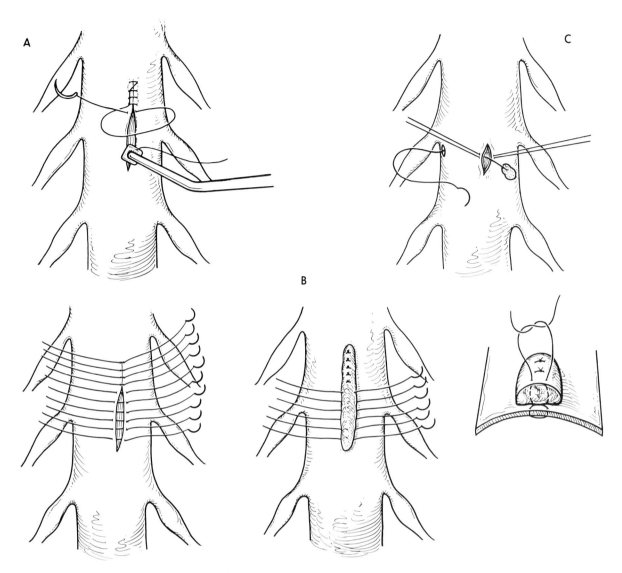

Fig. 84-28   A, Illustration of dural repair using running-locking dural suture on taper or reverse-cutting, one-half-circle needle. A smaller-sized suture should be used. Use of suction with sucker and small cotton pledgets is essential to protect nerve roots while operative field is kept dry of cerebrospinal fluid. **B,** Single dural stitches may be used to achieve closure, each suture end being left long. Second needle then is attached to free suture end, and ends of suture are passed through piece of muscle or fat, which is tied down over repaired tear to help to achieve watertight closure. Whenever dural material is inadequate to allow closure without placing excessive pressure on underlying neural tissues, a free graft of fascia or fascia lata, or freeze-dried dural graft, should be secured to margins of dural tear using simple sutures of appropriate size. **C,** For small dural defects in relatively inaccessible areas, transdural approach can be used to pull small piece of muscle or fat into defect from inside out, thereby sealing cerebrospinal fluid leak. Central durotomy should be large enough to expose defect from dural sac. Durotomy is then closed in standard watertight fashion. (From Eismont FJ, Wiesel SW, and Rothman RH: J Bone Joint Surg 63-A:1132, 1981.)

the buttock may be required to get sufficient fat to fill the defect.

Lumbar Root Anomalies

Lumbar nerve root anomalies (Figs. 84-29 to 84-32) are more common than may be expected, and they rarely

are correctly identified with myelography. Kadish and Simmons identified lumbar nerve root anomalies in 14% of 100 cadaver examinations. They noted nerve root anomalies in only 4% of 100 consecutive metrizamide myelograms. They identified four types of anomalies. Type I is an intradural anastomosis between rootlets at different levels. Type II is an anomalous origin of the

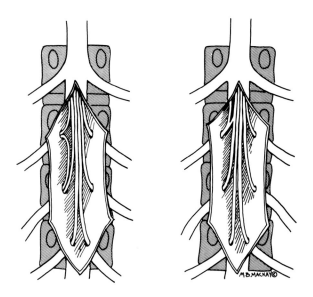

Fig. 84-29 Type I nerve root anomaly: intradural anastomosis. (From Kadish LJ and Simmons EH: J Bone Joint Surg 66-B:411, 1984.)

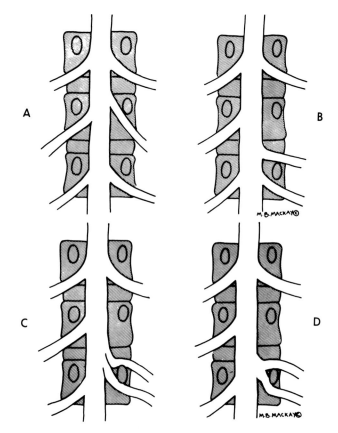

Fig. 84-30 Type II: anomalous origin of nerve roots. **A,** Cranial origin. **B,** Caudal origin. **C,** Closely adjacent nerve roots. **D,** Conjoined nerve roots. (From Kadish LJ and Simmons EH: J Bone Joint Surg 66-B:411, 1984.)

nerve roots. They separated this type into four subtypes: (1) cranial origin, (2) caudal origin, (3) combination of cranial and caudal origin, and (4) conjoined nerve roots. Type III is an extradural anastomosis between roots. Type IV is the extradural division of the nerve root. The surgeon must be aware of the possibility of anomalous roots hindering the disc excision. This may require a wider exposure. Sectioning of these roots results in irreversible neurologic damage. Traction on anomalous nerve roots has been suggested as a cause of sciatic symptoms without disc herniation.

Chemonucleolysis

Chemonucleolysis has been used experimentally in the United States for almost 30 years. The enzyme was released for general use by the Food and Drug Administration (FDA) in December of 1982. Before its release in the United States it was used extensively in Europe and Canada. A wealth of experimental and clinical information exists concerning the technique and the enzyme. Specific guidelines have been suggested by the FDA regarding the use of the enzyme in the United States. The initial enthusiasm for the use of chymopapain has all but vanished in the United States with fewer than 4000 such procedures performed in 1989. The use of this enzyme is still popular in Europe.

Because of the disclosure of the late development of transverse myelitis and other neurologic sequelae, the original guidelines issued in January of 1983 have been radically changed. The information presented regarding this technique reflects the most recent suggestions effective in January of 1985. Unlike other surgical procedures, this procedure requires certification of proficiency before the drug will be released to the treating physician.

Those interested in performing the technique are requested to contact the pharmaceutical companies producing the drug for information regarding training and certification in the technique. Treating physicians also are encouraged to frequently check the package insert accompanying the drug and the information bulletins sent out by the FDA and the pharmaceutical companies regarding any new changes in protocol or usage of the enzyme.

The indications for the use of chemonucleolysis are the same as for open surgery for disc herniation. Fraser reported the results of 60 patients treated for lumbar disc herniation in a 2-year double-blind study of chemonucleolysis. At 2 years 77% of the patients treated with chymopapain were improved, whereas only 47% of the saline injection group were improved. At 2 years from injection 57% of the chymopapain group were pain free compared with 23% of the placebo group. Numerous other studies of the efficacy of the drug place the good to excellent results between 40% and 89%, which is comparable to the clinical reports for open surgery (Table 84-8). As with open disc surgery, this technique is not applicable in all lumbar disc herniations. The use of the drug is limited to the lumbar spine. The patient optimally has

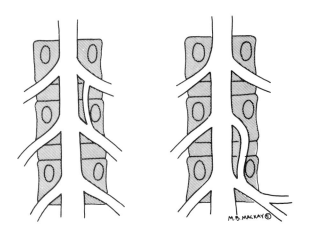

Fig. 84-31 Type III nerve root anomaly: extradural anastamosis. (From Kadish LJ and Simmons EH: J Bone Joint Surg 66-B:411, 1984.)

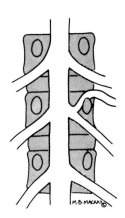

Fig. 84-32 Type IV nerve root anomaly: extradural division. (From Kadish LJ and Simmons EH: J Bone Joint Surg 66-B:411, 1984.)

predominantly unilateral leg pain and localizing neurologic findings consistent with confirmatory testing with CT or myelography. Patients with moderate lateral recess or foraminal stenosis may worsen after the procedure because of collapse of the disc space and narrowing of the foraminal opening. Large disc herniations may not shrink sufficiently to result in relief of symptoms, and sequestered discs may be untouched by the enzyme. Smith et al. reported cauda equina syndromes in three patients after chymopapain was injected after a myelogram revealed a complete block.

Dolan, Adams, and Hutton found that chymopapain did not affect the mechanical properties of the disc but did reduce the size of the nuclear material by 24% in 1 hour and 80% in 48 hours. Boumphrey et al. noted only 12% of patients had a decrease in the size of disc herniation by CT scan at 3 months. A much smaller number were also scanned at 6 months and 70% of those patients had a decreased disc herniation size. Suguro, Oegema, and Bradford noted a rapid removal of proteoglycans and matrix proteins after injection.

Chymopapain injection is specifically contraindicated in patients with a known sensitivity to papaya, papaya derivatives, or food containing papaya such as meat tenderizer. Other contraindications include severe spondylolisthesis; severe, progressive neurologic deficit or paralysis; and evidence of spinal cord tumor or a cauda equina lesion. The enzyme cannot be injected in a patient who has been previously injected, regardless of the level injected. Use of chymopapain is limited to the lumbar intervertebral discs. Relative contraindications include allergy to iodine or iodine contrast material; use of the enzyme in a previously operated disc; patients with elevated allergy studies such as radioallergosorbent (RAST), ChymoFast, and skin testing with the drug; and patients with a severe allergic history, especially with a previous anaphylactic attack. Recent clinical reports indicate that patients taking beta-blockers should not be considered for the procedure or should at least be taken off the drug for a time because these drugs may adversely affect epinephrine in the event of an anaphylactic reaction. It has also been suggested that the enzyme be injected without concomitant preinjection discography because of the intensification of neural damage if the en-

Table 84-8 Results and complications of chemonucleolysis and open disc excision

Technique	Year	Number performed	Results (percent)				Complications	Reoperation	Persistent back pain
			Excellent	Partial/good	None	Worse			
Open disc									
Semmes	1955	1440	53.6	43.3	1.7	1.4	NA*	6.3	
Spangfort	1972	2503	76.9	17.0	5.0	0.5	8.0		31.5
Weir	1979	100	73.0	22.0	3.0	1.0	NA	NA	
Rish	1984	57	74.0	17.0	9.0		4.0	18.0	
Chemonucleolysis									
Illinois trial	1982	273	90.0		10.0		1.1		
Javid	1983	40	82.0		18.0				
Nordby	1983	641	55.0	25.0	20.0		NA	NA	

*Not available.

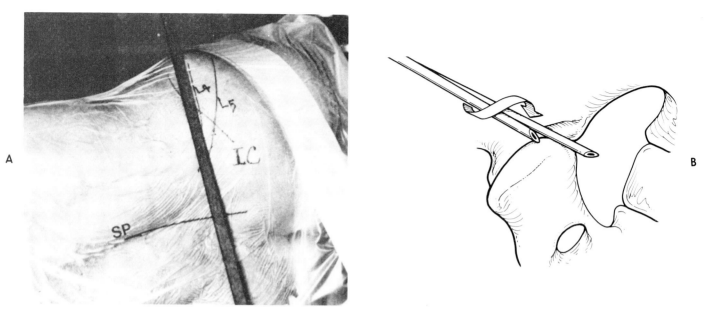

Fig. 84-33 **A,** Lines are drawn on skin parallel to disc space with metal bar or long ruler placed parallel to disc under image intensification. Lines are marked for L4-5 and L5-S1 discs. *IC,* Iliac crest. The smaller lines just below the iliac crest that transect the disc lines are the needle insertion points. Note the closeness of the L4-5 point to the L5-S1 point. **B,** Needle can be advanced over the facet by rotating the needle 180 degrees. Note that bevel of needle is pointing down in relation to position of insertion. (**A,** From Chung BU and **B,** from Thomas JC and Wiltse LL: In Brown JE, Nordby EJ, and Smith L: Chemonucleolysis, Thorofare, NJ, 1985, Slack.)

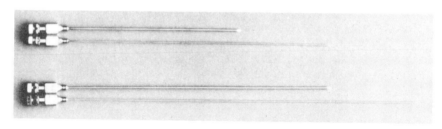

Fig. 84-34 Two sets of needles that are used in double-needle technique. Upper pair contains 4-inch, 18-gauge needle and 6-inch, 22-gauge needle. Lower pair contains 6-inch, 18-gauge needle and 8-inch, 22-gauge needle. The 22-gauge needle must be 2 inches longer than the 18-gauge needle. (From Thomas JC and Wiltse LL: In Brown JE, Nordby EJ, and Smith L: Chemonucleolysis, Thorofare, NJ, 1985, Slack.)

zyme is inadvertently injected intrathecally. All efforts should be made to prevent intrathecal leak or injection of the enzyme. At least 1 week should elapse between any intradural injection such as myelography and chymopapain injection. Injection should be further delayed if the patient is still experiencing a spinal headache. If spinal fluid is encountered in the process of needle placement, the procedure should be abandoned.

■ *TECHNIQUE.* The technique of chemonucleolysis (Figs. 84-33 and 84-34) begins with thorough patient preparation. This includes an explanation of the technique, possible adverse reactions, and usual postoperative occurrences and procedure. Testing for allergy or sensitivity to the enzyme is performed with adequate time to evaluate the results before the injection. The patient is started on cimetidine (Tagamet), 300 mg, and diphenhydramine (Benadryl), 50 mg, by mouth or intravenously every 6 hours for at least 24 hours before the procedure. Preoperative hydration also is suggested as an aid in the event of an anaphylactic reaction.

The procedure is done with the patient under local anesthesia with an anesthesiologist or an anesthetist in attendance administering oxygen and mild sedation as indicated. The injection of strong opiates is not recommended during the injection of the test dose and final injection because this may cause a drop in blood pressure, mimicking anaphylaxis. Constant monitoring of the blood pressure is essential. Insert a large-bore intravenous needle just before the initiation of the procedure. If there is any increased risk of anaphylaxis, insert an arterial line with the patient under local anesthesia. All materials for resuscitation in the event of anaphylaxis must be present in the room and available for immediate use. We presently use 1% lidocaine and 0.25% bupivacaine as the local anesthetic.

The technique requires image intensification capable of providing both anteroposterior and lateral projections. An operating platform capable of allowing the transmission of radiation also is required. The ability to provide roentgenographic documentation of needle placement also is suggested. Additional materials include 4-, 6-, and 8-inch (10, 15.2, and 20.3 cm) spinal needles in 18-, 20-, and 22-gauge sizes, a large metric ruler, several 5 or 10 ml syringes, and two 1 ml syringes for each level injected. The draping technique is variable and possibly dictated by the image intensification equipment. We presently use a large, clear plastic drape with an adhesive center that also is used in hip nailing procedures. Additional draping is not necessary with this method because a sterile barrier is maintained between the image intensifier and the operative field.

The anesthetist or anesthesiologist, having prepared the patient with a large-bore intravenous line and automatic blood pressure monitor or arterial line, instructs the patient to turn on the left side with the hips and knees flexed at 45 degrees. The procedure is performed on a table capable of allowing roentgen transmission and mobility of an image intensifier C-arm. The left iliac crest is elevated with a roll of towels or an inflatable bladder. This allows leveling the spine or opening the L5-S1 disc space if this level is to be injected. Absolute anteroposterior and lateral positioning of the patient is determined by image intensification. The patient is held in this position with tape if desired.

Prepare and drape the back in the standard surgical fashion. Using a long radiopaque object such as a steel ruler, identify the disc level of interest. Use a marking pen to draw a line on the back parallel with and at the level of each disc to be injected. Then make a mark about 8.5 cm lateral to the midline or spinous process, bisecting the disc lines. Remove the drape from the area to be injected. Infiltrate the skin with a local anesthetic agent at each level. Make a small stab wound with a No. 11 blade. Direct a spinal needle of at least 18-gauge and 4 to 6 inches (10 to 15.2 cm) in length parallel with the disc line drawn on the skin at about 45 to 55 degrees to the back, angling toward the spine. Inject additional anesthetic agent as the needle is advanced. Monitor proper alignment in both anteroposterior and lateral projections as you advance the needle.

When the disc level is reached, the needle should be at the outer border of the vertebral bodies and disc in the anteroposterior view and at the posterior edge of the bodies in the lateral view. If a double-needle technique is used, advance the larger needle (usually 18-gauge) only as far as the intertransverse ligament or lamina. Then insert the smaller needle (usually 22-gauge and at least 2 inches [5 cm] longer) into the larger needle and advance it into the disc. When the needle enters the disc, a distinct change in resistance and a "gritty" sensation are noted. The only pain that occurs during this maneuver is the result of nerve root irritation or penetration by the needle just lateral to the disc. Aspirate the needle if there is any question of dural penetration by the needle. *If the dura is penetrated, abandon the procedure.* Proper needle placement should put the needle in the center in the lateral view and dead center over the spinous process in the anteroposterior view. If there is any question regarding the needle position, perform a saline acceptance test using about 1 ml of sterile saline from a new container. The saline should enter easily. Check the level of injection and position of the needle with standard anteroposterior and lateral roentgenograms.

If resistance to the saline acceptance test is extreme, then the needle tip is in the anulus or the disc is normal. If the needle position is satisfactory, then carry out discography using metrizamide to be sure that the disc is normal. At this point if the injection is anular or the disc is normal, redirect the needle into the proper disc or direction. If the contrast leaks into the epidural space, it may be safer to abandon the procedure to avoid the potential of mixing contrast and chymopapain intradurally. When a nerve root is encountered repeatedly, injecting metrizamide into the root sleeve may be beneficial to demonstrate the nerve so as to position the needle to avoid it. Intradural injection demands termination of the procedure.

The most difficult needle placement is at L5-S1 (see Fig. 84-33). The usual entry point is about ¼-inch (6 mm) caudal to the L4-5 interspace. This needle is directed 45 to 60 degrees to the sagittal plane of the back and 30 degrees caudally. It must traverse the small opening formed by the iliac crest laterally, the ala of the sacrum caudally, and the transverse process of L5 cranially. Determine accurate placement by checking the anteroposterior view when the needle reaches the level of the lamina in the lateral view. At this point, the needle should be in the center of the triangle formed by the transverse process of L5, the ala of the sacrum, and the iliac crest as viewed in the anteroposterior view. The use of the double-needle technique with a small 22-gauge needle is of value here because it may be necessary to traverse the L5 root before entering the disc space. If a large needle is used, the nerve may be permanently damaged.

The recent availability of noncutting 18-gauge needles and prebent 22-gauge needles may diminish the risk of permanent nerve damage. If a prebent needle is used, the first needle must be advanced to the edge of the anulus. Further, a prebent needle will begin to turn immediately on exiting the first needle and there is little control. Therefore the surgeon is urged to practice with these needles before their use to master the eccentricities of the needle turning on exit from the first needle (see Fig. 84-34). Before initiating this procedure, check the lateral roentgenogram for a high iliac crest. This may indicate that entrance into the L5-S1 disc space will be difficult, and prebent needles may be necessary. Occasionally it is impossible to enter this space with a needle.

Pure oxygen is administered by the anesthesiologist for 3 minutes before injection, continuing to the end of the procedure. Inject a test dose of 0.2 ml of enzyme. Allow 15 to 20 minutes to elapse. Then inject the final dose of enzyme. The total dose injected should not exceed 1.5 ml or 4000 μl per disc or 8000 μl per patient. We suggest that only the one, symptomatic level be injected.

In the absence of any adverse reaction, the patient is transferred to the recovery room for 2 hours of constant monitoring before returning to his room. Narcotics and sedatives may be administered for the relief of back pain as indicated.

AFTERTREATMENT. Back pain and spasm are the most common occurrences after chemonucleolysis. When they occur, the patient should be placed in a position of rest such as the semi-Fowler or lateral decubitus position. Ice massage may be used for muscle spasm. Opiates and sedatives are provided as necessary. If the pain is mild, the patient is encouraged to walk wearing a lumbar corset. The patient is also instructed in the proper way to get out of bed without excessive spinal movement. The patient is discharged when the pain is easily controlled with mild pain medication and walking is comfortable. As after open disc surgery, the patient is to refrain from sitting, riding in vehicles, lifting, bending, and stooping. In uncomplicated injections discharge is within 1 to 2 days. The remaining postoperative care is similar to that for open disc surgery with the exception that patients with walking and sitting jobs involving minimal lifting may re-

Table 84-9   Reported severe complications of chemonucleolysis in 57,341 patients from Smith Laboratories postmarketing survey as of February 1, 1985

Complication	No. of patients	Percent
Mortality*	20	0.022
Anaphylaxis	5	
Cerebral hemorrhage	6	
Cardiorespiratory	4	
Infection	2	
Other	1	
Anaphylaxis	306	0.5
Male	106	0.3
Female	200	0.9
Neurologic complications	49	0.086
Cerebral hemorrhage	14	
Subarachnoid hemorrhage	1	
Paralysis	27	
Quadriplegia	1	
Hemiparesis	1	
Guillain-Barré	1	
Seizures	4	

From pp 23-25, Chemonucleolysis Resource Center Teaching Program, 1985, Smith Laboratories.
*Includes all reported deaths in 90,000 injections (0.022%).

turn to work sooner if they are pain free. Heavy laborers usually are able to return to work at 3 months.

COMPLICATIONS. The complications of chemonucleolysis (Table 84-9) have been well publicized, but similar complications of open disc surgery and myelography have received much less attention. Serious complications of chemonucleolysis are anaphylaxis (2.5% to 0.4% with five deaths in 50,000 injections), cerebral hemorrhage (eight patients in about 48,000 injections), paraplegia or paraparesis (20 patients in 48,000 injections), and disc space infection (two patients in 48,000 injections). Many of these complications can be prevented or minimized. Anaphylaxis must be considered and anticipated in all injections. Patients who could not tolerate any episode of hypotension should not be treated with this technique. Preoperative testing for sensitivity should pinpoint patients at risk. Testing with ChymoFast is 99.6% accurate with only a 0.4% false negative rate. The exact rates for the RAST test and skin testing are not known at this time. The evaluation of neurologic complications has implicated the use of a general anesthetic, dural puncture, injection of more than one level, and the concomitant use of radiopaque roentgenographic dyes as common denominators. Avoidance of these methods and meticulous attention to detail in the insertion of the needles should minimize the risk of neurologic complications. Infection can be minimized by using new sterile vials of saline for the saline acceptance test and the diluent enclosed with the drug.

Anaphylaxis from the injection is presently (1991) reported to occur in 0.24% of patients. Black females are the most susceptible, with a 1.72% incidence. White males are the least susceptible, with a 0.23% incidence. Death as a result of the anaphylaxis is reported at 1:30,000. Neurological complications have decreased dramatically since 1985. From 1982 to 1985, 116,329 procedures were reported with 57 adverse neurologic reactions, for a 0.05% reaction rate. From 1987 to 1989, 7616 procedures were performed with one reaction, for a 0.013% adverse neurologic reaction rate.

Patients who have had previous injections of chymopapain should not be reinjected. Other relative contraindications to the procedure are the presence of chymopapain-specific IgE antibodies, prior surgical procedures at the same level, progressive neurologic deficit, bowel or bladder symptoms, evidence of spinal cord tumor, spinal stenosis, spondylolisthesis, significant degenerative disc disease, serious concurrent illness, obesity, sequestrated disc fragment, and pregnancy.

Treatment of anaphylaxis. The most serious and life-threatening complication of chymopapain injection is anaphylaxis. The onset of anaphylaxis is within the first 20 minutes in 98% of the patients experiencing this complication. The risk of such a reaction is quite low 2 hours after injection. In the awake patient the first sign may be a generalized itch, a mild erythema over the trunk, respiratory difficulty, or a sinking, "dying" sensation. If an arterial line is in place there may be a sudden drop in pressure of 20 to 40 torr.

Immediate response is mandatory (see protocol below); intravenous fluids are opened fully, needles and drapes are removed, and the patient is moved to the supine position. Epinephrine is injected intravenously. The initial dosage is usually 0.5 to 1 ml of a 1/10,000 solution given every 1 to 5 minutes up to a total of 2 mg per hour. The patient should be intubated. Bicarbonate, diphenhydramine, cimetidine, and steroids also are given with large volumes of fluid. Cardiopulmonary resuscitation is instituted if necessary. Vigorous and prompt reaction to this complication is mandatory if death is to be prevented. Patients with severe systemic disease who could not tolerate the insult of hypotension, epinephrine injection, and massive volume expansion should not be considered candidates for the procedure.

The recommended treatment protocol for anaphylaxis follows*:

First priority:
Stop administration of antigen.
Administer 100% oxygen.
Stop administration of anesthetic.
Expand volume.
Give intravenous infusion of 0.5 to 1.0 ml of 1:10,000 epinephrine solution not to exceed 0.5 mg over 10

minutes or intravenous bolus of 0.5 to 5 ml 1:10,000 epinephrine solution (up to 2 mg/hr).
Obtain blood gases as soon as possible and treat acidosis appropriately or administer one 50 mEq ampule of bicarbonate prophylactically every 5 minutes for severe hypotension.
Second priority:
Give initial bolus of 1 g hydrocortisone IV.
Administer catecholamine if slow response in peripheral blood pressure.
Give loading dose of 5 to 9 mg/kg aminophylline over 20 to 30 minutes for bronchospasm.
Administer 50 mg diphenhydramine and 300 mg cimetidine (70 kg patient) IV.
After termination of reaction:
Check airway for laryngeal edema before extubation.

Percutaneous Lumbar Discectomy

Hijikata first published the results of percutaneous discectomy and noted that 80% of his patients were improved. Since that time many others have used the technique with variable results. New advancements have resulted in an automated form of the procedure. The procedure is limited to L4-5 and to a lesser degree to L5-S1 discs with subcapsular herniations or protrusions with predominant leg pain. Unlike chemonucleolysis there have been few controlled studies of this technique. Kahanovitz et al., in a multicenter study of the automated technique, reported a greater persistence of pain, weakness, and numbness in the percutaneous group when compared to a surgically treated group. Others (including Maroon, Onik, and Sternau; Shepperd, James, and Leach; Stern; Kambin and Schaffer; Onik et al.; and Schreiber, Suezawa, and Leu) have reported success rates ranging from 70% to 90%. There have been no blind controls in these studies. Although the frequency and types of complications encountered are unknown, reported complications include neurologic injury, vascular injury, and disc space infection. Injury to the abdominal contents and retroperitoneal structures is possible but has not been reported in the literature. We have no experience with this procedure.

SPINAL INSTABILITY FROM DEGENERATIVE DISC DISEASE

Farfan defines spinal instability (caused by degenerative disc disease) as a clinically symptomatic condition without new injury, in which a physiologic load induces abnormally large deformations at the intervertebral joint. Biomechanical studies have revealed abnormal motion at vertebral segments with degenerative discs and the transmission of the load to the facet joints. Numerous attempts at roentgenographic definition of spinal instability with disc disease have resulted in more controversy

---

*Modified from Whisler WW: Orthopedics 6:1628, 1983.

than agreement as to a standard method of measurement. The method described by Knutsson is simple and relatively efficient in determining anteroposterior motion. There is little controversy as to the surgical treatment of lumbar spinal instability — spinal fusion of the unstable segments. The type of fusion performed and the indications for fusion are areas of controversy.

The major problem in spinal instability is the correlation of the patient's symptoms of giving way, catching, and predominant back pain to the roentgenographic identification of instability. Other factors such as concomitant spinal stenosis, disc herniation, and psychologic problems only complicate any evaluation of spinal instability. Presently the decision for surgery for clinically significant lumbar spine instability caused by degenerative disc disease should be decided on an individual patient basis with all the factors and risks weighed carefully.

Disc Excision and Fusion

The necessity of lumbar fusion at the same time as disc excision was first suggested by Mixter and Barr. In the first 20 years after their discovery the combination of disc excision and lumbar fusion was common. More recent data comparing disc excision alone with the combination of disc excision and fusion by Frymoyer et al. and others indicate that there is little if any advantage to the addition of a spinal fusion to the treatment of simple disc herniation. These studies do indicate that spinal fusion does increase the complication rate and lengthen recovery. The indications for lumbar fusion should be independent of the indications for disc excision for sciatica.

Lumbar Vertebral Interbody Fusion

Anterior lumbar intervertebral fusion (ALIF) and posterior lumbar intervertebral fusion (PLIF) have been suggested as definitive procedures for lumbar disc disease. Biomechanically the lumbar interbody fusion offers the greatest stability. It also eliminates the disc segment as a further source of pain. The primary problems are the more involved and potentially dangerous dissection, the risk of graft extrusion, and pseudarthrosis.

Most series of these fusions include a significant number of salvage procedures and complex pathologic conditions, thus making direct comparison with primary disc surgery difficult. The routine use of such procedures for simple lumbar disc herniation with sciatica is not justified.

ANTERIOR LUMBAR INTERBODY FUSION

■ *TECHNIQUE.* Place the patient supine on an operating table capable of holding roentgenographic cassettes. Support the lumbar spine with a rolled sheet or inflatable bag. Prepare and drape the patient's abdomen from upper chest to groin, leaving the iliac crests exposed for obtaining bone grafts. Expose the lumbar spine through a transabdominal or retroperitoneal approach as desired. Mobilize the great vessels over the segment to be excised. Ligate the median artery and vein at the bifurcation of the aorta to prevent tearing this structure when exposing the disc at L4-5 or L5-S1.

Identify and inspect all major structures before and after disc excision and fusion. Obtain an anteroposterior roentgenogram to confirm the proper disc level. Then incise the anterior longitudinal ligament superiorly or inferiorly over the edge of the vertebral body. Elevate the ligament as a flap if possible. Next remove the anular and nuclear material of the disc. The use of magnification may be beneficial as the dissection nears the posterior longitudinal ligament. Remove all nuclear material from the posterior longitudinal ligament.

Techniques for fusion vary. Some prefer to use dowel grafts to fill the space. Others prefer to use tricortical iliac grafts (Fig. 84-35). Obtain the grafts from the iliac crest as described for anterior cervical fusions (p. 3750). Prepare the graft area for the desired grafting technique. We prefer tricortical grafts for this fusion. Good results using fibular grafts and banked bone have also been reported. Prepare the vertebrae by curetting the end plates to cancellous bone posteriorly. Then carefully make a slot in the vertebra to accommodate the grafts; use an osteotome slightly larger than the width of the disc space for this purpose and direct the cut toward the inferior vertebral body. Try to leave the upper and lower lips of the vertebral bodies intact. Remove enough tricortical iliac bone to allow insertion of at least three individual grafts. Fashion the grafts to fit snugly in the space with a laminar spreader in place. Insert the grafts so that the cancellous portions face the decorticated end plates. The grafts should be 3 to 4 mm shorter than the anteroposterior diameter of the vertebral body. Impact the grafts and seat them behind the anterior rim of the vertebral bodies. Usually three such grafts can be inserted. Add additional cancellous chips around the grafts. Suture the anterior longitudinal ligament. Close the retroperitoneum and abdomen in the usual manner.

AFTERTREATMENT. The patient is allowed to sit as soon as possible. Extension of the lumbar spine is prohibited for at least 6 weeks. Bracing or casting is left to the discretion of the surgeon after considering the stability of the grafts and reliability of the patient.

POSTERIOR LUMBAR INTERBODY FUSION

■ *TECHNIQUE (CLOWARD).* Position the patient in the prone or kneeling position as desired. Expose the spine through a midline incision centered over the level of the pathologic condition. Strip the muscle

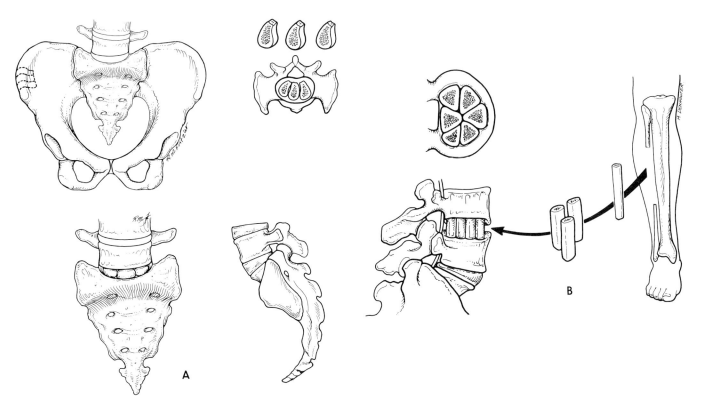

Fig. 84-35   Anterior lumbar intervertebral fusion (ALIF) can be performed using tricortical iliac crest graft, **A,** or fibular grafts, **B.** (**A,** From Ruge D and Wiltse LL: Spinal disorders: diagnosis and treatment, Philadelphia, 1977, Lea & Febiger; **B,** from Wiltse LL: AAOS Instr Course Lect 28:207, 1979.)

subperiosteally from the lamina bilaterally. Insert the laminar spreader between the spinous processes at the level of pathologic findings. Open and remove the ligamentum flavum from the midline laterally. Enlarge the opening laterally by removing the lower one third of the inferior facet and the medial two thirds of the superior facet (Fig. 84-36, *A*). The upper lamina may also be thinned by undercutting to increase the anteroposterior diameter of the canal. Retract the lower nerve root and dura to the midline and protect it with the self-retaining nerve root retractor. Cauterize the epidural vessels with bipolar cautery. Cut out the disc and vessels over the anulus laterally. Remove as much disc material as possible (Fig. 84-36, *B*). Remove a thin layer of the end plates posteriorly. Repeat this process on the opposite side. Remove the remaining anterior edges of the end plates to the anterior longitudinal ligament. This must be done under direct vision to avoid injury to the great vessels. Prepare a surface of bleeding cancellous bone on both vertebral bodies. Obtain tricortical iliac crest grafts as previously noted from the posterior iliac crest. (Cloward uses frozen human cadaver bone grafts.) Shape the grafts to be slightly shorter and the same height or slightly higher than the disc shape. Tamp the first graft in place and le-

ver it medially to allow insertion of the remaining grafts. Repeat the procedure on the opposite side (Fig. 84-36, *C*). Remove the laminar spreader and check the graft for stability. Close the wound in the usual fashion.

AFTERTREATMENT. Aftertreatment is the same as for lumbar discectomy (p. 3761). Early walking is encouraged.

FAILED SPINE SURGERY

One of the greatest problems in orthopaedic surgery and neurosurgery is the treatment of failed spine surgery. Numerous reasons for the failures have been advanced. The best results from repeat surgery for disc problems appear to be related to the discovery of a new problem or identification of a previously undiagnosed or untreated problem. Waddell et al. suggested that the best results from repeat surgery are when the patient had experienced 6 months or more of complete pain relief after the first procedure, when leg pain exceeded back pain, and when a definitie recurrent disc could be identified. They identified adverse factors such as scarring, previous infection, repair of pseudarthrosis, and adverse psychologic factors. Similar factors were identified by Lehmann

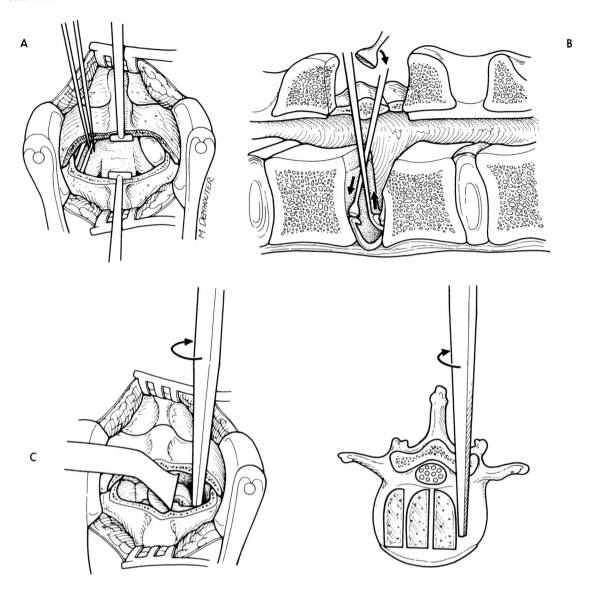

Fig. 84-36 Posterior lumbar interbody fusion technique. **A,** Bilateral laminotomy with preservation of facets. Control of epidural hemorrhage. Dipolar or insulated coagulation forceps are used on left side. On right side, epidural hemorrhage is controlled by impacted Surgicel tampons. Impacted Surgicel tampons also push nerve root medially and expose disc space without need for nerve root retractor. **B,** After intervertebral rims are removed, cleavage of disc attachment to cortical plate is identified. Curved up-bite curet is used to remove concave centrum of lower cartilaginous plate. Then detached large chunks of disc material are removed with ronguer. **C,** Medial graft advancement with single chisel. (From Cauthen JC: Lumbar spine surgery, Baltimore, 1983, Williams & Wilkins.)

and LaRocca and Finnegan et al. Satisfactory results from reoperation have been reported to be from 31% to 80%. Patients should expect improvement in the severity of symptoms rather than complete relief of pain. As the frequency of number of repeat back surgeries increases, the chance of a satisfactory result drops precipitously. Spengler et al. and Long et al. observed that the major cause of failure is improper patient selection.

The recurrence or intensification of pain after disc surgery should be treated with the usual conservative methods initially. If these methods fail to relieve the pain, a complete reevaluation should be performed. Frequently a repeat history and physical examination will give some indication of the problem. Additional testing should include psychologic testing, myelography, MRI to check for tumors or a higher disc herniation, and reformatted CT scans to check for areas of foraminal stenosis or for lateral herniation. The use of the differential spinal, root blocks, facet blocks, and discograms also may help identify the source of pain. The presence of abnormal psychologic test results or an abnormal differential spinal should serve as a modifier to any suggested treatment indicated by the other testing. Satisfactory nonoperative treatment of this problem should be attempted before additional surgery is performed, provided this surgery is elective. A distinct, surgically correctable, anatomic problem should be identified before surgery is contemplated. The surgery should be specifically tailored to the anatomic problem or problems identified.

Repeat Lumbar Disc Surgery

The technique of repeat lumbar disc surgery at the same level and side as the previous procedure is nearly the same as for initial surgery. The procedure will be longer and will involve more meticulous dissection.

■ *TECHNIQUE.* **Approach the spine using the method described previously. Identify normal tissue first. Use a curet to carefully remove scar from the edges of the lamina. Then remove additional bone as necessary to expose normal dura. Identify the pedicles superiorly and inferiorly if there is any question of position and status of the root. Carry the dissection from the pedicles to identify each root. This will allow the development of a normal plane between the dura and scar. Maintain meticulous hemostasis with bipolar cautery. Then remove disc material as indicated by the preoperative evaluation. Meticulously check the roots, dura, and posterior longitudinal ligament after removal of the offending disc herniation. Spinal fusion is not performed unless an unstable spine is created by the dissection or was identified preoperatively as a correctable and symptomatic problem.**

AFTERTREATMENT. **Aftertreatment is the same as for disc excision (p. 3761).**

REFERENCES

History

Aird R: Charles Lasègue. In Haymaker W and Sobiller F, editors: Founders of neurology, ed 2, Springfield, Ill, 1970, Charles C Thomas, Publisher.

Alajouanine TH: From the presidential address for Professor Jean Cauchoix before the Annual Meeting of the International Society for the Study of the Lumbar Spine, San Francisco, June 1978.

Aurelianus C: Acute diseases and chronic diseases, Chicago, 1950, University of Chicago Press, edited and translated by IE Drabkin.

Barr JS: Low-back and sciatic pain: results of treatment, J Bone Joint Surg 33-A:633, 1951.

Barr JS: Lumbar disc lesions in retrospect and prospect, Clin Orthop 129:4, 1977.

Barr JS, Hampton AO, and Mixter WJ: Pain low in the back and "sciatica" due to lesions of the intervertebral discs, JAMA 109:1265, 1937.

Cotugnio D: Treatise on the nervous sciatica or nervous hip gout, London, 1775, J Wilkie.

Dandy WE: Loose cartilage from the intervertebral disc simulating tumor of the spinal cord, Orthop Surg 19:1660, 1929.

Dandy WE: Concealed ruptured intervertebral disks: a plea for the elimination of contrast mediums in diagnosis, JAMA 117:821, 1941.

de Sèze S: Sciatique "banale" et disques lombo-sacrés, Presse Med 51-52:570, 1940.

de Sèze S: Histoire de la sciatique, Rev Neurol 138:1019, 1982.

Dimitrigevic DT: Historical note: Lasègue sign, Neurology 2:453, 1952.

Dyck P: Lumbar nerve root: the enigmatic eponyms, Spine 9:3, 1984.

Elsberg CA: Experiences in spinal surgery: observations upon 60 laminectomies for spinal disease, Surg Gynecol Obstet 16:117, 1913.

Forst JJ: Contribution a l'etude clinique de la sciatique, thesis, Lyon, France, 1881.

Goldthwait JE: The lumbosacral articulations: an explanation of many cases of "lumbago," "sciatica" and paraplegia, Bost Med Surg J 164:365, 1911.

Goldthwait JE: Backache, N Engl J Med 209:722, 1933.

Goldthwait JE: Low-back lesions, J Bone Joint Surg 19:810, 1937.

Hall GW: Neurologic signs and their discoverers, JAMA 95:703, 1930.

Kirkaldy-Willis WH and Hill RJ: A more precise diagnosis for low-back pain, Spine 4:102, 1979.

Kocher T: Die Verlitzungen der Wirbelsaule Zurleich Als Beitrag zur Physiologic des Menschichen Ruchenmarks, Mitt Grenzgeb Med Chir 1:415, 1896.

Lasègue C: Considerations sur la sciatique, Arch Gen Med 2:558, 1864.

Love JG: Removal of intervertebral discs without laminectomy, Proc Staff Meet Mayo Clin 14:800, 1939.

Mixter WJ: Rupture of the lumbar intervertebral disk: an etiologic factor for so-called "sciatic" pain, Ann Surg 106:777, 1937.

Mixter WJ and Barr JS: Rupture of the intervertebral disc with involvement of the spinal canal, N Engl J Med 211:210, 1934.

Nafziger HC, Inman V, and Saunders JB: Lesions of the intervertebral disc and ligamenta flava, J Surg Gynecol Obstet 66:288, 1938.

Oppenheim H and Krause F: Ueber Einklemmung bzw. Strangulation der Cauda equina, Deutsche Med Wchnschr 35:697, 1909.

Robinson JS: Sciatica and the lumbar disk syndrome: a historic perspective, South Med J 76:232, 1983.

Schmori G and Junghanns H: Archiv und Atlas der normalen und pathogischen Anatomie in typischen Röntgenbildern, Leipzig, 1932, Georg Thieme.

Semmes RE: Diagnosis of ruptured intervertebral discs without contrast myelography and comment upon recent experience with modified hemilaminectomy for their removal, Yale J Biol Med 11:433, 1939.

Sjöqvist O: The mechanism of origin of Lasègue's sign, Acta Psych Neurol 46(suppl):290, 1947.

Smith L, Garvin PJ, Gesler RM, et al: Enzyme dissolution of the nucleus pulposus, Nature 198:1131, 1963.

Sugar O: Charles Lasègue and his "Considerations on Sciatica," JAMA 253:1767, 1985.

Virchow R: Untersuchunger uber die Enwickelung die Schadeigrunder, Berlin, 1857, G Reimer.

Wartenberg R: Lasègue sign and Kernig sign: historical notes, Arch Neurol Psych 66:58, 1951.

Wartenberg R: On neurologic terminology, eponyms and the Lasègue sign, Neurology 6:853, 1956.

Wilkins RH and Brody IA: Lasègue's sign, Arch Neurol 21:219, 1969.

Wiltse LL: History of lumbar spine surgery. In White AA, editor: Lumbar spine surgery: techniques and complications, St Louis, 1987, Mosby–Year Book, Inc.

Wood MW: Sciatica and the herniated disc: a historical review, Memphis Mid-South Med J 37:12, 1966.

Epidemiology

Andersson GBJ: Epidemiologic aspects of low-back pain in industry, Spine 6:53, 1981.

Andersson GBJ, Svensson HO, and Oden A: The intensity of work recovery in low back pain, Spine 8:880, 1983.

Benn RT and Wood PHN: Pain in the back: an attempt to estimate the size of the problem, Rheumatol Rehab 14:121, 1975.

Berquist-Ullman M and Larsson U: Acute low back pain in industry: a controlled perspective study with special reference to therapy and confounding factors, Acta Orthop Scand (Suppl) 170:1, 1977.

Biering-Sorensen F and Hilden J: Reproducibility of the history of low-back trouble, Spine 9:280, 1984.

Buckle PW, Kember PA, Wood AD, and Wood SN: Factors influencing occupational back pain in Bedfordshire, Spine 5:254, 1980.

Chaffin DB: Human strength capability and low-back pain, J Occup Med 16:248, 1974.

Damkot DK, Pope MH, Lord J, and Frymoyer JW: The relationship between work history, work environment and low-back pain in men, Spine 9:395, 1984.

Deyo RA and Bass JE: Lifestyle and low-back pain: the influence of smoking and obesity, Spine 14:501, 1989.

Dillane JB, Fry J, and Kalton G: Acute back syndrome: a study from general practice, Br Med J 2:82, 1966.

Farfan HF and Sullivan JD: The relation of facet orientation to intervertebral disc failure, Can J Surg 10:179, 1967.

Frymoyer JW et al: Epidemiologic studies of low-back pain, Spine 5:419, 1980.

Frymoyer JW et al: Risk factors in low-back pain: an epidemiological survey, J Bone Joint Surg 65-A:213, 1983.

Frymoyer JW et al: Spine radiographs in patients with low-back pain: an epidemiological study in men, J Bone Joint Surg 66-A:1048, 1984.

Gardner RC: The lumbar intervertebral disc: a clinicopathological correlation based on over 100 laminectomies, Arch Surg 100:101, 1970.

Grabias S: Current concepts revue: the treatment of spinal stenosis, J Bone Joint Surg 62-A:308, 1980.

Gyntelberg F: One year incidence of low back pain among male residents of Copenhagen aged 40-59, Danish Med Bull 21:30, 1974.

Hult L: The Munkfors investigation, Acta Orthop Scand (Suppl) 16:1, 1954.

Jackson RP, Simmons EH, and Stripinis D: Incidence and severity of back pain in adult idiopathic scoliosis, Spine 8:749, 1983.

Johnsson K, Willner S, and Pettersson H: Analysis of operated cases with lumbar renal stenosis, Acta Orthop Scand 52:427, 1981.

Kelsey JL and White AA III: Epidemiology and impact of low-back pain, Spine 5:133, 1980.

Kelsey JL, White AA III, Pastides H, and Bisbee GE Jr: The impact of musculoskeletal disorders on the population of the United States, J Bone Joint Surg 61-A:959, 1979.

Kelsey JL et al: An epidemiologic study of lifting and twisting on the job and risk for acute prolapsed lumbar intervertebral disc, J Orthop Res 2:61, 1984.

Knutsson F: The instability associated with disk degeneration in the lumbar spine, Acta Radiol 25:593, 1944.

Kostuik JP and Bentivoglio J: The incidence of low-back pain in adult scoliosis, Spine 6:268, 1981.

Magora A: Investigation of the relation between low back pain and occupation: psychological aspects, Scand J Rehab Med 5:191, 1973.

Magora A: Investigation of the relation between low back pain and occupation: neurologic and orthopedic conditions, Scand J Rehab Med 7:146, 1975.

Manning DP and Shannon HS: Slipping accidents causing low-back pain in a gearbox factory, Spine 6:70, 1981.

Middleton GS and Teacher JH: Injury of the spinal cord due to rupture of an intervertebral disc during muscular effort, Glasgow Med J 76:1, 1911.

Mooney V and Robertson J: The facet syndrome, Clin Orthop 115:149, 1976.

Nachemson AL: The lumbar spine: an orthopaedic challenge, Spine 1:59, 1976.

Nachemson AL: Prevention of chronic back pain: the orthopaedic challenge for the 80's, Bull Hosp Jt Dis Orthop Inst 44:1, 1984.

Nag SZ, Riley LE, and Newby LG: A social epidemiology of back pain in a general population, J Chron Dis 26:769, 1973.

Ortengren R, Anderson G, Broman H, et al: Vocational electromyography: studies of localized muscle fatigue and the assembly line, Ergonomics 18:157, 1975.

Poulsen E.: Studies of back load tolerance limits during lifting of burdens, Scand J Rehabil Med (Suppl) 6:169, 1978.

Riihimaki H, Tola S, Videman T, and Hanninen K: Low-back pain and occupation: a cross-sectional questionnaire study of men in machine operating, dynamic physical work and sedentary work, Spine 14:204, 1989.

Rowe ML: Low back pain in industry: a position paper, J Occup Med 11:161, 1969.

Ryden LA, Molgaard CA, Bobbitt S, and Conway J: Occupational low-back injury in a hospital employee population and epidemiologic analysis of multiple risk factors of a high-risk occupational group, Spine 14:315, 1989.

Sandover J: Dynamic loading as a possible source of low-back disorders, Spine 8:652, 1983.

Sitken AP and Bradford CH: End results of ruptured intervertebral discs in industry, Am J Surg 73:365, 1947.

Snook SH: The costs of back pain in industry, Spine: State of the Art Reviews 2:11, 1987.

Snook SH and Webster BS: The cost of disability, Clin Orthop 221:77, 1987.

Stolley PD and Kuller LH: The need for epidemiologists and surgeons to cooperate in the evaluation of surgical therapies, Surgery 78:123, 1975.

Svensson HO and Andersson GBJ: Low back pain in forty to forty-seven year old men. I. Frequency of occurrence and impact on medical services, Scand J Rehab Med 14:47, 1982.

Svensson HO and Andersson GBJ: Low back pain in 40- to 47-year-old men: work history and work environment factors, Spine 8:272, 1983.

Svensson HO and Andersson GBJ: The relationship of low-back pain, work history, work environment and stress a retrospective cross-sectional study of 38- to 64-year-old women, Spine 14:517, 1989.

Svensson HO, Vedin A, Wilhelmsson C, and Andersson GBJ: Low-back pain in relation to other diseases and cardiovascular risk factors, Spine 8:277, 1983.

Troup JDG, Martin JW, and Lloyd DC: Back pain in industry: a prospective survey, Spine 6:61, 1981.

Waddell G, Main CJ, Morris EW, et al: Chronic low-back pain, psychologic distress, and illness behavior, Spine 9:209, 1984.

Webster BS and Snook SH: The cost of compensable low back pain, J Occup Med 32:13, 1990.

Weisz GM: Lumbar spinal canal stenosis in Paget's disease, Spine 8:192, 1983.

White AWM: Low back pain in men receiving workmen's compensation: a follow-up study, Can Med Assoc J 101:61, 1969.

Wilder DG, Woodworth BB, Frymoyer JW, and Pope MH: Vibration and the human spine, Spine 7:243, 1982.

General disc and spine anatomy

Adams MA and Hutton WC: The mechanical function of the lumbar apophyseal joints, Spine 8:327, 1983.

Bogduk N: The clinical anatomy of the cervical dorsal rami, Spine 7:319, 1982.

Bogduk N: The innervation of the lumbar spine, Spine 8:286, 1983.

Bogduk N and Engel R: The menisci of the lumbar zygapophyseal joints: a review of their anatomy and clinical significance, Spine 9:454, 1984.

Bogduk N and Macintosh JE: The applied anatomy of the thoracolumbar fascia, Spine 9:164, 1984.

Bose K and Balasubramaniam P: Nerve root canals of the lumbar spine, Spine 9:16, 1984.

Bradford FK and Spurling RG: The intervertebral disk, ed 2, Springfield, Ill, 1945, Charles C Thomas, Publisher.

Crock HV: Normal and pathological anatomy of the lumbar spinal nerve root canals, J Bone Joint Surg 63:487, 1981.

Cyriax J: Dural pain: mechanisms of symptoms, Lancet 1:919, 1978.

D'Avella D and Mingrino S: Microsurgical anatomy of lumbosacral spinal roots, J Neurosurg 51:819, 1979.

Edgar MA and Ghadially JA: Innervation of the lumbar spine, Clin Orthop 115:35, 1976.

Hasue M and Fujiwara M: Epidemiologic and clinical studies of long-term prognosis of low-back pain and sciatica, Spine 4:150, 1979.

Hasue M, Kikuchi S, Sakuyama Y, and Ito T: Anatomic study of the interrelation between lumbosacral nerve roots and their surrounding tissues, Spine 8:50, 1983.

Hirsch C and Schajowicz F: Studies on structural changes in the lumbar annulus fibrosus, Acta Orthop Scand 22:184, 1953.

Hollinshead WH: Anatomy of the spine: points of interest to orthopaedic surgeons, J Bone Joint Surg 47-A:209, 1965.

Inman VT and Saunders JB: Referred pain from skeletal structures, J Neurol Ment Dis 99:660, 1944.

Inoue H: Three-dimensional architecture of lumbar intervertebral discs, Spine 6:139, 1981.

Jayson MIV: Compression stresses in the posterior elements and pathologic consequences, Spine 8:338, 1983.

Jorgensen K: Back muscle strength and body weight as limiting factors for work in the standing slightly-stooped position, Scand J Rehab Med 2:149, 1970.

Keegan JJ: Dermatome hypalgesia associated with herniation of intervertebral disc, Arch Neurol Psych 50:67, 1943.

Keyes DC and Compere EL: The normal and pathological physiology of the nucleus pulposus of the intervertebral disc: an anatomical, clinical, and experimental study, J Bone Joint Surg 14:897, 1932.

Kikuchi S, Hasue M, Nishiyama K, and Ito T: Anatomic and clinical studies of radicular symptoms, Spine 9:23, 1982.

King AG: Functional anatomy of the lumbar spine, Orthopedics 6:1588, 1983.

Kirkaldy-Willis WH: The relationship of structural pathology to the nerve root, Spine 9:49, 1984.

Klausen K: The form and function of the loaded human spine, Acta Physiol Scand 65:176, 1965.

Knutsson F: The instability associated with disc degeneration in the lumbar spine, Acta Radiol 25:593, 1944.

Louis R: Topographic relationships of the vertebral column, spinal cord, and nerve roots, Anatomia Clinica 1:7, 1978.

Macrae IF and Wright V: Measurement of back movement, Ann Rheum Dis 28:584, 1969.

Magora A: Investigation of the relation between low back pain and occupation, Scand J Rehab Med 5:191, 1973.

Miller JAA, Haderspeck KA, and Schultz AB: Posterior element loads in lumbar motion segments, Spine 8:331, 1983.

Moll JMH and Wright V: Normal range of spinal mobility: an objective clinical study, Ann Rheum Dis 30:381, 1971.

Nachemson A: The lumbar spine and orthopaedic challenge, Spine 1:59, 1976.

Nachemson A, Lewin T, Maroudas A, et al: In vitro diffusion of dye through the end plates and the anulus fibrosus of human intervertebral discs, Acta Orthop Scand 4:589, 1970.

Pedersen H, Blunck CFJ, and Gardner E: The anatomy of lumbosacral posterior rami and meningeal branches of spinal nerves (sinuvertebral nerves), J Bone Joint Surg 38-A:2377, 1956.

Postacchini F, Urso S, and Ferro L: Lumbosacral nerve-root anomalies, J Bone Joint Surg 64-A:721, 1982.

Roofe PG: Innervation of annulus fibrosus and posterior longitudinal ligament, fourth and fifth lumbar level, Arch Neurol Psychiatr 44:100, 1940.

Rowe ML: Low back pain in industry, J Occup Med 11:161, 1969.

Rydevik B, Brown MD, and Lundborg G: Pathoanatomy and pathophysiology of nerve root compression, Spine 9:7, 1984.

Spencer DL, Irwin GS, and Miller JAA: Anatomy and significance of fixation of the lumbosacral nerve roots in sciatica, Spine 8:672, 1983.

Wall EJ, Cohen MS, Abitbol J, and Garfin SR: Organization of intrathecal nerve roots at the level of the conus medullaris, J Bone Joint Surg 72-A:1495, 1990.

Wall EJ, Cohen MS, Massie JB, et al: Cauda equina anatomy: intrathecal nerve root organization, Spine 15:1244, 1990.

Wilder DG, Pope MH, and Frymoyer JW: The functional topography of the sacroiliac joint, Spine 5:575, 1980.

Willis TA: Lumbosacral anomalies, J Bone Joint Surg 41-A:935, 1959.

Young A et al: Variations in the pattern of muscle innervation by the L5 and S1 nerve roots, Spine 8:616, 1983.

Natural history of disc disease

Biering-Sørensen F and Hilden J: Reproducibility of the history of low-back trouble, Spine 9:280, 1984.

Cyriax J: Dural pain: mechanisms of symptoms, Lancet 1:919, 1978.

Frymoyer JW, Pope MH, Constanza MC, et al: Epidemiological studies of low-back pain, Spine 5:419, 1980.

Gardner RC: The lumbar intervertebral disc: a correlation based on over 100 laminectomies, Arch Surg 100:101, 1970.

Gibson MJ, Szypryt EP, Buckley JH, et al: Magnetic resonance imaging of adolescent disc herniation, J Bone Joint Surg 69-B:699, 1987.

Goldthwait E: Low-back lesions, J Bone Joint Surg 19:810, 1937.

Hakelius A: Prognosis in sciatica, Acta Orthop Scand Suppl 129:1, 1970.

Hirsch C and Schajowicz F: Studies on structural changes in the lumbar annulus fibrosus, Acta Orthop Scand 22:184, 1953.

Jackson RP, Simmons EH, and Stripinis D: Incidence and severity of back pain in adult idiopathic scoliosis, Spine 8:749, 1983.

Jayson MIV: Compression stresses in the posterior elements and pathologic consequences, Spine 8:338, 1983.

Kelsey JL et al: An epidemiologic study of lifting and twisting on the job and risk for acute prolapsed lumbar intervertebral disc, J Orthop Res 2:61, 1984.

Kirkaldy-Willis WH and Hill RJ: A more precise diagnosis for low-back pain, Spine 4:102, 1979.

Miller JAA, Schmatz C, and Schultz AB: Lumbar disc degeneration: correlation with age, sex and spine level in 600 autopsy specimens, Spine 13:2173, 1988.

Nachemson A: The lumbar spine and orthopaedic challenge, Spine 1:59, 1976.

Naylor A: Intervertebral disc prolapse and degeneration, Spine 1:108, 1976.

Pope MH, Bevins T, Wilder DG, and Frymoyer JW: The relationship between anthropometric, postural, muscular, and mobility characteristics of males age 18-55, Spine 10:644, 1985.

Roland M and Morris R: A study of the natural history of back pain. I. Development of a reliable and sensitive measure of disability in low-back pain, Spine 8:141, 1983.

Rydevik B, Brown MD, and Lundborg G: Pathoanatomy and pathophysiology of nerve root compression, Spine 9:7, 1984.

Sandover J: Dynamic loading as a possible source of low-back disorders, Spine 8:652, 1983.

Scott JC: Stress factor in the disc syndrome, J Bone Joint Surg 37-B:107, 1955.

Takata K, Inoue S, Takahashi K, and Ohtsuka Y: Swelling of the cauda equina in patients who have herniation of a lumbar disc: a possible pathogenesis of sciatica, J Bone Joint Surg 70-A:3361, 1988.

Urban JPG and McMullin JF: Swelling pressure of the lumbar intervertebral discs: influence of age, spinal level, composition, and degeneration, Spine 13:2179, 1988.

Urovitz EPM and Fronasier VL: Autoimmunity in degenerative disc disease, Clin Orthop 142:215, 1979.

Varlotta GP, Brown MD, Kelsey JL, and Golden AL: Familial predisposition for herniation of a lumbar disc in patients who are less than twenty-one years old, J Bone Joint Surg 73-A:124, 1991.

Weber H: Lumbar disc herniation: a controlled, prospective study with ten years of observation, Spine 8:131, 1983.

Yasuma T, Koh S, Okamura T, and Yamauchi Y: Histological changes in aging lumbar intervertebral discs, J Bone Joint Surg 72-A:220, 1990.

Diagnostic studies

Abel MS, Smith GR, and Allen TNK: Refinements of the anteroposterior angled caudad view of the lumbar spine, Skel Radiol 7:113, 1981.

Abraham SR, Tedeschi AA, Partain CL, and Blumenkopf B: Differential diagnosis of severe back pain using MRI, South Med J 81:487, 1988.

Alemohammad S and Bouzarth WF: Intracranial subdural hematoma following lumbar myelography: case report, J Neurosurg 52:256, 1980.

Amundsen P: Cervical myelography with Amipaque: seven years experience, Radiologe 21:282, 1981.

Andersson G, Ortengren R, and Nachemson A: Quantitative studies of the load on the back in different working-postures, Scand J Rehabil Med Suppl 6:173, 1978.

Andersson GB and Schultz AB: Effects of fluid injection on mechanical properties of intervertebral discs, J Biomech 12:453, 1979.

Angiari P, Crisi G, and Merli GA: Aphasia and right hemiplegia after cervical myelography with metrizamide: a case report, Neuroradiology 26:61, 1984.

Asztely M, Kadziolka R, and Nachemson A: A comparison of sonography and myelography in clinically suspected spinal stenosis, Spine 8:885, 1983.

Barrow DL, Wood JH, and Hoffman JC Jr: Clinical indications for computer-assisted myelography, Neurosurgery 12:47, 1983.

Bell GR, Rothman RH, Booth RE, et al: A study of computer-assisted tomography. II. Comparison of metrizamide myelography and computed tomography in the diagnosis of herniated lumbar disc and spinal stenosis, Spine 9:552, 1984.

Bladé J, Gaston F, Montserrat E, et al: Spinal subarachnoid hematoma after lumbar puncture causing reversible paraplegia in acute leukemia: case report, J Neurosurg 58:438, 1983.

Bobest M, Furó I, Tompa K, et al: 1H nuclear magnetic resonance study of intervertebral discs: a preliminary report, Spine 11:709, 1986.

Boden SD, Davis DO, Dina TS, et al: Abnormal magnetic-resonance scans of the lumbar spine in asymptomatic subjects: a prospective investigation, J Bone Joint Surg 72-A:403, 1990.

Boden SD, McCowin PR, Davis DO, et al: Abnormal magnetic-resonance scans of the cervical spine in asymptomatic subjects, J Bone Joint Surg 72-A:1178, 1990.

Bohutova J, Vojir R, Kolar J, and Grepl J: Some unusual complications of myelography and lumbosacral radiculography, Diagn Imag 48:320, 1979.

Brady LP, Parker LB, and Vaughen J: An evaluation of the electromyogram in the diagnosis of the lumbar disc lesion, J Bone Joint Surg 51-A:539, 1969.

Brem SS, Hafler DA, Van Uitert RL, et al: Spinal subarachnoid hematoma: a hazard of lumbar puncture resulting in reversible paraplegia, N Engl J Med 304:1020, 1981.

Burton CV: Computed tomography scanning and the lumbar spine. I. Economic and historic review, Spine 4:353, 1979.

Charles MF, Byrd SE, Cohn ML, and Huntington CT: Metrizamide computer tomography of the postoperative lumbar spine, Orthop Rev 11(10):49, 1982.

Coin CG: Cervical disk degeneration and herniation: diagnosis by computerized tomography, South Med J 77:979, 1984.

Collier BD, Johnson RP, Carrera GF, et al: Painful spondylolysis or spondylolisthesis studied by radiography and single-photon emission computed tomography, Radiology 154:207, 1985.

Cook PL and Wise K: A correlation of the surgical and radiculographic findings in lumbar disc herniation, Clin Radiol 30:671, 1979.

Deburge A, Benoist M, and Boyer D: The diagnosis of disc sequestration, Spine 9:496, 1984.

Delamarter RB, Bohlman HH, Dodge LD, and Biro C: Experimental lumbar spinal stenosis: analysis of the cortical evoked potentials, microvasculature, and histopathology, J Bone Joint Surg 72-A:110, 1990.

Delamarter RB, Leventhal MR, and Bohlman HH: Diagnosis of recurrent lumbar disc herniation vs postoperative scar by gadolinium-DTPA enhanced magnetic resonance imaging (in press).

Dujovny M, Barrionuevo PJ, Kossovsky N, et al: Effects of contrast media on the canine subarachnoid space, Spine 3:31, 1978.

Dvonch V, Scarff T, Bunch WH, et al: Dermatomal somatosensory evoked potentials: their use in lumbar radiculopathy, Spine 9:291, 1984.

Edelstein WA, Schenck JF, Hart HR, et al: Surface coil magnetic resonance imaging, JAMA 253:828, 1985.

Eisen A and Hoirch M: The electrodiagnostic evaluation of spinal root lesions, Spine 8:98, 1983.

Eldevik OP: Side effects and complications of myelography with water soluble contrast agents, J Oslo City Hosp 32:121, 1982.

Fager CA: Evaluation of cervical spine surgery by postoperative myelography, Neurosurgery 12:416, 1983.

Firooznia H, Benjamin V, Kricheff II, et al: CT of lumbar spine disc herniation: correlation with surgical findings, AJR 142:587, 1984.

Fitzgerald RH, Reines HD, and Wise J: Diagnostic radiation exposure in trauma patients, South Med J 76:1511, 1983.

Ford LT and Goodman FG: X-ray studies of the lumbosacral spine, South Med J 10:1123, 1966.

Frymoyer JW, Hanley EN, and Howe J: A comparison of radiographic findings in fusion and nonfusion patients ten or more years following lumbar disc surgery, Spine 5:435, 1979.

Frymoyer JW, Newberg A, Pope MH, et al: Spine radiographs in patients with low-back pain: an epidemiological study in men, J Bone Joint Surg 66-A:1048, 1984.

Fullenlove TM and Williams AJ: Comparative roentgen findings in symptomatic and asymptomatic backs, Radiology 63:572, 1957.

Gershater R and Holgate RC: Lumbar epidural venography in the diagnosis of disc herniations, AJR 126:992, 1976.

Gibson MJ, Buckley J, Mulholland RC, and Worthington BS: The changes in the intervertebral disc after chemonucleolysis demonstrated by magnetic resonance imaging, J Bone Joint Surg 68-B:719, 1986.

Gibson MJ, Szypryt EP, Buckley JH, et al: Magnetic resonance imaging of adolescent disc herniation, J Bone Joint Surg 69-B:699, 1987.

Glasauer FE and Alker G: Metrizamide enhanced computed tomography: an adjunct to myelography in lumbar disc herniation, Comput Radiol 7:305, 1983.

Greenberg RP and Ducker TB: Evoked potentials in the clinical neurosciences, J Neurosurg 56:1, 1982.

Gulati AN, Guadognoli DA, and Quigley JM: Relationship of side effects to patient position during and after metrizamide lumbar myelography, Radiology 141:113, 1981.

Haldeman S: The electrodiagnosis evaluation of nerve root function, Spine 9:42, 1984.

Harrington H, Tyler HR, and Welch K: Surgical treatment of postlumbar puncture dural CSF leak causing chronic headache: case report, J Neurosurg 57:703, 1982.

Haughton VM, Eldevik OP, Magnaes B, and Amundsen P: A prospective comparison of computed tomography and myelography in the diagnosis of herniated lumbar disks, Radiology 142:103, 1982.

Hayes MA, Howard TC, Gruel CR, and Kopta JA: Roentgenographic evaluation of lumbar spine flexion-extension in asymptomatic individuals, Spine 14:327, 1989.

Hemminghytt S, Daniels DL, Williams AL, and Haughton VM: Intraspinal synovial cysts: natural history and diagnosis by CT, Radiology 145:375, 1982.

Herkowitz HN, Romeyn RL, and Rothman RH: The indications for metrizamide myelography: relationship with complications after myelography, J Bone Joint Surg 65-A:1144, 1983.

Herkowitz HN, Wiesel SW, Booth RE Jr, and Rothman RH: Metrizamide myelography and epidural venography: their role in the diagnosis of lumbar disc herniation and spinal stenosis, Spine 7:55, 1982.

Hirschy JC, Leue WM, Berninger WH, et al: CT of the lumbosacral spine: importance of tomographic planes parallel to vertebral end plate, AJR 136:47, 1981.

Hitselberger WE and Witten RM: Abnormal myelograms in asymptomatic patients, J Neurosurg 28:204, 1968.

Howie DW, Chatterton BE, and Hone MR: Failure of ultrasound in the investigation of sciatica, J Bone Joint Surg 65-B:144, 1983.

Hudgins WR: Computer-aided diagnosis of lumbar disc herniation, Spine 8:604, 1983.

Jajic I: The role of HLA-B27 in the diagnosis of low back pain, Acta Orthop Scand 50:411, 1979.

James AE Jr, Partain CL, Patton JA, et al: Current status of magnetic resonance imaging, South Med J 78:580, 1985.

Jepson K, Nada A, and Rymaszewski L: The role of radiculography in the management of lesions of the lumbar disc, J Bone Joint Surg 64-B:405, 1982.

Johansen JP, Fossgreen J, and Hansen HH: Bone scanning in lumbar disc herniation, Acta Orthop Scand 51:617, 1980.

Kambin P, Nixon JE, Chait A, and Schaffer JL: Annular protrusion: pathophysiology and roentgenographic appearance, Spine 13:671, 1988.

Kapoor W, Hemmer K, Herbert D, and Karpf M: Abdominal computed tomography: comparison of the usefulness of goal-directed vs non-goal-directed studies, Arch Intern Med 143:249, 1983.

Keller RH: Traumatic displacement of the cartilaginous vertebral rim: a sign of intervertebral disc prolapse, Radiology 110:21, 1974.

Kelsey JL, Githens PB, Walter SD, et al: An epidemiological study of acute prolapsed cervical intervertebral disc, J Bone Joint Surg 66-A:907, 1984.

Kieffer SA, Cacyorin ED, and Sherry RG: The radiological diagnosis of herniated lumbar intervertebral disk: a current controversy, JAMA 251:1192, 1984.

Kieffer SA, Sherry RG, Wellenstein DE, and King RB: Bulging lumbar intervertebral disk: myelographic differentiation from herniated disk with nerve root compression, AJR 138:709, 1982.

Kikuchi S, Macnab I, and Moreau P: Localisation of the level of symptomatic cervical disc degeneration, J Bone Joint Surg 63-B:272, 1981.

Killebrew K, Whaley RA, Hayward JN, and Scatliff JH: Complications of metrizamide myelography, Arch Neurol 40:78, 1983.

Liang M and Komaroff AL: Roentgenograms in primary care patients with acute low back pain: a cost-effectiveness analysis, Arch Intern Med 142:1108, 1982.

MacGibbon B and Farfan HF: A radiologic survey of various configurations of the lumbar spine, Spine 4:258, 1979.

Macnab I: The traction spur: an indicator of segmental instability, J Bone Joint Surg 53-A:663, 1971.

Macnab I, Cuthbert H, and Godfrey CM: The incidence of denervation of the sacrospinales muscles following spinal surgery, Spine 2:294, 1977.

Macnab I, St Louis EL, Grabias SL, and Jacob R: Selective ascending lumbosacral venography in the assessment of lumbar disc herniation, J Bone Joint Surg 58-A:1093, 1976.

Macon JB and Poletti CE: Conducted somatosensory evoked potentials during spinal surgery. I. Control conduction velocity measurements, J Neurosurg 57:349, 1982.

Macon JB, Poletti CE, Sweet WH, et al: Conducted somatosensory evoked potentials during spinal surgery. II. Clinical applications, J Neurosurg 57:354, 1982.

MacPherson P, Teasdale E, and MacPherson PY: Radiculography: is routine bed rest really necessary? Clin Radiol 34:325, 1983.

McNeill TW et al: A new advance in water-soluble myelography, Spine 1:72, 1976.

Meador K, Hamilton WJ, El Gammal TAM, et al: Irreversible neurologic complications of metrizamide myelography, Neurology 34:817, 1984.

Moufarrij NA, Hardy RW Jr, and Weinstein MA: Computed tomographic, myelographic, and operative findings in patients with suspected herniated lumbar discs, Neurosurgery 12:184, 1983.

Murphey F, Pascucci LM, Meade WH, and Van Zwaluwenburg BR: Myelography in patients with ruptured cervical intervertebral discs, Am J Roentgenol Radium Ther 56:27, 1946.

Nelson MA, Allen P, Clamp SE, et al: Reliability and reproducibility of clinical findings in low-back pain, Spine 4:97, 1979.

Paleari GL, Ballarati P, Gambrioli PL, and Paleari M: Recent progress in vertebral body section roentgenography in the study of the pathology of the lumbar vertebrae, Ital J Orthop Traumatol 8:109, 1982.

Peters ND and Ehni G: Xeroradiography in evaluation of cervical spine injuries, J Neurosurg 49:620, 1978.

Pope MH, Hanley EN, Matteri RE, et al: Measurement of intervertebral disc space height, Spine 2:282, 1977.

Post MJD, Brown MD, and Gargano FP: The technique and interpretation of lumbar myelograms, Spine 2:214, 1977.

Rab GT and Chao EY: Verification of roentgenographic landmarks in the lumbar spine, Spine 2:287 1977.

Raskin SP and Keating JW: Recognition of lumbar disk disease: comparison of myelography and computed tomography, AJR 139:349, 1982.

Risius B, Modic MT, Hardy RW Jr, et al: Sector computed tomographic spine scanning in the diagnosis of lumbar nerve root entrapment, Radiology 143:109, 1982.

Rockey PH, Tompkins RK, Wood RW, and Wolcott BW: The usefulness of x-ray examinations in the evaluation of patients with back pain, J Fam Pract 7:455, 1978.

Scavone JG, Latshaw RF, and Rohrer GV: Use of lumbar spine films: statistical evaluation of a university teaching hospital, JAMA 246:1105, 1981.

Schelkun SR, Wagner KF, Blanks JA, and Reinert CM: Bacterial meningitis following pantopaque myelography: a case report and literature review, Orthopedics 8(1):74, 1985.

Schutte HE and Park WM: The diagnostic value of bone scintigraphy in patients with low back pain, Skel Rad 10:1, 1983.

Sheldon JJ, Russin LA, and Gargano FP: Lumbar spinal stenosis: radiographic diagnosis with special reference to transverse axial tomography, Clin Orthop 115:53, 1976.

Shima F, Mihara K, and Hachisuga S: Angioma in the paraspinal muscles complicated by spinal epidural hematoma: case report, J Neurosurg 57:274, 1982.

Siddiqi TS and Buchheit WA: Herniated nerve root as a complication of spinal tap: case report, J Neurosurg 56:565, 1982.

Siqueira EB, Kranzler LI, and Schaffer L: Intraoperative myelography: technical note, J Neurosurg 58:786, 1983.

Smith GR: Nerve root cut-off on metrizamide-enhanced computerized tomography, South Med J 79:553, 1986.

Splithoff CA: Lumbosacral junction: roentgenographic comparison of patients with and without backaches, JAMA 152:1610, 1953.

Steiner RE: Nuclear magnetic resonance: its clinical application, J Bone Joint Surg 65-B:533, 1983.

Stokes IAF, Wilder DG, Frymoyer JW, and Pope MH: Assessment of patients with low-back pain by biplanar radiographic measurement of intervertebral motion, Spine 6:233, 1981.

Szypryt EP, Twining P, Wilde GP, et al: Diagnosis of lumbar disc protrusion, J Bone Joint Surg 70-B:717, 1988.

Tchang SPK, Howie JL, Kirkaldy-Willis WH, et al: Computed tomography versus myelography in diagnosis of lumbar disc herniation, J Can Assoc Radiol 33:15, 1982.

Teplick JG and Haskin ME: Intravenous contrast-enhanced CT of the postoperative lumbar spine: improved identification of recurrent disk herniation, scar, arachnoiditis, and diskitis, AJR 143:845, 1984.

Tibrewal SB and Pearcy MJ: Lumbar intervertebral disc heights in normal subjects and patients with disc herniation, Spine 10:452, 1985.

Torgerson WR and Dotter WE: Comparative roentgenographic study of the asymptomatic and symptomatic lumbar spine, J Bone Joint Surg 58-A:850, 1976.

Waddell G et al: Nonorganic physical signs in low-back pain, Spine 5:117, 1980.

Weiss T, Treisch J, Kazner E, et al: Intervenöse Kontrastmittelgabe bei der Computertomographie (CT) der operierten Lendenwirbelsäule, Fortschr Röntgenstr, 141:30, 1984.

Weiss T et al: CT of the postoperative lumbar spine: the value of intravenous contrast, Neuroradiology 28:241, 1986.

Whelan MA and Gold RP: Computed tomography of the sacrum. I. Normal anatomy, AJR 139:1183, 1982.

Whelan MA, Hilal SK, Gold RP, et al: Computed tomography of the sacrum. II. Pathology, AJR 139:1191, 1982.

Whiteleather JE, Semmes RE, and Murphey F: The roentgenographic signs of herniation of the cervical intervertebral disk, Radiology 46:213, 1946.

Wiesel S Tsourmas N, Feffer HL, et al: A study of computer-assisted tomography. I. The incidence of positive CAT scans in an asymptomatic group of patients, Spine 9:549, 1984.

Wilberger JE Jr and Pang D: Syndrome of the incidental herniated lumbar disc, J Neurosurg 59:137, 1983.

Williams AL, Haughton VM, Daniels DL, and Thornton RS: CT recognition of lateral lumbar disk herniation, AJR 139:345, 1982.

Williams PC: Reduced lumbosacral joint space: its relation to sciatic irritation, JAMA 99:1677, 1932.

Wiltse LL: The effect of the common anomalies of the lumbar spine upon disc degeneration and low back pain, Orthop Clin North Am 2:569, 1971.

Wiltse LL, Guyer RD, Spencer CW, et al: Alar transverse process impingement of the L5 spinal nerve: the far-out syndrome, Spine 9:31, 1984.

Winston K, Rumbaugh C, and Colucci V: The vertebral canals in lumbar disc disease, Spine 9:414, 1984.

Witt I, Vestergaard A, and Rosenklint A: A comparative analysis of x-ray findings of the lumbar spine in patients with and without lumbar pain, Spine 9:298, 1984.

Injection studies

Ahlgren EW, Stephen R, Lloyd EAC, and McCollum DE: Diagnosis of pain with a graduated spinal block technique, JAMA 195:125, 1966.

Angtuaco EJC, Holder JC, Boop WC, and Binet EF: Computed tomographic discography in the evaluation of extreme lateral disc herniation, Neurosurgery 14:350, 1984.

Benner B and Ehni G: Spinal arachnoiditis: the postoperative variety in particular, Spine 3:40, 1978.

Benoist M, Ficat C, Baraf P, and Cauchoix J: Postoperative lumbar epiduro-arachnoiditis: diagnostic and therapeutic aspects, Spine 5:432, 1980.

Berman AT, Garbarino JL, Jr, Fisher SM, and Bosacco SJ: The effects of epidural injection of local anesthetics and corticosteroids on patients with lumbosciatic pain, Clin Orthop 188:144, 1984.

Bogduk N and Long DM: The anatomy of the so-called "articular nerves" and their relationship to facet denervation in the treatment of low-back pain, J Neurosurg 51:172, 1979.

Brodsky AE: Cauda equina arachnoiditis: a correlative clinical and roentgenologic study, Spine 3:51, 1978.

Brodsky AE and Binder WF: Lumbar discography: its value in diagnosis and treatment of lumbar disc lesions, Spine 4:110, 1979.

Bromley JW et al: Double-blind evaluation of collagenase injections for herniated lumbar discs, Spine 9:486, 1984.

Brooks S, Dent AR, and Thompson AG: Anterior rupture of the lumbosacral disc: report of a case, J Bone Joint Surg 65-A:1186, 1983.

Brothers MA and Finlayson DC: Evaluation of low back pain by differential spinal block, Can Anaes Soc J 15:478, 1968.

Brown FW: Management of discogenic pain using epidural and intrathecal steroids, Clin Orthop 129:72, 1977.

Burton CV: Lumbosacral arachnoiditis, Spine 3:24, 1978.

Butt WP: Lumbar discography, J Can Assoc Radiol 14:172, 1963.

Cloward RB and Buzaid LL: Discography: technique, indications and evaluation of the normal and abnormal intervertebral disc, Am J Roentgenol 68:552, 1952.

Colhoun E, McCall IW, Williams L, and Pullicino VNC: Provocation discography as a guide to planning operations on the spine, J Bone Joint Surg 70-B:267, 1988.

Collins HR: An evaluation of cervical and lumbar discography, Clin Orthop 107:133, 1975.

Cuckler JM, Bernini PA, Wiesel SW, et al: The use of epidural steroids in the treatment of lumbar radicular pain: a prospective, randomized, double-blind study, J Bone Joint Surg 67-A:63, 1985.

Dandy WE: Concealed ruptured intervertebral disks: a plea for the elimination of contrast mediums in diagnosis, JAMA 117:821, 1941.

De La Porte C and Siegfried J: Lumbosacral spinal fibrosis (spinal arachnoiditis): its diagnosis and treatment by spinal cord stimulation, Spine 8:593, 1983.

Deburge A, Benoist M, and Rocolle J: La chirurgie dans les echecs de la nucleolyse des hernies discales lombaires, Rev Chir Orthop 70:637, 1984.

Destouet JM, Bilula LA, Murphy WA, and Monsees B: Lumbar facet joint injection: indication, technique, clinical correlation, and preliminary results, Radiology 145:321, 1982.

Dory MA: Arthrography of the lumbar facet joints, Radiology 140:23, 1981.

Eisenstein SM and Parry CR: The lumbar facet arthrosis syndrome, J Bone Joint Surg 69-B:3, 1987.

Eng RHK and Seligman SJ: Lumbar puncture-induced meningitis, JAMA 245:1456, 1981.

Feffer HL: Regional use of steroids in the management of lumbar intervertebral disc disease, Orthop Clin North Am 6:249, 1975.

Ford L: Personal communication, 1984.

Fox AJ: Lumbar discography: a dissenting opinion letter, J Can Assoc Radiol 34:88, 1983.

Fraser RD, Osti OL, and Vernon-Roberts B: Discitis after discography, J Bone Joint Surg 69-B:26, 1987.

Gentry WD, Newman MC, Goldner JL, and von Baeyer C: Relation between graduated spinal block technique and MMPI for diagnosis and prognosis of chronic low-back pain, Spine 2:210, 1977.

Ghia JN, Duncan GH, and Teeple E: Differential spinal block for diagnosis of chronic pain, Compr Ther 8:55, 1982.

Ghia JN, Mao W, Toomey TC, and Gregg JM: Acupuncture and chronic pain mechanisms, Pain 2:285, 1976.

Ghia JN, Duncan G, Toomey TC, et al: The pharmacologic approach in differential diagnosis of chronic pain, Spine 4:447, 1979.

Ghormley RK: Low back pain with special reference to the articular facets with presentation of an operative procedure, JAMA 101:1773, 1933.

Goldthwait E: Low-back lesions, J Bone Joint Surg 19:810, 1937.

Green PWB, Burke AJ, Weiss CA, and Langan P: The role of epidural cortisone injection in the treatment of diskogenic low back pain, Clin Orthop 153:121, 1980.

Hauelsen DC, Smith BS, Myers SR, and Pryce RL: The diagnostic accuracy of spinal nerve injection studies, Clin Orthop 198:179, 1985.

Haughton VM, Eldevik OP, Ho KC, et al: Arachnoiditis from experimental myelography with aqueous contrast media, Spine 3:65, 1978.

Hoffman GS, Ellsworth CA, Wells EE, et al: Spinal arachnoiditis. What is the clinical spectrum? II. Arachnoiditis induced by pantopaque/autologous blood in dogs, a possible model for human disease, Spine 8:541, 1983.

Hudgins WR: Diagnostic accuracy of lumbar discography, Spine 2:305, 1977.

Jackson RP, Jacobs RR, and Montesano PX: Facet joint injection in low-back pain: a prospective statistical study, Spine 13:966, 1988.

Johnson RG: Does discography injure normal discs? An analysis of repeat discograms, Spine 14:424, 1989.

Johnson RG and Macnab I: Localization of symptomatic lumbar pseudoarthroses by use of discography, Clin Orthop 197:164, 1985.

Johnston JDH and Matheny JB: Microscopic lysis of lumbar adhesive arachnoiditis, Spine 3:36, 1978.

Kahanovitz N, Arnoczky SP, Sissons HA, et al: The effect of discography on the canine intervertebral disc, Spine 11:26, 1986.

Kikuchi S, Macnab I, and Moreau P: Localisation of the level of symptomatic cervical disc degeneration, J Bone Joint Surg 63-B:272, 1981.

Krempen JF and Smith BS: Nerve-root injection: a method for evaluating the etiology of sciatica, J Bone Joint Surg 56-A:1435, 1974.

Krempen JF, Silver RA, and Hadley J: An analysis of differential epidural spinal anesthesia and pentothal pain study in the differential diagnosis of back pain: aids in avoiding unnecessary back surgery, Spine 4:452, 1979.

Laun A, Lorenz R, and Agnoli AL: Complications of cervical discography, J Neurosurg Sci 25:17, 1981.

Legré J, Louis R, Serrano R, and Debaene A: Anatomo-radiological considerations about lumbar discography: an experimental study, Neuroradiology 17:77, 1979.

Lindblom K: Diagnostic puncture of intervertebral discs in sciatica, Acta Orthop. Scand. 17:231, 1948.

Macnab I: Negative disc exploration: an analysis of the causes of nerve-root involvement in sixty-eight patients, J Bone Joint Surg 53-A:891, 1971.

Macnab I, Grabias SL, and Jacob R: Selective ascending lumbosacral venography in the assessment of lumbar-disc herniation: an anatomical study and clinical experience, J Bone Joint Surg 58-A:1093, 1976.

McCall IW, Park WM, and O'Brien JP: Induced pain referral from posterior lumbar elements in normal subjects, Spine 4:441, 1979.

McLaughlin RE, Miller WR, and Miller CW: Quadriparesis after needle aspiration of the cervical spine: report of a case, J Bone Joint Surg 58-A:1167, 1976.

Merriam WF and Stockdale HR: Is cervical discography of any value? Europ J Radiol 3:138, 1983.

Milette PC and Melanson D: A reappraisal of lumbar discography, J Can Assoc Radiol 33:176, 1982.

Mooney V: Alternative approaches for the patient beyond the help of surgery, Orthop Clin North Am 6:331, 1975.

Mooney V and Robertson J: The facet syndrome, Clin Orthop 115:149, 1976.

Murtagh FR: Computed tomography and fluoroscopy guided anesthesia and steroid injection in facet syndrome, Spine 13:6686, 1988.

Nachemson A: Lumbar discography: where are we today? Spine 14:555, 1989 (editorial comment).

Nelson MA, Allen P, Clamp SE, et al: Reliability and reproducibility of clinical findings in low-back pain, Spine 4:97, 1979.

Oudenhoven RC: The role of laminectomy, facet rhizotomy, and epidural steroids, Spine 4:145, 1979.

Park WM, McCall IW, O'Brien JP, and Webb JK: Fissuring of the posterior annulus fibrosus in the lumbar spine, Br J Radiol 53:382, 1979.

Quiles M, Marchisello PJ, and Tsairis P: Lumbar adhesive arachnoiditis: etiologic and pathologic aspects, Spine 3:45, 1978.

Quinnell RC and Stockdale HR: The significance of osteophytes on lumbar vertebral bodies in relation to discographic findings, Clin Radiol 33:197, 1982.

Quinell RC and Stockdale HR: Flexion and extension radiography of the lumbar spine: a comparison with lumbar discography, Clin Radiol 34:405, 1983.

Quinell RC, Stockdale HR, and Harmon B: Pressure standardized lumbar discography, Br J Radiol 53:1031, 1980.

Shealy CN: Facet denervation in the management of back and sciatic pain, Clin Orthop 115:157 1976.

Simmons EH and Segil CM: An evaluation of discography in the localization of symptomatic levels in discogenic disease of the spine, Clin Orthop 108:57, 1975.

Simmons JW, Aprill CN, Dwyer AP, and Brodsky AE: A reassessment of Holt's data on: "The question of lumbar discography," Clin Orthop 237:120, 1988.

Skalpe IO: Adhesive arachnoiditis following lumbar myelography, Spine 3:61, 1978.

Sneider SE, Winslow OP Jr, and Pryor TH: Cervical diskography: is it relevant, JAMA 185:163, 1963.

Stambough JL, Booth RE Jr, and Rothman RH: Transient hypercorticism after epidural steroid injection: a case report, J Bone Joint Surg 66-A:1115, 1984.

Steindler A and Luck JV: Differential diagnosis of pain low in the back: allocation of the source of pain by the procaine hydrochloride method, JAMA 110:106, 1938.

Sussman BJ, Bromley JW, and Gomez JC: Injection of collagenase for herniated lumbar disk: initial clinical report, JAMA 245:730, 1981.

Tajima T, Furukawa K, and Kuramochi E: Selective lumbosacral radiculography and block, Spine 5:68, 1980.

Teeple E, Scott DL, and Ghia JN: Intrathecal normal saline without preservative does not have a local anesthetic effect, Pain 14:3, 1982.

Walsh TR, Weinstein JN, Spratt KF, et al: Lumbar discography in normal subjects: a controlled, prospective study, J Bone Joint Surg 72-A:1081, 1990.

Weinberg JA: The surgical excision of psoas abscesses resulting from spinal tuberculosis, J Bone Joint Surg 39-A:17, 1957.

White AH, Derby R, and Wynne G: Epidural injections for the diagnosis and treatment of low-back pain, Spine 5:78, 1980.

Wilkinson HA: Field block anesthesia for lumbar puncture, JAMA 249:2177, 1983 (letter).

Yasuma T, Ohno R, and Yamauchi Y: False-negative lumbar discograms: correlation of discographic and histological findings in postmortem and surgical specimens, J Bone Joint Surg 70-A:1279, 1988.

Psychologic testing

Barnes D, Smith D, Gatchel RJ, and Mayer TG: Psychosocio-economic predictors of treatment success/failure in chronic low-back pain patients, Spine 14:427, 1989.

Bigos SJ, Battié MC, Spengler DM, et al: A prospective study of work perceptions and psychosocial factors affecting the report of back injury, Spine 16:1, 1991.

Caldwell AB and Chase C: Diagnosis and treatment of personality factors in chronic low back pain, Clin Orthop 129:141, 1977.

Carron H, DeGood DE, and Tait R: A comparison of low back pain patients in the United States and New Zealand: psychosocial and economic factors affecting severity of disability, Pain 21:77, 1985.

Cohen CA, Foster HM, and Peck EA III: MMPI evaluation of patients with chronic pain, South Med J 76:316 1983.

Colligan RC, Osborne D, Swenson WM, and Offord KP: The aging MMPI: development of contemporary norms, Mayo Clin Proc 59:377, 1984.

Cummings GS and Routan JL: Accuracy of the unassisted pain drawings by patients with chronic pain, J Orthop Sports Phys Ther 8:391, 1987.

Dennis MD, Greene RL, Farr SP, and Hartman JT: The Minnesota Multiphasic Personality Inventory: general guidelines to its use and interpretation of orthopedics, Clin Orthop 150:125, 1980.

Dennis MD, Rocchio PO, and Wiltse LL: The topographical pain representation and its correlation with MMPI scores, Orthopaedics 5:433, 1981.

Deyo RA and Diehl AK: Measuring physical and psychosocial function in patients with low-back pain, Spine 8:635, 1983.

Deyo RA, Walsh NE, Schoenfeld LS, and Ramamurthy S: Studies of the Modified Somatic Perceptions Questionnaire (MSPQ) in patients with back pain: psychometric and predictive properties, Spine 14:507, 1989.

Evanski PM, Carver D, Nehemkis A, and Waugh TR: The Burns' test in low back pain: correlation with the hysterical personality, Clin Orthop 140:42, 1979.

Gentry WD: Chronic back pain: does elective surgery benefit patients with evidence of psychologic disturbance? South Med J 75:1169, 1982.

Gentry WD, Shows WD, and Thomas M: Chronic low back pain: a psychological profile, Psychosomatics 15:174, 1974.

Herron LD and Pheasant HC: Changes in MMPI profiles after low-back surgery, Spine 7:591, 1982.

Leavitt F, Garron DC, McNeill TW, and Whisler WW: Organic status, psychological disturbance, and pain report characteristics in low-back-pain patients on compensation, Spine 7:398, 1982.

Long CJ, Brown DA, and Engelberg J: Intervertebral disc surgery: strategies for patient selection to improve surgical outcome, J Neurosurg 52:818, 1980.

Luck J: Psychosomatic problems in military orthopaedic surgery, J Bone Joint Surg 28:213, 1946.

Nehemkis AM, Carver DW, and Evanski PM: The predictive utility of the orthopaedic examination in identifying the low back pain patient with hysterical personality features, Clin Orthop 145:158, 1979.

Pheasant HC, Gilbert D, Goldfarb J, and Herron L: The MMPI as a predictor of outcome in low-back surgery, Spine 4:78, 1979.

Pincus T, Callahan LF, Bradley LA, et al: Elevated MMPI scores for hypochondriasis, depression and hysteria in patients with rheumatoid arthritis reflect disease rather than psychological status, Arthr Rheum 29:1456, 1986.

Rainsford AO, Cairns D, and Mooney V: The pain drawing as an aid to the psychologic evaluation of patients with low-back pain, Spine 1:127, 1976.

Rockwood CA and Eilert RE: Camptocormia, J Bone Joint Surg 51-A:533, 1969.

Southwick SM and White AA: The use of psychological tests in the evaluation of low-back pain, J Bone Joint Surg 65-A:560, 1983.

Sternback RA: Psychological aspects of chronic pain, Clin Orthop 129:150, 1977.

Udén A and Landin LA: Pain drawing and myelography in sciatic pain, Clin Orthop 216:124, 1987.

Waddell G, McCullouch JA, Kummel E, et al: Nonorganic physical signs in low-back pain, Spine 5:117, 1980.

Westrin C, Hirsch C, and Lindegard B: The personality of the back patient, Clin Orthop 87:209, 1972.

Wilfling BA, Klonoff H, and Kokan P: Psychological, demographic and orthopaedic factors associated with prediction of outcome of spinal fusion, Clin Orthop 90:153, 1973.

Wiltse LL and Rocchio P: Preoperative psychological tests as predictors of success of chemonucleolysis in the treatment of the low-back syndrome, J Bone Joint Surg 57-A:478, 1975.

Cervical disc disease

Aldrich F: Posterolateral microdiscectomy for cervical monoradiculopathy caused by posterolateral soft cervical disc sequestration, J Neurosurg 72:370, 1990.

Bailey RW and Badgley CE: Stabilization of the cervical spine by anterior fusion, J Bone Joint Surg 42-A:565, 1960.

Bernardo KL, Grubb RL, Coxe WS, and Roper CL: Anterior cervical disc herniation: case report, J Neurosurg 69:134, 1988.

Bloom MH, and Raney FL: Anterior intervertebral fusion of the cervical spine: a technical note, J Bone Joint Surg 63-A:842, 1981.

Boden SD, McCowin PR, Davis DO, et al: Abnormal magnetic-resonance scans of the cervical spine in asymptomatic subjects, J Bone Joint Surg 72-A:1178, 1990.

Boldrey EB: Anterior cervical decompression (without fusion). Paper presented to the twenty-fifth annual meeting of the American Academy of Neurological Surgery, Key Biscayne, Florida, November 12, 1964.

Braun IR, Pinto RS, De Fillip GJ, et al: Brain stem infarction due to chiropractic manipulation of the cervical spine, South Med J 76:1507, 1983.

Bucy PC, Heimburger RF, and Oberhill HR: Compression of the cervical spinal cord by herniated intervertebral discs, J Neurosurg 5:471, 1948.

Bull JWD: Rupture of the intervertebral disk in the cervical region, Proc R Soc Med 41:513, 1948.

Cloward RB: The treatment of ruptured lumbar intervertebral discs by vertebral body fusion. I. Indications, operative technique, after care, J Neurosurg 10:154, 1953.

Cloward RB: The anterior approach for removal of ruptured cervical discs, J Neurosurg 15:602, 1958.

Cosgrove GR and Théron J: Vertebral anteriovenous fistula following anterior cervical spine surgery: report of two cases, J Neurosurg 66:297, 1987.

Coventry MB, Ghormley RK, and Kernohan JW: The intervertebral disc: its microscopic anatomy and pathology. II. Changes in the intervertebral disc concomitant with age, J Bone Joint Surg 27:233, 1945.

Coventry MB, Ghormley RK, and Kernohan JW: The intervertebral disc: its microscopic anatomy and pathology. III. Pathological changes in the intervertebral disc, J Bone Joint Surg 27:460, 1945.

Davidson RI, Dunn EJ, and Metzmaker JN: The shoulder abduction test in the diagnosis of radicular pain in cervical extradural compressive monoradiculopathies, Spine 6:441, 1981.

De Palma AF and Cooke AJ: Results of anterior interbody fusion of the cervical spine, Clin Orthop 60:169, 1968.

Dunsker SB: Anterior cervical discectomy with and without fusion, Clin Neurosurg 24:516, 1976.

Evans DK: Anterior cervical subluxation, J Bone Joint Surg 58-B:318, 1976.

Farley ID, McAfee PC, Davis RF, and Long DM: Pseudarthrosis of the cervical spine after anterior arthrodesis, J Bone Joint Surg 72-A:1171, 1990.

Garcia A: Cervical traction, an ancient modality, Orthop Rev 13:429, 1984.

Harris RI and Macnab I: Structural changes in the lumbar intervertebral disc: their relationship to low back pain and sciatica, J Bone Joint Surg 36-B:304, 1954.

Hartman JT, Palumob F, and Hill BJ: Cineradiography of the braced normal cervical spine: a comparative study of five commonly used cervical orthoses, Clin Orthop 109:97, 1975.

Hirsch D: Cervical disc rupture: diagnosis and therapy, Acta Orthop Scand 30:172, 1960.

Horal J: The clinical appearance of low back disorders in the city of Gothenburg, Sweden: comparisons of incapacitated probands with matched controls, Acta Orthop Scand Suppl 116:1, 1969.

Jacobs B, Krueger EG, and Levy DM: Cervical spondylosis with radiculopathy: results of anterior diskectomy and interbody fusion, JAMA 211:2135, 1970.

Josey AI and Murphey F: Ruptured intervertebral disk simulating angina pectoris, JAMA 131:581, 1946.

Keegan JJ: Dermatome hypalgesia associated with herniation or intervertebral disc, Arch Neurol Psychiatr 50:67, 1943.

Kelsey JL et al: An epidemiological study of acute prolapsed cervical intervertebral disc, J Bone Joint Surg 66-A:907, 1984

Key CA: On paraplegia depending on the ligaments of the spine, Guy's Hosp Rep 7:1737, 1838.

Kikuchi S, Macnab I, and Moreau P: Localisation of the level of symptomatic cervical disc degeneration, J Bone Joint Surg 63-B:272, 1981.

Kikuchi S et al: Anatomic and clinical studies of radicular symptoms, Spine 9:23, 1984.

Koop SE, Winter RB, and Lonstein JE: The surgical treatment of instability of the upper part of the cervical spine in children and adolescents, J Bone Joint Surg 66-A:403, 1984.

Lindsey RW, Newhouse KE, Leach J, and Murphy MJ: Nonunion following two-level anterior cervical discectomy and fusion, Clin Orthop 223:155, 1987.

Lourie H, Shende MC, and Stewart DH: The syndrome of central cervical soft disk herniation, JAMA 226:302, 1973.

Lunsford LD, Bissonette DJ, Jannetta PJ, et al: Anterior surgery for cervical disc disease. I. Treatment of lateral cervical disc herniation in 253 cases, J Neurosurg 53:1, 1980.

Murphey F, Simmons JCH, and Brunson B: Surgical treatment of laterally ruptured cervical discs: a review of 648 cases, 1939 to 1972, J Neurosurg 38:679, 1973.

Murphey MG and Gado M: Anterior cervical discectomy without interbody bone graft, J Neurosurgg 37:71, 1972.

Odom GL, Finney W, and Woodhall B: Cervical disk lesion, JAMA 166:23, 1958.

O'Laoire SA and Thomas DGT: Spinal cord compression due to prolapse of cervical intervertebral disc (herniation of nucleus pulposus), J Neurosurg 59:847, 1983.

Pennecot GF, Gouraud D, Hardy JR, and Pouliquen JC: Roentgenographical study of the stability of the cervical spine in children, J Pediatr Orthop 4:346, 1984.

Rainer JK: Cervical disc surgery: a historical review, J Tenn Med Assoc 77:12, 1984.

Rath WW: Cervical traction: a clinical perspective, Orthop Rev 13:430, 1984.

Riley LH: Surgical approaches to the anterior structures of the cervical spine, Clin Orthop 91:16, 1973.

Robertson JT: Anterior removal of cervical disc without fusion, Clin Neurosurg 20:259, 1973.

Robertson JT and Johnson SD: Anterior cervical discectomy without fusion: long-term results, Clin Neurosurg 27:440, 1980.

Robinson JS: Sciatica and the lumbar disc syndrome: a historic perspective, South Med J 76:232, 1983.

Robinson RA and Southwick WO: Surgical approaches to the cervical spine, AAOS Instr Course Lect 17:299, 1960.

Roda JM et al: Intradural herniated cervical disc: case report, J Neurosurg 57:278, 1982.

Rosenorn J, Hansen EB, and Rosenorn MA: Anterior cervical discectomy with and without fusion, J Neurosurg 59:252, 1983.

Rothman RH and Marvel JP Jr: The acute cervical disk, Clin Orthop 109:59, 1975.

Scoville WB: Types of cervical disk lesions and their surgical approaches, JAMA 196:105, 1966.

Scoville WB, Whitcomb BB, and McLaurin R: The cervical ruptured disk: report of 115 operative cases, Trans Am Neurol Assoc 76th Ann Meet, 222, 1951.

Seddon HJ and Alexander GL: Discussion on spinal caries with paraplegia, Proc R Soc Med 39:723, 1946.

Semmes RE and Murphey F: The syndrome of unilateral rupture of the sixth cervical intervertebral disk, with compression of the seventh nerve root: a report of four cases with symptoms simulating coronary disease, JAMA 121:1209, 1943.

Sherk HH, Watters WC III, and Zeiger L: Evaluation and treatment of neck pain, Orthop Clin North AM 13:439, 1982.

Simmons EH and Bhalla SK: Anterior cervical discectomy and fusion: a clinical and biomechanical study with eight-year follow-up, with a note on discography: technique and interpretation of results by W.P. Butt, J Bone Joint Surg 51-B:225, 1969.

Simmons JCH: Rupture of cervical intervertebral discs. In Edmonson AS and Crenshaw AH, editors: Campbell's operative orthopaedics, ed 6, St Louis, 1980, Mosby-Year Book, Inc.

Smith GW and Robinson RA: Anterior lateral cervical disc removal and interbody fusion for cervical disc syndrome, Bull Johns Hopkins Hosp 96:223, 1955.

Spurling RG and Scoville WB: Lateral rupture of the cervical intervertebral discs: a common cause of shoulder and arm pain, Surg Gynecol Obstet 78:350, 1944.

Spurling RG and Segerberg LH: Lateral intervertebral disk lesions in the lower cervical region, JAMA 151:354, 1953.

Stookey B: Cervical chrondroma, Arch Neurol Psych 20:275, 1928.

Tamura T: Cranial symptoms after cervical injury: aetiology and treatment of the Barré-Lieou syndrome, J Bone Joint Surg 71-B:282, 1989.

Viikari-Juntura E, Porras M, and Laasonen EM: Validity of clinical tests in the diagnosis of root compression in cervical disc disease, Spine 14:253, 1989.

Welsh LW, Welsh JJ, and Chinnici JC: Dysphagia due to cervical spine surgery, Ann Otol Rhinol Laryngol 96:112, 1987.

White AA, Jupiter J, Southwick WO, and Panjabi MM: An experimental study of the immediate load bearing capacity of three surgical constructions for anterior spine fusions, Clin Orthop 91:21, 1973.

White AA et al: Relief of pain by anterior cervical spine fusion for spondylosis: a report of sixty-five cases, J Bone Joint Surg 55-A:525, 1973.

Whitecloud TS: Management of radiculopathy and myelopathy by the anterior approach: the cervical spine. The Cervical Spine Research Society, Philadelphia, 1983, JB Lippincott Co.

Thoracic disc disease

Albrand OW and Corkill G: Thoracic disc herniation: treatment and prognosis, Spine 4:41, 1979.

Antoni N: Fall av kronisk rotkompression med ovanlig orsak, hernia nuclei pulposi disci intervertebralis, Sv Lakartidn 28:436, 1931.

Arseni C and Nash F: Protrusion of thoracic intervertebral discs, Acta Neurochir 11:1, 1963.

Benson MKD and Byrnes DP: The clinical syndromes and surgical treatment of thoracic intervertebral disc prolapse, J Bone Joint Surg 57-B:471, 1975.

Bohlman HH and Zdeblick TA: Anterior excision of herniated thoracic discs, J Bone Joint Surg 70-A:1038, 1988.

Hochman MS, Pena C, and Ramirez R: Calcified herniated thoracic disc diagnosed by computerized tomography: case report, J Neurosurg 52:722, 1980.

Hulme A: The surgical approach to thoracic intervertebral disc protrusions, J Neurol Neurosurg Psychiat 23:133, 1960.

Logue V: Thoracic intervertebral disc prolapse with spinal cord compression, J Neurol Neurosurg Psychiat 15:227, 1952.

Love JG and Kiefer EJ: Root pain and paraplegia due to protrusions of thoracic intervertebral disks, J Neurosurg 15:62, 1950.

Maiman DJ, Larson SJ, Luck E, and El-Ghatit A: Lateral extracavity approach to the spine for thoracic disc herniation: report of 23 cases, Neurosurgery 14:178, 1984.

Martucci E, Mele C, and Martella P: Thoracic intervertebral disc protrusion, Ital J Orthop Traumatol 10:333, 1984.

Marzluff JM, Hungerford GD, Kempe LG, et al: Thoracic myelopathy caused by osteophytes of the articular process, J Neurosurg 50:779, 1979.

Muller R: Protrusion of thoracic intervertebral disks with compression of the spinal cord, Acta Med Scand 139:99, 1951.

O'Leary PF, Camins MB, Polifroni NV, and Floman Y: Thoracic disc disease: clinical manifestations and surgical treatment, Bull Hosp Jt Dis Orthop Inst 44:27, 1984.

Omojola MF, Cardoso ER, Fox AJ, et al: Thoracic myelopathy secondary to ossified ligamentum flavum: case report, J Neurosurg 56:448, 1982.

Otani K, Manzoku S, Shibasaki K, and Nomachi S: The surgical treatment of thoracic and thoracolumbar disc lesions using the anterior approach: report of six cases, Spine 2:266, 1977.

Panjabi MM, Krag MH, Dimnet JC, et al: Thoracic spine centers of rotation in the sagittal plane, J Orthop Res 1:387, 1984.

Perot PL Jr and Munro DD: Transthoracic removal of midline thoracic disc protrusions causing spinal cord compression, J Neurosurg 31:452, 1969.

Seddon HJ: Pott's paraplegia. In Platt H, editor: Modern trends in orthopaedics (second series), London, 1956, Butterworth & Co, Ltd.

Sekhar LN and Jannetta PJ: Thoracic disc herniation: operative approaches and results, Neurosurgery 12:303, 1983.

Tovi D and Strang RR: Thoracic intervertebral disk protrusions, Acta Chir Scand (Suppl) 267:1, 1960.

Lumbar disc disease: etiology, diagnosis, and conservative treatment

Alcoff J, Jones E, Rust P, and Newman R: Controlled trial of imipramine for chronic low back pain, J Fam Pract 14:841, 1982.

Anderson BJG and Ortengren R: Lumbar disc pressure and myoelectric back muscle activity during sitting. II, Scand J Rehab Med 6:115, 1974.

Anderson BJG, Ortengren R, Nachemson A, and Elfstrom G: Lumbar disc pressure and myoelectric back muscle activity during sitting. I, Scand J Rehab Med 6:104, 1974.

Atkinson JH, Kremer EF, and Garfin SR: Psychopharmaco-logical agents in the treatment of pain, J Bone Joint Surg 67-A:337, 1985.

Basmajian JV: Acute back pain and spasm: a controlled multicenter trial of combined analgesic and antispasm agents, Spine 14:438, 1989.

Bell GR and Rothman RH: The conservative treatment of sciatica, Spine 9:54, 1984.

Bergquist-Ullman M and Larsson U: Acute low back pain in industry: a controlled prospective study with special reference to therapy and confounding factors, Acta Orthop Scand (Suppl) 170:1, 1977.

Berman AT, Garbarino JL, Fisher ST, and Bosacco SJ: The effects of epidural injection of local anesthetics and corticosteroids on patients with lumbosciatic pain, Clin Orthop 188:144, 1984.

Bernard TN and Kirkaldy-Willis WH: Recognizing specific characteristics of nonspecific low back pain, Clin Orthop 217:266, 1987.

Berwick DM, Budman S, and Feldstein M: No clinical effects of back schools in an HMO: a randomized prospective trial, Spine 14:338, 1989.

Bigos SJ and Battié MC: Acute care to prevent back disability: ten years of progress, Clin Orthop 221:121, 1987.

Blower PW: Neurologic patterns in unilateral sciatica: a prospective study of 100 new cases, Spine 6:175, 1981.

Borgesen SE and Vang PS: Herniation of the lumbar intervertebral disk in children and adolescents, Acta Orthop Scand 45:540, 1974.

Bradford DS and Garcia A: Lumbar intervertebral disk herniations in children and adolescents, Orthop Clin North Am 2:583, 1971.

Breig A and Troup JDG: Biomechanical considerations in the straight-leg-raising test, Spine 4:242, 1979.

Brown FW: Management of diskogenic pain using epidural and intrathecal steroids, Clin Orthop 129:72, 1977.

Brown MD: Diagnosis of pain syndromes of the spine, Orthop Clin North Am 6:233, 1975.

Cauthen C: Lumbar spine surgery, Baltimore, 1983, Williams & Wilkins.

Charnley J: Orthopaedic signs in the diagnosis of disc protrusion, Lancet 1:186, 1951.

Christodoulides AN: Ipsilateral sciatica on femoral nerve stretch test is pathognomonic of an L4-5 disc protrusion, J Bone Joint Surg 71-B:88, 1989.

Clarke HA and Fleming ID: Disk disease and occult malignancies, South Med J 66:449, 1973.

Clarke NMP and Cleak DK: Intervertebral lumbar disc prolapse in children and adolescents, J Pediatr Orthop 3:202, 1983.

Coyer AB and Curwen IHM: Low back pain treated by manipulation, Br Med J 705, March 19, 1955.

Cuckler JM et al: The use of epidural steroids in the treatment of lumbar radicular pain, J Bone Joint Surg 67-A:63, 1985.

Cyriax J: Dural pain: mechanisms of symptoms, Lancet 1:919, 1978.

de Sèze S: Sciatique "banale" et disques lombo-sacrés, La Presse Medicale 51-52:570, 1940.

de Sèze S: Histoire de la sciatique, Rev Neurol 138:1019, 1982.

Deyo RA: Conservative therapy for low back pain: distinguishing useful from useless therapy, JAMA 250:1057, 1983.

Deyo RA, Diehl AK, and Rosenthal M: How many days of bed rest for acute low back pain? A randomized clinical trial, N Engl J Med 315:1064, 1986.

Deyo RA, Walsh NE, Martin DC, et al: A controlled trial of transcutaneous electrical nerve stimulation (TENS) and exercise for chronic low back pain, N Engl J Med 322:1627, 1990.

Dimitrigevic DT: Historical note: Laseègue sign, Neurology 2:453, 1952.

Dujovny M, Barrionuevo PJ, Kossovsky N, et al: Effects of contrast media on the canine subarachnoid space, Spine 3:31, 1978.

Dyck P: The stoop-test in lumbar entrapment radiculopathy, Spine 4:89, 1979.

Edgar MA and Park WM: Induced pain patterns on passive straight-leg raising in lower lumbar disc protrusion: a prospective clinical, myelographic and operative study in fifty patients, J Bone Joint Surg 56-B:658, 1974.

Estridge MN, Rouhe SA, and Johnson NG: The femoral stretching test: a valuable sign in diagnosing upper lumbar disc herniations, J Neurosurg 57:813, 1982.

Evanski PM, Carver D, Nehemkis A, and Waugh TR: The Burns' test in low back pain: correlation with the hysterical personality, Clin Orthop 140:42, 1979.

Fairbank JCT and O'Brien JP: The iliac crest syndrome: a treatable cause of low-back pain, Spine 8:220, 1983.

Farfan HF: The torsional injury of the lumbar spine, Spine 9:53, 1984.

Fisher RG and Saunders RL: Lumbar disc protrusion in children, J Neurosurg 54:480, 1981.

Friberg O: Clinical symptoms and biomechanics of lumbar spine and hip joint in leg length inequality, Spine 8:643, 1983.

Giles LGF and Taylor JR: Low back pain associated with leg length inequality, Spine 6:510, 1981.

Grabel JD, Davis R, and Zappulla R: Intervertebral disc space cyst simulating a recurrent herniated nucleus pulposus, J Neurosurg 69:137, 1988.

Hakelius A: Prognosis in sciatica, Acta Orthop Scand Suppl 129:6, 1970.

Hall GW: Neurologic signs and their discoverers, JAMA 95:703, 1930.

Hanman B: The evaluation of physical ability, N Engl J Med 258:986, 1958.

Hazard RG, Fenwick JW, Kalisch SM, et al: Functional restoration with behavioral support: a one-year prospective study of patients with chronic low-back pain, Spine 14:157, 1989.

Healy KM: Does preoperative instruction make a difference? Am J Nurs 68:62, 1968.

Herron LD and Pheasant HC: Prone knee-flexion provocative testing for lumbar disc protrusion, Spine 5:65, 1980.

Hirsch C: Reflections on the use of surgery in lumbar disc disease, Orthop Clin 2:493, 1971.

Hirsh LF and Finneson BE: Intradural sacral nerve root metastasis mimicking herniated disc: case report, J Neurosurg 49:764, 1978.

Hitselberger WE and Witten RM: Abnormal myelograms in asymptomatic patients, J Neurosurg 28:204, 1968.

Hollinshead WH: Anatomy of the spine: points of interest to orthopaedic surgeons, J Bone Joint Surg 47-A:209, 1965.

Kane RL, Olsen D, Leymaster C, et al: Manipulating the patient, Lancet 1:1333, 1974.

Keegan JJ: Dermatome hypalgesia associated with herniation of intervertebral disc, Arch Neurol Psych 50:67, 1943.

Kikuchi S, Hasue M, Nishiyama K, et al: Anatomic and clinical studies of radicular symptoms, Spine 9:23, 1984.

Kirkaldy-Willis WH and Hill RJ: A more precise diagnosis for low-back pain, Spine 4:102, 1979.

Klier I and Santo M: Low back pain as presenting symptoms of chronic granulocytic leukemia, Orthop Rev 11:111, 1982.

Kosteljanetz M, Bang F, and Schmidt-Olsen S: The clinical significance of straight-leg raising (Lasegue's sign) in the diagnosis of prolapsed lumbar disc: interobserver variation and correlation with surgical findings, Spine 13:393, 1988.

Kostuik JP and Bentivoglio J: The incidence of low-back pain in adult scoliosis, Spine 6:268, 1981.

Lidstrom A and Zachrisson M: Physical therapy on low back pain and sciatica, Scand J Rehab Med 2:37, 1970.

Macnab I: Management of low back pain. In Ahstrom JP Jr, editor: Current practice in orthopaedic surgery, St Louis, 1973, Mosby–Year Book, Inc.

Macnab I, Cuthbert H, and Godfrey CM: The incidence of denervation of the sacrospinales muscles following spinal surgery, Spine 2:294, 1977.

Melleby A and Kraus H: Chronic back pain: use of a YMCA-developed exercise regimen, J New Develop Clin Med 5:75, 1987.

Miller A, Stedman GH, Beisaw NE, and Gross PT: Sciatica caused by an avulsion fracture of the ischial tuberosity, J Bone Joint Surg 69-A:143, 1987.

Nachemson A: Physiotherapy for low back pain patients: a critical look, Scand J Rehab Med 1:85, 1969.

Nachemson AL: The lumbar spine: an orthopaedic challenge, Spine 1:59, 1976.

Nachemson AL: Adult scoliosis and back pain, Spine 4:513, 1979.

Nachemson AL: Prevention of chronic back pain: the orthopaedic challenge for the 80's, Bull Hosp Jt Dis Orth Inst 44:1, 1984.

Nachemson AL and Lindh M: Measurement of abdominal and back muscle strength with and without low back pain, Scand J Rehab Med 1:60, 1969.

Natchev E and Valentino V: Low back pain and disc hernia: observation during auto-traction treatment, Manual Med 1:39, 1984.

Nelson MA, Allen P, Clamp SE, et al: Reliability and reproducibility of clinical findings in low-back pain, Spine 4:97, 1979.

O'Brien JP: Anterior spinal tenderness in low-back pain syndromes, Spine 4:85, 1979.

Offierski CM and Macnab I: Hip-spine syndrome, Spine 8:316, 1983.

Onel D, Tuzlaci M, Sari H, and Demir K: Computed tomographic investigation of the effect of traction on lumbar disc herniations, Spine 14:82, 1989.

Oudenhoven RC: The role of laminectomy, facet rhizotomy, and epidural steroids, Spine 4:145, 1979.

Pheasant H, Bursk A, Goldfarb J, et al: Amitriptyline and chronic low-back pain: a randomized double-blind crossover study, Spine 8:552, 1983.

Postacchini F, Urso S, and Tovaglia V: Lumbosacral intradural tumours simulating disc disease, Inter Orthop (SICOT) 5:283, 1981.

Quinet RJ and Hadler NM: Diagnosis and treatment of backache, Semin Arthritis Rheum 8:261, 1979.

Ramamurthi B: Absence of limitation of straight leg raising in proved lumbar disc lesion: case report, J Neurosurg 52:852, 1980.

Robinson JS: Sciatica and the lumbar disk syndrome: a historic perspective, South Med J 76:232, 1983.

Rockwood CA and Eilert RE: Camptocormia, J Bone Joint Surg 51-A:533, 1969.

Rothman RH: The clinical syndrome of lumbar disc disease, Orthop Clin North Am 2:463, 1971.

Saal JA and Saal JS: Nonoperative treatment of herniated lumbar intervertebral disc with radiculopathy and outcome study, Spine 14:431, 1989.

Sandover J: Dynamic loading as a possible source of low-back disorders, Spine 8:652, 1983.

Shiqing X, Quanzhi Z, and Dehao F: Significance of the straight-leg-raising test in the diagnosis and clinical evaluation of lower lumbar intervertebral-disc protrusion, J Bone Joint Surg 69-A:517, 1987.

Simmons JW, Dennis MD, and Rath D: The back school: a total back management program, Orthopedics 7(9):1453, 1984.

Sjöqvist O: The mechanism of origin of Lasègue's sign, Acta Psych Neurol 46(suppl):290, 1947.

Solheim LF, Siewers P, and Paus B: The piriformis muscle syndrome: sciatic nerve entrapment treated with section of the piriformis muscle, Acta Orthop Scand 52:73, 1981.

Spurling RG: Lesions of the lumbar intervertebral disk, Springfield, Ill, 1953, Charles C Thomas, Publisher.

Steindler A and Luck JV: Differential diagnosis of pain low in the back: allocation of the source of pain by the procaine hydrochloride method, JAMA 110(2):106, 1938.

Tay ECK and Chacha PB: Midline prolapse of a lumbar intervertebral disc with compression of the cauda equina, J Bone Joint Surg 61-B:43, 1979.

Tonelli L, Falasca A, Argentieri C, et al: Influence of psychic distress on short-term outcome of lumbar disc surgery, J Neurosurg Sci 27:237, 1983.

Troup JDG: Straight-leg raising (SLR) and the qualifying tests for increased root tension: their predictive value after back and sciatic pain, Spine 6:526, 1981.

Ueyoshi A and Shima Y: Studies on spinal braces with special reference to the effects of increased abdominal pressure, Inte Orthop 9:255, 1985.

Verta MJ Jr, Vitello J, and Fuller J: Adductor canal compression syndrome, Arch Surg 119:345, 1984.

Waddell G: A new clinical model for the treatment of low-back pain, Spine 12:632, 1987.

Waddell G, Main CJ, Morris EW, et al: Chronic low-back pain, psychologic distress, and illness behavior, Spine 9:209, 1984.

Waddell G, McCullouch JA, Kummel E, et al: Nonorganic physical signs of low-back pain, Spine 5:117, 1980.

Ward NG: Tricyclic antidepressants for chronic low-back pain: mechanisms of action and predictors of response, Spine 11:661, 1986.

Wartenberg R: Lasègue sign and Kernig sign: historical notes, Arch Neurol Psych 66:58, 1951.

Wartenberg R: On neurologic terminology, eponyms and the Lasègue sign, Neurology 6:853, 1956.

Weber H: Lumbar disc herniation: a controlled, prospective study with ten years of observation, Spine 8:131, 1983.

Weise MD, Garfin SR, Gelberman RH, et al: Lower-extremity sensibility testing in patients with herniated lumbar intervertebral discs, J Bone Joint Surg 67-A:1219, 1985.

Weitz EM: The lateral bending sign, Spine 6:388, 1981.

White AA III and Gordon SL: Synopsis: workshop on idiopathic low-back pain, Spine 7:141, 1982.

White AH, Derby R, and Wynne G: Epidural injections for the diagnosis and treatment of low-back pain, Spine 5:78, 1980.

White AH, Taylor LW, Wynne G, and Welch RB: Appendix: a diagnostic classification of low-back pain, Spine 5(1):83, 1980.

Wilkins RH and Brody IA: Lasègue's sign, Arch Neurol 21:219, 1969.

Willis TA: Lumbosacral anomalies, J Bone Joint Surg 41-A:935, 1959.

Willner S: Effect of a rigid brace on back pain, Acta Orthop Scand 56:40, 1985.

Yoganandan N, Maiman DJ, Pintar F, et al: Microtrauma in the lumbar spine: a cause of low back pain, Neurosurgery 23:162, 1988.

Young A et al: Variations in the pattern of muscle innervation by the L5 and S1 nerve roots, Spine 8:616, 1983.

Zaleske DJ, Bode HH, Benz R, and Kirshnamoorthy KS: Association of sciatica-like pain and Addison's disease: a case report, J Bone Joint Surg 66-A:297, 1984.

Lumbar disc disease: surgical treatment and results

Aitken AP and Bradford CH: End results of ruptured intervertebral discs in industry, Am J Surg 73:365, 1947.

Andrews ET: A unique frame for back surgery, Orthopedics 2:130, 1979.

Arnoldi CC et al: Lumbar spinal stenosis and nerve root entrapment syndromes: definition and classification, Clin Orthop 115:4, 1976.

Barr JS: Low-back and sciatic pain: results of treatment, J Bone Joint Surg 33-A:633, 1951.

Barr JS et al: Evaluation of end results in treatment of ruptured lumbar intervertebral discs with protrusion of nucleus pulposus, J Surg 123:250, 1967.

Benner B and Ehni G: Degenerative lumbar scoliosis, Spine 4:548, 1979.

Blaauw G, Braakman R, Gelpke GJ, and Singh R: Changes in radicular function following low-back surgery, J Neurosurg 69:649, 1988.

Blower PW: Neurologic patterns in unilateral sciatica: a prospective study of 100 new cases, Spine 6:175, 1981.

Borgesen SE and Vang PS: Herniation of the lumbar intervertebral disk in children and adolescents, Acta Orthop Scand 45:540, 1974.

Bradford DS and Garcia A: Lumbar intervertebral disk herniations in children and adolescents, Orthop Clin North Am 2:583, 1971.

Bryant MS, Bremer AM, and Nguyen TQ: Autogeneic fat transplants in the epidural space in routine lumbar spine surgery, Neurosurgery 13:367, 1983.

Capanna AH et al: Lumbar discectomy — percentage of disc removal and detection of anterior annulus perforation, Spine 6:610, 1981.

Carruthers CC and Kousaie KN: Surgical treatment after chemonucleolysis failure, Clin Orthop 165:172, 1982.

Castellvi AE, Goldstein LA, and Chan DPK: Lumbosacral transitional vertebrae and their relationship with lumbar extradural defects, Spine 9:493, 1984.

Cauchoix J, Ficat C, and Girard B: Repeat surgery after disc excision, Spine 3:256, 1978.

Cauthen C: Lumbar spine surgery, Baltimore, 1983, Williams & Wilkins.

Charnley J: Orthopaedic signs in the diagnosis of disc protrusion, Lancet 1:186, 1951.

Choudhury AR, Taylor JC, Worthington BS, and Whitaker R: Lumbar radiculopathy contralateral to upper lumbar disc herniation: report of three cases, Br J Surg 65:842, 1978.

Chow SP, Leong JCY, and Yau AC: Anterior spinal fusion for deranged lumbar intervertebral disc: a review of 97 cases, Spine 5:452, 1980.

Clark K: Significance of the small lumbar spinal canal: cauda equina compression syndromes due to spondylosis. II. Clinical and surgical significance, J Neurosurg 31:495, 1969.

Clarke HA and Fleming ID: Disk disease and occult malignancies, South Med J 66:449, 1973.

Clarke NMP and Cleak DK: Intervertebral lumbar disc prolapse in children and adolescents, J Pediatr Orthop 3:202, 1983.

Compere EL: Spinal fusion following removal of intervertebral disk, South Med J 39:301, 1946.

Cook PL and Wise K: A correlation of the surgical and radiculographic findings in lumbar disc herniation, Clin Radiol 30:671, 1979.

Crawshaw C, Frazer AM, Merriam WF, et al: A comparison of surgery and chemonucleolysis in the treatment of sciatica: a prospective randomized trial, Spine 9:195, 1984.

Crock HV: Normal and pathological anatomy of the lumbar spinal nerve roots, J Bone Joint Surg 63-B:487, 1981.

Cyriax J: Dural pain: mechanisms of symptoms, Lancet 1:919, 1978.

Delamarter RB, Leventhal MR, and Bohlman HH: Diagnosis of recurrent lumbar disc herniation vs postoperative scar by gadolinium-DTPA enhanced magnetic resonance imaging (in press).

Di Lauro L, Poli R, Bortoluzzi M, and Marini G: Paresthesias after lumbar disc removal and their relationship to epidural hematoma, J Neurosurg 57:135, 1982.

Dvonch V et al: Dermatomal somatosensory evoked potentials: their use in lumbar radiculopathy, Spine 9:291, 1984.

Ebeling U, Kalbarcyk H, and Reulen HJ: Microsurgical reoperation following lumbar disc surgery: timing, surgical findings, and outcome in 92 patients, J Neurosurg 70:397, 1989.

Ebersold MJ, Quast LM, and Bianco AJ: Results of lumbar discectomy in the pediatric patient, J Neurosurg 67:643, 1987.

Eie N, Solgaard T, and Kleppe H: The knee-elbow position in lumbar disc surgery: a review of complications, Spine 8:897, 1983.

Eismont FJ, Wiesel SW, and Rothman RH: The treatment of dural tears associated with spinal surgery, J Bone Joint Surg 63-A:1132, 1981.

El-Gindi S, Aref S, Salama M, and Andrew J: Infection of the intervertebral discs after surgery, J Bone Joint Surg 58-B:114, 1976.

Epstein BS, Epstein JA, and Lavine L: The effect of anatomic variations in the lumbar vertebrae and spinal canal on cauda equina and nerve root syndromes, Am J Roentgenol Radium Ther Nucl Med 91:105, 1964.

Epstein JA, Carras R, Ferrar J, et al: Conjoined lumbosacral nerve roots, J Neurosurg 55:585, 1981.

Epstein JA, Epstein BS, and Jones MD: Symptomatic lumbar scoliosis with degenerative changes in the elderly, Spine 4:542, 1979.

Finneson BE and Cooper VR: A lumbar disc surgery predictive score card: a retrospective evaluation, Spine 4:141, 1979.

Fisher RG and Saunders RL: Lumbar disc protrusion in children, J Neurosurg 54:480, 1981.

Floman Y, Wiesel SW, and Rothman RH: Cauda equina syndrome presenting as a herniated lumbar disc, Clin Orthop 147:234, 1980.

Flynn JC and Price CT: Sexual complications of anterior fusion of the lumbar spine, Spine 9:489, 1984.

Frymoyer JW, Hanaley EN, and Howe J: A comparison of radiographic findings in fusion and nonfusion patients ten or more years following lumbar disc surgery, Spine 5:435, 1979.

Gardner RC: The lumbar intervertebral disk: a clinicopathological correlation based on over 100 laminectomies, Arch Surg 100:101, 1970.

Garrido E and Rosenwasser RH: Painless footdrop secondary to lumbar disc herniation: report of two cases, Neurosurgery 8:484, 1981.

Getty CJM, Johnson JR, Kirwan E, and Sullivan MF: Partial undercutting facetectomy for bony entrapment of the lumbar nerve root, J Bone Joint Surg 63-B:330, 1981.

Goald HJ: Microlumbar discectomy: followup of 147 patients, Spine 3:183, 1978.

Grant FC: Operative results in intervertebral discs, Ann Surg 124:1066, 1946.

Greenberg RP and Ducker TB: Evoked potentials in the clinical neurosciences, J Neurosurg 56:1, 1982.

Grobler LJ, Simmons EH, and Barrington TW: Intervertebral disc herniation in the adolescent, Spine 4:267, 1979.

Gurdjian ES and Webster JE: Lumbar herniations of the nucleus pulposus: an analysis of 196 operated cases, Am J Surg 76:235, 1948.

Hakelius A: Prognosis in sciatica, Acta Orthop Scand Suppl 129:6, 1970.

Hastings DE: A simple frame of operations of the lumbar spine, Can J Surg 12:251, 1969.

Healy KM: Does preoperative instruction make a difference? Am J Nurs 68:62, 1968.

Hirsch C: Reflections on the use of surgery in lumbar disc disease, Orthop Clin 2:493, 1971.

Hitselberger WE and Witten RM: Abnormal myelograms in asymptomatic patients, J Neurosurg 28:204, 1968.

Hodge CJ, Binet EF, and Kieffer SA: Intradural herniation of lumbar intervertebral discs, Spine 3:346, 1978.

Holmes HE and Rothman RH: The Pennsylvania plan: an algorithm for the management of lumbar degenerative disc disease, Spine 4:156, 1979.

Hurme M, Torma AT, and Einola S: Operated lumbar disc herniation: epidemiological aspects, Ann Chir Gynaecol 72:33, 1983.

Jacobs RR, McClain O, and Neff J: Control of postlaminectomy scar formation: an experimental and clinical study, Spine 5:223, 1980.

Jane JA, Haworth CS, Broaddus WC, et al: A neurosurgical approach to far-lateral disc herniation, J Neurosurg 72:143, 1990.

Kadish L and Simmons EH: Anomalies of the lumbosacral nerve roots and anatomical investigation and myelographic study, J Bone Joint Surg 66-B:411, 1984.

Kahanovitz N, Viola K, and Muculloch J: Limited surgical discectomy and microdiscectomy: a clinical comparison, Spine 14:79, 1989.

Kane RL, Olsen D, Leymaster C, et al: Manipulating the patient, Lancet 1:1333, 1974.

Kataoka O, Nishibayashi Y, and Sho T: Intradural lumbar disc herniation: report of three cases with a review of the literature, Spine 14:529, 1989.

Keller JT et al: The fat of autogenous grafts to the spinal dura, J Neurosurg 49:412, 1978.

Kelley JH, Voris DC, Svien HJ, and Ghormley RK: Multiple operations for protruded lumbar intervertebral disk, Mayo Clin Proc 29:546, 1954.

Key JA: Intervertebral-disk lesions in children and adolescents, J Bone Joint Surg 32-A:97, 1950.

Kieffer SA, Sherry RG, Wellenstein DE, and King RB: Bulging lumbar intervertebral disk: myelographic differentiation from herniated disk with nerve root compression, AJR 138:709, 1982.

Kikuchi S, Hasue M, Nishiyama K, et al: Anatomic and clinical studies of radicular symptoms, Spine 9:23, 1984.

Kirkaldy-Willis WH and Hill RJ: A more precise diagnosis for low-back pain, Spine 4:102, 1979.

Kiviluoto O: Use of free fat transplants to prevent epidural scar formation: an experimental study, Acta Orthop Scand Suppl 164:1, 1976.

Kostuik JP et al: Cauda equina syndrome and lumbar disc hernia, J Bone Joint Surg 68-A:386, 1986.

LaRocca H and Macnab I: The laminectomy membrane: studies in its evolution, characteristics, effects and prophylaxis in dogs, J Bone Joint Surg 56-B:545, 1974.

Leavitt F, Garron DC, Whisler WW, and D'Angelo CM: A comparison of patients treated by chymopapain and laminectomy for low back pain using a multidimensional pain scale, Clin Orthop 146:136, 1980.

Leong JCY et al: Long-term results of lumbar intervertebral disc prolapse, Spine 8:793, 1983.

Lewis PJ, Weir BKA, Broad RW, and Grace MG: Long-term prospective study of lumbosacral discectomy, J Neurosurg 67:49, 1987.

Lidstrom A and Zachrisson M: Physical therapy on low back pain and sciatica, Scand J Rehab Med 2:37, 1970.

Lindholm TS and Pylkkanen P: Discitis following removal of intervertebral disc, Spine 7:618, 1982.

Macnab I: Management of low back pain. In Ahstrom JP Jr, editor: Current practice in orthopaedic surgery, St Louis, 1973, Mosby–Year Book, Inc.

Macnab I, Cuthbert H, and Godfrey CM: The incidence of denervation of the sacrospinales muscles following spinal surgery, Spine 2:294, 1977.

Macon JB and Poletti CE: Conducted somatosensory evoked potentials during spinal surgery. I. Control, conduction velocity measurements, J Neurosurg 57:349, 1982.

Macon JB, Poletti CE, Sweet WH, et al: Conducted somatosensory evoked potentials during spinal surgery. II. Clinical applications, J Neurosurg 57:354, 1982.

Maroon JC, Kopitnik TA, Schulhoff LA, et al: Diagnosis and microsurgical approach to far-lateral disc herniation in the lumbar spine, J Neurosurg 72:378, 1990.

Martins AN, Ramirez A, Johnston J, and Schwetschenau PR: Double-blind evaluation of chemonucleolysis for herniated lumbar discs: late results, J Neurosurg 49:816, 1978.

Moll JMH and Wright V: Normal range of spinal mobility: an objective clinical study, Ann Rheum Dis 30:381, 1971.

Mullen JB and Cook WA Jr: Reduction of postoperative lumbar hemilaminectomy pain with marcaine, J Neurosurg 51:126, 1975.

Nachemson A: Physiotherapy for low back pain patients: a critical look, Scand J Rehab Med 1:85, 1969.

Nachemson A and Lindh M: Measurement of abdominal and back muscle strength with and without low back pain, Scand J Rehab Med 1:60, 1969.

Nachemson AL: Prevention of chronic back pain: the orthopaedic challenge for the 80's, Bull Hosp Jt Dis Orthop Inst 44:1, 1984.

Nachlas IW: End-result study of the treatment of herniated nucleus pulposus by excision with fusion and without fusion, J Bone Joint Surg 34-A:981, 1952.

Nafziger HC, Inman V, and Saunders JB: Lesions of the intervertebral disc and ligamenta flava, J Surg Gynecol Obstet 66:288, 1938.

Nakano N and Tomita T: Results of surgical treatment of low back pain: a comparative study of the anterior and posterior approach, Int Orthop (SICOT) 4:101, 1980.

Neidre A and Macnab I: Anomalies of the lumbosacral nerve roots, Spine 8:294, 1983.

Nielsen B, deNully M, Schmidt K, and Hansen RI: A urodynamic study of cauda equina syndrome due to lumbar disc herniation, Urol Int 35:167, 1980.

Nordby EJ and Lucas GL: A comparative analysis of lumbar disk disease treated by laminectomy or chemonucleolysis, Clin Orthop 90:119, 1973.

Pásztor E and Szarvas I: Herniation of the upper lumbar discs, Neurosurg Rev 4:151, 1981.

Pau A, Viale ES, Turtas S, and Zirattu G: Redundant nerve roots of the cauda equina, Ital J Orthop Traumatol 4:95, 1984.

Pheasant HC: Sources of failure in laminectomies, Orthop Clin North Am 6:319, 1975.

Pheasant HC, Bursk A, Goldfarb J, et al: Amitriptyline and chronic low-back pain: a randomized double-blind crossover study, Spine 8:552, 1983.

Posner I, White AA III, Edwards WT, and Hayes WC: A biomechanical analysis of the clinical stability of the lumbar and lumbosacral spine, Spine 7:374, 1982.

Postacchini F and Monttanaro A: Extreme lateral herniations of lumbar disks, Clin Orthop 138:222, 1979.

Postacchini F, Urso S, and Ferro L: Lumbosacral nerve-root anomalies, J Bone Joint Surg 64-A:721, 1982.

Rechtine GR, Reinert CM, and Bohlman HH: The use of epidural morphine to decrease postoperative pain in patients undergoing lumbar laminectomy, J Bone Joint Surg 66-A:1, 1984.

Rish BL: A critique of the surgical management of lumbar disc disease in a private neurosurgical practice, Spine 9:500, 1984.

Rosen J: Lumbar intervertebral disc surgery: review of 300 cases, Can Med Assoc J 101:317, 1969.

Rothman RH: The clinical syndrome of lumbar disc disease, Orthop Clin North Am 2:463, 1971.

Ruggieri F, Specchia L, Sabalat S, et al: Lumbar disc herniation: diagnosis, surgical treatment, and recurrence. A review of 872 operated cases, Ital J Orthop Traumatol 14:15, 1988.

Semmes RE: Diagnosis of ruptured intervertebral discs without contrast myelography and comment upon recent experience with modified hemilaminectomy for their removal, Yale J Biol Med 11:433, 1939.

Shinners BM and Hamby WB: The results of surgical removal of protruded laminar intervertebral discs, J Neurosurg 1:117, 1944.

Silvers HR: Microsurgical versus standard lumbar discectomy, Neurosurgery 22:837, 1988.

Simeone FA: The neurosurgical approach to lumbar disc disease, Orthop Clin 2:499, 1971.

Sitken AP and Bradford CH: End results of ruptured intervertebral discs in industry, Am J Surg 73:365, 1947.

Smith RV: Intradural disc rupture: report of two cases, J Neurosurg 55:117, 1981.

Solgaard T and Kleppe H: Long-term results of lumbar intervertebral disc prolapse, Spine 8:793, 1983.

Solheim LF, Siewers P, and Paus B: The piriformis muscle syndrome: sciatic nerve entrapment treated with section of the piriformis muscle, Acta Orthop Scand 52:73, 1981.

Spangfort EV: The lumbar disc herniation: a computer-aided analysis of 2,504 operations, Acta Orthop Scand 142(Suppl):1, 1972.

Spencer DL, Irwin GS, and Miller JA: Anatomy and significance of fixation of the lumbosacral nerve roots in sciatica, Spine 8:672, 1983.

Spengler DM: Lumbar discectomy: results with limited disc excision and selective foraminotomy, Spine 7:604, 1982.

Spengler DM and Freeman CW: Patient selection for lumbar discectomy: an objective approach, Spine 4:129, 1979.

Spurling RG and Grantham EG: The end-results of surgery for ruptured lumbar intervertebral disks, J Neurosurg 6:57, 1949.

Techakapuch S and Bangkok T: Rupture of the lumbar cartilage plate into the spinal canal in an adolescent, J Bone Joint Surg 63-A:481, 1981.

Vaughan PA, Malcolm BW, and Maistrelli GL: Results of L4-L5 disc excision alone versus disc excision and fusion, Spine 13:690, 1988.

Waddell G, Main CJ, Morris EW, et al: Chronic low-back pain, psychologic distress, and illness behavior, Spine 9:209, 1984.

Waddell G, Reilly S, Torsney B, et al: Assessment of the outcome of low back surgery, J Bone Joint Surg 70-B:723, 1988.

Wayne SJ: A modification of the tuck position for lumbar spine surgery: a 15-year follow-up study, Clin Orthop 184:212, 1984.

Weber H: Lumbar disc herniation: a controlled, prospective study with ten years of observation, Spine 8:131, 1983.

Weinstein J, Spratt KF, Lehmann T, et al: Lumbar disc herniation: a comparison of the results of chemonucleolysis and open discectomy after ten years, J Bone Joint Surg 68-A:43, 1986.

Weinstein JN, Scafuri RL, and McNeill TW: The Rush-Presbyterian-St. Luke's lumbar spine analysis form: a prospective study of patients with "spinal stenosis," Spine 8:891, 1983.

Weir BKA: Prospective study of 100 lumbosacral discectomies, J Neurosurg 50:283, 1979.

Weise MD, Garfin SR, Gelberman RH, et al: Lower-extremity sensibility testing in patients with herniated lumbar intervertebral discs, J Bone Joint Surg 67-A:1219, 1985.

Wilberger JE Jr and Pang D: Syndrome of the incidental herniated lumbar disc, J Neurosurg 59:137, 1983.

Wilkinson HA, Baker S, and Rosenfeld S: Gelfoam paste in experimental laminectomy and cranial trephination: hemostasis and bone healing, J Neurosurg 54:664, 1981.

Williams RW: Microlumbar discectomy: a conservative surgical approach to the virgin herniated lumbar disc, Spine 3:175, 1978.

Williams RW: Microcervical foraminotomy: a surgical alternative for intractable radicular pain, Spine 8:708, 1983.

Wiltberger BR: Surgical treatment of degenerative disease of the back, J Bone Joint Surg 45-A:1509, 1963.

Yong-Hing K, Reilly J, de Korompay V, and Kirkaldy-Willis WH: Prevention of nerve root adhesions after laminectomy, Spine 5(1):59, 1980.

Zamani MH and MacEwen GD: Herniation of the lumbar disc in children and adolescents, J Pediatr Orthop 2:528, 1982.

Chemonucleolysis

Agre K, Wilson RR, Brim M, and McDermott DJ: Chymodiactin postmarketing surveillance: demographic and adverse experience data in 29,075 patients, Spine 9:479, 1984.

Alexander AH: Debate: resolved — chemonucleolysis is the best treatment of the recalcitrant acute herniated nucleus pulposus. What's new and what's true in the Napa Valley, presented March 14, 1985.

Apfelbach HW: Technique for chemonucleolysis, Orthopedics 6:1613, 1983.

Barach EM, Nowak RM, Lee TG, and Tomlanovich MC: Epinephrine for treatment of anaphylactic shock, JAMA 251:2118, 1984.

Battit GE: Anaphylaxis associated with chymopapain injections, JAMA 253:977, 1985.

Benoist M et al: Treatment of lumbar disc herniation by chymopapain chemonucleolysis: a report on 120 patients, Spine 7:613, 1982.

Bernstein IL: Adverse effects of chemonucleolysis, JAMA 250:1167, 1983.

Boumphrey FRS, Bell GR, Modic M, et al: Computed tomography scanning after chymopapain injection for herniated nucleus pulposus: a prospective study, Clin Orthop 219:120, 1987.

Bradford DS, Cooper KM, and Oegema TR, Jr: Chymopapain, chemonucleolysis, and nucleus pulposus regeneration, J Bone Joint Surg 65-A:1220, 1983.

Brown MD and Tompkins JS: Pain response post-chemonucleolysis or disc excision, Spine 14:321, 1989.

Burkus JS, Alexander AH, and Mitchell JB: Evaluation and treatment of chemonucleolysis failures, Orthopaedics 11:1677, 1988.

Carruthers CC and Kousaie KN: Surgical treatment after chemonucleolysis failure, Clin Orthop 165:172, 1982.

Crawshaw C, Frazer AM, Merriam WF, et al: A comparison of surgery and chemonucleolysis in the treatment of sciatica: a prospective randomized trial, Spine 9:195, 1984.

Dolan P, Adams MA, and Hutton WC: The short-term effects of chymopapain on intervertebral discs, J Bone Joint Surg 69-B:422, 1987.

Eguro H: Transverse myelitis following chemonucleolysis: report of a case, J Bone Joint Surg 65-A:1328, 1983.

Fraser RD: Chymopapain for the treatment of intervertebral disc herniation: a preliminary report of a double-blind study, Spine 7:608, 1982.

Fraser RD: Chymopapain for the treatment of intervertebral disc herniation: the final report of a double-blind study, Spine 9:815, 1984.

Grammer LC, Ricketti AJ, Schafer MF, and Patterson R: Chymopapain allergy: case reports and identification of patients at risk for chymopapain anaphylaxis, Clin Orthop 188:139, 1984.

Hall BB and McCulloch JA: Anaphylactic reactions following the intradiscal injection of chymopapain under local anesthesia, J Bone Joint Surg 65-A:1215, 1983.

Hill GM and Ellis EA: Chemonucleolysis as an alternative to laminectomy for the herniated lumbar disc, Clin Orthop 225:229, 1987.

Leavitt F, Garron DC, Whisler WW, and D'Angelo CM: A comparison of patients treated by chymopapain and laminectomy for low back pain using a multidimensional pain scale, Clin Orthop 146:136, 1980.

Maciunas RJ and Onofrio BM: The long-term results of chymopapain: ten-year follow-up of 268 patients after chemonucleolysis, Clin Orthop 206:37, 1986.

Martins AN, Ramirez A, Johnston J, and Schwetschenau PR: Double-blind evaluation of chemonucleolysis for herniated lumbar discs: late results, J Neurosurg 49:816, 1978.

McCulloch JA: Chemonucleolysis: experience with 2000 cases, Clin Orthop 146:128, 1980.

McCulloch JA: Outpatient discolysis with chymopapain, Orthopedics 6:1624, 1983.

McCulloch JA and Ferguson JM: Outpatient chemonucleolysis, Spine 6:606, 1981.

Nachemson AL and Rydevik B: Chemonucleolysis for sciatica: a critical review, Acta Orthop Scand 59:56, 1988.

Naylor A, Earland C, and Robinson J: The effect of diagnostic radiopaque fluids used in discography on chymopapain activity, Spine 8:875, 1983.

Nordby EJ: Current concepts review: chymopapain in intradiscal therapy, J Bone Joint Surg 65-A:1350, 1983.

Nordby EJ and Lucas GL: A comparative analysis of lumbar disk disease treated by laminectomy or chemonucleolysis, Clin Orthop 90:119, 1973.

Parkinson D: Late results of treatment of intervertebral disc disease with chymopapain, J Neurosurg 59:990, 1983.

Schoendinger GR III and Ford LT Jr: The use of chymopapain in ruptured lumbar discs, South Med J 64:333, 1971.

Shields CB, Reiss SJ, and Garretson HD: Chemonucleolysis with chymopapain: results in 150 patients, J Neurosurg 67:187, 1987.

Simmons JW, Stavinoha WB, and Knodel LC: Update and review of chemonucleolysis, Clin Orthop 183:51, 1984.

Smith S, Leibrock LG, Gelber BR, and Pierson EW: Acute herniated nucleus pulposus with cauda equina compression syndrome following chemonucleolysis: report of three cases, J Neurosurg 66:614, 1987.

Suguro T, Oegema TR, and Bradford DS: Ultrastructural study of the short-term effects of chymopapain on the intervertebral disc, J Orthop Res 4:281, 1986.

Tsay Y-G et al: A preoperative chymopapain sensitivity test for chemonucleolysis candidates, Spine 9:764, 1984.

Wakano K, Kasman R, Chao EY, et al: Biomechanical analysis of canine intervertebral discs after chymopapain injection: a preliminary report, Spine 8:59, 1983.

Weinstein J, Spratt KF, Lehmann T, et al: Lumbar disc herniation: a comparison of the results of chemonucleolysis and open discectomy after ten years, J Bone Joint Surg 68-A:43, 1986.

Weitz EM: Paraplegia following chymopapain injection: a case report, J Bone Joint Surg 66-A:1131, 1984.

Whisler WW: Anaphylaxis secondary to chymopapain, Orthopedics 6:1628, 1983.

Willis J, editor: Chymopapain administration procedures modified, FDA Drug Bull, 14:14, 1984.

Wiltse LL, Widell EH, and Yuan HA: Chymopapain chemonucleolysis in lumbar disk disease, JAMA 231:474, 1975.

Percutaneous lumbar discectomy

Blankstein A, Rubinstein E, Ezra E, et al: Disc space infection and vertebral osteomyelitis as a complication of percutaneous lateral discectomy, Clin Orthop 225:234, 1987.

Davis GW and Onik G: Clinical experience with automated percutaneous lumbar discectomy, Clin Orthop 238:98, 1989.

Goldstein TB, Mink JH, and Dawson EG: Early experience with automated percutaneous lumbar discectomy in the treatment of lumbar disc herniation, Clin Orthop 238:77, 1989.

Graham CE: Percutaneous posterolateral lumbar discectomy: an alternative to laminectomy in the treatment of backache and sciatica, Clin Orthop 238:104, 1989.

Hijikata S: Percutaneous nucleotomy: a new concept of technique and 12 years' experience, Clin Orthop 238:9, 1989.

Hijikata S, Yamagishi M, Nakayama T, and Oomori K: Percutaneous nuclectomy: a new treatment method for lumbar disc herniation, J Toden Hosp 5:39, 1975.

Kahanovitz N, Viola K, and McCullough J: Limited surgical diskectomy and microdiskectomy: a clinical comparison, Spine 14:79, 1989.

Kahanovitz N, Viola K, Goldstein T, and Dawson E: A multicenter analysis of percutaneous diskectomy, Spine 15:713, 1990.

Kambin P and Brager MD: Percutaneous posterolateral discectomy: anatomy and mechanism, Clin Orthop 223:145, 1987.

Kambin P and Gellman H: Percutaneous lateral discectomy of the spine, Clin Orthop 174:127, 1983.

Kambin P and Schaffer JL: Percutaneous lumbar discectomy: review of 100 patients and current practice, Clin Orthop 238:24, 1989.

Maroon JC, Onik G, and Sternau L: Percutaneous automated discectomy: a new approach to lumbar surgery, Clin Orthop 238:64, 1989.

Monteiro A, Lefevre R, Pieters G, and Wilment E: Lateral decompression of a pathological disc in the treatment of lumbar pain and sciatica, Clin Orthop 238:56, 1989.

Morris J: Percutaneous discectomy, Orthopedics 11:1483, 1988.

Onik G, Helms CA, and Ginsburg L: Percutaneous lumbar discectomy using a new aspiration probe, Am J Radiol 144:1137, 1985.

Onik G, Maroon J, and Davis GW: Automated percutaneous discectomy at the L5-S1 level: use of a curved cannula, Clin Orthop 238:71, 1989.

Schreiber A, Suezawa Y, and Leu H: Does percutaneous nucleotomy with discoscopy replace conventional discectomy? Eight years of experience and results in treatment of herniated lumbar disc, Clin Orthop 238:35, 1989.

Schweigel J: Automated percutaneous discectomy: comparison with chymopapain. In Automated percutaneous discectomy, San Francisco, 1988, University of California Press.

Shepperd JAN, James SE, and Leach AB: Percutaneous disc surgery, Clin Orthop 238:43, 1989.

Stern MB: Early experience with percutaneous lateral discectomy, Clin Orthop 238:50, 1989.

Williams RW: Microlumbar discectomy: a conservative surgical approach to the virgin herniated lumbar disc, Spine 3:175, 1978.

Wilson D and Harbaugh R: Microsurgical and standard removal of protruded lumbar disc: a comparative study, Neurosurgery 8:422, 1986.

Complications of lumbar spine surgery

Aho AJ, Auranen A, and Pesonen K: Analysis of cauda equina symptoms in patients with lumbar disc prolapse, Acta Chir Scand 135:413, 1969.

Benoist M, Ficat C, Baraf P, and Cauchoix J: Postoperative lumbar epiduro-arachnoiditis: diagnostic and therapeutic aspects, Spine 5:432, 1980.

Bryant MS, Bremer AM, and Nguyen TQ: Autogeneic fat transplants in the epidural space in routine lumbar spine surgery, Neurosurgery 13:367, 1983.

Caplan LR, Norohna AB, and Amico LL: Syringomyelia and arachnoiditis, J Neurol Neurosurg Psychiatr 53:106, 1990.

Choudhury AR and Taylor JC: Cauda equina syndrome in lumbar disc disease, Acta Orthop Scand 51:493, 1980.

Clark K: Significance of the small lumbar spinal canal: cauda equina compression syndromes due to spondylosis. II. Clinical and surgical significance, J Neurosurg 31:495, 1969.

Di Lauro L, Poli R, Bortoluzzi M, and Marini G: Paresthesias after lumbar disc removal and their relationship to epidural hematoma, J Neurosurg 57:135, 1982.

Eismont FJ, Wiesel SW, and Rothman RH: The treatment of dural tears associated with spinal surgery, J Bone Joint Surg 63-A:1132, 1981.

El-Gindi S, Aref S, Salama M, and Andrew J: Infection of the intervertebral discs after surgery, J Bone Joint Surg 58-B:114, 1976.

Epstein BS, Epstein JA, and Lavine L: The effect of anatomic variations in the lumbar vertebrae and spinal canal on cauda equina and nerve root syndromes, Am J Roentgenol Radium Ther Nucl Med 91:105, 1964.

Floman Y, Wiesel SW, and Rothman RH: Cauda equina syndrome presenting as a herniated lumbar disc, Clin Orthop 147:234, 1980.

Harbison SP: Major vascular complications of intervertebral disc surgery, Ann Surg 140:342, 1954.

Holscher EC: Vascular complication of disc surgery, J Bone Joint Surg 30-A:968, 1948.

Javid MJ et al: Safety and efficacy of chymopapain (Chymodiactin) in herniated nucleus pulposus with sciatica: results of a randomized, double-blind study, JAMA 249:2489, 1983.

Jones AA, Stambough JL, Balderson RA, et al: Long-term results of lumbar spine surgery complicated by unintended incidental durotomy, Spine 14:443, 1989.

Keller JT et al: The fat of autogenous grafts to the spinal dura, J Neurosurg 49:412, 1978.

Kostuik JP et al: Cauda equina syndrome and lumbar disc hernia, J Bone Joint Surg 68-A:386, 1986.

May ARL, Brewster DC, Darling RC, et al: Arteriovenous fistula following lumbar disc surgery, Br J Surg 68:41, 1981.

Mayer PJ and Jacobsen FS: Cauda equina syndrome after surgical treatment of lumbar spinal stenosis with application of free autogenous fat graft: a report of two cases, J Bone Joint Surg 71-A:1090, 1989.

McLaren AC and Bailey SI: Cauda equina syndrome: a complication of lumbar discectomy, Clin Orthop 204:143, 1986.

Nielsen B, deNully M, Schmidt K, and Hansen RI: A urodynamic study of cauda equina syndrome due to lumbar disc herniation, Urol Int 35:167, 1980.

Puranen J, Makela J, and Lahde S: Postoperative intervertebral discitis, Acta Orthop Scand 55:461, 1984.

Salander JM, Youkey JR, Rich NM, et al: Vascular injury related to lumbar disc surgery, J Trauma 24:628, 1984.

Seeley SF, Hughes CW, and Jahnke EJ: Major vessel damage in lumbar disc operation, Surgery 35:421, 1954.

Shaw ED, Scarborough JT, and Beals RK: Bowel injury as a complication of lumbar discectomy: a case report and review of the literature, J Bone Joint Surg 63-A:478, 1981.

Zide BM, Wisoff JH, and Epstein FJ: Closure of extensive and complicated laminectomy wounds: operative technique, J Neurosurg 67:59, 1987.

Failed spine surgery

Aitken AP and Bradford CH: End results of ruptured intervertebral discs in industry, Am J Surg 73:365, 1947.

Blaauw G, Braakman R, Gelpke GJ, and Singh R: Changes in radicular function following low-back surgery, J Neurosurg 69:649, 1988.

Cauchoix J, Ficat C, and Girard B: Repeat surgery after disc excision, Spine 3:256, 1978.

Cauthen C: Lumbar spine surgery, Baltimore, 1983, Williams & Wilkins.

Ebeling U, Kalbarcyk H, and Reulen HJ: Microsurgical reoperation following lumbar disc surgery: timing, surgical findings, and outcome in 92 patients, J Neurosurg 70:397, 1989.

Frymoyer JW, Hanaley EN, and Howe J: A comparison of radiographic findings in fusion and nonfusion patients ten or more years following lumbar disc surgery, Spine 5:435, 1979.

Kelley JH, Voris DC, Svien HJ, and Ghormley RK: Multiple operations for protruded lumbar intervertebral disk, Mayo Clin Proc 29:546, 1954.

Long DM, Filtzer DL, BenDebba M, and Hendler NH: Clinical features of the failed-back syndrome, J Neurosurg 69:61, 1988.

Nachlas IW: End-result study of the treatment of herniated nucleus pulposus by excision with fusion and without fusion, J Bone Joint Surg 34-A:981, 1952.

Nakano N and Tomita T: Results of surgical treatment of low back pain: a comparative study of the anterior and posterior approach, Int Orthop (SICOT) 4:101, 1980.

Pheasant HC: Sources of failure in laminectomies, Orthop Clin North Am 6:319, 1975.

Quimjian JD and Matrka PJ: Decompression laminectomy and lateral spinal fusion in patients with previously failed lumbar spine surgery, Orthopaedics 2:563, 1988.

Spengler DM, Freeman C, Westbrook R, and Miller JW: Low-back pain following multiple lumbar spine procedures. Failure of initial selection? Spine 5:356, 1980.

Tria AJ, Williams JM, Harwood D, and Zawadsky JP: Laminectomy with and without spinal fusion, Clin Orthop 224:134, 1987.

CHAPTER 85

Infections of Spine

GEORGE W. WOOD II

Evidence of spinal infection in humans dates back to beyond the time of recorded history. Neolithic persons (c. 7000-300 BC) and Egyptian mummies (c. 3000 BC) have been found to have evidence of spinal deformity believed to be caused by tuberculosis. Hippocrates described the clinical condition of spinal infection and noted that the prognosis in this condition, believed to be tuberculosis, was better when the infection was below the diaphragm than when above it. In 1779 Percival Pott gave the first complete report of tuberculous infection of the spine. According to Wilensky, Nelaton coined the term *osteomyelitis* in 1854. The scientific understanding of osteomyelitis began with Rodet in 1884 when he described the development of osteomyelitis after injections of *Staphylococcus aureus* into the veins of animals. Early treatment for spinal infections was limited to abcess drainage, usually of tuberculosis infections. Unfortunately, secondary bacterial infection frequently caused death.

Before the use of antibiotics, mortality in patients with infections of the spine and contiguous tissues was 40% to 70%. Advances in chemotherapy over the past 40 years have dramatically altered the natural history of these diseases. Today spinal infections are relatively rare, accounting for only 2% to 4% of all osteomyelitis infec-

tions, and mortality is estimated to be 1% to 20%, depending on the patient group and the infecting agent. Paralysis is reported to occur in up to 50% of patients with spinal infections, depending on the patient population and the spinal segment involved. The primary problems today are the delay in diagnosis (estimated to average 3 months), the long recovery period (averaging 12 months or more), and the great cost of treating such infections.

Reconstructive surgery for spinal infection required the development of safe surgical and anesthetic techniques. In 1911 Hibbs and Albee independently developed posterior spinal fusion techniques for treating tuberculous spinal disease; these procedures decreased the degree of kyphosis and shortened the course of the disease. Both Hibbs and Albee chose the posterior approach because it avoided involvement of the area of active infection. Posterior spinal fusion remained the mainstay of treatment of spinal tuberculous infection until the advent of antibiotics. With the development of chemotherapeutic agents, surgical approaches became more aggressive in the direct treatment of both tuberculosis and apyogenic infections. Hodgson and Stock in 1956 pioneered radical anterior decompression for Pott's disease, and this procedure has been used with equal success in the treatment of other kinds of spinal infections.

BIOLOGY OF SPINAL INFECTION

A knowledge of the structure and composition of the spinal elements is essential to an understanding of spinal infections. The intervertebral disc has been identified as the most commonly infected spinal element, but more recent evidence now points to the metaphyses and cartilaginous end plates as the starting areas for blood-borne infections. The disc space is now considered the primary starting area only for infections resulting from direct inoculation.

Coventry, Ghormley, and Kernohan in 1945 described the microscopic anatomy of the intervertebral disc and its contiguous structures. They concluded that in adults older than 30 years the intervertebral disc receives its nutrition from tissue fluids rather than from direct blood supply. They noted multiple holes in the end plates of the vertebral bodies, which corresponded with the marrow cavities and were arranged in three distinct areas: (1) a central zone with numerous small holes, (2) a peripheral zone with a few large holes, and (3) an epiphyseal ring surrounding the end plate.

The epiphyseal ring overlaps the outer surface of the vertebral body and joins the more concave surface of the central and peripheral zones internally. Next to the bony end plate is the cartilaginous plate, which consists of hyaline cartilage and forms the inner base between the bone and the fibrous disc. Inoue in 1981 found that the disc was firmly adherent to the vertebral end plate: two thirds of its fibers were perpendicular to the end plate in this area. The central portion was less firmly attached, with fibers parallel to the end plate. This composition most likely allows the transport of nutrients through the holes and into the central portion of the disc without disturbing the structural integrity.

The arterial and venous supply to the vertebrae has been studied by numerous investigators for more than 100 years. In 1959 Wiley and Trueta found marked similarities in the arterial and venous supply in humans and rabbits at the cervical, thoracic, and lumbar levels. At the level of each vertebra, the vertebral artery, intercostal artery, or lumbar arteries provide nutrient vessels that enter the vertebral body (Fig. 85-1). Posterior spinal branch arteries enter the spinal canal through each neural foramen. These arteries separate into ascending and descending branches that anastomose with similar branches at each level (Fig. 85-2). This posterior network joins centrally to enter a large posterior nutrient foramen.

Whalen et al. investigated the microvasculature of the vertebral end plates in fetal cadavers and young rabbits and described vessels oriented obliquely in the cartilage toward the intervertebral disc. These vessels were found to originate from the circumferential vessels fed from the arterial plexus outside the perichondrium or from nearby metaphyseal marrow vessels. They noted that venous drainage was by a similar route. They concluded that the intervertebral disc was avascular, even in infants. In contrast, the surrounding cartilaginous material was highly vascular. They found no change in this relationship with growth unless a pathologic process was encountered (Fig. 85-3). The cartilaginous end plate, therefore, appears to be the anatomic area in which the arterial supply ends, regardless of age. The intervertebral disc is centrally avascular and dependent on diffusion for its nutrition.

The venous drainage of the pelvis and its relationship to spinal vasculature was first described by Breschet in 1819 and was later expanded by Batson in 1940 with the discovery that the pelvic veins drained into the spinal venous plexus. This explained the frequent metastasis of pelvic tumors and infections to the spine. In 1976 Crock and Yoshizawa described the microvascular circulation of the venous anatomy of the vertebral end plate.

DISC

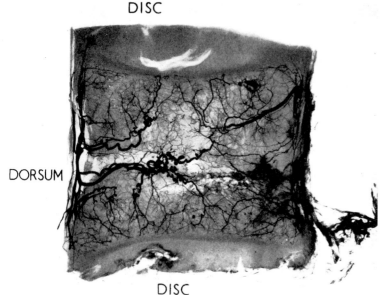

DORSUM

DISC

Fig. 85-1   Section through vertebral body after arterial injection. Nutrient vessels are visible on dorsal and ventral surfaces. (From Wiley AM and Trueta J: J Bone Joint Surg 41-B:796, 1959.)

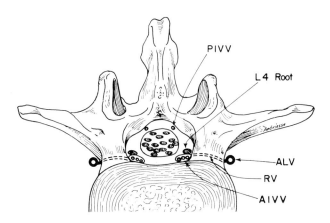

Fig. 85-2 Diagram of transverse section of lumbar vertebra. Anterior and internal vertebral arteries and veins are noted in canal. *PIVV,* posterior internal vertebral vein; *ALV,* ascending lumbar vein; *RV,* radicular vein; *AIVV,* anterior internal vertebral vein. (From Macnab I, St Louis EL, Grabias SL, and Jacob R: J Bone Joint Surg 58-A:1093, 1976.)

The venous microcirculation begins in the vertebral end plate where the arterial circulation ends. Attached to these are the large subvenous or venous channels oriented horizontally and parallel to the end plate. The horizontal system then drains through small vertical veins perforating the end plate and connecting with horizontal vessels in the cancellous bone adjacent to the end plate. Additional vertical veins drain to the basivertebral system and converge to form the anterior internal venous plexus as one or two major tributaries. These plexuses then drain externally into the external venous plexus. Externally these vessels join with the anterior internal vertebral, posterior internal vertebral, and posterior radicular veins. The internal vertebral veins course dorsal to the dural sac near the lamina. The anterior internal veins lie in the lateral aspect of the floor of the spinal canal bilaterally; these veins are sacrificed during disc excision. As the internal veins approach the midpoint of the body of the vertebra, they move centrally to drain the interosseous system through the nutrient foramen. The anterior internal veins also drain the articular vessels that course along the roots, joining the ascending lumbar veins outside the spinal canal. The series of interconnected veins continues from sacrum to skull (Figs. 85-2 and 85-4).

Spinal infection can occur by direct infection of the disc itself, usually through surgical manipulation directly or percutaneously, or by local spread from contiguous structures. Contiguous spread has been reported to occur from the colon via subphrenic abscesses and also from abdominal abscess extension from gunshot wounds without direct spinal injury. The most common method of spinal infection is through the arterial spread of pyogenic bacteria. This arterially spread infection originates in the end plate of the vertebra, probably in the venous channels, or in the vertebral body itself and spreads to the disc secondarily as the infection progresses.

On the other hand, because tuberculous spinal infection has only been reproduced by injecting the renal vein experimentally (Hodgson), it is believed that tuberculous infection results from venous spread, usually at the level of the renal veins. This is substantiated by the frequency of infection in tuberculous disease (Fig. 85-5). A similar frequency has not been noted with bacterial infection. Bacterial infections rapidly attack the intervertebral disc. Tuberculous and nonbacterial infections, on the other

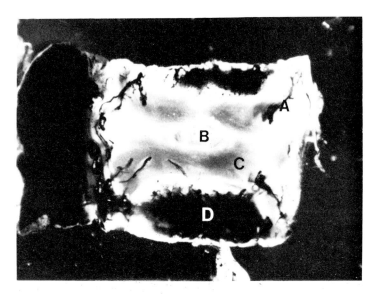

Fig. 85-3 Sagittal section of human fetal vertebra and intervertebral disc after arterial injection. Note oblique orientation of vessels to disc and absence of vessels penetrating disc. *A,* Neural canal; *B,* nucleus pulposus; *C,* hyaline cartilage end plate; *D,* ossified vertebral body. (From Whalen JL, Parke WW, Mazur JM, and Stauffer ES: J Pediatr Orthop 5:403, 1985.)

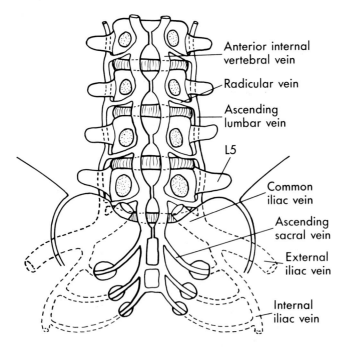

Fig. 85-4 Schematic diagram of vertebral venous system. (Modified from Macnab I, St Louis EL, Grabias SL, and Jacob R: J Bone Joint Surg 58-A:1093, 1976.)

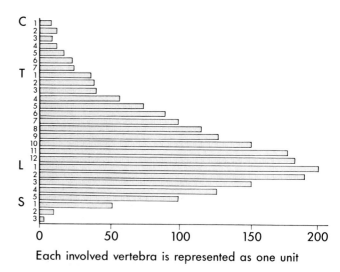

Each involved vertebra is represented as one unit

Fig. 85-5 Bar graph of 587 consecutive cases of spinal tuberculosis occurring in series of 1000 consecutive cases of bone and joint tuberculosis. (From Hodgson AR. In Rothman RH and Simeone FA, editors: The spine, Philadelphia, 1975, WB Saunders Co.)

NATURAL HISTORY

The natural history of pyogenic vertebral infections involves an infecting source or incident followed by a period of increased pain, with or without significant generalized sepsis. Generalized sepsis usually indicates a primary source of infection other than the spine. Blood-borne infection probably begins in the capillary loop or postcapillary venous channels in the end plate. Sludging in these channels results in suppurative inflammation, tissue necrosis, bony collapse, and spread of the infection into the adjacent intravertebral disc spaces. This eventually results in the end plate erosions that are the first roentgenographic findings. The infection can extend anteriorly to create a paravertebral abscess or posteriorly to cause an epidural abscess. Large paravertebral abscesses may extend down the psoas and into the groin. Likewise, epidural abscesses may cross the spinal epidural space and enter the meningeal space and spinal cord itself, although this occurs late in the course of pyogenic infections and rarely occludes the spinal arteries (Feldenzer et al.). As the bone becomes infected it softens and may collapse under the body weight and stress. Neurologic deficits appear as a result of (1) direct extension of the infection, in the form of abscess or bacterial communication with the spinal canal to the neural elements, or (2) by secondary compression from pathologic fracture

as a result of bone softening (Fig. 85-6). This progression of spinal infection is possible in both pyogenic and nonpyogenic infections. The course of the infection varies with the infecting organism and the patient's immune status. The infection itself may create a malnourished condition that compromises the immune system (Nichols). According to Waldvogel and Vasey, death occurs in 10% of patients with overwhelming spinal infections.

Individuals with a good immune response may actually overcome the infection with no treatment. This has been proven experimentally by Fraser, Osti, and Vernon-Roberts. They injected *Staphylococcus epidermidis* into sheep discs and noted that 6 weeks later only those discs injected with bacteria showed evidence of discitis; however, bacteria could not be cultured from those discs. This finding indicates that there is an optimum period for bacteriologic identification of disc space infections in otherwise healthy individuals. It also explains the widely varying clinical presentations of spinal infection and further compounds the difficulty of making an accurate and timely bacteriologic diagnosis.

Paralysis from spinal infection may occur early or late. Early onset of paralysis frequently suggests epidural extension of an abscess. Late paralysis may be caused by the development of significant kyphosis, vertebral collapse with retropulsion of bone and debris, or late abscess formation in more indolent infections. Eismont et al. identified four factors that indicate an increased predisposition to paralysis in pyogenic and fungal vertebral osteomyelitis. They noted that the incidence of paralysis increased with (1) age, (2) a higher vertebral level of infection (cervical), (3) the presence of debilitating disease

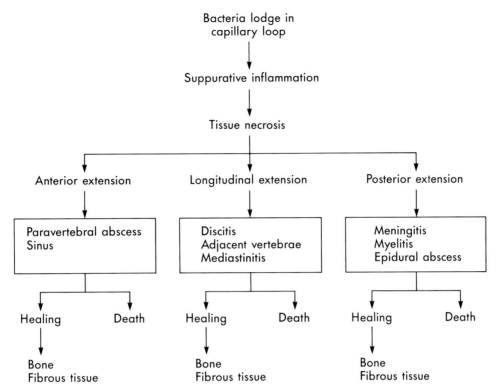

Fig. 85-6 Flow diagram of natural history of vertebral infection. (From Wood GW II. In Wood GW II, editor: State of the art and review, spine: spinal infections, vol 3, no 3, Philadelphia, 1989, Hanley & Belfus, Inc.)

such as diabetes mellitus, rheumatoid arthritis, or chronic steroid usage, and (4) *Staphylococcus aureus* infections. Paralysis from tuberculosis is not related to those factors.

EPIDEMIOLOGY

The vertebral end plate is the most commonly reported focus of vertebral infection, followed by inoculation of the disc space itself, epidural abscess formation, and paraspinal abscess formation. Other spinal elements, including the articular processes, facet joints, and even the odontoid, also have been reported as primary areas of infection, but generally these are isolated case reports. According to Waldvogel and Vasey, the thoracic and lumbar spinal vertebrae are the most common areas of pyogenic infection, and, according to Hodgson et al., the thoracolumbar junction is the most common area of tuberculous infection.

Numerous organisms have been reported to infect the spine (Table 85-1). Waldvogel and Vasey noted that *S. aureus* was the most common organism in pyogenic infection: this organism, and to a lesser degree *Staphylococcus epidermidis,* accounted for 60% of the infections in their review. The incidence of isolation of *S. aureus* varies from 40% to 90%. The present trend is a decrease in the frequency of *S. aureus* infections but an increase in the resistant strains of the organism. More recent reports indicate that over half of the isolates of the organism are resistant to penicillin and over one third of that group are resistant to methicillin. Roca and Yoshikawa reported that intravenous drug users are more commonly infected with *Pseudomonas aeruginosa. Mycobacterium tuberculosis* is the most common nonpyogenic infecting agent.

Spinal surgery is the most common cause of iatrogenic disc infection, whereas genitourinary infection is the most common predisposing factor for blood-borne infection. Respiratory and dermal infections are less frequently implicated in blood-borne infection. Postabortal and postpartum infections also have been reported to cause spinal infections. According to Eismont et al., patients with chronic diseases that decrease the natural immune response, such as diabetes, alcoholism, rheumatoid arthritis, and chronic renal disease, are more likely to develop a spinal infection and its complications.

The incidence of tuberculous spondylitis has been progressively declining since the advent of antituberculous medication but still accounts for more than one third of bone and joint infections (Table 85-2). Collert noted a marked decrease in tuberculous spondylitis since 1950, compared to a modest increase in pyogenic spondylitis. Other nonpyogenic infections are rare in healthy individuals but are much more common in immunocompromised patients.

Table 85-1 Infecting organisms in spinal osteomyelitis

Actinomyces	*Salmonella enteritidis*
Aerobacter aerogenes	*Salmonella oranienburg*
Bacteroides	*Salmonella panama*
Brucella	*Salmonella paratyphi A* and *B*
Corynebacterium	*Salmonella suipestifer*
Clostridium perfringens	*Salmonella typhimurium*
Enterobacter aerogenes	*Salmonella typhosa*
Escherichia coli	*Serratia marcescens*
Gonococcus	*Staphylococcus aureus*
Klebsiella	*Staphylococcus alba*
Micrococcus	*Staphylococcus epidermidis*
Proteus	*Streptococcus* (microaerophilic)
Pseudomonas	*Streptococcus* (alpha)
Pyocyaneus	

From Wood GW III, Edmonson AS: Osteomyelitis of the spine. In Wood GW III, editor: State of the art and review, spine: spinal infections, vol, 3, no 3, Philadelphia, 1989, Hanley and Belfus, Inc., p 461.

DIAGNOSIS

Physical Examination

The most common presenting symptom of spinal infection is pain. Ross and Fleming reported pain as the primary symptom in 85% of their patients with spinal infections. Pain occurs primarily with changes in position, ambulation, and other forms of activity. The intensity of the pain varies from mild to extreme. Constitutional symptoms include anorexia, malaise, night sweats, intermittent fever, and weight loss. Spinal deformity may be a late presentation of the disease. Paralysis is a serious complication but rarely is the presenting complaint. A history of an immune-suppressing disease and or a recent infection is not uncommon. Puig-Guri described four clinical syndromes that may be caused by the infection: (1) hip joint syndrome, with acute pain in the hip, flexion contracture, and limited motion; (2) abdominal syndrome, with symptoms and signs that may suggest acute appendicitis; (3) meningeal syndrome, with symptoms and signs that suggest acute suppurative or tuberculous meningitis; and (4) back pain syndrome, in which the onset of pain may be acute or insidious; pain may be mild or may be so severe that jarring the bed is agonizing.

Temperature elevation, if present, usually is minimal. Localized tenderness over the involved area is the most common physical sign. Sustained paraspinal spasm also is indicative of the acute process. Limitation of motion of the involved spinal segments because of pain is frequent. Torticollis may result from infection in the cervical spine, and bizarre posturing and physical positions that could be considered psychogenic in origin are not infrequent. Other possible findings include Kernig's sign, hamstring spasm, and generalized weakness. Clinical findings in elderly and immune-suppressed individuals may be minimal.

Table 85-2 Sites of tuberculous involvement of bones and joints in 99 cases,* British Columbia, 1967 through 1976

Site	No. of cases†	Site	No. of cases†
Joint	59	Spine	37
Wrist	8	C4-5	1
Elbow	7	C5-6	3
Shoulder	5	C6-7	1
Costosternal	1	T5-6	1
Sternoclavicular	1	T6-7	2
Sacroiliac	4	T7-8	2
Hip	16	T8-9	4
Knee	12	T9-10	3
Ankle	2	T10-11	5
Foot	3	T11-12	4
Bone (osteomyelitis)	9	T12-L1	3
Finger	1	L1-2	6
Sternum	1	L2-3	8
Rib	1	L3-4	8
Pelvis	4	L4-5	5
Fibula	1	L5-S1	6
Calcaneus	1	Unknown	2

From Enarson DA et al: Can Med Assoc J 120:139, 1979, with permission.
*In six cases there was tuberculous disease at two sites.
†The numbers in the left-hand column indicate the frequency of involvement of an individual site; the numbers to the right are the total number of cases.

Because of the depth of the spine, abscess formation is difficult to identify unless it points superficially. Frequently these areas of abscess pointing are some distance from the primary process. A paraspinal abscess not uncommonly presents as a swelling in the groin below Poupart's ligament (inguinal ligament) because of extension along the psoas muscle. Straight leg raising examination usually is not helpful because it may be negative or may elicit back or rarely leg pain. Neurologic findings are rarely radicular in nature and more frequently involve multiple nerve groups. Eismont et al. noted central cord syndrome in two thirds of patients with paralysis from cord compression, and anterior cord syndrome was found in one third. As might be expected, neurologic symptoms become more frequent at higher spinal levels; neurologic symptoms are most frequent with infections in the cervical and thoracic areas and are least common with infections in the thoracolumbar region.

Differentiation between pyogenic and caseating infections by physical examination is extremely difficult. The patient's history may suggest the etiologic factor. The development of neurologic signs should suggest the possibility of neural compression from abscess formation, bone collapse, or direct neural infection. Neurologic symptoms from arterial thrombosis are rare (Feldenzer et al.). In our experience, once neurologic symptoms appear they progress rapidly unless active decompression or drainage is undertaken.

Diagnostic Techniques

The purpose of diagnostic techniques is confirmation of the clinical impression. In spinal infection, no one diagnostic technique is 100% effective as a confirmatory test. Culture of the organism from the infected tissue is the most definitive test, but even under the most optimal conditions results may be negative. Likewise, all imaging and laboratory studies may be inconclusive, depending on the time at which they are done relative to the onset of infection.

ROENTGENOGRAMS. Plain roentgenograms of the involved area are the most common initial study in patients with spinal infection. According to Waldvogel and Vasey, roentgenographic findings appear from 2 weeks to 3 months after the onset of the infection. Roentgenographic findings include disc space narrowing, vertebral end plate irregularity or loss of the normal contour of the end plate, defects in the subchondral portion of the end plate, and hypertrophic (sclerotic) bone formation (Fig. 85-7). Occasionally, paravertebral soft tissue masses may be noted with involvement of nearby areas of the spine. Late roentgenographic findings may include vertebral collapse, segmental kyphosis, and finally bony ankylosis. The sequence of events may range from 2 to 8 weeks for early findings to more than 2 years for later findings. The only definable abnormality on plain roentgenograms and computed tomographic scans related specifically to tuberculosis is fine calcification in the paravertebral soft tissue space.

COMPUTED TOMOGRAPHY. Computed tomography (CT) adds another dimension to the plain roentgenograms. CT identifies paravertebral soft tissue swelling and abscesses much more readily and also can monitor changes in the size of the spinal canal. Some clinicians prefer CT to roentgenography for determining clinical progress. Findings with CT scanning are similar to those with plain roentgenograms, including lytic defects in the subchondral bone, destruction of the end plate with irregularity or multiple holes visible in the cross-sectional views, sclerosis near the lytic irregularities, hypodensity of the disc, flattening of the disc itself, disruption of the circumferential bone near the periphery of the disc, and soft tissue density in the epidural and paraspinal regions. Postmyelogram CT more clearly defines compression of the neural elements by abscess or bone impingement and helps determine whether the infection extends to the neural structures themselves.

MAGNETIC RESONANCE IMAGING. High-quality magnetic resonance imaging (MRI) is an accurate and rapid method for identifying spinal infection. It identifies infected and normal tissues and probably best determines the full extent of the infection. Unfortunately, MRI does

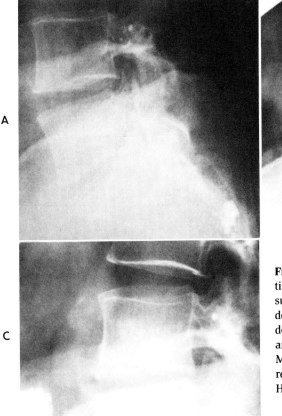

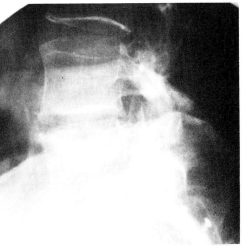

A

B

C

Fig. 85-7 Roentgenographic appearance of spinal osteomyelitis. **A,** Minimal disc space narrowing, but normal end plate and subchondral region. **B,** Reduction of disc height associated with destruction of end plate and development of subchondral lytic defects. **C,** After successful treatment, note sclerotic vertebra and large osteophyte. (From Acker JD, Wood GW II, Moinuddin M, and Eggers FM. In Wood GW II, editor: State of the art and review, spine: spinal infections, vol 3, no 3, Philadelphia, 1989, Hanley & Belfus, Inc.)

not differentiate between pyogenic and nonpyogenic infections and cannot eliminate the need for diagnostic biopsy. Modic, Masaryk, and Plaushtek noted an MRI sensitivity of 96%, a specificity of 92%, and an accuracy of 94% in 37 patients with disc space infections. To detect infection, both T1-intermediate and T2-weighted views in the sagittal plane should be obtained. Modic et al. described MRI findings in patients with vertebral osteomyelitis and noted that the T1-weighted images have a decreased signal intensity in the vertebral bodies and disc spaces. The margin between the disc and the adjacent vertebral body cannot be differentiated. In T2-weighted images, the signal intensity is increased in the vertebral disc and is markedly decreased in the vertebral body. Abscesses in the paravertebral soft tissue about the thecal sac can be readily identified as areas of increased uptake. Frequently, the delineation of infection in the paravertebral tissues with extension to the thecal tissues eliminates the need for additional myelography.

The addition of gadolinium-labeled diethylenetriamine pentacetic acid (Gd-DTPA) is being investigated for various pathologic processes, but it appears to enhance the delineation of epidural abscesses and to further delineate the extent of spinal infection. Our experience has been that this delineation is confined more to involvement of infected soft tissues than to the identification of true liquified abscess cavities. It is unclear at this time whether the added time, risk, and expense of this additional step yield significantly more information. This contrast material may be useful in older or questionable infections.

Although MRI appears to be the best test for delineating spinal infection, it does have some significant drawbacks. The most important is degradation from motion. Motion artifact is frequent in patients with spinal infections because pain makes it difficult for them to remain still in the supine position for long periods. Additionally, they must lie in an enclosed container, and claustrophobia is a frequent problem. Finally, many of these patients are elderly, and if they have a pacemaker, MRI is contraindicated. The small calcifications seen in the paravertebral abscesses of tuberculosis, which make it so characteristic on plain roentgenograms, are not identifiable with MRI.

RADIONUCLIDE SCANNING. Radionuclide studies are relatively effective in identifying spinal infection. These techniques include technetium 99 (Tc-99m) bone scan, gallium 67 (Ga-67) scan, and indium 111–labeled leukocyte (In-111 WBC scan). The technetium bone scan has three basic phases: angiogram, blood pool images, and delayed static images. In infection, diffuse activity is seen on the blood pool images; the diffuse activity becomes focal on delayed views. This marked reactivity may persist for months. Bone scans are almost always positive in patients with infection, but they are not specifically diagnostic of infection. The gallium 67 scan is a good adjunct to bone scanning for the detection of osteo-

myelitis. Modic et al. reported a sensitivity of 90%, specificity of 100%, and accuracy of 94% in patients having combined Tc-99 and Ga-67 scanning for infection. Gallium scans alone are not as accurate as the combination of bone scan and technetium scan for identifying infection. They also do not identify the type of organism involved. Because the gallium scan changes rapidly with the resolution of the acute active infection, it may be useful to document clinical improvement.

In-111 WBC scans are useful in detecting abscesses but do not differentiate between acute and chronic infections. False negative indium scans have been reported in chronic infections because the radionuclide accumulates with any inflammatory lesion. Likewise, neoplastic, noninfectious inflammatory lesions may lead to similar false-positive results with all scanning techniques. One major advantage of In-111 WBC scanning is that it differentiates noninfectious lesions such as hematomas and seromas, which may appear as a mass or an abscess like cavity on MRI or CT. Differentiation is important in the postoperative evaluation of potential infections.

LABORATORY STUDIES. The erythrocyte sedimentation rate (ESR) is the best laboratory study to identify or to evaluate and clinically monitor osteomyelitic disc space infection. Unfortunately, the ESR is not diagnostic and only indicates an inflammatory process, as do most of the roentgenographic findings. The ESR is elevated in 71% to 97% of children with vertebral osteomyelitis. In 37% of adults with osteomyelitis the rates exceed 100 mm/hr, and in 67% rates greater than 50 mm/hr are noted. However, the ESR normally is elevated after surgery (in the 25 mm/hr range), but usually falls to a nearly normal level at 4 weeks after surgery. Therefore persistent elevation of the ESR 4 weeks after surgery, with associated clinical findings, indicates a persistent infection.

Leukocytosis is not especially helpful in diagnosing spinal infection. White cell counts may actually drop in infants and debilitated patients. High white cell counts may indicate areas of infection other than the spine. Blood cultures are helpful if positive, which usually occurs in times of active sepsis with a febrile illness, and may be adequate for the diagnosis and treatment of osteomyelitis, but this occurrence is rare. Skin testing for microbacterial infections and organism-specific antibody testing may also give added information while the surgeon awaits biopsy results.

DIAGNOSTIC BIOPSY. Needle biopsy of the suspected lesion is the best method of determining infection and identifying the etiologic agent so that appropriate antibiotics can be administered. This technique is not foolproof, however. The administration of antibiotics before biopsy or a long period of time between the onset of the disease and the biopsy may result in a negative biopsy. Even open biopsy may not be positive in these situations.

An inflammatory process can be confirmed pathologically, although the etiologic agent cannot be isolated. Time, host resistance, bacterial virulence, prior antibiotic exposure, and culture of the proper anatomic part are all factors in successful isolation of the offending organism.

Needle biopsy for diagnosis should be and is the most common procedure performed for vertebral osteomyelitis. It frequently can be carried out with the patient under local anesthesia, with roentgenographic or CT scan control. Stoker and Kissin recommend general anesthesia only for biopsies in children. The reported success rates for percutaneous needle biopsy range from 71% to 96%; reported inadequate biopsy results range from 0% to 20%; and false negative results range from 4% to 20%. Up to 25% of infections have been reported to have negative biopsy results when patients were treated with antibiotics before biopsy.

Needle biopsy is not without risks. In 1975 Evarts warned against percutaneous biopsy in the thoracic spine because of damage to the vascular structures and the possibility of pneumothorax. With the development of new techniques and stronger and smaller needles, this is not as likely, but there is a definite risk of pneumothorax. Tube thoracostomy rarely is required to treat a pneumothorax, but chest roentgenograms and careful patient monitoring are mandatory after thoracic biopsy.

The use of CT guidance has improved the success rate of biopsy in both the thoracic and cervical spines. Presently, closed biopsy with CT guidance appears to have the highest success rate and the lowest complication rate. Even with this technique, however, percutaneous biopsy is not safe in all areas of the spine.

Differential Diagnosis

The differential diagnosis of spinal osteomyelitis should include primary and metastatic malignancies, metabolic bone diseases with pathologic fractures, and infections in contiguous and related structures, including the psoas muscle, hip joint, abdominal cavity, and genitourinary system. Charcot spinal arthropathy has been reported by Kalen et al. to resemble spinal osteomyelitis. Rheumatoid arthritis and ankylosing spondylitis also may cause findings resembling osteomyelitis of the spine. The acquired immunodeficiency syndrome (AIDS) may be another underlying factor in these infections. Crawfurd, Baird, and Clark reported five human immunodeficiency virus (HIV)-positive patients with spinal osteomyelitis who presented with radicular symptoms.

NONOPERATIVE TREATMENT

The traditional treatment of spinal infection has been bed rest and immobilization, and this is still the mainstay; however, the body cast now is often replaced with a removable body jacket in compliant patients. Antibiotic treatment for vertebral infection is the primary therapy. The antibiotic is chosen according to the positive stains, cultures, and sensitivities of the organism. Specific antibiotics, however, may not be adequate for spinal infections. Eismont et al. noted that 1 hour after injection cephalothin was not detectable in the disc and penetrated to less than 4% of serum values. Clindamycin and tobramycin levels were present at better than 50% of serum levels 1 hour after injection. Gibson et al. confirmed these conclusions in their study of fluocloxacillin and cephradine levels in the intravertebral discs of children during anterior spinal surgery. They found that neither antibiotic was identifiable in the discs even though high serum levels were present in other tissues.

The time for discontinuing antibiotic therapy also is variable. Collert suggests that antibiotic therapy should be continued until the ESR returns to normal. Intravenous antibiotics usually are continued for about 6 weeks and are followed by oral antibiotics as indicated by the ESR. Certainly a failure of improvement in the ESR or continued persistence of symptoms should initiate re-evaluation of the therapy, and possibly repeat biopsy or even open biopsy for cultures or to remove sequestered and infected material.

At present, with an adequate biopsy and a reliable patient who responds rapidly to antibiotics, hospitalization and bed rest usually are required only for the primary symptoms. Home intravenous antibiotic therapy may allow the patient to complete treatment out of the hospital. The only major risk to this technique is late pathologic fracture of the infected bone. The exact incidence of this complication with current therapy is unknown. Eismont et al. reported that staphylococcal infections appear to be more prone to cause paralysis than other types of infection, but their study did not include patients treated with ambulatory antibiotic therapy and immobilization. If ambulatory therapy is chosen, thorough education and close monitoring of the patient are mandatory. Long-term bed rest and cast immobilization are no longer necessary in most patients with spinal osteomyelitis or disc space infection, but they may be useful in recalcitrant infections that cannot be definitively diagnosed by standard techniques.

PROGNOSIS

Even if an absolute diagnosis is not made, most spinal infections resolve symptomatically and roentgenographically within 9 to 24 months of onset. Recurrence of the infection and periods of decreased immune response are always possible, as are delayed complications of kyphosis, paralysis, and myelopathy. These risks are greatest during the period when the infection is controlled but the bone is still soft, when the healing process has not advanced to the point where solid bone has formed around the infected tissue.

SPECIFIC INFECTIONS
Pyogenic Infections

The vertebrae are involved in from 0.15% to 3.9% of all osteomyelitic infections. Vertebral osteomyelitis has been reported by Digby and Kersley to occur in 1 of 250,000 inhabitants per year in a localized area of England. Males are affected more frequently than females, with a reported incidence from 55% to 75%. Adults are affected more frequently than children, with peak ages between 45 and 65 years. The most common organism reported is *S. aureus*. Drug abusers have been noted to be more likely to have *Pseudomonas aeruginosa* infections. Paralysis has been found by Eismont et al. to be the most common complication of *S. aureus* infection.

INFECTIONS IN CHILDREN. The syndrome of discitis in children is characterized by fever and an elevated ESR, followed by disc space narrowing on plain roentgenograms. The syndrome frequently is associated with difficulty in walking, malaise, irritability, and the sudden inability to stand or walk comfortably. Most reports indicate that the cause is bacterial infection, although trauma also has been implicated. Most culture reports are positive for *S. aureus*. The average age of onset is between 6 and 7 years. Symptoms usually are present for 4 weeks before hospitalization. Physical findings are limited. The child may refuse to walk or may cry when walking, and spinal flexion may be limited and painful so that the child holds himself erect. Physical findings directly related to the spine are rare. Neurologic findings are infrequent, but when present are ominous. In older children, abdominal pain may be a presenting symptom. Other, less frequent symptoms include hamstring tightness and spinal tenderness.

Diagnosing disc space infection (vertebral osteomyelitis) in children is difficult initially. Plain roentgenograms usually are negative. There may be a mild febrile reaction, but patients do not appear systemically ill. Laboratory investigation reveals only an elevated ESR in most patients. The best test to identify the infection probably is either MRI scanning or a combination of bone scanning and gallium scanning. These should give the earliest indication of possible infection, but are not totally diagnostic, and other possibilities, including inflammatory processes and tumors, may give false positive results. Blood cultures may be helpful if obtained during the initial febrile period of the illness.

The treatment of discitis in children varies considerably. Spiegel et al. and Boston, Bianco, and Rhodes do not recommend antibiotics and suggest bed rest and immobilization. On the other hand, Wenger, Bobechko, and Gilday recommend that the diagnosis be confirmed with blood cultures and that intravenous antibiotics be administered. They recommend placing the child at bed rest on intravenous antibiotics until he or she can walk and move about comfortably, and then switching to oral antibiotics for an additional arbitrary 3 weeks. They do not recommend cast or brace immobilization unless pain or difficulty in walking persists. They found immobilization most frequently needed in older children. Most patients are symptom free within several months. Spontaneous fusion occurs in about 25% of patients. Surgical procedures rarely are required, and persistent back pain rarely is a problem in children. Aggressive surgical treatment rarely is needed in children except in tuberculosis and other caseating diseases that have not responded well to antibiotics alone.

Special situations involving patients with immune suppression, suspected drug usage, tumorous conditions, or poor response to conservative treatment require more vigorous evaluation by needle aspiration biopsy for culture and sensitivity. CT scan control during the percutaneous biopsy, with the patient under a light general anesthesia, makes this a relatively safe procedure with high rates of positive culture. Definitive diagnosis and organism-specific antibiotic treatment constitute a more efficient method of dealing with these difficult situations.

In children younger than 6 years of age, the discitis may be viral in origin. Needle biopsy rarely is performed in these patients, and they may be the only group in which careful monitoring without antibiotics is reasonable.

The likelihood of paralysis depends on several factors. In the series of Eismont et al., no patient younger than 37 years of age developed paralysis. The higher the level of the infection in the spine, the greater the chance of paralysis.

DISC SPACE INFECTION IN ADULTS. In adults the intravertebral disc appears to be avascular, making it impossible for primary disc space infection to occur by a blood-borne route without first infecting bone. Therefore a true disc space infection in adults is most likely to be caused by penetrating trauma, the most common form of which is surgical manipulation. The reported incidences of disc space infection after disc surgery range from 1% to 2.8%. The reported incidence of disc space infection after discography is 1% when the single-needle technique is used and 0.5% with the double-needle technique. Postoperative disc space infection rarely is associated with a frank wound infection and wound drainage. The usual infecting organism is *S. aureus*, but other bacterial and fungal organisms have been reported.

The diagnosis of postoperative disc space infection is difficult and is almost always delayed. Pain is the most common complaint; however, persistence of back pain is not uncommon after surgical disc procedures. The most common diagnostic studies, including the ESR, bone scan, and gallium scan, are positive shortly after a spinal surgical procedure. MRI may be the best way to identify this complication rapidly. The ESR should return to nearly normal within 4 weeks after surgery. The persistence of back pain, muscle spasm, and difficulty in walking, along with an elevated ESR, 4 to 6 weeks after surgery should be highly indicative of a potential disc space infection. Disc space biopsy by closed-needle techniques or open biopsy, preferably before the administration of antibiotics, should allow identification of the offending organism in over 50% of patients.

Specific or empiric antibiotics have been suggested in most reports of postoperative disc space infection. Antibiotics should be continued until the ESR returns to normal. Immobilization in a body cast may be helpful to relieve pain, which usually lasts for 8 to 24 months. Spontaneous intervertebral fusion usually results in relief of pain. Occasionally spontaneous fusion does not occur. The indications for surgery are the same as for vertebral osteomyelitis.

EPIDURAL SPACE INFECTION. Spinal epidural infections have a low reported incidence of 0.2 to 1.2 cases per 10,000 hospital admissions per year. The incidence of this infection is increased in immunosuppressed patients. Morbidity and mortality are high with epidural infections. The causes of infection are the same as those for osteomyelitis and discitis. Epidural space infection may actually complicate a primary disc space infection. Trauma has been implicated as a causative factor in 25% of reported cases, presumably from secondary infection of an epidural hematoma. Feldenzer et al. noted that experimental epidural infection created physical signs from compression rather than from vascular thrombosis.

There are no biologic boundaries in the epidural space, and the infection frequently spans three to five vertebral segments, with the potential to cover the entire spinal canal. These infections occur more frequently in the thoracic and lumbar spine and are more frequently found on the dorsal and lateral portions of the epidural space. Ventral (anterior) infections are less frequent and are more likely to be related to a primary osteomyelitis or disc space infection. *S. aureus* is the most common infecting agent.

The clinical findings are similar to those of osteomyelitis but with several distinct differences: (1) a more rapid development of neurologic symptoms (days instead of weeks), (2) a more acute febrile illness, and (3) signs of meningeal irritation, including radicular pain with positive straight leg–raising test and neck rigidity. The classic progression of the disease is generalized spinal ache, root pain, weakness, and finally paralysis, all occurring within 7 to 10 days. Confirmatory testing is similar to that for osteomyelitis. MRI is critical to the determination of associated osteomyelitis.

Heusner noted that, even before antibiotics and at the dawn of the antibiotic age, with early decompression (before the development of paralysis or within 36 hours of onset) the chance of complete recovery was better than 50%. He also noted that the progression of the process was slow enough to allow evaluation and preparation without endangering the patient. Nonetheless, fail-

ure to provide prompt drainage can result in serious paralysis and possibly death. Some authors have reported successful treatment without surgical drainage, but these are few. Nonoperative management demands close observation and more active intervention if necessary.

The primary methods of treatment are surgical drainage and appropriate antibiotic therapy. The method of surgical treatment requires an accurate assessment of the location of the abscess and the presence of an associated osteomyelitis. Acute or chronic isolated dorsal (posterior), lateral, and some ventral (anterior) infections are best treated with total laminectomy for drainage, with closure over drains or secondary closure at a later date. Epidural infections associated with osteomyelitis are best exposed by anterior or posterolateral exposures that allow treatment of both the osteomyelitis and the epidural infection. Laminectomy in patients with ventral (anterior) osteomyelitis results in late deformity and collapse.

Other intraspinal infections include subdural abscess and spinal cord abscess. These infections are rare. Subdural abscesses progress at a slower pace than epidural abscesses and may be confused with tumors. Treatment requires durotomy without opening the arachnoid, thorough debridement, and dural closure if possible. Spinal cord abscesses cause pronounced incontinence and long tract signs. They frequently are confused with intramedullary tumors and transverse myelitis. In both of these conditions, the bone scan will be normal but the gallium scan should be positive. MRI, preferably with gadolinium contrast, is extremely helpful in defining the extent of the abscess. Some spinal cord abscesses may be successfully treated with antibiotics alone.

Brucellosis

Brucellosis results in a noncaseating, acid-fast, negative granuloma caused by a gram-negative capnophilic coccobacillus. This infection occurs most frequently in individuals involved in animal husbandry and meat processing. Pasteurization of milk and antibiotic treatment of animals have significantly decreased the incidence of this disease. Symptoms include polyarthralgia, fever, malaise, night sweats, anorexia, and headache. Psoas abscesses are found in 12% of patients. Bone involvement, most frequently the spine, occurs in 2% to 30% of patients. The lumbar spine is the most frequently involved spinal segment.

Roentgenographic changes of steplike erosions of the margin of the vertebral body require 2 months or more to develop. Disc space thinning and vertebral segment ankylosis by bridging are similar to changes in other forms of osteomyelitis (Fig. 85-8). CT scans and MRI may show soft tissue involvement. Moehring noted that gallium scanning is not helpful in sacroiliac infections. MRI may be helpful in the early identification of the disease but has not been reported for this specific infection. The diagnosis usually is indicated by brucella titers of

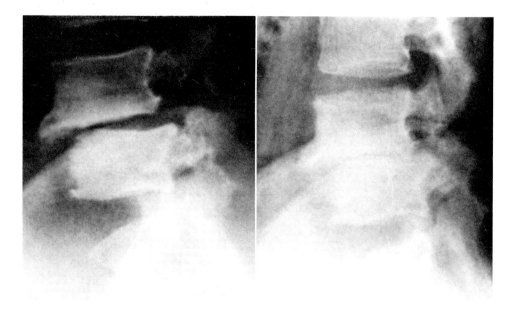

Fig. 85-8   Brucellosis of lumbar spine. Note vertebral sclerosis, spondylolisthesis, steplike irregularity in anterior vertebral body, and anterior osteophytes. (From Lifeso RM, Harder E, and McCorkell SJ: J Bone Joint Surg 67-B:345, 1985.)

1:80 or greater; confirmatory cultures also should be done, if possible using special techniques. Treatment usually consists of antibiotic therapy for 4 months and close monitoring of the brucella titers. Persistence of a titer of 1:160 or greater after 4 months of treatment may indicate recurrence or resistance of the infection. Indications for surgical treatment are the same as for tubercular spinal infections. Neurologic improvement after radical decompression and fusion is frequent. Because of the indolent nature of this disease it may be mistaken for a degenerative process.

Fungal Infections

Fungal infections generally are noncaseating, acid-fast, negative infections. They usually occur as opportunistic infections in immunocompromised patients. The development of symptoms usually is slow. Pain is less prominent as a physical symptom than in other forms of spinal osteomyelitis. Laboratory and roentgenographic findings are similar to those of pyogenic infections. Tubercular infection and tumors are the primary differential diagnoses. Direct culture by biopsy is the only method of absolute determination of the infecting organism.

Aspergillus and cryptococcal infections are of special note with regard to spinal infections.

Aspergillus is an opportunistic infecting agent in most reported cases. Barnwell, Jelsma, and Raff noted spinal involvement in 63% of 26 patients with apergillus infections. Pain, tenderness, and an elevated ESR were the most common symptoms. The diagnosis requires biopsy. Most patients do not require further surgery, but Ferris and Jones reported 10 patients who required radical de-

bridement. Their patients with paraplegia and epidural abscesses did not improve after surgery.

Cryptococcal infection is a less opportunistic, but more prevalent fungal infection. These organisms are found in avian excreta and usually infect the human respiratory system. Spinal infection is rare and usually is associated with generalized cryptococcal dissemination. The primary findings are pain, weakness, and a mildly elevated ESR. Roentgenograms show lytic lesions that on biopsy reveal non–acid-fast, caseating granulomas without pus. The indications for radical surgery are the same as for tuberculosis.

Tuberculosis

Tuberculosis was previously the primary cause of infectious spondylitis. Before the advent of effective chemotherapy, time and surgery for paralysis were the only treatment options. Laminectomy was initially performed for paralysis, but the results were disappointing until Ménard accidentally opened an abscess and the patient improved. Unfortunately, many patients treated in this manner died from secondary bacterial infection and the practice was abandoned. Posterior spinal fusion, as described by Hibbs and Albee, was the preferred operation to prevent deformity and promote healing by internal immobilization. Ito, Tsuchija, and Asami in 1934 reported the first radical debridement and bone grafting procedure for abscess formation. After the development of satisfactory chemotherapeutic agents, more aggressive surgery was attempted, including costotransversectomy with bone grafting and radical debridement with bone grafting as popularized by Hodgson.

Table 85-3 Mean annual incidence (per 100,000 population) of bone and joint tuberculosis according to age and sex, Canada, 1970 through 1974

Age (yr)	Sex	
	Male	Female
0-14	0.14	0.12
15-24	0.18	0.20
25-34	0.25	0.43
35-44	0.63	0.43
45-54	1.00	0.75
55-64	1.30	1.02
65+	1.60	1.40

From Enarson DA et al: Can Med Assoc J 120:139, 1979.

Presently tubercular bone and joint infections account for 2% to 3% of all reported cases of *Mycobacterium tuberculosis.* Spinal tubercular infections account for from one third to one half of the bone and joint infections. The thoracolumbar spine is the most commonly infected area (see Fig. 85-5). The incidence of infection appears to increase with age, but males and females are almost equally infected (Table 85-3).

Pathologically, the infection is characterized by acid-fast, positive, caseating granulomas with or without pus. Tubercles composed of monocytes and epithelioid cells, forming minute masses with central caseation in the presence of Langerhans-type giant cells, are typical on microscopic examination. Abscesses expand, following the path of least resistance, and contain necrotic debris. Skin sinuses form, drain, and spontaneously heal. Bone reaction to the infection varies from intense reaction to no reaction. In the spine the infection spares the intervertebral discs and spreads beneath the anterior and posterior longitudinal ligaments. Epidural infection is more likely to result in permanent neurologic damage.

Slowly progressive constitutional symptoms are predominant in the early stages of the disease, including weakness, malaise, night sweats, fever, and weight loss. Pain is a late symptom associated with bone collapse and paralysis. Cervical involvement may cause hoarseness because of recurrent laryngeal nerve paralysis, dysphagia, and respiratory stridor (known as Milar's asthma). These symptoms may result from anterior abscess formation in the neck. Sudden death has been reported with cervical disease after erosion into the great vessels. Neurologic signs usually occur late and may wax and wane. The presence of motor function and rectal tone are good prognostic predictors. Seddon reported that 60% to 90% of patients with Pott's paraplegia recovered with prolonged bed rest in an open-air hospital.

Laboratory studies suggest chronic disease. Findings include anemia, hypoproteinemia, and mild ESR elevation. Skin testing may be helpful but is not diagnostic. The test is contraindicated in patients with prior tuberculous infection because of the risk of skin slough from an intense reaction and is therefore not of use in patients with suspected reactivation of the disease.

Early roentgenographic findings include a subtle decrease in one or more disc spaces and localized osteopenia. Later findings include vertebral collapse, called "concertina collapse" by Seddon because of its resemblance to an accordion. Soft tissue swelling and its late calcification are highly predictable roentgenographic findings. CT scanning, with or without contrast, allows better evaluation of the pathologic process and the degree of neural compromise. MRI permits further delineation of the pathologic process. None of these tests, however, are confirmatory for tuberculosis. Gorse et al. noted that gallium scanning was most useful in patients with disseminated tuberculosis.

Definitive diagnosis is dependent on culture of the organism and requires biopsy of the lesion. Percutaneous techniques with roentgenographic or CT control usually are adequate. Open biopsy may be required if the needle biopsy is dangerous or nonproductive or if other open procedures are required.

Delayed diagnosis and missed diagnosis are common. Differential diagnoses include pyogenic and fungal infections, secondary metastatic disease, primary tumors of bone (such as osteosarcoma, chondrosarcoma, myeloma, eosinophilic granuloma, and aneurysmal bone cyst), sarcoidosis, giant cell tumors of bone, and bone deformities such as Scheuermann's disease.

TREATMENT OF TUBERCULAR SPINAL INFECTION. Definitive diagnosis by biopsy culture is important because of the toxicity of the chemotherapeutic agents and the length of treatment required. If open biopsy is required, Hodgson suggests definitive debridement and grafting at the same time. In 1960 Hodgson et al. reported 412 patients treated by radical removal of the diseased area and anterior spinal arthrodesis. Their technique requires a more extensive excision of bone than that of Roaf, Kirkaldy-Willis, and Cathro, but their mortality was only 2.9%, and no deaths occurred in patients who had disease of limited extent or of short duration and who had no pulmonary involvement. No patient developed paraplegia after surgery. Hodgson et al. advise this method for all patients with early tuberculosis of the spine and believe that it should supplant conservative treatment in most patients. They have operated on all patients, even those in whom the disease was far advanced, and of the first 100 patients observed from 2 to 4 years, 93 had solid arthrodeses consisting of an uninterrupted bridge of mature bone and healing of the tuberculous focus.

Nonoperative and operative methods have been extensively evaluated by the Medical Resource Council Working Party. Their reports indicate better results with regard to deformity, recurrence, development of paralysis, and resolution when radical surgery is performed with chemotherapeutic coverage. The resolution of paraplegia was not dependent on surgical intervention. Long-term bed rest, with or without cast immobilization, was ineffective. When the facilities for radical surgery are not available, ambulatory chemotherapy is the treatment of choice.

The indications for surgery in the absence of neurologic symptoms vary widely. Involvement of more than one vertebra significantly increases the risk of kyphosis and collapse. Open biopsy for diagnosis, debridement, and grafting may offer the most direct approach in these patients. Resistance to chemotherapy and recurrence of the disease are other indications for radical surgical treatment. Yau et al. listed the indications for surgery in early or late disease as severe kyphosis with active disease, signs and symptoms of cord compression, progressive impairment of pulmonary function, and progression of the kyphotic deformity. Primary contraindications to surgery are cardiac and respiratory failure.

Posterior fusion, with or without spinal instrumentation, is indicated after anterior decompression and grafting to prevent late collapse and stress fracture of the graft when more than two vertebrae are involved. Posterior fusion alone rarely is indicated at this time. High incidences of failure and late progression of kyphotic deformity, with or without fatigue fracture of the fusion, have followed posterior fusion alone. Tricortical iliac crest is the preferred bone graft material for all levels provided it is long enough. If the ribs are strong, autogenous rib grafts may be used in the thoracic region, although Rajasekaran and Shanmugasundaram and others reported frequent failure with the use of ribs as grafts. Fibular grafts may be required if the area of debridement is extensive and the available iliac crest graft is too short or if the ribs are not strong enough. The use of fibular or rib grafts results in an increased incidence of late stress fracture (Table 85-4). External immobilization is mandatory whenever debridement and grafting are performed. Halo (vest, cast, or pelvic) immobilization for up to 3 months is used after cervical and cervicothoracic procedures. Removable or nonremovable thoracolumbar immobilization is used after thoracic and thoracolumbar procedures until the grafts have completely healed (9 to 12 months or longer). Lumbosacropelvic immobilization is used after low lumbar procedures and should include from the hip to the knee of at least one leg for 6 to 8 weeks, followed by thoracolumbosacral immobilization until the graft has healed and the infection is resolved.

Cervical tuberculosis is a rare disease with a high complication rate. Hsu and Leong reported a 42.5% spinal cord compression rate in 40 patients. Children younger than 10 years of age were more likely to develop abscesses, whereas older children were more likely to develop paraplegia. Drainage and chemotherapy were adequate for the younger children. They recommend for older patients radical anterior debridement and strut grafting followed by chemotherapy. Cervical laminectomy resulted in increased kyphosis, subluxation, and neurologic deficits. Posterior cervical fusion resulted in persistent pain, kyphosis, and neurologic deficits that required anterior debridement and strut grafting. Subluxation was treated with skull traction for reduction, followed by anterior decompression and strut grafting.

Lifeso recommended various treatments for three different stages of C1-2 tubercular infection. Stage 1 infections involve minimal bone and ligamentous destruction. Surgical treatment for this consists of transoral biopsy, decompression, and immobilization in an orthosis. Stage 2 infections involve ligamentous destruction, minimal bone loss, and anterior displacement of C1 on C2. The suggested treatment for this is transoral biopsy and decompression, followed by reduction with halo traction and later C1-2 posterior fusion. Stage 3 infections exhibit

Table 85-4 Analysis of results in relation to type of graft

Type of graft	No.	No follow-up	Non-union or incomplete fusion	Body fusion	Average time to fusion (mo)	Decreased	Static	Increased (and average)
Autologous rib	63	8	21	34 (62%)	24	1	30	24 (13°)
Autologous ilium* Series I	23	—	6	17 (74%)	14	1	21	1 (nil)
Autologous ilium Series II	18	—	1	17 (94.5%)	10	2	11	5 (7°)
Homologous rib	1	—	—	1	24	—	1	—
Homologous tibia	7	—	2	5 (71%)	28	—	5	2
Heterologous Kiel bone, 4 Kiel bone–ilium, 1	5	—	1	4 (80%)	18.5	—	3	2

From Kemp HBS et al: J Bone Joint Surg 55-B:715, 1973.
*Autologous ilium: Series I denotes full-thickness ilium used as an inlay graft. Series II denotes full-thickness ilium crossing the coronal diameters of the affected vertebrae. The difference between the rate of fusion for autologous rib and autologous ilium was statistically significant (P < 0.001).

marked ligamentous and bone destruction with C1-2 displacement. The suggested treatment here is transoral biopsy and decompression, followed by reduction with halo traction and later occiput to C3 posterior fusion.

The thoracic and lumbar spines are more commonly involved with tubercular infection. Rajasekaran and Shanmugasundaram compared the development of kyphosis with the degree of collapse at the time of presentation of tubercular disease and the institution of antibiotic treatment. They developed a formula to predict the degree of final gibbus deformity that was 90% accurate: y = a + bx, where *y* is the measurement of the final angle of gibbus deformity, *x* is the initial loss of vertebral body, and a and b are constants 5.5 and 30.5, respectively. Initial vertebral loss was determined by dividing the vertebra into tenths for each involved vertebra (Figs. 85-9 and 85-10). They suggest that this formula may be used to identify patients most likely to develop significant kyphosis.

POTT'S PARAPLEGIA. The development of neurologic deficit is a strong indication for surgical treatment. Seddon noted that 70% to 95% of patients with Pott's paralysis recovered. He noted a poorer prognosis in paralysis caused by vascular embarrassment, penetration of the dura by the infection, and transection of the cord by a bony ridge. Paralysis persisting longer than 6 months was unlikely to improve.

Hodgson et al. (1964) described two basic groups: group A, paraplegia with active disease, which included subtypes 1 (external pressure on the cord) and 2 (penetration of the dura by infection); and group B, paraplegia of healed disease, which included subtypes 1 (transection of the cord by a bony ridge) and 2 (constriction of the cord by granulation and fibrous tissue). Hodgson et al. recommend early surgery to prevent the development of dural invasion by the infection, resulting in irreversible paralysis. A thorough preoperative examination, using MRI and CT scans of the involved segment, allows a complete evaluation of the extent of the disease and thus the development of a satisfactory approach for complete debridement and grafting. Late paralysis with inactive disease and significant kyphosis is much less responsive to treatment.

ABSCESS DRAINAGE BY ANATOMIC LEVEL

Any abscess cavity about the spine and pelvis can be drained by the following techniques.

Cervical Spine

If the cervical spine is involved, the abscess may be present retropharyngeally in the posterior triangle of the neck or supraclavicular area, or the tuberculous detritus may gravitate downward under the prevertebral fascia to form a mediastinal abscess.

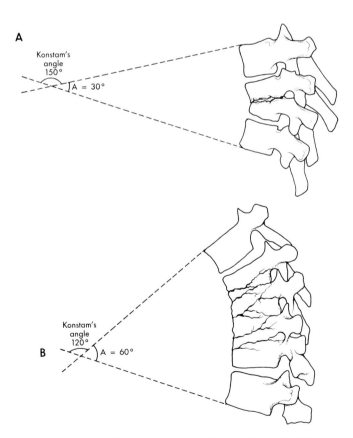

Fig. 85-9 Line diagrams showing Konstam's angle *(K)* and angle *A* (see text). (Redrawn from Rajasekaran S and Shanmugasundaram K: J Bone Joint Surg 69-A:503, 1987.)

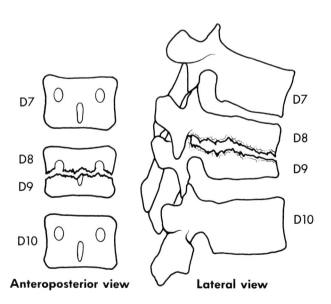

Fig. 85-10 Line diagram showing method of assessment of loss of vertebral body. (Redrawn from Rajasekaran S and Shanmugasundaram K: J Bone Joint Surg 69-A:503, 1987.)

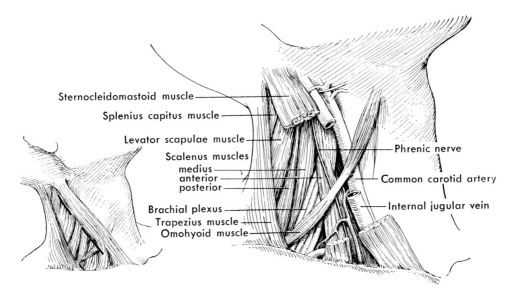

Sternocleidomastoid muscle

Splenius capitus muscle

Levator scapulae muscle

Scalenus muscles
medius
anterior
posterior

Brachial plexus

Trapezius muscle

Omohyoid muscle

Phrenic nerve

Common carotid artery

Internal jugular vein

Fig. 85-11   Drainage of tuberculous abscess of cervical spine.

DRAINAGE OF RETROPHARYNGEAL ABSCESS. Drainage of a retropharyngeal abscess through an incision in the posterior wall of the pharynx is warranted only in an emergency, as indicated by cyanosis and respiratory difficulty. Usually drainage should be through an extraoral approach (Fig. 85-11).

■ *TECHNIQUE.* Make a 7.5 cm incision along the posterior border of the sternocleidomastoid muscle at the junction of its middle and upper thirds. Incise the superficial layer of cervical fascia and protect the spinal accessory nerve that pierces the sternocleidomastoid muscle and runs obliquely across the posterior triangle. Retract the sternocleidomastoid muscle medially or divide it transversely. Using blunt dissection, expose the levator scapulae and splenius muscles, displace the internal jugular vein anteriorly, and palpate the abscess in front of the transverse processes and bodies of the vertebrae. Puncture the abscess wall with a hemostat, enlarge the opening, and gently but thoroughly evacuate the abscess. If the abscess is unusually large and symptoms are severe, do not close the wound; if not, close the wound in layers. A tracheostomy set should be available should the patient develop respiratory difficulty from edema of the larynx or should the abscess rupture into the pharynx.

DRAINAGE OF ABSCESS OF POSTERIOR TRIANGLE OF NECK

■ *TECHNIQUE.* Incise obliquely the skin and superficial fascia for 6.3 cm along the posterior border of the sternocleidomastoid muscle. Retract this muscle medially, but carefully protect the superficial nerves and external jugular vein. Identify the scaleni muscles without injuring the phrenic nerve. Locate and divide the line of cleavage between the scalenus anterior and longus colli muscles by blunt dissection

obliquely inward to the abscess beneath the paravertebral fascia. Evacuate the cavity and close the wound.

ALTERNATIVE APPROACH FOR DRAINAGE OF RETROPHARYNGEAL ABSCESS. Expose the anterior aspect of the cervical vertebrae as for standard anterior disc excision. This technique allows exposure from C2 to C7. A transverse incision is possible if only two or three vertebrae are involved. A longitudinal incision is made along the lateral border of the sternocleidomastoid muscle if longer exposure is necessary.

■ *TECHNIQUE.* Place the patient supine on the operating table with endotracheal anesthesia administered through a noncollapsible tube. Position the head turned to the right 10 to 20 degrees. The insertion of a small nasogastric tube may facilitate the positive identification of the esophagus. Place a small roll between the scapulas; the shoulders may be pulled downward with tape to allow easy roentgen exposure. Slightly extend the neck over a small roll placed beneath it. Then place a head halter on the mandible and occiput and apply several pounds of traction. Prepare and drape the area from the mandible to the upper chest. It may be necessary to suture the initial drapes in place.

Undermine the subcutaneous tissue both above and below and divide the platysma muscle longitudinally in the direction of its fibers. Open the cervical fascia along the anteromedial border of the sternocleidomastoid muscle. Develop a plane between the sternocleidomastoid laterally and the omohyoid and sternohyoid medially. Palpate the carotid artery in this plane and gently retract it laterally with a finger. With combined blunt and sharp dissection develop a relatively avascular plane between the carotid sheath laterally and the thyroid, trachea, and esophagus medially. Insert hand-held retractors initially. Identify the esophagus by palpation of the nasogastric tube. Dissect free the filmy connective tissue on the posterolateral aspect of the esophagus along the entire exposed wound to prevent ballooning of the esophagus above and below the retractor. Expose the prevertebral fascia and open the abscess cavity. Insert a hypodermic needle into this material and obtain a lateral roentgenogram to confirm the proper level. Drain the wound in a standard fashion. Do not close the neck fascia but let it fall together. The skin may be loosely closed or left open for delayed closure.

Dorsal Spine

COSTOTRANSVERSECTOMY. Most abscesses caused by disease of the dorsal spine may be evacuated by costotransversectomy (Fig. 85-12). This procedure, originally performed by Haidenhaim, was described by Ménard in 1894.

■ *TECHNIQUE.* Make a midline incision over three spinous processes. Reflect the periosteum and soft tissues laterally from the spinous processes and laminae on the side containing the abscess. Expose fully the middle transverse process and resect it at its base. After reflecting the periosteum from the contiguous rib, resect its medial end by division 5 cm from the tip of the transverse process. Bevel the end of the rib, taking care to avoid puncture of the pleura. Open the abscess by blunt dissection close to the vertebral body. The opening should be large enough to permit thorough exploration of the cavity and removal of all debris. If resection of more than one rib is necessary, enlarge the initial incision accordingly. After resecting the ribs, doubly ligate and divide the intervening neurovascular bundle. Close the wound in layers.

■ *TECHNIQUE (SEDDON).* Begin a semicircular skin incision in the midline about 10 cm proximal to the

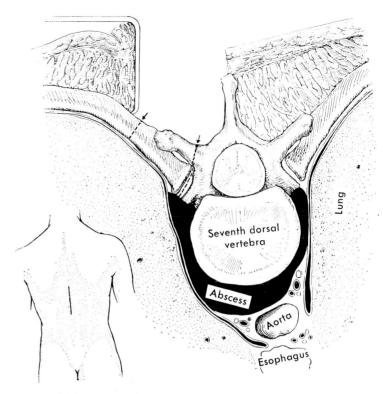

Fig. 85-12 Costotransversectomy to drain tuberculous abscess of dorsal spine.

apex of the kyphos, curve it distally and laterally to a point 10 cm from the midline at this apex, and continue distally and medially to the midline at a point 10 cm distal to the apex (Fig. 85-13). If the infection is pyogenic without a kyphosis, a midline incision can be used. Elevate the skin flap and retract it medially. Cut the superficial muscles and turn them in whatever direction is appropriate for the particular level. Divide the erector spinae muscles transversely opposite the apex of the deformity. Using diathermy dissection, expose the medial 8.3 cm

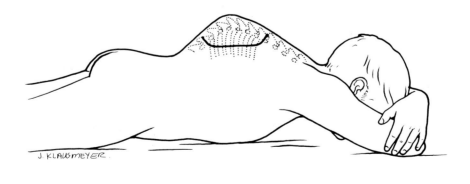

Fig. 85-13 Incision for costotransversectomy or anterolateral decompression. (From Seddon HJ. In Platt H, editor: Modern trends in orthopedics, second series, London, 1956, Butterworth & Co, Ltd.)

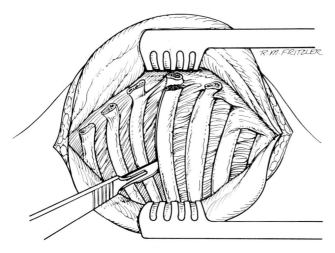

Fig. 85-14 Exposure of ribs and resection of transverse processes. (From Seddon HJ. In Platt H, editor: Modern trends in orthopedics, second series, London, 1956, Butterworth & Co, Ltd.)

of not less than three ribs, the corresponding transverse processes, and the lateral third of the laminae (Fig. 85-14).

Resect the rib that roentgenograms show to be level with the widest bulge of the abscess as follows. After dividing the costotransverse ligaments, remove the transverse process in one piece with large bone-cutting forceps. Using subperiosteal dissection, expose the rib, being careful not to perforate the pleura. If such a perforation occurs, place a small swab over it and try to close it as soon as the rib has been removed. The use of a Carlen tube will allow deflation of the lung. Transect the rib at a point not less than 6.8 cm (in adults) lateral to the costotrans-

verse joint. Use a curved gouge to free the medial end of the rib, pushing the gouge gently anteriorly and medially until it strikes the head of the rib or the vertebral column. Gently rotate the medial end of the rib and use the gouge to divide any remaining attachment. If the operation is successful, pus will pour out of the hole; remove it immediately with a sucker. Explore the abscess with a finger, reaching the vertebral bodies, opening small cavities, and dislodging necrotic material. If the abscess is unusually large, remove a second transverse process and rib for more exposure. Remove the tuberculous material from the abscess cavity and superficial tissues. After dusting the wound and the cavity with streptomycin powder, close the muscles and skin without a drain.

Lumbar Spine and Pelvic Drainage

DRAINAGE OF PARAVERTEBRAL ABSCESS

■ *TECHNIQUE.* Make a 7.5 to 10 cm longitudinal incision 5 to 7.5 cm lateral to the midline parallel to the spinous processes. Divide the lumbodorsal fascia in line with the incision and pass a hemostat bluntly around the lateral and anterior borders of the erector spinae muscles to the transverse processes (Fig. 85-15). Usually the abscess is encountered immediately; if not, puncture the layer of lumbodorsal fascia that separates the quadratus lumborum muscle from the erector spinae group and force the hemostat along the anterior border of the transverse processes. After thorough evacuation of the abscess, close the incision in layers.

DRAINAGE OF PSOAS ABSCESS. Psoas abscesses are

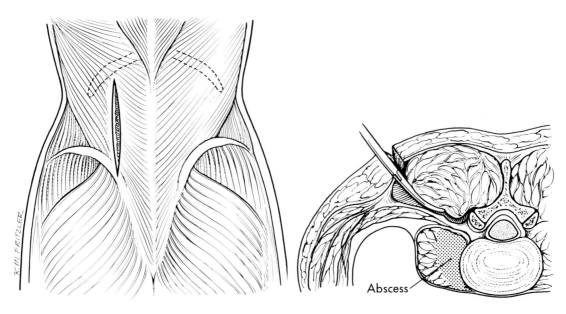

Abscess

Fig. 85-15 Drainage of paravertebral abscess.

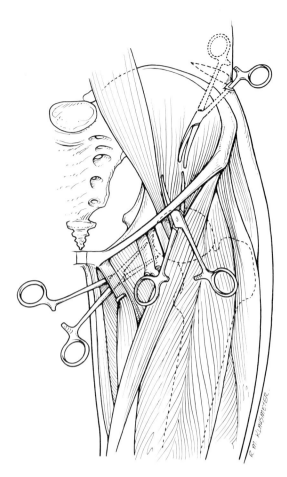

Fig. 85-16   Drainage of psoas abscess. Hemostat in adductor region is pointed toward inferior edge of acetabulum; abscess is usually located nearer junction of femoral head and neck. (Adapted from Freiberg JA and Perlman R: J Bone Joint Surg 18:417, 1936.)

entirely extraperitoneal and follow the course of the iliopsoas muscle. Drainage may be accomplished posteriorly through Petit's triangle, by a lateral incision along the crest of the ilium, or anteriorly under Poupart's ligament, depending on the size of the abscess and the area in which it appears. Occasionally an abscess burrows beneath Poupart's ligament and is seen subcutaneously in the proximal third of the thigh in the adductor region (Fig. 85-16).

Drainage through Petit's triangle. The sides of Petit's triangle are formed by the lateral margin of the latissimus dorsi muscle and the medial border of the obliquus externus abdominis muscle and its base by the crest of the ilium. The floor of the triangle is the obliquus internus abdominis muscle.
- *TECHNIQUE.* Make a 7.5 cm incision 2.5 cm proximal to and parallel with the posterior crest of the ilium, beginning lateral to the erector spinae group of muscles (Fig. 85-17). After exposure of Petit's triangle, bluntly dissect through the obliquus internus abdominis muscle directly into the abscess. After

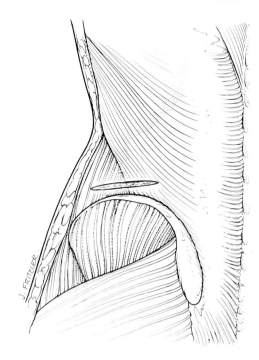

Fig. 85-17   Drainage of pelvic abscess through Petit's triangle.

thorough evacuation of the abscess close the incision in layers.

AFTERTREATMENT. Since flexion contracture of the hip usually accompanies a psoas abscess, Buck's traction should be employed to correct the deformity and relax the spastic muscles until the hip is fully extended.

Drainage by lateral incision

- *TECHNIQUE.* Make a 10 cm incision along the middle third of the crest of the ilium and free the attachments of the internal and external obliquus abdominis muscles. Puncture with a hemostat the abscess, which may be palpated as a fluctuant extraperitoneal mass on the inner surface of the wing of the ilium. Avoid rupture of the peritoneum.

Drainage by anterior incision

- *TECHNIQUE.* Begin a longitudinal skin incision at the anterosuperior spine and continue it distally for 5 to 7.5 cm on the anterior aspect of the thigh. Identify the sartorius muscle and carry the dissection deep to its medial border to the level of the anteroinferior spine. Protect the femoral nerve, which lies just medial to this area. Now insert a long hemostat along the medial surface of the wing of the ilium under Poupart's ligament and puncture the abscess. Separate the blades of the hemostat to enlarge the opening and permit complete evacuation. Close the incision in layers.

Drainage by Ludloff's incision. When a psoas abscess

points subcutaneously in the adductor region of the thigh, drainage is accomplished by Ludloff's incision, as described on p. 70.

Weinberg described a method of excising a psoas abscess when simpler treatment has failed or is likely to fail because of the size of the abscess, its chronicity, or involvement with mixed bacterial infection. He removes the abscess and also any bony or cartilaginous sequestra lodged in the tract or in the diseased vertebrae. The reader is referred to his work for details of technique and aftertreatment.

COCCYGECTOMY FOR DRAINAGE OF PELVIC ABSCESS. Lougheed and White noted that when tuberculosis involves the lower lumbar and lumbosacral areas, soft tissue abscesses may gravitate into the pelvis, forming a large abscess anterior to the sacrum. These soft tissue abscesses may point to the skin on the anterior surface of the thigh or above the iliac crest, but drainage at these sites alone is insufficient, resulting only in a chronically draining sinus despite antibacterial therapy. The pelvic abscess usually can be demonstrated roentgenographically by retrograde injection of an opaque medium. Lougheed and White devised a method of establishing dependent drainage posteriorly by coccygectomy. Their results in treatment of 10 patients by this method have been uniformly good. The wound usually healed within 6 to 8 weeks, and the spinal lesions all became inactive.

■ *TECHNIQUE (LOUGHEED AND WHITE)*. Make a 15 cm elliptical incision over the coccyx, removing a strip of skin. After freeing the coccyx from soft tissues, disarticulate it from the sacrum. With careful

hemostasis carry the dissection upward, staying close to the sacrum until the resulting pyramidal tunnel communicates with the abscess cavity. After evacuating the purulent matter, insert an irrigating catheter to the top of the cavity and pack the wound with iodoform gauze.

AFTERTREATMENT. For 2 to 3 weeks the wound is irrigated through the catheter several times daily with a solution of streptomycin. The packing is changed at intervals until the wound has healed by granulation tissue from within.

SURGICAL TREATMENT FOR TUBERCULOSIS OF SPINE
Radical Debridement and Arthrodesis

■ *TECHNIQUE (HODGSON ET AL.)*. Approach the *upper cervical area* (C1 and C2) through either the transoral or transthyrohyoid approach. In either approach perform a tracheostomy before operation. Have the anesthesia given through the tracheostomy opening, thus leaving the pharynx free of endotracheal tubing that would obstruct the view.

In the transoral approach, place the head in hyperextension and pack the hypopharynx. Turn back the soft palate on itself and anchor it with stay sutures exposing the nasopharynx. Next in the posterior pharyngeal wall make a midline incision 5 cm long with its center one fingerbreadth inferior to the anterior tubercle of the atlas that is palpable (Fig. 85-18, *A*). Carry the incision down to bone. Now

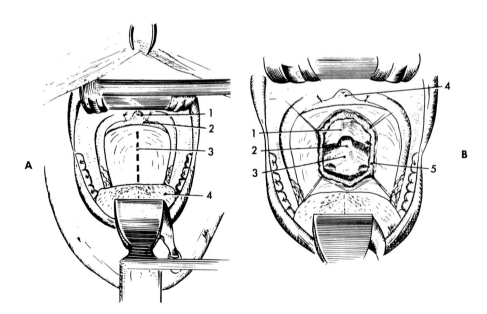

Fig. 85-18 Transoral approach to upper cervical area. **A,** Incision in posterior pharyngeal wall. *1,* Uvula; *2,* soft palate; *3,* incision in posterior pharyngeal wall; *4,* tongue. **B,** Atlas and axis exposed. *1,* Atlas; *2,* odontoid process; *3,* axis; *4,* uvula; *5,* edge of posterior pharyngeal wall retracted. (From Fang HSY and Ong GB: J Bone Joint Surg 44-A:1588, 1962.)

strip the posterior pharyngeal wall subperiosteally as far laterally as the lateral margin of the lateral masses of the atlas and the axis. Retract the raised soft tissue flaps with long stay sutures (Fig. 85-18, *B*) and control any oozing of blood by packing. The anterior arch of the atlas, the body of the axis, and the atlantoaxial joints on either side now are exposed.

For the transthyrohyoid approach, make a collar incision along the uppermost crease of the neck between the hyoid bone and the thyroid cartilage extending as far laterally as the carotid sheaths (Fig. 85-19, *A*). Divide the sternohyoid and thyrohyoid muscles, exposing the thyrohyoid membrane. Detach this membrane as near to the hyoid bone as possible to avoid damaging the internal laryngeal nerve and the superior laryngeal vessels that pierce it from the side nearer to its inferior attachment (Fig. 85-19, *B*). Next enter the hypopharynx by cutting into the exposed mucous membrane from the side to avoid damaging the epiglottis. Expose the posterior pharyngeal wall by retracting the hyoid bone and the epiglottis; make a midline incision in it down to bone (Fig. 85-19, *C*). Raise subperiosteally soft tissue flaps on either side and retract them to expose the bodies of C2, C3, and C4 (Fig. 85-19, *D*).

As an alternative, approach the *upper cervical* vertebrae (anterior base of the skull and C1-4) through a transmaxillary approach (Chapter 79).

Approach the *lower cervical* vertebrae (C3

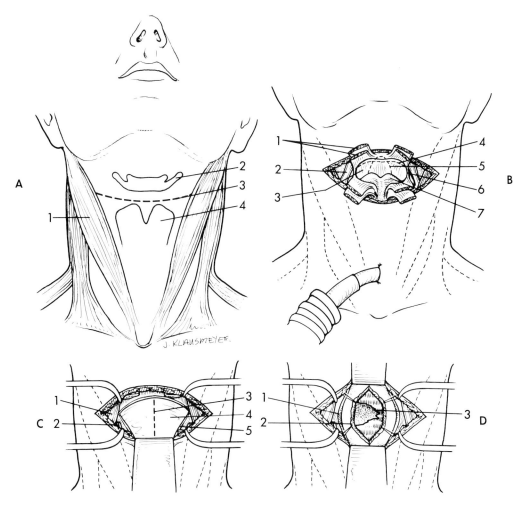

Fig. 85-19 Transthyrohyoid approach to upper cervical area. **A,** Skin incision. *1,* Sternocleidomastoid muscle; *2,* hyoid bone; *3,* skin incision; *4,* thyroid cartilage. **B,** Incision in thyrohyoid membrane. *1,* Cut ends of sternohyoid and thyrohyoid muscles; *2,* omohyoid muscle; *3,* thyrohyoid membrane; *4,* incision in thyrohyoid membrane; *5,* epiglottis; *6,* internal laryngeal nerve and superior laryngeal artery; *7,* thyroid cartilage. **C,** Incision in posterior pharyngeal wall. *1,* Omohyoid muscle; *2,* cut ends of sternohyoid and thyrohyoid muscles; *3,* incision; *4,* posterior pharyngeal wall; *5,* cut edges of thyrohyoid membrane and hypopharyngeal mucosa. **D,** Vertebral bodies exposed. *1,* Cut edges of thyrohyoid membrane and hypopharyngeal mucosa; *2,* retracted edge of posterior pharyngeal wall; *3,* bodies of C2, C3, and C4 are exposed. (From Fang HSY, Ong GB, and Hodgson AR: Clin Orthop 35:16, 1964.)

through C7) through a collar incision or one along the anterior or posterior border of the sternocleidomastoid muscle (Chapter 79). Incise the abscess longitudinally, exposing the spine.

Approach the *lower cervical* and *upper thoracic* vertebrae (C7 through T3) on the side with the larger abscess through a periscapular incision similar to that used for a first-stage thoracoplasty. Elevate the scapula with a mechanical retractor and resect the third rib. The pleura usually is opened, but if it is adherent, or if for other reasons it is necessary, make an extrapleural approach. Divide the superior intercostal artery at its origin, along with the accompanying vein.

Approach the *midthoracic* vertebrae (T4 through T11) usually from the left side. Select the rib that in the midaxillary line lies opposite the maximum convexity of the kyphos. It usually is two ribs superior to the center of the vertebral focus. Make an incision along this rib, resect it, and do a standard thoracotomy. The abscess usually is seen immediately, or there may be adhesions between it and the adjacent lung. Mobilize the lung and push it anteriorly. Now make a longitudinal incision in the pleura close to the aorta in the groove between the aorta and the abscess. Displace the aorta anteriorly and medially, revealing the intercostal vessels; secure and divide these for the entire length of the abscess cavity. Divide also elements of the splanchnic nerves. Now displace the aorta anteriorly away from the spine and palpate the abscess across the anterior aspects of the vertebrae. Make a T-shaped incision through the abscess wall: the first incision is transverse and opposite the center of the disease process, and the second is longitudinal and medial to the distally placed ligatures on the intercostal vessels. Now raise the two triangular flaps, revealing the diseased area, including the inside of the abscess cavity (Fig. 85-20).

Approach the *thoracolumbar area* (T12 through L2) through an incision along the left eleventh rib. Keep the dissection extrapleural and retroperitoneal and separate the diaphragm from the spine. Divide the psoas muscle transversely and turn it distally. Ligate the lumbar arteries and veins, as just described for the intercostals, and proceed with the approach as for the middorsal area.

Expose the *lower lumbar* vertebrae (L3 and L4) through a renal approach, using a left twelfth rib incision. The psoas muscle usually is divided transversely at a more distal level, often going through an ill-defined abscess between the muscle fibers. Avoid the trunks of the lumbar plexus posterior to the muscle.

Expose the *fifth lumbar* and *first sacral* vertebrae through an extraperitoneal approach. Start the incision in the midline midway between the symphysis

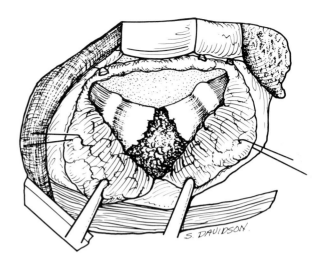

Fig. 85-20 Abscess opened with T-shaped incision through its wall. (From Hodgson AR and Stock FE: In Rob C and Smith R, editors: Operative surgery service, vol 9, London, 1960, Butterworth & Co, Ltd.)

pubis and the umbilicus and carry it to the left in a lazy-**S** fashion to a point midway between the iliac crest and the lowest rib in the flank (Fig. 85-21, *A*). Divide the skin, superficial fascia, and deep fascia in line with the incision. Divide the obliquus internus abdominis muscle in the same line but across its fibers. Divide also the transversus abdominis muscle and fascia in the same line. Then expose and dissect the peritoneum from the lateral wall of the abdomen, the left psoas muscle, and the lower lumbar spine. If the bifurcation of the aorta is high, the easiest approach to the lumbosacral region is between the common iliac vessels. The only vessels encountered are the middle sacral artery and vein; cauterize and divide these (Fig. 85-21, *B*). Retract or divide any fibers of the presacral plexus as necessary. If the bifurcation of the aorta is low, make the approach lateral to the aorta, the vena cava, and the common iliac vessels. Ligate and divide the iliolumbar and ascending lumbar veins to mobilize adequately the left common iliac vein (Fig. 85-21, *C*). If necessary, ligate and divide the fifth lumbar artery and vein and, if a higher approach is required, the fourth lumbar artery and vein as well. Then displace the large vessels to the right side and protect them with retractors.

The technique of excision of the diseased tissue and of anterior arthrodesis is about the same at all levels of the spine. Remove debris, pus, and sequestrated bone or disc by suction or with a pituitary rongeur. If possible, pass the sucker anterior to or between diseased vertebrae into the abscess cavity on the opposite side, and evacuate all material. Remove with an osteotome, rongeur, or chisel all diseased bone, both soft and sclerotic, exposing the spinal canal for the whole length of the disease. Also remove with a knife or rongeur the posterior common ligament and tuberculous granulation and fibrous tissue, exposing the dura. Excise the entire vertebral body affected by the disease, since collections of pus or sequestrated bone or disc material are often found in the spinal canal posterior to ap-

parently normal posterior parts of diseased bodies. If there is a definite indication, open the dura for inspection of the cord.

Now remove the disc at each end of the cavity, exposing normal bleeding bone (Fig. 85-22, *A*). Partially correct the kyphosis by direct pressure poste-

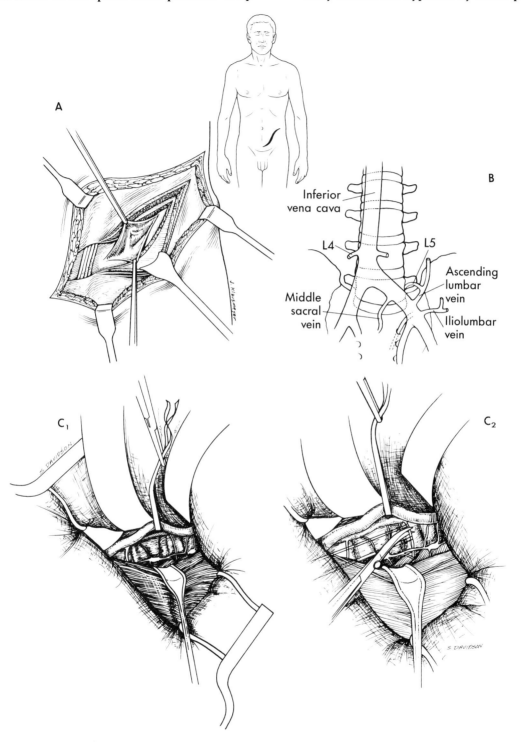

Fig. 85-21   A, Extraperitoneal approach to fifth lumbar and first sacral vertebrae (see text). *Inset,* Skin incision. **B,** In high bifurcation of aorta, middle sacral artery and vein are cauterized and divided. In low bifurcation of aorta, iliolumbar and ascending lumbar veins are cauterized and divided. **C1,** Exposed vertebrae are crossed by ascending lumbar vein. **C2,** Ascending lumbar vein is ligated and divided. (From Hoover NW: J Bone Joint Surg 50-A:194, 1968.)

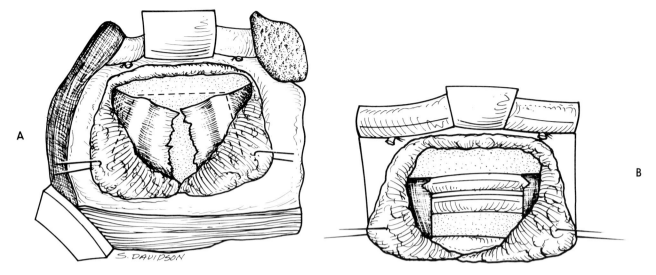

Fig. 85-22   A, Excision of diseased bone. **B,** Grafts inserted, keeping vertebrae sprung apart. (From Hodgson AR and Stock FE: In Rob C and Smith R, editors: Operative surgery service, vol 9, London, 1960, Butterworth & Co, Ltd.)

riorly on the spine. After cutting a mortise in the vertebrae at each end, insert one or more strut grafts of the correct length, keeping the vertebrae sprung apart (Fig. 85-22, *B*). For the dorsal area, fashion the grafts from the rib removed during thoracotomy (Fig. 85-23); bone bank grafts may be added. For the cervical area obtain the grafts from the bone bank or from the iliac crest. For the lum-

bar area take a massive graft from the iliac crest (Figs. 85-24 and 85-25).

Put streptomycin and isoniazid into the cavity before closure. After thoracotomy, close the chest in the usual way and maintain suction drainage of the pleural space for 2 or 3 days.

AFTERTREATMENT. The patient is placed in a plaster bed consisting of anterior and posterior shells

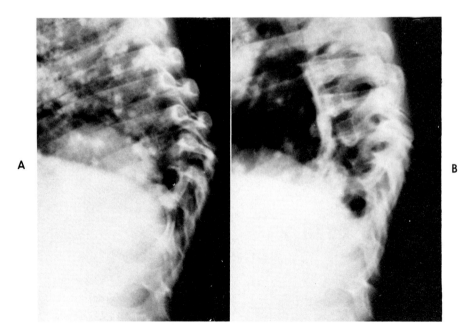

Fig. 85-23   Tuberculosis of spine without paraplegia in 4-year-old girl. **A,** Destruction of vertebral bodies before surgery. **B,** Six months after a thoracotomy approach, excision of diseased bone, and anterior fusion from D6 to D11 using resected ribs for grafts; 4½ years later, pain and evidence of activity are absent.

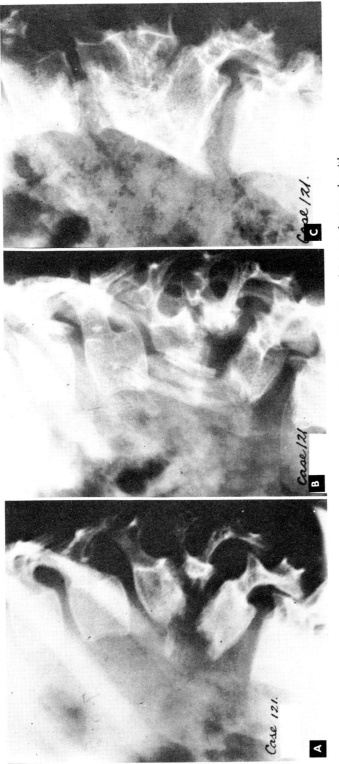

Fig. 85-24   Tuberculosis of spine in 13-year-old girl. **A,** L2, L3, and L4 are destroyed, with resulting kyphosis. **B,** One month after excision of diseased bone and grafting of bone between L1 and L4 from resected twelfth rib and from iliac crest. **C,** Three years after operation. Fusion is almost complete. (Courtesy Professor AR Hodgson.)

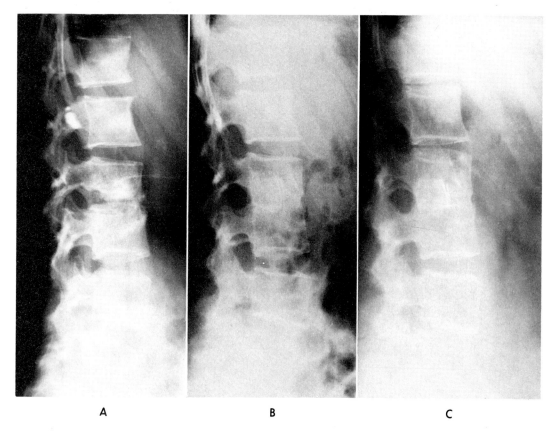

A   B   C

Fig. 85-25 Tuberculosis of bodies of L2 and L3 without paraplegia in 23-year-old woman. **A,** Before surgery. **B,** Six months after debridement and anterior arthrodesis through left extraperitoneal approach; grafts were from ilium. **C,** Four years after surgery; fusion is complete.

and remains there until the spine is judged to have united clinically. The time of immobilization after surgery averages about 3½ months. Mobilization is then gradually started and is continued for 6 to 8 weeks, the patient being carefully watched for increasing kyphosis or other signs of disease activity.

Dorsolateral Approach to Dorsal Spine

■ *TECHNIQUE (ROAF, KIRKALDY-WILLIS, AND CATH-RO).* Expose the dorsal spine through a dorsolateral approach. Maintain careful hemostasis throughout. Select the side with the larger abscess shadow, or in the absence of an abscess use the left side, and make a curved incision. Begin posteriorly 3.8 cm from the midline, 7.5 cm proximal to the center of the lesion, and curve distally and laterally to a point 12.5 cm from the midline at the center of the lesion; continue medially and distally, ending 3.8 cm from the midline 7.5 cm distal to the center of the lesion (Fig. 85-26). Divide the superficial and deep fascia and the underlying muscles down to the ribs in the line of the incision. Retract the flap of the skin and muscle medially. Now locate the rib opposite the center of the focus and remove 7.5 to 10 cm of this

rib and the one proximal and distal in the following manner. Free the ribs with a periosteal elevator and divide them with rib shears 7.5 to 10 cm from the tips of the transverse processes. Now resect each at the tip of the transverse process. Divide under direct vision the ligaments and muscles attached to the rib heads and transverse processes and resect these bony parts. Identify two and preferably three intercostal nerves and trace them medially to the intervertebral foramina. These nerves, as they pass into the foramina, indicate the level of the cord in the spinal canal. Expose the intercostal vessels near the spinal column and cut them between clamps. Divide the intercostal muscles near the vertebral column. Separate the pleura from the spinal column by blunt dissection, exposing the lateral and anterolateral aspects of the vertebral bodies. Take care to avoid perforating the pleura, as it is often adherent and thickened; if a perforation should occur, suture it at once. Locate the center of the lesion by passing a finger into the wound anterior to the vertebral bodies. Remove all pus, granulation tissue, and necrotic matter. Occasionally one or more vertebral bodies may be sequestrated and lying free in the abscess cavity. Usually two or three small bony sequestra and

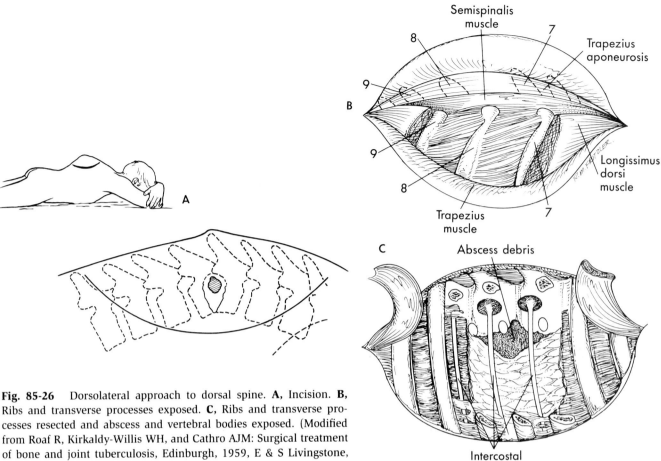

Fig. 85-26 Dorsolateral approach to dorsal spine. **A,** Incision. **B,** Ribs and transverse processes exposed. **C,** Ribs and transverse processes resected and abscess and vertebral bodies exposed. (Modified from Roaf R, Kirkaldy-Willis WH, and Cathro AJM: Surgical treatment of bone and joint tuberculosis, Edinburgh, 1959, E & S Livingstone, Ltd.)

pieces of necrotic disc material are found. If the paravertebral shadow, thought to be an abscess, is found to be mainly fibrous tissue, it is more difficult to find the lesion. Under these circumstances using roentgenographic control, explore the bone with a fine gouge, burr, and rongeur. After thorough debridement decide whether bone grafts are advisable. The simplest method of grafting is to pack the cavity with bone chips. Or a more extensive procedure may be undertaken: with a chisel or gouge roughen the lateral and anterolateral aspects of the diseased vertebral bodies and if possible of one healthy vertebra above and below and cut a groove in them, passing from healthy bone above to healthy bone below. Wedge a full-thickness rib graft into the groove and sink it deeply within the vertebral bodies. Place cancellous bone chips obtained from the remaining portion of the resected ribs in the groove and laterally along the roughened surface of the vertebral bodies. If the pleura has been accidentally opened, drain the pleural cavity with a chest tube inserted through a small stab incision in the eighth intercostal space in the midaxillary line and connected to an underwater seal for 48 hours after surgery.

Costotransversectomy

Costotransversectomy is discussed on p. 3807.

Anterolateral Decompression (Lateral Rhachotomy)

In 1933 Capener originated a procedure that he called lateral rhachotomy and that is now popularly known as anterolateral decompression, in which the spine is opened from its lateral side. This affords access to the front and side of the cord, permitting decompression by the removal of bony spurs, granulation tissue, and sequestra or the evacuation of abscesses. Since the procedure entails resection of one or more pedicles, it is contraindicated if the spine is unstable. The operation, at best difficult, is easiest when there is a sharp kyphos.

■ *TECHNIQUE (CAPENER)*. If the disease is in the mid-dorsal region, begin the incision in the midline at a point 10 cm proximal to the lesion, gently curve it laterally a distance of 7.5 cm, and return to the midline at a point 10 cm distal to the lesion (Fig. 85-27). Reflect the skin and superficial and deep fasciae as a thick flap. Now incise and retract laterally the origin

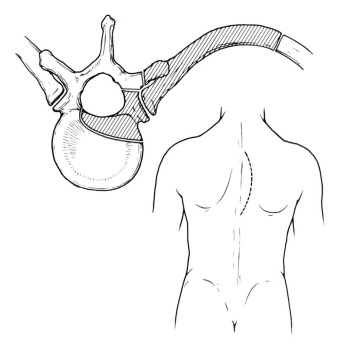

Fig. 85-27 Capener anterolateral decompression for tuberculous abscess of dorsal spine. *Stippled areas,* Extent of bone resection. *Inset,* Skin incision.

of the trapezius muscle; divide the erector spinae muscles transversely over the rib leading to the affected intervertebral space and retract them proximally and distally. After exposing the rib subperiosteally, resect it from its angle to the transverse process; if necessary, resect the rib proximal and distal in the same manner. Now separate the intercostal nerve from its accompanying vessels and divide it, using the proximal end as a guide to further dissection and later for traction on the cord. Carefully retract the pleura along with the intercostal vessels and remove the medial end of the rib and the transverse process and pedicle of the vertebra with a rongeur; a sphenoid punch and a motor-driven burr are of assistance at this stage. The dura and the posterolateral aspect of the vertebral body are seen after anterior depression of the pleura and the intercostal vessels and traction on the intercostal nerve. Now work from the more normal tissues in the vertebral canal toward the site of compression. Gently remove diseased bone with a curet; also remove all impinging and encroaching tissues so carefully that the dura is not even momentarily dented. Thoroughly evacuate a paravertebral abscess if present. Close the wound in layers.

AFTERTREATMENT. Anterior and posterior plaster shells, prepared before surgery, are applied; when the lesion is in the cervical or upper dorsal region, skeletal traction should be employed.

• • •

Alexander has recommended that three or more ribs be widely resected to provide better exposure; Griffiths, Seddon, and Roaf, Kirkaldy-Willis, and Cathro also endorsed the more extensive approach.

■ *TECHNIQUE (SEDDON).* The approach and the method of rib resection are as described for costotransversectomy on p. 3807. Resect not less than three and not more than four ribs. Isolate the intercostal nerves and trace them medially to the intervertebral foramina; now cut away the intervening intercostal muscles (Fig. 85-28, *A*). Gently push the pleura anteriorly with the fingers and determine by palpation the position of the two or three pedicles to be resected. To increase exposure, cut away small parts of the overhanging neural arches. Remove as little bone as possible dorsal to the pedicles, since anything in the least approaching hemilaminectomy is likely to be followed by a lateral subluxation of the spine. Now resect the pedicles by nibbling away from their lateral surfaces with a rongeur (Fig. 85-28, *B*). Use utmost care to avoid tearing the dura, which may be adherent to the inner surface of the pedicles. If a rent occurs, suture it as soon as possible.

Remove the offending material such as a caseous mass, granulation tissue, a necrotic disc, or a nest of sequestra. This may be accomplished easily, but the removal of a ridge of living bone is difficult. Do not retract the cord, but leave it untouched and attack the bony ridge from the side or from beneath. Drill the ridge in several places with a slowly rotating hand drill and then nibble away from the side and below with a small rongeur. The mass may be further broken up with an osteotome. The cord now rests on a shell of bone; gently push this bone anteriorly with a blunt instrument. Be sure to leave no offending ridges. Now pass a probe along the anterior surface of the cord both proximally and distally to locate any secondary cause of compression inside the spinal canal, such as an encapsulated caseous mass. Wash the wound with saline solution and dust it with streptomycin. Suture the muscles and skin without drainage.

AFTERTREATMENT. Aftertreatment is the same as for the Capener technique.

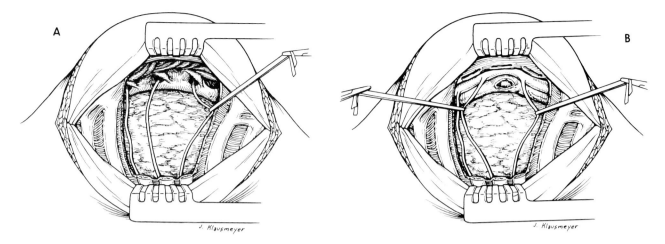

Fig. 85-28 **A,** Intercostal nerves isolated and pedicles exposed. **B,** Exposure of spinal cord after resection of three pedicles. Material anterior to cord may now be removed. Sequestrum is shown within abscess. (From Seddon HJ. In Platt H, editor: Modern trends in orthopedics, second series, London, 1956, Butterworth & Co, Ltd.)

REFERENCES

Biology, diagnosis, and treatment of spinal infection

Batson OV: The function of the vertebral veins and their role in the spread of metastases, Ann Surg 112:138, 1940.

Batson OV: The vertebral vein system as a mechanism for the spread of metastases, Am J Roentgenol Radium Ther 48:715, 1942.

Batson OV: The vertebral vein system. Caldwell Lecture, 1956, Am J Roentgenol Radium Ther Nucl Med 78:195, 1957.

Brant-Zawadzki M, Burke VD, and Jeffrey RB: CT in the evaluation of spine infection, Spine 8:358, 1983.

Breschet G: Essai sur les veines der rachis, Paris, 1819, Mequigon-Morvith.

Collert S: Osteomyelitis of the spine, Acta Orthop Scand 48:283, 1977.

Coventry MB, Ghormley RK, and Kernohan JW: The intervertebral disc: its microscopic anatomy and pathology. I. Anatomy, development, and physiology, J Bone Joint Surg 27-A:105, 1945.

Coventry MB, Ghormley RK, and Kernohan JW: The intervertebral disc: its microscopic anatomy and physiology. III. Pathological changes in the intervertebral disc, J Bone Joint Surg 27:460, 1945.

Crawfurd EJ, Baird PR, and Clark AL: Cauda equina and lumbar nerve root compression in patients with AIDS, J Bone Joint Surg 69-B:36, 1987.

Crock HV and Yoshizawa H: The blood supply of the lumbar vertebral column, Clin Orthop 115:6, 1976.

Crock HV, Yoshizawa H, and Kame SK: Observations on the venous drainage of the human vertebral body, J Bone Joint Surg 55-B:528, 1973.

Digby JM and Kersley J: Pyogenic non-tuberculous spinal infection, J Bone Joint Surg 61-B:47, 1979.

Dommisse GF: The blood supply of the spinal cord, J Bone Joint Surg 56-B:225, 1974.

Eismont FJ, Wiesel SW, Brighton CT, and Rothman RH: Antibiotic penetration into rabbit nucleus pulposus, Spine 12:254, 1987.

Evarts CM: Diagnostic technique: closed needle biopsy, Clin Orthop 107:100, 1975.

Feldenzer JA, McKeever PE, Schaberg DR, et al: The pathogenesis of spinal epidural space abscess: microangiographic studies in an experimental model, J Neurosurg 69:110, 1988.

Fraser RD, Osti OL, and Vernon-Roberts B: Discitis following chemonucleolysis: an experimental study, Spine 11:679, 1986.

Gibson MJ, Karpinski MRK, Slack RCB, et al: The penetration of antibiotics into the normal intervertebral disc, J Bone Joint Surg 69-B:784, 1987.

Golimbu C, Firooznia H, and Rafii M: CT of osteomyelitis of the spine, AJR 142:159, 1984.

Grollmus J, Perkins RK, and Russel W: Erythrocyte sedimentation rate as a possible indicator of early disc space infection, Neurochirurgia 17:30, 1974.

Hassler O: The human intervertebral disc: a microangiographical study on its vascular supply at various ages, Acta Orthop Scand 40:765, 1969.

Hodgson AR and Stock FE: Anterior spinal fusion: a preliminary communication on the radical treatment of Pott's disease and Pott's paraplegia, Br J Surg 44:266, 1956.

Inoue H: Three-dimensional architecture of lumbar intervertebral discs, Spine 6:139, 1981.

Kalen V, Isono SS, Colin SC, and Perkash I: Charcot arthropathy of the spine in long-standing paraplegia, Spine 12:480, 1987.

Kapp JP and Sybers WA: Erythrocyte sedimentation rate after uncomplicated lumbar disc operations, Surg Neurol 12:329, 1979.

Kattapuram SV, Phillips WC, and Boyd R: Computed tomography in pyogenic osteomyelitis of the spine, AJR 140:1199, 1983.

Keyes DC and Compere EL: The normal and pathological physiology of the nucleus pulposus of the intervertebral disc, J Bone Joint Surg 14:897, 1932.

Konnberg M: Erythrocyte sedimentation rate following lumbar discectomy, Spine 11:766, 1986.

Macnab I, St Louis EL, Grabias SL, and Jacob R: Selective ascending lumbosacral venography in the assessment of lumbar-disc herniation, J Bone Joint Surg 58-A:1093, 1976.

Modic T, Masaryk T, and Plaushtek D: Magnetic resonance imaging of the spine, Radiol Clin North Am 14:229, 1986.

Nelaton A: Elemens de pathologie chirurgicle, Paris, 1844, Bailliere.

Norris SH, Ehrlich MG, and McKusick K: Early diagnosis of disc space infection with 67-Ga in an experimental model, Clin Orthop 144:2983, 1979.

Norris SH, Ehrlich MG, McKusick K, and Provine H: The radioisotopic study of an experimental model of disc space, J Bone Joint Surg 60-B:281, 1978.

Ogata K and Whiteside LA: Nutritional pathways of the intervertebral disc, Spine 6:211, 1981.

Pott P: Remarks on that kind of palsy of the lower limbs which is frequently found to accompany a curvature of the spine, London, 1779, J Johnson.

Puig-Guri J: Pyogenic osteomyelitis of the spine: differential diagnosis through clinical and roentgenographic observations, J Bone Joint Surg 28:29, 1946.

Roca RP and Yoshikawa TT: Primary skeletal infections in heroin users: a clinical characterization, diagnosis and therapy, Clin Orthop 144:238, 1979.

Rodet A: Etude experimentale sur l'osteomyelite infectieuse, Compt Rend Acad Sci, pp 569-571, 1884.

Ross PM and Fleming JL: Vertebral body osteomyelitis: spectrum and natural history: a retrospective analysis of 37 cases, Clin Orthop 118:1890, 1976.

Ryan LM, Carrera GF, Lightfoot RW Jr, et al: The radiographic diagnosis of sacroiliitis: a comparison of different views with computed tomograms of the sacroiliac joint, Arthritis Rheum 26:760, 1983.

Stoker DJ and Kissin CM: Percutaneous vertebral biopsy: a review of 135 cases, Clin Radiol 36:569, 1985.

Waldvogel FA, Medoff G, and Swartz MN: Osteomyelitis: a review of clinical features, therapeutic considerations and unusual aspects (first of three parts), N Engl J Med 282:198, 1976.

Waldvogel FR and Vasey H: Osteomyelitis: the past decade, N Engl J Med 303:360, 1980.

Whalen JL, Parke WW, Mazur JM, and Stauffer ES: The intrinsic vasculature of developing vertebral end plates and its nutritive significance to the intervertebral discs, J Pediatr Orthop 5:403, 1985.

Whelan MA, Schonfeld S, Post JD, et al: Computed tomography of nontuberculous spinal infection, J Comp Assist Tomog 9:280, 1985.

Wilensky AO: Osteomyelitis of the vertebra, Ann Surg 89:561, 1929.

Wiley AM and Trueta J: The vascular anatomy of the spine and its relationship to pyogenic vertebral osteomyelitis, J Bone Joint Surg 41-B:796, 1959.

Pyogenic infections

Altemeier WA and Largen T: Antibiotic and chemotherapeutic agents in infections of the skeletal system, JAMA 150:1462, 1952.

Ambrose GB, Alpert M, and Neer CS: Vertebral osteomyelitis: a diagnostic problem, JAMA 197:619, 1966.

Avila L Jr: Primary pyogenic infections of the sacro-iliac articulation: a new approach to the joint, J Bone Joint Surg 23:922, 1941.

Badgley CE: Osteomyelitis of the ilium, Arch Surg 28:83, 1934.

Bonfiglio M, Lange TA, and Kim YM: Pyogenic vertebral osteomyelitis: disk space infections, Clin Orthop 96:234, 1973.

Bosworth DM: Surgery of the spine, AAOS Instr Course Lect 14:39, 1957.

Calot F: L'Orthopedie Indispensable aux Practiciens, Paris, 1909.

Collert S: Osteomyelitis of the spine, Acta Orthop Scand 48:283, 1977.

Digby JM and Kersley JB: Pyogenic non-tuberculous spinal infection, J Bone Joint Surg 61-B:47, 1979.

Eismont FJ, Bohlman HH, Soni PL, et al: Pyogenic and fungal vertebral osteomyelitis with paralysis, J Bone Joint Surg 65-A:19-29, 1983.

El-Gindi S, Aref S, Salama M, and Andrew J: Infection of intervertebral discs after operation, J Bone Joint Surg 58-B:114, 1976.

Emery SE, Chan DPK, and Woodward HR: Treatment of hematogenous pyogenic vertebral osteomyelitis with anterior debridement and primary bone grafting, Spine 14:284, 1989.

Frank TJF: Osteomyelitis of the odontoid process of the axis (dens of the epistropheus), Aust Med J 1:198, 1944.

Frederickson B, Yuan H, and Olans R: Management and outcome of pyogenic vertebral osteomyelitis, Clin Orthop 131:160, 1978.

Freehafer AA, Heiser DP, and Saunders AP: Infection of the lower lumbar spine with *Neisseria meningitidis*, J Bone Joint Surg 60-A:1001, 1978.

Garcia A Jr and Grantham SA: Hematogenous pyogenic vertebral osteomyelitis, J Bone Joint Surg 42-A:429, 1960.

Ghormley RK, Bickel WH, and Dickson DD: A study of acute infectious lesions of the intervertebral disks, South Med J 33:347, 1940.

Gleckman R: Afebrile bacteremia: a phenomenon in geriatric patients, JAMA 248:1478, 1982.

Griffiths HED and Jones DM: Pyogenic infection of the spine: a review of twenty-eight cases, J Bone Joint Surg 53-B:383, 1971.

Hale JE and Aichroth P: Vertebral osteomyelitis: a complication of urological surgery, Br J Surg 61:867, 1974.

Halpern AA, Rinsky LA, Fountain S, and Nagel DA: Coccidioidomycosis of the spine: unusual roentgenographic presentation, Clin Orthop 140:78, 1979.

Harris HN and Kirkaldy-Willis WH: Primary subacute pyogenic osteomyelitis, J Bone Joint Surg 47-B:526, 1965.

Hartman JT and Phalen GS: Needle biopsy of bone: report of three representative cases, JAMA 200:201, 1967.

Hazlett JW: Pyogenic osteomyelitis of the spine, Can J Surg 1:243, 1958.

Heberling JA: A review of two hundred and one cases of suppurative arthritis, J Bone Joint Surg 23:917, 1941.

Henson SW Jr and Coventry MB: Osteomyelitis of the vertebrae as the result of infection of the urinary tract, Surg Gynecol Obstet 102:207, 1956.

Holzman RS and Bishko F: Osteomyelitis in heroin addicts, Ann Intern Med 75:693, 1971.

Jackson JW: Surgical approaches to the anterior aspect of the spinal column, Ann R Coll Surg Engl 48:83, 1971.

Kelly PJ, Martin WJ, and Coventry MB: Bacterial (suppurative) arthritis in the adult, J Bone Joint Surg 52-A:1595, 1970.

Kemp HBS, Jackson JW, Jeremiah JD, and Cook J: Anterior fusion of the spine for infective lesions in adults, J Bone Joint Surg 55-B:715, 1973.

Kemp HBS, Jackson JW, Jeremiah JD, and Hall AJ: Pyogenic infections occurring primarily in intervertebral discs, J Bone Joint Surg 55-B:698, 1973.

Kemp HBS, Jackson JW, and Shaw NC: Laminectomy in paraplegia due to infective spondylosis, Br J Surg 61:66, 1974.

King DM and Mayo KM: Infective lesions of the vertebral column, Clin Orthop 96:248, 1973.

Kirkaldy-Willis WH and Thomas TG: Anterior approaches in the diagnosis and treatment of infections of the vertebral bodies, J Bone Joint Surg 47-A:87, 1965.

Lame EL: Vertebral osteomyelitis following operation on the urinary tract or sigmoid: the third lesion of an uncommon syndrome, Am J Roentgenol Radium Ther Nucl Med 75:938, 1956.

Leach RE, Goldstein H, and Younger D: Osteomyelitis of the odontoid process, J Bone Joint Surg 49-A:369, 1967.

Lindholm TS and Pylkkänen P: Discitis following removal of intervertebral disc, Spine 7:618, 1982.

Ling CM: Pyogenic osteomyelitis of the spine, Orthop Rev 4:23, September 1975.

Makins GH and Abbot FC: An acute primary osteomyelitis of the vertebrae, Ann Surg 23:150, 1896.

Malawski SK: Pyogenic infection of the spine, Inte Orthop 1:125, 1977.

Morrey BF, Kelly PJ, and Nichols DR: Viridans streptococcal osteomyelitis of the spine, J Bone Joint Surg 62-A:1009, 1980.

Nagel DA, Albright JA, Keggi KJ, and Southwick WO: Closer look at spinal lesions: open biopsy of vertebral lesions, JAMA 191:975, 1965.

Nichols BL: Nutrition and infection, South Med J 71:705, 1978.

Paus B: Tumor, tuberculosis and osteomyelitis on the spine: differential diagnostic aspects, Acta Orthop Scand 44:372, 1973.

Pott P: Remarks on that kind of palsy of the lower limbs which is frequently found to accompany a curvature of the spine, London, 1779, J Johnson.

Puranen J, Mäkelä J, and Lähde S: Postoperative intervertebral discitis, Acta Orthop Scand 55:461, 1984.

Ray MJ and Bassett RL: Pyogenic vertebral osteomyelitis, Orthopedics 8:506, 1985.

Robertson RC and Ball RP: Destructive spine lesions: diagnosis by needle biopsy, J Bone Joint Surg 17:749, 1935.

Roca RP and Yoshikawa TT: Primary skeletal infections in heroin users: a clinical characterization, diagnosis and therapy, Clin Orthop 144:238, 1979.

Shaw NE and Thomas TG: Surgical treatment of chronic infective lesions of the spine, Br Med J 1:162, 1963.

Shehadi WH: Primary pyogenic osteomyelitis of the articular processes of the vertebrae, J Bone Joint Surg 34:343, 1936.

Sherman M and Schneider GT: Vertebral osteomyelitis complicating postabortal and postpartum infection, South Med J 48:333, 1955.

Siebert WT, Moreland N, and Williams TW Jr: Methicillin-resistant *Staphylococcus epidermidis*, South Med J 7:1353, 1978.

Speed JS and Boyd HB: Bone syphilis, South Med J 29:371, 1936.

Stauffer RN: Pyogenic vertebral osteomyelitis, Orthop Clin North Am 6:1015, 1975.

Stern WE and Balch RE: Surgical aspects of nonspecific inflammatory and suppurative disease of the vertebral column, Am J Surg 122:314, 1966.

Stone JL, Cybulski GR, Rodriguez J, and Gryfinski ME: Anterior cervical debridement and strut-grafting for osteomyelitis of the cervical spine, J Neurosurg 70:879, 1989.

Sullivan CR, Bickel WH, and Svien HJ: Infections of vertebral interspaces after operations on the intervertebral disks, JAMA 166:1973, 1958.

Sullivan CR and Symmonds RE: Disk infections and abdominal pain, JAMA 188:655, 1964.

Waldvogel FA, Medoff G, and Swartz MN: Osteomyelitis: a review of clinical features, therapeutic considerations and unusual aspects. I, N Engl J Med 282:198, 1976.

Waldvogel FA and Vasey H: Osteomyelitis: the past decade, N Engl J Med 303:360, 1980.

Wedge JH, Oryschak AF, Robertson DE, and Kirkaldy-Willis WH: Atypical manifestations of spinal infections, Clin Orthop 123:155, 1977.

Wilensky AO: Osteomyelitis of the vertebra, Ann Surg 89:561, 1929.

Wiltberger BR: Resection of the vertebral bodies and bone-grafting for chronic osteomyelitis of the spine, J Bone Joint Surg 34-A:215, 1952.

Infections in children

Blanche DW: Osteomyelitis in infants, J Bone Joint Surg 34-A:71, 1952.

Boston HC Jr, Bianco AJ Jr, and Rhodes KH: Disk space infections in children, Orthop Clin North Am 6:953, 1975.

Menelaus MB: Discitis: an inflammation affecting the intervertebral discs in children, J Bone Joint Surg 46-B:16, 1964.

Nade S: Acute haematogenous osteomyelitis in infancy and childhood, J Bone Joint Surg 65-B:109, 1983.

Saenger EL: Spondylarthritis in children, Am J Roentgenol Radium Ther 64:20, 1950.

Scoles PV and Quinn TP: Intervertebral discitis in children and adolescents, Clin Orthop 162:31, 1982.

Spiegel PG, Kengla KW, Isaacson AS, and Wilson JC Jr: Intervertebral disc-space inflammation in children, J Bone Joint Surg 54-A:284, 1972.

Wenger DR, Bobechko WP, and Gilday DL: The spectrum of intervertebral disc-space infection in children, J Bone Joint Surg 60-A:100, 1978.

Epidural space infection

Feldenzer JA, McKeever PE, Schaberg DR, et al: The pathogenesis of spinal epidural abscess: microangiographic studies in an experimental model, J Neurosurg 69: 110, 1988.

Heusner AP: Nontuberculous spinal epidural infection, N Engl J Med 239:845, 1948.

Mampalam TJ, Rosegay H, Andrews BT, et al: Nonoperative treatment of spinal epidural infections, J Neurosurg 71: 208, 1989.

Brucellosis

Aguilar JA and Elvidge AR: Intervertebral disk disease caused by the *Brucella* organism, J Neurosurg 18:27, 1961.

Goodhart GL, Zakem JF, Collins WC, and Meyer JD: Brucellosis of the spine: report of a patient with bilateral paraspinal abscesses, Spine 12:414, 1987.

Lifeso RM, Harder E, and McCorkell SJ: Spinal brucellosis, J Bone Joint Surg 67-B:345, 1985.

Moehring HD: Brucella sacroiliitis: a case report, Orthopedics 8:499, 1985.

Samra Y, Hertz M, Shaked Y, et al: Brucellosis of the spine: a report of three cases, J Bone Joint Surg 64-B:429, 1982.

Torres-Rojas J, Taddonio RF, and Sanders CV: Spondylitis caused by *Brucella abortus*, South Med J 72:1166, 1979.

Fungal infections

Barnwell PA, Jelsma LF, and Raff MJ: Aspergillus osteomyelitis: report of a case and review of the literature, Diagn Microbiol Infect Dis 3:515, 1985.

Eismont FJ, Bohlman HH, Soni PL, et al: Pyogenic and fungal vertebral osteomyelitis with paralysis, J Bone Joint Surg 65-A:19, 1983.

Ferris B and Jones C: Paraplegia due to aspergillosis: successful conservative treatment of two cases, J Bone Joint Surg 67-B:800, 1985.

Halpern AA, Rinsky LA, Fountain S, and Nagel DA: Coccidioidomycosis of the spine: unusual roentgenographic presentation, Clin Orthop 140:78, 1979.

Matsushita T and Suzuki K: Spastic paraparesis due to cryptococcal osteomyelitis: a case report, Clin Orthop 196:279, 1985.

Mawk JR, Erickson DL, Chou SN, and Seljeskog EL: *Aspergillus* infections of the lumbar disc spaces: report of three cases, J Neurosurg 58:270, 1983.

Mazet R Jr: Skeletal lesions of coccidioidomycosis, Arch Surg 70:633, 1955.

Winter WG Jr, Larson RK, Zettas JP, and Libke R: Coccidioidal spondylitis, J Bone Joint Surg 60-A:240, 1978.

Tuberculosis

Acker JD, Wood GW II, Moinuddin M, and Eggers FM: Radiologic manifestations of spinal infection. In Wood GW II, editor: Spinal infections, Philadelphia, 1989, Hanley & Belfus.

Ahn BH: Treatment of Pott's paraplegia, Acta Orthop Scand 39:145, 1968.

Albee FH: Transplantation of a portion of the tibia into the spine for Pott's disease: a preliminary report, JAMA 57:885, 1911.

Alexander GL: Neurological complications of spinal tuberculosis, Proc R Soc Med 39:730, 1945-1946.

Allen AR and Stevenson AW: A ten-year follow-up of combined drug therapy and early fusion in bone tuberculosis, J Bone Joint Surg 49-A:1001, 1967.

Arct W: Operative treatment of tuberculosis of the spine in old people, J Bone Joint Surg 50-A:255, 1968.

Bailey HL, Gabriel M, Hodgson AR, and Shin JA: Tuberculosis of the spine in children: operative findings and results in one hundred consecutive patients treated by removal of the lesion and anterior grafting, J Bone Joint Surg 54-A:1633, 1972.

Bakalim G: Tuberculosis spondylitis: a clinical study with special reference to the significance of spinal fusion and chemotherapy, Acta Orthop Scand, suppl 47, 1960.

Bakalim G: Results of radical evacuation and arthrodesis in sacroiliac tuberculosis, Acta Orthop Scand 37:375, 1966.

Bickel WH: Tuberculosis of bones and joints, Mayo Clin Proc 28:370, 1953.

Bosworth D: Tuberculosis of the osseous system. IV. Operative methods, Q Bull Sea View Hosp 5:441, 1940.

Bosworth DM: Surgery of the spine, AAOS Instr Course Lect 14:39, 1957.

Bosworth DM: Treatment of bone and joint tuberculosis in children, J Bone Joint Surg 41-A:1255, 1959.

Bosworth DM: Treatment of tuberculosis of bone and joint, Bull NY Acad Med 35:167, 1959.

Bosworth DM, Della Pietra A, and Rahilly G: Paraplegia resulting from tuberculosis of the spine, J Bone Joint Surg 35-A:735, 1953.

Brashear HR Jr and Rendleman DA: Pott's paraplegia, South Med J 71:1379, 1978.

Butler RW: Paraplegia in Pott's disease with special reference to the pathology and etiology, Br J Surg 22:738, 1934-1935.

Calot F: L'Orthopedie Indispensable aux Practiciens, Paris, 1909.

Calot F and Pierre I: Est-il permis, dans l'etat actuel de la science d'operer des malades atteints de paralysie du mal de Pott? Rev Orthop 6:249, 1895.

Campos OP: Bone and joint tuberculosis and its treatment, J Bone Joint Surg 37-A:937, 1955.

Capener N: Personal communication to Girdlestone GR, 1934. Cited in Platt H, editor: Modern trends in orthopaedics, New York, 1950, Paul B Hoeber, Inc.

Capener N: The evolution of lateral rhachotomy, J Bone Joint Surg 36-B:173, 1954.

Chu C-B: Treatment of spinal tuberculosis in Korea, using focal debridement and interbody fusion, Clin Orthop 50:235, 1967.

Compere EL and Garrison M: Correlation of pathologic and roentgenologic findings in tuberculosis and pyogenic infections of the vertebrae, Ann Surg 104:1038, 1936.

Davies PDO et al: Bone and joint tuberculosis: a survey of notifications in England and Wales, J Bone Joint Surg 66-B:326, 1984.

Dickson JA: Spinal tuberculosis in Nigerian children: a review of ambulant treatment, J Bone Joint Surg 49-B:682, 1967.

Dott NM: Skeletal traction and anterior decompression in the management of Pott's paraplegia, Edinburgh Med J 54:620, 1947.

Dove J, Hsu LCS, and Yau ACMC: The cervical spine after halo-pelvic traction: an analysis of the complications in 83 patients, J Bone Joint Surg 62-B:158, 1980.

Eighth report of the Medical Research Council Working Party on Tuberculosis of the Spine. A 10-year assessment of a controlled trial comparing debridement and anterior spinal fusion in the management of tuberculosis of the spine in patients on standard chemotherapy in Hong Kong, J Bone Joint Surg 64-B:393, 1982.

Enarson SA, Fujii M, Nakielna EM, and Grzybowski S: Bone and joint tuberculosis: a continuing problem, Can Med Assoc J 120:139, 1979.

Erlacher PJ: The radical operative treatment of bone and joint tuberculosis, J Bone Joint Surg 17:536, 1935.

Evans ET: Tuberculosis of the bones and joints, J Bone Joint Surg 34-A:267, 1952.

Fang D, Leong JC, and Fang HS: Tuberculosis of the upper cervical spine, J Bone Joint Surg 65-B:47, 1983.

Fang HSY, Ong GB, and Hodgson AR: Anterior spinal fusion, the operative approaches, Clin Orthop 35:16, 1964.

Felländer M: Radical operation in tuberculosis of the spine, Acta Orthop Scand, suppl 19, 1955.

Fifth report of the Medical Research Council Working Party on Tuberculosis of the Spine, Brompton Hospital, London, England. A five-year assessment of controlled trials of in-patient and out-patient treatment and of plaster-of-Paris jackets for tuberculosis of the spine in children on standard chemotherapy: studies in Masan and Pusan, Korea, J Bone Joint Surg 58-B:399, 1976.

First report of the Medical Research Council Working Party on Tuberculosis of the Spine. A controlled trial of ambulant out-patient treatment and in-patient rest in bed in management of tuberculosis of the spine in young Korean patients on standard chemotherapy: a study in Masan, Korea, J Bone Joint Surg 55-B:678, 1973.

Fountain SS, Hsu LCS, Yau ACMC, and Hodgson AR: Progressive kyphosis following solid anterior spine fusion in children with tuberculosis of the spine: a long term study, J Bone Joint Surg 57-A:1104, 1975.

Fourth report of the Medical Research Council Working Party on Tuberculosis of the Spine. A controlled trial of anterior spinal fusion and debridement in the surgical management of tuberculosis of the spine in patients on standard chemotherapy: a study in Hong Kong, Br J Surg 61:853, 1974.

Garceau GJ and Brady TA: Pott's paraplegia, J Bone Joint Surg 32-A:87, 1950.

Girdlestone GR: The operative treatment of Pott's paraplegia, Br J Surg 19:121, 1931.

Girdlestone GR: Tuberculosis of bones and joints. In Platt H, editor: Modern trends in orthopaedics, New York, 1950, Paul B Hoeber, Inc.

Girdlestone GR and Somerville EW: Tuberculosis of bone and joint, ed 2, New York, 1952, Oxford University Press.

Goel MK: Treatment of Pott's paraplegia by operation, J Bone Joint Surg 49-B:674, 1967.

Gorse GJ, Pais MP, Kusske JA, and Cesario TC: Tuberculous spondylitis: a report of six cases and a review of the literature, Medicine 62:178, 1983.

Griffiths DL: Pott's paraplegia and its operative treatment, J Bone Joint Surg 35-B:487, 1953.

Guirguis AR: Pott's paraplegia, J Bone Joint Surg 49-B:658, 1967.

Hallock H and Jones JB: Tuberculosis of the spine, J Bone Joint Surg 36-A:219, 1954.

Hibbs RA: An operation for progressive spinal deformities, NY Med J 93:1013, 1911.

Hodgson AR, Skinsnes OK, and Leong CY: The pathogenesis of Pott's paraplegia, J Bone Joint Surg 49-A:1147, 1967.

Hodgson AR and Stock FE: Anterior spinal fusion: a preliminary communication on the radical treatment of Pott's disease and Pott's paraplegia, Br J Surg 44:266, 1956.

Hodgson AR and Stock FE: Anterior fusion. In Rob C and Smith R, editors: Operative surgery service, vol 9, London, 1960, Butterworth & Co, Ltd.

Hodgson AR and Stock FE: Anterior spine fusion for the treatment of tuberculosis of the spine: the operative findings and results of treatment of the first one hundred cases, J Bone Joint Surg 42-A:295, 1960.

Hodgson AR, Stock FE, Fang HSY, and Ong GB: Anterior spinal fusion: the operative approach and pathological findings in 412 patients with Pott's disease of the spine, Br J Surg 48:172, 1960.

Hodgson AR, Yau A, Kwon JS, and Kim D: A clinical study of 100 consecutive cases of Pott's paraplegia, Clin Orthop 36:128, 1964.

Hoover MJ Jr: The treatment of the tuberculous psoas abscess, South Surg 16:729, 1950.

Hoover NW: Methods of lumbar fusion, J Bone Joint Surg 50-A:194, 1968.

Hsu LCS and Leong JCY: Tuberculosis of the lower cervical spine (C2 to C7) a report on 40 cases, J Bone Joint Surg 66-B:1, 1984.

Hsu LCS, Cheng CL, and Leong JCY: Pott's paraplegia of late onset: the cause of compression and results after anterior decompression, J Bone Joint Surg 70-B:534, 1988.

Ito H, Tsuchija J, and Asami G: A new radical operation for Pott's disease, J Bone Joint Surg 16:449, 1934.

Janeway T and Moseberg WH Jr: Tuberculous paraplegia with lateral vertebral dislocation: a case report, J Bone Joint Surg 59-A:554, 1977.

Jenkins DHR et al: Stabilization of the spine in the surgical treatment of severe spinal tuberculosis in children, Clin Orthop 110:69, 1975.

Johnson RW Jr, Hillman JW, and Southwick WO: The importance of direct surgical attack upon lesions of the vertebral bodies, particularly in Pott's disease, J Bone Joint Surg 35-A:17, 1953.

Jones AR: The influence of Hugh Owen Thomas on the evolution of treatment of skeletal tuberculosis, J Bone Joint Surg 35-B:309, 1958.

Jones BS: Pott's paraplegia in the Nigerian, J Bone Joint Surg 40-B:16, 1958.

Kaplan CJ: Conservative therapy in skeletal tuberculosis: an appraisal based on experience in South Africa, Tubercle 40:355, 1959.

Karlén A: Early drainage of paraspinal tuberculous abscesses in children: a preliminary report, J Bone Joint Surg 41-B:491, 1959.

Kemp HBS, Jackson JW, Jeremiah JD, and Cook J: Anterior fusion of the spine for infective lesions in adults, J Bone Joint Surg 55-B:715, 1973.

Key JA: The pathology of tuberculosis of the spine, J Bone Joint Surg 22:799, 1940.

Kite JH: Tuberculosis of the spine with paraplegia, South Med J 29:883, 1936.

Kohli SB: Radical surgical approach to spinal tuberculosis, J Bone Joint Surg 49-B:668, 1967.

Kondo E and Yamada K: End results of focal débridement in bone and joint tuberculosis and its indications, J Bone Joint Surg 39-A:27, 1957.

Konstam PG and Blesovsky A: The ambulant treatment of spinal tuberculosis, Br J Surg 50:26, 1962-1963.

Langenskiöld A and Riska EB: Pott's paraplegia treated by anterolateral decompression in the thoracic and lumbar spine: a report of twenty-seven cases, Acta Orthop Scand 38:181, 1967.

Li J-Q: Operative treatment of 183 cases of tuberculosis of the cervical spine, Chinese J Orthop 3:231, 1983.

Lifeso R: Atlanto-axial tuberculosis in adults, J Bone Joint Surg 69-B:183, 1987.

Lougheed JC and White WG: Anterior dependent drainage for tuberculous lumbosacral spinal lesions: coccygectomy and dependent drainage in treatment of tuberculous lesions of the lower spine with associated soft-tissue abscesses, Arch Surg 81:961, 1960.

Martin NS: Tuberculosis of the spine: a study of the results of treatment during the last twenty-five years, J Bone Joint Surg 52-B:613, 1970.

Martin NS: Pott's paraplegia: a report of 120 cases, J Bone Joint Surg 53-B:596, 1971.

Medical Resource Council Working Party on Tuberculosis of the Spine. Five-year assessments of controlled trials of ambulatory treatment, debridement and anterior spinal fusion in the management of tuberculosis of the spine: studies in Bulawayo (Rhodesia) and in Hong Kong, J Bone Joint Surg 60-B:163, 1978.

Ménard V: Étude pratique sur le mal du Pott, Paris, 1900, Masson et Cie.

Naim-Ur-Rahman: Atypical forms of spinal tuberculosis, J Bone Joint Surg 62-B:162, 1980.

Neal SL, Kearns MA, Seelig JM, and Harris JP: Manifestations of Pott's disease in the head and neck, Laryngoscope 96:494, 1986.

Neville CH Jr and Davis WL: Is surgical fusion still desirable in spinal tuberculosis? Clin Orthop 75:179, 1971.

O'Connor BT, Steel WM, and Sanders R: Disseminated bone tuberculosis, J Bone Joint Surg 57-A:537, 1970.

Paus B: Tumor, tuberculosis and osteomyelitis on the spine: differential diagnostic aspects, Acta Orthop Scand 44:372, 1973.

Rajasekaran S and Shanmugasundaram TK: Prediction of the angle of gibbus deformity in tuberculosis of the spine, J Bone Joint Surg 69-A:503, 1987.

Risko T and Novoszel T: Experiences with radical operations in tuberculosis of the spine, J Bone Joint Surg 45-A:53, 1963.

Roaf R, Kirkaldy-Willis WH, and Cathro AJM: Surgical treatment of bone and joint tuberculosis, Edinburgh, 1959, E & S Livingstone, Ltd.

Seddon HJ: Pott's paraplegia, Br J Surg 22:769, 1935.

Seddon HJ: The pathology of Pott's paraplegia, Proc R Soc Med 39:723, 1945-1946.

Seddon HJ: Antero-lateral decompression of Pott's paraplegia, J Bone Joint Surg 33-B:461, 1951.

Seddon HJ: Treatment of Pott's paraplegia by anterolateral decompression, Mém Acad Chir 79:281, 1952.

Seddon HJ: Pott's paraplegia and its operative treatment, J Bone Joint Surg 35-B:487, 1953.

Seddon HJ: Pott's paraplegia. In Platt H, editor: Modern trends in orthopaedics (second series), London, 1956, Butterworth & Co, Ltd.

Seddon HJ and Alexander GL: Discussion of spinal caries with paraplegia, Proc R Soc Med 39:723, 1946.

Sixth report of the Medical Research Council Working Party on Tuberculosis of the Spine. Five-year assessments of controlled trials of ambulatory treatment, debridement and anterior spinal fusion in the management of tuberculosis of the spine studies in Bulawayo (Rhodesia) and in Hong Kong, J Bone Joint Surg 60-B:163, 1978.

Smith AD: The treatment of bone and joint tuberculosis, J Bone Joint Surg 37-A:1214, 1955.

Smith AD: Tuberculosis of the spine: results in 70 cases treated at the New York Orthopaedic Hospital from 1945 to 1960, Clin Orthop 58:171, 1968.

Smith TK and Livermore NB: Hoarseness accompanying Pott's paraplegia, J Bone Joint Surg 63-A:159, 1981.

Steindler A: Posterior mediastinal abscess in tuberculosis of the dorsal spine, Illinois Med J 50:201, 1926.

Steindler A: On paraplegia in Pott's disease, Lancet 54:281, 1934.

Tuli SM: Tuberculosis of the craniovertebral region, Clin Orthop 104:209, 1974.

Tuli SM: Results of treatment of spinal tuberculosis by "middle-path" regimen, J Bone Joint Surg 57-B:13, 1975.

Tuli SM, Sprivastava TP, Varma BP, and Sinha GP: Tuberculosis of spine, Acta Orthop Scand 38:445, 1967.

Weinberg JA: The surgical excision of psoas abscesses resulting from spinal tuberculosis, J Bone Joint Surg 39-A:17, 1957.

Wilkinson MC: The treatment of tuberculosis of the spine by evacuation of the paravertebral abscess and curettage of the vertebral bodies, J Bone Joint Surg 37-B:382, 1955.

Yau ACMC and Hodgson AR: Penetration of the lung by the paravertebral abscess in tuberculosis of the spine, J Bone Joint Surg 50-A:243, 1968.

Yau ACMC, Hsu LCS, O'Brien JP, and Hodgson AR: Tuberculous kyphosis: correction with spinal osteotomy, halo-pelvic distraction, and anterior and posterior fusion, J Bone Joint Surg 56-A:1419, 1974.

Other Disorders of Spine

GEORGE W. WOOD

In this chapter are discussed spondylolisthesis, spinal stenosis, congenital anomalies of the spine, rheumatoid arthritis of the spine, ankylosing spondylitis, tumors of the spine, and spinal deformity after late treatment.

SPONDYLOLISTHESIS

Spondylolisthesis is generally defined as an anterior or posterior slipping or displacement of one vertebra on another. A unilateral or bilateral defect of the pars interarticularis without displacement of the vertebra is known as spondylolysis or, less frequently, spondyloschisis.

The first description of spondylolisthesis is attributed to Herbinaux, a Belgian obstetrician who noted a bony protuberance that hindered delivery. The term spondylolisthesis was coined by Kilian in 1854 from the Greek "spondylo" meaning vertebra and "olisthesis" meaning slip. In 1855 Robert of Koblenz noted the location of the defect in the pars but misidentified it as a subluxation of the facets. Lambi in the same year correctly identified the nature of the defect.

Classification

Wiltse, Newman, and Macnab have developed the following classification of spondylolisthesis and spondylolysis:

1. Dysplastic — in this type congenital abnormalities of the upper sacrum or the arch of L5 permit the slipping to occur.
2. Isthmic — the lesion is in the pars interarticularis. Three types can be recognized.
   a. Lytic — fatigue fracture of the pars interarticularis
   b. Elongated but intact pars interarticularis
   c. Acute fracture of the pars interarticularis
3. Degenerative — this lesion results from intersegmental instability of long duration.
4. Traumatic — this type results from fractures in areas of the bony hook other than pars interarticularis.
5. Pathologic — generalized or localized bone disease is present.

This classification is based on the cause of the defect as described by other authors.

Dysplastic spondylolisthesis results from congenital dysplasia of the upper sacrum. The sacrum is not strong enough to withstand the weight and stress; thus the pars and inferior facets of L5 are deformed. If the pars elongates, it becomes impossible to differentiate it roentgenographically from the isthmic elongated (type IIB) spondylolisthesis. If the pars separates, it becomes impossible to differentiate it roentgenographically from the isthmic lytic (type IIA) spondylolisthesis. Differentiation of this type must be made at surgery by the identification of an abnormal L5-S1 facet relationship. This type also is associated with sacral and neural arch deficiencies. It appears to be more common in girls than in boys and has a high familial tendency.

Isthmic spondylolisthesis is characterized by bilateral defects in the pars interarticularis of a vertebra and the resultant anterior displacement of the body of this vertebra and the superincumbent spine on the vertebra below. Alterations in the shape of the upper sacrum and L-5 are not present in this type. The lytic subtype A results from the separation or dissolution of the pars. It is a fatigue fracture rarely seen in patients younger than 5 years of age. The incidence of this type of spondylolisthesis increases from less than 1% in children 5 years of age to 4.5% in children 7 years of age. The remaining 0.8% to 1% increase occurs between the ages of 11 and 16 years, presumably because of stress fractures caused by athletic activity. Although this subtype has a strong hereditary tendency, it comprises only half of the dysplastic group. The elongated pars (subtype B) is believed to result from microfractures that heal with an elongated pars rather than from a lytic lesion. Acute pars fractures (subtype C) always result from significant trauma; these are rare and most frequently occur with spondylolysis rather than with spondylolisthesis.

Degenerative spondylolisthesis results from long-standing intersegmental instability, with remodeling of the articular processes at the level of the lesion. Multiple small compression fractures of the inferior articular process of the vertebra that slips forward also have been postulated as a cause. The articular proscesses change direction to a more horizontal position as the slip progresses. This lesion is four times more frequent in females than in males and is six times more likely to occur at L4-5 than at the adjacent levels. This lesion is not seen in patients younger than 40 years of age and does not slip any more than 33% without surgical intervention.

Traumatic spondylolisthesis results from an acute fracture in some other portion of the vertebra that allows a slip to occur. An isolated pars fracture is *not* seen with this lesion.

Pathologic spondylolisthesis is a slip that results from a local or generalized bone disease that allows the vertebra to slip forward. This type is extremely rare. It has been reported in Albers-Schönberg disease, arthrogryposis, Paget's disease, and syphilitic bone disease.

Etiology and Pathology

Normally the inferior articular facets of the fifth lumbar vertebra prevent the body of this vertebra from being displaced anteriorly on the sacrum. Hutton, Stott, and Cyron showed mathematically and Cyron, Hytton and Troup confirmed experimentally that repeated stress on the L5-S1 complex results in fracture of the pars. In addition, Rosenberg, Bargar, and Friedman reviewed the roentgenograms of a large number of patients who had never ambulated and noted no spondylolisthesis or

spondylolysis, further supporting the fatigue fracture hypothesis. Bilateral defects in the pars interarticularis make the neural arch a loose fragment, causing a loss in osseous continuity between the inferior articular facets and the body of the fifth lumbar vertebra, and allowing the body of the vertebra to gradually become displaced anteriorly. Hambley et al. produced a spondylolytic defect experimentally and demonstrated a significant decrease in bending stiffness in flexion and extension with this defect. Gill, Manning, and White have consistently found at the defects fibrocartilaginous masses that they believe cause pressure on the nerve roots. In addition, as the slip progresses, the foramen elongates and flattens, resulting in a foraminal stenosis. When the loose neural arch is removed, the reparative attempts by bone are evidenced in the hypertrophy of the cephalad pars stump. This overgrowth or elongation results in a "hook" that may rest directly on the nerve roots. This "hook" must be removed if the patient is to be relieved of his radicular complaints.

Terminology

Spondylolisthesis has been classified into grades I, II, III, or IV, depending on the severity of the displacement of the vertebra above on the vertebra below. In grade I the displacement is 25% or less of the anteroposterior diameter of the vertebra below; in grade II, between 25% and 50%; in grade III, between 50% and 75%; in grade IV, greater than 75%.

Boxall et al. in 1979 and later Wiltse and Winter have preferred standard measurement and terminology to describe the anterior displacement of the lumbar vertebra as a percentage of the widest anteroposterior diameter of the body below, usually the first sacral (Figs. 86-1 and 86-2, A). This method of slip measurement is much more sensitive in detecting the progression of slip over time.

The analysis of spondylolisthesis has resulted in numerous methods to quantify the problem and the resultant effects of surgery. Wiltse and Winter have catalogued these terms. *Sacral inclination* or sacral tilt refers to the relationship of the sacrum to the vertical plane (Fig. 86-2, B). This measurement requires an erect lateral roentgenogram, including the sacrum. *Sagittal rotation* expresses the angular relationship between the sacrum and the fifth lumbar vertebra (Fig. 86-3). It is also known as sagittal roll, lumbosacral kyphosis, or slip angle. *Rounding of the cranial border of the first sacral vertebra* is described as the percentage of the depth of the rounding compared to the width of the sacrum (Fig. 86-4). *Wedging of the olisthetic vertebra* is the percentage resulting from the division of the posterior body height to the anterior body height (Fig. 86-5). *The angle of lumbar lordosis* is calculated from a standing lateral roentgenogram. This is the angular relationship between a line drawn across the top of the first lumbar vertebra and a

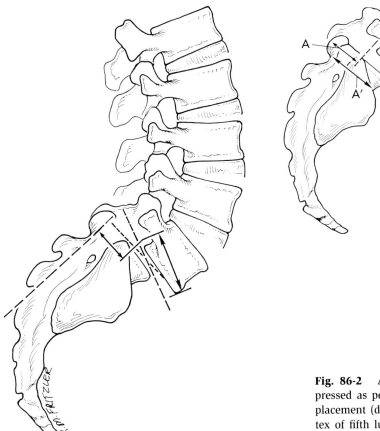

Fig. 86-1 Percentage of slipping calculated by measuring distance from line parallel to posterior portion of first sacral vertebral body to line parallel to posterior portion of body of fifth lumbar vertebra; anteroposterior dimension of fifth lumbar vertebra inferiorly is used to calculate percentage of slipping. (Redrawn from Boxall D, Bradford DS, Winter RB, and Moe JH: J Bone Joint Surg 61-A:479, 1979.)

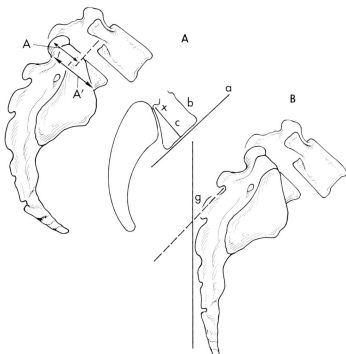

Fig. 86-2 **A,** Extent of anterior displacement or slip is expressed as percentage obtained by dividing *A,* amount of displacement (determined by relationship of posterior part of cortex of fifth lumbar vertebra to posterior part of cortex of first sacral vertebra), by *A1,* maximum anteroposterior diameter of first sacral vertebra, and multiplying by 100. Smaller drawing shows how to determine posteroinferior tip of body of fifth lumbar vertebra, which is often indistinct. Line *a* is drawn parallel to front of body of fifth lumbar vertebra. Line *b* is drawn perpendicular to line *a,* to posterosuperior tip of body of fifth lumbar vertebra. Line *c* is drawn parallel to line *b* and is exactly same length. Point at which line *c* intersects inferior body of fifth lumbar vertebra is point *x,* relative constant used in measuring percentage of slip. **B,** Sacral inclination, *g,* is determined by drawing line along posterior border of first sacral vertebra and measuring angle created by this line intersecting true vertical line. (From Wiltse LL and Winter RB: J Bone Joint Surg 65-A:768, 1983.)

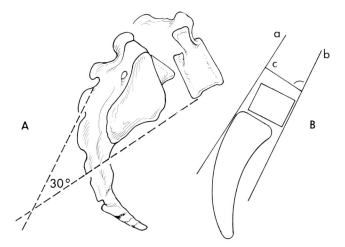

Fig. 86-3 **A,** Sagittal rotation expresses angular relationship between fifth lumbar and first sacral vertebrae. It is determined by extending line along anterior border of body of fifth lumbar vertebra until it intersects line drawn along posterior border of body of first sacral vertebra. **B,** Alternative method of measuring sagittal rotation, used when degree of olisthesis is small and lines *a* and *b* do not intersect; third line, *c,* is added perpendicular to line *a.* Lines *c* and *b* intersect to form angle of sagittal rotation. (From Wiltse LL and Winter RB: J Bone Joint Surg 65-A:768, 1983.)

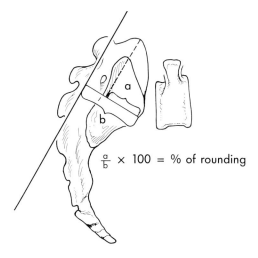

Fig. 86-4 Rounding of top of centrum of first sacral vertebra is expressed as relationship between lines *a* and *b,* drawn as shown. When multipled by 100, result is percentage of rounding of first sacral vertebra. (From Wiltse LL and Winter RB: J Bone Joint Surg 65-A:768, 1983.)

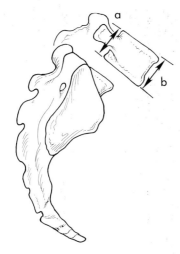

Fig. 86-5 Wedging of olisthetic vertebra is expressed as percentage determined by dividing line *a* by line *b*, drawn as shown, and multiplying by 100. (From Wiltse LL and Winter RB: J Bone Joint Surg 65-A:768, 1983.)

similar line drawn across the top of the fifth lumbar vertebra (Fig. 86-6). The *sacrohorizontal angle* is the angle formed by a line drawn across the top of the sacrum to the horizontal (Fig. 86-7). This measurement requires a standing lateral roentgenogram. It is also known as the sacral angle, sacrolumbosacral angle, lumbosacral angle,

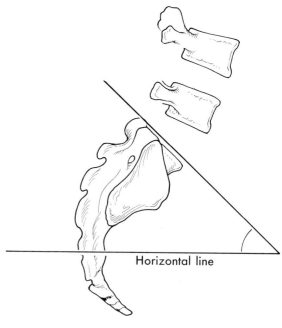

Fig. 86-7 Sacrohorizontal angle is angle between horizontal and line drawn across cranial border of body of first sacral vertebra. (From Wiltse LL and Winter RB: J Bone Joint Surg 65-A:768, 1983.)

and Ferguson's angle. The *lumbosacral joint angle* is the angle formed by the longitudinal axes of the bodies of the fifth lumbar vertebra and the sacrum (Fig. 86-8). The *lumbosacral angle* is the angle formed by the long axis of

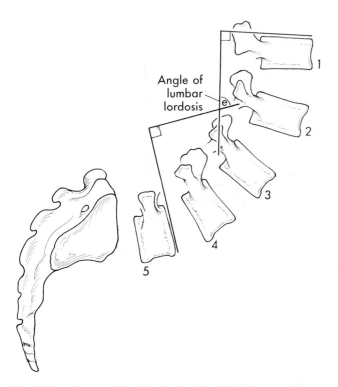

Fig. 86-6 Degree of lumbar lordosis is defined as angle *e*, as shown. With significant sagittal rotation of fifth lumbar vertebra, lordosis may extend well up into thoracic spine, in which case "total spinal lordosis" should be distinguished from "lumbar lordosis." (From Wiltse LL and Winter RB: J Bone Joint Surg 65-A:768, 1983.)

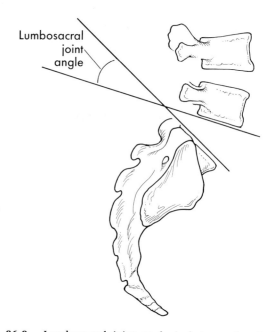

Fig. 86-8 Lumbosacral joint angle is between longitudinal axes of bodies of fifth lumbar and first sacral vertebrae. In normal spine, lines across caudal and cranial borders of centra of these vertebrae can be used. Angle between lines is lumbosacral joint angle. (From Wiltse LL and Winter RB: J Bone Joint Surg 65-A:768, 1983.)

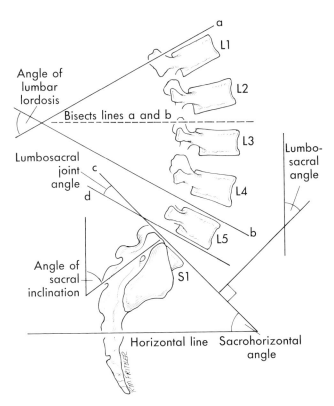

Fig. 86-9 To determine lumbosacral angle as defined here, longitudinal axis of lumbar spine must be established by bisecting angle of lumbar lordosis and then drawing line perpendicular to this. Angle formed by this line and longitudinal axis of first sacral vertebra is lumbosacral angle. For convenience, line is drawn across cranial border of first sacral vertebra. Line perpendicular to this is longitudinal axis of first sacral vertebra. (From Wiltse LL and Winter RB: J Bone Joint Surg 65-A:768, 1983.)

the lumbar part of the vertebral column and the sacrum (Fig. 86-9).

Spondylolisthesis in Children

Children may have either the dysplastic or isthmic type of spondylolisthesis. The former is secondary to congenital defects at the lumbosacral joint, and the latter usually results from a fatigue fracture combined with a hereditary element. Fredrickson et al. noted a strong association of spina bifida occulta with spondylolisthesis in children. They also noted a gradual increase in the incidence of spondylolysis from 4.4% at age 6 to 6% by adulthood.

Spondylolisthesis in children is characteristically different from that in adults. Periodic follow-up during the patient's growth is necessary to search for further slipping. If severe slipping occurs (75% to 100%), compensatory mechanisms of pelvic flexion with hyperlordosis of the spine above results in a kyphotic deformity at L5 and S1. This abnormal anatomy produces the peculiar gait because of tight hamstrings as described by Phalen and

Dickson. The flattening of the sacrum and loss of lumbar lordosis result in a forward rotation of the pelvis, which effectively decreases hip extension and thus adds to the distinctive posture and gait. Laurent and Einola reported an increase in displacement in 23 of 52 children and adolescents. According to them, displacement is usually slight before the age of 10 years, and progression of displacement is most common between the ages of 10 and 15 years. Fredrickson et al. noted the average progression of slip to be 14% to 16% before and during adolescence. During adulthood an increase in displacement is rare.

Further slippage will occur in more than 50% of those with a trapezoid-shaped L5 and a dome-shaped upper sacrum. Therefore those patients with the dysplastic type are more likely to need surgical stabilization. When slippage exceeds 25% and the child is symptomatic, or with slippage of 50% or more in the growing child regardless of symptoms, fusion should be performed. A bilateral lateral fusion from L4 to the sacrum is best for most children with spondylolisthesis.

Reduction of Spondylolisthesis

Reduction of severe spondylolisthesis has gained increasing attention since the publications of Jenkins in 1936 and Harris in 1951. Later Harrington proposed open reduction with instrumentation. The technique of Scaglietti, Frontino, and Bartolozzi of closed reduction and casting by traction and hyperextension allows the abnormal anatomy to accommodate the changes during 4 months before fusion is performed. Reduction of 75% to over 100% slips have been reported in relatively small numbers by several surgeons using both skeletal traction and several types of posterior instrumentation. Most techniques include an anterior interbody fusion and frequently also a posterolateral fusion. Bradford has used halo-femoral traction in bed for reduction, followed by a first-stage Gill procedure and decompression with posterolateral fusion (Fig. 86-10, *A*). Through an anterior transperitoneal approach, an interbody fusion with a strut graft or with iliac wedge grafts is performed as a second stage (Fig. 86-10, *B*). Because of the neurologic risk, Bradford and Gotfried recommend that posterior decompression be done first and the spine extended only after full length has been obtained. McPhee and O'Brien (1979) of England reported success with basically the same approach. More recently, Bradford, Dick and Schnebel, Herman and Pouliquen, Sijbrandij, and Steffee and Sitkowski have all reported series of patients treated by closed reduction or by operative reduction with and without instrumentation. Each of these series includes a small number of patients who developed neurologic deficits that not infrequently persisted. Most of these authors believe that significant improvements in posture, cosmesis, and pain relief after reduction outweigh the risk of neurologic injury. The danger of producing a neurologic deficit is ever present, and thus we agree with Wiltse that reduction of a spondylolisthesis must accomplish two objectives to justify the added danger and effort: (1) extension of the flat buttocks to improve cosmesis, and (2) lengthening of the torso.

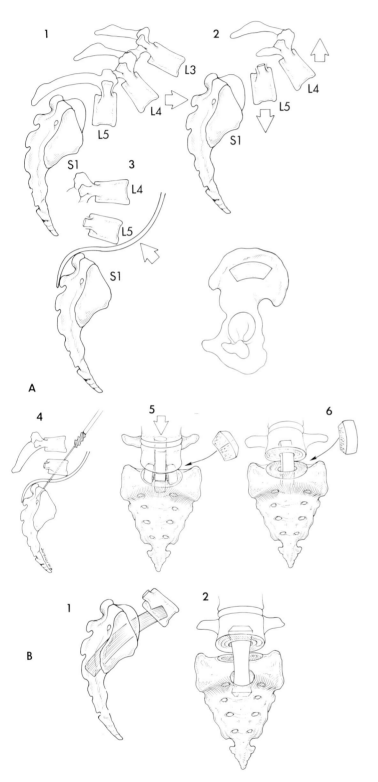

Fig. 86-10 Steps in technique of reduction of spondylolisthesis by combined posterior and anterior approach. (Redrawn from Bradford DS: Spine 4:423, 1979.)

Most patients will do well with an in situ fusion. Peek et al. and Freeman and Donati reported high rates of fusion, pain relief, and improvements in ambulation and cosmesis in children and adults after in situ fusion of high-grade spondylolisthesis. They noted improvement in the preoperative neurologic status, and no neurologic deficits resulted from the in situ fusion. Sixteen patients with cauda equina syndrome after in situ fusion for high-grade spondylolisthesis, with and without concomitant decompression, have been reported by Maurice and Morley and Schoenecker et al. Schoenecker et al. noted that some of their 12 patients had preoperative sacral nerve dysfunction, and they suggested that decompression be combined with the fusion in such patients. Immediate decompression, including resection of the posterior dome of the sacrum, along with reduction and instrumentation when possible, is their suggested treatment for this complication.

Symptoms and Signs in Adults

In spondylolysis symptoms are often absent, and the defects are then discovered only incidentally on roentgenograms made for other purposes. In spondylolisthesis injury may aggravate any symptoms, but rarely does a single injury cause symptoms in a patient who previously had none. Usually symptoms begin insidiously during the second or third decade as an intermittent dull ache in the lower back, present with increasing frequency during walking and standing. Later, pain may develop in the buttocks and thighs, and still later unilateral sciatica may develop. Unilateral sciatica accompanied by sensory or motor disturbances may be caused by protrusion of an intervertebral disc, most often the one between L4 and L5. In explorations of the lumbar spine in 45 patients with spondylolisthesis, Laurent found a protruded disc in only 2 (about 4%). However, Henderson, in a review of 216 patients operated on for spondylolisthesis, reported that of 157 in whom the nerve roots were explored, a definitely abnormal intervertebral disc was found in 46 (about 29%). According to Gill, Manning, and White, the L5 and S1 nerve roots are compressed by or attached by adhesions to the fibrocartilaginous mass at the defects in the pars interarticularis, and consequently movement of the loose laminae may irritate them. Hamstring spasm, flattening of the back, and a spinous process step-off also may be present. Claudication symptoms may signal the development of lateral recess stenosis, foraminal stenosis, or far-out compression of the L5 root by pressure between a large L5 transverse process and the sacrum.

Lumbosacral spondylolisthesis associated with scoliosis presents special problems. When it is associated with a major thoracic curve, there are two treatments with separate indications: the spondylolisthesis should be fused on the basis of symptom severity, and the thoracic curve should be treated as required by its severity. When the spondylolisthesis is associated with a thoracolumbar or lumbar curve, the lumbosacral joint must be fused in a corrected position.

Evaluation

Plain roentgenograms are the best way to make the diagnosis of spondylolisthesis or spondylolysis. Standing roentgenograms in spondylolisthesis have been advised by Lowe et al. Twenty-six percent of their group of 50 patients showed increased displacement on standing. Therefore an apparent spondylolysis in recumbent roentgenograms may be revealed as a spondylolisthesis in standing roentgenograms. Defects in the pars are best defined by oblique views of the lumbar spine. Tomography is most useful in the identification of facet fractures and obscure pars defects. Bone scans are helpful in identifying acute fractures and pseudarthrosis in old spinal fusions. Computerized axial tomographic (CAT) scans are not as effective in identifying spondylolisthesis or spondylolysis as plain films are, but multiplanar CAT scans are helpful. The sagittal and coronal views allow the identification of nerve root compression by soft tissue and bone inside and outside the canal. Myelography may be necessary to rule out intraspinal problems, but alone it adds little to the evaluation of spondylolisthesis and spondylolysis. Myelography followed by multiplanar CAT scans offers the greatest assistance in identifying the intraspinal and extraspinal effects of spondylolisthesis that may be of surgical significance. Magnetic resonance imaging (MRI) is similar to postmyelogram multiplanar CT. This technique also allows the evaluation of disc degeneration, which may be helpful in determining the upper extremes of fusion. Unfortunately, MRI does not clearly delineate all the soft tissues.

Treatment

Surgery is not always necessary in spondylolisthesis. Often restriction of the patient's activities, spinal and abdominal muscular rehabilitation, and other conservative measures, including the intermittent use of a rigid back brace, are sufficient. Bell, Ehrlich, and Zaleske reported that 23 patients treated an average of 25 months in antilordodic braces were pain free with decreased lumbar lordosis. Gramse, Sinaki, and Ilstrup reported significant clinical improvement in patients treated with flexion exercises, whereas those treated with extension exercises did not improve. In general, the younger the patient with painful spondylolisthesis, the more definite is the indication for surgery, and the more likely is surgery to be successful. Persistent pain in the lower back, buttocks, and thighs without sciatica is often sufficient to incapacitate a laborer for heavy work or a homemaker for chores and thus to be an indication for surgery. For sedentary workers, on the other hand, sciatica is more often the reason for surgery because any less severe pain in the lower

back and buttocks may not be disabling. For adolescents severe hamstring tightness is often an indication for fusion; for them progression of displacement is another indication for surgery. In general, about 20% of patients with symptomatic spondylolisthesis require surgery.

Patient selection is extremely important in the use of decompression or fusion in adults with spondylolisthesis. Hanley and Levy noted that satisfactory results were significantly fewer in compensation cases (39%), patients with radicular symptoms (50%), and smokers (48%). Pseudarthrosis correlated with poor results. An educational level of less than the twelfth grade also is related to a poor prognosis for pain relief and return to work.

FUSION. Opinions vary as to the proper operation in spondylolisthesis. Fixation of the unstable spine by posterolateral fusion is the treatment that most surgeons prefer. A successful fusion in situ usually relieves symptoms enough to allow the patient to work. Posterior rather than anterior fusion is preferred by most because its technique is more flexible; it permits exploration of the defects, nerve roots, and intervertebral discs. In addition, it is relatively safe. Spinal fusion should not be undertaken lightly, however, because it is more difficult to perform in spondylolisthesis than in other conditions. The fusion mass should extend as far proximally and distally as necessary to stabilize the affected vertebrae and interspaces. In the absence of sciatica and with an absolutely normal L4 disc and joint, fusion between L5 and S1 is sufficient but is rarely done. However, when the neural arch of L5 has been excised or when both the fourth and fifth interspaces have been explored to relieve sciatica, the fusion should extend from L4 to S1. In most instances it should extend over this longer area, that is, from L4 to S1. Details of technique vary with the preference of the surgeon. Several techniques for spinal fusion are described in this chapter and in Chapter 81. When symptoms of pressure on nerve roots are present, the fifth lumbar and first sacral roots should be inspected, and any protruding intervertebral discs and all fibrocartilaginous tissue about them should be excised before posterior fusion is performed, because otherwise radiating pain may persist even after the fusion becomes solid. The pedicle may require excision if the nerve root angulates acutely around it. When symptoms of nerve root compression are absent, posterior fusion with or without excising the loose neural arch of L5 is reasonable.

The rate of fusion in spondylolisthesis varies considerably. Prothero, Parkes, and Stinchfield reported a 26% pseudarthrosis rate after fusions for spondylolisthesis and noted that the pseudarthrosis rate after bilateral lateral fusion technique was 10%. The rate of pseudarthrosis also increases as the number of levels fused increases. The use of bone stimulators and internal fixation has been advocated by some to decrease the incidence of pseudarthrosis.

Posterolateral or bilateral lateral fusion using the tech-

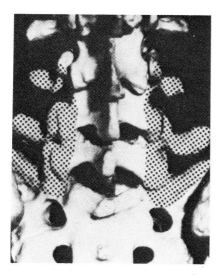

Fig. 86-11 Intertransverse fusion for spondylolisthesis. Stippled area indicates bed prepared for grafting. (From Macnab I and Dall D: J Bone Joint Surg 53-B:628, 1971.)

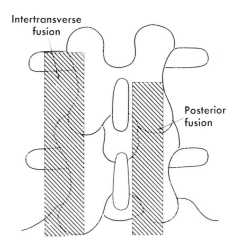

Fig. 86-12 Comparison of beds prepared for intertransverse and posterior fusions. (From Macnab I and Dall D: J Bone Joint Surg 53-B:628, 1971.)

nique of Watkins (Chapter 81) or a modification of it, with or without excision of the loose neural arch of L5, is now often used in spondylolisthesis. Rombold reported successful fusion in 96% of 73 patients treated by posterolateral fusion and resection of the arch. A high rate of successful fusion by the posterolateral technique has also been reported by Watkins, Wiltse, and others. In their study of the blood supply of the lumbar spine as applied to intertransverse fusion, Macnab and Dall showed a lower pseudarthrosis rate than with other methods in a group with degenerative disc disease. They think that the intertransverse technique has special value in the treatment of spondylolisthesis, since it is easily limited to one segment, and that it is the technique of choice for stabilization after extensive posterior decompression and foraminotomy. According to them, there are three reasons for a lower incidence of pseudarthrosis: (1) the graft bed includes the lateral aspects of the superior articular facets, the pars interarticularis, and the transverse process as a continuous raw bony surface (Fig. 86-11); (2) the zygoapophyseal joints are included in the fusion mass; and (3) because the graft extends to the transverse process of the most superior vertebra, this vertebral segment is more firmly incorporated in the fusion mass than with the standard posterior technique, in which the graft extends only to the spinous process and laminae of the most superior vertebra (Fig. 86-12). Kiviluoto et al. in Helsinki reported solid fusion in 78 of 80 adolescents and adults after posterolateral arthrodesis; Dawson, Lotysch, and Urist in Los Angeles reported 92% successful fusion, and Boccanera et al. in Bologna found that posterolateral fusion produced a high percentage of success with low risk.

Several surgeons have reported successful interbody fusion through either an anterior or a posterior approach in spondylolisthesis. The anterior technique of Freebody, Bendall, and Taylor has been highly successful in their

hands, but we have had no experience with it (Fig. 86-13). When the fifth lumbar vertebra is so severely displaced on the sacrum that the fifth interspace cannot be exposed and curetted, Kellogg Speed's technique of

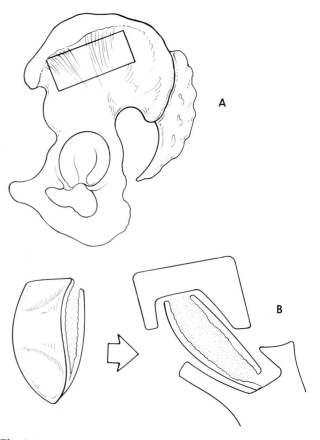

Fig. 86-13 Freebody, Bendall, and Taylor technique for anterior interbody fusion in lower lumbar spine for spondylolisthesis. **A,** Full-thickness graft of iliac bone, centered over lateral convexity, is removed. **B,** Shaped graft, convex anteriorly, is slotted in adjacent vertebral bodies. (Redrawn from Freebody D, Bendall R, and Taylor RD: J Bone Joint Surg 53-B:617, 1971.)

anterior fusion (p. 3835), in which a graft is inserted through the fifth lumbar vertebra and into the sacrum, has been recommended. Recently modifications of this technique in combination with posterior arthrodesis, instrumentation, or both have been used by spine surgeons such as DeWald et al., Bradford et al. and others.

In 1955, Gill, Manning, and White recommended that both the loose neural arch and the dense fibrocartilaginous tissue at the defects in the pars interarticulares be excised to free the fifth lumbar and first sacral nerve roots and to thus relieve pain without spinal fusion. They pointed out that on motion of the spine, especially extension, the proximal border of the loose neural arch might tilt anteriorly and press on the fifth lumbar roots or by this tilting stretch the first sacral roots. In 14 patients who before surgery had back pain, radiating pain, and positive neurologic signs and who had been followed after surgery from 16 to 56 months, only three had occasional mild back pain. The neurologic findings had completely disappeared in all but two, and all patients had been able to return to their former occupations. This treatment was supported in 1957 by the experience of King, Baker, and McHolick; they reported that, of 29 patients in whom only the loose neural arch had been excised, the nerve roots had been explored, and fusion had not been performed, only three had any significant recurrence of pain. In 1962 Gill and White reported further results of the operation they had recommended in 1955; they followed 43 patients ages 14 to 57 years for 4 months to about 12 years (average about 5 years). Although some increase in anterior displacement occurred in 19, they rated the result as excellent (the patient asymptomatic) in 18, good in 12, and fair in 7; or, to put it another way, in a total of 37 or 86.1% they considered the result satisfactory, and in 13.9% a failure. They state that any increase in displacement after surgery is self-limiting, does not necessarily cause symptoms, and in their experience is not related to excision of the loose neural arch. A Gill procedure without fusion should not be performed in children with spondylolisthesis. Further slipping following the procedure has been observed by us and other investigators.

Numerous methods of internal fixation have been used to enhance the fusion or repair the spondylolysis or spondylolisthesis defect. Buck described a method of repair of the pars defect with a bone screw directed across the defect from the inferior facet region to the superior region and augmented with a bone graft to the lesion. He reported 16 fusions with one failure and two reoperations. Pedersen and Hagen more recently reported 83% satisfactory results in 18 patients using the Buck method. Bradford and Iza reported 80% excellent results and 90% fusion in 22 patients treated with tension band wiring around the transverse process of the affected vertebra and directed around the spinous process of that vertebra (Fig. 86-14). Hambley et al. reported a 92% success rate and a 100% fusion rate in a series of 13 patients with spondylolysis or minimal spondylolisthesis treated with a similar tension band wiring technique.

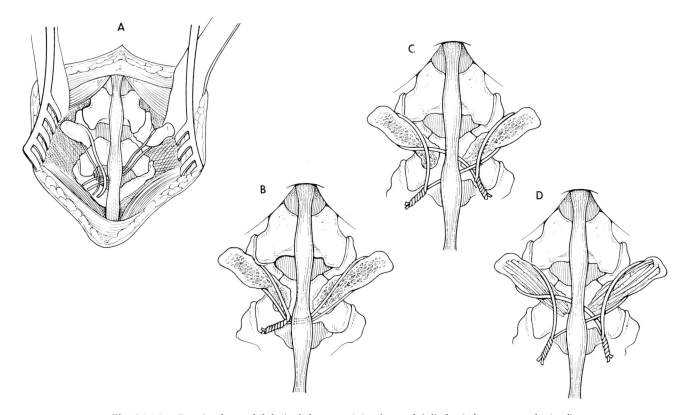

Fig. 86-14   Repair of spondylolytic defect or minimal spondylolisthesis by segmental wire fixation and bone grafting. (Redrawn from Bradford DS and Iza J: Spine 10:673, 1985.)

Degenerative spondylolisthesis is a special problem. According to Newman, degenerative spondylolisthesis produces the symptoms of stenosis of either the canal or the lateral recesses. Surgical management involves decompression of the appropriate roots by laminectomy. Foraminotomy may also be necessary, but extensive excision of the neural arch may result in further spinal instability, in which case the addition of a spinal fusion would be advisable. Cauchoix, Benoist, and Chassaing reported immediate postoperative relief in 25 of 26 patients after this technique. Follow-up (average 3¼ years) showed 22 still leading a normal life. Four patients developed a secondary slip. Herron and Trippi reported the results of decompression only for the spinal stenosis variants occurring with degenerative spondylolisthesis. They rated the results in all but four of their 26 patients as good. They did note that postoperative progression of the slip was no more than 4 mm. Fitzgerald and Newman suggested that fusion should be used when decompression results in destabilization of the spine or when the patient is young.

Wiltse and Hutchinson have outlined the following reasonable policy for the surgical treatment of spondylolisthesis:

1. For most patients with backache and little if any leg pain, a bilateral posterolateral fusion from L4 to S1 is performed; only when there are signs of nerve root compression is the loose neural arch of L5 excised and the affected root traced into the soft tissues.
2. For young adults with little if any leg pain, with minimal displacement of L5, and with large transverse processes of L5, a bilateral posterolateral fusion from L5 to S1 is performed through one or two skin incisions but using bilateral muscle splitting fascial incisions (Chapter 81).
3. For young adults with signs of nerve root compression, with minimal anterior displacement of L5, and with large transverse processes of L5, the loose neural arch is excised, and a bilateral posterolateral fusion from L5 to the sacrum is performed through a midline incision.
4. For patients with failure of previous posterior fusion, an anterior fusion through a left extraperitoneal approach is performed.
5. For patients over 60 years of age with good stability of the L5 vertebral body but with signs and symptoms of nerve root compression, the loose neural arch is excised, care being taken to avoid traumatizing the nerve roots; fusion is omitted.

Thus opinions differ as to whether spinal fusion is necessary or whether simply excising the loose neural arch and any protruded intervertebral discs and freeing the nerve roots are sufficient. Although we have treated a few patients surgically without arthrodesing the spine, we still believe that spinal fusion is indicated after any exploration of the nerve roots in spondylolisthesis.

Fusion in children and adolescents. Posterolateral and posterior fusion in situ for spondylolisthesis in children and adolescents is recommended by many surgeons, including Sherman, Rosenthal, and Hall, and Stanton, Meehan, and Lovell. Pain, other symptoms, and slipping of 50% or greater are consistent indicators for surgical treatment. Stanton et al. recommended bed rest and a pantaloon cast to prevent further slipping postoperatively, but they are in the minority; in contrast, Sherman et al. stated that additional slipping was not related to postoperative ambulation.

Harris and Weinstein compared the results of high-grade slips treated with and without fusion. Of 11 patients treated nonoperatively, 36% were asymptomatic, and 55% had mild symptoms; in 22 patients treated operatively, 57% were asymptomatic, and 38% had mild symptoms. They concluded that, with an 18-year average follow-up, there was little difference between the results of operative and nonoperative treatment. Pseudarthrosis did not affect the results. Seitsalo et al. reported a similar comparison of 56 patients. They also noted no difference in the operated and unoperated patients with regard to pain. In their series girls had more severe displacement and earlier worsening of the deformity than did boys.

Verbiest of the Netherlands described an extensive anterior fusion, including a strut-graft after a posterior laminectomy and foraminotomy without reduction in adolescents with 100% slips. As in all reports of in situ fusion, neurologic complications are rare, and this is stressed.

Sevastikoglou, Spangfort, and Aaro from Stockholm reported nine patients on whom an extraperitoneal anterior interbody fusion was done also without reduction. Solid fusion and relief of symptoms were obtained in all.

Ohki et al. of Japan and Balderston and Bradford of Minneapolis have used posterior traction wires through the spinous processes to attach to tightening devices (on a cast or a halo-pelvic traction apparatus) to pull the lower lumbar vertebrae into place before fusion.

Sijbrandij of the Netherlands has reduced five severe slips with posterior devices, using screws inserted into the lumbar vertebrae to pull them into a reduced position.

Attempts at reduction of severe slips carry a risk of neurologic deficit whether traction or instrumentation is being used. Only skillful and experienced spinal surgeons should attempt procedures of this magnitude in medical centers equipped for maximum support.

Bilateral lateral fusion

■ *TECHNIQUE (WILTSE, MODIFIED).* Induce anesthesia and insert an endotracheal tube, Foley catheter, and arterial intravenous line as indicated by the clinical status of the patient. Place the patient on a spinal frame that allows the abdomen to hang free. Make a midline skin incision extending one spinous process above and one below the levels to be fused.

Elevate the subcutaneous tissue off the fascia for a distance of 3 to 4 fingerbreadths bilaterally; include exposure of the posterosuperior iliac crest on the side to be used for the bone graft donor site. Make a fascial incision 2 fingerbreadths lateral to the midline, extending over the area to be fused. Bluntly dissect the paraspinal muscles down to the facet joint capsules. Carry the dissection down to the transverse processes to be fused. Clean the muscle subperiosteally to expose the transverse process and intertransverse ligament. Denude the facet joints by removing the fascia over them and then stripping them clean by subperiosteal dissection. Carry the dissection around the pars articularis. Prepare the opposite side in a similar manner. Do not denude the superior facets of the most cephalad level to be fused.

Obtain the bone graft from the donor site before denuding the recipient site. Incise the fascia over the iliac crest with sharp or electocautery dissection. Carry the dissection from the posterosuperior iliac spine to about 3 to 4 cm lateral on the iliac crest. Strip the gluteal musculature from the crest laterally. Remove a corticocancellous bone graft from the exposed portions of the crest down to the inner table. Close the wound over closed suction drainage.

Prepare the recipient site for grafting by first placing cortico-cancellous strips beneath the transverse processes, bridging the interspinous ligament. Place the grafts with the cortical side toward the ligament. Remove all cartilage from the facets to be fused. Place cancellous bone grafts in the facet defects. Denude all areas of exposed bone, including the ala of the sacrum, the transverse processes, and the exposed pars interarticularis. Carefully pack the remaining bone in the gutters bilaterally from the pars interarticularis to the tips of the transverse processes.

Close the wound in layers. Place closed suction drains in the subcutaneous tissue bilaterally.

AFTERTREATMENT. The patient is allowed to be up the next day wearing a rigid lumbosacral brace but is strongly advised to refrain from smoking until the fusion is solid. Asprin and nonsteroidal medication are discontinued, and bracing is continued until the fusion is solid.

Modifications of bilateral lateral fusion. Spinal decompression can be performed through a midline exposure of the spine over the areas to be decompressed. This decompression is closed before starting the lateral approach.

Pedicle screw instrumentation to improve the fusion rate is rapidly increasing in popularity. This instrumentation is especially important if a reduction has been performed. The pedicles usually are identified after the pri-

mary exposure is complete. They may be identified at the point formed by the intersection of an imaginary line bisecting the transverse process and another line bisecting the superior facet. This area is denuded, and the pedicle is probed with special instruments or guide wires. The pedicles are then tapped to receive the screws after the postition of the probes or guide wires has been confirmed by roentgenograms. The placement of the screws and plates varies with the type of instrumentation used. Pedicle screw instrumentation has not yet been approved by the FDA for use in the spine.

Posterior lumbar interbody fusion. A posterior lumbar interbody fusion method was devised by Cloward in 1943 and has been used extensively by him and others for treatment of spondylolisthesis. It is best suited for displacements of grades I and II and generally unsuited for displacements of grade III or higher unless reduction is accomplished by posterior Harrington or similar instrumentation as advocated by Vidal et al. in France. Bohlman and Cook of Cleveland and Takeda of Japan combine the posterior interbody fusion with other posterior fusion techniques: Bohlman and Cook, a posterolateral fusion, and Takeda, a Bosworth H-graft fusion. Retraction of nerve roots and the dural sac is necessary to insert the grafts, and cauda equina deficits are reported (Cloward reported 4% incidence of footdrop), although they usually are not permanent. This technique frequently requires internal fixation methods to prevent displacement of the graft and further slip. Cloward uses spinous process wiring. Steffee and Sitkowski and others suggest the use of pedicle screws and plates for this type of fixation.

Anterior lumbar interbody fusion

■ *TECHNIQUE (SPEED).* Make a midline incision from the umbilicus to the pubis and fully expose the sacral promontory. Then raise the foot of the table and pack the intestines out of the way. Palpate the relations of the fifth lumbar vertera with the sacrum and confirm the roentgenographic findings. If the bifurcation of the aorta is low, retract it with the left common iliac vein. Just to the right of the midline and avoiding the midsacral nerve and artery and the sympathetic ganglia, incise the peritoneum from the fourth lumbar interspace to the sacrum. Then determine the proper angle and depth for a drill to be inserted to pass obliquely through the body of the fifth lumbar vertebra and into the sacrum; with the patient supine, the direction is almost perpendicular to the floor. Then pass a large drill through the fifth lumbar vertebra and into the sacrum; as the drill passes from the body of the fifth lumbar vertebra and into the intervertebral space, advancing the drill is easier until the body of the sacrum is reached, when it becomes more difficult. From the tibia take a cortical graft and insert it into the hole,

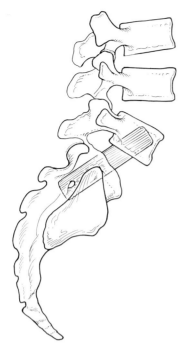

Fig. 86-15 Kellogg Speed anterior fusion for spondylolisthesis. (Redrawn from Speed K: Arch Surg 37:715, 1983.)

transfixing the fifth lumbar vertebra to the sacrum (Fig. 86-15).

AFTERTREATMENT. The patient is placed on a moderately firm bed that permits nursing care without flexing the spine. At 8 weeks a rigid back brace is fitted, and the patient is allowed up.

Gill procedure

■ *TECHNIQUE (GILL ET AL.).* Place the patient prone on the operating table and through a midline incision expose subperiosteally the spinous processes of the fourth and fifth lumbar and the first sacral vertebrae (Fig. 86-16, *A).* Demonstrate the mobility of the fifth lumbar neural arch and with a rongeur resect the spinous processes of all three vertebrae (Fig. 86-16, *B).* Also with a rongeur resect the middle part of the loose fifth lumbar neural arch (Fig. 86-16, *C).* Then bite away the inferior aspect of the laminae of the fourth lumbar vertebra until the ligamentum flavum has been freed. By sharp dissection excise the ligamentum flavum from between the fourth and fifth vertebrae. Again by sharp dissection excise on one side the lateral part of the loose fifth lumbar arch, freeing it from its articulation with the sacrum and from the tissues in the defect in the pars interarticularis (Fig. 86-16, *E);* dissect close to bone to avoid damaging the fifth lumbar nerve root. Next retract this root superiorly and medially. Carefully dissect it from the fibrocartilaginous tissue and free it laterally until it passes through the intervertebral foramen (Fig. 86-16, *F* and *G).* Resect bone from the

pedicle as necessary to free the root. Then examine the exposed fourth and fifth lumbar discs and, if indicated, excise one or both. Carry out the same procedure on the opposite side.

AFTERTREATMENT. No support is necessary at any time after surgery. The patient is encouraged to move about in bed as desired and to sit as soon as he is able. At 3 days walking is allowed, and straight leg raising exercises are begun. If by the fifth day straight leg raising is restricted to less than 75 degrees, a solution of 0.2% procaine or 0.2% lidocaine is injected extradurally through the caudal foramen. The exercises are then continued.

SPINAL STENOSIS

Before the development of roentgenograms, there were scattered reports of paralysis caused by narrowing of the spinal canal. The first verifiable report of lumbar spinal stenosis relieved by two-level laminectomy was that of Sachs and Fraenkel in 1900. Bailey and Casamajor in 1911 and Elsberg in 1913 wrote similar adequate descriptions of the symptoms, pathologic findings, and relief following surgery.The syndrome was not widely diagnosed until Verbiest in 1954 described the classic findings of middle-aged and older adults with back and lower extremity pain precipitated by standing and walking and aggravated by hyperextension. He delineated congenital narrowing of the spinal canal as a contributing factor in many and the secondary development of degenerative changes to further narrow the lumbar canal and precipitate symptoms. Myelographic block in the midlumbar region with the characteristic degenerative hypertrophic changes about the discs, facets, and ligamentous structures was described in detail. A subsequent article by Verbiest on lumbar spondylosis documented detailed measurements of the spinal canal obtained during surgery with an appropriate instrument for obtaining these operative measurements. Since that time the syndrome has been well recognized, and numerous well-documented series have been reported. An excellent four-part review of the entire topic was published by Ehni et al. in 1969.

Classification

Spinal stenosis can be categorized according to the anatomic area of the spine affected, the region of each vertebral segment affected, and the specific pathologic entity involved (Table 86-1). Stenosis can be generalized or localized to specific anatomic areas of the cervical, thoracic, or lumbar spine. It is most common in the lumbar region, but cervical stenosis is recognized. It has been rarely reported in the thoracic spine. Spinal stenosis can be localized, affecting only one segment or a portion of one segment. The most recent terminology for regional

Fig. 86-16 Operation of Gill, Manning, and White for spondylolisthesis (see text). (From Gill GG, Manning JG, and White HL: J Bone Joint Surg 37-A:493, 1955.)

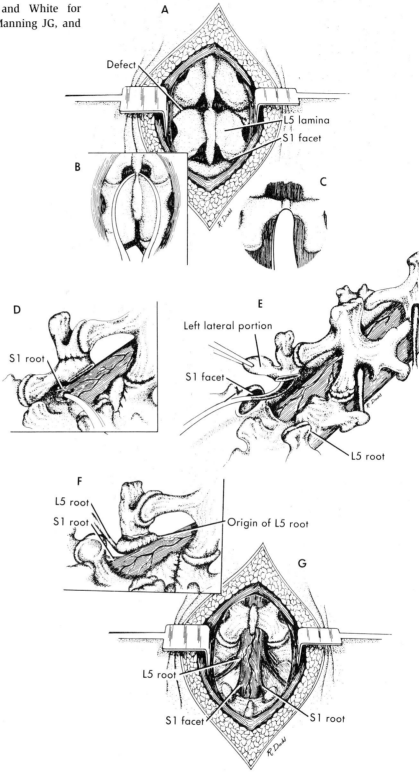

localized stenosis is central, lateral recess, foraminal, and far-out. This terminology deals primarily with the regional area of root compression at each vertebral level. It is most frequently used to describe lumbar spinal stenosis, but it can be applied to all areas of the spine. Finally, spinal stenosis can be categorized by the pathologic process.

Arnoldi et al. proposed a classification scheme for the lumbar spine based on pathologic processes (see Box). This classification separates spinal stenosis into congenital stenosis and acquired stenosis. Congenital stenosis is subdivided into achondroplastic and idiopathic forms. Acquired stenosis is subdivided into degenerative, com-

Table 86-1 Classification of spinal stenosis

ANATOMIC

Anatomic area	Anatomic region (local segment)
Cervical	Central
	Foraminal
Thoracic	Central
Lumbar	Central
	Lateral recess
	Foraminal
	Extraforaminal (far-out)

PATHOLOGIC

Congenital
  Achondroplastic (dwarfism)
  Congenital forms of spondylolisthesis
  Scoliosis
  Kyphosis
  Idiopathis
Degenerative & inflammatory
  Osteoarthritis
  Inflammatory arthritis
  Diffuse idiopathic skeletal hyperostosis (DISH)
  Scoliosis
  Kyphosis
  Degenerative forms of spondylolisthesis
Metabolic
  Paget's disease
  Fluorosis

CLASSIFICATION OF SPINAL STENOSIS BASED ON SPINAL PROCESSES

 I. Congenital-developmental stenosis
    A. Idiopathic
    B. Achondroplastic
 II. Acquired stenosis
    A. Degenerative
       1. Central portion of spinal canal
       2. Peripheral portion of canal
          a. Lateral recess
          b. Foraminal
    B. Combined
       Any combination of all types
    C. Spondylolisthetic/spondylolytic
       May also include lateral recess, foraminal and far-out forms
    D. Iatrogenic
       1. Postlaminectomy
       2. Postfusion (anterior or posterior)
    E. Post-traumatic, late changes
    F. Miscellaneous (metabolic/inflammatory)
       1. Paget's disease
       2. Fluorosis
       3. Forester's disease
       4. DISH

MODIFIERS

 I. Segmental disease
 II. Generalized disease

Adapted from Arnoldi CC, et al: Clin Orthop 115:4, 1976.

bined, spondylolisthetic or spondylolytic, iatrogenic, post-traumatic, and miscellaneous groups. Although this classification was developed for the lumbar spine, it can be applied to all other areas of the spine as well. The anatomic and pathologic classification of spinal stenosis is helpful in the proper selection of both treatment modality and prognosis. Tile et al. added segmental and generalized disease and found that patients with the generalized type tended to have less relief of pain after surgery than did those with the segmental type.

The most common type of spinal stenosis is caused by degenerative arthritis of the spine, including Forestier's syndrome, ankylosing disease of the spine characterized by hyperostosis, and spinal rigidity in elderly patients. Congenital forms caused by such disorders as achondroplasia and congenital spondylolisthesis are much less frequent. Finally, other processes such as Paget's disease, fluorosis, kyphosis, scoliosis, and fracture with canal narrowing have been reported to result in spinal stenosis. Hypertrophy and ossification of the posterior longitudinal ligament in the cervical spine (diffuse idiopathic skeletal hyperostosis [DISH] syndrome) is another example of a disease that may result in an acquired form of spinal stenosis. This disease is usually confined to the cervical spine.

Direct anatomic measurement of dried human spines has been reported by several authors. Most recently,

Eisenstein in 1977 reported a direct analysis of spinal canal measurements in 433 dried spines. In his study the lower limit of the midsagittal diameter was 15 mm and of the transverse diameter 20 mm. This measurement technique does not include the most common cause of stenosis: degenerative bulging of the annulus of the disc combined with hypertophy of the facets and ligamentum flavum. Anatomic measurements therefore are only rough indicators of spinal narrowing.

The radiographic identification and confirmation of lumbar spinal stenosis has improved with the development of new imaging techniques. Initially only central spinal stenosis was recognized. Canal narrowing to 10 mm was considered diagnostic. This could be measured using roentgenograms or preferably myelography. In 1985 Schonstrom, Bolender, and Spengler reported a comparison of the identification of central spinal stenosis with anteroposterior canal measurement by computed tomography to the measurement of the dural sac with myelography in patients undergoing surgery for spinal stenosis. They found no correlation between the transverse area of the bony canal in normal patients and patients with spinal stenosis. A dural sac transverse area of 100 mm^2 or less did correlate with symptomatic spinal

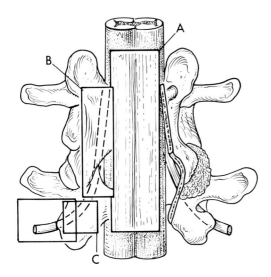

Fig. 86-17 Three dimensional illustration of segmental stenoses. **A,** Anatomic; **B,** segmental; **C,** pathologic. (Redrawn from Ciric I, Mikhael MA, Tarkington JA, and Vic NA: J Neurosurg 53:433, 1980.)

stenosis. This method allows the inclusion of soft tissue in the determination of spinal stenosis. The analysis of this area can be easily and relatively inexpensively calculated using standard personal computers.

REGIONAL CLASSIFICATION. Ciric et al. and others have used computed tomography to further define lateral recess stenosis and foraminal stenosis. These types of stenosis are rarely identified with myelography. The lateral recess is anatomically the area bordered laterally by the pedicle, posteriorly by the superior articular facet, and anteriorly by the posterolateral surface of the vertebral body and the adjacent intervertebral disc. The superior and rostral border of the corresponding pedicle is the narrowest portion of the lateral recess. Measurement of the recess in this area using the tomographic cross section is usually 5 mm or greater in normal patients, but in symptomatic patients the diagnosis is confirmed if the height is 2 mm or less (Fig. 86-17). The foramen is the area of the spine bordered by the inferior edge of the pedicle cephalad, the pars interarticularis with the associated inferior articular facet and the superior articular facet from the lower segment dorsally, the superior edge of the pedicle of the next lower vertebra caudally, and the vertebral body and disc ventrally. This area can rarely be seen with myelography. Standard computed tomography in the cross-sectional mode can suggest narrowing. This is suggested when the foraminal space immediately after the pedicle cut is only present for one or two more cuts (provided the cuts are close together). The best way to appreciate foraminal narrowing is to reformat the lumbar scan. This technique can create sagittal views through the pedicles and structures situated laterally. MRI also allows excellent evaluation of all forms of

stenosis, especially foraminal stenosis, and is an excellent method of confirming the diagnosis of degenerative disease when infection or tumor is suspected.

Wiltse et al. have described a far-out compression of the root seen predominantly in spondylolisthesis when the root is compressed by a large L5 transverse process subluxed below the root and pressing the root against the ala of the sacrum. This diagnosis is best confirmed with a reformatted computed tomography scan with coronal cuts (Fig. 86-18).

PATHOLOGIC CLASSIFICATION. Differentiation between the pathologic processes causing spinal stenosis is relatively simple. Congenital spinal stenosis is usually central. In achondroplasia the canal is narrowed in both the anteroposterior measurement (pedicle height) and lateral width (distance between the pedicles) in addition to showing other stigmata of achondroplasia. Idiopathic congenital narrowing usually involves one dimension of canal measurement, and the patient is otherwise normal.

Acquired forms of spinal stenosis are caused by degenerative arthritis, spondylolisthesis, post-traumatic deformity, and other disease processes. Degenerative forms of stenosis are usually localized to the facet joints, with additional evidence of roentgenographically visible changes in the joints. Frequently these abnormalities are symmetric. The L4-5 level is the most commonly involved, followed by L5-S1 and L3-4. Disc herniation and spondylolisthesis may further increase the narrowing. Spondylolisthesis and spondylolysis rarely cause spinal stenosis in the young. The combination of degenerative change, aging, and spondylolisthesis or spondylolysis in patients 50 years old or older frequently results in stenosis of the lateral recess or foraminal variety. Paget's disease and fluorosis have been reported to result in central or lateral spinal stenosis. Paget's disease causes one form of spinal stenosis that responds well to treatment with calcitonin.

Etiology of Degenerative Stenosis

Dunlop et al. have experimentally identified the presence of a significant increase in pressure on the facet joints with disc space narrowing and increasing angles of extension. Degenerative spinal stenosis has been attributed to simple hypertrophic overgrowth of the superior articular facets that is the result of a progressive degeneration of the disc with resultant instability or hypermobility in the facet joints. As joint destruction progresses, the hypertrophic process finally results in local ankylosis. Calcification and hypertrophy of the ligamentum flavum and venous hypertension resulting in generalized bone overgrowth may also be factors in this disease. Mild trauma and occupational activity do not appear to significantly affect the development of this disease, but they may exacerbate a preexisting condition. Liyang et al. measured the canal size in 10 lumbar spine cadaver

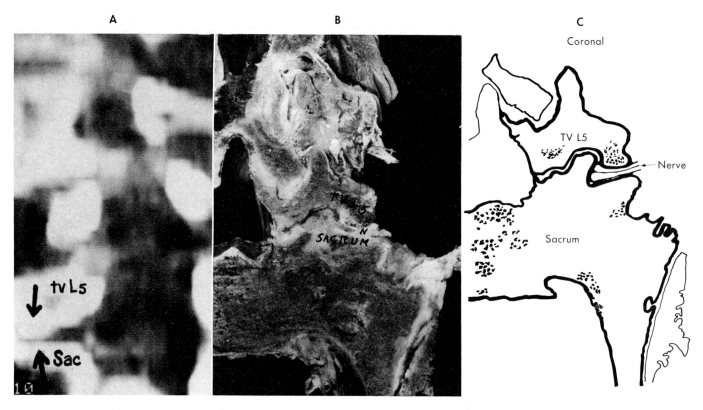

Fig. 86-18 **A,** Coronal view of computed tomography scan showing impingement of transverse process of L5 on sacrum. **B,** Coronal section showing right transverse process. **C,** Line drawing of coronal section. (From Wiltse LL, Guyer RD, Spencer CW, et al: Spine 9:31, 1984.)

specimens and determined that the canal size was greater in flexion than in extension.

Natural History and Clinical Symptoms

The natural course of patients with all forms of spinal stenosis is the insidious development of symptoms occasionally exacerbated by trauma or heavy activity. Many patients have significant roentgenographic findings with minimal complaints and physical findings. Porter et al. note that most patients can be treated conservatively for many years. The physical complaints of lumbar spinal stenosis vary. Most patients complain of back pain relieved by rest and increased by activity. Radicular symptoms do occur, but they are infrequent. Most pain may be centered in the buttocks and thigh, making differentiation from hip disease mandatory. The pain is eased with sitting or recumbency and increased with standing and walking. Staying in any position for any length of time may be uncomfortable. About one third of the patients complain of increasing leg pain with walking. Neurogenic claudication of this type usually begins very rapidly, intensifies with walking, and is not relieved by standing. On the other hand, vascular claudication usually begins after walking some distance and is relieved by standing. Claudication is more frequent in central or advanced stenosis and rare in foraminal stenosis. Moderate lateral recess stenosis and foraminal stenosis may

mimic osteoarthritis of the hip. Failure of a vascular or joint replacement procedure to relieve symptoms should alert one to the possibility of spinal stenosis.

Nelson noted two types of clinical presentation attributable to spinal stenosis: claudicant and sciatic. He describes patients with the claudicant type as having no symptoms at rest, but having back pain with progressive walking, leg pain that develops early, paresthesias, and numbness that progresses with distance. Sitting down and crouching significantly decrease the pain. Physical examination is normal in these patients. Patients with the sciatic type have a long history of low back pain, followed by a short period of unilateral leg pain with segmental paresthesias and numbness. Physical examination in these patients is normal and without sciatic tension signs.

Physical Findings

The physical findings with all forms of spinal stenosis are vague. Distal pulses should be strong, and internal and external rotation of the hips in extension should be full and painless. Straight leg raising and sciatic tension tests are usually normal. The neurologic examination is usually normal, but some abnormality may be detected if the patient is allowed to walk to the limit of pain and is then reexamined. The gait and posture after walking may reveal a positive "stoop test." This test is performed

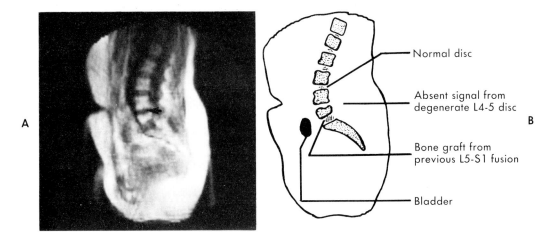

Fig. 86-19 Sagittal section showing normal discs above L4-5 with abnormal disc at this level (reduced signal). Fusion site is also demonstrated. (From Crawshaw C, Kean DM, Mulholland RC, et al: J Bone Joint Surg 66-B:711, 1984.)

by asking the patient to walk briskly. As the pain intensifies, the patient may complain of sensory symptoms followed by motor symptoms. If the patient is asked to continue to walk, he may assume a stooped posture, and the symptoms may be eased; or, if he sits in a chair bent forward, the same resolution of symptoms will occur. In reviewing patients with combined vascular and spinal claudication, Dodge, Bohlman, and Rhodes noted that the failure to relieve symptoms should alert one to the presence of a dual problem. Spinal surgery in patients with these combined diseases relieved paresthesias, but the cramplike leg pain was difficult to attribute to a specific cause. The absence of peripheral pulses should not eliminate the possibility of coexistent spinal stenosis. Primary osteoarthritis of the hip also is frequently a combined finding. Guo-Xiang, Wei-Dong, and Ai-Hao reported seven of 11 patients with meralgia paresthetica symptoms that were relieved by L3-4 decompression.

Conservative Treatment

The conservative treatment of symptomatic spinal stenosis is similar that for disc disease. Rest, nonsteroidal anti-inflammatory medication (usually aspirin), and decreased activity may be all that is necessary to relieve the initial attack. A back support that decreases lumbar motion and increases lumbar flexion may also help. Strong narcotics and sedatives are rarely necessary. Epidural steroids may also produce significant symptomatic relief if combined with decreased activity. As in disc disease, the Back School is essential to teach good posture and body mechanics. When spinal stenosis is present with coexistent degenerative arthritis in the hips or knees, some permanent limitation in activity may be necessary, regardless of the treatment.

Porter, Hibbert, and Wellman reported 249 patients over 40 years old with constant leg pain without significant physical abnormalities. These patients accounted for 11% of those seen at a chronic back pain clinic and were assumed to have lateral recess or foraminal stenosis. Over 1 to 4 years, 80% to 90% were treated conservatively. Spengler notes that the quality of the patient's life is the key determining factor when deciding between conservative and surgical treatment. The patient must understand that surgery may not relieve the symptoms.

Confirmation of Diagnosis

The best method of confirming the diagnosis is with *metrizamide*, thoracic and lumbar myelography, and a reformatted computed tomography scan of the suspected lumbar segments. Magnetic resonance imaging (MRI) is helpful in identifying other disease processes such as tumors and infections. Crawshaw et al. reported 21 patients with lateral canal entrapment identified by MRI. They identified the entrapment by a reduction of epidural fat around the nerve root in the foraminal sagittal reconstructions. This abnormality was identified by myelography in only seven of the patients (Fig. 86-19). Schnebel et al. noted a 96.6% agreement in pathologic anatomy defined by contrast CT (postmyelogram) and MRI. They noted the greatest disagreement in the MRI L5-S1 axial cuts because of the inability of the cut to be aligned parallel to the disc space. A disadvantage of MRI is the cost. Radiation exposure of 4.8 to 7 rads and the need for an invasive procedure with dye injection are disadvantages of contrast CT.

Wiesel et al. evaluated 52 patients without low back symptoms or spinal disease and discovered that 50% of the patients over 40 years old had abnormal CT scans. They identified herniated nucleus pulposus in 29.2%, facet degeneration in 81.5%, and spinal stenosis in 48.1%. Boden et al. noted similar findings in 67 asymptomatic patients evaluated by MRI. In those patients who were 60 years old or older, 57% of MRI scans were abnormal, including 36% with herniated nucleus pulposus and 21% with spinal stenosis.

Frequently multiple areas are affected with stenosis as indicated by imaging techniques, but usually the symptoms are unilateral. The use of a lumbar root block with or without contrast may indicate the symptomatic root if all pain is relieved with one block. As with disc disease, psychologic testing is of benefit as a predictor of outcome.

Indications for Surgery

The primary indication for surgery in spinal stenosis is increasing pain resistant to conservative measures. Since the primary complaint is back and some leg pain, the relief after surgery may only be in degrees. The results of most series show about a 70% rate of improvement, and most patients still have some minor complaints usually referable to the pre-existing degenerative arthritis of the spine. When neurologic findings are present, they rarely decrease after surgery. Roentgenographic findings alone are never an indication for surgery, as clearly indicated in the studies by Wiesel et al. and Boden et al. The best results in most reported series are with localized lesions without general involvement. Ganz reported 86% good results in his series of 33 patients treated by decompressive surgery. In those patients whose preoperative symptoms were relieved by postural change, the success rate was 96%, compared to only 50% in those unchanged by postural change.

The patient's inability to tolerate the decreased lifestyle necessitated by the disease and failure of a good conservative treatment should be the primary determining factors in a well-informed patient. The patient should weigh the potential for the operation to fail to relieve pain or to actually worsen it, in addition to the general risks of spinal surgery, against his degree of symptoms and life-style. Lumbar spinal stenosis does not result in paralysis, only decreased ambulatory capacity. Cervical and thoracic spinal stenoses, on the other hand, are associatied with painless paralysis in the form of cervical and thoracic myelopathy.

LUMBAR SPINAL STENOSIS

Principles of spinal stenosis surgery. Whenever possible, the source of pain should be localized preoperatively using root blocks. At surgery specific attention should be directed to that area. If radical decompression of only one root is necessary, additional stabilization is not needed. The removal of two or more facet joints usually requires some additional stabilization unless the patient is elderly or has a narrow disc at that level. It is advisable to prepare the patient for a fusion in case the findings at surgery require a more radical approach than anticipated. Positioning the patient in the kneeling position minimizes bleeding. As in disc surgery, the use of magnifying loupes and a head lamp is helpful. When pro-

ceeding with the decompression, care should be taken to watch for adhesions that may result in dural tears. Frequently the narrowing in the lateral recess and foramen is so great that the use of a Kerrison rongeur may be impossible without damaging the root. Dissection in the lateral recess and foramen usually requires a small, sharp osteotome or preferably a chisel. Unlike disc surgery, the lateral gutter is best seen from the opposite side of the table. The operating surgeon may find it necessary to switch sides during the operation to better view the pathology and nerve root. When the lamina is extremely thick, the use of a high-speed drill with a diamond burr may decrease the thickness of the lamina to afford easier removal with a Kerrison rongeur or chisel. Blunt probes with increasing diameters are also useful to determine adequate foraminal enlargement. McLaren and Bailey reviewed six patients with postoperative cauda equina syndrome. In five of these a disc was removed from a stenotic spine without adequate decompression of the stenosis. Spinal stenosis should be treated at the same time as the disc herniation.

Midline decompression (neural arch resection)

■ *TECHNIQUE.* **Perform the procedure with the patient under general endotracheal anesthesia. Position the patient kneeling using the frame of choice. Make the incision in the midline centered over the level of stenosis. Localizing roentgenograms should be taken if the level of dissection is in question. Carry the incision vertically to the fascia. Strip the fascia and muscle subperiosteally from the spinous processes and laminae to the facet joints. Take care to avoid damaging facet joints that are not involved in the bony dissection. Identify and remove the spinous processes of the levels to be decompressed. Then clear the soft tissue with a sharp curet. Dissect the lower edge of ligamentum flavum from the lamina with a curet and remove the lamina with a Kerrison rongeur. If the lamina is extremely thick, a high-speed drill with a diamond burr may be used to thin the outer cortex to allow easier removal of the inner portion with a Kerrison rongeur. Take special care in removal of the lamina and ligamentum flavum. The neural structures will be found compressed, and the usual space for instrument insertion may not be available. Remove the lamina until the pedicles can be seen. Using the pedicle as a guide, identify the nerve root and trace it out to the foramen. With a chisel, carefully remove the medial portion of the superior facet that forms the upper portion of the lateral recess. Check the foramen for patency with a Murphy ball elevator or graduated probes. If there is further restriction, carry the dissection laterally and open the foramen. Inspect the disc and remove gross herniations. Usually the disc is bulging, and the annulus is firm. Remove the annulus and bony ridge ventrally if it is kinking the**

OTHER DISORDERS OF SPINE **3843**

nerve. This procedure involves some risk of nerve injury and requires a bloodless field. If safety is in question, a more radical removal of the facet may be better. Complete the dissection at all symptomatic levels. Carefully advance a red rubber catheter caudally and cranially to check for central obstructions. If no obstructions are noted and all areas have been adequately decompressed, close the wound, or, if desired, take a large fat graft from the wound or buttock and place it over the laminectomy defect and then close the wound.

Selective decompression (Getty et al.)

■ *TECHNIQUE.* Expose the spine as described above. Localize the dissection to the level of compression unilaterally near the foramen previously identified as the source of painful constriction. Confirm the level of resection with roentgenograms if in doubt. Remove the lamina in the standard fashion and identify the pedicle. Place an osteotome (or preferably a chisel) over the medial portion of the inferior articular facet. Advance the bone cut in an oblique direction as noted. Identify the nerve root proximally. Make the initial cut in the direction of the nerve root. This line is roughly parallel to the longitudinal axis of the spinal canal where the root passes under the facet joint before turning outward below the pedicle. Possible damage to the nerve root is minimized with such a cut. If possible, interpose a Penfield elevator between root and facet to provide additional safety. Advance the osteotome or chisel with the percussion effect of rapid blows to reduce further the risk of sudden uncontrolled advance. Make the initial osteotomy through the inferior articular process of the facet. When the articular process of the superior facet is reached, twist the osteotome to free the osteotomized fragment and then ease it out with a rongeur. Advance the osteotome into the superior articular facet in the same direction. Remove this fragment in the same careful manner. Perform a complete facetectomy if further restriction is present. Check the disc and canal for herniations and obstructions. If no obstructions are found, apply a fat graft over the laminar defect if desired. Close the wound in layers.

AFTERTREATMENT. Special considerations are not necessary after a simple decompression. The patient should be examined carefully for the first few days for new neurologic changes that may indicate the formation of an epidural hematoma. The patient is encouraged to walk on the first day. Sutures are removed at 14 days. The same limitations as after disc surgery (Chapter 84) apply to decompressions. For patients engaged in heavy manual labor, a permanent job change may be required. Return to work is also similar to disc surgery.

Surgical results. The results of decompression for spinal stenosis vary with the extent of disease and the primary diagnosis. Patients with extensive disease, central stenosis, and degenerative joint disease do not improve as much as patients with localized, segmental, central, and lateral stenosis. In many instances the age of the patient, an already decreased activity level, disc space narrowing at the operated level, and an absence of motion at this level preoperatively make fusion unnecessary.

Spinal fusion with decompression. The indications for spinal fusion with decompression for spinal stenosis are not clearly defined. The exact incidence of postoperative problems related to instability is highly variable, possibly because of the great variations in the extent of the surgical decompression. Shenkin and Hash noted a 6% incidence of postoperative spondylolisthesis in patients with bilateral facetectomy and a 15% incidence when three or more facets were removed. White and Wiltse noted subluxation after decompression in 66% of patients with degenerative spondylolisthesis. They suggested that a fusion be performed in conjunction with decompression in (1) patients younger than 60 years of age with instability caused by the loss of an articular process on one side; (2) patients younger than 55 years of age with a midline decompression for degenerative spondylolisthesis that preserves the facets; and (3) patients younger than 50 years of age with isthmic spondylolisthesis. Others have suggested that patients with scoliosis and spinal stenosis should be treated with fusion. The complete removal of one facet does not result in instability. Generalized spinal stenosis that requires extensive decompression with the loss of multiple articular processes may require fusion. When the facetectomies are bilateral at the same level, the addition of a lateral fusion may be difficult, and the bone graft may impinge on the exposed neural elements. In this instance an anterior interbody fusion may be necessary at a later date if symptoms of instability are noted. Some surgeons suggest performing this procedure 2 weeks after an extensive destabilizing procedure. New segmental fixation instrumentation may decrease the high incidence of pseudarthrosis with these long lumbar fusions.

The complications of this procedure are similar to those of disc surgery. However, the risk of nerve root damage and dural laceration is greater. The rate of infection, thrombophlebitis, and pulmonary embolism is also slightly greater. When a facet has been narrowed, later facet or pars fracture may account for any recurrence of symptoms. However, Getty et al. found that the most important reason for failure to relieve symptoms in their series was inadequate decompression.

CERVICAL SPINAL STENOSIS. Cervical spinal stenosis is frequently referred to by its neurologic presentation of cervical myelopathy. Hypertrophic arthritis, both segmental and more generalized, is the most common cause of acquired spinal stenosis. Ossification of the posterior longitudinal ligament, a manifestation of diffuse idiopathic skeletal hyperostosis (DISH) syndrome, is another infrequent cause of diffuse cervical spinal stenosis.

The treatment of diffuse cervical spinal stenosis is extremely difficult. Treatments have varied from radical anterior decompression of multiple vertebral bodies with fibular strut or iliac crest grafting to expansive cervical laminoplasty posteriorly. Extensive cervical laminectomies lead to late deformity or instability or both in young people. A long-term study by Crandall and Gregorius revealed late worsening of symptoms in patients treated by multiple level laminectomy. They noted only 31% improvement after this method compared with 71% improvement after anterior disc excision and fusion at multiple levels. The greatest improvement occurred in patients who were symptomatic for less than 12 months. Boni et al. reported 39 patients with spondylotic myelopathy treated by multiple subtotal somatectomy with 51% good and 47% moderate improvement. Kimura, Oh-Hama, and Shingu reported 24 patients treated with expansive laminaplasty. They noted 16% excellent and 75% good results.

Many patients with cervical spinal stenosis become symptomatic after trauma or minor repeated trauma. The presenting symptoms may be multiple and varied, including pain, weakness, and spasticity. Some patients may complain of sharp, tingling sensations on neck extension similar to Lhermitte's sign of multiple sclerosis. Physical findings may include signs of root compression, clonus, Babinski's sign, hyperactive reflexes, muscle wasting, and generalized sensory loss.

Myelography to rule out an intradural lesion is mandatory in the evaluation of this problem. Magnetic resonance imaging (MRI) may replace myelography for this purpose. Cervical spinal canal measurement in the lateral dimension on standard roentgenograms is helpful in the identification of this disorder. The normal cervical spinal canal on the lateral view measures about 17 mm in the adult. The spinal cord at this level measures about 10 mm. When the canal is narrowed to 10 mm, significant symptoms of myelopathy are usually present. Edwards and LaRocca observed that narrowing of 13 mm or more on the lateral cervical spine view was predictive of myelopathy or a premyelopathic state.

Subtotal somatectomy

■ *TECHNIQUE.* Position and prepare the patient in the supine position as for an anterior cervical disc excision. Approach the spine from the left. Because of the extent of the exposure, a longitudinal incision is recommended. Continue the approach as described for anterior cervical disc excision (Chapter 84). Elevate or excise the anterior longitudinal ligament over the segments involved. Remove the central portion of the vertebral bodies. Boni et al. use the Cloward drill to remove the bone and disc at each level

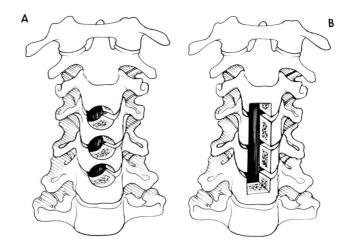

Fig. 86-20 Multiple subtotal somateotomy. Excision of multiple anterior cervical vertebral bodies using Cloward instrumentation. **A,** Initial excision of discs at symptomatic levels. **B,** Final trough. (Redrawn from Boni M, Cherubino P, Denaro V, and Benazzo F: Spine 9:358, 1984.)

indicated (Fig. 86-20, *A).* The remaining areas of bone are then removed, leaving a trough down to the posterior longitudinal ligament (Fig. 86-20, *B).* Another method is to create a trough in the involved vertebral bodies using a high-speed burr. Depending on the length of the trough, use a tricortical iliac crest graft or a fibular strut graft. Prepare the ends of the caudal and cranial end plates by drilling down to cancellous bone centrally. Then trim the graft to allow insertion into the holes in the end plates. We prefer to shape the graft to resemble a keystone. Boni et al. describe making a notch in the graft so the cortical edge of the vertebral bodies has a place to rest in the notch.

AFTERTREATMENT. The patient is placed in a Philadelphia collar with a chest extension initially. Boni et al. recommend the use of a minerva cast followed by a SOMI brace. A halo vest or cast may be substituted for the minerva cast. Bracing should be continued until early evidence of union is noted. Immobilization should be determined by the reliability of the patient and the graft fixation.

Expansive laminaplasty

■ *TECHNIQUE (TSUJI).* Position the patient prone with the head in a cervical rest. Retract the shoulders with tape to allow satisfactory roentgenographic exposure. Then prepare and drape the patient in the usual manner. Expose the cervical (or thoracic) spine in the usual manner bilaterally. Remove the spinous processes at the involved vertebral levels. Clear the remaining soft tissue from the laminae to the lateral edge of the facet joints. Make a longitudinal groove bilaterally at the point of intersection of the lamina and the facet (Fig. 86-21, *B).* Use a power

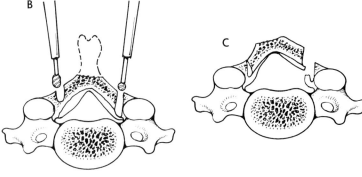

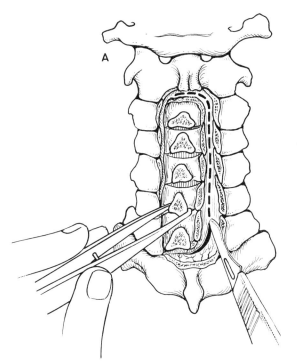

Fig. 86-21 Technique of expansive laminaplasty. **A,** Laminotomy from C3 to C7 with cutting of yellow ligaments with gentle rolling-reelevation maneuver of floated lamina. Knife should be used as shown. **B,** Position and direction of air drills. Long steel burr can only be used until internal cortex is exposed. Internal cortex is to be chiseled with a small-tipped diamond burr in perforator fashion. **C,** Horizontal view of completion of widening of spinal canal. Note opposite cut surfaces of laminae contact each other in one side of groove at which site bony union can easily be obtained. (Redrawn from Tsuji H: Spine 7:28, 1982.)

drill with a diamond burr to make the grooves. Lengthen the grooves to include all involved segments. Deepen them until the ligamentum flavum is identified. Then on both sides widely expose the ligamentum flavum at the caudal and cranial ends of the dissection (usually C3 and C7). Carefully open the ligamentum flavum caudally, cranially, and on one side laterally. Mobilize the laminae by gently rolling them up and peeling them off the dura (Fig. 86-21, *A* and *C).* The flap resulting should float and pulsate with the dura at this point. Suture the flap slightly open with nonabsorbable sutures from the ligamentum flavum to the muscle and fascia on the side of the ligamentous hinge. Then close the wound in the usual fashion.

AFTERTREATMENT. The patient is kept supine with the neck in the neutral position for 2 to 3 weeks. A Philadelphia collar or SOMI brace is then worn for 6 to 12 weeks as indicated by symptoms.

CONGENITAL ANOMALIES OF SPINE

Segmentation of the mesoderm about the neural tube occurs early in the third week of gestation and comes to lie dorsal and lateral to the notochord. At 4 to 5 weeks of gestation, fusion of the mesenchymal tissue occurs in the cephalocaudal direction. Hemivertebrae are formed and fuse to form the vertebral bodies at 6 weeks. Other mesenchymal cells migrate dorsolaterally to form two ossification centers, giving rise to the laminae and pedicles. At birth there are three primary ossification centers — one in the body and one in each half of the neural arch —

that unite during the first year of life. This process starts in the lumbar region and progresses cephalad.

Zimbler and Belkin studied this development and the many problems that may result. Among them are the following nine anomalies:

1. *Basilar impression.* This is characterized by a cephalad displacement of the cervical spine on the skull and an occipital indentation of the posterior foramen magnum. Symptoms usually begin in the second decade because of pressure on vital structures such as the brain stem, cerebellar tonsils, and vertebral arteries. These symptoms include ataxia, nystagmus, headache, neck pain, spasticity, hyperreflexia, weakness, syncope, seizures, difficulty with speech and deglutition, and intellectual impairment. There is an association with Morquio's syndrome, Klippel-Feil syndrome, and cleidocranial dysostosis.

The diagnosis of basilar impression is based on the roentgenographic evaluation of the dens with respect to Chamberlain's line. Chamberlain's line is drawn from the hard palate to the inner aspect of the posterior rim of the foramen magnum. McGregor's line is similar to Chamberlain's line except that it is drawn to the outer cortex of the posterior rim of the foramen magnum. Whenever the dens protrudes above Chamberlain's line, some degree of basilar impression is present (Fig. 86-22). Symptomatic basilar impression usually requires significant dens protrusion. Menezes et al. suggest the addition of air contrast myelography and lateral tomography to identify indention of the brain stem. They also suggest measurement of the clivus-canal angle, which is the angle formed by a line bisecting the clivus and the cervical vertebral bodies. This angle should be greater

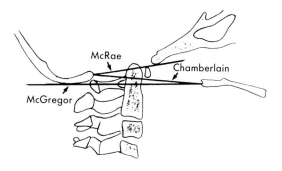

Fig. 86-22 Line drawing of base of skull and upper spine showing McGregor's line and Chamberlain's line. (From Hensinger RN: Section 23, Cervical Spine: pediatric. In American Academy of Orthopaedic Surgeons: Orthopaedic knowledge update I: Home study syllabus, 1984.)

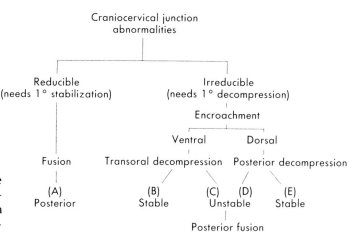

Fig. 86-23 Approach to abnormalities of the cervicobasilar junction. (From Menezes A, et al: J Neurosurg 3:444, 1980.)

than 130 degrees. Basilar impression should not be confused with platybasia. Platybasia is a benign flattening of the base of the skull.

The symptoms and signs of basilar impression are many and varied. They include signs and symptoms of cord compression, cranial nerve palsies, sudden syncope, and visual and vestibular dysfunction.

Menezes et al. outlined a logical approach to the treatment of craniocervical abnormalities based on stability, reducibility, and area of compression (Fig. 86-23). They suggest posterior occipitocervical fusion for lesions that become reduced in tong traction. Nonreducible lesions are decompressed at the area of encroachment. Ventral encroachment is decompressed through a transoral approach with removal of the anterior rim of the foramen magnum, the ring of C1, and the odontoid. The transmaxillary approach described by Cocke et al. (Chapter 79) gives wider exposure. Posterior encroachment is decompressed through a posterior approach with removal of the ring of C1 and the posterior edge of the foramen magnum. If instability is demonstrated after the decompression, a posterior occiput to C3 fusion is performed.

2. *Congenital atlantoaxial instability.* Because of ligamentous laxity of the transverse ligament of the atlas or bony anomalies of the odontoid, C1-2 instability results as in Down syndrome. Roentgenographic diagnosis includes a measurement from the anterior ring of the atlas to the odontoid. This space is greater than 4 mm in children and 3 mm in adults. The distance from the posterior aspect of the odontoid to the anterior edge of the arch of the atlas is abnormal if it is less than 14 mm. This space is also called the space available for the spinal cord (SAC) (Fig. 86-24).

Treatment in these patients consists of reduction of the atlantoaxial displacement by traction and C1-2 or occiput to C2 cervical fusion. Irreducible situations demand decompression of the spinal cord and brain stem at that level, using the rationale of Menezes et al.

3. *Atlantooccipital fusion.* In this anomaly partial or complete synostosis is present between the ring of the at-

las and the occiput, resulting in a short-neck appearance with a low hairline. These individuals have a 20% incidence of associated anomalies. Treatment of this condition, if symptomatic, may require decompression and suboccipital craniectomy combined with fusion of the occiput to C2 or C3 if unstable.

4. *Congenital anomalies of odontoid.* Aplasia or hyperplasia of the odontoid or os odontoideum may produce atlantoaxial instability. The separate ossification centers of the odontoid should be fused by the age of 5 years. The diagnostic problem persists in differentiating the os odontoideum from a post-traumatic nonunion of a fracture of the odontoid (Fig. 86-25). Patients with congenital odontoid dysplasia may have normal atlantoaxial stability. However, in those with generalized ligamentous laxity, atlantoaxial instability may lead to a chronic compressive myelopathy of the cervical spinal cord (Fig. 86-

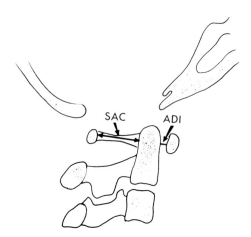

Fig. 86-24 Line drawing of lateral upper cervical spine showing space available for the cord *(SAC)* and atlanto-dens interval *(ADI)*. (From Hensinger RN: Section 23, Cervical Spine: pediatric. In American Academy of Orthopaedic Surgeons: Orthopaedic knowledge update I: Home study syllabus, 1984.)

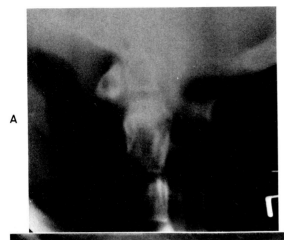

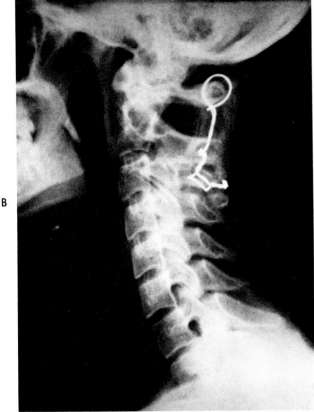

Fig. 86-25 Congenital pseudarthrosis of odontoid process. **A,** Laminagram showing pseudarthrosis and os odontoideum. **B,** After fusion of arches of C1, C2, and C3.

26). In a study by Perovic, Kopits, and Thompson, gas myelography revealed loss of the subarachnoid space mainly on the ventral aspect; this was caused by a thick mass of soft tissue posterior to the dysplastic odontoid at a point where the posterior longitudinal ligament blended with the transverse atlantal ligament. They thought that this structure underwent hypertrophy resulting from the abnormal motion because an atlantoaxial fusion, suppressing the motion, resulted in atrophy of this tissue and an increase in the space provided for the spinal canal. It was also noted that this mass of tissue

produced a flattening in the sagittal dimension and displaced it laterally, thus explaining the predominance of lateralizing neurologic signs. An atlantoaxial fusion is indicated when motion is painful or transitory neurologic signs are present. If the neural arch of C1 is intact and not malformed, arthrodesis of C1 and C2 is sufficient. With a deficient neural arch of C1, an occipitocervical arthrodesis is done (Fig. 86-27).

Aplasia of the odontoid (Fig. 86-28) has been studied in 21 patients by the Piedmont Orthopaedic Society. A neurologic deficit was present in nine; its onset was sudden in three and gradual in six. The remaining 12 patients had no neurologic abnormality, but symptoms after an injury were sufficient to justify roentgenographic evaluation. Associated congenital defects at the base of the skull were found in four. Six patients were treated by fusions of the cervical spine, three from the occiput to C3, and three between C1 and C2. Those from the occiput to C3 were all successful; those between C1 and C2 failed, but sufficiently strong fibrous union developed to stabilize the spine. It was concluded that fusion is indicated when any patient with aplasia of the odontoid develops neurologic signs or symptoms, either transient or permanent.

Care should be taken in the choice of C1-2 fusion technique to avoid fusion in a hyperextended position.

Morgan, Onofrio, and Bender reported familial os odontoideum associated with a Klippel-Feil fusion of C2-3 and noted the inheritance pattern to be autosomal dominant.

5. *Congenital laxity of the transverse atlantal ligament.* There is a reported 20% incidence of this abnormality in Down syndrome. Instability shown on flexion-extension roentgenograms in the symptomatic patient requires fusion from the occiput to C2 or C3.

6. *Klippel-Feil syndrome.* Congenital cervical synostosis was first described by Klippel and Feil in 1912 and consisted of a short neck, low hairline, and decreased range of motion of the cervical spine. Webbing of the neck and torticollis may also be seen. Neurologic symptoms may include radiculopathy, myelopathy, or quadraplegia, usually caused by instability or spondylosis. If symptoms ensue, they usually occur in young adulthood. This is often associated with Sprengel's deformity (30%), deafness (30%), urinary tract abnormality (30%), or scoliosis or kyphosis. Congenital heart disease and synkinesia are common. Roentgenographic studies show fusion of two or more cervical vertebrae and a decreased number of vertebral bodies. Treatment is directed toward investigation of any neurologic abnormality, instability, and spondylosis. Elster and Hall et al. recommend that all patients with Klippel-Feil syndrome be screened for instability and that prophylactic fusion of any unstable segments be considered.

7. *Diastematomyelia.* Diastematomyelia is discussed in Chapter 48.

8. *Lumbar and sacral agenesis.* This is a rare anomaly;

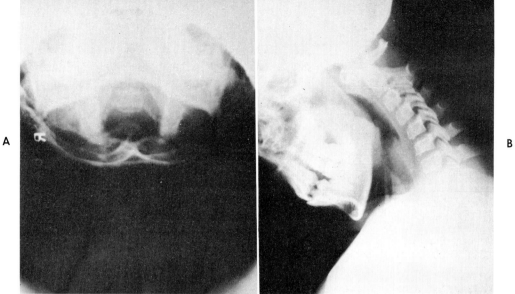

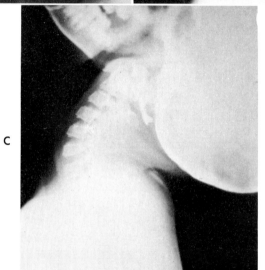

Fig. 86-26 Congenital pseudarthrosis of odontoid. **A,** This basal view of skull demonstrates os odontoideum better than routine open-mouth view because occiput is not superimposed. **B** and **C,** Roentgenograms in flexion and extension demonstrate marked subluxation of atlas on axis. (Courtesy Dr. CH Herndon; from Garber JN: J Bone Joint Surg 46-A:1782, 1964.)

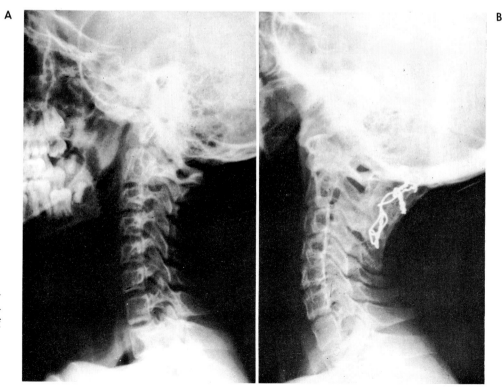

Fig. 86-27 Congenital pseudarthrosis of odontoid. **A,** Before surgery. **B,** After fusion of occiput to C1, C2, C3, and C4.

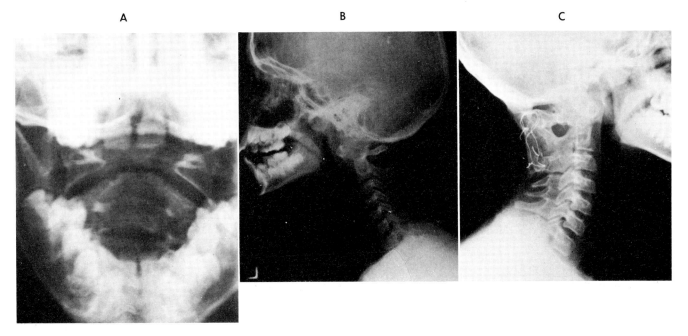

Fig. 86-28.   Aplasia of odontoid process in boy 10 years of age. **A,** Open-mouth roentgenogram shows absence of odontoid process. **B,** Lateral roentgenogram shows anterior displacement of atlas on axis. **C,** Lateral roentgenogram made 4 years after fusion of C1, C2, and C3; spontaneous fusion occurred between atlas and occiput. (From Garber JN: J Bone Joint Surg 46-A:1782, 1964.)

about 18% occur with diabetic mothers. There is motion between the last lumbar vertebra and the pelvis. Motor loss corresponds to the last vertebra present, and the anus is usually patulous and horizontal. The lower extremities may have flexed and abducted hips, flexed knees, and equinovarus feet. There is a 35% incidence of

association with visceral anomalies. Renshaw studied 23 patients with sacral agenesis and provided a working classification:

Type I — Either total or partial unilateral sacral agenesis (Fig. 86-29, *A)*

Type II — Partial sacral agenesis with partial but bilat-

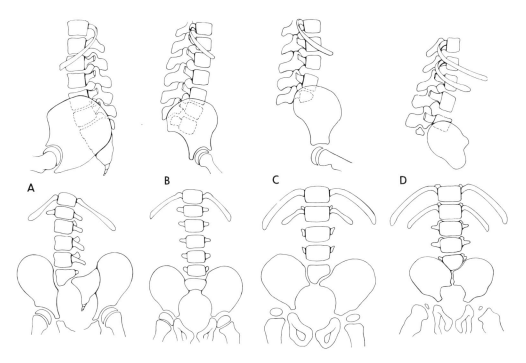

Fig. 86-29   Types of sacral agenesis (see text). **A,** Type 1; **B,** type II; **C,** type III; **D,** type IV. (Redrawn from Renshaw TS: J Bone Joint Surg: 60-A:373, 1978.)

erally symmetric defect in the stable articulation be-tween the ilia and a normal or hypoplastic first sac-ral vertebra (Fig. 86-29, *B)*

Type III — Variable lumbar and total sacral agenesis with the ilia articulating with the sides of the lowest vertebra present (Fig. 86-29, *C)*

Type IV — Variable lumbar and total sacral agenesis with caudal end plate of the lowest vertebra resting above either fused ilia or an iliac amphiarthrosis (Fig. 86-29, *D)*

The type II defect is the most common, and type I the least common: type IV is the most severe. Type I and II defects usually have a stable vertebropelvic articulation, whereas types III and IV show instability and possibly a progressive kyphosis. The clinical picture ranges from one of severe deformities of the pelvis and lower extremities to those with no deformity or weakness whatsoever.

Scoliosis is the most common associated spinal abnormality. Progressive scoliosis or kyphosis necessitates surgical stabilization as indicated, and occasionally stabilization is required for spinopelvic instability. In addition, lower extremity abnormalities will require treatment.

9. *Congenital kyphosis and scoliosis.* See Chapters 82 and 83.

Other congenital abnormalities of the spine involving segmentation are usually asymptomatic. These include absence of pedicles or of the posterior arch. The significance of these abnormalities is their association with more serious congenital abnormalities. Absence of a pedicle in children is usually congenital. This abnormality has been reported in all areas of the spine. In the lumbar spine it is associated with urologic defects. Absence of the arch or portions of the arch is not associated with instability of the spine or other significant abnormalities. The techniques of occipitocervical, atlantoaxial fusion, and subaxial posterior cervical fusions are described in Chapter 81.

RHEUMATOID ARTHRITIS OF THE SPINE

Cervical instability is the most serious and potentially lethal manifestation of rheumatoid arthritis. Three basic types of cervical instability occur in this disease: (1) basilar impression or atlantoaxial impaction, (2) atlantoaxial instability, and (3) subaxial subluxation. Lipson (1984) notes that the incidence of all types of cervical instability in rheumatoid arthritis is 43% to 86%. The incidence of neck pain is 40% to 88%, and the incidence of neurologic findings is from 7% to 34%. He also notes that, once cervical myelopathy is established, mortality is common. The incidence of sudden death from the combination of basilar impression and atlantoaxial instability is about 10%. Patients with rheumatoid arthritis have a shorter life expectancy than the normal population. Pellicci et al. reported a mortality rate 10% higher than the normal rate for comparable ages in patients with rheumatoid ar-

thritis, even though none died as a result of cervical disease.

Basilar impression, vertical settling, or atlantoaxial impaction (AAI) is the settling of the skull onto the atlas and the atlas onto the axis from erosive arthritis and bone loss. This settling can result in vertebral arterial thrombosis. As in congenital basilar impression, atlanto-axial impaction is measured using McGregor's line (Fig. 86-22). Atlantoaxial impaction is considered present in men when the tip of the odontoid is 8 mm above the line and in women when it is 9.7 mm above. Ranawat et al. described a method of determining the degree of settling using the minimum distance between the line from the center of the anterior arch to that of the posterior arch of the atlas and the center of the pedicles. They reported that the normal value was 15 mm for females and 17 mm for males (Fig. 86-30). Redlund-Johnell and Petters-son reported still another method of determining vertebral settling (Fig. 86-31). Their method uses the minimum distance between the McGregor line and the midpoint of the inferior margin of the body of the axis in the

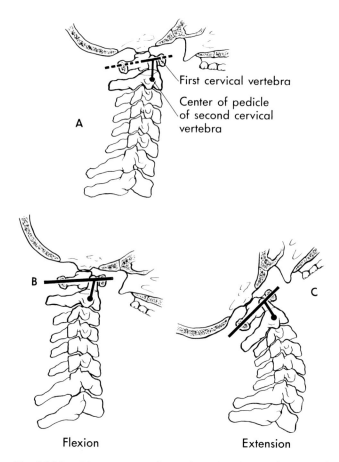

Fig. 86-30 Measurement of superior migration in rheumatoid arthritis. **A,** Diameter of ring of first cervical vertebra and distance from center of pedicle of second cervical vertebra to this diameter are measured. **B** and **C,** Measurement of superior migration is not changed in flexion or extension of spine. (Modified from Ranawat CS, O'Leary P, Pellicci P, et al: J Bone Joint Surg 61-A:1003, 1979.)

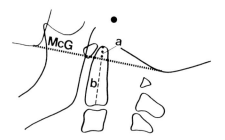

Fig. 86-31 Determination of vertebral settline in rheumatoid arthritis. (From Redlund-Johnell I and Pettersson H: Acta Radiol [Diagn] 25:23, 1984.)

lateral roentgenogram in the neutral position. They noted the normal value for males to be 34 mm or more and 29 mm or more for females (100 patients each). Kawaida, Sakou, and Morizono compared the predictive power of these screening methods and reported that they found the Redlund-Johnell method best for diagnosing basilar impression. Menezes et al. suggest the use of air myelography with lateral tomography to confirm the medullary compression. This also allows the determination of the point of primary compression. Kawaida et al. noted that MRI identified 100% of the cases of vertical settling. MRI is presently the most definitive test for this problem, but its cost limits its use as a screening test.

Atlantoaxial subluxation (AAS) can be anterior, posterior, or lateral. Anterior atlantoaxial subluxation is the most common instability, with a reported incidence of 11% to 46% of cases at necropsy. This instability results from erosive synovitis of the atlantoaxial, atlantoodontoid, and atlanto-occipital joints. It is usually determined by measuring the distance between the posterior edge of the ring of C1 and the anterior edge of the odontoid. This distance is called the atlantodens interval (ADI), and normally it should not be greater than 3.5 mm in the adult. Subluxation greater than 10 to 12 mm is clinically significant and indicative of complete ligamentous disruption. Posterior subluxation is best determined by acute angulation of the cord and upper cervical spine as identified by sagittal reformatted computed tomography, lateral air contrast tomography, and now preferably by MRI. Lateral subluxation implies some rotation of the atlas. It is present when the lateral masses of C1 lie 2 mm or more laterally on those of C2. Menezes et al. suggest the use of air myelography and lateral tomography to confirm the cord and medullary compression from these instabilities. MRI is useful in the identification of cord size and the degree of compression, especially basilar impression and, when available, is preferable to air myelography for determining cord encroachment.

Subaxial subluxations (SAS) are more subtle and frequently multiple. They are believed to result from synovitis of the facet joints accompanied by erosion of the ventral end plates. They may result in root compression from foraminal narrowing. Myelography, postmyelogra-

phy reformatted CAT scans, and MRI all show root cut off and partial or complete block. Postmyelography reformatted CAT scans and MRI are clearly superior in identifying soft tissue obstructions and cord compression. Absolute subluxation distances of clinical significance are not available for this problem.

The signs and symptoms of these instability patterns include findings of pyramidal tract involvement, vertebrobasilar insufficiency, root findings, and symptoms similar to Lhermitte's sign in multiple sclerosis. Menezes et al. suggest air or metrizamide myelography to confirm medullary or cord compression. The availability of MRI has eliminated the need for this uncomfortable and dangerous confirmatory testing.

The indication for surgery in these problems is the development of neurologic impairment and to a lesser degree severe pain. Menezes et al. suggest fusion for instabilities that are reducible and decompression anteriorly or posteriorly combined with fusion if indicated. Lipson, on the other hand, recommends decompression only when the instability is not reducible. In atlantoaxial impression a trial of halo or tong traction for reduction is suggested. If reduction is accomplished, a posterior occipitocervical fusion is performed. If reduction is not possible, posterior fusion is performed after anterior transoral decompression or posterior decompression. Cocke et al. have described an excellent transmaxillary approach to the upper cervical vertebra and the foramen magnum that facilitates this excision (Chapter 79). Atlantoaxial subluxation is best treated by posterior C1 and C2 fusion. Lipson suggests halo traction followed by occipitocervical fusion reinforced with metal mesh, wire, and polymethylmethacrylate to treat posterior subluxation at C1 and C2. Symptomatic subaxial subluxation is probably best treated by posterior fusion. The results of anterior cervical decompression and fusion for this problem reported by Ranawat et al. were not satisfactory. Decompression is occasionally necessary when reduction is not possible and clinically significant narrowing of the space available for the cord is present. Four of five patients treated this way in their series did not improve. Stabilization may be increased by the use of polymethylmethacrylate placed around the wires. A bone graft is placed laterally to provide long-term stability. The mortality associated with surgery for these problems is 8% to 20%. The complication rate is also high, including a nonunion rate of 20% to 33%.

Kudo, Iwano, and Yoshizawa identified extradural granulation tissue as a cause of myelopathy in five patients with rheumatoid arthritis and mild subaxial subluxations of the cervical spine. They suggested longitudinal division of the dura and a fascial patch graft; three of the five patients improved after this treatment. Similar compressive myelopathies have been reported with synovial swelling caused by gout. MRI is the test of choice for clearly identifying these types of soft tissue compression.

The techniques for occipitocervical, atlantoaxial, and subaxial posterior cervical fusion are described in Chapter 81.

Osteotomy of Lumbar Spine

Smith-Petersen, Larson, and Aufranc in 1945 described an osteotomy of the spine to correct the flexion deformity that develops often in Marie-Strümpell arthritis and sometimes in rheumatoid arthritis. Since then, LaChapelle, Herbert, Wilson, Law, Simmons, and others have reported similar procedures. The technique described by Smith-Petersen et al. is carried out in one stage. Others have described methods in two stages, one consisting of division of the anterior longitudinal ligament under direct vision instead of allowing it to rupture when the deformity is corrected by gentle manipulation as in the method of Smith-Petersen et al.

When the flexion deformity is severe, the patient's field of vision is limited to a small area near his feet, and walking is extremely difficult. Respiration becomes almost completely diaphragmatic, and gastrointestinal symptoms resulting from pressure of the costal margin on the contents of the upper abdomen are common. Needless to say, in addition to improvement in function, the improvement in appearance made by correcting the deformity is of great importance to the patient. When extreme, the deformity should be corrected in two or more stages because of contracture of soft tissues and the danger of damaging the aorta, the inferior vena cava, and the major nerves to the lower extremities. Lichtblau and Wilson reported one instance of transverse rupture of the aorta caused by manipulating the spine for Marie-Strümpell arthritis with severe flexion deformity. The patient had previously received 2000 units of roentgen therapy. These authors think that the roentgen therapy once used for this type of arthritis, not the arthritis itself, causes the aorta to adhere to the anterior longitudinal ligament and makes it subject to rupture during manipulation or osteotomy. They advocate a procedure in two stages in which the aorta is freed from the anterior longitudinal ligament in the first and the osteotomy is made in the second. They point out that in all of their patients, regardless of the number of levels at which osteotomies were made, all correction took place at only one level. Law reported a series of 114 patients and Herbert one of 50 in which the patients were treated by osteotomy; in each series the mortality was about 10%, but in each most of the deaths occurred early in the series, and both surgeons believed that the rate in the future should be lower. In fact, Goel has since reported a series of 15 patients in whom no deaths or serious complications occurred. According to Law, 25 to 45 degrees of correction can usually be obtained, resulting in marked improvement both functionally and cosmetically.

Adams suggests that the operation be carried out with the patient lying on the side. This lateral position has several advantages: it is easier to place the grossly deformed patient on the table, danger of injuring the ankylosed cervical spine by pressure of the forehead against the table is eliminated, the anesthesia is easier to manage because maintaining a clear airway and free respiratory exchange is less difficult, and the operation is easier because any blood will flow out from the depth of the wound rather than into it. We agree that this is the safest and most efficient position for this procedure. Adams hyperextends the spine with an ingenious three-point pressure apparatus. Simmons performs surgery with the patient on his side and under local anesthesia. When the osteotomy is complete, the patient is turned prone, carefully fracturing the anterior longitudinal ligament with the patient briefly under nitrous oxide and fentanyl anesthesia.

Osteotomy is usually made at the upper lumbar level because the spinal canal here is large and the osteotomy is distal to the end of the cord. A lumbar lordosis is created to compensate for the thoracic kyphosis; motion of the spine is not increased. Osteotomy methods include resection of the spinous processes from the laminae to the pedicles, simple wedge resection of the spinous processes into the neural foramina (Fig. 86-32, A and B), chevron excision of the laminae and spinous processes (Fig. 86-32, C and D), or combined anterior opening wedge osteotomy following posterior resection of the spinous processes and laminae (Fig. 86-32, E). We usually perform this surgery with somatosensory-evoked potential monitoring to avoid a wake-up test or light anesthesia.

Styblo, Bossers, and Slot in 1985 reported an average correction from 80 degrees to 44 degrees after upper lumbar osteotomy; correction was maintained by internal fixation. Manual osteoclysis worked best in patients with calcified ligaments. They noted seven different types of spinal disruption caused by the manual osteoclysis. Complications from this procedure included hypertension, gastrointestinal problems, neurologic defects, urinary infections, psychologic problems, dural tears with leakage, and retrograde ejaculation. One rupture of the aorta was reported by Lichtblau and Wilson.

■ *TECHNIQUE (SMITH-PETERSEN ET AL.) (Fig. 86-32, C and D).* **Place the patient prone on the operating table. Expose the spinous processes and laminae of three or more vertebrae subperiosteally through a midline incision; the extent of exposure will depend on whether the osteotomy is to be made at one, two, or three levels. Carefully maintain hemostasis throughout the operation. Resect the spinous processes and cut them into small strips for grafting later. At the level of osteotomy detach the ligamentum flavum from the inferior margin of the lamina and the inferior articular facet with a small periosteal elevator. Carefully insert the elevator beneath the lamina and inferior articular facet and bring it out through the intervertebral foramen laterally.**

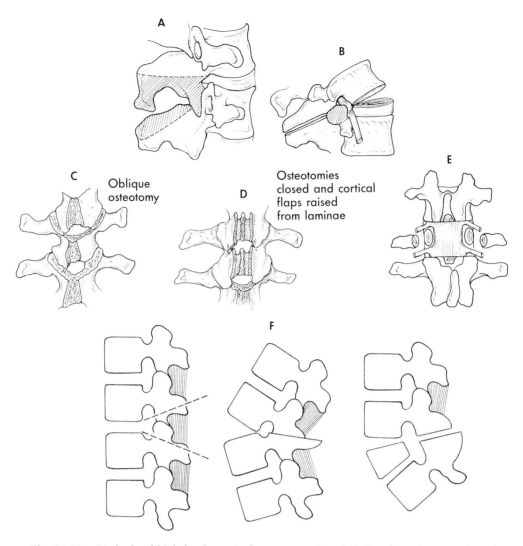

Fig. 86-32   Methods of high lumbar spinal osteotomy. **A** and **B,** Simple wedge resection of spinous processes into neural foramina. **C** and **D,** Chevron excision of laminae and spinous processes. **E,** Total laminectomy. **F,** Schematic representation of effects of total laminectomy and spinous process resection. (**A, B, E,** and **F,** Redrawn from Thomasen E: Clin Orthop 194:142, 1984; **C** and **D,** redrawn from Smith-Petersen MN, Larson CB, and Aufranc OE: J Bone Joint Surg 27:1, 1945.)

The elevator now serves as a guide for the osteotomy through the superior articular facet of the vertebra below and the inferior facet of the vertebra above. Make the osteotomy oblique, its angle approximately 45 degrees with the coronal plane. Widen the osteotomy with small osteotomes, gouges, and rongeurs to at least 6.2 to 9.4 mm. When the ligaments are ossified, take great care to avoid injuring the dura and nerves. Now repeat the procedure on the opposite side. The osteotomy may be made at two or three levels if necessary. Simmons emphasizes preplanning the amount of wedge to be removed so that proper coaptation of the osteotomy results and the patient achieves an optimum functional upright position.

After completing the osteotomy (or osteotomies),

extend the spine by raising the head and foot of the operating table very slowly. The obliquity of the osteotomy ensures locking of the vertebrae and prevents serious displacement. Raise flaps of bone from the laminae adjacent to the osteotomy and bridge the defect with the bone grafts obtained from the spinous processes. Now carefully close the wound with interrupted sutures and apply a plaster shell to maintain the corrected position.

AFTERTREATMENT. The plaster is removed at 4 to 6 weeks, and a plaster jacket or back brace for walking is fitted. A back support is worn continuously for at least a year. To prevent recurrence of the deformity, the patient must wear the brace part of the time for 2 or 3 years more. Postural and deep breathing exercises are carried out regularly.

Goel uses no bone grafts or internal fixation and reports that abundant callus may be seen on the roentgenograms made as early as 3 weeks after surgery. He discards the final plaster jacket at 6 months and uses no external support thereafter.

Osteotomy of Cervical Spine

In patients with severe cervicodorsal kyphosis in rheumatoid arthritis, often the mandible is so near the sternum that opening the mouth and chewing properly are difficult. Law reported a series of 14 patients treated by osteotomy of the cervical spine for this deformity. He points out that cervicodorsal kyphosis can usually be treated satisfactorily by lumbar osteotomy, which provides a compensatory lumbar lordosis and results in an erect posture. But, according to him, cervical osteotomy may be indicated (1) to elevate the chin from the sternum, thus improving the appearance, the ability to eat, and the ability to see ahead; (2) to prevent atlantoaxial and cervical subluxations and dislocations, which result from the weight of the head being carried forward by gravity; (3) to relieve tracheal and esophageal distortion, which causes dyspnea and dysphasia; and (4) to prevent irritation of the spinal cord tracts or excessive traction on the nerve roots, which cause neurologic disturbances. The appropriate level for osteotomy is determined by the deformity and the degree of ossification of the anterior longitudinal ligament. Law has successfully performed osteotomies at the levels of C3 and C4, C5 and C6, and C6 and C7. He prefers to fix the spine internally with the plates devised by Wilson and Straub for use in lumbosacral arthrodesis. However, wiring of the spinal processes as described by Rogers (Chapter 80) should also be effective. Correcting the deformity too much must be avoided because otherwise the trachea and esophagus could be overstretched and become obstructed. Law usually obtained correction of 20 to 30 degrees. After surgery he supports the neck either by skeletal traction with Crutchfield tongs, a Minerva plaster jacket, or a halo attached to a plaster jacket. There were two deaths among his 14 patients, one at 3 weeks after surgery and one at 2 months.

Freeman reported treating by skeletal traction a patient with severe cervicodorsal kyphosis who could not actively lift his chin from the sternum but in whom minimal passive motion of the cervical spine was demonstrated by skeletal traction. The traction reduced a subluxation of C4 on C5 but failed to restore acceptable alignment. The Crutchfield tongs were then removed, and a plaster jacket with an attached halo was applied. The neck was gradually extended until some of the cervical lordosis had been restored. Then, with the halo still in place and the patient under a local anesthesia, an arthrodesis from the occiput to T3 was carried out successfully.

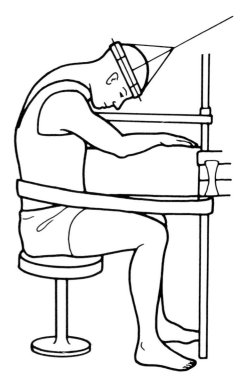

Fig. 86-33 Position of patient for cervical osteotomy: sitting on stool with head suspended by halo and traction. (Redrawn from Simmons EH: Clin Orthop 86:132, 1972.)

■ *TECHNIQUE (SIMMONS).* Simmons applies a plaster body jacket incorporating halo supports 2 to 3 days preoperatively. The operation is carried out with the patient sitting in a dental chair and inclined forward with the arms resting on an operating table (Fig. 86-33).

Apply a halo to the skull with local anesthesia and support the skull by 9 pounds (4 kg) of traction along the axis of neck deformity. Carry out the exposure with local anesthesia and identify the bifid spinous process of C6. Remove the spinous process and laminae of C7 together with the inferior portion of C6 and the upper portion of D1. Remove bone laterally through the fused posterior joints, exposing the eighth nerve root. Remove approximately 1.25 to 1.5 cm of bone bilaterally to thoroughly decompress the eighth nerve root, leaving beveled edges to oppose later (Fig. 86-34). After decompression is complete, the patient is given nitrous oxide and halothane (Fluothane) and the spine is fractured. As the gap closes posteriorly, the dura will buckle as the lateral masses come together. Verify the absence of root compression and close the wound routinely over a suction drain. Then stabilize the head by connection of the halo to the previously applied cast. The fully conscious patient is checked for neurologic function in all extremities and can be assisted in ambulation to the CircOlectric bed.

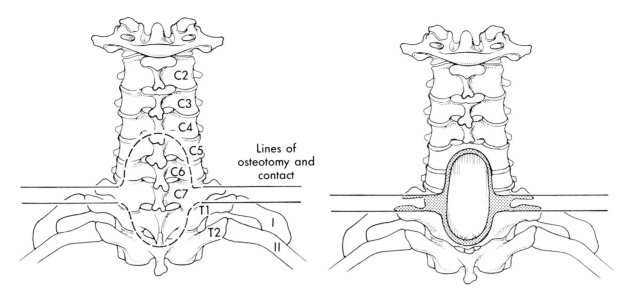

Fig. 86-34 Extent of resection of cervical laminae for safe osteotomy. Lateral resections are beveled toward each other so that opposing surfaces are parallel and in apposition after extension osteotomy. (Redrawn from Simmons EH: Clin Orthop 86:132, 1972.)

AFTERTREATMENT. The patient is allowed to walk and move about but remains immobilized in the halo and cast until healing is complete at approximately 4 months after operation.

TUMORS
Benign Tumors
POSTERIOR ELEMENT TUMORS

Osteoid osteoma. The osteoid osteoma, first described by Jaffe in 1935, may be seen in the spine, involves males more commonly than females, and is most common in the second decade. The lumbar spine is the most common location, the cervical next, and the thoracic last, and the lesion is almost invariably located in the posterior elements. Only nine osteoid osteomas of vertebral bodies have been reported.

Pain is usually the patient's primary complaint, is worse at night, and often is relieved by aspirin. A painful scoliosis may result, with the concavity of the curve on the side of the lesion. Various curve types may result and usually demonstrate poor flexibility on side bending.

Diagnosis may be difficult since early roentgenograms may look normal. Later the usual configuration of a central nidus with surrounding sclerosis may be found, but in only half the patients will it be typical in appearance. Oblique roentgenograms may be helpful when the pedicle, facet, and pars interarticularis are studied. A radioisotopic bone scan will be most helpful in accurate localization.

Treatment should consist of surgical excision of the lesion. If the spine is considered unstable by virtue of facet or pedicle removal, we prefer to perform a one-level fusion at the same time. Complete excision should result in improvement in the angular degree of the scoliosis. Brace management may be necessary in the immature patient, and regular follow-up is advised.

Osteoblastoma. Osteoblastoma is a rare tumor, but over 40% of those reported have been in the spine. It may be misdiagnosed as an osteosarcoma. Radical excision is the treatment of choice. The tumor can recur as late as nine years after resection.

VERTEBRAL BODY TUMORS. Lesions such as aneurysmal bone cyst, giant cell tumor, and others were once considered inaccessible surgically when found in the vertebrae. The older literature recommended irradiation or chemotherapy. Although this treatment still may apply in special circumstances such as in highly radiosensitive malignant tumors, angular deformity with potential paraplegia may result because of subsequent spinal instability. Benign tumors are best treated without irradiation to avoid secondary sarcomatous change. With other tumors, however, optimum treatment may be anterior resection of the tumor to effect a cure or for tumor debulking.

Significant advances in anterior spinal surgery have made possible the resection of vertebral bodies with minimal morbidity. A clearer understanding of the meaning of spinal instability has led to improvements in results. As reported by Stener and Johnsen, we have resected up to three thoracic vertebral bodies but have emphasized the achievement of spinal stability to avoid the late angulatory deformity they described. Our experience has included giant cell tumors, aneurysmal bone cysts, and lymphomas. One giant cell tumor recurred after initial resection of one vertebral body along with the tumor. The fibular graft was eroded by the recurrent tumor that then involved the adjacent cephalad and caudad vertebral bodies. At reoperation three bodies were resected and replaced using a construction of two rib grafts and one fibular strut graft.

Ultimate spinal stability to allow ambulation has been

our goal. This we have achieved by first-stage tumor resection and fibular strut grafting followed in 10 to 14 days by posterior Harrington instrumentation and fusion (Fig. 86-35) in thoracic and lumbar lesions. Proper bone graft selection is essential for a predictable fusion without complications. Tricortical iliac crest bone graft gives the most reproducible and trouble-free results, whereas rib strut grafts frequently break. Fibular strut grafts are useful when the area of excision and grafting exceeds the

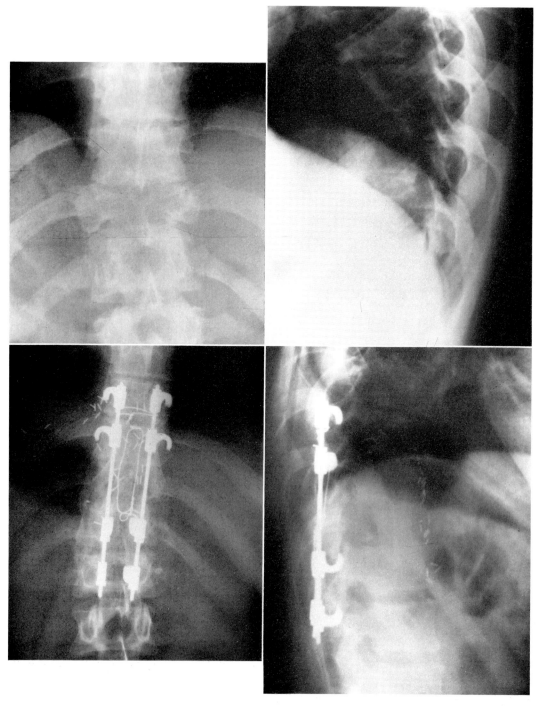

Fig. 86-35 Tumor resection and fibular strut grafting, followed by posterior Harrington instrumentation and fusion. Polymethylmethacrylate was added for stability.

width of the iliac crest. Fibular grafts are prone to late fracture or collapse. Whenever the stability of the anterior construct is in quesion, a posterior fusion with instrumentation should be carried out.

The symptoms of vertebral body tumors may include paraparesis that has been treated by a neurosurgeon with a laminectomy. The combination of anterior instability from tumor destruction of the body and that resulting from the laminectomy produces a most unstable situation. The surgeon must be prepared to properly decompress such a spine via the anterior route and stabilize the spine with a strut graft while preserving the only stability the patient has remaining, that is, the posterior arch and ligament complex. This approach will achieve complete removal of the tumor, decompression of the spinal cord, and stabilization of the spine. Since there are exceptions, each case must be considered on its own merits and involve oncologists, radiotherapists, and other interested specialists.

Primary Malignant Tumors

OSTEOSARCOMA OF THE SPINE. Primary osteosarcoma of the spine is rare and frequently lethal. Pain is the most common presenting complaint, but neurologic symptoms are frequently present. Intensive radiation therapy and chemotherapy are the primary treatment. Radical surgery has been suggested, but the efficacy of this approach has yet to be proven.

Metastatic Tumors

Recent advances in chemotherapy, radiation therapy, and other cancer therapies have resulted in a significant improvement in survival for many types of cancer. With the improved survival, previously silent spinal metastases are becoming clinically apparent and significantly impairing the quality of life. The standard methods of treatment for benign tumors involving excision and grafting are usually insufficient for the early mobilization of the patient. Siegal, Tiqva, and Siegal estimate that 5% of patients with metastatic cancer will develop spinal cord compression. Kawabata et al. noted that 2% of 3880 patients autopsied with the diagnosis of metastatic cancer had previous clinical evidence of spinal metastasis but that at autopsy the rate of metastasis varied from 21% to 48%. Schaberg and Gainor analyzed 322 patients with metastatic cancer. The rate of spinal metastases varied from 2.2% to 31%. Breast, lung, and prostate tumors were the most frequent. Of patients with spinal metastases, 36% did not have back pain. Spinal cord compression was noted in 20% of the patients. Prostatic tumors were the most common cause of epidural impingement. Hypernephroma was the most common malignancy to present, with neurologic impairment as the first sign of malignancy.

CLASSIFICATION. DeWald et al. suggested a classification of patients with spinal metastases. Class I is destruction without collapse but with pain. This class is further divided into (a) less than 50% destruction, (b) greater than 50% destruction, and (c) pedicle destruction. In this class they considered surgery only in *b* and *c.* Class II is the addition of moderate deformity and collapse with immune competence. This class is considered a good risk for surgery. Class III is the addition of immune incompetence. This class carries greater risk for surgery. Class IV adds paralysis with immune competence. This class is considered a relative surgical emergency. Class V adds immune incompetence with paralysis. This class is not considered a good surgical risk.

SURGICAL TREATMENT. Laminectomy has been shown to be of little value in progressive paralysis caused by malignant spinal tumors in the anterior column. Nicholls and Jarecky reported no benefit in 70% of patients treated with decompressive laminectomy. They did note limited improvement in 30% of patients, but their average survival was 18 weeks. Radial laminectomy for posterior tumor resection is of value. Scoville et al. in 1967 were the first to use polymethylmethacrylate to fill defects in the vertebral bodies. Keggi, Southwick, and Keller reported the use of polymethylmethacrylate as an adjunct to internal fixation in situations in which bone fixation is questionable. There have been numerous reports on the efficacy of this material as an adjunct to internal fixation and bone grafting. Fear of neural injury from this technique has been a frequent concern. Wang et al. have shown that, although the temperature of the curing cement may reach 176° to 194° F, the temperature measured beneath an intact lamina and under gelfoam covering the dura at a laminar defect were significantly less (45° F). Later examination of the spinal cord in test animals did not show evidence of neural injury. Clinically we have noted a fall in amplitude of somatosensory-evoked potentials during the curing phase that returns to normal within 20 to 30 minutes of insertion of polymethylmethacrylate. Injury after the use of the material near the spinal cord has not been reported.

Numerous methods have been devised to provide additional stability with polymethylmethacrylate. Wang et al. tested 11 different methods of anterior and posterior fixation in the cervical spine. They concluded that anterior fixation with chain, screws, and cement provided the greatest rigidity in extension. The addition of a posterior wiring with cement further improved the degree of rigidity. Clark, Keggi, and Panjabi have recommended the use of polymethylmethacrylate, incorporating the wires in a posterior fusion, leaving the lateral edges of the spine, the lateral two thirds of the bone graft, and the tops of the spinous processes for revascularization and fusion. Anteriorly they suggest the use of a wire mesh against the dura or posterior longitudinal ligament and threaded Steinmann pins drilled into the vertebral bodies as additional fixation with the cement. This popular anterior construction was not included in the group tested by Wang et al.

In a postmortem biomechanical evaluation Panjabi et al. concluded that the initial rigidity decreased with time. The spontaneous fusion that occurred in their patient enhanced the long-term stability. Whitehill et al. compared posterior cervical fusions in dogs with and without polymethylmethacrylate. Fusions with the cement showed loosening by the second month, whereas fusions with bone grafting were mechanically equal to or stronger than controls at the same time. McAfee et al. reported that the mean time to failure of methylmethacrylate in their retrospective series of 24 patients was about 200 days. They stressed the use of this method only for the treatment of tumors and with adequate posterior fusion augmentation. It is our practice to use this technique acutely and perform the standard posterior fusion without methylmethacrylate within 6 months if the patient improves and has a good prognosis for survival.

Harrington reported excellent results in 77 patients treated by anterior corpectomy and replacement with an anterior Knott rod distraction device encased in polymethylmethacrylate. More than two thirds of those with neurologic compromise improved or completely recovered. He noted only five failures of fixation in 77 patients with a 42- to 146-month follow-up. Six patients developed instability after tumor recurrence. Excellent results with significant neurologic improvement have been reported in numerous patients. This technique allows debilitated patients to walk immediately with minimal or no external spinal support. In addition, significant pain relief is obtained in almost all patients. Further pain relief can be obtained with additional radiation or chemotherapy. This method of treatment is rapidly replacing simple laminectomy in patients with neural involvement from metastatic cancer.

The indications for the use of the technique are varied and will probably expand as further experience is acquired. The primary indications are (1) the development of a neural deficit and (2) intractable pain. Before surgery is performed, the patient should be evaluated for (1) additional areas of metastasis, (2) general medical condition, (3) efficacy or use of nonoperative methods, (4) location and extent of the metastatic lesion, and (5) estimation of the expected life span (Clark et al. suggested a minimum of 4 to 6 weeks) considering current therapy, tumor type, and aggressiveness. Each patient should be considered on his own merits in relation to this evaluation. A careful preoperative evaluation is mandatory since multiple spinal lesions with skip areas are common.

Lesions situated in the vertebral bodies are best approached anteriorly. Frequently the excision of one or more vertebral bodies is involved. One should be prepared to extend the dissection in the event of the discovery of additional metastatic disease. If the predominant

lesion is posterior, the posterior approach for that region of the spine should be used. Cement-augmented internal fixation should be considered if the spine is unstable (Fig. 86-35). Autogenous bone grafting is performed only if considerable longevity is assumed. Some case reports and clinical series have used the posterior approach exclusively to prevent or reduce anterior collapse, dislocation, or both. This may be a consideration in the severely debilitated patient with a short anticipated life span. Clark et al. suggest a combined anterior and posterior resection with polymethylmethacrylate and metal fixation. They suggest posterior decompression and cement fusion first to prevent anterior implant displacement or turning postoperatively.

■ *TECHNIQUE (ANTERIOR).* **Approach the spinal segment using the standard anterior approach for that spinal segment, but choose an approach that allows for more radical or extensive exposure if necessary. Identify normal bone cranially and caudally. Then excise the tumor mass. Remove all disc and central end plate material in the normal caudal and cranial vertebral bodies. Prepare the normal cancellous bone in these vertebral bodies as desired for the method of fixation desired. (We presently use threaded Steinmann pins.) Cover the exposed dura or anterior longitudinal ligament or both with gelfoam. Insert the polymethylmethacrylate in a semiliquid or doughy state. (We presently use a small amount of cement to line the floor of the cavity before inserting the threaded Steinmann pins superiorly and inferiorly, in conjunction with a Harrington or Knott distraction apparatus that engages the vertebral bodies and is totally covered with polymethylmethacrylate to provide a smooth external surface.) Remove excess cement. (This is especially important in the cervical spine where a large mass of cement may cause dysphagia.) Take care to avoid pushing the cement against the dura and spinal cord. As soon as the cement has been trimmed, begin continuous irrigation of the wound with normal saline. (We presently prefer the irrigation solution used for arthroscopy that comes in 3-liter bags.) Continue the irrigation for at least 20 minutes. Test the construction for stability before closing. Remove and replace the cement and metal fixation if it is loose. Close the wound in the standard fashion.**

■ *TECHNIQUE (POSTERIOR).* **Approach the spine using the standard posterior approach for the spinal segment involved. Allow for extension of the exposure if indicated. Then perform laminectomies as indicated by the pathology. Clean the remaining normal lamina and spinous processes of all soft tissue for at *least* two segments above and below the pathologic process. Pass wires through the remaining spinous processes. Clark et al. suggest wiring two spinous processes above and below large laminar defects. Cover the exposed dura with gelfoam. Then** insert other internal fixation as indicated by the spinal level. (We usually add Harrington compression rods in the thoracic region, Harrington distraction rods at the thoracolumbar junction, and pedicle screw and plate instrumentation in the lower lumbar region. Others have used the Luque instrumentation.) Reserve polymethylmethacrylate for patients with a limited life expectancy. Apply the cement in a semiliquid or doughy consistency. Never apply cement directly on the dura. Allow the tips of the spinous processes to be exposed. If autogenous bone grafting is performed, place the grafts laterally and allow the cement to cover only their inner one third or add the grafts laterally after application of the cement. Close the wound in the standard fashion.

AFTERTREATMENT. Rigid immobilization is not necessary if the surgical construction is deemed solid. Clark et al. suggest only soft collar immobilization of the cervical spine until soft tissue healing is complete. In the thoracic and lumbar spine we have allowed immediate sitting and early walking in a long Thomas back brace. The use of radiation or chemotherapy after the procedure is left to the judgment of the oncologist.

• • •

The use of polymethylmethacrylate as an adjunct to spinal fusion is also applicable in other pathologic conditions in which the rate of successful fusion is low or the patient is unable to tolerate prolonged immobilization. Such conditions include fusions for cervical instability in rheumatoid arthritis, instability in renal osteodystrophy, and selected fractures or spondylosis in elderly and debilitated patients.

LATE DEFORMITY AFTER TREATMENT
Intraspinal Tumors in Childhood

Although they are rare, spinal tumors in children may lead to significant spinal deformity, instability, or paraplegia. The orthopaedic surgeon may be presented with this problem, both early and for long-term management, and must be aware of its symptoms and management.

The diagnosis of intraspinal tumors should be considered whenever an otherwise healthy, active child has symptoms of back pain, especially at night. Pain radiating to an extremity, a limp with demonstrated atrophy or weakness but no local cause, and sphincter disturbance are other symptoms. Fraser, Paterson, and Simpson, reporting on 40 children, recorded 67% presenting with weakness of a limb, 60% with back or radiating extremity pain, and 22% with sphincter disturbance.

Presenting clinical signs may include painful scoliosis, muscle weakness, sensory loss, or pathologic reflexes. Definite paravertebral muscle spasm may also be seen.

Fraser et al. reported that 30% of their patients were first seen with paraparesis or paraplegia.

The initial diagnosis is often missed, and the symptoms and signs are minimized. Diagnoses such as back strain, discitis, osteomyelitis, and others may be made. Again it must be emphasized that, since back pain in children is so rare, special attention must be paid to those having the above complaints, and a thorough investigation must be made.

Plain roentgenograms should be taken and carefully scrutinized for erosion of the neural arch or vertebral body, erosions, widened interpedicular distances, and paraspinal masses of calcifications. Myelography is then indicated with laboratory investigation of the cerebrospinal fluid. An elevated protein determination in the cerebrospinal fluid is the most significant finding in support of intraspinal tumors. A wide variety of tumors is possible, and specific information should be sought in articles dealing with this subject.

Neurosurgeons will primarily care for these children, but the orthopaedic surgeon will be presented with the long-term problems inherent with the necessary laminectomy. Fraser et al. emphasize that, the higher the laminectomy is in the spine, the more likely is instability or deformity. Yasuoka, Peterson, and MacCarty reviewed 58 patients who had extensive laminectomies before the age of 25. Spinal deformity developed in 46% of the patients ages 12 to 24 years. The incidence of cervical deformity in this group was 100%, and the incidence of thoracic deformity was 36%. There was no deformity after lumbar laminectomy. Swan-neck deformity occurs in the cervical area, and scoliosis and kyphosis in the thoracic area, whereas the lumbar area is relatively free of deformity.

Treatment of any resulting deformity must follow the guidelines for paralytic or nonparalytic spinal deformity discussed elsewhere. As pointed out by Ingraham and Matson in 1954, it must be remembered that a childhood laminectomy might result in spinal deformity. Anterior or posterior fusion and appropriate bracing are necessary, depending on the specific deformity.

Spinal Irradiation in Childhood

Despite studies of the effect of irradiation on the growing spine, little is really known regarding growth retardation. Probert, Parker, and Kaplan are presently using a prospective protocol at Stanford University to further delineate this problem. Their previous studies suggest periods of accelerated growth under 6 years of age and at puberty and an increased sensitivity to irradiation. Neuhauser et al. suggest a dosage and age relationship with the ultimate effect on the vertebral bodies. Studies continue to lower the irradiation dose to protect growth while still remaining effective on the primary tumor pathology.

Probert et al. and Riseborough et al. reported vertebral body abnormalities following irradiation, consisting of subcortical osteoporosis in the mildest type to complete cessation of growth in the most severe. Growth arrest lines, end plate irregularity, altered trabecular pattern, decreased vertebral body height, contour abnormalities, and asymmetric or symmetric body maldevelopment were listed by Riseborough et al. in their study of 81 patients. They also showed a 70% incidence of scoliosis, 26% of kyphosis, and 27% with no abnormality in axial alignment.

Riseborough et al. found a statistically significant correlation between the amount of irradiation, the severity of the spinal changes, the age of the patient, and the type of deformity. Those patients receiving more than 3070 rads had a higher rate of scoliosis; those receiving less than 3070 rads had a lower than expected rate of scoliosis. If irradiation occurred before the age of 5 years, more than 2600 rads resulted in deformity. Their data also showed that the younger the patient, the greater the deformity.

The deformities progress rapidly during the adolescent growth period. The curves are rigid and frequently are associated with kyphosis; hence bracing is of little value. Surgical stabilization is necessary and is best accomplished by a two-stage anterior and posterior fusion as in other kyphoscoliotic deformities.

Spinal Deformity in Acquired Spinal Cord Injury

Mayfield, Erkkila, and Winter report that spinal cord injury before the adolescent growth spurt is associated with a 100% rate of deformity, of which 96% is progressive. Conservative bracing is difficult. They recommend bracing with a bivalved underarm polypropylene body jacket for curves of 20 to 30 degrees until the age of 10 to 12 years. Surgery is then performed using a staged anterior and posterior fusion. They suggest fusion from the upper thoracic spine to the sacrum.

KYPHOSIS
Scheuermann's Juvenile Kyphosis

Scheuermann first noted wedging of vertebral bodies in kyphosis. This common disorder is thought to occur in approximately 10% of the population. It occurs almost equally in males and females. In 1964 Sorenson suggested that the diagnosis be made if the three central vertebrae are wedged 5 degrees or more. Winter, however, does not believe that wedging is necessary for diagnosis, and believes other signs, especially a relatively fixed deformity, are sufficient for diagnosis.

Although its true cause remains unknown, there are many theories, including endocrine abnormalities, hereditary characteristics, malnutrition, osteoporosis, and mechanical factors. In the past Scheuermann's deformity has been labeled as "epiphysitis," but no evidence of in-

flammatory changes has been reported. Histologic examinations have revealed marked irregularity of the end plates and perforations of nuclear material into the vertebral bodies. DiGiovanni, Scoles, and Latimer reported a distinct anterior elongation of the vertebral body in individuals with Scheuermann's deformity. This elongation is not a vertebral osteophyte and was not found in normal individuals. It appears to result from an alteration of normal growth in the immature spine that produces a triangular extension of cancellous bone along the anterior border of the vertebral body. More recently (1991), Scoles et al. in cadaver studies found additional support for the mechanical theory. They found the apex vertebra (T8) to be the most wedged, to have the most prominent anterior extension, and to have the highest incidence of Schmorl's nodes. They postulate that during mid to late adolescence, when iliac apophyseal excursion is nearly complete and when the majority of posterior and posterolateral end plate growth has occurred, increased pressures generated by abnormal round back cause a disruption of endochondral ossification in the anterior end plate, producing the histologic, roentgenographic, and clinical signs of Scheuermann's kyphosis.

A normal spine viewed laterally shows a continuous smooth arc from the sacrum to the cervical area when the patient bends forward. However, the kyphotic patient will show a hump or angulation in the middle or lower thoracic area. Tight hamstrings and pectoral muscles are commonly seen in this disorder. Roentgenographic evaluation uses a 2 m standing lateral film taken with the patient's arms horizontal. Usual roentgenographic findings include narrowing of the disc spaces, increased anteroposterior diameter of the apical thoracic vertebrae, loss of normal height of the involved vertebra, irregularity of the end plates, and wedging of one or more apical vertebrae. Schmorl's nodules may or may not be present. A mild scoliotic curve is seen in 30% of these patients. Moe et al. consider a thoracic kyphosis greater than 40 degrees in the growing child to be abnormal.

Scheuermann's kyphosis may cause neither pain nor deformity, but more often it causes a significant clinical or cosmetic problem. Pain subsides at the end of growth in most patients, but lower back and neck pain may result from hyperlordosis in these segments in later years. The deformity can also be psychologically quite important to the patient.

Treatment in adolescents has used serial casts, but in 1965 Moe reported the Milwaukee brace to be of greater benefit. Bradford et al. later studied 194 patients with kyphosis and vertebral body wedging and 29 patients with kyphosis but no wedging deformities. It was found that with kyphosis greater than 35 degrees and with at least one vertebra wedged more than 5 degrees, correction was obtained within 6 to 12 months. The curve correction improved 40% overall, with the wedging improving 41% and the lordosis 36%. If a kyphosis exceeds 65 degrees and the wedging of vertebral bodies is greater than

10 degrees, and if the patient is near or past maturity, the results are much poorer. It is therefore recommended that patients with a kyphosis that is supple and without wedging be placed on exercises and observed. If the kyphosis angle increases or if wedging of vertebral bodies appears, then a Milwaukee brace is indicated. Those patients with vertebral body wedging when first examined must be braced immediately. Surgery rarely should be necessary with this approach. It is reserved for a severe deformity after completion of growth for severe pain in the kyphotic area that has been unresponsive to long-term rehabilitative efforts and for those patients with neurologic signs or symptoms.

Posterior instrumentation and fusion in Scheuerman's kyphosis has been reported to result in progressive correction at long-term follow-up, with pseudarthrosis rates as high as 40%. Anterior interbody fusion alone does not provide adequate correction. Moe et al. recommended anterior surgical decompression of the spinal canal, where indicated, and anterior strut grafting. Kostuik et al. reported the use of anterior distraction instrumentation (Kostuik-Harrington) in 279 kyphotic deformities, 36 of which were Scheuermann's kyphosis. Preliminary results in these 36 patients were good, and complications were minimal. His indications for anterior distraction instrumentation of kyphosis in skeletally mature patients are pain, deformity of 75 degrees or more, spinal cord compression (rare), and progression of kyphosis. In skeletally immature patients, indications are failure of bracing and deformity of 65 degrees or more. Significant complications have been reported by other authors using anterior instrumentation for kyphosis correction. (See Chapter 83 for further discussion of instrumentation for kyphosis).

Congenital Kyphosis

In a study of 130 patients, Winter, Moe, and Wang classified congenital kyphosis in three types. In type I vertebral bodies are absent; in type II a failure of vertebral body segmentation is present; and in type III both of these conditions exist. The histories of these patients revealed an average progression of 7 degrees per year. Treatment with a Milwaukee brace has proved to be ineffective, and correction is difficult and perhaps dangerous to obtain. It is recommended that progression be halted by a posterior fusion in patients less than 3 years old. Exploration 6 months after surgery with the addition of more bone grafts is also recommended to develop a large posterior fusion. A spine with a kyphosis of 50 degrees or less of types I and II can be treated by a posterior fusion alone, and type III deformities occasionally require both anterior and posterior fusions. An anterior osteotomy is necessary if correction is sought. In the study of Winter et al. the pseudarthrosis rate was as high as 50% after posterior fusion alone, but it dropped significantly after combined anterior and posterior fusions. Ex-

cept in quite flexible curves, halofemoral traction carries a high risk of causing paraplegia, since the spinal cord is stretched tightly over the rigid kyphotic deformity.

Somewhat later, Winter, Moe, and Lonstein reviewed 77 patients operated on for congenital kyphosis with an average age of 5 years and an average kyphosis of 75 degrees. Approximately two thirds had combined anterior and posterior fusions, and one third had posterior fusion alone. Combined anterior and posterior fusions produced better correction and better maintenance of correction than posterior fusion alone. They offer the following recommendations.

Posterior arthrodesis alone is adequate for congenital anterior failure of segmentation when no correction is needed and for an adolescent or younger patient with mild deformity (less than 55 degrees).

A combination of anterior and posterior arthrodeses is best in all other surgery for congenital kyphosis. Skeletal traction is not recommended for correction because of the risk of neurologic damage.

For anterior strut grafting of kyphosis, Bradford has reported using a segment of an adjacent rib as a vascularized graft by rotating it on its intact intercostal blood supply. With the vascularized graft, fracture of the strut should be less common and union more rapid than with ordinary strut grafts.

TECHNIQUE (WINTER ET AL). **Expose the spine through an anterior approach appropriate for the vertebral level sought. Ligate the segmental vessels and expose the spine by subperiosteal stripping. Divide the thickened anterior longitudinal ligament at one or more levels. Divide one or more vertebral bodies at the foraminal level using gouges first and progressing posteriorly, curets. Take great care as the area of the posterior longitudinal ligament is reached, for the ligament may be absent. If it is present, resect it to see the dura. Widen this exposure superiorly, inferiorly, and laterally, removing all anteriorly compressing bone. A Blount spreader aids exposure. Once the osteotomy and decompression are complete, insert strut grafts, slotting them into bodies above and below the area of decompression. Hollow out the cancellous bone of each body with a curet. Using rib, fibula, tibia, or iliac crest grafts of sufficient length, insert the upper end in the slot first. Now apply manual pressure from posteriorly against the kyphos and use an impactor to tap the lower end of the graft in place. Place additional grafts in the disc space defects and close the pleura over them if possible.**

Postlaminectomy kyphosis

In normal spine, the deforming force of gravity is resisted by the posterior ligament complex. Radical laminectomy removes some or all of these supporting structures, and kyphotic deformity occurs. The younger the child at the time of laminectomy and the more support-ing structures removed, the more severe the kyphotic de-formity becomes. Usually anterior and posterior arthro-deses are required for correction, but high failure rates have been reported after posterior fusion alone and after combined fusions.

REFERENCES
Spondylolisthesis

Adkins EWO: Spondylolisthesis, J Bone Joint Surg 37-B:148, 1955.

Apel DM, Lorenz MA, and Zindrick MR: Symptomatic spondylolis-thesis in adults: four decades later, Spine 14:345, 1989.

Balderston RA and Bradford DS: Technique for achievement and maintenance of reduction for severe spondylolisthesis using spinous process traction wiring and external fixaton of the pelvis, Spine 10:376, 1985.

Barash HL, Galante JO, Lambert CN, and Ray RD: Spondylolisthesis and tight hamstrings, J Bone Joint Surg 52-A:1319, 1970.

Barr JS: Spondylolisthesis (editorial), J Bone Joint Surg 37-A:878, 1955.

Beeler JW: Further evidence on the acquired nature of spondylolysis and spondylolisthesis, Am J Roentgenol Radium Ther Nucl Med 108:796, 1970.

Bell DF, Ehrlich MG, and Zaleske DJ: Brace treatment for symptom-atic spondylolisthesis, Clin Orthop 236:192, 1988.

Blackburne JS and Velikas EP: Spondylolisthesis in children and ad-olescents, J Bone Joint Surg 59-B:490, 1977.

Boccanera L, Pellicioni S, Laus M, and Lelli A: Surgical treatment of isthmic spondylolisthesis in adults (review of 44 cases with long term control), Ital J Orthop Traumatol 8:271, 1982.

Bohlman HH and Cook SS: One-stage decompression and postero-lateral and interbody fusion for lumbosacral spondyloptosis through a posterior approach: report of two cases, J Bone Joint Surg 64-A:415, 1982.

Bosworth DM: Technique of spinal fusion in the lumbosacral region by the double clothespin graft (distraction graft; H graft) and re-sults, AAOS Instr Course Lect 9:44, 1952.

Bosworth DM, Fielding JW, Demarest L, and Bonaquist M: Spondylolisthesis: a critical review of a consecutive series of cases treated by arthrodesis, J Bone Joint Surg 37-A:767, 1955.

Boxall D, Bradford DS, Winter RB, and Moe JH: Management of se-vere spondylolisthesis in children and adolescents, J Bone Joint Surg 61-A:479, 1979.

Bradford, D.S.: Treatment of severe spondylolisthesis: a combined approach for reduction and stabilization, Spine 4:423, 1979.

Bradford DS: Closed reduction of spondylolisthesis and experience in 22 patients, Spine 13:580, 1988.

Bradford DS and Gotfried Y: Staged salvage reconstruction of grade-IV and V spondylolisthesis, J Bone Joint Surg 69-A:191, 1987.

Bradford DS and Iza J: Repair of the defect in spondylolysis or min-imal degrees of spondylolisthesis by segmental wire fixation and bone grafting, Spine 10:673, 1985.

Buck JE: Direct repair of the defect in spondylolisthesis preliminary report, J Bone Joint Surg 52-B:432, 1970.

Burns BH: Two cases of spondylolisthesis, Proc R Soc Med 25:571, 1932.

Burns BH: An operation for spondylolisthesis, Lancet 2:1233, 1933.

Capener N: Spondylolisthesis, Br J Surg 19:374, 1932.

Cauchoix J, Benoist M, and Chassaing V: Degenerative spondylolis-thesis, Clin Orthop 115:122, 1976.

Chandler FA: Lesions of the "isthmus" (pars interarticularis) of the laminae of the lower lumbar vertebrae and their relation to spondylolisthesis, Surg Gynecol Obstet 53:273, 1931.

Cheng CL, Fang F, Lee PC, and Leong JCY : Anterior spinal fusion for spondylolysis and isthmic spondylolisthesis long-term results in adults, J Bone Joint Surg 71-B:264, 1989.

Cloward RB: Spondylolisthesis: treatment by laminectomy and pos-terior interbody fusion: review of 100 cases, Clin Orthop 154:74, 1981.

Cyron BM, Hutton WC, and Troup JDG: Spondylolytic fractures, J Bone Joint Surg 58-B:462, 1976.

Davis IS and Bailey RW: Spondylolisthesis: long-term follow-up study of treatment with total laminectomy, Clin Orthop 88:46 1972.

Davis IS and Bailey RW: Spondylolisthesis: indications for lumbar nerve root decompression and operative technique, Clin Orthop 117:129, 1976.

Dawson EG, Lotysch M III, and Urist MR: Intertransverse process lumbar arthrodesis with autogenous bone graft, Clin Orthop 154:90, 1981.

DeWald RL, Faut MM, Taddonio RF, and Neuwirth MG: Severe lumbosacral spondylolisthesis in adolescents and children: reduc-tion and staged circumferential fusion, J Bone Joint Surg 63-A:619, 1981.

Dick WT and Schnebel B: Severe spondylolisthesis reduction and internal fixation, Clin Orthop 232:70, 1988.

Eisenstein S: Spondylolysis: a skeletal investigation of two popula-tion groups, J Bone Joint Surg 60-B:488, 1978.

Farfan HF, Osteria V, and Lamy C: The mechanical etiology of spondylolysis and spondylolisthesis, Clin Orthop 117:40, 1976.

Fitzgerald JAW and Newman PH: Degenerative spondylolisthesis, J Bone Joint Surg 58-B:184, 1976.

Flynn JC and Hoque MA: Anterior fusion of the lumbar spine: end-result study with long-term follow-up, J Bone Joint Surg 61-A:1143, 1979.

Fredrickson B, Baker D, McHolick W, et al: The natural history of spondylolysis and spondylolisthesis, J Bone Joint Surg 66-A:699, 1984.

Freebody D, Bendall R, and Taylor RD: Anterior transperitoneal lumbar fusion, J Bone Joint Surg 53-B:617, 1971.

Freeman BL and Donati NL: Spinal arthrodesis for severe spondylolisthesis in children and adolescents, J Bone Joint Surg 71-A:594, 1989.

Gill GG: Treatment of spondylolisthesis and spina bifida, Exhibit, American Academy of Orthopaedic Surgeons' Meeting, Chicago, January 1952.

Gill GG and White HL: Surgical treatment of spondylolisthesis with-out spine fusion: a long term follow-up of operated cases, pre-sented at the Western Orthopaedic Association, San Francisco, November 1962.

Gill GG, Manning JG, and White HL: Surgical treatment of spondylolisthesis without spine fusion, J Bone Joint Surg 37-A:493, 1955.

Goldstein LA, Haake PW, Devanney JR, and Chan DPK: Guidelines for the management of lumbosacral spondylolisthesis associated with scolosis, Clin Orthop 117:135, 1976.

Gramse RR, Sinaki M, and Ilstrup DM: Lumbar spondylolisthe-sis — a rational approach to conservative treatment, Mayo Clin Proc 55:681, 1980.

Hambley M, Lee CK, Gutteling E, et al: Tension band wiring bone grafting for spondylolysis and spondylolisthesis: a clinical and bi-omechanical study, Spine 14:455, 1989.

Hammond G, Wise RE, and Haggart GE: Review of seventy-three cases of spondylolisthesis treated by arthrodesis, JAMA 163:175, 1957.

Hanley EN and Levy JA: Surgical treatment of isthmic lumbosacral spondylolisthesis analysis of variables influencing results, Spine 14:148, 1989.

Harrington PR and Dickson JH: Spinal instrumentation in the treat-ment of severe progressive spondylolisthesis, Clin Orthop 117:157, 1976.

Harrington PR and Tullos HS: Spondylolisthesis in children: obser-vations and surgical treatment, Clin Orthop 79:75, 1971.

Harris IE and Weinstein SL: Long-term follow-up of patients with grade-III and IV spondylolsithesis, J Bone Joint Surg 69-A:960,1987.

Harris RI: Spondylolisthesis. In Essays in surgery (presented to Dr. W.E. Gallie), Toronto, 1950, University of Toronto Press.

Harris RI: Spondylolisthesis, Ann R Coll Surg Engl 8:259, 1951.

Haukipuro K, Keranen N, Koivisto E, et al: Familial occurrence of lumbar spondylolysis and spondylolisthesis, Clin Genet 13:471,1978.

Henderson ED: Results of the surgical treatment of spondylolisthesis, J Bone Joint Surg 48-A:619, 1966.

Herman S and Pouliquen JC: Spondylolisthesis with severe displacement in children and adolescents — results of posterior reduction and fixation in 12 cases, French J Orthop Surg 2:512, 1988.

Herron LD and Trippi AC: L4-5 degenerative spondylolisthesis: the results of treatment by decompressive laminectomy without fusion, Spine 14:534, 1989.

Howorth B.: Low backache and sciatica: results of surgical treatment. Part III. Surgical treatment of spondylolisthesis, J Bone Joint Surg 46-A:1515, 1964.

Hutton WC, Stott JR, and Cyron BM: Is spondylolysis a fatigue fracture? Spine 2:202, 1977.

Inoue S, Wantanabe T, Goto S, et al: Degenerative spondylolisthesis: pathophysiology and results of anterior interbody fusion, Clin Orthop 227:90, 1988.

Jackson AM, Kirwan EO, and Sullivan MF: Lytic spondylolisthesis above the lumbosacral level, Spine 3:260, 1978.

Jenkins JA: Spondylolisthesis Br J Surg 24:80, 1936.

Johnson JR and Kirwan EO'G.: The long-term results of fusion in situ for severe spondylolisthesis, J Bone Joint Surg 65-B:43, 1983.

Jones AA, McAfee PC, Robinson RA, et al: Failed arthrodesis of the spine for severe spondylolisthesis: salvage by interbody arthrodesis, J Bone Joint Surg 70-A:25, 1988.

Kaneda K, Satoh S, Nohara Y, and Oguma T: Distraction rod instrumentation with posterolateral fusion in isthmic spondylolisthesis: 53 cases followed for 18-89 months, Spine 10:383, 1985.

King AB, Baker DR, and McHolick WJ: Another approach to the treatment of spondylolisthesis and spondyloschisis, Clin Orthop 10:257, 1957.

Kirkaldy-Willis WH, Wedge JH, Yong-Hing K, and Reilly J: Pathology and pathogenesis of lumbar spondylosis and stenosis, Spine 3:319, 1978.

Kiviluoto O, Santavirta S, Salenius P, et al: Postero-lateral spine fusion; a 1-4 year follow-up of 80 consecutive patients, Acta Orthop Scand 56:152, 1985.

Laurent LE: Spondylolisthesis: a study of 53 cases treated by spine fusion and 32 cases treated by laminectomy, Acta Orthop Scand 35(suppl):1, 1958.

Laurent LE and Einola S: Spondylolisthesis in children and adolescents, Acta Orthop Scand 31:45, 1961.

Laurent LE and Ôsterman K: Operative treatment of spondylolisthesis in young patients, Clin Orthop 117:85, 1976.

Lowe RW, Hayes TD, Kaye J, et al: Standing roentgenograms in spondylolisthesis, Clin Orthop 117:80, 1976.

Macnab I: Spondylolisthesis with an intact neural arch — the so-called pseudo-spondylolisthesis, J Bone Joint Surg 32-B:325,1950.

Macnab I and Dall D: The blood supply of the lumbar spine and its application to the technique of intertransverse lumbar fusion, J Bone Joint Surg 53-B:628, 1971.

Marmor L and Bechtol CO: Spondylolisthesis: complete slip following the Gill procedure: a case report, J Bone Joint Surg 43-A:1068, 1961.

Mau H: Scoliosis and spondylolysis-spondylolisthesis, Arch Orthop Trauma Surg 99:129, 1981.

Maurice HD and Morley TR: Cauda equina lesions following fusion in situ and decompressive laminectomy for severe spondylolisthesis four case reports, Spine 14:214, 1989.

McAfee PC and Yuan HA: Computed tomography in spondylolisthesis, Clin Orthop 166:62, 1982.

McPhee IB and O'Brien JP: Reduction of severe spondylolisthesis: a preliminary report, Spine 4:430, 1979.

McPhee IB and O'Brien JP: Scoliosis in symptomatic spondylolisthesis, J Bone Joint Surg 62-B:155, 1980.

Mercer W.: Spondylolisthesis: with a description of a new method of operative treatment and notes of ten cases, Edinburgh Med J 43:545, 1936.

Meyerding HW: Low backache and sciatic pain associated with spondylolisthesis and protruded intervertebral disc: incidence, significance and treatment (symposium), J Bone Joint Surg 23:461, 1941.

Nachemson A: Repair of the spondylolisthetic defect and intertransverse fusion for young patients, Clin Orthop 117:101, 1976.

Newman PH: Stenosis of the lumbar spine in spondylolisthesis, Clin Orthop 115:116, 1976.

Newman PH: Surgical treatment for spondylolisthesis in the adult, Clin Orthop 117:106, 1976.

Newman PH and Stone KH:The etiology of spondylolisthesis, J Bone Joint Surg 45-B:39, 1963.

Österman K, Lindholm TS, and Laurent LE: Late results of removal of the loose posterior element (Gill's operation) in the treatment of lytic lumbar spondylolisthesis, Clin Orthop 117:121, 1976.

Ohki I, Inoue S, Murata T, et al: Reduction and fusion of severe spondylolisthesis using halo-pelvic traction with a wire reduction device, Int Orthop (SICOT) 4:107, 1980.

Pedersen AK and Hagen R: Spondylolysis and spondylolisthesis: treatment by internal fixation and bone grafting of the defect, J Bone Joint Surg 70-A:15, 1988.

Peek RD, Wiltse LL, Reynolds JB, et al: In situ arthrodesis without decompression for grade-III or IV isthmic spondylolisthesis in adults who have severe sciatica, J Bone Joint Surg 71-A:62, 1989.

Pellicci PM, Ranawat CS, Tsairis P, and Beyan WJ: A prospective study of the progression of rheumatoid arthritis of the cervical spine, J Bone Joint Surg 63-A:342, 1981.

Phalen GS and Dickson JA: Spondylolisthesis and tight hamstrings, J Bone Joint Surg 43-A:505, 1961.

Prothero SR, Parkes JC, and Stinchfield FE: Complications after low-back fusion in 1000 patients, J Bone Joint Surg 48-A:157, 1966.

Raugstad TS, Harbo K, Ogberg A, and Skeie S: Anterior interbody fusion of the lumbar spine, Acta Orthop Scand 53:561, 1982.

Ravichandran G: Multiple lumbar spondylolyses, Spine 5:552, 1980.

Rombold C: Treatment of spondylolisthesis by posterolateral fusion, resection of the pars interarticularis, and prompt mobilization of the patient: an end-result study of seventy-three patients, J Bone Joint Surg 48-A:1282, 1966.

Rosenberg NJ, Bargar WL, and Friedman B: The incidence of spondylolysis and spondylolisthesis in nonambulatory patients, Spine 6:135, 1981.

Rosomoff HL: Neural arch resection for lumbar spinal stenosis, Clin Orthop 154:83, 1981.

Scaglietti O, Frontino G, and Bartolozzi P: Technique of anatomical reduction of lumbar spondylolisthesis and its surgical stabilization, Clin Orthop 117:164, 1976.

Schoenecker PL, Cole HO, Herring JA, et al: Cauda equina syndrome after insitu arthrodesis for severe spondylolisthesis at the lumbosacral junction, J Bone Joint Surg 72-A:369, 1990.

Seitsalo S, Osterman K, Poussa M, and Laurent L: Spondylolisthesis in children under 12 years of age: long-term results of 56 patients treated conservatively or operatively, J Pediatr Orthop 8:516, 1988.

Semon RL and Spengler D: Significance of lumbar spondylolysis in college football players, Spine 6:2172, 1981.

Sevastikoglou JA, Spangfort E, and Aaro S: Operative treatment of spondylolisthesis in children and adolescents with tight hamstrings syndrome, Clin Orthop 147:192, 1980.

Sherman FC, Rosenthal RK, and Hall JE: Spine fusion for spondylolysis and spondylolisthesis in children, Spine 4:59, 1979.

Sienkiewicz PJ and Flatley TJ: Postoperative spondylolisthesis, Clin Orthop 221:172, 1987.

Sijbrandij S: A new technique for the reduction and stabilisation of severe spondylolisthesis: a report of two cases, J Bone Joint Surg 63-B:266, 1981.

Sijbrandij S: Reduction and stabilisation of severe spondylolisthesis: a report of three cases, J Bone Joint Surg 65-B:40, 1983.

Smith MD and Bohlman HH: Spondylolisthesis treated by a single-stage operation combining decompression with in situ posterolateral and anterior fusion: an analysis of eleven patients who had long-term follow-up, J Bone Joint Surg 72-A:415, 1990.

Sørensen KH: Anterior interbody lumbar spine fusion for incapacitating disc degeneration and spondylolisthesis, Acta Orthop Scand 49:269, 1978.

Speed K: Spondylolisthesis: treatment by anterior bone graft, Arch Surg 37:175, 1938.

Stanton RP, Meehan P, and Lovell WW: Surgical fusion in childhood spondylolisthesis, J Pediatr Orthop 5:411, 1985.

Steffee A and Sitkowski D: Reduction and stabilization of grade IV spondylolisthesis, Clin Orthop 227:82, 1988.

Taillard WF: Etiology of spondylolisthesis, Clin Orthop 117:30, 1976.

Tajima T, Furukawa K, and Kuramochi E: Selective lumbosacral radiculography and block, Spine 5:168, 1980.

Takeda M: A newly devised "three-one" method for the surgical treatment of spondylolysis and spondylolisthesis, Clin Orthop 147:228, 1980.

Todd EM Jr and Gardner WJ: Simple excision of the unattached lamina for spondylolysis, Surg Gynecol Obstet 106:724, 1958.

Troup JD: The etiology of spondylolysis, Orthop Clin North Am 8:157, 1977.

Turner RH and Bianco AJ Jr: Spondylolysis and spondylolisthesis in children and teen-agers, J Bone Joint Surg 53-A:1298, 1971.

van den Oever M, Merrick MV, and Scott JHS: Bone scintigraphy in symptomatic sponylolysis, J Bone Joint Surg 69-B:453, 1987.

Velikas EP and Blackburne JS: Surgical treatment of spondylolisthesis in children and adolescents, J Bone Joint Surg 63-B:67, 1981.

Verbiest H: The treatment of spondyloptosis or impending lumbar spondyloptosis accompanied by neurologic deficit and/or neurogenic intermittent claudication, Spine 4:68, 1979.

Vidal J, Fassio B, Fuscayret Ch, and Allieu Y: Surgical reduction of spondylolisthesis using a posterior approach, Clin Orthop 154:156, 1981.

Watkins MB: Posterolateral fusion in pseudarthrosis and posterior element defects of the lumbosacral spine, Clin Orthop 35:80, 1964.

Wiltse LL: Spondylolisthesis in children, Clin Orthop 21:156, 1961.

Wiltse LL: The etiology of spondylolisthesis, J Bone Joint Surg 44-A:539, 1962.

Wiltse LL: Common problems of the lumbar spine: spondylolisthesis and its treatment, J Cont Ed Orthop 7:713, 1979.

Wiltse LL and Hutchinson RH: Surgical treatment of spondylolisthesis, Clin Orthop 35:116, 1964.

Wiltse LL and Jackson DW: Treatment of spondylolisthesis and spondylolysis in children, Clin Orthop 117:92, 1976.

Wiltse LL and Winter RB: Terminology and measurement of spondylolisthesis, J Bone Joint Surg 65-A:768, 1983.

Wiltse LL, Newman PH, and Macnab I: Classification of spondylolisis and spondylolisthesis, Clin Orthop 117:23, 1976.

Wiltse LL, Bateman JG, Hutchinson RH, and Nelson WE: The paraspinal sacrospinalis-splitting approach to the lumbar spine, J Bone Joint Surg 50-A:919, 1968.

Wiltse LL, Widell EH Jr, and Jackson DW: Fatigue fracture: the basic lesion in isthmic spondylolisthesis, J Bone Joint Surg 57-A:17, 1975.

Woolsey RD: The mechanism of neurological symptoms and signs in spondylolisthesis at the fifth lumbar, first sacral level, J Neurosurg 11:67, 1954.

Wynne-Davies R and Scott JH: Inheritance and spondylolisthesis: a radiographic family survey, J Bone Joint Surg 61-B:301,1979.

Spinal stenosis

Arnoldi CC, Brodsky AE, Cauchoix J, et al: Lumbar spinal stenosis and nerve root entrapment syndromes: definition and classification, Clin Orthop 115:4, 1976.

Bailey P and Casamajor L: Osteoarthritis of spine compressing cord, J Nerv Ment Dis 38:588, 1911.

Bell GR and Rothman RH: The conservative treatment of sciatica, Spine 9:54, 1984.

Bell GR, Rothman RH, Booth RE, et al: A study of computer-assisted tomography. II. Comparison of metrizamide myelography and computed tomography in the diagnosis of herniated lumbar disc and spinal stenosis, Spine 9:552, 1984.

Boden SD, Davis DO, Dina TS, et al: Abnormal magnetic-resonance scans of the lumbar spine in asymptomatic subjects, J Bone Joint Surg 72-A:403, 1990.

Bohl WR and Steffee AD: Lumbar spinal stenosis: a cause of continued pain and disability after total hip arthroplasty, Spine 4:168, 1979.

Ciric I, Mikhael MA, Tarkington JA, and Vick NA: The lateral recess syndrome: a variant of spinal stenosis, J Neurosurg 53:433, 1980.

Claussen CD, Lohkamp FW, and v Bazan UB: The diagnosis of congenital spinal disorders in computed tomography (CT), Neuropadiatrie 8:405, 1977.

Cranston PE, Patel RB, and Harrison RB: Computed tomography for metastatic lesions of the osseous pelvis, South Med J 76:1503, 1983.

Crawshaw C, Kean DM, Mulholland RC, et al: The use of nuclear magnetic resonance in the diagnosis of lateral canal entrapment, J Bone Joint Surg 66-B:711, 1984.

Dodge LD, Bohlman HH, and Rhodes RS: Concurrent lumbar spinal stenosis and peripheral vascular disease, Clin Orthop 230:141, 1988.

Dunlop RB, Adams MA, and Hutton WC: Disc space narrowing and the lumbar facet joints, J Bone Joint Surg 66-B:706, 1984.

Dyck P: The stoop-test in lumbar entrapment radiculopathy, Spine 4:89, 1979.

Ehni G, Clark K, Wilson CB, and Alexander E Jr: Significance of the small lumbar spinal canal cauda equina compression syndromes due to spondylosis, Parts 1 to 4), J Neurosurg 31:490, 1969.

Eisenstein S: The morphometry and pathological anatomy of the lumbar spine in South African negroes and caucasoids with specific reference to spinal stenosis, J Bone Joint Surg 59-B:173,1977.

Elsberg CA: Experiences in spinal surgery, Surg Gynecol Obstet 16:117, 1913.

Farfan HF: The pathological anatomy of degenerative spondylolisthesis: a cadaver study, Spine 5:412, 1980.

Foley RK and Kirkaldy-Willis WH: Chronic venous hypertension in the tail of the wistar rat, Spine 4:251, 1979.

Forestier J and Rotes-Querol J: Senile ankylosing hyperostosis of the spine, Ann Rheum Dis 9:321, 1950.

Ganz JC: Lumbar spinal stenosis: postoperative results in terms of preoperative posture-related pain, J Neurosurg 72:71,1990.

Getty CJM: Lumbar spinal stenosis: the clinical spectrum and the results of operation, J Bone Joint Surg 62-B:481, 1980.

Getty CJM, Johnson JR, Kirwan E, and Sullivan MF: Partial undercutting facetectomy for bony entrapment of the lumbar nerve root, J Bone Joint Surg 63-B:330, 1981.

Gokalp HZ and Ozkai E.: Intradural tuberculomas of the spinal cord: report of two cases, J Neurosurg 55:289, 1981.

Grabias S.: The treatment of spinal stenosis: current concepts review, J Bone Joint Surg 62-A:308, 1980.

Guo-Xiang J, Wei-Dong X, and Ai-Hao W: Spinal stenosis with meralgia paresthetica, J Bone Joint Surg 70-B:272, 1988.

Herkowitz HN, Garfin SR, Bell G, et al.: The use of computerized tomography in evaluating nonvisualized vertebral levels caudad to a complete block on a lumbar myelogram, J Bone Joint Surg 69-A:218, 1987.

Herron LD and Pheasant HC: Bilateral laminotomy and discectomy for segmental lumbar disc disease: decompression with stability, Spine 8:86, 1983.

Hirsh LF and Finneson BE: Intradural sacral nerve root metastasis mimicking herniated disc; case report, J Neurosurg 49:764, 1978.

Johnsson K, Willner S, and Pettersson H: Analysis of operated cases with lumbar spinal stenosis, Acta Orthop Scand 52:427, 1981.

Karayannacos PE, Yashon D, and Vasko JS: Narrow lumbar spinal canal with "vascular" syndromes, Arch Surg 111:803, 1976.

Kimura I, Oh-Hama M, and Shingu H: Cervical myelopathy treated by canal-expansive laminaplasty: computed tomographic and myelographic findings, J Bone Joint Surg 66-A:914, 1984.

Kirkaldy-Willis WH: The relationship of structural pathology to the nerve root, Spine 9:49, 1984.

Kirkaldy-Willis WH, Wedge JH, Yong-Hing K, et al: Lumbar spinal nerve lateral entrapment, Clin Orthop 169:171, 1982.

Kirkaldy-Willis WH, Paine KWE, Cauchoix J, and McIvor G: Lumbar spinal stenosis, Clin Orthop 99:30, 1974.

Kirkaldy-Willis WH, Wedge JH, Yong-Hing K, and Reilly J: Pathology and pathogenesis of lumbar spondylosis and stenosis, Spine 4:319, 1978.

Lipson SJ: Spinal stenosis definitions, Semin Spine Surg 1:135, 1989.

Liyang D, Yinkan X, Wenming Z, and Zhihua Z: The effect of flexion-extension motion of the lumbar spine on the capacity of the spinal canal: an experimental study, Spine 14:523, 1989.

Macnab I: Cervical spondylosis, Clin Orthop 109:69, 1975.

Messersmith RN, Cronan J, and Esparza AR: Computed tomography-guided percutaneous biopsy: combined approach to the retroperitoneum, Neurosurgery 14:218, 1984.

Nelson MA: Lumbar spinal stenosis, J Bone Joint Surg 55-B: 506, 1973.

Paine KWE: Clinical features of lumbar spinal stenosis, Clin Orthop 115:77, 1976.

Porter RW, Hibbert C, and Evans C: The natural history of root entrapment syndrome, Spine 9:418, 1984.

Porter RW, Hibbert C, and Wellman P: Backache and the lumbar spinal canal, Spine 5:99, 1980.

Posner I, White AA III, Edwards WT, and Hayes WC: A biomechanical analysis of the clinical stability of the lumbar and lumbosacral spine, Spine 7:374, 1982.

Postacchini F, Pezzeri G, Montanaro A, and Natali G: Computerized tomography in lumbar stenosis: a preliminary report, J Bone Joint Surg 62-B:78, 1980.

Raskin SP: Degenerative changes of the lumbar spine: assessment by computed tomography, Orthopedics 4:186, 1981.

Rinaldi I, Mullins WJ, Delandy WF, et al: Computerized tomographic demonstration of rotational atlanto-axial fixation: case report, J Neurosurg 50:115, 1979.

Rydevik B, Brown MD, and Lundborg G: Pathoanatomy and pathophysiology of nerve root compression, Spine 9:7, 1984.

San Martino A, D'Andria FM, and San Martino C: The surgical treatment of nerve root compression caused by scoliosis of the lumbar spine, Spine 8:261, 1983.

Schnebel B, Kingston S, Watkins R, and Dillin W: Comparison of MRI to contrast CT in the diagnosis of spinal stenosis, Spine 14:332, 1989.

Schonstrom NSR, Bolender N, and Spengler DM: The pathomorphology of spinal stenosis as seen on CT scans of the lumbar spine, Spine 10:806, 1985.

Shenkin HA and Hash CJ: Spondylolisthesis after multiple bilateral laminectomies and facetectomies for lumbar spondylosis, J Neurosurg 50:45, 1979.

Spengler DM: Current concepts review: degenerative stenosis of the lumbar spine, J Bone Joint Surg 69-A:305, 1987.

Styblo K, Bossers GThM, and Slot GH: Osteotomy for kyphosis in ankylosing spondylitis, Acta Orthop Scand 56: 294, 1985.

Surin V, Hedelin E, and Smith L: Degenerative lumbar spinal stenosis: results of operative treatment, Acta Orthop Scand 53:79, 1982.

Tile M: The role of surgery in nerve root compression, Spine 9:57, 1984.

Tile M, McNeil SR, Zarins RK, et al: Spinal stenosis: results of treatment, Clin Orthop 115:104, 1976.

Verbiest H: Pathological influence of developmental narrowness of bony lumbar vertebral canal, J Bone Joint Surg 37-B:576, 1954.

Verbiest H: Results of surgical treatment of idiopathic developmental stenosis of the lumbar vertebral canal: a review of twenty-seven years' experience, J Bone Joint Surg 59-B:181, 1977.

Verbiest H: The significance and principles of computerized axial tomography in idiopathic developmental stenosis of the bony lumbar vertebral canal, Spine 4:369, 1979.

Walpin LA and Singer FR: Paget's disease: reversal of severe paraparesis using calcitonin, Spine 4:213, 1979.

Weinstein JM, Scafuri RL, and McNeill TW: The Rush-Presbyterian-St. Luke's lumbar spine analysis form: a prospective study of patients with "spinal stenosis," Spine 8:891, 1983.

Weisz M.: Lumbar spinal canal stenosis in Paget's disease, Spine 8:192, 1983.

White AH and Wiltse LL: Postoperative spondylolisthesis. In Weinstein PR, Ehni G, and Wilson CB, eds: Lumbar spondylosis: diagnosis, management and surgical treatment, St. Louis, 1977, Mosby–Year Book, Inc.

Wiesel SW, Tsourmas N, Feffer HL, et al: A study of computer-assisted tomography. 1. The incidence of postitive CAT scans in an asymptomatic group of patients, Spine 9:549, 1984.

Wiesz GM: Stenosis of the lumbar spinal canal in Forestier's disease, Int Orthop 7:61, 1983.

Wilson PD and Straub LR: Operative indications in trauma to the low back, Am J Surg 74:270, 1947.

Wiltse LL: Common problems of the lumbar spine: degenerative spondylolisthesis and spinal stenosis, J Cont Ed Orthop 7:17,1979.

Wiltse LL, Kirkaldy-Willis WH, and McIvor GWD: The treatment of spinal stenosis, Clin Orthop 115:83, 1976.

Wiltse LL, Guyer RD, Spencer CW, et al: Alar transverse process impingement of the L5 spinal nerve: the far-out syndrome, Spine 9:31, 1984.

Congenital anomalies of spine

Abraham E: Lumbosacral coccygeal agenesis: autopsy case report, J Bone Joint Surg 58-A:1169, 1976.

Abraham E: Sacral agenesis with associated anomalies (caudal regression syndrome): autopsy case report, Clin Orthop 145:168, 1979.

Andrish J, Kalamchi A, and MacEwen GD: Sacral agenesis: a clinical evaluation of its management, heredity, and associated anomalies, Clin Orthop 139:52, 1979.

Bassett FH III: Aplasia of the odontoid process (Piedmont Orthopaedic Society), personal communication, 1969.

Cattell JS and Filtzer DL: Pseudosubluxation and other normal variations in the cervical spine in children, J Bone Joint Surg 47-A:1295, 1965.

Coventry MB and Harris LE: Congenital muscular torticollis in infancy, some observations regarding treatment, J Bone Joint Surg 41-A:815, 1959.

Dalinka MK, Rosenbaum AE, and Van Houten F: Congenital absence of the posterior arch of the atlas, Radiology 103:581, 1972.

Dawson EG and Smith L: Atlanto-axial subluxation in children due to vertebral anomalies, J Bone Joint Surg 61-A:582, 1979.

Denton JR: The association of congenital spinal anomalies with imperforate anus, Clin Orthop 162:91, 1982.

Elster AD: Quadriplegia after minor trauma in the Klippel-Feil syndrome, J Bone Joint Surg 66-A:473, 1984.

Fielding JW, Hawkins RJ, and Ratzen SA: Spine fusion for atlanto-axial instability, J Bone Joint Surg 58-A:400, 1976.

Fielding JW, Hensinger RN, and Hawkins RJ: Os odontoideum, J Bone Joint Surg 62-A:376, 1980.

Guthkelch AN: Diastematomyelia with median septum, Brain 97:729, 1974.

Hall JE, Simmons ED, Danylchuk K, and Barnes PD: Instability of the cervical spine and neurologic involvement in Klippel-Feil syndrome, J Bone Joint Surg 72-A:460, 1990.

Hawkins RJ, Fielding JW, and Thompson, WJ: Os odontoideum: congenital or acquired—a case report, J Bone Joint Surg 58-A:413, 1976.

Herring JA: Rapidly progressive scoliosis in multiple epiphyseal dysplasia: a case report, J Bone Joint Surg 58-A:703, 1976.

Hilal SK, Marton D, and Pollack E: Diastematomyelia in children: radiographic study of 34 cases, Radiology 112:609, 1974.

Huick VC, Hopkins CE, and Savara BS: Sagittal diameter of the cervical spinal canal in children, Radiology 79:971, 1962.

Hukuda S, Ota H, Okabe N, and Tazima K: Traumatic atlantoaxial dislocation causing os odontoideum in infants, Spine 5:207, 1980.

James CCM and Lassman LP: Spinal dysraphism: the diagnosis and treatment of progressive lesions in spina bifida occulta, J Bone Joint Surg 44-B:828, 1962.

Klippel M and Feil A: Un cas d'absence des vertebres cervicales, Bull Mem Soc Anat Paris 87:185, 1912.

Lee PC, Chun SY, and Leong JCY: Experience of posterior surgery in atlanto-axial instability, Spine 9:231, 1984.

Ling CM and Low HS: Sternomastoid tumor and muscular torticollis, Clin Orthop 86:144, 1972.

Menezes AH, VanGilder JC, Graf CJ, and McDonnell DE: Craniocervical abnormalities: a comprehensive surgical approach, J Neurosurg 53:444, 1980.

Micheli LJ, Hall JE, and Watts HG: Spinal instability in Larsen's syndrome: report of three cases, J Bone Joint Surg 58-A;562, 1976.

Mongeau M and Leclaire R: Complete agenesis of the lumbosacral spine: a case report, J Bone Joint Surg 54-A:161, 1972.

Morgan MK, Onofrio BM, and Bender CE: Familial os osontoideum, J Neurosurg 70:636, 1989.

Nordt JC and Stauffer ES: Sequelae of atlantoaxial stabilization in two patients with Down's syndrome, Spine 6:437, 1981.

Perovic MN, Kopits SE, and Thompson RC: Radiological evaluation of the spinal cord in congenital atlanto-axial dislocation, Radiology 109:713, 1973.

Perry J, Bonnett CA, and Hoffer MM: Vertebral pelvic fusions in the rehabilitation of patients with sacral agenesis, J Bone Joint Surg 52-A:288, 1970.

Polga JP and Cramer GG: Cleft anterior arch of atlas simulating odontoid fracture, Radiology 113:341, 1974.

Pueschel SM, Herndon JH, Gelch MM, et al: Symptomatic atlanto-axial subluxation in persons with Down syndrome, J Pediatr Orthop 4:682, 1984.

Renshaw TS: Sacral agenesis: a classification and review of twenty-three cases, J Bone Joint Surg 60-A:373, 1978.

Ricciardi JE, Kaufer H, and Louis DS: Acquired os odontoideum following acute ligament injury: report of a case, J Bone Joint Surg 58-A:410, 1976.

Richardson EG, Boone SC, and Reid RL: Intermittent quadriparesis associated with a congenital anomaly of the posterior arch of the atlas: case report, J Bone Joint Surg 57-A:853, 1975.

Roach JW, Duncan D, Wenger DR, et al: Atlanto-axial instability and spinal cord compression in children: diagnosis by computerized tomography, J Bone Joint Surg 66-A:708, 1984.

Scatliff JH, Till K, and Hoare RD: Incomplete, false, and true diastematomyelia: radiological evaluation by air myelography and tomography, Radiology 116:349, 1975.

Sherk HH and Dawoud S: Congenital os odontoideum with Klippel-Feil anomaly and fatal atlanto-axial instability: report of a case, Spine 6:42, 1981.

Shikata J, Yamamuro T, Mikawa Y, et al: Surgical treatment of symptomatic atlantoaxial subluxation in Down's syndrome, Clin Orthop 220:111, 1987.

Spierings ELH and Braakman R: The management of os odontoideum: analysis of 37 cases, J Bone Joint Surg 64-B:422, 1982.

Stanley JK, Owen R, and Koff S: Congenital sacral anomalies, J Bone Joint Surg 61-B:401, 1979.

Winter RB, Moe JH, and Eikers VE: Congenital scoliosis: a study of 234 patients treated and untreated, J Bone Joint Surg 50-A:1, 1968.

Winter RB, Moe JH, and Lagaard SM: Diastematomyelia and congenital spine deformities, J Bone Joint Surg 56-A:27, 1974.

Wolf JW Jr and Kahler SG: Atlanto-axial rotary fixation associated with the 18q-syndrome, J Bone Joint Surg 62-A:295, 1980.

Wollin DG: The os odontoideum: separate odontoid process, J Bone Joint Surg 45-A:1459, 1963.

Zimbler S and Belkin S: Birth defects involving the spine, Orthop Clin North Am 7:303, 1976.

Rheumatoid arthritis

Abe H, Tsuru M, Ito T, et al: Anterior decompression for ossification of the posterior longitudinal ligament of the cervical spine, J Neurosurg 55:108, 1981.

Adams JC: Technic, dangers and safeguards in osteotomy of the spine, J Bone Joint Surg 34-B:226, 1952.

Alenghat JP, Hallett M, and Kido DK: Spinal cord compression in diffuse idiopathic skeletal hyperostosis, Radiology 142:119, 1982.

Boni M, Cherubino P, Denaro V, and Benazzo F: Multiple subtotal somatectomy: technique and evaluation of a series of 39 cases, Spine 9:358, 1984.

Calabro JJ and Maltz BA: Current concepts: ankylosing spondylitis, N Engl J Med 282:606, 1970.

Clark CR: Occipitocervical fusion for the unstable rheumatoid neck, Orthopedics 12:469, 1989.

Clark CR, Goetz DD, and Menezes AH: Arthrodesis of the cervical spine in rheumatoid arthritis, J Bone Joint Surg 71-A:381, 1989.

Cocke EW, Robertson JH, Robertson JT, and Crook JP Jr: The extended maxillotomy and subtotal maxillectomy for excision of skull base tumors, Arch Otolaryngol Head Neck Surg 116:92, 1990.

Conlon PW, Isdale IC, and Rose BS: Rheumatoid arthritis of the cervical spine: an analysis of 333 cases, Ann Rheum Dis 25:120, 1966.

Crandall PH and Gregorius FK: Long-term followup of surgical treatment of cervical spondylotic myelopathy, Spine 2:139, 1977.

de los Reyes RA, Malik GM, Wu KK, and Ausman JI: A new surgical approach to stabilizing C1-2 subluxation in rheumatoid arthritis, Henry Ford Hosp Med J 29:127, 1981.

Detenbeck LC: Rheumatoid arthritis of the spinal column: pathologic aspects and treatment, Orthop Clin North Am 2:679, 1971.

Detwiler KN, Loftus CM, Godersky JC, and Menezes AH: Management of cervical spine injuries in patients with ankylosing spondylitis, J Neurosurg 72:210, 1990.

Edwards WC and LaRocca H: The developmental segmental sagittal diameter of the cervical spinal canal in patients with cervical spondylosis, Spine 8:20, 1983.

Epstein JA, Carras R, Hyman RA, and Costa S: Cervical myelopathy caused by developmental stenosis of the spinal canal, J Neurosurg 51:362, 1979.

Fang D, Leong JCY, Ho EKW, et al: Spinal pseudarthrosis in ankylosing spondylitis: clinicopathological correlation and the results of anterior spinal fusion, J Bone Joint Surg 70-B:443, 1988.

Fehring TK and Brooks AL: Upper cervical instability in rheumatoid arthritis, Clin Orthop 221:137, 1987.

Floyd AS, Learmonth ID, Mody SAG, and Meyers OL: Atlantoaxial instability and neurologic indicators in rheumatoid arthritis, Clin

Orthop 241:177, 1989. Freeman GE Jr: Correction of severe deformity of the cervical spine in ankylosing spondylitis with the halo device, J Bone Joint Surg 43-A:547, 1961.

Goel MK: Vertebral osteotomy for correction of fixed flexion deformity of the spine, J Bone Joint Surg 50-A:287, 1968.

Govoni AF: Developmental stenosis of a thoracic vertebra resulting in narrowing of the spinal canal, Am J Roentgenol Radium Ther Nucl Med 112:401, 1971.

Gui L, Merlini L, Savini R, and Davidovits P: Cervical myelopathy due to ossification of the posterior longitudinal ligament, Ital J Orthop Traumatol 9:269, 1983.

Hadley MN, Spetzler RT, and Sonntag VKH: The transoral approach to the cervical spine: a review of 53 cases of extradural cervicomedullary compression, J Neurosurg 71:16, 1989.

Harta S, Tohno S, and Kawagishi T: Osteoarthritis of the atlanto-axial joint, Int Orthop 5:277, 1981.

Helfet AJ: Spinal osteotomy, S Afr Med J 26:773, 1952.

Herbert JJ: Vertebral osteotomy, technique, indications, and results, J Bone Joint Surg 30-A:680, 1948.

Herbert JJ: Vertebral osteotomy for kyphosis, especially in Marie-Strümpell arthritis: a report on fifty cases, J Bone Joint Surg 41-A:291, 1959.

Heywood AWB, Learmonth ID, and Thomas M: Cervical spine instability in rheumatoid arthritis, J Bone Joint Surg 70-B:702, 1988.

Hirabayashi K, Watanabe K, Wakano K, et al: Expansive open-door laminoplasty for cervical spinal stenotic myelopathy, Spine 8:693, 1983.

Hoff J, Nishimura M, Pitts L, et al: The role of ischemia in the pathogenesis of cervical spondylotic myelopathy: a review and new microangiographic evidence, Spine 2:100, 1977.

Hukuda S, Mochizuki T, Ogata M, and Shichikawa K: The pattern of spinal and extraspinal hyperostosis in patients with ossification of the posterior longitudinal ligament and the ligamentum flavum causing myelopathy, Skeletal Radiol 10:79, 1983.

Jacobs B, Krueger EG, and Leivy DM: Cervical spondylosis with radiculopathy, JAMA 211:2135, 1970.

Kawaida H, Sakou T, and Morizono Y: Vertical settling in rheumatoid arthritis: diagnositic value of the Ranawat and Redlund-Jonell methods, Clin Orthop 239:128, 1989.

Kimura I, Oh-hama M, Shingu H, and Shingu H: Cervical myelopathy treated by canal-expansive laminaplasty, J Bone Joint Surg 66-A:914, 1984.

Kubota M, Baba I, and Sumida T: Myelopathy due to ossification of the ligamentum flavum of the cervical spine: a report of two cases, Spine 6:553, 1981.

Kudo H, Iwano K, and Yoshizawa H: Cervical cord compression due to extradural granulation tissue in rheumatoid arthritis, J Bone Joint Surg 66-B:426, 1984.

LaChapelle EH: Osteotomy of the lumbar spine for correction of kyphosis in a case of ankylosing spondylarthritis, J Bone Joint Surg 28:851, 1946.

Law WA: Osteotomy of the spine and the treatment of severe dorsal kyphosis: four cases, Proc R Soc Med 42:594, 1949.

Law WA: Arthritis: surgical treatment of chronic arthritis. In Carling ER and Ross JP, editors: British surgical practice, surgical progress, London, 1952, Butterworth Publishers.

Law WA: Surgical treatment of the rheumatic diseases, J Bone Joint Surg 34-B:215, 1952.

Law WA: Lumbar spinal osteotomy, J Bone Joint Surg 41-B:270, 1959.

Law WA: Osteotomy of the spine, J Bone Joint Surg 44-A:1199, 1962.

Law WA: The spine in rheumatoid spondylitis, Clin Orthop 36:35, 1964.

Lichtblau PO and Wilson PD: Possible mechanism of aortic rupture in orthopaedic correction of rheumatoid spondylitis, J Bone Joint Surg 38-A:123, 1956.

Lipson SJ: Rheumatoid arthritis of the cervical spine, Clin Orthop 182:143, 1984.

Lipson SJ: Rheumatoid arthritis in the cervical spine, Clin Orthop 239:121, 1989.

Lourie H and Stewart WA: Spontaneous atlantoaxial dislocation: a complication of rheumatoid disease, N Engl J Med 265:677, 1961.

Lunsford LD, Bissonette DJ, and Zorub DS: Anterior surgery for cervical disc disease. Part 2. Treatment of cervical spondylotic myelopathy in 32 cases, J. Neurosurg 53:12, 1980.

Martel W and Page JW: Cervical vertebral erosions and subluxations in rheumatoid arthritis and ankylosing spondylitis, Arthritis Rheum 3:546, 1960.

Matthews JA: Atlanto-axial subluxation in rheumatoid arthritis: a five-year follow-up study, Ann Rheum Dis 33:526, 1974.

Mayfield FH: Cervical spondylosis: a comparison of the anterior and posterior approaches, Clin Neurosurg 13:181, 1966.

McCarron RF and Robertson WW: Brooks fusion for atlantoaxial instability in rheumatoid arthritis, South Med J 81:474, 1988.

McLaren AC and Bailey SI: Cauda equina syndrome: a complication of lumbar dissectomy, Clin Orthop 204:143, 1986.

McMaster PE: Osteotomy of the spine for fixed flexion deformity, J Bone Joint Surg 44-A:1207, 1962.

Ono K, Ota H, Tada K, and Yamamoto T: Cervical myelopathy secondary to multiple spondylotic protrusions: a clinicopathologic study, Spine 2:109, 1977.

Ranawat CS, O'Leary P, Pellicci P, et al: Cervical spine fusion in rheumatoid arthritis, J Bone Joint Surg 61-A:1003, 1979.

Ranawat CS, O-Leary P, Pellicci P, et al: Cervical spine fusion in rheumatoid arthritis, J Bone Joint Surg 61-A:1003, 1979.

Redlund-Johnell I and Pettersson H: Radiographic measurements of the cranio-vertebral region, designed for evaluation of abnormalities in rheumatoid arthritis, Acta Radio (Diagn) (Stockh) 25:23, 1984.

Robinson RA, Afeiche N, Dunn EJ, and Northrup BE: Cervical spondylotic myelopathy: etiology and treatment concepts, Spine 2:89, 1977.

Sachs B and Fraenkel J: Progressive ankylotic rigidity of the spine (spondylose rhizomelique), J Nerv Ment Dis 27:1, 1900.

Santavirta S, Sandelin J, and Slatis P: Posterior atlanto-axial subluxation in rheumatoid arthritis, Acta Orthop Scand 56:298, 1985.

Santavirta S, Slatis P, Kankaanpaa U, et al: Treatment of the cervical spine in rheumatoid athritis, J Bone Joint Surg 70-A: 658, 1988.

Sharp J and Purser DW: Spontaneous atlanto-axial dislocation in ankylosing spondylitis and rheumatoid arthritis, Ann Rheum Dis 20:47, 1961.

Simmons EH: Surgery of the spine in rheumatoid arthritis and ankylosing spondylitis. In Cruess RL and Mitchell NS, editors: Surgery of rheumatoid arthritis, Philadelphia, 1971, JB Lippincott Co.

Simmons EH: The surgical correction of flexion deformity of the cervical spine in ankylosing spondylitis, Clin Orthop 86:132, 1972.

Slatis P, Santavirta S, Sandelin J, and Konttinen YT: Cranial subluxation of the odontoid process in rheumatoid arthritis, J Bone Joint Surg 71-A:189, 1989.

Smith HP, Challa VR, and Alexander E Jr: Odontoid compression of the brain stem in a patient with rheumatoid arthritis: case report, J Neurosurg 53:841, 1980.

Smith-Petersen MN, Larson CB, and Aufranc OE: Osteotomy of the spine for correction of flexion deformity in rheumatoid spondylitis, J Bone Joint Surg 27:1, 1945.

Stern WE and Balch RE: Surgical aspects of nonspecific inflammatory and suppurative disease of the vertebral column, Am J Surg 112:314, 1966.

Styblo K, Bossers GThM, and Slot GH: Osteotomy for kyphosis in ankylosing spondylitis, Acta Orthop Scand 56:294, 1985.

Thomas WH: Surgical management of the rheumatoid cervical spine, Orthop Clin North Am 6:793, 1975.

Thomasen E: Vertebral osteotomy for correction of kyphosis in ankylosing spondylitis, Clin Orthop 194:142, 1985.

Tsuji H: Laminoplasty for patients with compressive myelopathy due to so-called spinal canal stenosis in cervical and thoracic regions, Spine 7:28, 1982.

Veidlinger OF, Colwill JC, Smyth HS, and Turner D: Cervical myelopathy and its relationship to cervical stenosis, Spine 6:550, 1981.

Weinstein PR, Karpman RR, Gall EP, and Pitt M: Spinal cord injury, spinal fracture, and spinal stenosis in ankylosing spondylitis, J Neurosurg 57:609, 1982.

Wilson MJ and Turkell JH: Multiple spinal wedge osteotomy: its use in a case of Marie-Strumpell spondylitis, Am J Surg 77:777, 1949.

Wilson PD: Surgical reconstruction of the arthritic cripple, Med Clin North Am 21:1623, 1937.

Wilson PD and Osgood RB: Reconstructive surgery in chronic arthritis, N Engl J Med 209:117, 1933.

Winfield J, Cooke D, Brook AS, and Corbett M: A prospective study of the radiological changes in the cervical spine in early rheumatoid disease, Ann Rheum Dis 40:109, 1981.

Zanasi R, Fioretta G, Rotolo F, and Zanasi L: "Open door" operation to raise the vertebral arch in myelopathy due to cervical spondylosis, Ital J Orthop Traumatol 10:21, 1984.

Zhang Z, Yin H, Yang K, et al: Anterior intervertebral disc excision and bone grafting in cervical spondylotic myelopathy, Spine 8:16, 1983.

Tumors

Akbarnia BA and Rooholamini SA: Scoliosis caused by benign osteoblastoma of the thoracic or lumbar spine, J Bone Joint Surg 63-A:1146, 1981.

Asnis SE, Lesniewski P, and Dowling T Jr: Anterior decompression and stabilization with methylmethacrylate and a bone bolt for treatment of pathologic fractures of the cervical spine: a report of two cases, Clin Orthop 187:139, 1984.

Bahalla SK: Metastatic disease of the spine, Clin Orthop 73: 52, 1970.

Bohlman HH, Sachs BL, Carter JR, et al: Primary neoplasms of the cervical spine: diagnosis and treatment of twenty three patients, J Bone Joint Surg 68-A:483, 1986.

Calderoni P, Gusella A, and Martucci E: Multiple osteoid osteoma in the 7th dorsal vertebra, Ital J Orthop Traumatol 10:257, 1984.

Capanna R, Albisinni U, Picci P, et al: Aneurysmal bone cyst of the spine, J Bone Joint Surg 67-A:527, 1985.

Chadduck WM and Boop WC Jr: Acrylic stabilization of the cervical spine for neoplastic disease: evolution of a technique for vertebral body replacement, Neurosurgery 13:23, 1983.

Clark CR, Keggi KJ, and Panjabi MM: Methylmethacrylate stabilization of the cervical spine, J Bone Joint Surg 66-A:40, 1984.

Clarke HA and Fleming ID: Disk disease and occult malignancies, South Med J 66:449, 1973.

Conley RK, Britt RH, Hanbery JW, and Silverberg GD: Anterior fibular strut graft in neoplastic disease of the cervical spine, J Neurosurg 51:677, 1979.

Constans JP, et al: Spinal metastases with neurological manifestations: review of 600 cases, J Neurosurg 59:111, 1983.

Cross GO, White HL, and White LP: Acrylic prosthesis of the fifth cervical vertebra in multiple myeloma: technical note, J Neurosurg 35:112, 1971.

Cusick JF, Larson SJ, Walsh PR, and Steiner RE: Distraction rod stabilization in the treatment of metastatic carcinoma, J Neurosurg 59:861, 1983.

DeWald RL, Bridwell KH, Prodromas C, and Rodts MF: Reconstructive spinal surgery as palliation for metastatic malignancies of the spine, Spine 10:21, 1985.

Dunn EJ: The role of methyl methacrylate in the stabilization and replacement of tumors of the cervical spine, Spine 2:15, 1977.

Ferris RA, Pettrone FA, McKelvie AM, et al: Eosinophilic granuloma of the spine: an unusual radiographic presentation, Clin Orthop 99:57, 1974.

Fett HC and Russo VP: Osteoid osteoma of a cervical vertebra: report of a case, J Bone Joint Surg 41-A:948, 1959.

Fidler MW: Pathological fractures of the cervical spine: pallative surgical treatment, J Bone Joint Surg 67-B:352, 1985.

Fielding JW, Fietti VG, Hughes JEO, and Gabrielian JZ: Primary osteogenic sarcoma of the cervical spine: a case report, J Bone Joint Surg 58-A:892, 1976.

Flatley TJ, Anderson MH, and Anast GT: Spinal instability due to malignant disease: treatment by segmental spinal stabilization, J Bone Joint Surg 66-A:47, 1984.

Fornasier VL and Czitrom AA: Collapsed vertebrae: a review of 659 autopsies, Clin Orthop 131:261, 1978.

Fountain SS: A single-stage combined surgical approach for vertebral resections, J Bone Joint Surg 61-A:1011, 1979.

Fraser RD, Paterson DC, and Simpson DA: Orthopaedic aspects of spinal tumours in children, J Bone Joint Surg 59-B:143, 1977.

Gelberman RH and Olson CO: Benign osteoblastoma of the atlas: a case report, J Bone Joint Surg 56-A:808, 1974.

Glenn JN, Reckling FW, and Mantz FA: Malignant hemangioendothelioma in a lumbar vertebra: a rare tumor in an unusual location, J Bone Joint Surg 56-A:1279, 1974.

Gore DR and Mueller HA: Osteoid-osteoma of the spine with localization aided by 99 mTc-polyphosphate bone scan: case report, Clin Orthop 113:132, 1975.

Griffin JB: Benign osteoblastoma of the thoracic spine: case report with fifteen-year follow-up, J Bone Joint Surg 60-A:833, 1978.

Guarnaschelli JJ, Wehry SM, Serratoni FT, and Dzenitis AJ: Atypical fibrous histiocytoma of the thoracic spine: case report, J Neurosurg 51:415, 1979.

Hamby WB and Glaser HT: Replacement of spinal intervertebral discs with locally polymerizing methyl methacrylate: experimental study of effects upon tissues and report of a small clinical series, J Neurosurg 16:311, 1959.

Hansebout RR and Blomquist GA Jr: Acrylic spinal fusion: a 20-year clinical series and technical note, J Neurosurg 53:606, 1980.

Harrington KD.: Anterior decompression and stabilization of the spine as a treatment for vertebral collapse and spinal cord compression from metastatic malignancy, Clin Orthop 233:177, 1988.

Heiman ML, Cooley CJ, and Bradford DS: Osteoid osteoma of a vertebral body, Clin Orthop 118:159, 1976.

Hejgaard N and Larsen E: Value of early attention to spinal compression syndromes, Acta Orthop Scand 55:234, 1984.

Ingraham FD and Matson DD: Neurosurgery of infancy and childhood, Springfield, Ill, 1954, Charles C Thomas, Publisher.

Jaffe HL: "Osteoidosteoma": benign osteoblastic tumour composed of osteoid and atypical bone, Arch Surg 31:709, 1935.

Kagan AR: Diagnostic oncology case study: lytic spine lesion and cold bone scan, AJR 136:129, 1981.

Katzman H, Waugh T, and Berdon W: Skeletal changes following irradiation of childhood tumors, J Bone Joint Surg 51-A:825, 1969.

Kawabata M, Sugiyama M, Suzuki T, and Kumano K: The role of metal and bone cement fixation in the management of malignant lesions of the vertebral column, Int Orthop 4:177, 1980.

Keggi KJ, Southwick WO, and Keller DJ: Stabilization of the spine using methylmethacrylate (abstr), J Bone Joint Surg 58-A:738, 1976.

Ker NB and Jones CB: Tumours of the cauda equina: the problem of differential diagnosis, J Bone Joint Surg 67-B:358, 1985.

Kirwan EOG, Hutton PAN, Pozo JL, and Ransford AO: Osteoid osteoma and benign osteoblastoma of the spine: clinical presentation and treatment, J Bone Joint Surg 66-B:21, 1984.

Lindholm TS, Snellman O, and Osterman K: Scoliosis caused by benign osteoblastoma of the lumbar spine: a report of three patients, Spine 2:276, 1977.

Manabe S, Tateishi A, Abe M, and Ohno T: Surgical treatment of metastatic tumors of the spine, Spine 14:41, 1989.

Marymont JV: Spinal osteoblastoma in an 11-year-old boy, South Med J 81:922, 1988.

McAfee PC, Bohlman HH, Ducker T, and Eismont FJ: Failure of stabilization of the spine with methylmethacrylate, J Bone Joint Surg 68-A:1145, 1986.

Nagashima C, Iwasaki T, Okada K, and Sakaguchi A: Reconstruction of the atlas and axis with wire and acrylic after metastatic destruction: case report, J Neurosurg 50:668, 1979.

Nicholls PJ and Jarecky TW: The value of posterior decompression by laminectomy for malignant tumors of the spine, Clin Orthop 201:210, 1985.

O'Neil J, Gardner V, and Armstrong G: Treatment of tumors of the thoracic and lumbar spinal column, Clin Orthop 227: 103, 1988.

Palmer FJ and Blum PW: Osteochondroma with spinal cord compression: report of three cases, J Neurosurg 52:842, 1980.

Panjabi MM, Goel VK, Clark CR, et al: Biomechanical study of cervical spine stabilization with methylmethacrylate, Spine 10:198, 1985.

Postacchini F, Urso S, and Tovaglia V: Lumbosacral intradural tumours simulating disc disease, Int Orthop 5:283, 1981.

Ransford AO, Pozo JL, Hutton PAN, and Kirwan EOG: The behaviour pattern of the scoliosis associated with osteoid osteoma or osteoblastoma of the spine, J Bone Joint Surg 66-B:16, 1984.

Raycroft JF, Hockman RP, Albright JA, and Southwick WO: Surgery of malignant tumors of the cervical spine, J Bone Joint Surg 54-A:1794, 1972.

Raycroft JF, Hockman RP, and Southwick WO: Metastatic tumors involving the cervical vertebrae: surgical palliation, J Bone Joint Surg 60-A:763, 1978.

Savini R, Martucci E, Prosperi P, et al: Osteoid osteoma of the spine, Ital J Orthop Traumatol 14:233, 1988.

Schaberg J and Gainor BJ: A profile of metastatic carcinoma of the spine, Spine 10:19, 1985.

Scoville WB, Palmer AH, Samra K, and Chong G: The use of acrylic plastic for vertebral replacement or fixation in metastatic disease of the spine, J Neurosurg 27:274, 1967.

Sherk HH, Nolan JP, and Mooar P: Treatment of tumors of the cervical spine, Clin Orthop 233:163, 1988.

Shives TC, Dahlin DC, Sim FH, et al: Osteosarcoma of the spine, J Bone Joint Surg 68-A:660, 1986.

Siegal T and Siegal T.: Current considerations in the management of neoplastic spinal cord compression, Spine 14:223, 1989.

Siegal T, Tiqva P, and Siegal T: Vertebral body resection for epidural compression by malignant tumors: results of forty-seven consecutive operative procedures, J Bone Joint Surg 67-A:375, 1985.

Silverberg IJ and Jacobs EM: Treatment of spinal cord compression in Hodgkin's disease, Cancer 27:308, 1971.

Simmons EH and Grobler LJ: Acute spinal epidural hematoma: a case report, J Bone Joint Surg 60-A:395, 1978.

Stener B: Total spondylectomy in chondrosarcoma arising from the seventh thoracic vertebra, J Bone Joint Surg 53-B:288, 1971.

Stener B and Gunterberg B: High amputation of the sacrum for extirpation of tumors: principles and technique, Spine 3:351, 1978.

Stener B and Johnsen OE: Complete removal of three vertebrae for giant-cell tumour, J Bone Joint Surg 53-B:278, 1971.

Stevens WW and Weaver EN: Giant cell tumors and aneurysmal bone cysts of the spine: report of four cases, South Med J 63:218, 1970.

Stillwell WT and Fielding JW: Aneurysmal bone cyst of the cervicodorsal spine, Clin Orthop 187:144, 1984.

Suit HD, Goitein M, Munzenrider J, et al: Definitive radiation therapy for chordoma and chondrosarcoma of base of skull and cervical spine, J Neurosurg 56:377, 1982.

Symeonides PP: Osteoid osteoma of the lumbar spine, South Med J 63:975, 1970.

Tigani D, Pignati G, Picci P, et al: Vertebral osteosarcoma, Ital J Orthop Traumatol 14:5, 1988.

Turner ML, Mulhern CB, and Dalinka, MK: Lesions of the sacrum: differential diagnosis and radiological evaluation, JAMA 245:275, 1981.

Wang G, Lewish GD, Reger SI, et al.: Comparative strengths of various anterior cement fixations of the cervical spine, Spine 8:717, 1983.

Wang G, Wilson CS, Hubbard SL, et al: Safety of anterior cement fixation in the cervical spine: in vivo study of dog spine, South Med J 77:178, 1984.

Wang G, Reger SI, McLaughlin RE, et al: The safety of cement fixation in the cervical spine: studies of a rabbit model, Clin Orthop 139:276, 1979.

White WA, Patterson RH Jr, and Bergland RM: Role of surgery in the treatment of spinal cord compression by metastatic neoplasm, Cancer 27:558, 1971.

Whitehill R, Reger SI, Fox E, et al: Use of methylmethacrylate cement as an instantaneous fusion mass in posterior cervical fusions: a canine in vivo experimental model, Spine 9:246, 1984.

Wilkinson RH and Hall JE: The sclerotic pedicle: tumor or pseudo-tumor? Radiology 111:683, 1974.

Young RF, Post EM, and King GA: Treatment of spinal epidural metastases: randomized prospective comparison of laminectomy and radiotherapy, J Neurosurg 53:741, 1980.

Growth problems

Cattell HS and Clark GL: Cervical kyphosis and instability following multiple laminectomies in children, J Bone Joint Surg 49-A:713, 1967.

Dawson WB: Growth impairment following radiotherapy in childhood, Clin Radiol 19:241, 1968.

DeSousa AL, Kalsbeck JE, Mealey J Jr, et al: Intraspinal tumors in children: a review of 81 cases, J Neurosurg 51:437, 1979.

Mayfield JK, Erkkila JC, and Winter RB: Spine deformity subsequent to acquired childhood spinal cord injury, J Bone Joint Surg 63-A:1401, 1981.

Neuhauser EBD, et al.: Irradiation effects of roentgen therapy on the growing spine, Radiology 59:637, 1952.

Probert JC, Parker BR, and Kaplan HS: Growth retardation in children after megavoltage irradiation of the spine, Cancer 32:634, 1973.

Riseborough EJ, Grabias SL, Burton RI, and Jaffe N: Skeletal alteration following irradiation for Wilms' tumor, with particular reference to scoliosis and kyphosis, J Bone Joint Surg 58-A:526, 1976.

Tachdjian MO and Matson DD: Orthopaedic aspects of intraspinal tumors in infants and children, J Bone Joint Surg 47-A:223, 1965.

White WA, Patterson RH Jr, and Bergland RM: Role of surgery in the treatment of spinal cord compression by metastatic neoplasm, Cancer 27:558, 1971.

Yasuoka S, Peterson HA, and MacCarty CS: Incidence of spinal column deformity after multilevel laminectomy in children and adults, J Neurosurg 57:441, 1982.

Miscellaneous anomalies

Bernard TN Jr, Burke SW, Johnston CE III, and Roberts JM: Congenital spine deformities: a review of 47 cases, Orthopedics 8:777, 1985.

Bethem D, Winter RB, Lutter L, et al: Spinal disorders of dwarfism: review of the literature and report of eighty cases, J Bone Joint Surg 63-A:1412, 1981.

Kahanovitz N, Rimoin DL, and Sillence DO: The clinical spectrum of lumbar spine disease in achondroplasia, Spine 7:137, 1982.

Mattews LS, Vetter WL, and Tolo VT: Cervical anomaly simulating hangman's fracture in a child: case report, J Bone Joint Surg 64-A:299, 1982.

Kyphosis

Bjekreim I, Magnaes B, and Semb G: Surgical treatment of severe angular kyphosis, Acta Orthop Scand 53:913, 1982.

Bradford DS: Anterior vascular pedicle bone grafting for the treatment of kyphosis, Spine 5:318, 1980.

Bradford DS, and Moe JH: Scheuermann's juvenile kyphosis: a histologic study, Clin Orthop 110:45, 1975.

Bradford DS, Ahmed KB, Moe JH, et al: The surgical management of patients with Scheuermann's disease: a review of twenty-four cases managed by combined anterior and posterior spine fusion, J Bone Joint Surg 62-A:705, 1980.

Bradford DS, Moe JH, Montalvo FJ, and Winter RB: Scheuermann's kyphosis and roundback deformity: results of Milwaukee brace treatment, J Bone Joint Surg 56-A:740, 1974.

Bradford DS, Moe JH, Montalvo FJ, and Winter RB: Scheuermann's kyphosis: results of surgical treatment by posterior spine arthrodesis in 22 patients, J Bone Joint Surg 57-A:439, 1975.

Bradford DS, et al: Anterior strut-grafting for the treatment of kyphosis: review of experience with forty-eight patients, J Bone Joint Surg 64-A:680, 1982.

Cloward RB: Treatment of ruptured intervertebral discs by vertebral body fusion: indications, operative technique and aftercare, J Neurosurg 10:154, 1953.

DeWald RL, et al: Severe lumbosacral spondylolisthesis in adolescents and children: reduction and staged circumferential fusion, J Bone Joint Surg 63-A:619, 1981.

DiGiovanni BF, Scoles PB, and Latimer BM: Anterior extension of the thoracic vertebral bodies in Scheuermann's kyphosis, Spine 14:712, 1989.

Fountain SS, Hsul CS, Yau ACMC, and Hodgson AR: Progressive kyphosis following solid anterior spine fusion in children with tuberculosis of the spine: a long-term study, J Bone Joint Surg 57-A:1104, 1975.

Freebody D, Bendall R, and Taylor RD: Anterior transperitoneal lumbar fusion, J Bone Joint Surg 53-B:617, 1971.

Herndon WA, Emans JB, Micheli LJ, and Hall JE: Combined anterior and posterior fusion for Scheuermann's kyphosis, Spine 6:125, 1981.

Kostuik JP: Anterior Kostuik-Harrington distraction systems for the treatment of kyphotic deformities, Spine 15:169, 1990.

Kostuik JP, Maurais GR, Richardson WF, and Okajima Y: Combined anterior and posterior osteotomy for correction of iatrogenic lumbar kyphosis, Spine 13:257, 1988.

Lonstein JE, et al: Neurologic deficits secondary to spinal deformity: a review of the literature and report of 43 cases, Spine 5:331, 1980.

Moe JH: Treatment of adolescent kyphosis by nonoperative and operative methods, Manitoba Med Rev 45:481, 1965.

Moe JH, Winter RB, Bradford DS, and Lonstein JE: Scoliosis and other spinal deformities, Philadelphia, 1978, W.B. Saunders Co.

Montgomery SP and Hall JF: Congenital kyphosis, Spine 7:360, 1982.

Ohtani K, Nakai S, Fujimura Y, et al: Anterior surgical decompression of thoracic myelopathy as a result of ossification of the posterior longitudinal ligament, Clin Orthop 166:82, 1982.

Ryan MD, and Taylor TKF: Acute spinal cord compression in Scheuermann's disease, J Bone Joint Surg 64 B:409, 1982.

Scheuermann H: Kyphosis dorsalis juvenile, Ztschr Orthop Chir 41:305, 1921.

Scoles PV, Latimer BM, DiGiovanni BF, et al: Vertebral alterations in Scheuermann's kyphosis, Spine 16:509, 1991.

Sorenson KH: Scheuermann's juvenile kyphosis, Copenhagen, 1964, Munksgaard.

Swischuk LE: The beaked, notched, or hooked vertebra: its significance in infants and young children, Radiology 95:661, 1970.

Taylor TC, Wenger DR, Stephen J, et al: Surgical management of thoracic kyphosis in adolescents, J Bone Joint Surg 61-A:496, 1979.

Winter RB, and Swayze C: Severe neurofibromatosis kyphoscoliosis in a Jehovah's Witness: anterior and posterior spine fusion without blood transfusion, Spine 8:39, 1983.

Winter RB, Lovell WW, and Moe JH: Excessive thoracic lordosis and loss of pulmonary function in patients with idiopathic scoliosis, J Bone Joint Surg 57-A:972, 1975.

Winter RB, Moe JH, and Lonstein JE: The surgical treatment of congenital kyphosis: a review of 94 patients age 5 years or older with 2 years or more follow-up in 77 patients, Spine 10:224, 1985.

Winter RB, Moe JH, and Wang JF: Congenital kyphosis: its natural history and treatment as observed in a study of one hundred and thirty patients, J Bone Joint Srug 55-A:223, 1973.

Index

Anterior compartment — cont'd
  of knee
    approaches to, 46-47
    meniscectomy and, 1517
Anterior cord syndrome, 3522
Anterior cruciate ligament
  acute injury of, 1565-1581
    augmentation of repair of,
      1576-1581
    lateral compartment injury and,
      1561
  arthroscopic augmentation of repair
    of, 1839-1840
  arthroscopy of knee and, 1798
  combined instabilities of, 1660-1661
  knee stability and, 1587
  lateral compartment reconstruction
    and, 1610-1686
    allograft ligament replacement for,
      1683-1686
    anterolateral femorotibial ligament
      tenodesis and, 1619-1620
    arthroscopy and, 1686
    combined instabilities and,
      1660-1661
    extraarticular procedures for,
      1611-1620
    general considerations in,
      1610-1611
    iliotibial band tenodesis for,
      1611-1619
    iliotibial band through
      intercondylar notch and,
      1649-1652
    intraarticular procedures for,
      1620-1661
    patellar tendon for, 1622-1647
    patelloquadriceps tendon
      substitution for, 1647-1649
    semitendinosus or gracilis and,
      1652-1660
    synthetic augmentation for, 1668,
      1670-1683
    synthetic materials for, 1661-1668
  reconstruction of, arthroscopic,
    1835-1840
Anterior decompression of spinal
  fracture, 3555
Anterior dislocation
  of hip, 949, 1355, 1356
    old, unreduced, 1375
  of radial head, 1389
  of shoulder, 1414-1434
    Bankart operation for, 1415-1418
    Bristow operation for, 1424-1427
    capsular shift procedure for,
      1429-1434
    Magnuson and Stack operation
      for, 1422-1424
    old, unreduced dislocation of,
      1381-1383
    Putti-Platt operation for, 1422
    staple capsulorrhaphy of du Toit
      and Roux for, 1418-1422
    Weber subcapital osteotomy for,
      1427-1429
  of sternoclavicular joint, 1357

Anterior drainage for septic arthritis
  hip and, 158-159
  knee and, 154
  shoulder and, 164
Anterior drawer test
  ankle injury and, 1467
  knee ligament injury and, 1537,
    1539
Anterior glenoid labrum, 1874
Anterior hip release in
  myelomeningocele, 2443-2444
Anterior impingement syndrome of
  ankle, 1478
Anterior instability of knee, 1548
Anterior instrumentation, scoliosis
  and, 3690-3697
Anterior internal fixation of spinal
  fracture, 3571-3572
Anterior interosseous syndrome,
  pronator teres and, 2265
Anterior lumbar interbody fusion,
  3835-3836
Anterior lumbar vertebral interbody
  fusion, 3772
Anterior margin of tibia, fracture of,
  794
Anterior oblique meniscal tear, 1812
Anterior occipitocervical arthrodesis,
  3589
Anterior portal for arthroscopy
  elbow and, 1888-1889
  shoulder and, 1869-1871
Anterior radial collateral artery, 2542
Anterior rotary drawer test, Slocum's,
  1541
Anterior shoulder release, 2452-2453
Anterior spinal fusion
  kyphosis and, 3699
  myelomeningocele and, 3702
Anterior talofibular ligament rupture,
  1467, 1470
Anterior tarsal tunnel syndrome, 2781
Anterior technique for spinal tumor,
  3858
Anterior thoracic nerve, injury to,
  2244
Anterior tibial artery
  arthroscopy and, 1783
  occlusion of, 1988
Anterior transfer
  of long toe flexors for spastic
    equinus and equinovarus, 2312
  of tibialis posterior tendon,
    2399-2401
    muscular dystrophy and, 2478
  of triceps muscle, 2427-2428
Anterocentral portal for arthroscopy of
  ankle, 1846
Anteroinferior portal for arthroscopy
  of shoulder, 1871
Anterolateral approach
  to femur, 53-54
    fracture and, 857
  to hip, 60-61
  to humerus, 96-97
  to knee, 37, 38
  to tarsus and ankle, 28

Anterolateral capsule
  extraarticular knee ligament and,
    1492
  knee anatomy and, 1492
Anterolateral decompression of spine,
  3817-3818
Anterolateral dislocation of proximal
  tibiofibular joint, 1353
Anterolateral drainage for septic
  arthritis of ankle, 152-153
Anterolateral femorotibial ligament
  tenodesis, 1619-1620
Anterolateral portal for arthroscopy
  ankle and, 1846, 1852
  elbow and, 1887-1888
  knee and, 1791-1792
  shoulder and, 1872
Anterolateral release of
  myelomeningocele, 2437
Anterolateral rotary instability of
  knee, 1548, 1609-1610
Anterolateral-anteromedial rotary
  instability of knee, 1549
Anterolateral-posteromedial rotary
  instability of knee, 1549
Anteromedial approach
  hip and, 71
    dislocation and, 2170
  knee and, 37, 38
  shoulder and, 88-89
Anteromedial bundle of knee
  ligament, 1567
Anteromedial capsule
  extraarticular knee ligament and,
    1492
  knee anatomy and, 1492
Anteromedial drainage for septic
  arthritis of ankle, 153
Anteromedial portal for arthroscopy
  of ankle, 1846
  elbow and, 1888
  of knee, 1792
Anteromedial rotary instability of
  knee, 1547
Anteromedial-posteromedial rotary
  instability, of knee, 1549
Anteroposterior stress test, ankle
  injury and, 1467
Anterosuperior iliac spine graft, Lee,
  839
Anteversion
  of acetabulum, 542-544
  femoral neck, hip arthroplasty and,
    560
Antibiotic
  arthroplasty cement and, 380
  bite injury and, 3486
  culture and, 125
  diabetic ulcer and, 2820-2821
  gas gangrene and, 777
  hand infection and, 3479-3480
  hip arthroplasty and, 575
  knee arthroplasty and, 397, 424
  nonunion of fracture and, 1301
  open fracture and, 772, 774
  prophylactic, 120-121
    arthroplasty and, 382

Peter Evans

Senior Lecturer

1992